Review of Sleep Medicine

Fourth Edition

Alon Y. Avidan, MD, MPH

Professor and Vice Chair
Department of Neurology
Director, UCLA Sleep Disorders Center
David Geffen School of Medicine at UCLA
University of California, Los Angeles
Los Angeles, California

ELSEVIER

Philadelphia, PA

ELSEVIER

1600 John F. Kennedy Blvd.
Ste 1800
Philadelphia, PA 19103-2899

Previous editions copyrighted 2012, 2007, and 2003.

Library of Congress Cataloging-in-Publication Data
Names: Avidan, Alon Y., editor.
Title: Review of sleep medicine / [edited by] Alon Y. Avidan.
Description: Fourth edition. | Philadelphia, PA : Elsevier, [2018] | Includes bibliographical references and index.
Identifiers: LCCN 2017015432 | ISBN 9780323462167 (pbk.)
Subjects: | MESH: Sleep Wake Disorders | Sleep–physiology | Examination Questions | Outlines
Classification: LCC RC547 | NLM WL 18.2 | DDC 616.8/4980076–dc23 LC record available at
    https://lccn.loc.gov/2017015432

Executive Content Strategist: Dolores Meloni
Content Development Specialist: Angie Breckon
Publishing Services Manager: Patricia Tannian
Senior Project Manager: Cindy Thoms
Book Designer: Brian Salisbury

Printed in China

Last digit is the print number: 9 8 7 6 5 4 3 2 1

Working together
to grow libraries in
developing countries

www.elsevier.com • www.bookaid.org

Review of Sleep Medicine

Contributors

Sabra M. Abbott, MD, PhD
Assistant Professor, Department of Neurology, Northwestern University, Feinberg School of Medicine, Chicago, Illinois

Qanta A. Ahmed, MD
NYU Winthrop University Hospital, Sleep Disorders Center, Garden City, New York

Cathy A. Alessi, MD
Geriatric Research, Education, and Clinical Center, VA Greater Los Angeles Healthcare System; David Geffen School of Medicine at UCLA, Los Angeles, California

Richard P. Allen, PhD
Associate Professor, Neurology, Johns Hopkins University, Baltimore, Maryland

Zahreddin Alsheikhtaha, MD, RPSGT
Polysomnography Technician, Cleveland Clinic Sleep Disorders Center, Cleveland, Ohio

Dennis Auckley, MD
Associate Professor of Medicine, Case Western Reserve University; Director, MetroHealth's Center for Sleep Medicine, Division of Pulmonary, Critical Care and Sleep Medicine, MetroHealth Medical Center, Cleveland, Ohio

Alon Y. Avidan, MD, MPH
Professor and Vice Chair, Department of Neurology; Director, UCLA Sleep Disorders Center, David Geffen School of Medicine at UCLA, University of California, Los Angeles, Los Angeles, California

Carl W. Bazil, MD, PhD
Professor, Neurology, Columbia University, New York, New York

Richard B. Berry, MD
Professor of Medicine, Division of Pulmonary, Critical Care, and Sleep Medicine, University of Florida, Gainesville, Florida

Sushanth Bhat, MD
JFK Neuroscience Institute, Edison, New Jersey; Seton Hall University, South Orange, New Jersey

Matt T. Bianchi, MD, PhD
Director, Sleep Division, Neurology, Massachusetts General Hospital, Boston, Massachusetts

Rita Brooks, MEd, RST, RPSGT, REEG/EPT
Diagnostic Services, Capital Health, Trenton, New Jersey

Nic Butkov, RPSGT
Education Coordinator, Asante Sleep Center, Medford, Oregon

Sean M. Caples, DO, MSc
Division Pulmonary and Critical Care Medicine, Center for Sleep Medicine, Mayo Clinic, Rochester, Minnesota

Paul R. Carney, MD
Professor, Department of Neurology, University of North Carolina at Chapel Hill, Chapel Hill, North Carolina

Sudhansu Chokroverty, MD
Professor and Director of Research for Sleep Medicine, Co-Chair Emeritus of Neurology, Seton Hall University, South Orange, New Jersey; JFK Neuroscience Institute, Edison, New Jersey

Derek J. Chong, MD, MSc
Vice-Chair; Director, Division of Epilepsy, Neurology, Lenox Hill Hospital System, New York, New York

Christopher S. Colwell, PhD
Department of Psychiatry and Biobehavioral Sciences, Laboratory of Circadian Sleep Medicine, University of California—Los Angeles, Los Angeles, California

Deirdre A. Conroy, PhD
Clinical Associate Professor, Department of Psychiatry, University of Michigan, Ann Arbor, Michigan

Emmanuel H. During, MD
Clinical Assistant Professor, Stanford Center for Sleep Sciences and Medicine, Palo Alto, California

Joseph M. Dzierzewski, PhD
Department of Psychology, Virginia Commonwealth University, Richmond, Virginia

Nancy Foldvary-Schaefer, DO, MS
Professor of Medicine, Cleveland Clinic Lerner College of Medicine; Director, Sleep Disorders Center, Staff, Epilepsy Center, Cleveland Clinic, Cleveland, Ohio

James D. Geyer, MD
Chief Medical Science Officer, NeuroTexion, LLC; Medical Director of Sleep Medicine and Clinical Neurophysiology, Alabama Neurology and Sleep Medicine, Tuscaloosa, Alabama

Namni Goel, PhD
Associate Professor, Division of Sleep and Chronobiology, Department of Psychiatry, Perelman School of Medicine, University of Pennsylvania, Philadelphia, Pennsylvania

Cathy Goldstein, MD
Assistant Professor, Department of Neurology, University of Michigan, Ann Arbor, Michigan

Nalaka Gooneratne, MD, MSc
Associate Professor of Medicine, Associate Director, Masters of Translational Research, Division of Geriatric Medicine and the Center for Sleep and Circadian Neurobiology, Perelman School of Medicine, University of Pennsylvania, Philadelphia, Pennsylvania

Kara S. Griffin, MA
Research Associate, Sleep Medicine and Research Center, St. Luke's Hospital, Chesterfield, Missouri

Madeleine M. Grigg-Damberger, MD
Professor of Neurology, Department of Neurology, University of New Mexico School of Medicine; Medical Director, Pediatric Sleep Medicine Services, University of New Mexico Sleep Center; Associate Medical Director, Clinical Neurodiagnostic Laboratory, University of New Mexico Medical Center, Albuquerque, New Mexico

Shelby F. Harris, PsyD, CBSM
Associate Professor, Department of Neurology and Department of Psychiatry and Behavioral Sciences, Albert Einstein College of Medicine; Director, Behavioral Sleep Medicine Program, Sleep-Wake Disorders Center, Montefiore Medical Center, Bronx, New York

Ron D. Hays, PhD
Professor of Medicine, Department of Medicine, Department of Health Policy and Management, University of California—Los Angeles, RAND Health Program, RAND, Santa Monica, California

John Herman, PhD
Adjunct Professor, Departments of Psychiatry and Psychology, University of Texas Southwestern Medical Center, Dallas, Texas

Max Hirshkowitz, PhD
Consulting Professor, Division of Public Mental Health and Population Sciences, School of Medicine, Stanford University, Stanford, California; Professor Emeritus, Department of Medicine, Baylor College of Medicine, Houston, Texas

Timothy F. Hoban, MD
Professor of Pediatrics and Neurology, Director, Pediatric Sleep Medicine, University of Michigan, Ann Arbor, Michigan

Michael Howell, MD
Associate Professor, Neurology, University of Minnesota, Minneapolis, Minnesota

Benjamin H. Hughes, MD
Assistant Professor of Pediatrics in Pulmonary and Sleep Medicine, Department of Pediatrics, Children's Hospital Colorado, University of Colorado Anschutz Medical Campus, Aurora, Colorado

Marcel Hungs, MD, PhD
Adjunct Assistant Professor, Department of Neurology, University of Minnesota, Minneapolis, Minnesota; Director, Sleep Clinic, Neurological Associates of St. Paul, Maplewood, Minnesota

Vikas Jain, MD, CCSH
Sleep Physician, Health System Clinician, Pulmonary and Sleep Medicine, Northwestern Medicine, Winfield, Illinois; Adjunct Clinical Instructor, The Stanford Center for Sleep Sciences and Medicine, Stanford University, Redwood City, California

Sharon A. Keenan, PhD, REEGT, RPSGT, D
The School of Sleep Medicine, Inc., Palo Alto, California

Ian Kestin, MD, FRCA
Emeritus Consultant Anaesthetist, Western Infirmary, Glasgow, Scotland, United Kingdom

Douglas Benjamin Kirsch, MD
Medical Director, Carolinas HealthCare System; Associate Professor, Department of Medicine, UNC School of Medicine, Charlotte, North Carolina

Suresh Kotagal, MD
Professor, Department of Neurology, Consultant, Departments of Neurology, Pediatrics, and the Center for Sleep Medicine, Mayo Clinic, Rochester, Minnesota

Clete A. Kushida, MD, PhD
Professor of Psychiatry and Behavioral Sciences, Stanford University Medical Center, Redwood City, California

Teofilo Lee-Chiong, MD
Professor of Medicine, Department of Medicine, National Jewish Health, University of Colorado, Denver, Colorado; Chief Medical Liaison, Philips Respironics, Monroeville, Pennsylvania

Joyce K. Lee-Iannotti, MD
Assistant Professor, Neurology, Banner University Medical Center, Phoenix, Arizona

Laura A. Linley, RST, RPSGT, CRTT
VP of Clinical Operations, Advanced Sleep Management, LLC, Richardson, Texas

Honghu Liu, PhD
Division of General Internal Medicine and Health Services Research, David Geffen School of Medicine at UCLA, Los Angeles, California

Robin Lloyd, MD
Department of Pediatrics, Center for Sleep Medicine, Rochester, Minnesota

Cindy Mack, RPSGT
Advanced Sleep Center, Delgado Community College, New Orleans, Louisiana

Raman K. Malhotra, MD
Co-Director, SLUCare Sleep Disorders Center, Associate Professor, Neurology, Saint Louis University, St. Louis, Missouri

Emmanuel Mignot, MD, PhD
Director, Stanford Center for Sleep Sciences and Medicine, Palo Alto, California

Kimberly Nicole Mims, MD
Charlotte Medical Clinic, Carolinas HealthCare System, Charlotte, North Carolina

Silvia Neme-Mercante, MD
Staff, Sleep Disorders Center, Epilepsy Center, Cleveland Clinic, Cleveland, Ohio

David N. Neubauer, MD
Johns Hopkins Bayview Medical Center, Baltimore, Maryland

Shalini Paruthi, MD
Adjunct Associate Professor, Pediatrics, Saint Louis University; Co-Medical Director, Sleep Medicine and Research Center, St. Luke's Hospital, Chesterfield, Missouri

Brandon R. Peters, MD
Clinical Faculty Affiliate, Department of Psychiatry and Behavioral Sciences, Stanford University, Palo Alto, California

Grace W. Pien, MD, MSCE
Assistant Professor of Medicine, Division of Pulmonary and Critical Care Medicine, Johns Hopkins University School of Medicine, Baltimore, Maryland

David T. Plante, MD
Assistant Professor, Department of Psychiatry, University of Wisconsin—Madison, Madison, Wisconsin

Melanie Pogach, MD, MMSc
Medicine/Pulmonary, Critical Care, and Sleep Division, Harvard Medical School, Beth Israel Deaconess Medical Center, Boston, Massachusetts

Charles A. Polnitsky, MD
Associate Clinical Professor, Frank H. Netter MD School of Medicine, Quinnipiac University, Hamden, Connecticut

Kathryn J. Reid, PhD
Research Associate Professor, Department of Neurology, Northwestern University Feinberg School of Medicine, Chicago, Illinois

Timothy V. Roehrs, PhD
Senior Bioscientist, Sleep Disorders and Research Center, Henry Ford Health System, Wayne State University, Detroit, Michigan

Ilene M. Rosen, MD, MSCE
Assistant Dean for Graduate Medical Education, Program Director, Sleep Medicine Fellowship, Division of Sleep Medicine, Perelman School of Medicine, University of Pennsylvania, Philadelphia, Pennsylvania

Richard S. Rosenberg, PhD
Department of Psychology, California State University, Long Beach, California

Thomas Roth, PhD
Sleep Disorders and Research Center, Henry Ford Hospital, Department of Psychiatry and Behavioral Neuroscience, School of Medicine, Wayne State University, Detroit, Michigan

Chad M. Ruoff, MD
Adjunct Clinical Assistant Professor, The Stanford Center for Sleep Sciences and Medicine, Stanford University, Redwood City, California

Scott Ryals, MD
Clinical Assistant Professor, Division of Pulmonary, Critical Care, and Sleep Medicine, University of Florida, Gainesville, Florida

Paula K. Schweitzer, PhD
Director of Research, Sleep Medicine and Research Center, St. Luke's Hospital, Chesterfield, Missouri

Denise Sharon, MD, PhD
Assistant Professor of Medicine, Tulane University School of Medicine, New Orleans, Louisiana; Clinical Director, Advanced Sleep Center, Metairie, Louisiana

Anita V. Shelgikar, MD
Director, Sleep Medicine Fellowship, Clinical Assistant Professor of Neurology, University of Michigan, Ann Arbor, Michigan

Jerome M. Siegel, PhD
Professor, Psychiatry and Biobehavioral Sciences, University of California—Los Angeles; Chief, Neurobiology Research, Veterans Affairs Greater Los Angeles Healthcare System, Los Angeles, California

Virend K. Somers, MD, PhD
Division of Cardiovascular Diseases, Mayo Clinic College of Medicine, Rochester, Minnesota

Shannon S. Sullivan, MD
Clinical Assistant Professor, Stanford Center for Sleep Medicine, Palo Alto, California

Leslie M. Swanson, PhD
Clinical Assistant Professor, Department of Psychiatry, University of Michigan, Ann Arbor, Michigan

Todd Swick, MD
Clinical Assistant Professor of Neurology, University of Texas Health Sciences Center—Houston, McGovern School of Medicine; Senior Physician, Neurology and Sleep Medicine Consultants, Houston, Texas

Ronald Szymusiak, PhD
Research Service, VA Greater Los Angeles Healthcare System, Departments of Medicine and Neurobiology, David Geffen School of Medicine at UCLA, Los Angeles, California

Juan Carlos Rodriguez Tapia, MD
Geriatric Research, Education, and Clinical Center, VA Greater Los Angeles Healthcare System; David Geffen School of Medicine, University of California, Los Angeles, California; Department of Medicine, Pontificia Universidad Catolica de Chile, Santiago, Chile

Robert Thomas, MD, MMSc
Associate Professor of Medicine, Medicine/Pulmonary, Critical Care, and Sleep Division, Beth Israel Deaconess Medical Center, Boston, Massachusetts

Michael J. Thorpy, MD
Professor of Clinical Neurology, Albert Einstein College of Medicine; Director, Sleep-Wake Center, Montefiore Medical Center, Bronx, New York

Lynn Marie Trotti, MD, MSc
Emory Sleep Center and Department of Neurology, Emory University School of Medicine, Atlanta, Georgia

Sheila C. Tsai, MD
Associate Professor of Medicine, National Jewish Health, Denver, Colorado; Associate Professor of Medicine, University of Colorado Denver School of Medicine, Aurora, Colorado

Sigrid C. Veasey, MD
Professor of Medicine, Perelman School of Medicine, University of Pennsylvania, Philadelphia, Pennsylvania

Andrew Vosko, PhD
Transdisciplinary Studies Program, Claremont Graduate University, Claremont, California

Kevin A. Walker, MD
Program Director, Sleep Medicine Fellowship, University of Utah and Affiliated Hospitals, Salt Lake City, Utah

Arthur S. Walters, MD
Professor of Neurology, Vanderbilt University Medical Center, Nashville, Tennessee

Christopher J. Watson, PhD
Department of Anesthesiology, University of Michigan, Ann Arbor, Michican

Michael Weinstein, MD
NYU Winthrop University Hospital, Sleep Disorders Center, Garden City, New York

Rochelle Zak, MD
Sleep Disorders Center, University of California, San Francisco, California

Foreword

I am deeply honored with the opportunity to write this foreword for the *Review of Sleep Medicine*. The fourth edition of this highly successful volume is published by Elsevier. Alon Y. Avidan, MD, MPH, has again served as the editor, after co-editing the previous two editions with Teri J. Barkoukis, MD, FCCP.

The *Review of Sleep Medicine* has become a premier resource for anyone learning sleep medicine, and especially for those approaching board exams. Practice questions and concise, referenced answers have long made this volume invaluable to many of the fellows training here at the University of Michigan. With each subsequent edition, the initial chapters – concise but well-illustrated information on sleep disorders, from diagnosis to treatment – have grown substantially. The fourth edition now features an entire section on normal sleep, likely to leave readers better prepared to tackle subsequent sections on sleep disorders and practice exams. The newest version provides comprehensive reviews in an outline format, along with assessment tools likely to prove useful to anyone who wishes to expand his or her knowledge base in sleep medicine. With this growth, the expanded list of contributing authors still features many of the most accomplished clinicians and educators in the field. Many have been responsible for development of sleep medicine itself into an age where the Accreditation Council for Graduate Medical Education (ACGME) and the American Board of Medical Specialties (ABMS) recognize it as an independent specialty.

Among the exceptional academic clinicians who provide educational leadership in sleep medicine, few have contributed as much as Dr. Alon Avidan. After a fellowship in sleep medicine under the mentorship of Nancy Foldvary-Schaefer, DO, MS, at the Cleveland Clinic, Alon arrived to his first academic faculty position here at the University of Michigan in 1999. From the start, he was excited by opportunities to introduce our field to fellows and residents. He assisted Michael S. Aldrich, MD, in an NIH-sponsored Sleep Academic Award to develop new, more effective teaching tools. Alon took over that project when health challenges impaired Mike's ability to complete it, and this proved to be a transformative experience. From that point on, Alon embraced sleep medicine education as his calling, and never looked back. At this point he has led key national courses on sleep medicine for the American Academy of Sleep Medicine and the American Academy of Neurology, lectured around the country, written countless chapters, developed educational modules focusing on sleep disorders, and edited several books in sleep medicine. After leaving the University of Michigan for the University of California, Los Angeles (UCLA) in 2006, Alon directed the neurology residency, co-directed and then directed the UCLA Sleep Disorders Center, and secured external funding to develop online sleep education resources. Demand for his lectures has risen across the country, probably because they are characteristically enlightening, but at the same time highly animated, humorous, and entertaining in a manner that makes them memorable. In 2014, the deep respect and highest regard of his peers led to Alon's receipt of the American Academy of Sleep Medicine Excellence in Education Award.

Alon has now applied his considerable talent and expertise to the new, fourth edition of *Review of Sleep Medicine*, likely to prove the most successful yet. As an educator myself in sleep medicine for 22 years now, I know that some of the most rewarding moments arrive beyond the point where your mentees have proven beyond doubt to be successful clinical colleagues in the effort to address challenges with sleep and alertness. At some point, if you are lucky, you may witness the achievement of your mentees as well-recognized educators themselves. The University of Michigan programs in sleep medicine have been the home, at some point in training or faculty years, for many of the *Review of Sleep Medicine*, fourth edition authors. Mike Aldrich, as one of the early pioneers who helped to develop the American Board of Sleep Medicine and establish a culture in our field that prioritizes education, would no doubt be proud, as am I, to see this volume come to life under the exceptional guidance, dedication, energy, and passion for education in sleep medicine that Alon Avidan brings to the task. I eagerly await my own printed copy of the newest version of *Review of Sleep Medicine*, which at this moment is in press. If history is any guide, it will again serve as an invaluable resource in board preparation, prove useful for any student of sleep medicine, and perhaps contribute to the knowledge and enthusiasm of our next generation of clinical sleep medicine educators.

Ronald D. Chervin, MD, MS
Professor of Neurology and Michael S. Aldrich Collegiate
Professor of Sleep Medicine
Director, University of Michigan Sleep Disorders Center
Ann Arbor, Michigan

Preface

It is my honor to serve as Editor for a fourth edition of *Review of Sleep Medicine*. The specific aim of this textbook is to provide a complete but succinctly organized updated review of sleep medicine. The textbook has a dual purpose: (a) it may be used by physicians and health care providers to expand their sleep medicine competency skills, and (b) it can also be used as an educational resource in preparing for the sleep medicine board examination.

Sleep medicine has experienced a renaissance of growth in new research findings about disease pathology, assessment tools, and management strategies. This explosion of new knowledge has helped catalyze a convergence of new ideas, which exemplify the importance of the multidisciplinary foundation of sleep medicine. This knowledge needs to be mastered from the fields of neurology, pulmonology medicine, endocrinology, pediatrics, psychiatry, psychology, anesthesiology, otolaryngology, and dental sleep medicine. It is impossible to condense this volume of knowledge in a manner that fulfils the needs of all stakeholders. Yet I believe that the aims of this volume have been met, since I have restricted the specific focus of this book to serve as a high-impact review and an assessment tool as opposed to an encyclopedia or comprehensive textbook of sleep medicine. As in the previous three editions, the book is divided into a review and an assessment section. However, in this fourth edition, I have asked the authors to present the material utilizing an outline format and have also included high-yield educational resources such as tables and high-impact diagrams and illustrations to help drive educational messages. Here is a brief introduction to and an overview of the fourth edition of the *Review of Sleep Medicine*:

- *Review Section*: Consisting of 27 chapters, this is the core section that provides the readers a fundamental background knowledge base in sleep medicine covering the main sleep disorders presented in the International Classification of Sleep Medicine, Third Edition (ICSD III). The section also covers sleep stage scoring, published by the American Academy of Sleep Medicine (AASM), polysomnography and sleep technology, assessment of sleep, sleep physiology, sleep neuroanatomy and pharmacology, sleep evolution, ontogeny and phylogeny, sleep deprivation, circadian systems, the genetics of sleep, and sleep through the life cycle.
- *Assessment Section*: This remains a unique focus of the book with practice multiple-choice questions followed by comprehensive detailed answers. There are new and expanded chapters on clinical cases in neurology, pulmonary medicine, medical disorders, special populations, pediatrics, and psychiatry as well as specific assessment chapters focusing on major sleep diagnoses.
- New in this edition is the use of color illustrations The ability to utilize color in this textbook will certainly enhance its educational value, will bring another dimension to neuroanatomical plates and complex polysomnographic tracings, and would enhance opportunities for learning.
- The online version of the textbook allows us to also store and make available previous assessment questions from the previous editions of the Review of Sleep Medicine. This means that readers have the opportunity to access hundreds of assessment questions, gauge knowledge, and remedy potential gaps.

It is my hope that this key resource will continue to be utilized as an important educational tool among physicians wishing to expand and build their knowledge base in sleep medicine as well as when preparing for sleep medicine board examinations. While this textbook was first developed as a board review resource, it has undergone transformation to include review and assessment as well as exam preparation by anyone who wishes to build upon and enhance his or her knowledge base in sleep medicine. Historically, this book also serves a critical role in challenging the mind of the sleep trainee by providing questions drawn from actual clinical practice and engaging the reader in active thinking. We therefore hope that this critical educational exercise will improve, enhance, and stimulate the minds of our colleagues, leading to overall better care of their patients.

I would like to conclude by thanking all of the authors for their exceptional contributions. I have had the pleasure of working with many of them as colleagues and friends in this ever-evolving and exciting field. I would like to thank many of my colleagues at UCLA, in particular, Dr. S. Thomas Carmichael, Chair, UCLA Department of Neurology, for his exceptional support and Dr. Barbara Giesser, Clinical Director of the UCLA MS Program, for her gracious support and mentorship. I appreciate the help of many other faculty members in the Department of Neurology and colleagues at the UCLA Sleep Disorders Center. Special recognition goes to the many support staff of the UCLA Sleep Disorders Center and the Neurology Department who provide exceptional services advocating our patients. I would also like to thank the following individuals at Elsevier whose help made our work both successful and enjoyable: Angie Breckon, Nancy Duffy, Kellie Heap, Russell Gabbedy, Maureen Iannuzzi, Dolores Meloni, and Cindy Thoms.

Last, but not least, I thank my family for their patience and enthusiastic support of this book project.

Alon Y. Avidan
Los Angeles, California
June, 2017

I would like to dedicate this volume to Dr. Michael S. Aldrich. Dr. Aldrich was founder of the University of Michigan Sleep Disorders Laboratory and a prominent clinical and basic sleep researcher. Dr. Aldrich was considered a pioneer sleep neurologist. Some of the authors of this textbook have had the privilege to meet and work with Michael in the past and remember him as quiet, brilliant, humble, and magnificent; a true giant in the field of sleep medicine. In 1999, when Mike became ill, he asked me to carry through his efforts on a National Institutes of Health–sponsored Sleep Academic Award to develop new and innovative teaching tools to catalyze sleep education in the United States. Nearly two decades later, I have no doubt in my mind that Mike was the reason for fueling my desire to fulfil the duty and privilege to educate. This textbook is dedicated to him and for his memory as a consummate physician educator.

Alon Y. Avidan
Los Angeles, California
June, 2017

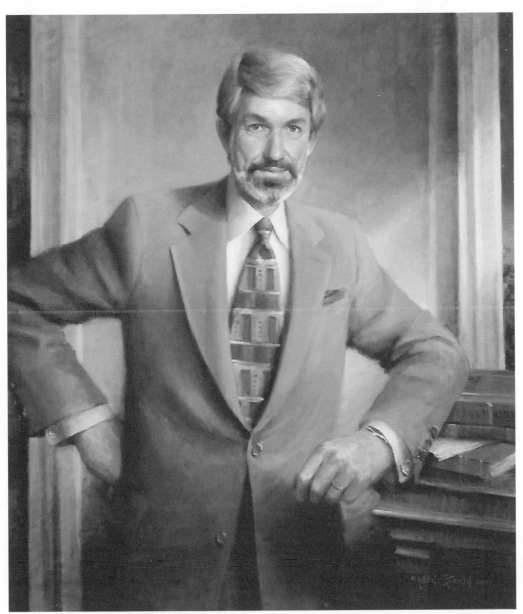

Dr. Michael S. Aldrich, a pioneer sleep researcher and educator and founder of the University of Michigan Sleep Disorders Center, Ann Arbor, Michigan. (Portrait by Kevin Gordon, From the Collection of Michigan Medicine at the University of Michigan.)

Contents

Abbreviations

A	auricle
AASM	American Academy of Sleep Medicine
ABG	arterial blood gas
ABIM	American Board of Internal Medicine
ABPN	American Board of Psychiatry and Neurology
ABSM	American Board of Sleep Medicine
ACGME	Accreditation Council for Graduate Medical Education
Ach	acetylcholine
ACT	acid clearance time
ACTH	adrenocorticotropic hormone
ADHD	attention-deficit hyperactivity disorder
AHI	apnea-hypopnea index
ALTE	apparent life-threatening episode
ANP	atrial natriuretic peptide
ANS	autonomic nervous system
APAP	autotitrating positive airway pressure
APOE	apolipoprotein E
ARAS	ascending reticular activating system
ASD	autistic spectrum disorder
ASPS	advanced sleep phase syndrome
ASPT	advanced sleep phase type
BETS	benign epileptiform transients of sleep
BF	basal forebrain
BMI	body mass index
BP	blood pressure
BPAP	bilevel positive airway pressure
BRS	baroreceptor sensitivity
BZ	benzodiazepine
BZRA	benzodiazepine receptor agonist
CAD	coronary artery disease
CAHS	central alveolar hypoventilation syndrome
CBF	cerebral blood flow
CBT	cognitive behavioral therapy
CCHS	congenital central hypoventilation syndrome
CHF	congestive heart failure
CNS	central nervous system
CO	cardiac output
COPD	chronic obstructive pulmonary disease
COX	cyclooxygenase
CPAP	continuous positive airway pressure
CPBS	central periodic breathing in sleep
cps	cycles per second (or Hertz or Hz)
CRH	corticotropin-releasing hormone
CRP	C-reactive protein
CRSD	circadian rhythm sleep disorder
CRY	cryptochrome
CSA	central sleep apnea
CSF	cerebral spinal fluid
CSR	Cheyne-Stokes respiration
CYP	cytochrome P-450
D	decrease
DA	dopamine
DLB	dementia with Lewy bodies
DLMO	dim light melatonin onset
DRG	dorsal respiratory group
DRN	dorsal raphe nucleus
DSIP	delta sleep-inducing peptide
DSPD	delayed sleep phase disorder
DSPS	delayed sleep phase syndrome (or DSPD)
dsRNA	double stranded RNA
Dx	diagnosis
ECG	electrocardiogram
EDS	excessive daytime sleepiness
EEG	electroencephalogram
EKG	electrokardiogram (or electrocardiogram or ECG)
EMG	electromyogram
EOG	electrooculogram
ePAP	expiratory positive airway pressure
EPSP	excitatory postsynaptic potentials
ESS	Epworth Sleepiness Score
F	frontal
FDA	Food and Drug Administration
FFI	fatal familial insomnia
FGF	fibroblast growth factor
FIRDA	frontal intermittent rhythmic delta activity
Fpz	nasion on EEG mapping
FRC	functional residual capacity
FSH	follicle-stimulating hormone
FSS	Fatigue Severity Scale
GABA	gamma aminobutyric acid
GBS	Guillain-Barré syndrome
GER	gastroesophageal reflux
GH	growth hormone
GHB	gamma hydroxybutyrate
GHRH	growth hormone–releasing hormone
GHT	geniculohypothalamic tract
GLU	glutamate
GND	ground
GnRH	gonadotropin-releasing hormone
GTC	generalized tonic-clonic (seizures)
H	histamine
Hcrtr2	hypocretin receptor 2 gene
HFF	high-frequency filters
HLA	human leukocyte antigen
HR	heart rate

HRV	heart rate variability		P	parietal
HSAT	Home Sleep Apnea Testing		PAC	premature atrial contraction
HT	hydroxytryptamine (serotonin)		PACAP	pituitary adenyl cyclase–activating peptide
5-HT	5-hydroxytryptamine		PB	periodic breathing
5-HTP	5-hydroxytryptophan		PCO_2 or $PaCO_2$	arterial partial pressure of carbon dioxide
Hz	Hertz (or cycles per second or cps)		PDR	posterior dominant rhythm
I	increase		PER	period
ICSD	*International Classification of Sleep Disorders*		PFA	paroxysmal fast activity
IFN	interferon		PG	prostaglandin
IGF-1	insulin-like growth factor-1		PGO	ponto-geniculo-occipital
IGL	intergeniculate leaflet		PH	pulmonary hypertension
IH	idiopathic hypersomnia		PLEDS	periodic lateralized epileptiform discharges
IL	interleukin		PLMD	periodic limb movement disorder
IMT	intima-media thickness		PLMI	periodic limb movement index
iPAP	inspiratory positive airway pressure		PLMS	periodic limb movements during sleep
IPSP	inhibitory postsynaptic potential		PO_2 or PaO_2	arterial partial pressure of oxygen
LC	locus caeruleus		POA	preoptic area
LDT	laterodorsal tegmental nucleus		PPT	pedunculopontine tegmental nucleus
LFF	low-frequency filters		PRC	phase response curve
LGN	lateral geniculate nucleus		PRF	pontine reticular formation
LH	luteinizing hormone		PSG	polysomnogram/polysomnography
L-NAME	*N*-nitro-L-arginine methyl ester		PT	pars tuberalis
LOC	outer canthus of the left eye		PTSD	post-traumatic stress disorder
m	meter		PVC	premature ventricular complex
MAD	mandibular advancement device		PWS	Prader-Willi syndrome
MAO-I	monoamine oxidase inhibitor		RBD	REM sleep behavior disorder
m-CPP	meta-chlorophenylpiperazine		rCBF	regional cerebral blood flow
Mflo	mask flow channel		RDI	respiratory disturbance index
mm Hg	millimeters of mercury		REM	rapid eye movement
MRA	mandibular repositioning appliance		RERA	respiratory effort-related arousal
MRI	magnetic resonance imaging		RGC	retinal ganglion cells
MSH	melanocyte-stimulating hormone		RHT	retinohypothalamic tract
MSL	mean sleep onset latency		RLS	restless legs syndrome
MSLT	Multiple Sleep Latency Test		RMD	rhythmic movement disorder
MWT	maintenance of wakefulness test		RME	rapid maxillary expansion
NA	noradrenaline		RNT	reticular nucleus of the thalamus
NBM	nucleus basalis of Meynert		ROC	outer canthus of the right eye
NE	norepinephrine		RPO	reticularis pontis oralis
NFκB	nuclear factor kappa B		SA	sleep apnea
NIMV	noninvasive mechanical ventilation		SaO_2	arterial oxyhemoglobin saturation
NIPPV	noninvasive positive pressure ventilation		SCN	suprachiasmatic nucleus
NMDA	*N*-methyl-D-aspartate		SDB	sleep-disordered breathing
NO	nitric oxide		SIDS	sudden infant death syndrome
N/O	nasal-oral		SL	sleep latency
NPD	nocturnal paroxysmal dystonia		SO	sleep onset
NPSG	nocturnal polysomnography		SOAD	sleep-onset association disorder
NPT	nocturnal penile tumescence		SOREMP	sleep onset REM period(s)
NPY	neuropeptide Y		SpO_2	pulse oximetry saturation
NREM	non–rapid eye movement sleep		SPZ	subparaventricular zone
NSAID	nonsteroidal antiinflammatory drug		SRBD	sleep-related breathing disturbances
NSF	National Sleep Foundation		SRED	sleep-related eating disorder
NTS	nucleus tractus solitarius		SREs	sleep related erections
O	occipital		SSI	Stanford Center for Narcolepsy Sleep Inventory
OA	obstructive apnea			
ODI	oxygen-desaturation index		SSRI	selective serotonin reuptake inhibitor
OH	obstructive hypopnea		SSS	Stanford Sleepiness Scale
OHS	obesity-hypoventilation syndrome		SubC	subcoeruleus
OSA	obstructive sleep apnea		SVR	systemic vascular resistance
OSAH	obstructive sleep apnea–hypopnea		SWS	slow wave sleep
OSAHS	obstructive sleep apnea–hypopnea syndrome		T	temporal
OSAS	obstructive sleep apnea syndrome		TCA	tricyclic antidepressant
Oz	inion on EEG mapping		TCS	Treacher Collins syndrome

Th1	T-helper 1	UARS	upper airway resistance syndrome
TIB	time in bed	UPPP	uvulopalatopharyngoplasty
TMN	tuberomammillary nucleus	VLPO	ventrolateral preoptic nucleus
TMS	transcranial magnetic stimulation	VRG	ventral respiratory group
TNF	tumor necrosis factor	VT	ventricular tachycardia
TRH	thyrotropin-releasing hormone	VTA	ventral tegmental area (of the midbrain)
TSH	thyroid-stimulating hormone	WASO	wake after sleep onset
TST	total sleep time	WSN	warm-sensitive neurons
TWT	total wake time		

1

Introduction to Sleep Medicine

ALON Y. AVIDAN

Organization of the Review of Sleep Medicine

- *Section 1*: Provides an overview of sleep covering the definition, ontogency, phylogeny, architecture, staging and scoring of sleep, sleep habits and requirements, neurobiology of sleep and wakefulness, circadian rhythm, chronobiology, physiology, genetics and functions of sleep, sleep deprivation, the approach to a patient with sleep complaints, and review of the ways in which sleep disorders are classified.
- *Section 2*: Utilizes question and answer format to reinforce the phenomenology of sleep and its disorders, using specific cases and integrating polysomnographic markers, laboratory assessment, and treatment of selected sleep disorders.
- The textbook also provides the reader with key illustrations, tables detailing diagnostic criteria, up-to-date treatment recommendations, as well as key highlights. The appendix consists of key tools that would help the readers with statistics methods, electrocardiogram (EKG) guides, and other high utility resources to assist with clinical care and polysomnography interpretation.
- While this textbook would be helpful to provide the fundamental knowledge base in sleep medicine and can be utilized as a reference guide and for review purposes, the reader is referred to other in-depth major textbooks and atlases to gain information about the order and disorders of sleep. This list is provided at the end of this chapter under "Recommended Sleep Medicine Textbooks."[1–10]

Brief Historical Overview

- Sleep is necessary, but its function, physiology, and pathophysiology have only been unfolding this century. Sleep research has opened the doors to and propelled the field of sleep medicine as we know it today.
- Since ancient times, two fundamental questions have intrigued scholars, scientists, and philosophers: (i) What is sleep? and (ii) Why do we sleep?
- The historical highlights that helped evolve the field are summarized in Table 1.1, which outlines chronologically important milestones in sleep research that have had a major impact on the development of sleep medicine.[11–16,18–24,26]
- Titus Lucretius Carus (40–50 BCE) proposed that sleep is an absence of wakefulness.

TABLE 1.1	Sleep Medicine History at a Glance		
Year	**Investigator/Author**	**Discovery**	**References**
1729	Jean Jacques d'Ortous de Mairan	Chronobiology of heliotrope plant	11
1875	R. Caton	EEG waves in dogs	11
1880	Jean Baptiste Edouard Gelineau	Narcolepsy named and described	11
1928–1930	H. Berger	Human brain surface: Alpha waves EEG to differentiate wake versus sleep	11,12
1935	F. Bremer	Two cat preps: Cerveau isole and encephale isole	11
1937	Loomis, Harvey, and Hobart	Stages of sleep reflected in the EEG	12
1949	G. Moruzzi and H. Magoun	Brainstem reticular formation to describe EEG wake versus sleep	11
1951–1955	N. Kleitman and E. Aserinsky	REM sleep discovery	11,12
1957	N. Kleitman and W. Dement	Described sleep stages	11
1959–1962	M. Jouvet	REM EMG suppression; pontine brainstem source of REM	11
1960	O. Pompeiano	Cat REM atonia mechanisms	11
1960	G. Vogel	Sleep onset REM periods	11
1960–1964	R. Hodes and W. Dement	Depressed "H" reflexes in REM sleep	11
1964	W. Dement and S. Mitchell	First narcolepsy clinic	11
1965	R. Jung and W. Kuhlo Gastaut, Tassinari, and Duron	First clear recognition and description of obstructive sleep apnea	11,12
1965	Oswald and Priest	First sleep tests to evaluate sedatives	11
1966–1971	A. Kales et al.	Sleep lab to study hypnotics; other illness	11
1968	A. Rechtschaffen and A. Kales	Standard method for scoring sleep stages	13
1970	R. Yoss, N. Moyer, and R. Hollenhorst	Pupillometry	14
1970–1978	E. Lugaresi et al.	Signs, symptom, and pathophysiology of sleep apnea	11
1972	J. Holland and Stanford et al.	Polysomnography	11
1973	E. Hoddes et al.	Stanford Sleepiness Scale	15
1977	C. Guilleminault and W. Dement	Dx/Classification of EDS	16
1976–1978	M. Carskadon et al.	Studies of sleep latency; MSLT developed	11
1975	Association of Sleep Disorders Centers	Now American Academy of Sleep Med.	11
1980	S. Fujita et al.	Introduction of UPPP for the treatment of sleep apnea	17
1981	C. Sullivan et al.	CPAP for treatment of sleep apnea	18
1986	C. Scheck and M. Mahowald	Description of RBD in humans	19
1991	M. Thorpy	Creation of the first ICSD	20
1993	S. Redline and T. Young	First community epidemiology data on sleep apnea	21
1999	E. Van Cauter	Sleep restriction may contribute to the metabolic syndrome.	22
1999	E. Mignot and J. Siegel	Abnormal hypocretin gene expression in narcolepsy. (+) HLA-DQB1*0602 are associated with loss of CSF hypocretin	23,24
2003	G. Tononi and C. Cirelli	SHY	25
2005	National Institutes of Health (NIH)	NIH Consensus Conference statement on Manifestations and Management of Chronic Insomnia in Adults	26
2007	J. Winkelman and D. Rye	Polygenetic association in RLS and PLMs	27,28
2007	AASM	New AASM Sleep Stage Classification: Reclassifies stages of non-REM sleep into three categories.	29–31

TABLE 1.1	Sleep Medicine History at a Glance—cont'd		
Year	Investigator/Author	Discovery	References
2008	Young et al.	Untreated sleep-disordered breathing leads to increased risk of mortality.	32
2009–2011	J. Bass, M.A. Lazar et al.	Circadian desynchrony leads to metabolic pathologies. CLOCK genes polymorphism may increase risk for tumorigenesis.	Multiple Authors
2010	Redline et al.	Sleep heart health study: Obstructive sleep apnea is associated with increased stroke risk for men.	33
2013	G.S. Perry et al. (CDC)	Establishes sleep duration as a public health epidemic in the publication "Raising Awareness of Sleep as a Healthy Behavior"	34
2013	L Xie et al.	Sleep is established to have a critical function in ensuring metabolic homeostasis via augmented removal of waste products that accumulate in the awake central nervous system.	35
2015–2016	AASM, SRS	AASM Consensus Statements detailing recommended amount of sleep for adult and pediatric populations	36,37

AASM, American Academy of Sleep Medicine; *CDC*, Centers for Disease Control; *CLOCK*, Circadian Locomotor Output Cycles Kaput; *CPAP*, continuous positive airway pressure; *CSF*, cerebrospinal fluid; *Dx*, diagnosis; *EDS*, excessive daytime sleepiness; *EEG*, electroencephalogram; *EMG*, electromyogram; *HLA*, human leukocyte antigen; *ICSD*, International Classification of Sleep Disorders; *MSLT*, multiple sleep latency test; *PLMs*, periodic limb movements; *RBD*, REM behavior disorder; *REM*, rapid eye movement; *RLS*, restless legs syndrome; *SA*, sleep apnea; *UPPP*, uvulopalatopharyngoplasty.

- In "The Philosophy of Sleep," in 1830 Robert Macnish revised Lucretius's theory, defining *sleep* as "suspension of sensorial power in which the voluntary functions are absent but the involuntary functions, such as circulation, respiration, and other functions controlled by the autonomic nervous system, remain intact."
- However, we know that sleep neither is the absence of wakefulness nor is it simply the suspension of sensorial power. Sleep proceeds from a combination of passive withdrawal of afferent stimuli to the brain and the simultaneous activation of discrete neurons in selective brain areas.
- The golden age of sleep medicine was ushered in 1929 by the invention of the electroencephalogram (EEG), which propelled key physiological studies to unravel consciousness, sleep, and wakefulness in the 1930s and 1940s.
- The discovery of rapid eye movement (REM) sleep in 1953 (by Aserinsky and Kleitman) ushered in the golden age of sleep medicine.
- Since the second half of the last century, significant advances were made in the scientific understanding of sleep and its disorders, which galvanized the establishment of sleep medicine as an important clinical discipline. Recognition of the importance of sleep and its disorders is increasing among the medical profession and the public.
- The 2014 *International Classification of Sleep Disorders, 3rd edition* (ICSD-III) published by the American Academy of Sleep Medicine (AASM) organizes and classifies the sleep disorders in the field of sleep medicine.[38]
- Medical schools and residency programs have not always aligned educational curriculum with the rapid growth of sleep medicine or consistently integrated it in their curriculum.[39]

Ontogeny of Sleep

- Newborns: Sleep is characterized by a polyphasic pattern with 16 hours of sleep per day. About 50% of the time is spent in REM sleep, or active sleep is accompanied by restless movements of the arms, legs, and facial muscles.
- Age 3 months: The nonrapid eye movement (NREM)–REM cyclical pattern of adult sleep is established, but with a shorter duration. Sleep spindles begin to appear.
- Age 6 months: Appearance of K complexes.
- Age 3–5 years: Sleep requirement diminishes to about 10 hours per day. Time spent in REM sleep decreased to the normal adult pattern of 25%.
- Preschool children: Sleep assumes a biphasic pattern.
- Adults exhibit a monophasic sleep pattern, with an average duration of 7.5–8 hours per night.
- Older age:
  - Amplitude and percentage of slow waves (delta) sleep are attenuated.
  - Sleep is characterized by frequent awakenings, including a predisposition to early morning awakenings.
  - REM sleep percentage remains relatively constant.
  - Total sleep duration within 24 hours: Compares with that of a young adults, but is characterized by napping during the daytime.

Definition of Sleep

- Modern researchers define sleep on the basis of both behavioral and physiological criteria (Table 1.2).
  - The behavioral criteria consist of immobility or slight mobility, closed eyes, a characteristic species-specific sleeping posture, decreased response to external stimulation, quiescence, increased reaction time, elevated arousal threshold, and attenuated cognitive function in the setting of reversible unconscious state.
  - Physiological criteria are based on EEG, electrooculography (EOG), and electromyography (EMG) findings, as well as unique physiological changes such as unique ventilation and circulation.
- Transition to sleep and sleep onset is highlighted by progressive changes in key behavioral and physiological characteristics consisting of rhythms, cognition, and mental processing.

TABLE 1.2	Behavioral and Physiological Criteria of Wakefulness and Sleep		
Criteria	Awake	Nonrapid Eye Movement Sleep	Rapid Eye Movement Sleep
Posture	Erect, sitting, or recumbent	Recumbent	Recumbent
Mobility	Normal	Slightly reduced or immobile; postural shifts	Moderately reduced or immobile; myoclonic jerks
Response to stimulation	Normal	Mildly to moderately reduced	Moderately reduced to no response
Level of alertness	Alert	Unconscious but reversible	Unconscious but reversible
Eyelids	Open	Closed	Closed
Eye movements	Waking eye movements	Slow rolling eye movements	Rapid eye movements
EEG	Alpha waves; desynchronized	Synchronized	Theta or sawtooth; desynchronized
EMG (muscle tone)	Normal	Mildly reduced	Moderately to severely reduced or absent
EOG	Waking eye movements	Slow rolling eye movements	Rapid eye movements

EEG, Electroencephalogram; *EMG,* electromyogram; *EOG,* electrooculogram.

- Sleep onset is subjectively characterized by heaviness and drooping of the eyelids; clouding of the sensorium; and loss of the ability to see, hear, or perceive things in a rational or logical manner. The person at this moment has no control of his brain and cannot respond logically and adequately.
- Sleep offset, or awakening, is similarly marked by a gradual process similar to the moment of sleep onset.

Proposed Biological Functions of Sleep

1. Body and brain tissue restoration
2. Facilitation of waste clearance of the central nervous system via the glymphatic system (Fig. 1.1)
3. Energy conservation
4. Adaptation
5. Memory reinforcement and consolidation
6. Synaptic neuronal network integrity
7. Gene expression in sleep/wakefulness (Fig. 1.2)
8. Thermoregulation

Dreams

- Sigmund Freud called dreams the "royal road to the unconscious," representing repressed feelings that emerge psychologically suppressed in the unconscious mind.
- In the modern era, sleep scientists, however, interpret dreams within a neurophysiological domain.
- The discovery in 1953 of REM sleep by Aserinsky and Kleitman has catalyzed dream research, shifting it to a new direction. In 1957 Dement and Kleitman discovered that REM coincided with the appearance of dreams.
- Approximately 80% of dreams occur during REM sleep and 20% during NREM sleep.
- Dreams occurring during REM sleep are characterized by complex, bizarre, and highly emotionally charged dreams, for which there is good recollection. This is particularly true if the subject is awakened immediately after the onset of REM dreams.
- Dreams occurring during NREM sleep are somewhat more rational and realistic, but recollection is more difficult.

- In general, people are oriented when awakening from REM sleep, but disorientation and confusion typically characterizes awakening from NREM sleep.
- The neurobiological significance of dreams remains an enigma, but might allow the brain to optimize its generative model of the world during wakefulness.[40]
  - Monophasic potentials within the pontine region are generated and can be recorded on the lateral geniculate body and in the occipital cortex; hence the name of ponto-geniculo-occipital waves (PGO).
  - The PGO spread to the oculomotor system to provoke the REMs of REM sleep and possibly give rise to visual hallucinatory phenomena.
  - PGO also stimulate limbic structures related to emotion and memory and are activated by these potentials, generating the mnemonic and emotional components of dreams.
- The important clinical corollary is dream-enacting behavior associated with abnormal movements during sleep, which constitutes an important REM sleep parasomnia.
- Some suggest that dreaming results in activation of the neural networks in the brain, restructuring and reinterpretation of data stored in memory, and removal of unnecessary and useless information from the brain of a dreamer.

Sleep Architecture Sleep Stages

- Table 1.3 outlines EEG sleep stage based on EEGH frequencies, duration, voltage, and origin within the brain.
- From a physiological perspective, sleep is segregated into two independent states: NREM sleep and REM sleep.
- Based on EEG criteria, NREM sleep consists of three stages: stage N1, N2, and N3 sleep.
- The 1968 Rechtschaffen and Kales (R&K) sleep stage scoring divided NREM sleep into stages 1, 2, 3, and 4.
- The 2007 AASM Task Force divided NREM into three stages: N1, N2, and N3 (slow-wave sleep). The latter was previously divided into stage 3 and 4 sleep, but this dichotomy is of unclear clinical significance.
- NREM and REM sleep alternate, with each cycle lasting for approximately 90–100 min, with about four to six such cycles noted during a normal sleep period.

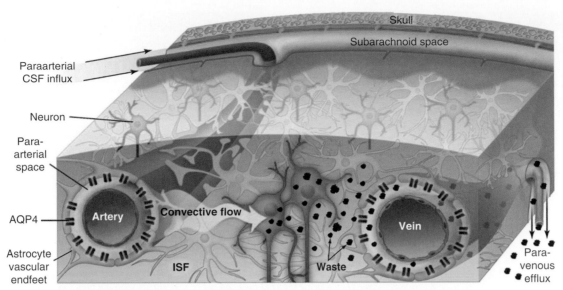

• **Figure 1.1** Pathway to Clear Cellular Waste from the Brain Using the Glymphatic System. Cerebrospinal fluid (CSF) enters the paraarterial space surrounding the arteries (*top part* of the figure). This space is bound by the nonluminal surface of the blood vessel and the apical processes of astrocytes. Aquaporin-4 (AQP4) is a water channel that facilitates convective flow out of the paraarterial space into the interstitial space. CSF exchanges with interstitial fluid (ISF) and generates a convective flow that clears the waste using a paravenous route. (Reproduced with permission from American Association for the Advancement of Science, from Nedergaard. Romero R, Badr MS. A role for sleep disorders in pregnancy complications: challenges and opportunities. *Am J Obstet Gynecol.* 2014;210[1]:3–11.)

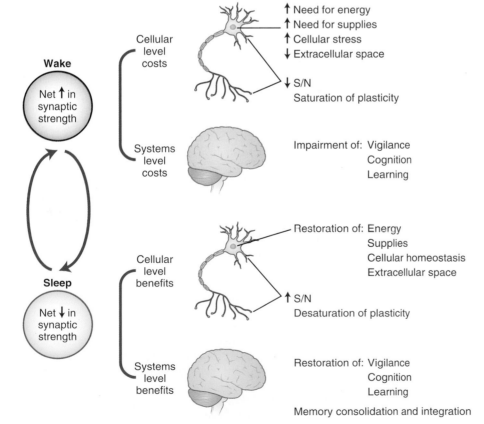

• **Figure 1.2** Synaptic Homeostasis Hypothesis. The Synaptic Homeostasis Hypothesis (SHY): SHY postulates that the fundamental function of sleep is the restoration of synaptic homeostasis, which is challenged by synaptic strengthening triggered by learning during wake and by synaptogenesis during development. To put plainly, sleep is "the price we pay for plasticity." Increased synaptic strength has various costs at the cellular and systems level including higher energy consumption, greater demand for the delivery of cellular supplies to synapses leading to cellular stress, and associated changes in support cells such as glia. Increased synaptic strength also reduces the selectivity of neuronal responses and saturates the ability to learn. By renormalizing synaptic strength, sleep reduces the burden of plasticity on neurons and other cells while restoring neuronal selectivity and the ability to learn, and in doing so enhances signal-to-noise ratios, leading to the consolidation and integration of memories. *S/N*, Signal-to-noise ratios. (From Tononi G, Cirelli C. Sleep and the price of plasticity. Synaptic and cellular homeostasis to memory consolidation and integration. *Neuron.* 2014;81[1]:12–34.)

TABLE 1.3 **Key Brain Wave Frequencies and Landmarks Used in Sleep Staging**

Sample	Label	Definition
	Alpha activity	8–13 Hz rhythm, usually most prominent in occipital loads. Thought to be generated by cortex, possibly via dipole located in layers 4 and 5. Used as a marker for relaxed wakefulness and CNS arousals.
	Theta activity	4–8 Hz waves, typically prominent in central and temporal leads. Sawtooth activity (shown in figure) is a unique variant of theta activity (containing waveforms with a notched or *sawtooth-shaped* appearance) frequently seen during REM sleep.
	Vertex sharp waves	Sharply contoured, negative-going bursts that stand out from the background activity and appear most often in central leads placed near the midline.
	Sleep spindle	A phasic burst of 11–16 Hz activity, prominent in central scalp leads; typically last for 0.5–1.5 sec. Spindles are a scalp representation of thalamocortical discharges; the name derives from their shape (which is spindle-like).
	K complex	Recently redefined in the AASM manual as *an EEG event consisting of a well-delineated negative sharp wave immediately followed by a positive component standing out from the background EEG with total duration ≥0.5 sec, usually maximal in amplitude over the frontal regions.*
	Slow waves	High-amplitude (≥75 µV) and low-frequency (≤2 Hz) variants of delta (1–4 Hz) activity. Slow waves are the defining characteristics of stage N3 sleep.
	REM	Rapid eye movements are conjugate saccades occurring during REM sleep correlated with the dreamer's attempt to look at the dream sensorium. They are sharply peaked with an initial deflection usually less than 0.5 sec in duration.
	SEM	Slow eye movements are conjugate, usually rhythmic, rolling eye movements with an initial deflection usually ≥0.5 sec in duration.

AASM, American Academy of Sleep Medicine; *CNS*, central nervous system; *EEG*, electroencephalogram; *REM*, rapid eye movements.
Modified from Kryger MH, Avidan A, Berry R. *Atlas of Clinical Sleep Medicine.* 2nd ed. Philadelphia, PA: Saunders/Elsevier; 2013.

- Stage N3 sleep dominates the initial two cycles, diminishing later at night, while REM sleep cycles progressively increase from the first to the last cycle, and toward the end of the night.
- Thus the first third of a normal sleep episode is dominated by slow-wave sleep, and REM sleep dominates the last third.
- Human adult-NREM sleep accounts for 75%–80% of total sleep time.
- Stage N1 sleep:
  - Makes up approximately 3%–8% of sleep time.
  - Marked by decrease in alpha rhythms (8–13 Hz), to less than 50% in a 30 sec epoch (segment of a polysomnogram [PSG]), an admixture of slower frequency theta rhythms (4–7 Hz) and appearance of beta waves (>13 Hz).
  - EMG activity diminishes.
  - Towards the end of N1 sleep, slow rolling eye movements and vertex sharp waves are noted.
- Stage N2 sleep:
  - Characterized by two key EEG findings: sleep spindles (12–18 Hz, most often 14 Hz) and biphasic K complexes intermixed with vertex sharp waves.

- The EEG recording contains theta activity and fewer than 20% slow waves (0.5–2 Hz).
- It lasts for approximately 30–60 min.
- Stage N3 sleep:
  - Slow waves; delta activity occupies 20%–100% of the epoch.
  - Body movements are registered as artifacts in the PSG recordings.
- REM sleep (R sleep):
  - Occurs 60–90 min after the onset of sleep.
  - Accounts for 20%–25% of total sleep time.
  - Further subdivided into two stages: tonic and phasic (based on EEG, EMG, and EOG features).
  - EEG is characterized by fast rhythms and theta activity, some assuming sawtooth morphology.
    - *Tonic REM sleep:* Characterized by desynchronized EEG, hypotonia, or atonia of the major skeletal muscle groups and depression of monosynaptic and polysynaptic reflexes.
    - *Phasic REM sleep*: Characterized by REM in all directions, as well as phasic fluctuations in autonomic activity (blood

pressure, heart rate, irregular respiration), spontaneous middle-ear muscle activity, and tongue movements.

Prevalence of Sleep Disorders

- More than 80 different types of sleep disorders are currently defined.
- Inadequate sleep is the most common sleep problem in the United States.
- In 2009 the National Sleep Foundation (NSF; http://www.sleepfoundation.org/) reported that 46% of people reported inadequate sleep. Furthermore, they also stated, "54% of drivers (105 million) have driven while drowsy at least once in the past year, and 28% (54 million) do so at least once per month."[41]
- Drowsiness, fatigue, and insomnia are prevalent in our culture and are the primary symptoms leading to sleep medicine consultation.
- Table 1.4 provides a compilation of the prevalence rates for the key sleep disorders, if data is known.[38,42]

Circadian Clock Systems and Sleep Habits

- The circadian clock system is regulated by transcriptional and translational negative feedback loops of multiple clock genes in a tissue-specific manner and is a major regulator of cellular metabolism, stress response, and other key physiologic functions.[43]
- The Circadian Locomotor Output Cycles Kaput (CLOCK) gene polymorphism is associated with human diurnal preference.[44]
- Two groups of individuals are recognized based on sleep habits, evening types and morning types, and this is likely determined by genetic factors.
  - Evening types ("owls") have difficulty getting up early and feel tired in the morning. They tend to feel more energetic and perform best in the evening; they go to sleep late and wake up late.
  - Morning types ("larks") wake up early, feel rested, and work efficiently in the morning.
- The body temperature rhythm shows two different curves in these two circadian phenotypes; it reaches the evening peak an hour earlier in morning types than in evening types.
- Genetic variations at the CLOCK locus have been linked with lifestyle-related conditions including obesity, metabolic syndrome, and cardiovascular diseases.[45]
- Dysregulation of the 'period' (PER) clock genes, which have tumor suppressor properties, has been associated with sleep disorders, differences in diurnal hormone secretion, and increased susceptibility to certain cancer risk.[46–48]

Sleep Requirements

- *Sleep requirement* is defined as the optimal amount of sleep required to remain alert and fully awake and to function adequately throughout the day.
- Sleep requirement for an average adult is approximately 7.5–8 hours regardless of environment or cultural differences.
- Sleep need is determined by heredity rather than by different personality traits or other psychological factors. Social or biological factors may also play a role.

- Both excessively long and short sleep periods may be risk factors for high blood pressure, with a stronger association in women than men.[36]

Sleep Duration Consensus

- In 2015 members of the AASM and the Sleep Research Society (SRS) published a consensus statement regarding the recommended amount of sleep to promote optimal health in adults.[49]
- The report coincides with the goals of the National Healthy Sleep Awareness Project (NHSAP) together with a Sleep Health Objective of Healthy People 2020 to "increase the proportion of adults who get sufficient sleep."[50]
- The paper examined 2391 young adults, 20–39 years of age, in whom the associations of sleep duration with Health Related Quality of Life (HRQOL) and sleep health disparities were reviewed. The data demonstrates the following trends in the sample population[40]:
  - Sleep duration less than 7 hours is more likely to be associated with poor general health and low overall physical and mental HRQOL than those sleeping ≥7 hours.
  - Sleep duration less than 7 hours is associated with poorer general health (typically assessed by HRQOL measures) and increased risk or presence of disease compared with 7–8 hours of sleep.
  - Less solid evidence was found for an association of longer sleep duration and adverse health status, with only a few studies demonstrating an association of poorer general health or increased risk/presence of disease with ≥9 hours of sleep.
  - Higher risk for both overall cardiovascular disease and hypertension was associated with sleep durations less than 6 hours, (possibly for sleep durations of 6–7 hours), compared with sleep durations of 7–8 hours (Table 1.5).
  - Sleep duration of 6 hours or less was not sufficient to support optimal health in adults.
  - Sleep duration of 7–9 hours of sleep were appropriate to support optimal health in adults.
  - Sleep duration of 9 or more hours of sleep on optimal adult health could not be ascertained with certainty.
  - Consensus regarding the appropriateness of sleep durations in the 6–7-hour range could not be reached, but the median vote of consensus members suggested that this duration was in the inappropriate range.
- In 2016 the AASM members developed consensus recommendations for the proper amount of sleep per 24 hours needed to promote optimal health in children and adolescents using a modified RAND Appropriateness Method. The recommendations are summarized in Table 1.6.
- A poll by the NSF in 2000, 2001, and 2002 indicated that the average sleep duration for Americans had fallen to 6.9–7.0 hours.
- Across the board, over the last half of the 20th century, sleep duration has diminished by 1.5–2 hours, leading to an epidemic of sleep deprivation, where most people are in bed for only 5–6 hours per night on a regular basis.
- In 2014 the NSF utilized the Sleep Health Index, a new annual general population poll that tracks Americans' sleep behaviors and trends. The data reported that 45% of Americans say that poor or insufficient sleep affected their daily activities at least once in the past 7 days.[51]

TABLE 1.4 Estimated Prevalence Rates for Major Sleep Disorders[42]	
Sleep Disorder	Prevalence[a,b]
Adjustment Insomnia	15%–20% approximate
Advanced Sleep Phase Disorder	About 1% middle-age adults or older
Behavioral Insomnia of Childhood	10%–30% of children
Cheyne-Stokes Breathing Pattern	25%–40% of heart failure; 10% of stroke
Circadian: Delayed Sleep Phase Disorder	7%–16% of adolescents/young adults
Circadian: Free-running type	Likely in over half of blind subjects
Circadian: Shift Work Sleep Disorder	2%–5% or more
Confusional Arousals	17.3% of age 3–13; 2.9%–4.2% ≥ age 15
Congenital Central Alveolar Hypoventilation	Rare with 160–180 living children reported
Hypersomnolence-no substance/condition	5%–7% of hypersomniacs
Idiopathic Insomnia	0.7% adolescents; <10% sleep patients
Inadequate Sleep Hygiene	5%–10% of sleep clinic insomniacs
Infant Sleep Apnea	<31 weeks 50%–80%; >32 weeks 12%–15%
Insomnia due to Mental Disorder	3% general population
Long Sleeper	2% of men; 1.5% of women sleep ≥ 10 hours/night
Narcolepsy with Cataplexy	0.02%–0.18% United States/Western Europe
Narcolepsy without Cataplexy	Unknown overall; 10%–50% of narcoleptics
Obstructive Sleep Apnea, Adult	4%–24% men; 2%–9% women; depends on study
Obstructive Sleep Apnea, Pediatric	2% of children, usually preschool age
Paradoxical Insomnia	<5% of insomniacs
Periodic Limb Movement Disorder	Up to 34% > age 60; 1%–15% of insomniacs
Primary Sleep Apnea of Infancy	25% of babies <2.5 kg; <0.5% full-term
Psychophysiological Insomnia	1%–2% population; 12%–15% sleep patients
Recurrent Hypersomnia	Rare with 200 reported subjects; male predominance
Recurrent Isolated Sleep Paralysis	5%–6% adults; 15%–40% < age 30 of ≥1 episode
Rapid Eye Movement Sleep Behavior Disorder	About 0.5% of elderly; 0.38% general population
Restless Legs Syndrome	10% of N. European adults
Short Sleeper	3.6% of men; 4.3% of women sleep ≤5 hours/night
Sleep Enuresis	30% of age 4; 10% of age 6; 5% of age 10
Sleep-Related Bruxism	14%–15% of children; 8% young to middle-age adults
Sleep-Related Eating Disorder	3/4 female; 4.6% of college students in a study
Sleep-Related Leg Cramps	7% of children; nearly all adults > age 50
Sleep-Related Rhythmic Movement Disorder	59% of babies; 5% by age 5
Sleep Starts	60%–70%
Sleep Talking	1/2 of young children; 5% of adults
Sleep Terrors	1%–6.5% children; 2.2% adults
Sleep Walking	Up to 17% children; up to 4% adults
Sleep-Related Epilepsy	10%–45% of epileptics
Snoring (habitual)	10%–12% of children; 24% adult women; 40% men

[a]Prevalence may not be known for unlisted diagnoses.
[b]Unless otherwise specified, prevalence rates are for the general population.

TABLE 1.5	Joint Consensus Statement of the American Academy of Sleep Medicine and Sleep Research Society on the Recommended Amount of Sleep for a Healthy Adult: Methodology and Discussion[48]
Adults	Sleep duration appropriate to support optimal health in adults
18–60 years of age	7–9 hours

TABLE 1.6	American Academy of Sleep Medicine Consensus Statement Outlining Recommended Amount of Sleep for Pediatric Populations: Data Is Listed Per 24 Hours, Including Naps, on a Regular Basis to Promote Optimal Health[37]
Age Group	Amount of Sleep Recommended Per 24 Hours
Infants <4 months of age:	NA*
Infants: (4–12 months):	12–16 hours
Children:	
• 1–2 years of age	11–14 hours
• 3–5 years of age	10–13 hours per 24 hours
• 6–12 years of age	9–12 hours
Teenagers: 13–18 years of age	8–10 hours

*Specific recommendations are not part of the consensus due to the extensive range of normal variation in duration and patterns of sleep and lack of insufficient evidence for associations with health outcomes.

TABLE 1.7	New Recommendations for Appropriate Sleep Durations Sleep Health: The National Sleep Foundation, Along With a Multi-Disciplinary Expert Panel, Issued a Report That Recommends Wider Appropriate Sleep Ranges for Most Age Groups
Newborns (0–3 months):	Sleep range narrowed to 14–17 hours each day (previously it was 12–18)
Infants (4–11 months):	Sleep range widened 2 hours to 12–15 hours (previously it was 14–15)
Toddlers (1–2 years):	Sleep range widened by 1 hour to 11–14 hours (previously it was 12–14)
Preschoolers (3–5):	Sleep range widened by 1 hour to 10–13 hours (previously it was 11–13)
School age children (6–13):	Sleep range widened by 1 hour to 9–11 hours (previously it was 10–11)
Teenagers (14–17):	Sleep range widened by 1 hour to 8–10 hours (previously it was 8.5–9.5)
Younger adults (18–25):	Sleep range is 7–9 hours (new age category)
Adults (26–64):	Sleep range did not change and remains 7–9 hours
Older adults (65+):	Sleep range is 7–8 hours (new age category)

- Americans report sleeping an average of 7 hours and 36 min a night, on average going to bed at 10:55 PM and waking at 6:38 AM.
- On workdays, sleep duration was roughly 40 min longer that on nonworkdays or weekends.
- In February 2017, the NSF issued the first report detailing sleep quality recommendations stratified by specific age group, summarized in Table 1.7.[52]

Symptoms of Sleep Disorders

Excessive Daytime Sleepiness

- The overall prevalence of sleepiness is somewhat variable depending on how the survey is completed and the size of the population, geography, but is estimated to be from 0.3%–36% overall.[53]
- Excessive sleepiness must be differentiated from fatigue or tiredness.
  - Based on the behavioral definition, fatigue can be differentiated by absence of the previously mentioned criteria for the presence of sleep.

- *Fatigue* defines a state of sustained lack of energy, such as one would observe in patients suffering from multiple sclerosis, coupled with a lack of motivation and drive, but without the behavioral criteria of sleepiness such as heaviness or drooping of the eyelids, sagging or nodding of the head, and yawning.
- In a Swedish study of 10,216 participants, excessive daytime sleepiness (EDS) was approximately five times more prevalent in the elderly with poor health versus good health.[54] That same year in 1996 was published a Finnish study of 11,354 adults, 33–60 years old that showed 11% of women and 6.7% of men had EDS nearly every day.[55] A Japanese study published in 2005 studied 28,714 subjects that revealed EDS in 2.5% of participants.[56] More recently, of 959 American women respondents, 21% reported having daytime sleepiness.[57]
- The youth have had an excess of problems with sleepiness as well. The NSF reports on March 28, 2006, that 45% of adolescents, ages 11–17, sleep less than 8 hours on school nights and at least 14% oversleep and 28% fall asleep in school at least once per week. Fifty-one percent of adolescent drivers have also admitted to driving drowsy within the year preceding this poll.
- Fig. 1.3 provides a flow diagram describing the potential causes of EDS, based on the possibility that it could originate from sleep deprivation, primary sleep disorders, medical and psychiatric comorbidities, and could be confused with but should be differentiated from fatigue.

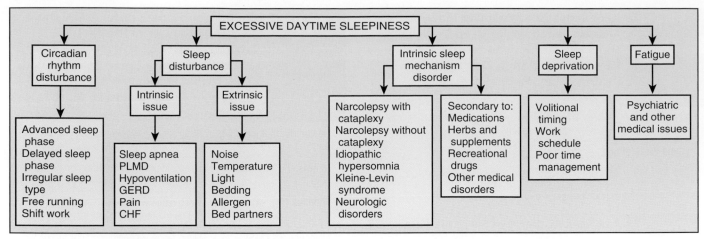

• **Figure 1.3** Diagnostic Flow Chart to Approach Excessive Daytime Sleepiness. *CHF*, Congestive heart failure; *GERD*, gastroesophageal reflux disease; *PLMD*, periodic limb movement disorder. (From Kryger MH, Roth T, Dement WC, eds. *Principles and Practice of Sleep Medicine.* 6th ed. Philadelphia, PA: Elsevier; 2017:577.)

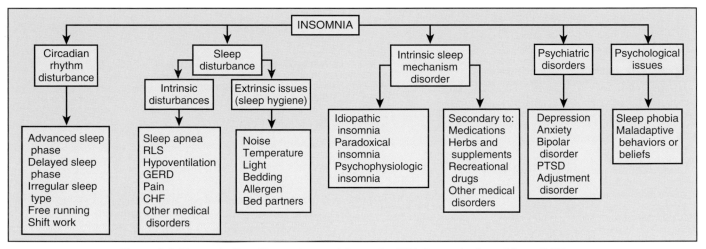

• **Figure 1.4** Diagnostic Flow Chart to Approach Insomnia. *CHF*, Congestive heart failure; *GERD*, gastroesophageal reflux disease; *PTSD*, posttraumatic stress disorder; *RLS*, restless legs syndrome. (From: Kryger MH, Roth T, Dement WC, eds. *Principles and Practice of Sleep Medicine.* 6th ed. Philadelphia, PA: Elsevier; 2017:577.)

Insomnia

- Insomnia has traditionally been discussed separately than EDS in terms of diagnosis, surveys, and epidemiology and has been thought to be more of a 'hyper-aroused' state rather than EDS.
- Insomnia prevalence has varied, depending on the patient population and type of insomnia evaluated. Prevalence appears to range from 1%–2% for chronic insomnia in the general population to 15%–20% for acute insomnia.[41]
- Usually women report more insomnia than men.
- Recently a study of 4188 employees were surveyed about sleep patterns and classified into four categories of insomnia, insufficient sleep syndrome, at-risk, and good sleep. The highest rate of sleep medication use was in the insomnia group.[58]
- Fig. 1.4 outlines a diagnostic approach to the evaluation of insomnia based on underlying primary sleep disorders, medical, psychiatric, and psychological comorbidities, and due to circadian rhythm disturbances.

Abnormal and Complex Nocturnal Behaviors

- Nocturnal events may be categorized into simple behaviors (repetitive or periodic movements, rhythmical movements) and complex behaviors (sleep talking, sleep walking, sleep terrors, dream enactment behavior).
- Simple movements, such as rhythmic movements, occur during the transition from wake to sleep or sleep to wake or during light, NREM sleep.
- Complex nocturnal behaviors can result from incomplete oscillation and disruptions of the control mechanisms of the three normal states of being: wakefulness, NREM sleep, and REM sleep.
- The differential diagnosis is extensive and includes nocturnal seizures, NREM, and REM parasomnias, dissociative psychiatric events, or physiological states such as hypoglycemia.
- A detailed history, including a clear description from the patient and ideally a bed partner or family witness, is the cornerstone of establishing clues about the underlying etiology. The challenge

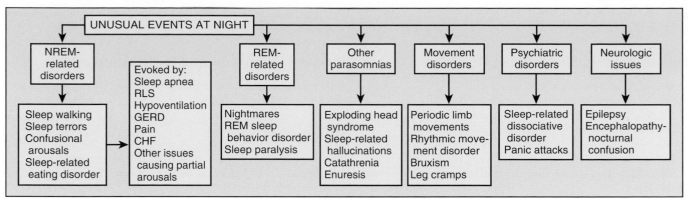

• **Figure 1.5** Diagnostic Flow Chart to Approach Unusual Nocturnal Events. *CHF,* Congestive heart failure; *GERD,* gastroesophageal reflux disease; *NREM,* nonrapid eye movement; *REM,* rapid eye movement; *RLS,* restless legs syndrome. (From Kryger MH, Roth T, Dement WC, eds. *Principles and Practice of Sleep Medicine.* 6th ed. Philadelphia, PA: Elsevier; 2017:577.)

for the clinician is to recognize when certain nocturnal events signal an underlying, treatable disorder, an emerging neurological abnormality, or a benign age-appropriate episode.
• Fig. 1.5 provides a flow chart to approach unusual nocturnal events. CHF, Congestive heart failure; GERD, gastroesophageal reflux disease; RLS, restless legs syndrome.

International Classification of Sleep Disorders

The third edition of the ICSD-III (published by AASM)[38] includes seven major categories of sleep disorders:
1. Insomnia
2. Sleep-related breathing disorders
3. Central disorders of hypersomnolence
4. Circadian rhythm sleep–wake disorders
5. Parasomnias
6. Sleep-related movement disorders
7. Other sleep disorders

Each of the seven major categories can be further divided as follows:

Insomnia

1. Disorders
   a. Chronic insomnia disorder
   b. Short-term insomnia disorder
   c. Other insomnia disorder
2. Isolated symptoms and normal variants
   a. Excessive time in bed
   b. Short sleeper

Sleep-Related Breathing Disorders

Sleep-related breathing disorders are characterized by abnormal respiration during sleep; they occur in both adults and children. There are four major sleep-related breathing disorders:
1. Central sleep apnea syndromes
   a. Central sleep apnea with Cheyne-Stokes

   b. Central apnea due to a medical disorder without Cheyne-Stokes breathing
   c. Central sleep apnea due to high altitude periodic breathing
   d. Central sleep apnea due to a medication or substance
   e. Primary central sleep apnea
   f. Primary sleep apnea of infancy
   g. Primary central sleep apnea of prematurity
   h. Treatment-emergent central sleep apnea (previously noted as "Complex sleep apnea")
2. Obstructive sleep apnea syndromes (OSASs)
   The OSASs include adult obstructive sleep apnea and pediatric obstructive sleep apnea.
3. Sleep-related hypoventilation disorders
   a. Obesity hypoventilation syndrome
   b. Congenital central alveolar hypoventilation syndrome
   c. Late-onset central hypoventilation with hypothalamic dysfunction
   d. Idiopathic central alveolar hypoventilation
   e. Sleep-related hypoventilation due to a medication or substance
   f. Sleep-related hypoventilation due to a medical disorder
4. Sleep-related hypoxemia disorder
   a. Sleep-related hypoxemia
5. Isolated symptoms and normal variants
   a. Snoring
   b. Catathrenia

Central Disorders of Hypersomnolence

   a. Narcolepsy type 1 (previously referred to as narcolepsy with cataplexy)
   b. Narcolepsy type 2 (previously referred to as narcolepsy without cataplexy)
   c. Idiopathic hypersomnia (IH)
   d. Kleine–Levin syndrome (KLS)
   e. Hypersomnia due to a medical disorder
   f. Hypersomnia due to a medication or substance
   g. Hypersomnia associated with a psychiatric disorder
   h. Insufficient sleep syndrome

1. Isolated symptoms and normal variants
   a. Long sleeper

Circadian Rhythm Sleep–Wake Disorders

   a. Delayed sleep–wake phase disorder
   b. Advanced sleep–wake phase disorder
   c. Irregular sleep–wake rhythm disorder
   d. Non-24-hour sleep–wake rhythm disorder
   e. Shift work disorder
   f. Jet lag disorder
   g. Circadian sleep–wake disorder not otherwise specified (NOS)

Parasomnias

1. NREM-related parasomnias
   a. Disorders of arousal (from NREM sleep)
   b. Confusional arousals
      (i) Subtype: Sexsomnias
   c. Sleepwalking
      (i) Subtype: Sleep-related eating disorder (SRED)
   d. Sleep terrors
2. REM-related parasomnias
   a. REM sleep behavior disorder (RBD)
   b. Recurrent isolated sleep paralysis
   c. Nightmare disorder
3. Other parasomnias
   a. Exploding head syndrome
   b. Sleep-related hallucinations
   c. Sleep enuresis
   d. Parasomnia due to a medical disorder
   e. Parasomnia due to a medication or substance
   f. Parasomnia, unspecified
4. Isolated symptoms and normal variants
   a. Sleep talking

Sleep-Related Movement Disorders

   a. RLS, a.k.a. Willis-Ekbom Disease (WED)
   b. Periodic limb movement disorder (PLMD)
   c. Sleep-related leg cramps
   d. Sleep-related bruxism
   e. Sleep-related rhythmic movement disorder
   f. Benign sleep myoclonus of infancy
   g. Propriospinal myoclonus at sleep onset
   h. Sleep-related movement disorder due to a medical disorder
   i. Sleep-related movement disorder due to a medication or substance
   j. Sleep-related movement disorder, unspecified
1. Isolated symptoms and normal variants
   a. Excessive fragmentary myoclonus
   b. Hypnagogic foot tremor and alternating leg muscle activation
   c. Sleep starts (hypnic jerks)

Other Sleep Disorders

This category includes sleep disorders that cannot be appropriately classified elsewhere in the ICSD-III, either because the disorder overlaps with more than one category or when insufficient data have been collected to firmly establish another diagnosis.

Isolated Symptoms and Normal Variants

Other sleep-related symptoms or events do not meet the standard definition of a sleep disorder.

Appendices

The third edition of the ICSD-III includes two appendices:
   Appendix A includes diagnoses that can be classified as medical or neurologic disorders.
1. Disorders
   a. Fatal familial insomnia
   b. Sleep-related epilepsy
   c. Sleep-related headaches
   d. Sleep-related laryngospasm
   e. Sleep-related gastroesophageal reflux
   f. Sleep-related myocardial ischemia
   Appendix B is a guide to ICD-10-CM coding for substance-induced sleep disorders.

Key Tools for the Evaluation of Sleep Disorder

- Diagnostic workup for the primary or comorbid condition causing sleep disturbance.

Laboratory Tests for the Diagnosis and Monitoring of Sleep Disorders

- Overnight polysomnography (PSG): Sleep apnea, PLMD, narcolepsy
- High-definition video PSG: Complex nocturnal events (seizures, parasomnias, movement disorders)
- Multiple sleep latency tests (MSLTs): Evaluation of hypersomnia
- Maintenance of wakefulness test (MWT): Assessment of patients for whom inability to remain awake constitutes safety issue (e.g., patient is a truck driver, pilot) and for the assessment of patient's response to treatment
- Actigraphy: Circadian rhythm sleep disorders; insomnia where sleep–wake patterns are thought to play a role
- Video-PSG with multiple expanded electromyographic (EMG) montage (complex nocturnal behaviors-parasomnias, nocturnal seizures, motor disorders of sleep including periodic limb movements)

Laboratory Tests for Suspected Seizure Disorders

- Standard electroencephalography (EEG)
- Video-EEG monitoring for suspected seizure disorders
- Video-PSG with multiple expanded electroencephalography (EEG) montage

Imaging Studies

- Upper airway imaging: Surgical and dental assessment of obstructive sleep apnea

- Neuroimaging studies: Computed tomography, magnetic resonance imaging (MRI) in cases of suspected neurological illness causing sleep disorder (KLS, nocturnal seizures, secondary narcolepsy, secondary RBD)
- Fiberoptic endoscopy and cephalometric radiographs of the cranial base and facial bones: Utilized to locate site of the upper airway collapse, and to assess posterior airway space in obstructive sleep apnea (OSA) patients

Miscellaneous Tests

- Standard blood and urine analysis
- Pulmonary function tests, including arterial blood gases (ABGs) in cases of suspected bronchopulmonary and neuromuscular disorders causing sleep-disordered breathing and nocturnal hypocentillation
- Histocompatibility leukocyte antigen for suspected narcolepsy (HLA DQB1*0602)
- Cerebrospinal fluid (CSF) hypocretin-1 levels in suspected narcolepsy
- Urine toxicology: Prior to MSLT in the assessment of narcolepsy
- Serum ferritin, total iron binding capacity (TIBC) levels for patients with RLS/WED
- EMG and nerve conduction studies to exclude comorbid or secondary RLS/WED
- Cardiological investigations including EKG, Holter EKG, and echocardiogram (prior to the use of analeptics)
- Endocrine tests (particular, hyper/hypothyroidism in the setting of fatigue, insomnia)
- Autonomic function tests in patients with suspected autonomic dysfunction; hypothalamic lesions with secondary narcolepsy and sleep-related breathing disorders

Indications for home sleep apnea testing (HAST): May be an alternative for the initial diagnosis of OSA in patients with a high pretest probability for the conditions.

Contraindications for HSAT:
1. Patient is 18 years old or younger
2. Moderate or severe chronic obstructive pulmonary disease (COPD)—FEV1/FVC less than or equal to 0.7 and FEV1 less than 80% of predicted
3. Moderate or severe CHF—NYHA class III or IV
4. Cognitive impairment (inability to follow simple instructions)
5. Neuromuscular impairment
6. Suspicion of a sleep disorder other than OSA (e.g. central sleep apnea, narcolepsy, restless leg syndrome, circadian rhythm disorder, parasomnias, PLMD)
7. Previous technically suboptimal home sleep study (2 nights of study attempted)
8. Previous 2-night home sleep study which did not diagnose OSA in a patient with ongoing clinical suspicion of OSA
9. Patient is oxygen dependent for any reason
10. History of cerebrovascular accident (CVA) within the preceding 30 days
11. History of ventricular fibrillation or sustained ventricular tachycardia

Specific Indications for Overnight Polysomnography

- A polysomnography (PSG) study is routinely indicated:
  - For the diagnosis of sleep-related breathing disorders
  - For continuous positive airway pressure (CPAP) titration in patients with sleep-related breathing disorders
  - Before undergoing uvulopalatopharyngoplasty (UPPP)
  - For assessment of treatment results after an oral appliance treatment for OSAS
  - For parasomnias if these are unusual or atypical or if the behaviors are violent or otherwise potentially injurious to the patient or others
  - For diagnosis of RBD
- An overnight PSG, preferably video-PSG with multiple channels of electroencephalography (EEG), is indicated in patients suspected of having nocturnal seizures.
- A PSG study may be indicated for patients whose insomnia has not responded satisfactorily to a comprehensive behavioral or pharmacological treatment program for the management of insomnia. However, if a sleep-related breathing disorder or associated periodic limb movements in sleep (PLMS) is strongly suspected in a patient with insomnia, a PSG study is indicated.
- A follow-up PSG is indicated:
  - When the clinical response is inadequate or when symptoms reappear despite a good initial treatment with CPAP
  - After substantial weight loss or weight gain, which may have occurred in patients previously treated successfully with CPAP
- Overnight PSG followed by MSLT the next day is routinely indicated in patients with suspected narcolepsy. An overnight PSG is required in persons with suspected PLMS or PLMD, but is not routinely performed to diagnose RLS/WED.

Suggested Reading

Berry RB, Wagner MH. *Sleep Medicine Pearls*. 3rd ed. Philadelphia, PA: Elsevier/Saunders; 2015:xii, 690.

Chervin RD. *Common Pitfalls in Sleep Medicine: Case-Based Learning*. Cambridge: Cambridge University Press; 2014:xvii, 352.

Chokroverty S, Billiard M. *Sleep Medicine: A Comprehensive Guide to its Development, Clinical Milestones, and Advances in Treatment*. New York, NY: Springer; 2015:xix, 584.

Chokroverty S, Thomas RJ. *Atlas of Sleep Medicine*. 2nd ed. Philadelphia, PA: Elsevier/Saunders; 2014:xviii, 397.

Colwell CS. *Circadian Medicine*. Hoboken, NJ: John Wiley & Sons Inc.; 2015:xviii, 353.

Kryger MH, Roth T, Dement WC. *Principles and Practice of Sleep Medicine*. 6th ed. Philadelphia, PA: Elsevier; 2017:xlv, 1730.

Kryger MHA, Avidan AY, Berry R. *Atlas of Clinical Sleep Medicine*. 2nd ed. Philadelphia, PA: Elsevier/Saunders; 2013:xxiii, 511.

Mindell JA, Owens JA. *A Clinical Guide to Pediatric Sleep: Diagnosis and Management of Sleep Problems*. 3rd ed. Philadelphia, PA: Wolters Kluwer/Lippincott Williams & Wilkins; 2015:xii, 291.

Sheldon SH, Ferber R, Kryger MH. *Principles and Practice of Pediatric Sleep Medicine*. 2nd ed. London: Elsevier Saunders; 2014:xv, 425.

Spriggs WH. *Essentials of Polysomnography: A Training Guide and Reference for Sleep Technicians*. 2nd ed. Burlington, MA: Jones & Bartlett Learning; 2015:x, 385.

2

Sleep Phylogenic Evolution and Ontogeny

JEROME M. SIEGEL

The central scientific issue in sleep research is "Why do we sleep?" We all know we sleep to keep from being sleepy; however, this is like saying we eat to keep from being hungry. In the case of eating, we have an understanding of the need for food, including energy acquisition and the ingestion of vital nutrients. But we do not have a comparable understanding of why we sleep.

The seemingly straightforward way to investigate sleep function is by deprivation. However, deprivation necessarily involves stress. We know that awakening is accompanied by cortisol release[1–4] and phasic activation of a large number of neuronal groups.[5,6] Human studies rarely control for the stress of maintaining awakening and alertness. The controls used in animal deprivation studies frequently involve stimulating a control animal in the same pattern as the animal being deprived, but confining this stimulation to periods of spontaneous waking. But an animal that is awake will not show the autonomic or hormonal response to the awakening stimulus seen in the sleeping experimental animal. Long-term deprivation of rats can require more than 1000 awakenings a day.[7] So this leaves the investigator studying the effect of repeated awakening plus sleep loss, not just the effect of sleep loss.

Another approach is to correlate spontaneous sleep duration with a variety of physiological variables. Do people who sleep a lot learn faster than people who sleep less? Are they healthier? Recent studies contradict both of these assertions.[8,9] Other human studies have demonstrated that there is considerable interindividual variation in the response to sleep deprivation. Some individuals are able to be relatively vigilant and functional when their sleep is reduced, whereas others are not. These groups do not greatly differ in baseline sleep amounts.[10]

Rapid Eye Movement Sleep

One key unknown in sleep function is the role of rapid eye movement (REM) sleep. Why do animals vary in the amount of REM sleep they have? The discovery of REM sleep and its link to dreaming in 1953[11] led to considerable speculation that this was a uniquely human aspect of sleep and was presumably related to higher cognitive functions, even to schizophrenia and other mental disorders. But further phylogenetic work revealed that REM sleep was present in the most "primitive" mammals, including the platypus and echidna, and in these species it was quite intense, with rapid eye movements and neuronal activation comparable with that seen in cats, rats, and humans.[12,13]

The platypus has more than 7 hours/day of REM sleep, compared with the approximately hour and a half in humans (Fig. 2.1). Recent work has shown that the ostrich, considered a relatively primitive (plesiomorphic) bird, also has large amounts of REM sleep and "sleeps like the platypus."[14]

Marine Mammals

- Although most land mammals have a REM sleep-like state, this had not been seen in certain marine mammals. Early work in dolphins indicated that these animals had a very unusual electroencephalogram (EEG) pattern. They show slow waves, similar to those seen in deep (stage N3) human sleep. But these waves appear in only one hemisphere at a time, never bilaterally.[15] This pattern has been labeled unihemispheric slow waves or unihemispheric slow wave sleep (USWS).
- In contrast, all land mammals show bilateral high voltage EEG during sleep. Although this has been termed "unihemispheric sleep," it could be argued that these animals do not meet the conventional behavioral definition of sleep. They remain responsive during this EEG pattern and are able to time their breaths to avoid aspiration of water as waves break around them, a task not required in land mammals. Their posture is

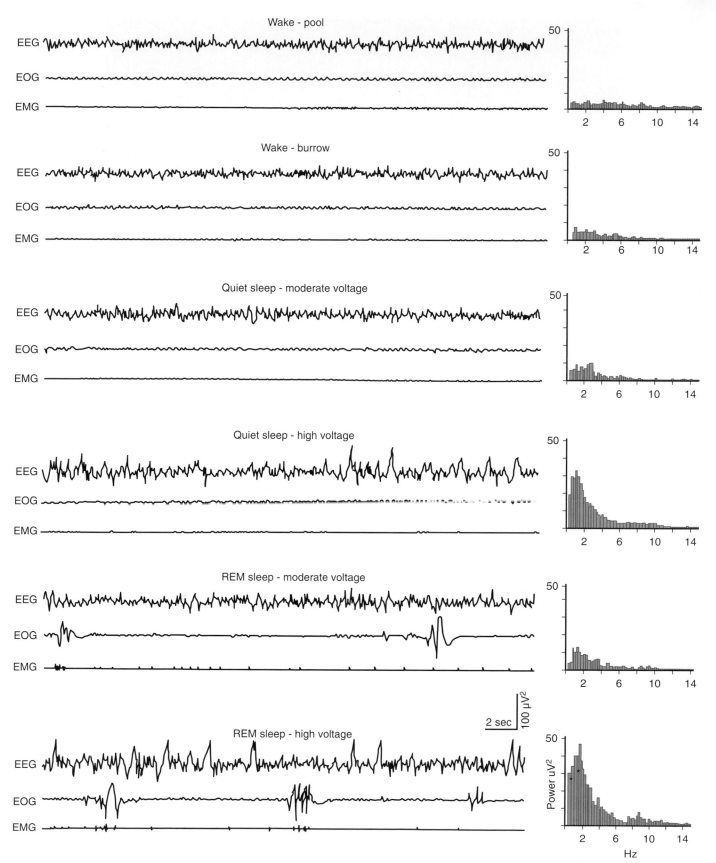

• **Figure 2.1** The platypus has the largest amount of REM sleep yet reported. This graph shows power spectra of EEG in each trace. *EEG,* Electroencephalogram; *EMG,* electromyogram; *EOG,* electrooculogram; *REM,* rapid eye movement. (Copyright Jerome M. Siegel.)

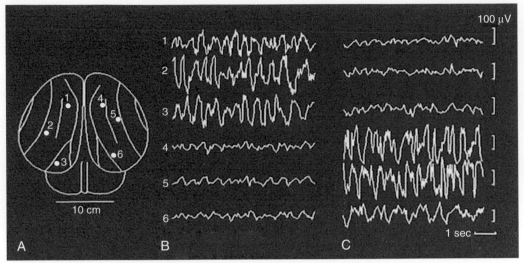

• **Figure 2.2** Unihemispheric Slow Waves in the Dolphin. The dolphin never shows the bilateral high voltage slow waves that characterize slow wave sleep in mammals. Their electroencephalogram state is not consistently correlated with the behavioral quiescence of sleep.[16,45] **A,** Indicates location of recording electrodes. **B** and **C,** Indicate left and right hemisphere sleep. (Modified from Mukhametov LM, Supin AY, Polyakova IG. Interhemispheric asymmetry of the electroencephalographic sleep patterns in dolphins. *Brain Res.* 1977;134:581–584.)

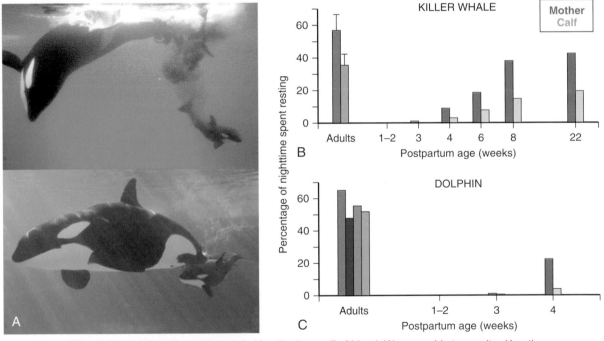

• **Figure 2.3 A,** Birth of the killer whale Kasatka in a puff of blood. We were able to monitor Kasatka and Nakai's activity for more than 7 weeks postpartum, finding continuous activity throughout that period. **B,** Postpartum activity of Nakai *(yellow)* and his mother Kasatka *(red)* in comparison to control adult killer whales *(blue and green)* housed at the same facility. Resting time is absent for months after birth in both mother and calf, with no rebound after this period. **C,** A similar pattern is seen in dolphins. (**A,** Photo courtesy of SeaWorld, San Diego.)

symmetrical, and the presence of USWS cannot be easily identified by observation of the animal's posture or activty (Fig. 2.2).[16,17]

• A further peculiarity of sleep in cetaceans (whales and dolphins) is that there had been no reports of REM sleep in this clade. We know that sleep duration and the percentage of sleep time devoted to REM sleep are maximal at birth.[18] So if REM sleep is present in cetaceans, it should be readily detectable at birth. Therefore we undertook studies of newborn killer whales and dolphins in an attempt to identify REM sleep (Fig. 2.3).

• We were very surprised to find no evidence for REM sleep in the newborn killer whale. Even more surprising was that there was no evidence for sleep of any kind in the calf for at least 3 weeks. The mother also stopped sleeping during this period. Mother and calf remained in constant motion, coordinating their movement to stay in formation, avoiding obstacles and breathing normally. We saw the same pattern in dolphins.[19] A further surprise was that although periods of inactivity returned to baseline levels by about 5 months of age, there was no "rebound" of inactivity beyond baseline levels in either mother or calf. The ecological literature indicates that this period of continuous activity coincides with migrations in the wild. This migration period is particularly dangerous for newborn cetaceans. Killer whale calves can be killed by sharks and by other killer whales. So the continuous 24 hours/day alertness the mother and calf exhibit has obvious adaptive value not required in most land mammals.

- Further work showed that this ability to be active and responsive for many days was not confined to the postpartum period. It was shown that adult male and female dolphins can perform an auditory or visual discrimination task (the latter presented to either eye) for 24 hours a day for as long as 15 days, with no decrement in responsiveness during the period and no rebound of inactivity after the task was removed. Cetaceans do not sleep as this term is understood in humans.
- Periods of extended waking are not unique to cetaceans (whales and dolphins). Although the walrus and fur seal exhibit both non-REM and REM sleep (Fig. 2.4), they frequently stop sleeping, spontaneously, for more than 3 days,[20] unlike land mammals. Such behavioral patterns may be common in marine mammals because their environmental opportunities and risks are more linked to the tides than the day-night cycle. Fish may show a similar flexibility in sleep duration and timing.[21]
- Another marine mammal that we have studied is the fur seal. The fur seal may well deserve the distinction of having the most unusual and perhaps most informative sleep pattern seen in mammals. When the fur seal, which is related to the dog and other carnivores, sleeps on land, it has both REM and non-REM sleep, as seen in other carnivores. However, when it is in water, where it spends most of its life, it switches to unihemispheric EEG patterns resembling those of dolphins.
- REM sleep amounts are greatly reduced. In contrast to dolphins, this unihemispheric sleep pattern is accompanied by quiescence

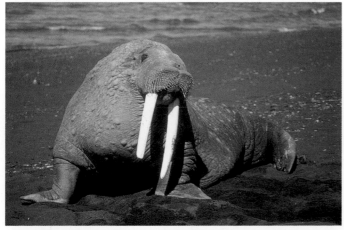

• **Figure 2.4** Walrus. The walrus (*Odobenus rosmarus divergens*) shows spontaneous periods of waking lasting more than 3 days. (Copyright Jerome M. Siegel.)

of the limbs controlled by the "sleeping" hemisphere. Therefore, whereas the label "unihemispheric sleep" is questionable in dolphins, which show no motor or postural asymmetry during their EEG asymmetry, the designation "unihemispheric sleep" fits the pattern seen in the fur seal.[22–24]

- The absence of REM sleep in the dolphin and its near elimination in water in the fur seal suggests that REM sleep serves a function not required when alertness and responsiveness is not reduced bilaterally.
- Bilateral sleep is associated with sleep inertia upon awakening.[25] The arousal linked to REM sleep,[26,27] its prevalence near the time of awakening,[26,28] and its relative absence following unihemispheric slow waves is consistent, with a role for REM sleep in reversal of sleep inertia.

The Neurochemistry of Electroencephalogram Control

We took advantage of the interhemispheric EEG pattern seen in fur seals to investigate the neurochemical substrates of this pattern. In land mammals we know that the release of a number of waking neurotransmitters is reduced in sleep.

However, we do not know if these changes in release are related to the changes in the cortical EEG, or whether they are simply secondary to the reduction in movement or sensory experience or of motivational drive in waking. Are the transmitters linked to waking asymmetrically release in unihemispheric sleep? To our surprise, we found that norepinephrine, serotonin, and histamine were symmetrically released in asymmetric sleep.[29,30] But acetylcholine release was greatly asymmetric, being maximal in the waking hemisphere.[31] In contrast, the release of all of these transmitters was comparably increased from quiet waking to active waking. This work identifies a unique role for acetylcholine in EEG activation.

Birds

Birds show great seasonal changes in sleep duration. The white crowned sparrow greatly reduces REM and non-REM sleep time during migrating season, acting in a "manic" manner, even when prevented from migrating. During this period, they do not show impairment in learning ability. After this period, they do not exhibit a rebound of lost sleep, similar to the lack of rebound in dolphins and killer whales after the postpartum period of sleep suppression.[32] Yet another example of this phenomenon has been observed in male polygynous pectoral sandpipers (Fig. 2.5). These birds have a virtually complete suppression of sleep during the annual mating period, with the birds that sleep the least producing the most offspring. During the 3-week period of sleep suppression they fought off rivals and showed little or no sleep, and no decrease in the effectiveness of their behavior.[32] Birds show no relationship between sleep duration and any of the parameters considered in mammals.[33]

Land Mammals

There is seasonal heterogeneity in the daily activity pattern of land mammals, particularly those living in regions with great seasonal changes in food availability. The arctic reindeer *Rangifer tarandus* spends 43% more time active in the summer than in the winter, likely accompanied by a great decrease in sleep and drowsy states relative to winter (Fig. 2.6).[34] Other mammals such as the ground squirrel and bear hibernate, entering the hibernation state through sleep.[35–37]

Phylogenetic Correlates of Sleep Duration

- When one compares the sleep of animals with their other attributes, it is clear that sleep duration is not correlated with brain size or brain–body weight ratio (Fig. 2.7).
- Closely related species can have widely divergent sleep durations. Statistical manipulations calculating REM sleep as total time versus percent of sleep time do not clarify the issue. Some striking examples of this can be seen in Figs. 2.8 and 2.9.[38,39] The guinea pig has precisely the same amount of REM sleep as the baboon. The eastern American mole has the same sleep

durations as those reported in humans. The golden mantled ground squirrel has more than twice the sleep duration of the degu, a rodent of similar size. The house cat has approximately double the sleep duration of the genet, a related feline carnivore. Brain size is not correlated with total sleep or REM sleep duration (Fig. 2.10).

- These many examples are drawn from the set of 70 or so mammals whose sleep has been systematically studied (i.e. they are not rare exceptions to rules derived from some larger set).
- One analysis showed that big animals sleep less.[40] This is a relatively weak correlation, but implies a relation between sleep and mass specific metabolic rate, since metabolic rate is linked to mass. However, closer analysis reveals that the body mass–sleep duration relationship is only present in herbivores.[17,41]
- Big animals like the tiger and giant armadillo sleep a lot, undermining the likelihood that metabolic rate determines sleep time. This same analysis also showed that carnivores sleep more than omnivores, who sleep more than herbivores (Fig. 2.11).
- These data suggest that the ecological niche and particularly the caloric density of the customary food is a major determinant of sleep duration. If an animal eats grass and leaves, they have to spend a lot of time collecting, ingesting, and chewing their food. In contrast if a carnivore kills its prey, it need not spend time hunting again for as long as several days, and it is most adaptive for it to sleep and stay with its offspring as it digests and metabolizes its kill. The big brown bat (Fig. 2.12) is the current sleep champion, sleeping 20 hours a day, awake only at dusk and in the early evening when its insect prey are airborne.
- Another reasonable conjecture is that lifespan might be related to sleep duration across species. However, this is not the case.[40] A common misconception is that there is a linear relation between sleep duration and lifespan in humans. In fact, the relation forms a U-shaped curve, with a self-report of 7 hours optimal for survival, and both higher and lower amounts of sleep being correlated with reduced lifespan. A surprising but consistent finding of these very large epidemiological studies is that sleeping more than 7 hours is correlated with a shorter

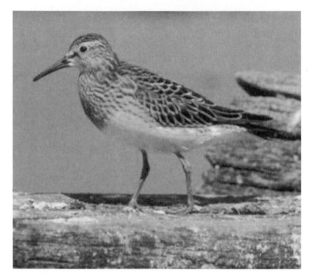

• **Figure 2.5** The polygynous pectoral sandpiper shows 3-week-long periods of no sleep and high mating performance levels during the arctic summer. (Copyright Jerome M. Siegel.)

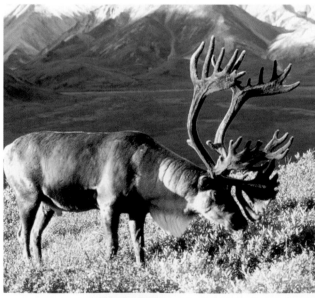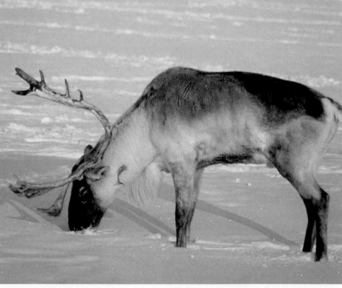

• **Figure 2.6** Reindeer (*Rangifer tarandus*) show 43% more activity in the summer, when food is available, than in the winter. (Copyright Jerome M. Siegel.)

Same phylogenetic order, different sleep times

Golden mantled ground squirrel	Degu
Spermophilus lateralis	*Octodon degu*

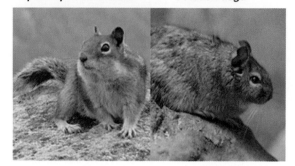

Total sleep	15.9 Hours	7.7 Hours
REM sleep	3.0 Hours	0.9 Hours

Cat	Genet
Felis catus	*Genetta genetta*

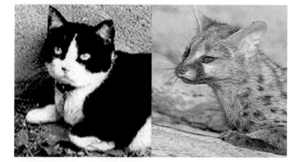

Total sleep	12.5 Hours	6.3 Hours
REM sleep	3.2 Hours	1.3 Hours

Owl monkey	Man
Aotus trivirgatus	*Homo sapiens sapiens*

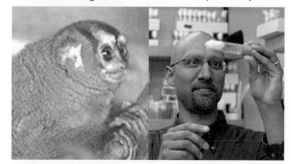

Total sleep	17.0 Hours	8.0 Hours
REM sleep	1.9 Hours	1.9 Hours

Different phylogenetic order, similar sleep times

Guinea pig	Baboon
Cacia porcellis	*Papio papio*

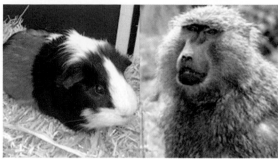

Total sleep	9.4 Hours	9.4 Hours
REM sleep	0.8 Hours	1.0 Hours

Goat	Eastern tree hyrax
Caprihircus	*Dendro hyrax validus*

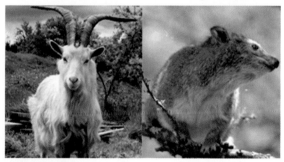

Total sleep	5.3 Hours	5.3 Hours
REM sleep	0.6 Hours	0.5 Hours

Eastern american mole	Man
Scalopus aquaticus	*Homo sapiens sapiens*

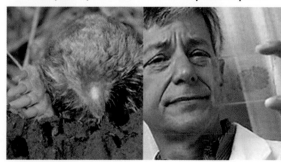

Total sleep	8.4 Hours	8.0 Hours
REM sleep	2.1 Hours	1.9 Hours

• **Figure 2.7** Closely related animals do not have similar sleep patterns. *REM,* Rapid eye movement.[38,50] (Copyright Jerome M. Siegel.)

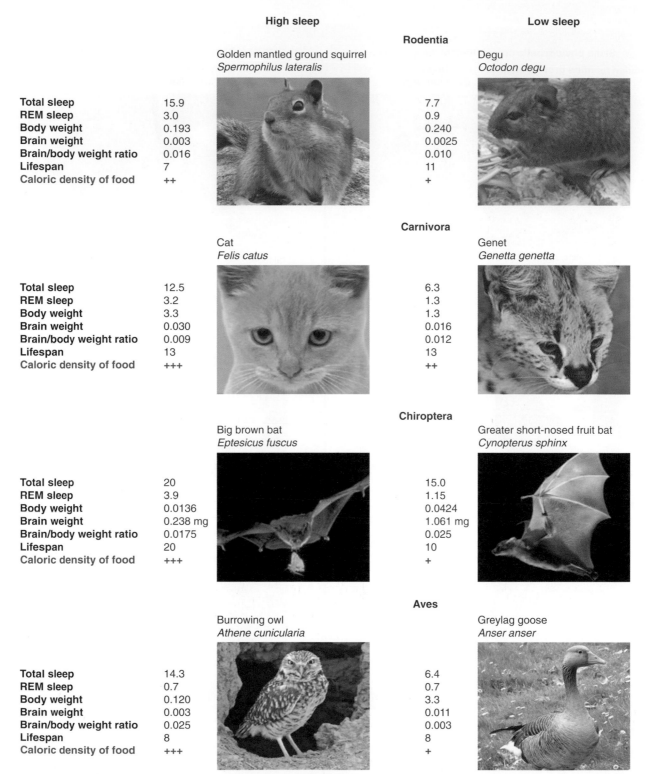

	High sleep		Low sleep
	Rodentia		
	Golden mantled ground squirrel *Spermophilus lateralis*		Degu *Octodon degu*
Total sleep	15.9		7.7
REM sleep	3.0		0.9
Body weight	0.193		0.240
Brain weight	0.003		0.0025
Brain/body weight ratio	0.016		0.010
Lifespan	7		11
Caloric density of food	++		+
	Carnivora		
	Cat *Felis catus*		Genet *Genetta genetta*
Total sleep	12.5		6.3
REM sleep	3.2		1.3
Body weight	3.3		1.3
Brain weight	0.030		0.016
Brain/body weight ratio	0.009		0.012
Lifespan	13		13
Caloric density of food	+++		++
	Chiroptera		
	Big brown bat *Eptesicus fuscus*		Greater short-nosed fruit bat *Cynopterus sphinx*
Total sleep	20		15.0
REM sleep	3.9		1.15
Body weight	0.0136		0.0424
Brain weight	0.238 mg		1.061 mg
Brain/body weight ratio	0.0175		0.025
Lifespan	20		10
Caloric density of food	+++		+
	Aves		
	Burrowing owl *Athene cunicularia*		Greylag goose *Anser anser*
Total sleep	14.3		6.4
REM sleep	0.7		0.7
Body weight	0.120		3.3
Brain weight	0.003		0.011
Brain/body weight ratio	0.025		0.003
Lifespan	8		8
Caloric density of food	+++		+

• **Figure 2.8** Physiological variables are not strongly correlated with sleep duration, even in related species. *REM,* Rapid eye movement.[50] (Copyright Jerome M. Siegel.)

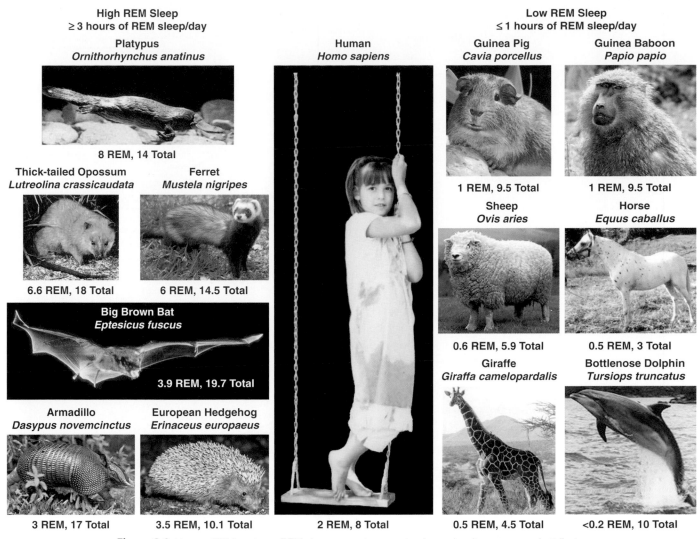

High REM Sleep
≥ 3 hours of REM sleep/day

Platypus
Ornithorhynchus anatinus

8 REM, 14 Total

Thick-tailed Opossum
Lutreolina crassicaudata

6.6 REM, 18 Total

Ferret
Mustela nigripes

6 REM, 14.5 Total

Big Brown Bat
Eptesicus fuscus

3.9 REM, 19.7 Total

Armadillo
Dasypus novemcinctus

3 REM, 17 Total

European Hedgehog
Erinaceus europaeus

3.5 REM, 10.1 Total

Human
Homo sapiens

2 REM, 8 Total

Low REM Sleep
≤ 1 hours of REM sleep/day

Guinea Pig
Cavia porcellus

1 REM, 9.5 Total

Guinea Baboon
Papio papio

1 REM, 9.5 Total

Sheep
Ovis aries

0.6 REM, 5.9 Total

Horse
Equus caballus

0.5 REM, 3 Total

Giraffe
Giraffa camelopardalis

0.5 REM, 4.5 Total

Bottlenose Dolphin
Tursiops truncatus

<0.2 REM, 10 Total

• **Figure 2.9** Human REM and non-REM sleep amounts are not unique, despite our unusual attributes. *REM,* Rapid eye movement.[51] (Copyright Jerome M. Siegel.)

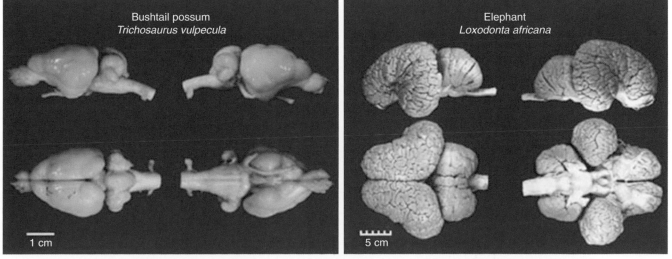

Bushtail possum
Trichosaurus vulpecula

1 cm

18 hours of sleep, 6.6 hours of REM

Elephant
Loxodonta africana

5 cm

3.9 hours of sleep, 1.8 hours of REM

• **Figure 2.10** Brain size is not correlated with total sleep or REM sleep duration. *REM,* Rapid eye movement.[51] (Copyright Jerome M. Siegel.)

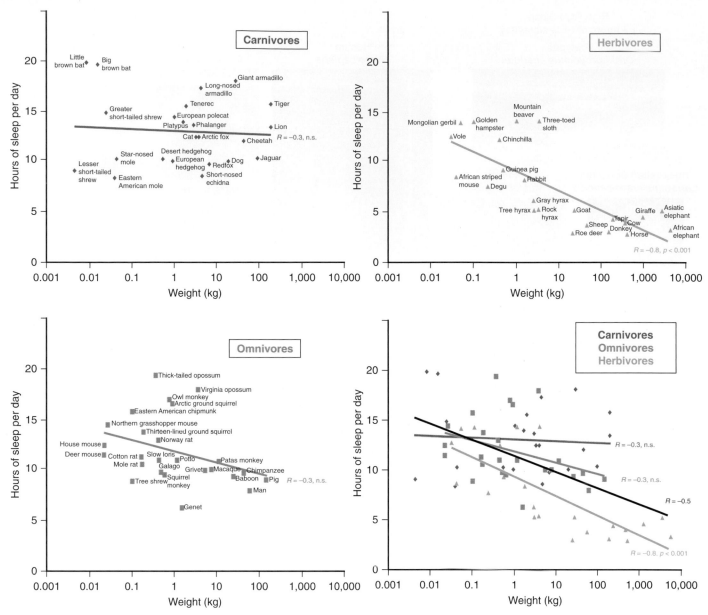

• **Figure 2.11** Carnivores sleep more than herbivores. Sleep duration is correlated with body size only in herbivores. The correlation is negative.[17] (Copyright Jerome M. Siegel.)

lifespan than sleeping less than 7 hours. This finding is robust, even after exclusion of subjects inclined toward sleep apnea or other pathologies.[42-44]

Clinical Significance

- These findings are of clinical significance, since the argument that the more you sleep the longer you will live is used to sell sleeping pills, including hypnotics acting on the benzodiazepine receptor.
- Although chronic use of sleeping pills only produces a small elevation of sleep duration, at least 15 studies have shown that chronic use substantially shortens the lifespan, whereas untreated insomnia does not.[42] There is, to my knowledge, no study showing increased lifespan with chronic use of sleeping pills

(see https://www.semel.ucla.edu/sleepresearch/publication/newspaper-article/2010/huffington-post-are-sleeping-pills-good-you).

- One of the main factors driving sleeping pill use is the idea that sleeping times have greatly decreased in "modern" societies because of the use of artificial light, television, and most recently the Internet. However, the evidence for this is scant. Tools for accurately quantifying sleep time were developed long after the invention of electric lights. Although we cannot go back in time, several groups of hunter-gatherers still exist. These groups lack electricity and battery-powered devices. Some of them live in the very regions in which *Homo sapiens* evolved. If the supposition that modern life has greatly reduced sleep time is correct, these individuals should go to sleep at sunset and sleep 9, 10, or 11 hours. This is not what we found (Fig. 2.13).[45]

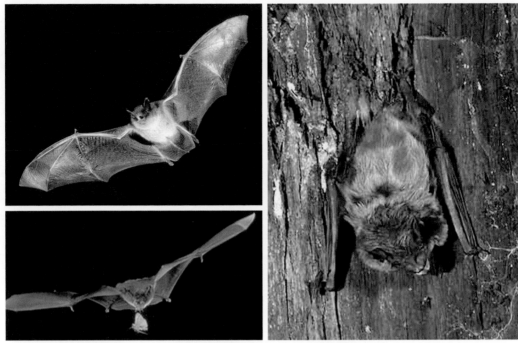

• **Figure 2.12** The big brown bat has the highest amount of sleep yet documented, at 20 hours/day.[52] (Copyright Jerome M. Siegel.)

Sleep in Preindustrial People

- None of the individuals in the three groups studied habitually go to sleep at sunset. Rather, sleep onset occurred, on average, 3.3 hours after sunset. The average sleep period duration was 7.7 hours, an amount at the low end of those reported using identical actigraph measurements and scoring algorithms. Winter sleep durations are an hour longer than summer durations.
- Most important, in all seasons, sleep onset occurs during a period of falling environmental temperature. Sleep continues, without long interruptions, until temperature hits the daily nadir, when awakening occurs. Sleeping during the coldest part of the day is consistent with an energy conservation role. To use a phrase popularized by Desmond Morris, the "naked ape" would be at a great disadvantage if it was active during the coldest part of the day. Metabolically costly heat loss is minimized by allowing body temperature and brain energy consumption to fall, as occurs in sleep.
- The daily rhythm of temperature experienced by hunter-gatherers, and also by the primate ancestors of all humans, has largely been abolished in "modern" civilizations. Given the extent to which this rhythm is so tightly linked to temperature (rather than light), it may be hypothesized that the removal of this rhythm in "modern" society may contribute to sleep pathology.
- Although sleep disorder centers routinely recommend a reduction in the thermostat setting at night, the magnitude and time course of this reduction may not resemble the time course of temperature that our ancestors may have experienced. It is also important to appreciate that this temperature variation is experienced by hunter-gatherers from birth, and may induce physiological changes that cannot be simply transferred by exposing adults to such changes. Further work is necessary to fully understand and therapeutically exploit the dynamics of this relationship.
- We see no data to support the assumption that human sleep has been greatly reduced by the amenities of modern life. A more recent study of sleep over the last 50 years has also found no change, consistent with our study and conflicting with the notion that recent technological developments have reduced sleep.[46]
- Habitual napping and insomnia are nearly nonexistent in all three of the groups examined. It is well known that daily napping is a common cause of insomnia.[47,48] Napping is correlated with shorter lifespan.[49]

Conclusions

- Sleep and sleep-like states vary greatly across the animal kingdom.
- Most mammals and birds have not been systematically studied. But both REM and non-REM sleep have been seen in most land mammals that have been polygraphically investigated.
- Marine mammals provide important insights into the nature of sleep. Cetaceans (dolphins and whales) are able to maintain a vigilant state, even while having unihemispheric slow waves. Dolphins do not appear to have REM sleep and can remain vigilant and responsive for more than 15 days with no evidence of rebound sleep.
- Sleep depth and duration vary across species and seasons.
- Sleep duration across species is not correlated with brain size or brain–body weight ratio.
- The strongest correlate of sleep duration across species is diet, suggesting that herbivores have evolved to sleep very little so they can spend large amounts of time eating and chewing.

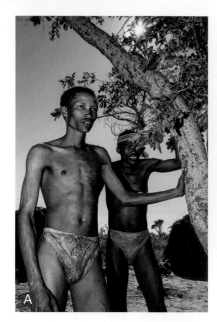

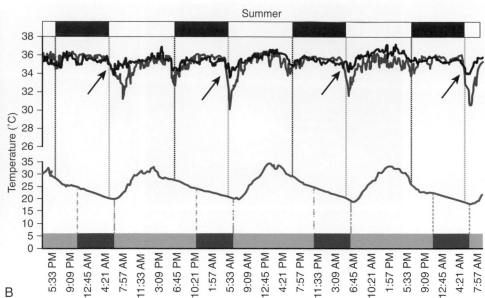

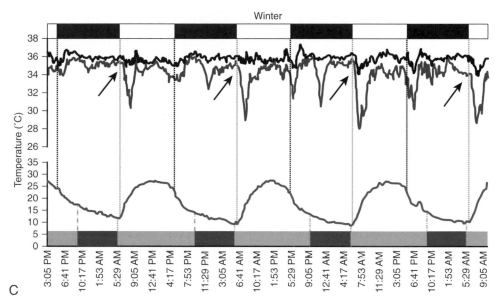

• **Figure 2.13** **A,** Hunter-gatherers of Namibia. **B** and **C,** Sleep in hunter-gatherers of Namibia. *Black* and *white* bars indicate the period of night and day. *Blue* and *orange* bars indicate periods of sleep and waking. *Violet* color indicates environmental temperature. Note that sleep occurs during a period of falling temperature and terminates when temperature hits the daily minimum. Sleep onset occurs 3.3 hours after sunset, on average. Sleep durations are near the low end of what has been reported in "modern" societies. Vasoconstriction, indicated by cooling of the fingers, occurs at wake onset in both summer and winter.[45] (**A,** Photo courtesy of Josh Davimes.)

- Preindustrial humans sleep nearly 1 hour more in the winter than in the summer. Their average amount of sleep does not exceed average sleep amounts reported in industrial societies.
- Insomnia and napping are rare in preindustrial groups.
- Awakening during the night is also rare in these groups, with wake after sleep onset not differing from that of "modern" populations.
- The daily temperature rhythm is a potent regulator of sleep in preindustrial societies, suggesting that the loss of this rhythm by artificial temperature regulation in modern societies may be a factor in sleep disorders.

Suggested Reading

Lesku JA, Meyer LC, Fuller A, et al. Ostriches sleep like platypuses. *PLoS ONE.* 2011;6:e23203.

Lyamin O, Pryaslova J, Lance V, Siegel J. Animal behaviour: continuous activity in cetaceans after birth. *Nature.* 2005;435:1177.

Siegel JM. Clues to the functions of mammalian sleep. *Nature.* 2005;437:1264-1271.

Siegel JM. Sleep viewed as a state of adaptive inactivity. *Nat Rev Neurosci.* 2009;10:747-753.

Yetish G, Kaplan H, Gurven M, et al. Natural sleep and its seasonal variations in three pre-industrial societies. *Curr Biol.* 2015;25:2862-2868.

3

Normal Human Sleep-Wake Patterns

SHEILA C. TSAI

What Is Sleep?

- Definition of sleep: Sleep is a reversible state of unconsciousness. It is an active state achieved by stimulating sleep-promoting neurons and inhibiting wake-promoting regions. It is an essential physiologic process that appears important in maintaining homeostasis. It is controlled both by the body's internal clock and by external forces.
- Sleep patterns and changes: Sleep patterns and sleep requirements change as one ages. In addition, gender differences are noted. In this chapter, normal human sleep-wake patterns, gender differences in sleep, and changes that occur during aging will be discussed.

Role of Sleep

- Functions of sleep: Sleep is important in homeostasis, memory, learning, and well-being. Sleep is essential to survival.
- Sleep deprivation: Sleep deprivation studies in animals result in death.[1] In humans, sleep deprivation results in impaired performance and attention, which occurs in a dose-dependent fashion with greater sleep deprivation, resulting in greater lapses in vigilance.[2]
- Sleep in memory and learning: Sleep is important in memory and learning. Local increases in slow wave activity (SWA) after learning a task have been associated with improved performance of the task.[3] Although the mechanism is not entirely clear, numerous studies support the instrumental role sleep plays in memory consolidation and learning.[4]
- Sleep and other organ systems: Metabolic, hormonal, and cardiovascular impairments have all been associated with sleep deprivation.

- Chronic sleep deprivation has been associated with alterations in glucose metabolism; abnormalities in leptin and ghrelin, which are important in appetite and satiety; and the development of obesity.
- Sleep disorders have been linked to cardiovascular problems. For example, untreated obstructive sleep apnea is associated with the development of cardiovascular disorders, particularly hypertension.[5] In addition, short and long sleep, described as less than 4–5 hours and greater than 9 hours of sleep nightly, respectively, have been associated with greater cardiovascular disease risk and all-cause mortality.[6,7]
- Sleep in immunity: An important interplay occurs between sleep and infection. During illness, fatigue and a strong desire to sleep occur.[8]
- There are associations of infection with sleepiness, such as in viral infections; poststreptococcal infection[9]; trypanosomiasis, or African sleeping sickness; and exposure to bacterial endotoxin.[10]
- The lipopolysaccharide component of cell wall endotoxin increases the sleep observed during sepsis. Cytokines, such as IL-1 and TNF, are increased with viral and bacterial infections. IL-1 and TNF infusion induces sleepiness and fatigue. Furthermore, sleep assists in recovery from illness, which is supported by studies on sleep loss. Severely sleep-deprived rats die of septicemia.[11] Furthermore, with sleep deprivation there is less antibody response to vaccination.[12]

Normal Sleep and Wake Timing

- Control of sleep: Sleep and wakefulness are under both homeostatic and circadian control. Sleep propensity increases with the amount of wakefulness.
- Circadian factors affect the timing and duration of sleep. Different models of sleep exist. In the two-process model of sleep,[13] as depicted in Fig. 3.1, a homeostatic process (process S) rises during waking and decreases with sleep. This is dependent on prior sleep and waking.
- Adenosine has been proposed to be this process S, since levels of adenosine increase during prolonged wakefulness and decrease during sleep.[14] Furthermore, caffeine, an adenosine receptor antagonist, reduces the sleep propensity increase that occurs during wakefulness.[15]
- Process S interacts with a circadian process (process C). As a consequence of these two processes, sleepiness peaks and alertness tends to nadir in the middle of the usual sleep period, between 2 AM and 6 AM, with a second peak

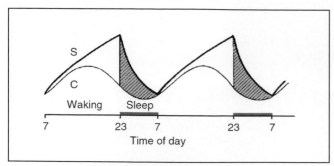

• **Figure 3.1** In the two-process model of sleep, homeostatic (S) and circadian (C) processes regulate sleep and wakefulness. Process S increases with increasing wake time.

in sleep propensity in the midafternoon between 2 PM and 6 PM.[16]

- The suprachiasmatic nucleus:
  - The timing of sleep and wakefulness is determined by the master clock of the body, the suprachiasmatic nuclei (SCN), found in the anterior hypothalamus.[17]
  - At the molecular level, the circadian clock appears to be controlled by the precise expression of genes and their protein products.
    - These genes include *CLOCK*; period circadian clock genes, *PER1, PER2, PER3*; and *BMAL1*. They affect mammalian "eveningness" or "morningness."
    - Mutations and polymorphisms of the genes have been associated with circadian rhythm dysfunction. For example, advanced sleep phases syndrome may result from a mutation of the PER2 gene.[18]
    - Light affects the suprachiasmatic nucleus: The SCN are a pair of nuclei that respond to light and dark, which are the key environmental signals that impact the circadian rhythm. Light exposure is linked to melatonin secretion: melatonin secretion increases in the evening and is stimulated by darkness, whereas light rapidly suppresses melatonin production.
  - Fig. 3.2 demonstrates how the SCN sends timing information to the brain and periphery. Light hits the retina, which then sends signals to the SCN via the retinal hypothalamic tract (RHT). The SCN inhibits the superior cervical ganglion (SCG), which in turn provides excitatory input to the pineal gland. This excitatory input suppresses melatonin release from the pineal gland. Melatonin activates the SCN at the melatonin type 1 (MT1) and type 2 (MT2) receptors, thereby affecting sleep.
  - The SCN also receives input from the raphe nucleus, which provides serotonergic input to the serotonin receptor 5-HT2C. In addition, the SCN receives input from activity, behaviors, and scheduling cues to coordinate the circadian rhythm and synchronize it to the 24-hour clock.
  - The SCN provides timing information to various parts of the brain and provides signals to peripheral tissue, via the autonomic nervous system and hormones, to coordinate more complex behaviors and control the peripheral circadian oscillators, as demonstrated in Fig. 3.3.[19]
- Influences on the circadian pacemaker: The average circadian pacemaker period is 24.15 hours.[20] It is slightly shorter in women at 24.1 hours versus that of men at 24.2 hours.

- In order to maintain synchronization with the 24-hour day, external factors help regulate circadian patterns.
- Factors such as light exposure, meals, and timing of activity such as work and exercise all influence the circadian rhythm.
- These external cues are *zeitgebers*, factors that help synchronize and entrain the circadian rhythm. However, light and dark are the key environmental signals. We can override signals for sleep with exposure to light, either purposefully or unintentionally, such as through overt bright light exposure or via electronics usage, respectively. This suppression of sleep signals may contribute to sleep loss and health consequences as a result of sleep deprivation.
- The SCN regulates temperature and hormones:
  - The master clock regulates the body's rhythms such as temperature and hormones. As a result of light, darkness, and SCN signals, melatonin levels are at their highest during nighttime sleep. Core temperature also varies over the course of 24 hours, declining during sleep.
  - Core body temperature is at its lowest during nighttime sleep, with the nadir occurring about 2.3 hours prior to normal waking. Fig. 3.4 demonstrates melatonin and body temperature levels over the course of 24 hours, and the associated sleep propensity in relation to the sleep period.
- Light influences the circadian rhythm:
  - Blue spectrum light with a wavelength of about 450–500 nm is the most potent suppressor of melatonin production and a strong signal for phase shifting.[21,22] Light exposure, if timed appropriately, can phase shift the circadian rhythm. For example, if the light exposure occurs before the minimum core body temperature, a phase delay occurs.
  - Light late in the day or early in the night causes a phase delay. Conversely, a phase advance occurs if the light exposure occurs after the core body minimum. Light late in the biologic night or early in the biologic day causes phase advancement.[17]
- Dampening of circadian amplitudes with age: With increasing age, the circadian clock moves earlier, on average, and the amplitude of rhythms decreases.[23] The melatonin amplitude decreases, with a more notable decrease in men than in women.[24] These changes in rhythm amplitude may partially explain the increase in sleep complaints with age. Although the majority of people over 65 years old complain of at least one chronic sleep problem, they may be able to tolerate sleep loss better.[25]

Normal Sleep Patterns

- Sleep staging: Sleep staging is discussed in subsequent chapters. However, in brief, sleep is divided into stages N1, N2, N3, and R sleep.[26] Arousal threshold increases with increasing stages of nonrapid eye movement (NREM) sleep. Stage N1 sleep may be considered drowsy or transitional sleep, with a lower arousal threshold. During stage N2 sleep, high-voltage SWA appears, with K-complexes and spindles being the hallmarks of N2 sleep. N3, or slow wave sleep (SWS), is characterized by a greater percentage of high-amplitude slow (delta) waves and a high arousal threshold. Stage R sleep is characterized by rapid eye movements (REMs); low-voltage, mixed-frequency electroencephalogram (EEG); and muscle atonia.
- Sleep evolves with CNS development: The EEG and sleep-wake states evolve as the central nervous system (CNS) develops.

Organization

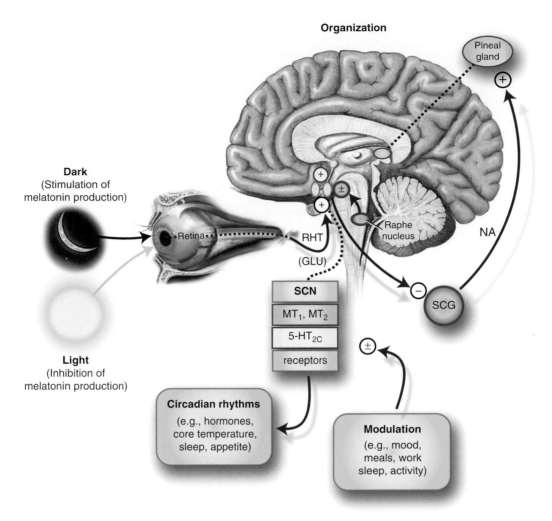

• **Figure 3.2** The circadian pacemaker, the SCN sends timing information to the brain and periphery. The SCN receives information from the retina via the retinohypothalamic tract, which allows synchronization with the external environment. *GLU,* Glutamate; *NA,* noradrenaline; *RHT,* retinal hypothalamic tract; *SCG,* superior cervical ganglion; *SCN,* suprachiasmatic nucleus. (From Chokroverty S, Avidan AY. Sleep and its disorders. In: Daroff RB, Jankovic J, Mazziota JC, Pomeroy SL, eds. *Bradley's Neurology in Clinical Practice.* 7th ed. Vol 1. London: Elsevier, 2016:1615–1685.)

During infancy, sleep occupies the majority of the 24-hour day. Infant sleep is categorized as either active sleep or quiet sleep.

- Active sleep is characterized by continuous EEG activity with REM and eventually develops into REM sleep.
- Quiet sleep, characterized by discontinuous EEG activity without REM, becomes NREM sleep.
- Sleep that is not clearly active or quiet sleep is called *indeterminate.* The normal NREM EEG develops over the course of the first 2–6 months of life.
- Spindles begin to appear around 4–8 weeks of age.[27,28]
- In general, K complexes are seen by 4–6 months.[29] These are hallmarks used to define N2 sleep.
- Newborns begin their sleep period with active sleep and then transition to quiet sleep, with cycles occurring in about 50-min intervals. In newborns, active and quiet sleep each occupy about 50% of the sleep period.
- Infants enter sleep through REM sleep until about 3 months of age, and over the next 2 years of development, the percent of active/REM sleep decreases to about 20–25% of the sleep

period.[30] In 2–5-year-olds, about seven NREM/REM cycles occur over the nocturnal sleep period.[29]

- Sleep in childhood: By childhood, sleep-onset REM should not occur and may suggest pathology. It is abnormal for an adult to enter sleep through REM sleep. When sleep-onset REM sleep does occur, potential etiologies include sleep deprivation, travel across multiple time zones, acute withdrawal of REM suppressant medications, shift work, narcolepsy, and other sleep disorders, such as untreated sleep apnea.[31,32] Normal latency to REM sleep is 80–100 min.[30] REM periods are longest in the last ⅓ of the sleep periods. The NREM/REM cycle occurs at about 90-min intervals at around 10 years of age and older. In young adulthood, about 4–5 REM periods occur during a night's sleep. The percentages of each sleep stage change somewhat over time. NREM and REM sleep occur in fairly equal amounts in infancy, but by later childhood, the percent of REM sleep decreases to 20%–25%.
- Sleep in adolescence: SWS declines significantly during adolescence.[33] Delta SWA decreases by about 50% between 10 and

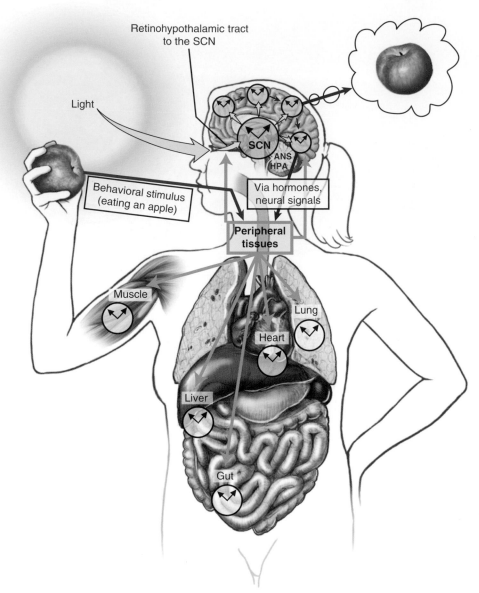

• **Figure 3.3** Light cues provide information to the SCN, which provides timing information to the brain via nuclei, the autonomic nervous system, and hormones. This influences such rhythms as sleep–wake and feeding–fasting. *ANS*, Autonomonic nervous system; *HPA*, hypothalamic pituitary adrenal axis; *SCN*, suprachiasmatic nucleus. (From Chokroverty S, Avidan AY. Sleep and its disorders. In: Daroff RB, Jankovic J, Mazziota JC, Pomeroy SL, eds. *Bradley's Neurology in Clinical Practice*. 7th ed. Vol 1. London: Elsevier, 2016:1615–1685.)

20 years old. This decrease in SWS may be due in part to decreased amplitude and/or decrease in growth hormones with increasing age. SWA, and N3 sleep predominates in the first ⅓ of the night. The amount of SWS appears to be related to the previous level of wakefulness. Partial or total sleep deprivation results in increased SWS on the recovery night of sleep. Naps decrease the trend of slow wave propensity. In adults, normal percentages of sleep stages are as follows: N1 (2%–5%), N2 (45%–55%), N3 (10%–20%), R (20%–25%).[30,34] Table 3.1 summarizes the age-related changes that occur in human sleep patterns.

• Sleep architecture changes with aging: With aging, increased sleep latency and more frequent nocturnal awakenings may be noted. As a result, the total sleep time and sleep efficiency

(SE) decrease. There is another drop in N3 sleep around 36–50 years of age and a more gradual decline in REM sleep over time.[35] As a result, N1 and N2 sleep increase. In women, more issues with insomnia may occur, with an increase in hypnotic usage.[33,36–38] Medical comorbidities can disrupt sleep architecture and contribute to sleep complaints. Fig. 3.5 demonstrates the changes in sleep time and sleep stages that occur with aging.

Normal Sleep Duration

• Sleep needs decrease into adulthood: Normal sleep needs decrease from birth to adulthood. This amount of sleep allows a person to remain alert, awake, and able to function throughout the

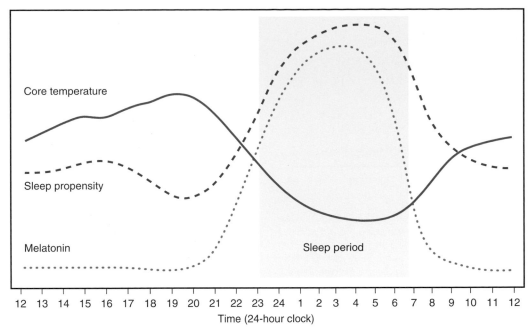

• **Figure 3.4** Plasma melatonin levels rise with darkness and peak during nighttime sleep. Core temperature declines during sleep and reaches its nadir about 2.3 hours prior to normal waking. (From Lack LC, Gradisar M, Van Someren EJ, Wright HR, Lushington K. The relationship between insomnia and body temperatures. *Sleep Med Rev*. 2008;12(4):307–317.)

TABLE 3.1 Normal Sleep Patterns in Humans[29,30,35,36]			
	Infants	**Young Adults**	**Elderly**
Wake after sleep onset (%)	<5	<5	10–25
Sleep efficiency (%)	>90	>90	75–85
Stage N1 (%)	Quiet sleep*	2–5	5–10
Stage N2 (%)	Quiet sleep	45–55	55–6
Stage N3 (%)	Quiet sleep	10–20	2–10
Stage R (%)	50	20–25	15–20
Stage R/NREM ratio	50:50	20:80	20:80
Time of stage R, NREM cycle (min)	45–60	90–110	90–110
Total sleep time (hours)	14–16	7–8	7

*Quiet sleep collectively is about 50% of sleep alternating with about 50% of active sleep (later developing into stage R).

day. Sleep needs are determined by behavioral and genetic components and by length of prior waking.

- A newborn spends the majority of the 24-hour day sleeping. The nocturnal sleep period becomes consolidated during the first year, with 6 months being the average age at which an infant sleeps through the night.[39]
- By 9 months about 80% of children are sleeping through the night.[40] A long night's sleep period occurs, with discrete daytime naps occurring. Napping during the day can be culturally related, but many children stop napping once they reach school age. Naps can be normal in some societies and are not uncommon in the elderly.[41] The average infant requires about 14–16 hours of sleep. This sleep requirement decreases to about 10–14 hours at 1 year, 12 hours at 2 years, and 10–11 hours at 4 years.[42]
- A school age child's sleep needs average about 9–10 hours per night. By adolescence, this sleep duration is about 8–10 hours.[43]
- In adulthood, the average sleep requirement is 7–8 hours. Fig. 3.6 demonstrates the changes in sleep needs with aging.
- Quantifying sleep need: Attempts have been made to quantify sleep needs and determine "normal" levels of sleepiness. A person's sleep need is the amount of sleep needed to perform optimally and without decrements in performance and vigilance.
- Semiobjective measures, such as the Epworth Sleepiness Scale (ESS)[44] and Stanford Sleepiness Scale (SSS)[45] assess sleepiness

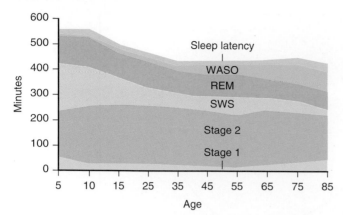

• **Figure 3.5** Changes in Sleep with Age. Sleep time (in minutes), wake time, sleep latency, and sleep stages change with aging. *REM,* Rapid eye movement; *SWS,* slow wave sleep; *WASO,* wake after sleep onset. (From Carskadon MA, Dement WC. Normal human sleep. In: Kryger MH, Roth T, Dement WC, eds. *Principles and Practice in Sleep Medicine.* 6th ed. Philadelphia, PA: Elsevier, 2017:15–24.)

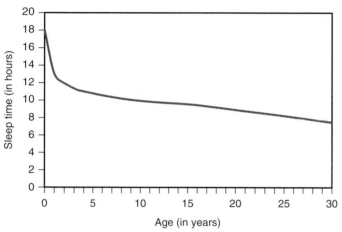

• **Figure 3.6** Average Sleep Needs Decrease with Age. A newborn spends the majority of 24 hours asleep. The average sleep need of an adult is 7–8 hours of sleep. (From Tsai SC. Excessive sleepiness. *Clin Chest Med.* 2010;31(2):341–351.)

by self-rating a person's sleep propensity in various situations. Normal sleep needs are determined based on averages and surveys/questionnaires. Sleep duration is somewhat under voluntary control. Many people do not obtain an adequate amount of sleep, with an increasing number of people in developed countries reporting decreasing sleep amounts.[46]

• There are differences in ability to tolerate sleep loss, which is in part due to baseline sleepiness and genetic differences. However, with enough sleep restriction, when normal subjects are sleep deprived, there are decrements in motor performance and cognitive functioning and increases in sleepiness.[47,48]

Gender Differences

• Boys are poorer sleepers than girls: In infancy, boys are more likely to be poor sleepers, and girls tend to have a longer sleep period. Boys have increased arousability in quiet sleep.[49] Sudden infant death syndrome (SIDS) has a male predominance. In children, girls sleep longer (via actigraphy data), have higher

SE, and more N3 sleep. During adolescence, girls have increased SE and fewer awakenings. They experience an earlier decrease in sleep delta power, possibly related to puberty. Girls report a longer ideal sleep duration.[50]

• Women report more sleep difficulties than men: In adulthood, women need more sleep, spend more time in bed, and sleep longer. They report more sleep difficulties, but by actigraphy, women have a longer sleep duration and better sleep quality than men.[33] By polysomnography monitoring, women appear to also have more SWA. When comparing sleep in men to women, in general men have more N1 and N2 sleep, with an increase in arousal index and a decrease in SE. Men appear to objectively have poorer sleep architecture. Men have less N3 sleep, with a more significant decrease with age in men versus women.

• Increased risk of insomnia in women: In adolescence, insomnia risk increases with menses.[51] Despite better sleep objectively, women describe more sleep problems, more issues with insomnia, and greater hypnotic use than men.[33] In women, the increased risk of insomnia is 1.4 : 1, with the greatest risk occurring in the elderly.[52] Furthermore, with increased age, women's risks of sleep disordered breathing (SDB) nearly equal those of age-matched males.[53,54]

Sleep and Menses

• Menarche: In adolescence, menses increases the risk for insomnia and possibly depression.[51]

• Sleep and the menstrual cycle: In the menstrual cycle, day 1 marks the 1st day of menses. There is the preovulatory follicular phase, followed by the postovulatory luteal phase, which ends with decreased progesterone and estrogen. More sleep disturbances and poorer subjective sleep quality are noted during the premenstrual week and the 1st few days of menstruation.[55] Menstrual-related hypersomnia may be noted with premenstrual hypersomnia the week before or during menses. During the luteal phase, N3 sleep is unchanged, but there is a decrease in REM sleep and a decreased body temperature rhythm. Severe dysmennorhea may also contribute to wakefulness.[56]

Sleep and Pregnancy

• Hormonal changes in pregnancy: The increase in progesterone has a hypnotic effect, with an increase in NREM sleep, a decrease in sleep-onset latency, and decreased upper airway collapsibility. The increase in estrogen contributes to decreased REM sleep and increased vasodilation, which can cause nasal congestion and lower extremity edema. Increased prolactin levels may enhance SWS. Prolactin may also contribute to decreased dopamine release resulting in worsened restless legs syndrome (RLS) symptoms.[57]

• Mechanical changes affect sleep: The growing belly and discomfort of pregnancy disrupt sleep. More frequent nocturnal awakening and decreased SE are noted.

• The 1st trimester: During the 1st trimester, sleepiness, fatigue, and total sleep time increase. This is attributable to hormones and physical discomfort, such as urinary frequency and breast tenderness.

• The 2nd trimester: Sleep tends to improve during the 2nd trimester, with many women noting more energy.

• The 3rd trimester: By the 3rd trimester, 54%–74% of women report insomnia symptoms.[58] Most women report sleep disturbances, which include poor SE, significantly exacerbated by

TABLE 3.2	**Sleep in Female Humans** *In General, Females Have More Subjective Sleep Complaints but Better Objective Sleep*						
Infancy*	**Childhood***	**Adolescence***	**Adulthood***	**Menses**	**Pregnancy**	**Postmenopausal**
• Risk of SIDS • Arousability	• TST • SE • N3 sleep • Awakenings • Report longer sleep need	• Risk of insomnia • Earlier in delta SWA • Report longer sleep duration	• TST • SE • N3 sleep • Awakenings • Report poorer quality sleep • Hypnotic usage	• Sleepiness in the luteal phase • May experience recurrent hypersomnia related to menses • Sleep disruption due to discomfort	• TST • SE • Sleepiness and fatigue • Sleep disorders (e.g., RLS, cramps, GERD) • Sleep disruption due to gravid uterus • Insomnia	• Greatest risk of insomnia • Sleep disruption due to vasomotor symptoms • Advancement in circadian phase • Risk of other sleep disorders and medical comorbidities (e.g., SDB, depression)

*When compared with male counterparts.
SE, Sleep efficiency; *SIDS,* sudden infant death syndrome; *SWA,* slow wave activity.

the mechanical effects of a gravid uterus, such as gastroesophageal reflux, dyspnea, leg cramps, and RLS.[57] Leg cramps are noted in up to ¾ of pregnant women.[59,60] In addition, RLS peaks in the 3rd trimester, exacerbated by a decrease in iron and folate, with about 1 in 4 reporting RLS during pregnancy.[61] These leg symptoms often resolve after delivery, although they may predict the future risk of RLS.

Sleep and Menopause

• Changes in sleep during menopause: Women note more sleep difficulties as they transition to menopause.[62] An increase in sleep maintenance issues is noted. Important factors include significant hormonal changes contributing to vasomotor symptoms and hot flashes, depression, stress, and life changes.[63] In addition, the change in estrogen levels may affect the circadian control of sleep, resulting in an advance in the sleep phase.[64] Increased medical comorbidities, including risk for sleep disordered breathing, occur in the postmenopausal period, with resultant sleep disruption.[53,54] Table 3.2 summarizes the gender differences in sleep between females and males and the specific sleep issues attributable to female hormonal changes.

Suggested Reading

Bliwise DL, Scullin MK. Normal aging. In: Kryger MH, Roth T, Dement WC, eds. *Principles and Practice in Sleep Medicine.* 6th ed. Philadelphia, PA: Elsevier; 2017:25-38.

Carskadon MA, Dement WC. Normal human sleep. In: Kryger MH, Roth T, Dement WC, eds. *Principles and Practice in Sleep Medicine.* 6th ed. Philadelphia, PA: Elsevier; 2017:15-24.

Chokroverty S, Avidan AY. Sleep and its disorders. In: Daroff RB, Jankovic J, Mazziota JC, Pomeroy SL, eds. *Bradley's Neurology in Clinical Practice.* Vol. 1. 7th ed. London: Elsevier; 2016:1615-1685.

Czeisler CA, Buxton OM. Human circadian timing systems and sleep-wake regulation. In: Kryger MH, Roth T, Dement WC, eds. *Principles and Practice in Sleep Medicine.* 6th ed. Philadelphia, PA: Elsevier; 2017:362-376.

Reyner LA, Horne JA, Reyner A. Gender- and age-related differences in sleep determined by home-recorded sleep logs and actimetry from 400 adults. *Sleep.* 1995;18:127-134 [erratum in: *Sleep.* 1995;18(5):391].

4

Highlights of Sleep Neuroscience

RONALD SZYMUSIAK

Introduction

- Rapid progress is being made in understanding the cellular/molecular mechanisms and the organization of brain circuits that regulate sleep and wakefulness. This progress has been fueled, in part, by the creation of genetically engineered tools that allow neuroscientists to manipulate neuronal activity and to functionally map brain circuits with unprecedented specificity and precision.
- Application of these tools to the study of arousal state regulation is rapidly expanding and is revealing new and unexpected findings about brain regions and circuits previously implicated in sleep-wake control, as well as identifying novel mechanisms and circuits.
- This chapter will review the current status of knowledge about the functional organization of brain systems that regulate sleep and arousal, with a focus on findings published during the past 5 years. Sleep-wake regulatory mechanisms discovered in rodents are highly conserved, and the rapidly expanding understanding of these mechanisms being gained from the study of genetically engineered mice promises to improve our understanding of sleep disturbance in human disorders.

Regulation of Arousal

- Electrographic, behavioral, and autonomic activation during waking arises from the activity of several neurochemically specified arousal systems located in the brainstem, hypothalamus, and basal forebrain (BF).
- Neurons involved in modulating arousal use histamine (HA), serotonin (5-HT), noradrenalin (NA), dopamine (DA), acetylcholine (ACH), glutamate (GLU), and hypocretin/orexin (HCT) as neurotransmitters (Fig. 4.1). Arousal systems can impact neocortical activity indirectly through projections to thalamus, the lateral hypothalamus, or BF, as well as through direct projections to cortex.

Monoaminergic Neurons

- HA neurons in the hypothalamic tuberomammillary nucleus (TMN), 5HT neurons in the dorsal raphe nucleus (DRN), and NA neurons in the locus coeruleus (LC) are characterized by aggregated cell bodies in distinct nuclei with projections to widespread forebrain and brainstem targets.[1-3] All three nuclei target the thalamus, the hypothalamus, and BF and send direct projections to cortex. Descending projections target visceromotor and somatic motor cranial nerve nuclei.
- HA, 5HT, and NA neurons also share a "rapid eye movement (REM) off" discharge pattern (Table 4.1), characterized by tonic slow discharge rates during waking, reductions in discharge during non-REM sleep (NREM), and cessation of activity during REM sleep.[4-6]
- Drugs that promote release or inhibit reuptake of one or more monoaminergic systems promote waking. Drugs that antagonize the postsynaptic actions of the monoamines can be sedating.[5]
- Optogenetic and other genetic targeting of NA and HA neurons have provided novel perspectives on mechanisms of arousal regulation. Optogenetic methods involve genetically targeting neuronal expression of light-sensitive proteins, channel rhodopsin2 (ChR2) or haplorhodopsin (NpHR), to excite or inhibit neuronal activity.[6] Neurons expressing ChR2 are excited when

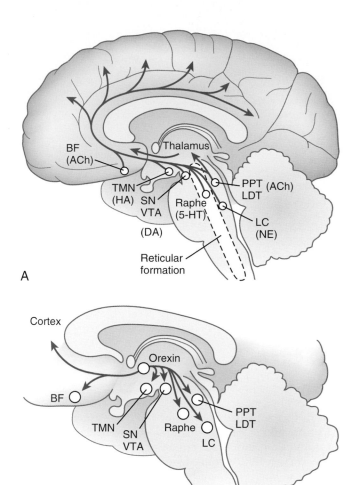

A

B

Figure 4.1 Sagittal views (**A** and **B**) of the human brain, indicating the location of arousal regulatory neuronal groups as described in the text and in Table 4.1. *ACh*, Acetylcholine; *BF*, basal forebrain; *DA*, dopamine; *5-HT*, serotonin; *LC*, locus coeruleus; *LDT*, laterodorsal tegmentum; *NE*, norepinephrine; *PPT*, pedunculopontine tegmentum; *Raphe,* dorsal and median raphe nuclei; *SN*, substantia nigra; *VTA*, ventral tegmental area. Orexin is referred to as hypocretin (HCT) in text and in Table 4.1. (Modified from Espana RA, Scammell TE. Sleep neurobiology for the clinician. *Sleep.* 2004;27:811–820.)

exposed to pulses of blue light at approximately 473 nm (photo-excitation). Neurons expressing NpHR are inhibited when exposed to pulses of yellow light at approximately 590 nm (photo-inhibition).

- Carter et al.[7] genetically targeted NA neurons in the LC by stereotaxically injecting a Cre-recombinase dependent adeno-associated virus (AAV) containing transgenes for ChR2 or NpHR in tyrosine hydroxylase-Cre-knock-in mice. NA neurons could then be excited or silenced *in vivo* by the delivery of light pulses via optic fibers positioned dorsal to the LC. In agreement with pharmacologic studies, photo-inhibition of the LC resulted in decreased waking and increased non-REM sleep.[7] Photo-inhibition of LC neurons also reduced the duration of wakefulness.
- Acute photo-excitation of the LC with low-frequency (3–5 Hz) trains of light pulses delivered during non-REM sleep produced arousal with short latency, indicating that activation of NA neurons is sufficient to induce awakening from sleep. Tonic

photo-excitation at 3 Hz for 1 hour during the rest phase caused reduced sleep followed by a sleep rebound.
- Paradoxically, high-frequency (10–15 Hz) photo-excitation produced a sequence in which mice were initially activated for 20–30 seconds, followed by a behavioral arrest.[7] During arrests, mice were immobile and the EEG exhibited prominent theta activity, but no EEG signs of seizures. Arrests bore some resemblance to cataplexy, and the findings suggest that excessive activation NA neuronal may cause both arousal and motor suppression.
- In addition to HA, many TMN neurons also contain GABA,[8] and co-release of GABA can modulate HA-mediated arousal. Both knockdown of the vesicular GABA transporter (*vgat*) with small interfering RNA and genetic deletion of *vgat* in HA neurons produces hyperactive mice that display increased wakefulness.[9]
- Optogenetic stimulation of HA axon terminals in the cortex evokes $GABA_A$ receptor Cl currents in pyramidal neurons that are prevented by deletion of *vgat* in the TMN.[9] It can be hypothesized that release of GABA by wake-active HA neurons modulates cortical and subcortical arousal induced by TMN neuronal activation.

Dopamine Neurons

- DA is inactivated primarily through reuptake by the DA transporter. The alerting drugs amphetamine and modafinil block the DA transporter and raise extracellular DA levels,[10] suggesting that the net effect of global elevations in DA signaling is arousal. Several antipsychotic medications that block DA receptors are sedating.[5]
- Several DA neuronal groups have been implicated in the control of arousal, including those in the ventral periaqueductal gray (vPAG), the ventral tegmental area (VTA), and the substantia nigra pars compacta (SNc).
- DA neurons in the vPAG have been identified as wake-active based on state-dependent patterns of c-Fos expression (see Table 4.1), and selective lesions of these DA neurons result in 20% reduction in waking.[11] DA neurons in the vPAG project to other brain regions involved in sleep and arousal regulation, including the thalamus, lateral hypothalamus, and preoptic area.[11]
- The role of SNc and VTA DA neurons in arousal regulation is unclear. SNc DA neurons do not exhibit sleep-related c-Fos expression,[11] and their neuronal discharge is not strongly sleep-wake state dependent.[12] DA neurons in the VTA exhibit bursts of action potentials during REM sleep, and during some waking behaviors (e.g., consumption of palatable food[13]), suggesting an involvement in cortical and hippocampal activation (see Table 4.1).
- VTA neurons project to the nucleus accumbens (NAC) in the ventral striatum, the medial prefrontal cortex, and the hippocampus. DA release in the prefrontal cortex and the NAC in rats is elevated during arousing stimuli, such as exposure to novel objects and handling.[14] Lesions of the NAC eliminate the wake-promoting effects of modafinil.[15]
- The arousing effects of VTA DA neurons that project to the NAC may be primarily related to reward-seeking behavior. Optogenetic activation of DA neurons in the VTA enhanced food-seeking behavior in an operant task.[16] No behavioral activation in response to photo-stimulation of DA neurons was observed in the absence of a food reward.

TABLE 4.1 Summary of Arousal Systems

Brain Nuclei	Neurotransmitter	NEURONAL DISCHARGE			Sleep-Wake Discharge Profile
		Wake	NREM	REM	
Tuberomammillary nucleus (TMN) in the posterior hypothalamus	Histamine (HA)	+++	+	–	Wake active, REM off
Dorsal raphe nucleus (DRN) in the midbrain	Serotonin (5-HT)	+++	+	–	Wake active, REM off
Locus coeruleus (LC) in the rostral pons	Norepinephrine (NE)	+++	+	–	Wake active, REM off
Perifornical lateral hypothalamus (PFLH)	Hypocretin/orexin (HCT)	++++	+	–	Wake active, REM off
Basal forebrain (BF) and laterodorsal/pedunculopontine tegmentum (LDT/PPT)	Acetylcholine (ACh)	++++	+	++++	Wake/REM active
Ventral tegmental area (VTA) in the midbrain	Dopamine (DA)	+++	+	+++	Wake/REM active
Ventral periaqueductal gray (vPAG) in the midbrain	Dopamine (DA)	+++	+	?	Unknown
Parabrachial nucleus/precoeruleus (PB/PC) in the pons and thalamocoritical neurons	Glutamate (GLU)	++++	+	++++	Wake/REM active

NREM, Non rapid eye movement; *REM*, rapid eye movement.

Cholinergic Neurons

- ACH-containing neurons are localized in the dorsolateral[17] ponto-mesencephalic reticular formation, including the pedunculopontine tegmental (PPT) and laterodorsal tegmental (LDT) nuclei and in the BF.[17] ACH neurons in the LDT/PPT project to the thalamus and hypothalamus; those in the BF project to the limbic system and neocortex. Neurons in both groups exhibit higher rates of discharge in both waking and REM than in nonrapid eye movement (NREM) sleep (see Table 4.1).[17,18]
- In mice expressing ChR2 in BF ACH neurons, photo-excitation during NREM sleep evokes short-latency EEG and behavioral arousal.[19]
- Recent studies using optogenetic and chemogenetic (also called pharmacogenetic) methods are forcing a reevaluation of the organization of BF control of EEG and behavioral arousal.
- Chemogenetics involves targeted neuronal expression of mutant G-protein coupled muscarinic receptors. These designer receptors activated by designer drugs (DREADDs) are not responsive to ACH but do have a high affinity for the ligand clozapine-n-oxide (CNO), which is otherwise inert in mammals.[20] G_i-DREADDs (M_2- and M_4-mutant muscarinic receptors) cause neuronal inhibition in the presence of CNO, and G_q-DREAADs (M_1-, M_3-, and M_5-mutant muscarinic receptors) are excitatory.[20]
- In mice expressing hM3Dq excitatory DREADD in BF cholinergic neurons, administration of CNO caused reductions of EEG slow wave activity (SWA) (0.3–4 Hz) during NREM sleep, but no change in time spent asleep or awake.[21] In contrast, CNO administration in mice expressing excitatory DREADDs in BF GABAergic neurons evoked short latency suppression of NREM and REM sleep and increased gamma band oscillations (30–80 Hz) in the waking EEG. CNO induced activation of inhibitory hM4Di DREADD expressed in BF GABAergic neurons, increased NREM sleep, and suppressed gamma band oscillations.[21]

- In further support of a role for BF GABAergic neurons in high-frequency EEG oscillations, optogenetic excitation of GABAergic neurons that project to cortex, those that express parvalbumin (PARV), caused increased gamma band oscillations in the waking EEG, and photo-inhibition of this neuronal population suppressed gamma oscillations.[22]
- Cortical activation mediated by BF cholinergic neurons may involve local actions on GABAergic neurons as well as direction actions in the cortex. BF ACH neurons exhibit local axonal connections with PARV-containing GABA neurons in the BF, and in vitro application of cholinergic agonists excites this subset of GABA neurons.[23] The optogenetic activation of BF ACH neurons that was associated with behavioral and EEG arousal from NREM sleep was accompanied by local increases in extracellular ACH levels in the BF.[24] The local perfusion of cholinergic receptor antagonists in the BF blocked the behavioral and EEG activating effects of photo-excitation of BF cholinergic neurons.[24]

Glutamate

- GLU is the most prevalent excitatory neurotransmitter in the brain, and GLU-containing neurons are found throughout pontine and midbrain reticular formation. Specifically, GLU neurons in the parabrachial/precoeruleus (PB/PC) region of the pons have been implicated in regulation cortical arousal. Cell-specific lesions of the PB/PC disrupt desynchronized EEG patterns during waking and in response to arousing stimuli.[25] Projections of GLU neurons in the PB/PC to cortically projecting neurons in the BF may be important in mediating PB/PC effects on cortical activation.
- Thalamic neurons that project to cortex contain GLU.[26] Similar to ACH, extracellular levels of GLU in the cortex are elevated during waking and REM sleep, compared to NREM sleep,[27,28] suggesting that GLU and ACH neurotransmission contribute to brain activation in both states. In mice expressing excitatory

hM3Dq DREADD in GLU neurons in the thalamus, CNO administration increased high-frequency EEG activity during waking and NREM sleep.[21]

Hypocretin/Orexin

- The HCTs are peptides expressed by neurons in the perifornical lateral hypothalamus (PFLH). HCT neurons have extensive projections to other hypothalamic nuclei, the limbic system, the thalamus, the cortex, and to the brainstem and spinal cord (see Fig. 4.1B).[29] HCT neurons occupy a powerful position among arousal systems in that they target the monoaminergic cell groups, ACH neurons in the brainstem, and BF and DA neurons in the VTA.[30,31]

- Acting through HCT-1 and/or HCT-2 receptors, the neuropeptides exert predominately excitatory effects.

- Given their central position among the arousal circuits, integrity of the HCT system is critical for consolidated arousal states. Knockout of HCT peptides or HCT receptors in mice yields a narcolepsy-like phenotype that includes fragmented wakefulness.[32] Central or systemic administration of dual antagonists of HCT-1 and HCT-2 receptors have been shown to promote sleep and EEG synchrony in several species.[33]

- Discharge of HCT neurons is highest during waking, declines dramatically during NREM sleep, and remains low during REM sleep (see Table 4.1).[17] Discharge during waking is phasic, often occurring during vigorous waking movements. Studies in mice and humans suggest that the maximal activity of HCT neurons occurs when working for positive reinforcement (mice), and during positive emotions and social interactions (humans).[34,35]

- Optogenetic targeting of HCT neurons confirm their critical role in arousal regulation. In mice expressing ChR2 in HCT neurons, trains of blue light pulses at 5–50 Hz evoked short-latency awakenings from NREM and REM sleep.[36] Photo-excitation induced arousals were blocked by treatment with an HCT-1 receptor antagonist. In transgenic mice expressing the inhibitory opsin, archaerhodopsin in HCT neurons,

photo-inhibition increased time spent in NREM sleep and the number of sleep-wakefulness transitions during the dark phase.[37]

Sleep-Promoting Mechanisms

Brain mechanisms that promote sleep must be able to achieve a coordinated suppression of multiple arousal-promoting neuronal systems over a period of seconds to minutes during the wake to sleep transition, and maintain that suppression over the subsequent sleep period. The onset and maintenance of sleep are accomplished through interactions among three cellular/molecular and neurochemical mechanisms: (1) systems of sleep-promoting neurons, many of which use GABA as a neurotransmitter, located in the preoptic hypothalamus, lateral hypothalamus, and rostral medulla, which exert inhibitory control over key arousal systems; (2) production of endogenous sleep-regulatory substances, principally adenosine (AD), during waking that regulates homeostatic sleep drive by targeting both wake- and sleep-regulatory circuits in multiple brain regions; and (3) output of the circadian clock in the suprachiasmatic nucleus that functions to promote wakefulness and sleep at different times of day. The topic of the circadian control of sleep is beyond the scope of this article, and the reader is referred to recent reviews of the subject.[38–40]

Preoptic Hypothalamic Neurons

- Sleep regulatory neurons have been identified by direct neuronal recording during sleep and wakefulness (Fig. 4.2)[41] and by sleep-related expression of the protein product of the *c-Fos* gene, an anatomical marker of neuronal activity (Fig. 4.3).[42] The functional importance of sleep-active neurons is confirmed by the loss of function lesion studies.

- Two subregions of the preoptic hypothalamus contain high densities of functionally important sleep-active neurons: the ventrolateral preoptic area (VLPO)[42,43] and the median preoptic nucleus (MnPN).[44] VLPO and MnPO neurons exhibit elevated discharge rates during NREM and REM sleep compared to waking (see Fig. 4.2). MnPO and VLPO neurons are dynamically

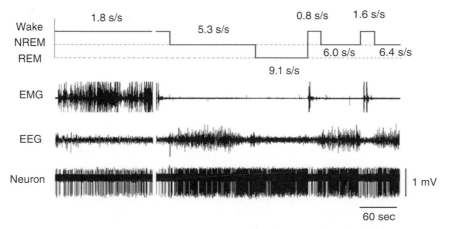

• **Figure 4.2** Example of sleep-related neuronal activity recorded in the rat preoptic hypothalamus. The top panel is a histogram indicating time spent in wake, nonrapid eye movement (NREM), and rapid eye movement (REM) sleep. The numbers indicate the discharge rate of the cell during each state in spikes per second (s/s). The bottom panel (neuron) shows the extracellular action potentials of the recorded neuron. Note the increases in neuronal discharge during both NREM and REM sleep in comparison to waking; *EEG*, Electroencephalogram; *EMG*, electromyogram. (Modified from Suntsova N, Szymusiak R, Alam MN, et al. Sleep-waking discharge patterns of median preoptic nucleus neurons. *J Physiol.* 2002;543:665–677.)

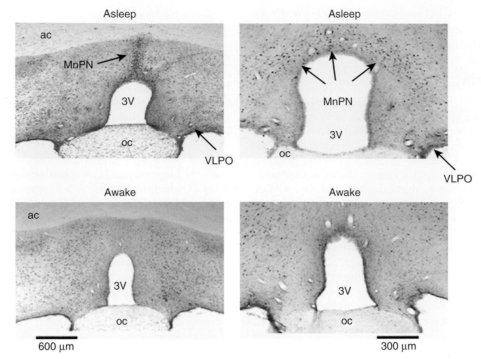

• Figure 4.3 Examples of c-Fos protein staining in the preoptic hypothalamus in one rat that was asleep *(top panels)* and another rat that was awake *(bottom panels)* during the 2 hours before sacrifice. c-Fos protein is a marker of neuronal activity. The nuclei of c-Fos–positive cells are stained black. In the sleeping animal note the presence of Fos staining in the median preoptic nucleus (MnPN) on the midline *(top left)* and dorsal to the third ventricle (3V) in a more rostral section *(top right)*. Sleep-related Fos staining is also present in the ventrolateral preoptic (VLPO) area. Note the absence of Fos staining in these nuclei in the awake rat brain. *ac*, Anterior commissure; *oc*, optic chiasm. (Modified from Gong H, Szymusiak R, King J, et al. Sleep-related c-Fos protein expression in the preoptic hypothalamus: effects of ambient warming. *Am J Physiol.* 2000;279:R2079–R2088.)

responsive to changes in homeostatic sleep pressure induced by sleep deprivation.[45]

- Sleep-related c-Fos expression is co-localized with GABA in the MnPO[44] and with GABA and the inhibitory neuropeptide, galanin, in the VLPO.[42,46] VLPO neurons project to HA neurons in the TMN and to the DRN, LC, and the PPT/LDT.[47] MnPO neurons project to the DRN and LC. MnPO and VLPO neurons that express sleep-related c-Fos project to the HCT neuronal field in the lateral hypothalamus.[48]

- These findings support the hypothesis that VLPO/MnPO neurons promote sleep through monosynaptic GABAergic inhibition of monoamine ACH and HCT neurons. To date there are no published studies using optogenetics or chemogenetics to probe sleep regulatory functions of GABA or galanin neurons in the preoptic hypothalamus.

- VLPO GABA/galanin neurons are inhibited by ACH, 5-HT, and NE. In vitro optogenetic activation of HA neuronal terminals in the VLPO evokes membrane hyperpolarization and increases inhibitory synaptic input to the VLPO neurons.[49] Reciprocal inhibitory interactions between sleep and arousal regulatory neurons are hypothesized to function as a bistable sleep-wake switch.[31]

Melanin Concentrating Hormone Neurons

- Neurons expressing the inhibitory neuropeptide melanin concentrating hormone (MCH) are located in the posterior lateral hypothalamus, where they are intermingled with HCT neurons.[50] A majority of MCH neurons also express GABA. MCH neurons project to hypothalamic and brainstem nuclei implicated in sleep-wake regulation.[51]

- Increased c-Fos expression is observed in MCH neurons during REM enriched sleep following 72 hours of sleep deprivation. REM sleep-related Fos expression is found in MCH neurons projecting to brainstem nuclei implicated in REM sleep control.[52]

- In a small sample of MCH neurons recorded in rats, discharge rates were elevated during REM sleep, compared to waking and NREM sleep,[53] consistent with a hypothesized role in REM regulation.

- Optogenetic excitation of MCH during NREM sleep promoted transitions to REM sleep,[54] while photo-excitation during REM sleep prolonged REM bout duration.[55] The release of GABA by MCH neurons during photo-stimulation may contribute to REM enhancement.[55]

- Other genetic targeting studies of MCH neurons point to a role in sleep onset and sleep maintenance.

- Continuous optogenetic excitation of MCH neurons (light pulses delivered for 1 minute every 5 minutes at 10 Hz) at the start of the dark (active) phase in mice reduced sleep latency, reduced duration of waking episodes by 50%, and increased NREM and REM sleep time.[56]

- Widespread, conditional ablation of the MCH neuronal population by cell-specific expression of diphtheria toxin A increased wakefulness and decreased NREM sleep without affecting REM sleep.[54] These findings are consistent with prior reports that ICV administration of MCH promotes both NREM and REM sleep[57] and that MCH levels in human cerebrospinal fluid are elevated at sleep onset.[35]

- While the state regulatory functions of MCH neurons is not entirely clear, findings suggest a heterogeneity of MCH neuronal function, with some neurons principally interacting with circuits that control REM sleep, and a population of MCH neurons functioning to promote sleep onset and maintenance.

Rostral Medullary Neurons

- Recent findings have identified a sleep regulatory neuronal group in the rostral medulla of rats and mice, located lateral and dorsal to the facial nerve in the parafacial zone (PZ).[58,59] PZ neurons express c-Fos during sleep but not during waking, and sleep-related c-Fos is co-localized with markers for GABA.[58]
- Excitotoxic lesions of the PZ result in persistent sleep loss,[58] and acute chemogenetic activation of PZ GABAergic neurons results in increases in NREM sleep and suppression of waking and REM sleep.[59]
- PZ neurons project rostrally to the PB/PC[58] nuclei that contain arousal-promoting GLU neurons.[25]
- Optogenetic activation of GABAergic neurons in the PZ evokes GABA-mediated inhibition of PB/PC neurons that project to the BF.[59] The ascending circuit of GABAergic PZ neurons evoking sleep-related inhibition of PB/PC neurons complements the descending sleep-related inhibition of arousal systems that originates in the MnPO/VLPO.

Sleep Regulatory Substances

Adenosine

- Homeostatic sleep pressure accumulates slowly during periods of sustained waking and dissipates slowly during subsequent sleep. It has long been hypothesized that accumulation and dissipation of endogenous somnogenic substances during waking and sleep, respectively, underlie the dynamics of sleep homeostasis.[60]
- AD is an inhibitory neuromodulator in the CNS, whose role in sleep is suggested by the arousal-producing effects of caffeine, an antagonist of A_1 and A_{2A} AD receptors.[61]
- Sleep deprivation is accompanied by elevated AD levels in the BF, cortex, and other brain areas, followed by a decline during recovery sleep.[4,62] AD and its analogues promote sleep after systemic and central administration, and AD-induced sleep is accompanied by increased EEG SWA, as is sleep that follows sleep deprivation.[4,61]
- A conditional knockout of the A_1-R gene in mice attenuates EEG SWA in NREM sleep following sleep deprivation.[63]
- AD release by astrocytes is functionally important in homeostatic sleep regulation. Genetically inhibiting the release of gliotransmitters by astrocytes, including ATP, which is converted to AD extracellularly, diminishes homeostatic responses to sleep deprivation.[64]
- Mice deficient for glial adenosine kinase (ADK), the primary catabolizing enzyme for AD, exhibit enhanced homeostatic responses to sleep deprivation; the knockout of ADK in neurons has no effect on sleep homeostasis.[65]
- ACH and non-ACH neurons in the BF are important targets of the sleep-promoting effects of AD acting on A_1 receptors.[66]

Local perfusion of A_1 receptor agonists in the rat lateral hypothalamus suppresses waking c-Fos expression in HCT neurons.[67]

- Complementary actions of AD on excitatory A_{2A} receptors also impact sleep. Central administration of A_{2A} agonists promote sleep and activate VLPO neurons.[68] Administration of A_{2A} agonists into the subarachnoid space ventral to the preoptic area increases sleep and increases c-Fos expression in GABAergic neurons in the MnPO and VLPO.[69]
- A_{2A} receptors in the shell of the NAC have also been implicated in sleep regulation and in mediating the arousing effects of caffeine.[70]

Cytokines

- Cytokines, including interleukin-1β (IL-1β) and tumor necrosis factor-α (TNF-α), are sleep promoting.[60] Antagonism of IL-1β and TNF-α can disrupt normal sleep and impair homeostatic responses to sleep deprivation.[60,71]
- The expression of IL-1β and TNF-α is elevated in multiple brain regions in response to waking neuronal activity.[71] Cellular mechanisms of cytokine-mediated sleep generation are not completely understood, but may involve a combination of arousal system inhibition and activation of preoptic sleep-regulatory neurons.[72–75]

Rapid Eye Movement Sleep-Generating Mechanisms

Brainstem GABA-Glutamate Neuronal Interactions

- Recent findings in rodents emphasize interactions among GABAergic and glutamatergic neurons in the caudal midbrain and pons (Fig. 4.4). A population of "REM-on" neurons (i.e., neurons with elevated discharge during REM sleep compared with waking and NREM sleep) is located ventral to the LC.[18,76,77] This part of the rostral pons has been variously called the subcoeruleus nucleus, pontine inhibitory area, and peri LCα, but sublaterodorsal tegmental nucleus (SLD) is currently the most widely used designation.
- In addition to the SLD, expression of c-Fos during augmented REM sleep in rats has identified REM-on neurons in the precoeruleus region and medial parabrachial nucleus.[78,79]
- REM-off GABAergic neurons in the ventrolateral periaqueductal gray (vlPAG) and lateral pontine tegmentum (LPT) inhibit the activity of REM-on neurons in the SLD.[80]
- One model of NREM-REM switching involves reciprocal inhibitory interactions among GABAergic vlPAG/LPT neurons and GABAergic REM-on neurons in the SLD.[50]
- The ventral SLD contains glutamatergic REM-on neurons that project to GABA/glycine neurons in the ventromedial medulla and spinal cord, and regulates muscle atonia of REM sleep.[77,80]
- Cell-specific lesions or inhibition of the vlPAG/LPT increase the amount of REM sleep and produce cataplexy-like periods of atonia during wakefulness; SLD lesions and medial medulla lesions can result in REM sleep without atonia.[77]
- Another set of GLU neurons in the PB/PC nuclei project to the BF and regulate EEG phenomena of REM sleep. Current evidence suggests that most ACH neurons in the LDT/PPT are wake/REM active,[18] and through ascending projections

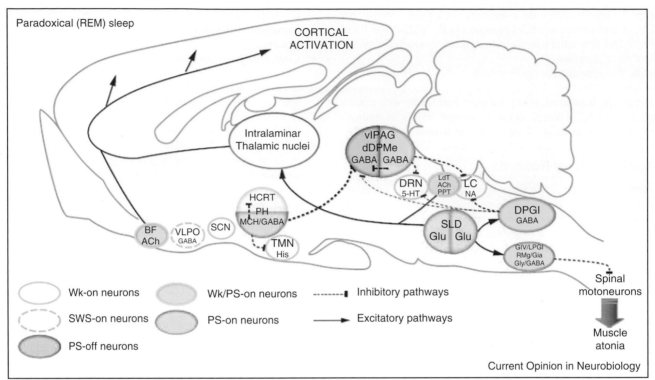

• **Figure 4.4** Neuronal network responsible for REM (paradoxical; PS) sleep during waking. *5-HT*, 5-Hydroxytryptamine (serotonin); *ACh*, acetylcholine; *BF*, basal forebrain; *DPGi*, dorsal para-gigantocellular reticular nucleus; *dDPMe*, deep mesencephalic reticular nucleus; *DRN*, dorsal raphe nucleus; *GABA*, gamma-aminobutyric acid; *Gia*, alpha gigantocellular reticular nucleus; *GiV*, ventral gigantocellular reticular nucleus; *Gly*, glycine; *HCRT*, hypocretin (orexin)-containing neurons; *His*, histamine; *LC*, locus coeruleus; *LDT*, laterodorsal tegmental nucleus; *LPGi*, lateral para-gigantocellular reticular nucleus; *MCH*, melanin concentrating hormone-containing neurons; *NA*, noradrenaline; *PH*, posterior hypothalamus; *PPT*, pedunculopontine tegmental nucleus; *PS*, paradoxical sleep; *REM*, rapid eye movement; *SCN*, suprachiasmatic nucleus; *SLD*, sublaterodorsal nucleus; *SWS*, slow-wave sleep; *TMN*, tuberomamillary nucleus; *vlPAG*, ventrolateral periaqueductal gray; *VLPO*, ventrolateral preoptic nucleus; *Wk*, waking. (From Luppi PH, Clement O, Fort P. Paradoxical (REM) sleep genesis by the brainstem is under hypothalamic control. *Curr Opin Neurobiol.* 2013;23:786–792.)

to the thalamus promote thalamocortical activation during REM sleep.

Cholinergic and Monoaminergic Modulation of Rapid Eye Movement Sleep

• In humans, anticholinergic drugs have potent REM suppressing effects, as do drugs that promote monoamine signaling (e.g., selective serotonin reuptake inhibitors).[5]
• Cholinergic LDT/PPT and monoaminergic neurons in the TMN, DRN, and LC appear to be modulatory of the core REM generating circuitry, with ACH signaling facilitating REM sleep and monoaminergic neuronal activation suppressing REM sleep, although exact sites of modulatory control are not well understood.
• In mice expressing ChR2 in ACH neurons of the LDT/PPT, photo-stimulation during NREM sleep causes more frequent transitions to REM sleep without changing REM bout duration.[81] This indicates that activation of the LDT/PPT is sufficient to generate REM sleep from a background of NREM sleep.
• Other studies suggest that LDT/PPT activation is not required for REM sleep generation. Drug micro-perfusion studies targeting

REM-on neurons in the SLD demonstrate that the perfusion of GABA agonists eliminates REM sleep, indicating that activation of the SLD is required for REM generation.[82]
• However, REM sleep persists during SLD microperfusion of the cholinergic antagonist, scopolamine, indicating that ACH signaling in the SLD is not necessary for REM generation. Scopolamine perfusion did result in more aborted or brief transitions from NREM to REM, consistent with a modulatory role for ACH neurotransmission.[83,84]
• Future studies of targeted optogenetic/chemogenetic neuronal excitation and silencing will be required to better understand the core and modulatory components of REM generating circuitry.

Forebrain-Brainstem Interactions and the Generation of the Nonrapid Eye Movement/Rapid Eye Movement Cycle

Hypocretin/Orexin

• While the core REM-generating circuits reside in the brainstem, REM sleep is normally expressed from a background of NREM sleep. Forebrain-brainstem interactions are involved in orchestrating this aspect of sleep architecture.

- Descending inputs from sleep- and arousal-regulatory hypothalamic neuronal systems are sources of modulatory control of REM sleep circuits.
- The HCT peptides have REM suppressing effects. HCT receptor antagonists augment REM sleep.[33] The knockout of HCT proteins or receptors in mice yields a narcolepsy phenotype, including cataplexy.[32] Optogenetic activation of HCT neurons during either NREM or REM sleep evokes waking.[36]
- HCT neurons target and excite key REM-off neuronal populations in the brainstem, including GABAergic neurons in the vlPAG/LPT, and monoaminergic neurons in the TMN, DRN, and LC.
- Activation of HCT neurons during waking suppresses REM sleep and its components (e.g., muscle atonia), and REM-generating circuits are disinhibited during NREM sleep when HCT neuronal activity is low.

Preoptic Neurons

- Sleep-active GABAergic neurons in the VLPO target many of the REM-off neuronal populations that impact the SLD, including the vlPAG, DRN, and LC.[47]
- The majority of VLPO neurons exhibit elevated discharge during both NREM and REM sleep, and a population of REM-on neurons are located in the dorsal extended VLPO.[41,45]
- Inhibitory effects of VLPO neurons on the REM-off neuronal populations can be hypothesized to facilitate transitions to REM sleep from a background of NREM sleep through disinhibition of the SLD.
- REM-off neurons in the extended VLPO are activated in response to sleep deprivation and may be involved homeostatic aspects of REM sleep regulation.[45]

Melanin-Concentrating Hormone Neurons

- As discussed previously, evidence suggests a role for MCH/GABA neurons in the lateral hypothalamus in promoting both

sleep and REM sleep. Included among the targets of MCH neurons are the TMN LC, DRN, and vlPAG.

- Optogenetic activation of MCH neurons during NREM sleep significantly increases the probability of transitions to REM sleep.[55] As hypothesized for VLPO neurons, mechanisms of MCH REM sleep enhancement involve disinhibition of SLD REM-on neurons via MCH/GABA inhibition of REM-off neurons in the TMN, vlPAG, DRN, and LC.[52,56]
- While activation of MCH neurons during NREM sleep is sufficient to promote REM sleep, it is not necessary. Photo-inhibition of MCH neurons during NREM sleep has no effect on the frequency of REM transitions or REM bout duration.[55,56]
- Critical knowledge gaps exist in understanding the dynamics of MCH neuronal discharge across the sleep-wake cycle, as only a handful of MCH neurons in one portion of the MCH neuronal field have been shown to have a REM-off discharge pattern.[54]
- Optogenetic targeting of MCH neurons suggests functional heterogeneity with respect to NREM and REM sleep control. This may be reflected in heterogeneity of neuronal discharge patterns across different subpopulations of MCH neurons.

Suggested Reading

Brown RE, Basheer R, McKenna JT, et al. Control of sleep and wakefulness. *Physiol Rev.* 2012;92:1087-1187.

de Lecea L. Hypocretins and the neurobiology of sleep-wake mechanisms. *Prog Brain Res.* 2012;198:15-24.

Espana RA, Scammell TE. Sleep neurobiology from a clinical perspective. *Sleep.* 2011;34:845-858.

Luppi PH, Clement O, Fort P. Paradoxical (REM) sleep genesis by the brainstem is under hypothalamic control. *Curr Opin Neurobiol.* 2013;23:786-792.

Saper CB, Fuller PM, Pedersen NP, et al. Sleep state switching. *Neuron.* 2011;68:1023-1042.

5

Normal Sleep Physiology (Including Respiratory and Cardiac Physiology)

SUDHANSU CHOKROVERTY, SUSHANTH BHAT

Introduction

- Physiologic changes during sleep affect virtually every system in the body.
- The two distinct stages of sleep, *nonrapid eye movement (NREM)* sleep and *rapid eye movement (REM)* sleep, differ from each other, and from wakefulness, in specific physiologic, molecular, and functional aspects.
- This chapter provides a brief overview of the physiologic changes associated with sleep in various systems and its impact in certain disease states.

Changes in the Central Nervous System During Sleep

- The brain does not simply "deactivate" during sleep. Intracellular electrophysiologic studies, c-Fos activation (shown by immunohistochemical observations), and positron emission tomographic (PET) scans of the brain demonstrate that many distinct and specific areas of the central nervous system (CNS) show excitation or inhibition during NREM and REM sleep.
- *During NREM sleep*, there is activation of the vetrolateral preoptic (VLPO) and the median preoptic (MnPO) anterior hypothalamic nuclei, and to a certain extent also lower brainstem nucleus tractus solitarius (NTS); in contrast, the wake-promoting regions such as the ascending reticular activating system (ARAS), the histaminergic, aminergic, and orexinergic neurons of the hypothalamus, as well as most of the cerebral cortical regions are deactivated.
- *During REM sleep*, there is activation of most cortical regions and pontine areas controlling REM sleep (the pedunculopontine, laterodorsal tegmental, and sublaterodorsal [SDL] nuclei).

In addition, there are changes in certain neural reflexes during sleep:

- *H-reflex*, the electrical counterpart of the *monosynaptic* muscle stretch reflex, is decreased in amplitude because of motor neuron hyperpolarization, presynaptic inhibition, and disfacilitation of brainstem aminergic neurons and lateral hypothalamic orexinergic neurons projecting to brainstem motor neurons and to the ventral horn cells of the spinal cord.
- *Polysynaptic blink reflex*: There is marked reduction in amplitude and excitability of the R2 component (and to a lesser extent of the R1 component) of the *polysynaptic* blink reflex during all stages of NREM sleep, with significant recovery during REM sleep; the R2 excitability in REM sleep is almost the same as that seen during wakefulness.[1]
- *The flexor reflex (FR)*, seen in lower limbs in humans, is another *polysynaptic* spinal reflex with early and late components. Long latency FR (R3 component) is mediated by high-threshold nociceptive A-delta and C fibers. Sandrini et al.[2] examined the effects of NREM and REM sleep on the FR3 (i.e., the nociceptive component in the lower limbs of healthy humans). The FR3 threshold is increased in all stages of NREM sleep, with further increase in REM sleep. They also noted prolonged latency during slow wave sleep (SWS), with further prolongation in REM sleep. However, the maximal amplitude and duration were seen during REM sleep. The prolonged latency indicated reduced excitability, whereas the prolonged duration reflected temporal and spatial summation causing changes in the interneuron excitability.

Cortical potential responses are also altered by sleep. There is increased intracortical inhibition of interneurons in NREM sleep and decreased intracortical facilitation in REM sleep as determined by paired brain magnetic stimulation technique.

- *Somatosensory cortical evoked potential amplitudes* attenuate during sleep, particularly during deeper stages of sleep.
- *Motor evoked potential amplitudes* following magnetic brain stimulation also show attenuation in all stages of sleep

Clinical Relevance

In patients with restless legs syndrome (RLS, also known as Willis-Ekbom disease [WED]), both primary and secondary (comorbid with chronic renal failure), spinal FR study during sleep shows hyperexcitability (a low threshold, more easily excitable, and widely distributed response), suggesting the release of spinal motor centers from supraspinal inhibition.[3,4] In addition, enhancement of FR components during sleep in patients with RLS indicates state dependence of flexor response in these patients.

Changes in the Autonomic Nervous System and Its Changes During Sleep

- A central autonomic nervous system (ANS) network located in the brainstem with its reciprocally connected ascending and descending projections has been shown to control cardiovascular, respiratory, gastrointestinal, and genitourinary systems during sleep and wakefulness.
- The NTS may be considered a central station in the central autonomic network. It is located in the dorsal region of the medulla and is influenced by higher brainstem, diencephalon, forebrain, and neocortical regions.
- Afferent fibers from the cardiovascular, respiratory, and gastrointestinal systems project to the NTS, which in turn sends efferent ascending projections to the supramedullary structures and descending efferent projections to the ventral medulla, and

---

• **BOX 5.1** **Central Autonomic Network**

- Nucleus tractus solitarius (NTS), the major central station of the CAN
  - Afferents
    - Cardiovascular
    - Respiratory
    - Taste
    - Gastrointestinal
    - Descending projections from cerebrum and upper brainstem
  - Efferents
    - Ventral medulla
    - Intermediolateral neurons
    - Inspiratory neurons
    - Vagal efferents to cardiovascular, respiratory, and gastrointestinal systems
    - Ascending projections to upper brainstem and cerebrum

• **BOX 5.2** **Autonomic Nervous System Changes During Sleep**

- NREM sleep
  - Increased parasympathetic activity
  - Decreased sympathetic activity
  - Decreased LF components reflecting decreased sympathetic tone but increased HF components reflecting increased respiratory vagal tone
- REM sleep
  - Further increase in parasympathetic activity
  - More marked decrease in sympathetic activity
  - Intermittent bursts of sympathetic activity in phasic rapid eye movements
  - Profound increase in sympathetic activity in skin and muscle vessels (microneurographic recordings)
  - Variable LF and HF with decreased HF and intermittent increment of LF components

HF, High frequency; *LF*, low frequency; *NREM*, nonrapid eye movement; *REM*, rapid eye movement.

---

then to the intermediolateral neurons of the spinal cord (Box 5.1).
- The final common pathways from the NTS through the vagus nerve and sympathetic fibers orchestrate the central autonomic network for integrating autonomic functions that maintain internal homeostasis.[5]
- The lower brainstem hypnogenic and central respiratory neurons are also located near the region of the NTS, and therefore a dysfunction of the ANS may have a serious implication on human sleep and breathing. Fig. 5.1 schematically shows the visceral afferents to and efferents from the NTS.

Alterations in Autonomic Nervous System Activity During Sleep (Box 5.2)

- There is increase in the parasympathetic tone and a decrease in the sympathetic activity during NREM sleep; this is accentuated during REM sleep (Fig. 5.2).
- During phasic REM sleep, however, sympathetic activity increases intermittently, resulting in fluctuations in blood pressure (BP) and heart rate, causing bradytachyarrhythmias.

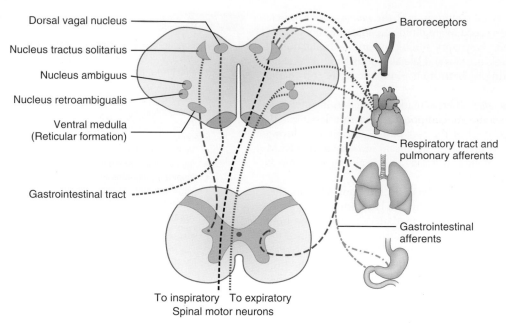

• **Figure 5.1** The visceral afferents to and efferents from the nucleus tractus solitarius. (Reprinted with permission from Chokroverty S. *Sleep Disorders Medicine: Basic Science, Technical Considerations and Clinical Aspects.* 3rd ed. Philadelphia, PA: Saunders/Elsevier; 2009).

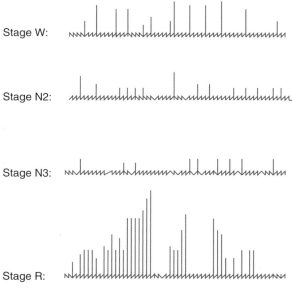

• **Figure 5.2** Sympathetic nerve activity (SNA) during wakefulness (*W*), NREM sleep (*Stages N2 and N3*) and REM sleep (*Stage R*) in a normal subject shown schematically. Progressive decrement of SNA from W to Stage N2 and Stage N3 but marked increment in Stage R. (Modified from Hornyak M, Cejnar M, Elam M, Matousek M, Wallin BG. Sympathetic muscle nerve activity during sleep in man. *Brain*. 1991;114:1281.)

As a result of these autonomic changes, there are alterations in the activity of the heart, circulation, respiration, thermoregulation, and pupils.

• Pupillary constriction occurs during NREM sleep and is maintained during REM sleep due to tonic parasympathetic drive. Pupilodilation during phasic REM sleep results from a central inhibition of parasympathetic outflow to the iris.

• Sympathetic activity in muscle and skin blood vessels, as measured by the microneurographic technique,[6–9] shows a reduction in muscle sympathetic nerve activity during NREM sleep but an increment above waking levels during REM sleep, particularly during phasic REM sleep (see Box 5.2 and Fig. 5.2). In addition, there are transient bursts of sympathetic activity during arousals in NREM sleep.

• The ANS changes in the cardiovascular system during sleep can be assessed by measuring heart rate variability (HRV).[10] A power spectrum analysis of HRV by using fast Fourier transform shows power in mainly two bands: high frequency (HF) ranging from 0.15–0.4 Hz and low frequency (LF), with power ranging between 0.04 and 0.15 Hz. Respiratory vagal activity contributes mainly to the HF component, whereas the LF component is thought to be a marker of sympathetic modulation, but some authors consider this to contain both sympathetic and parasympathetic activities.

• The LF/HF ratio is thought to reflect sympathovagal balance.[11,12] The heart rate changes precede electroencephalographic (EEG) changes during transitions to sleep states. NREM sleep can be considered a state of relative cardiorespiratory stability, while REM sleep is a state of profound instability with an intense autonomic dysregulation. Based on a greater increment in LF/HF power, Richard et al.[13] pointed out that NREM-to-REM excitatory cardiorespiratory responses are more marked among women compared with men.

Clinical Relevance

• Profound neurophysiologic changes in the ANS may adversely affect patients with cardiorespiratory disorders, as well as those with neurologic and other medical illnesses. Furthermore, patients with primary autonomic failure (e.g., multiple system atrophy, familial dysautonomia) and conditions causing secondary autonomic failure are exquisitely sensitive to adverse impact of autonomic dysregulation on cardiorespiratory functions during sleep.

- The significant sleep-related changes in the ANS affecting various systems have important clinical implications in patients with central or peripheral autonomic failure (e.g., sleep-related respiratory dysrhythmias, cardiac arrhythmias, gastrointestinal dysmotility, and urogenital disorders). Chronic sympathetic hyperactivity in patients with obstructive sleep apnea (OSA) is thought to play a major role linking OSA with hypertension, cardiac ischemia, congestive cardiac failure, and stroke,[14,15] although additional inflammatory mechanisms also likely play a role.[16]

Control of Respiration During Sleep and Wakefulness

- The function of breathing is to maintain arterial homeostasis (i.e., normal partial pressure of oxygen [PO_2] and carbon dioxide [PCO_2]), which requires optimal gas exchange (elimination of carbon dioxide and extraction of oxygen from the atmospheric air) through alveolar ventilation.
- The PCO_2 depends predominantly on the central chemoreceptors, with some influence from the peripheral chemoreceptors, whereas PO_2 depends entirely upon the peripheral chemoreceptors. The metabolic respiratory system uses mainly the peripheral and central chemoreceptors, but also to some extent the body's metabolism and the intrapulmonary receptors to maintain internal homeostasis. Hypoxia and hypercapnia both stimulate breathing. In normal individuals, the hypoxic ventilatory responses are hyperbolic, showing a sudden increase in ventilation when PO_2 falls below 60 mm Hg. In contrast, hypercapnic ventilatory responses are linear. When PCO_2 falls below a certain minimal level (called apnea threshold), ventilation is inhibited.
- There are three interrelated components for control of breathing (Box 5.3): central controllers located in the medulla aided by the supramedullary structures, including the influence of the forebrain providing volitional control, central and peripheral chemoreceptors, and pulmonary and upper airway receptors; the thoracic bellows, consisting of respiratory and other thoracic muscles, their innervations, and bones; and the lungs, including the airways.
- The thoracic bellows consist of the diaphragm, the intercostal and other respiratory muscles in addition to bones, connective tissues, the nerves, and blood vessels that support them. The main inspiratory muscle is the diaphragm innervated by the phrenic nerve (C3, C4, and C5 roots of anterior horn cells), assisted by the external intercostal muscles innervated by the thoracic motor roots and nerves (T1–T12 segments). Expiration is passive, but during effortful breathing, accessory muscles of respiration assist the breathing (Box 5.4). A dysfunction anywhere within these three major components of the respiratory control systems results in respiratory failure.

- Two principal groups of neurons located in the medulla are responsible for central control of ventilation:
  - The *dorsal respiratory group* located in the region of the NTS is responsible principally for inspiration, and
  - The *ventral respiratory group* located in the region of the nucleus ambiguus and retroambigualis is responsible for both inspiration and expiration.
- The ventral group, in addition, contains the Bötzinger complex in the rostral region, and the pre-Bötzinger region immediately below the Bötzinger complex is responsible mainly for the respiratory rhythmicity by virtue of intrinsic pacemaker activities of these neurons (Fig. 5.3).[17,18]
- The rostral pontine group of neurons located in the region of parabrachial and Kolliker-Fuse nuclei (pneumotaxic center) and the lower pons (apneustic center) exerts strong influence on the medullary respiratory neurons.
- The dorsal and ventral groups of medullary respiratory neurons send axons that decussate below the obex (the point where the central canal widens to form the fourth ventricle) and descend with the reticulospinal tracts in the ventrolateral cervical spinal cord to synapse with the spinal respiratory motor neurons, innervating the various respiratory muscles (see Fig. 5.3).
- The rate, rhythm, and frequency of breathing and internal homeostasis are regulated by the peripheral and central afferents to the medullary neurons. These afferents include the parasympathetic vagal fibers from the respiratory tracts, the carotid and aortic body peripheral chemoreceptors, and the central chemoreceptors (located on the ventrolateral surface of the medulla lateral to the pyramids), as well as other central regions (forebrain, midbrain, and pontine areas) and the ARAS.

Two independent systems—the metabolic (or automatic) and voluntary (or behavioral) systems—control respiration.[19-23]

• BOX 5.3   Respiratory Components for Control of Breathing

- Central controllers (brainstem) aided by:
  - Central and peripheral chemoreceptors
  - Forebrain and limbic cortex
  - Pulmonary and upper airway receptors
- Thoracic bellows
  - Respiratory pump muscles, bones, and tissues
- The lungs
  - Including the airways

• BOX 5.4   The Respiratory Muscles

- Inspiratory muscles
  - Diaphragm
  - External intercostal
- Accessory inspiratory muscles
  - Sternocleidomastoideus
  - Scalenus (anterior, middle, posterior)
  - Pectoralis major
  - Pectoralis minor
  - Serratus anterior
  - Serratus posterior superior
  - Latissimus dorsi
  - Alae nasi
  - Trapezius
- Expiratory muscles (silent during quiet breathing but contract during moderately severe airway obstruction or during forceful and increased rate of breathing)
  - Internal intercostal
  - Rectus abdominis
  - External and internal oblique

- Both metabolic and voluntary systems operate during wakefulness, whereas only the metabolic system operates during NREM sleep.
- The voluntary control system for breathing originates in the forebrain and limbic system and descends with the corticobulbar and corticospinal tracts, descending partly to the medullary respiratory neurons, and traveling to the spinal respiratory motor neurons in the high cervical spinal cord, where the fibers finally integrate with the reticulospinal fibers originating from the

medullary respiratory neurons for smooth, coordinated functioning of respiration during wakefulness.

Changes in Breathing During Sleep

- During sleep, changes are noted in respiratory rate and rhythm, alveolar ventilation, tidal volume, blood gases, chemosensitivity, respiratory muscle tone, as well as the upper airway reflexes and resistance (Table 5.1).
- During both NREM and REM sleep, respiratory neurons in the pontomedullary regions show decreased firing rates.
- Respiratory rate decreases during NREM sleep, whereas in REM sleep the respiration becomes irregular, especially during phasic REM, where there may be a few periods of brief apneas.
- Periodic breathing resembling Cheyne-Stokes breathing due to waxing and waning of the tidal volume is often noted at the onset of sleep.[24] This periodic breathing may be related to sudden loss of wakefulness stimulus, reduced chemosensitivity at sleep onset, and transient arousal.
- During stage N3, respiration becomes stable and rhythmic and depends entirely upon the metabolic system. Breathing during stage N3 (SWS) is slower than in wakefulness and more regular, whereas during REM sleep, respiration shows large breath-to-breath variability in rate, volume, and duration, and is often interrupted by transient quiescent periods (fractionations) of about 50 msec, which may result in overt clinical central apneas that are physiologic.
- Minute ventilation progressively decreases during all stages of NREM and REM sleep. Minute ventilation falls by 0.5–1.5 L/min as a result of reduction of tidal volume.
- In addition, during REM sleep there is marked variability in ventilation, and minute ventilation is about 40% lower in REM as compared with ventilation in wakefulness.
- The following factors in combination appear to be responsible for alveolar hypoventilation during sleep: reduced metabolic rate (basal metabolic rate falls during sleep causing a reduction in ventilation and ventilatory responses); absence of wakefulness stimulus; increased airway resistance as a result of muscle hypotonia of the upper airway dilator muscles; diminished

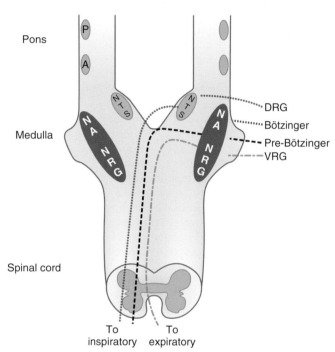

- **Figure 5.3** Schematic representation of central respiratory neurons in Pons and Medulla. *A*, Apneustic center; *DRG*, dorsal respiratory group with projections to contralateral predominantly inspiratory muscles; *P*, pneumotaxic center; *VRG*, ventral respiratory group with projections to contralateral inspiratory and expiratory muscles.

TABLE 5.1	Summary of Physiologic Changes in Breathing During Sleep		
Parameters	**Wakefulness**	**NREM Sleep**	**REM Sleep**
Respiratory rate	Normal	Decreases	Variable, apnea may occur
Minute ventilation	Normal	Decreases	Decreases further
Alveolar ventilation	Normal	Decreases	Decreases further
PaCO$_2$	Normal	Increases slightly	Increases further slightly
PaCO$_2$	Normal	Decreases slightly	Decreases further slightly
SaO$_2$	Normal	Decreases slightly	Decreases further slightly
Hypoxic ventilator response	Normal	Decreases	Decreases further
Hypercapnic ventilatory response	Normal	Decreases	Decreases further
Upper airway muscle tone	Normal	Decreases slightly	Decreases markedly or is absent
Upper airway resistance	Normal	Increases	Increases further

NREM, Nonrapid eye movement; *REM*, rapid eye movement.

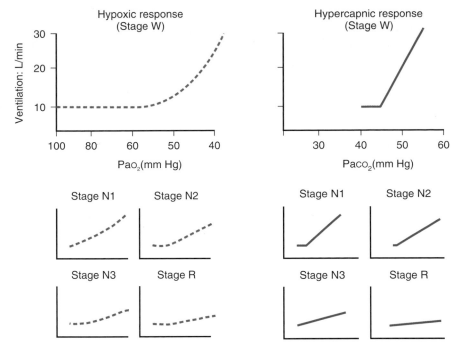

• **Figure 5.4** Hypoxic and hypercapnic ventilatory responses during wakefulness, nonrapid eye movement (*Stages N1, N2,* and *N3*) and rapid eye movement (REM; Stage R) sleep in a normal man shown schematically. There is progressive decrement of responses with shift to the right from wakefulness to Stages N1, N2, N3, and REM state (Stage R). (Modified from Douglas NJ, White DP, Weil JV, et al. Hypoxic ventilatory response decreases during sleep in normal men. *Am Rev Respir Dis.* 1982;125:286; Douglas NJ, White DP, Weil JV, Pickett CK, Zwillich CW. Hypercapnic ventilatory response in sleeping adults. *Am Rev Respir Dis.* 1982;126:758.)

thoracic movements due to intercostal muscle hypotonia; and diminished ventilatory drive due to decreased hypoxic and hypercapnic ventilatory responses, as well as a decreased number of functioning medullary respiratory neurons.

• As a result of these changes, in normal individuals, there is mild hypoxemia (PO_2 decreases by 3–10 mm Hg and oxygen saturation decreases by < 2%) and mild hypercapnia (PCO_2 rises by 2–8 mm Hg) due to mild alveolar hypoventilation during sleep.

• Hypoxic ventilatory response decreases slightly during NREM sleep in adult men but not in women, whereas hypoxic ventilatory response during REM sleep is decreased in both men and women (Fig. 5.4).[25,26] These findings result from decreased chemosensitivity and increased upper airway resistance to air flow.

• Hypercapnic ventilatory response also decreases 20%–50% during NREM sleep and decreases further during REM sleep (see Fig. 5.4).[27,28] Thus the CO_2 response curve shifts to the right so that increasing amounts of PCO_2 are needed to stimulate ventilation resulting from a decreased number of functioning medullary respiratory neurons, decreased chemosensitivity of central chemoreceptors subserving medullary respiratory neurons, and increased upper airway resistance during sleep.

Upper Airway Reflexes and Resistance

• In wakefulness, the activity of the upper airway inspiratory dilator muscles reflexively increases at the onset of inspiration due to the negative intrathoracic pressure, to prevent upper airway collapse.

• Such reflex responses, however, are decreased during sleep, making the upper airway susceptible to suction collapse.

• The role of the upper airway reflexes in maintaining the upper airway resistance is strengthened by the observation of increased frequency of obstructive apneas and hypopneas in normal subjects during sleep following upper airway anesthesia,[29] as well as increased apnea index after upper airway anesthesia in snorers.[30]

• Patients with OSA, however, do not show an increase in their apnea index after upper airway anesthesia.[31]

• Alcohol, benzodiazepines, and age clearly cause a decrement in upper airway reflex response.[32]

Sleep-Related Changes in the Upper Airway and Related Muscles

• The limb and cranial muscles show marked alteration of tone during sleep. Muscle tone is maximal during wakefulness, slightly decreased in NREM sleep, and markedly decreased or absent in REM sleep.[5] There is hypotonia of the intercostal muscles during NREM sleep and near-atonia in REM sleep. During REM sleep, the tonic activity of the diaphragm is reduced, but the phasic activities are maintained.

• Upper airway patency is maintained by the coordinated activity of the upper airway dilator muscles (e.g., muscles of the soft palate, tongue, and hyoid, as well as intrinsic laryngeal muscles). The collapse caused by the inspiratory intrathoracic pressure is counterbalanced by the tone of the upper airway dilator muscles. Inspiratory-related genioglossus muscle activity is associated with forward protrusion of the tongue and increased upper airway size. Genioglossus electromyographic activities consisting of phasic and tonic discharges are decreased during NREM sleep and further decreased during REM sleep. Alcohol, diazepam, and many anesthetic agents cause selective reduction of hypoglossal nerve activity. In contrast, protriptyline and strychnine selectively increase such activity.

- Changes in the function of the upper airway muscle during sleep have important clinical implications, particularly for patients with OSA. During NREM sleep, there is decrement of muscle tone, with further decrement in REM sleep, causing increased upper airway resistance due to decreased pharyngeal volume. This is a critical factor in patients with OSA, most of which already have small upper airway space.

Mechanism of Muscle Hypotonia in Nonrapid Eye Movement Sleep

- Mild muscle hypotonia during NREM sleep most likely results from a combination of disfacilitation of brainstem motor neurons controlling muscle tone (e.g., slight reduction of activity of locus coeruleus noradrenergic and midline raphe serotonergic neurons) and mild hyperpolarization of brainstem and spinal motor neurons.[33]
- In addition, the paired pulse transcranial magnetic brain stimulation technique showing significant enhancement of intracortical inhibition during SWS suggests a direct cerebral cortical mechanism for mild muscle hypotonia in NREM sleep.[34]

Mechanism of Muscle Atonia or Hypotonia in Rapid Eye Movement Sleep

- During REM sleep, there is complete suppression of voluntary muscle tone in the presence of highly active forebrain (paralyzed body with an activated brain) with inhibition of the mesencephalic locomotor region.
- The mechanism of muscle atonia during REM sleep includes an activation of a polysynaptic descending pathway from perilocus ceruleus alpha in the region of the nucleus pontis oralis in the dorsolateral region of the pontine reticular formation. Axons from this region transmitted along the lateral tegmentoreticular tract through the ventromedial medulla (nucleus reticularis magnocellularis and gigantocellularis in the medial medulla) and via the ventral tegmentoreticular and reticulospinal tracts terminate on the spinal inhibitory interneurons and spinal motor neurons, causing hyperpolarization and muscle atonia (Fig. 5.5).[35]
- A key element in the REM sleep-generating mechanism in the pons is activation of the GABAergic neurons, located in a subgroup of pontine reticular formation, as well as GABAergic neurons in the lateral pontine tegmentum and ventrolateral periaqueductal gray region in mesencephalon. Activation of GABAergic neurons causes an excitation or a disinhibition of cholinergic neurons, and inhibition of noradrenergic and serotonergic neurons in the pons. The cholinergic neurons, in turn, excite pontine glutamatergic neurons projecting to the glycinergic premotor neurons in the medullary reticular formation, causing hyperpolarization of the brainstem and spinal motor neurons, and motor paralysis during REM sleep.
- The GABAergic mechanism also plays an important role in motor neuron hyperpolarization. Disfacilitation of motor

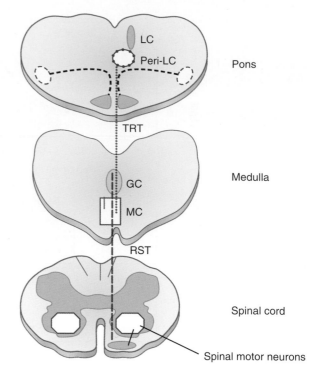

• **Figure 5.5** Schematic diagram to explain the mechanism of muscle atonia in rapid eye movement sleep. *GC,* Gigantocellularis; *LC,* locus ceruleus; *MC,* magnocellularis; *Peri-LC,* peri-locus ceruleus alpha; *RST,* reticulospinal tract; *TRT,* tegmentoreticular tract. (Reprinted with permission from Chokroverty S. *Sleep Disorders Medicine: Basic Science, Technical Considerations and Clinical Aspects.* 3rd ed. Philadelphia, PA: Saunders/Elsevier; 2009).

neurons as a result of reduction of the release of midline raphe serotonin and locus ceruleus norepinephrine partially contributes to muscle atonia.

- Finally, a cerebral cortical mechanism may also contribute to the inhibition of spinal motor neurons in REM sleep, as evidenced by decreased intracortical facilitation in the paired-pulse transcranial magnetic brain stimulation technique.
- In summary, three principal mechanisms are responsible for muscle atonia in REM sleep: inhibitory postsynaptic potentials (IPSPs), causing postsynaptic inhibition of motor neurons (major mechanism); disfacilitation of brainstem motor neurons controlling muscle tone; and decreased intracortical facilitation. As a result, motor neurons are hyperpolarized by 2–10 mV during REM sleep. Intracellular recordings reveal an increased number and appearance of REM sleep-specific IPSPs in the lumbar motor neurons of cats, which are derived from inhibitory interneurons, possibly located either in the spinal cord or in the brainstem, from which long axons project to the spinal motor neurons.
- Intermittently during REM sleep, there are bursts of excitatory postsynaptic potentials (EPSPs), causing motor neuron depolarization shifts and giving rise to transient myoclonic bursts during REM sleep. Muscle movements caused by these excitatory drives during REM sleep are abrupt, jerky, and purposeless, somewhat different from the movements noted during wakefulness. Facilitatory reticulospinal fibers are responsible for transient EPSPs (phasic or transient discharges), causing muscle twitches

in REM sleep. Corticospinal or rubrospinal tracts are not responsible for these twitches, because destruction of these fibers in cats does not affect these twitches.

- The elegant work of Chase and Morales[33] suggested that glycine is the main neurotransmitter responsible for motor neuron hyperpolarization and IPSPs. The REM-specific IPSPs are reversed after strychnine (a glycine antagonist), but picrotoxin and bicuculline (a GABA antagonist) did not abolish these IPSPs. Recent evidence, however, suggests an important role for GABA in addition to glycine.[36,37]
- Brooks and Peever challenged this concept and stated that glycinergic and GABA-mediated postsynaptic inhibition is not exclusively responsible for REM muscle atonia, but is one of the many biochemical pathways responsible for controlling muscle tone in REM sleep.[38] In a subsequent paper[39] these authors concluded, based on their experimental results, that GABA(B) receptors, acting in concert with GABA(A) and glycine receptors, do indeed play a role in mediating REM sleep–related upper airway muscle atonia. These authors have subsequently published research in rats that supports the idea that a powerful GABA and glycine drive triggers REM paralysis by switching off motor neuron activity, targeting both metabotropic GABA(B) and ionotropic GABA(A)/glycine receptors, with REM paralysis only reversed when motor neurons are cut off from GABA(B), GABA(A), and glycine receptor–mediated inhibition.[40] They also demonstrated that impaired GABA and glycine transmission triggers the cardinal features of REM sleep behavior disorder (RBD) in mice.[41]
- It is also known that hypocretinergic neurons located in the lateral hypothalamus play a facilitatory role in the motor system through direct projections to motor neurons and indirectly through projections to the monoaminergic, histaminergic, and cholinergic neurons; withdrawal of their activities contributes in part to muscle atonia in REM sleep.[42] Despite these considerable recent advances, much research remains to be done with regard to the mechanisms underlying REM atonia.

Clinical Relevance

- The decreased tone in the upper airway dilator muscles during NREM sleep, with further reduction in REM sleep, causing increased upper airway resistance and decreased upper airway space, plays a significant role in contributing to upper airway obstruction in patients with OSA, particularly because these patients have smaller upper airways than normal controls.
- In wakefulness, patients with OSA have increased genioglossal muscle activity as a compensatory mechanism to prevent upper airway collapse. Most cases of OSA show occlusion at the level of the soft palate, and therefore decreased activity in the palatal muscles causes increased upper airway resistance and the onset of OSA. In about half the cases, the obstruction extends caudally to the region of the tongue, with further caudal extension during REM sleep.
- Sleep-related alveolar hypoventilation also predisposes such individuals to upper airway occlusion and obstructive apneas. Patients with neuromuscular disorders, chronic obstructive pulmonary disease, and bronchial asthma may be affected adversely by such hypoventilation. Asthmatic attacks may also be exacerbated at night as a result of bronchoconstriction, which is a normal physiologic change during sleep.[43,44]

TABLE 5.2	Summary of Physiologic Changes in the Heart and Circulation		
Physiologic Characteristics		NREM	REM
Heart rate		↓	↓↑
• Cardiac output		↓	↓↑
• Systematic arterial BP		↓	↓↑
	• Dippers		
	• Extreme dippers		
	• Nondippers		
	• Reverse dippers		
• Pulmonary arterial BP		↑	↑
• Peripheral vascular resistance		—↓	↓
• Systematic blood flow			
	• Cutaneous	—	↓
	• Muscular	—	↓
	• Mesenteric	—	↑
	• Renal	—	↑
• Cerebral blood flow		↓	↑

NREM, Nonrapid eye movement; *REM*, rapid eye movement; ↓, decreased; ↑, increased; ↓↑, uncertain; —, unchanged.

Changes in the Cardiovascular System During Sleep

- The dynamic interaction in sleep between the sympathetic and parasympathetic divisions of the ANS controlling the heart rate and rhythm, cardiac output, peripheral vascular resistance (PVR), systemic and pulmonary arterial pressure, as well as systemic and cerebral blood flow (CBF) result in profound cardiovascular changes (Table 5.2).

Heart Rate and Rhythm

- The heart rate slows by about 5%–8% during NREM sleep due to tonic increase in parasympathetic activity (sympathetic activity has little effect).[45–48]
- During REM sleep, the heart rate slows further due to a combination of persistence of parasympathetic predominance and additional decrease of sympathetic activity. However, heart rate becomes highly variable during phasic REM sleep, causing bradytachyarrhythmia.
- HRV can be assessed by the spectral analysis of cardiac beat-to-beat intervals. The documentation of increased HF component of electrocardiogram (EKG) clearly indicates the predominance of parasympathetic activity during both NREM and REM sleep. These studies also show intermittent increases of LF components in the EKG, indicating intermittent sympathetic nervous system activation during REM sleep. In addition, studies also show that the heart rate acceleration occurs at least 10 beats before EEG arousals.[49–51]
- The effect of sleep on cardiac rhythm has been studied in normal individuals using Holter monitors.[52] Sinus arrhythmias are the most frequent nocturnal dysrhythmia, noted in 50% of young

individuals. In another study using 24-hour continuous EKG recordings, sinus pauses lasting from 1.8–2 sec were noted in half of 50 male medical students without any apparent heart disease, and episodes of atrioventricular block were observed in another 6%.[53] Sinus arrest in REM sleep lasting up to 9 sec has been described in young healthy adults without any associated apneas or significant oxygen desaturation.[54]

- Although there are contradictory reports of the effects of sleep on ventricular arrhythmia, in the majority of patients, there is an antiarrhythmic effect of sleep on ventricular premature beats as a result of increased parasympathetic tone. Ventricular arrhythmias, however, have been reported to occur during arousal from sleep due to increased sympathetic activity. An important observation is prolongation of QT interval in some normal men during sleep, posing a risk factor for susceptible individuals with long QT syndrome, as well as a risk of sudden death in the elderly.[55]

Cardiac Output

- There is a progressive fall of cardiac output during sleep, with maximum decrement during early morning, particularly during the last REM cycle.[56]

Systemic and Pulmonary Arterial Pressure

- During NREM sleep, systemic blood pressure (SBP) decreases by 5%–9% in stages N1 and N2, and 8%–14% in SWS.[57] This fall of BP is most likely due to the reduction in cardiac output.[58]
- In REM sleep, BP swings up and down, with an overall increase in pressure by about 5% above that noted in NREM sleep. In addition to decreased cardiac output, BP changes in REM sleep appear to be secondary to decreased PVR.[58]
- There is a sharp rise in BP around the time of awakening.
- The pulmonary arterial pressure rises slightly to 23/12 mm Hg above the mean waking value of 18/8 mm Hg.[59]

Systemic Blood Flow and Peripheral Vascular Resistance

- Cutaneous, muscular, and mesenteric vascular blood flow shows little change during NREM sleep, but during REM sleep, there is profound vasodilation in these splanchnic beds resulting in increased blood flow in the mesenteric and renal vascular beds. As a result, in general PVR remains unchanged during NREM sleep but falls significantly during REM sleep.[60]

Systolic Blood Pressure

- Physiologically, there is a fall of systolic BP of 10%–20% during sleep, as compared with the waking value, and this phenomenon is called "dipping."
- In some individuals, this does not occur, and these individuals are known as "nondippers." Nondippers have higher supine brachial and central systolic BP, significantly different central hemodynamics, and elevated left ventricular mass index compared with dippers.[61]
- In contrast, there are individuals in whom systolic BP actually increases during sleep periods, and they are called "reverse dippers."

Cerebral Blood Flow

- CBF and cerebral metabolic rates are lower in postsleep wakefulness, compared with the values noted in presleep wakefulness, and also lower at the end of the night compared with those at the beginning of the night.
- CBF and cerebral metabolic rates for glucose and oxygen decrease during all stages of NREM sleep, whereas during REM sleep, CBF and cerebral metabolic rates increase.[62–67] The largest increases during REM sleep are noted in the hypothalamus and the brainstem structures, and the smallest increases are in the cerebral cortex and white matter.
- Studies using PET scanning have shown major differences in brain activation during wakefulness, REM, and NREM sleep.[68–72] In addition to a global decrease in CBF during NREM sleep, there is a regional decrement of CBF in the dorsal pons, mesencephalon, thalami, basal ganglia, basal forebrain, anterior hypothalamus, prefrontal cortex, anterior cingulate cortex, and precuneus. These observations correlate with the electrophysiologic findings of hyperpolarization of the thalamic neurons generating sleep spindles, K-complexes, and delta and waves, and modulating very slow oscillations.[73,74] Very slow EEG oscillations appear to be of neocortical origin and an intrinsic state of the neocortex.[75]
- The pattern of deactivation during NREM sleep is not, however, homogeneous, and the dorsolateral prefrontal (DLPF) and orbito-frontoparietal regions are seen to be the least active areas.
- During REM sleep, there is increased neuronal activity and CBF in the pontine tegmental, thalamus, amygdala, anterior cingulate cortex, hippocampus, temporal and occipital regions, basal forebrain, cerebellum and caudate nucleus, and activation of limbic and paralimbic structures, including the amygdala, hippocampal formation, and anterior cingulate cortex, supporting the modulatory role of these structures in REM sleep mechanism and participation of REM sleep in memory processing. The DLPF, precuneus, posterior cingulate cortex, temporoparietal region, and inferior parietal lobule show regional deactivation during REM sleep.[76]
- CBF is controlled by cerebral autoregulation, cerebral metabolism, and respiratory blood gases. Cerebral autoregulation is determined by the intrinsic properties of the muscles of the cerebral arterioles and is normally maintained between mean arterial pressure of 60 and 150 mm Hg.[77] As the SBP falls, cerebral blood vessels dilate in response to changes in transmural pressure, whereas in cases of a rise in BP, the cerebral vessels constrict, thus protecting the brain from fluctuation in SBP.

Clinical Relevance

- Profound hemodynamic changes consisting of unstable BP and heart rate, progressive decrease in cardiac output causing maximum oxygen desaturation and periodic breathing, and sympathetic alteration during REM sleep may explain increasing mortality during early morning hours, especially in patients with cardiopulmonary disease.
- The most susceptible period for myocardial infarction, stroke, and sudden cardiac death is in the morning between 6 AM and 11 AM. The reason is not definitively known, but appears to be multifactorial and may include increased platelet aggregability, sympathetic surge during REM sleep in the early morning hours just before the final awakening from sleep, attenuation of endothelial function leading to vascular disease, as well as

increased morning plasma catecholamines. These factors are particularly lethal in those with preexisting coronary arterial or other cardiovascular disease.

- *Circadian patterns of calculability:* There is increased coagulability during sleep as a result of increased tissue plasminogen activator (tPA) inhibitor 1 (PAI 1) and a decrease in tPA. This increased platelet aggregation and coagulability, and endothelial dysfunction in the early morning hours, plays a major role in the early morning increased incidence of cardiovascular events and sudden cardiac death.[55]
- Individuals who are considered "extreme dippers" (in whom BP falls excessively), as well as nondippers and reverse dippers, are at higher risk for stroke than dippers.[78]
- Cerebral autoregulation may break down in disease such as a stroke, encephalitis, hypertensive crisis, acute head injury, and excessive antihypertensive therapy.[79]

Changes in Endocrine Secretions During Sleep

Circadian Changes in Endocrine Function

- The rhythmic, pulsatile nature of most neuroendocrine secretions (occurring every 1–2 hours) is governed by both the internal biologic clock located in the suprachiasmatic nuclei (SCN) and the sleep state.
- Adrenocorticotrophic hormone (ACTH), cortisol, and melatonin rhythms are determined by the circadian clock, whereas growth hormone (GH), prolactin, thyroid stimulating hormone (TSH), and renin are sleep-related.[80,81]
- The patterns of endocrine secretion in an adult human are schematically shown in Fig. 5.6.

Adrenocorticotrophic Hormone and Cortisol

- The ACTH-cortisol rhythm is mainly controlled by circadian rhythmicity but clearly modulated by the sleep-wake state.
- Sleep onset is associated with a decrease in cortisol secretion, but with a rapid elevation in the later part of the sleep at night and with subsequent decline throughout the day.[81,82]
- Daytime sleep fails to significantly inhibit cortisol secretion, suggesting that sleep suppresses cortisol release only within a limited range of entrainment.[83]
- During sleep deprivation, the effect of sleep on cortisol levels is absent.
- The inhibitory influence of early nocturnal sleep on ACTH-cortisol levels is most marked during SWS.[84]

Growth Hormone

- Two-thirds of GH secretion during sleep is associated with SWS.[85,86] Thus the largest GH secretory pulse occurs shortly after sleep onset. Although GH secretion also occurs during daytime sleep onset, there is an increased propensity for GH secretion at night. Nocturnal GH secretion can, however, occur in absence of SWS.
- If SWS is decreased, GH secretion also decreases, and if SWS is increased, GH secretion is increased. The sleep-related release of GH is reduced in old age, and there is no sleep-related release of GH before the age of 3 months.[87]

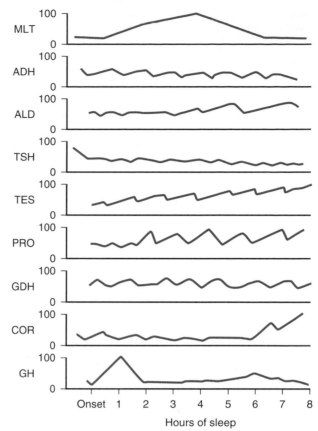

• **Figure 5.6** Schematic representation of the plasma levels of hormones in an adult during 8 hours of sleep. Zero indicates the lowest secretory episode and 100 indicates the peak. *ADH,* Antidiuretic hormone; *ALD,* aldosterone; *COR,* cortisol; *GDH,* gonadotropic hormone; *GH,* growth hormone; *MLT,* melatonin; *PRO,* prolactin; *TES,* testosterone; *TSH,* thyroid stimulating hormone. (Reprinted with permission from Chokroverty S. *Sleep Disorders Medicine: Basic Science, Technical Considerations and Clinical Aspects.* 3rd ed. Philadelphia: Saunders/Elsevier; 2009).

- Although in general the major peak in plasma GH occurs during the early part of nocturnal sleep, in about one-fourth of healthy men, peaks in GH secretion occur before sleep onset.[88]
- There is some evidence of possible circadian influences on the regulation of GH secretion from a study on jet lag by Goldstein et al., who showed increased GH secretion after flights both eastward and westward.[89]
- In acromegaly, a disorder of unregulated GH synthesis, the relationship between sleep and hormone secretion is lost.[90]
- Hypothalamic GH releasing hormone (GHRH) stimulates release of GH from the anterior pituitary, whereas hypothalamic somatostatin inhibits release of GH. Ghrelin, an appetite-stimulant gastric peptide, also stimulates GH secretion. Sleep, especially SWS, is associated with increased GH, GHRH, and ghrelin levels.
- Agents promoting SWS (e.g., gamma hydroxybutyrate) will promote GH secretion. An activation of hypothalamic GHRH neurons promotes both the onset of SWS and the peak GH levels, suggesting a direct link between SWS and GH secretion. Furthermore, the GHRH gene is found in the

mouse in the same region regulating NREM sleep in the hypothalamus.[91,92]

Prolactin

- The pulsatile plasma prolactin (PRL) secretion is sleep dependent but is not related to any specific sleep stage.
- The PRL secretion shows a rise about 60–90 min after sleep onset and peaks in the early morning hours around 5–7 AM.[93]
- A sleep independent circadian pattern has also been postulated for prolactin secretion in subsequent studies,[94] contradicting some earlier observations of an entirely sleep-dependent pattern.
- Prolactin secretion is suppressed by dopamine but stimulated by thyrotropin-releasing hormone.[95]
- It is notable that the secretory pattern of prolactin does not decline with age, unlike that of GH.[96]

Thyroid Stimulating Hormone

- TSH levels are low during the daytime, increase rapidly in the early evening, peak shortly before sleep onset, and are followed by a progressive decline during sleep.
- Sleep deprivation is associated with nocturnal rise of TSH levels.[97]
- It is, however, observed that during SWS rebound following prior sleep deprivation, there is marked inhibition of nocturnal rise of TSH, suggesting that the sleep-associated fall in TSH is related to SWS.
- TSH secretion is not suppressed significantly during daytime sleep, but sleep-related inhibition of TSH secretion occurs following nighttime elevation of TSH, indicating an interaction between circadian timing and sleep for the control of TSH secretion.[98]

Gonadotropic Hormone

- The gonadotropin-releasing hormone of the hypothalamus controls the secretion of the anterior pituitary luteinizing hormone (LH) and follicle stimulating hormone (FSH). LH is responsible for the secretion of testosterone by the testes in men, and FSH stimulates spermatogenesis. LH and FSH are the stimuli for the ovarian hormones, estrogen, and progesterone, which are responsible for menstrual cycle changes.
- There has not been a clear relationship between LH and FSH plasma levels and the sleep-wake cycle or sleep stages, nor any distinct circadian rhythms. However, they show a pulsatile rise at sleep onset in prepuberty (both sexes), whereas in pubertal boys and girls, gonadotropin levels increase during sleep.[99–101]
- Plasma testosterone levels show an increase at sleep onset and are consistent with the sleep-associated rise of LH levels in normal men.[102] Some studies link the nocturnal rise of testosterone to REM sleep.[103] The sleep-related rise in testosterone is reduced in older men, and the relationship to REM sleep is lost.[104]
- In women, sleep-related inhibitory effect on LH secretion has been found in the early parts of the follicular and luteal phases of the menstrual cycle.[105]

Renin-Angiotensin-Aldosterone Activity

- Renin is an enzyme secreted by the juxtaglomerular cells of the kidneys that acts upon angiotensinogen, which is then converted

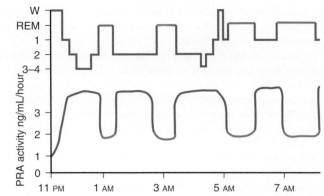

- **Figure 5.7** Schematic representation of plasma renin activity (PRA) profiles in a normal subject during sleep from 11 PM–7 AM. Note synchronized oscillations of PRA to nonrapid eye movement–rapid eye movement cycling, showing the lowest values during REM sleep. (Reprinted with permission from Chokroverty S. *Sleep Disorders Medicine: Basic Science, Technical Considerations and Clinical Aspects.* 3rd ed. Philadelphia, PA: Saunders/Elsevier; 2009).

into angiotensin II; the latter acts upon the zona glomerulosa of the adrenal cortex to stimulate aldosterone secretion.
- Plasma renin activity (PRA) is synchronized with the NREM-REM cycles in an ultradian rhythm, with higher values during NREM sleep associated with a fall in BP, and the lowest values during REM sleep associated with fluctuating BP and intermittently enhanced sympathetic activity (Fig. 5.7).[106]
- Sleep-related aldosterone levels are related to PRA oscillations, whereas during daytime wakefulness, aldosterone levels parallel cortisol pulses. Aldosterone levels are increased during sleep, but sleep deprivation prevents the rise of nocturnal sleep-related aldosterone release, causing an alteration of overnight hydromineral balance.[107]

Parathormone Secretion

- Plasma parathyroid hormone (PPH) or parathormone shows a significant increase during night time sleep in normal young men, but there is no significant association with sleep stages or plasma ionized calcium and phosphate levels.[108] These findings contradict the earlier observations of PPH peaks related to SWS.[109]

Antidiuretic Hormone

- Antidiuretic hormone (ADH) shows episodic secretion without any relationship to sleep, sleep stages, or circadian system; however, there appears to be a slight increase in the second half of the night.[110]

Melatonin

- Melatonin, the hormone of darkness, is synthesized by the pineal gland from the precursor amino acid L-tryptophan, which is then converted to 5-hydroxytryptophan by the enzyme tryptophan hydroxylase, followed by decarboxylation to serotonin. The latter is then catalyzed by the enzymes acetyltransferase and hydroxyindole-o-methyltransferase into melatonin, which is then released directly into the blood stream or cerebrospinal fluid.

- The daily rhythm of melatonin production is controlled by the environmental light-dark cycle and the SCN. Melatonin secretion is controlled by a complex polysynaptic pathway, with impulses originating from the retinal ganglion cells transmitting via the retinohypothalamic tract to the SCN, which then sends efferent fibers to the superior cervical ganglia. The latter in turn transmits impulses via the postganglionic efferent fibers to the pineal gland. This pathway is activated during the night, triggering melatonin production, which is suppressed by exposure to bright light. The melatonin circadian rhythm is driven by the SCN through activation of two major melatonin receptors (MT_1 and MT_2).
- Melatonin begins to rise in the evening, reaching maximum values between 3 AM and 5 AM and decreasing to low levels during the day. The maximum nocturnal secretion of melatonin has been noted in young children ages 1–3 years; secretion then begins to fall around puberty and decreases significantly in the elderly.[111]

Clinical Relevance

- Neuroendocrine secretions and sleep are tightly linked, and hence sleep disturbances may result in the disruption of the endocrine functions. A disturbance of the link between GH secretion and SWS may cause sleep disturbance in OSA, narcolepsy, older age, some cases of insomnia, depression (although results are contradictory), Cushing's syndrome, alcoholism, schizophrenia, and thyrotoxicosis.[112–116] Nocturnal release of GH and PRL is decreased in untreated OSA patients, but is increased following continuous positive airway pressure (CPAP) treatment.[117] In OSA patients, sodium and urinary output normalizes following CPAP treatment, which may be related to restoration of normal PRA and aldosterone oscillations, as well as the decreased release of atrial natriuretic peptide.
- The age-related decrease in GH and PRL and linear increase of cortisol in old age may be related to the age-related reduction of SWS and increased sleep fragmentation. These changes may impair anabolic function of sleep in the elderly.[117]
- Glucose tolerance and thyrotropin concentrations are reduced, whereas evening cortisol concentrations and sympathetic nervous system activity increase after sleep debt resulting from partial sleep deprivation. These effects are similar to those noted in normal aging, suggesting that sleep debt may increase the severity of age-associated chronic disorders.
- Similarly, age-related sleep fragmentation may cause increased nocturnal corticotrophic activities.[117] Shift work-related increased incidence of infertility in women is thought to be related to the sleep-associated inhibitory effect on gonadotropin release during the follicular phase of the menstrual cycle.[118]
- The hypnotic effect of melatonin has been noted in several reports, which led to the development and availability of a melatonin receptor agonist (ramelteon) for the treatment of sleep-onset insomnia.
- The administration of melatonin has been shown to have some beneficial effects on symptoms of jet lag and some primary circadian rhythm sleep disorders such as delayed sleep phase syndrome and non-24-hour sleep-wake syndrome.[119] In a subgroup of elderly insomniacs with reduced melatonin secretion at night, the beneficial effects of melatonin on sleep disturbances were noted.[120]

Changes in the Alimentary System During Sleep

- The activity of the alimentary system during sleep is controlled by the ANS, as well as by enteric nervous system (ENS), which is an intrinsic system within the walls of the visceral organs working closely with the ANS.
- Sleep-related physiologic changes in the alimentary system are summarized in Table 5.3.

Esophageal Function

- Gastroesophageal reflux (GER) may be exacerbated by sleep through various mechanisms. Although during wakefulness, salivary flow ensures rapid (within 1–2 min) clearing of reflux events, during sleep, swallowing is suppressed and the flow of saliva is decreased, causing prolongation of acid clearance and increased mucosal contact with refluxed acid.[121] This predisposes individuals to the development of esophagitis.
- In addition, esophagitis is exacerbated by decreased esophageal peristaltic contractions in sleep, particularly SWS, and proximal migration of gastric contents in the distal esophagus.[122]
- Refluxed acid contents are harmful not only to the esophagus but also the tracheobronchial tree.[123] The three barriers to reflux that must be overcome to cause gastroesophageal and pharyngoesophageal reflux aspirating into the lungs and paranasal sinuses are the upper esophageal sphincter (UES), the lower esophageal sphincter (LES), and the epiglottis. The LES acts

TABLE 5.3	Physiologic Changes During Normal Wakefulness and Sleep in the Gastrointestinal System	
Physiologic Characteristics	**Wakefulness**	**Sleep**
Swallowing frequency	Normal	Decreased
Salivary flow	Normal	Decreased
Esophageal acid clearance time	Normal	Prolonged
Lower and upper esophageal sphincter pressure	Normal	Decreased
Esophageal peristaltic contractions	Normal	Decreased
Gastric motility	Normal	Decreased
Gastric acid secretion	Depends on food ingestion	Peak secretion between 10 PM and 2 AM
Migrating motor complex (MMC) recurs every 90 min	Normal velocity	Reduced velocity
Colonic motility	Normal	Decreased
Rectal motor activity and anal periodic canal pressure	Normal	Increased activity with propagation and higher anal canal pressure

as the primary barrier to GER, and both the UES and the LES act as barriers to pharyngoesophageal reflux. The UES pressure is generated mainly by the cricopharyngeus, and to a certain extent, the inferior pharyngeal constrictor muscles. LES pressure is generated by contractions of the esophageal smooth muscles and the diaphragm.

- Pandolfino et al.,[124] in contrast with other authors,[125] noted that the majority of postprandial transient relaxations are associated with brief periods of UES relaxations.

Gastric Acid Secretion and Gastric Motility

- Gastric acid secretion increases considerably during the day and night, with a peak period of secretion between 10 PM and 2 AM (Fig. 5.8).
- In patients with duodenal ulcers, there is failure of inhibition of acid secretion during the first 2 hours of sleep.[121–123] Acid secretion shows no clear relationship between different stages of NREM and REM sleep.
- There is an absence of circadian rhythm for gastric acid secretion following vagotomy, suggesting the importance of vagal stimulation for such control.[126]
- There are contradictory reports in the literature about the effects of sleep on gastric motility, with both inhibition and enhancement of gastric motility having been described[127,128] and one group reporting that gastroduodenal motility during sleep was related to sleep-stage shifts and body movements.[129]

Intestinal Motility and Secretions

- ENS-mediated sleep-related changes are responsible for alterations of motor and secretory function of the entire gastrointestinal tract. The results of intestinal motility studies during sleep, however, have been contradictory.[122]
- Migrating motor complex (MMC) is a special type of intestinal motor activity pattern consisting of four phases that recurs every 90 min in the stomach and small intestine.[130]

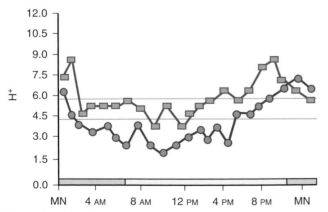

- **Figure 5.8** Mean 24-hour values for gastric acid secretion shown schematically from a group of patients with active peptic ulcer disease *(rectangles)* and normal controls *(circles)*. The ordinate shows hydrochloric acid secretion in milliequivalents. *MN,* midnight. (Reprinted with permission from Chokroverty S. *Sleep Disorders Medicine: Basic Science, Technical Considerations and Clinical Aspects.* 3rd ed. Philadelphia, PA: Saunders/Elsevier; 2009).

- The periodicity of the gut motor activity superficially resembles a cyclic REM-NREM sleep; however, MMC distribution does not relate to REM or NREM sleep stages.[131–133]
- There is decreased velocity of MMC, as well as colonic motility and myoelectric activity during sleep with increment on awakening. This sleep-wake change in colonic motility explains the well-known and universally experienced urge for defecation in the morning. During sleep there is increased periodic rectal motor activity, but the majority of these contractions are propagated in a retrograde fashion, and at the same time the anal canal pressure remains consistently above the rectal pressure, thus preventing the passive escape of the rectal contents during sleep.[134]

Clinical Relevance

- Sleep is a highly vulnerable time for patients with GERD because of decreased swallowing and salivation, as well as decreased esophageal peristaltic waves causing prolonged acid clearance.
- The proximal migration of acid gastric contents into the distal esophagus and decreased LES pressure and absence of response to heartburn, which is a waking conscious phenomenon, coupled with a reduction of UES pressure during sleep may promote esophagitis, laryngopharyngitis, pulmonary aspiration, and exacerbation of bronchial asthma. Laryngopharyngeal reflux is the most dreaded complication of sleep-related GER.[135,136] OSA also predisposes to nocturnal GERD.
- Sleep disturbances characterized by repeated arousals and awakenings may occur in patients with peptic ulcer disease because of the failure of the inhibition of gastric acid secretion that occurs after sleep onset.
- Measuring MMC may be important for the diagnosis of gastrointestinal disorders; its absence has been associated with gastroparesis, intestinal pseudo-obstruction, and bacterial overgrowth in the small intestine.[132]
- Increased sleep complaints may occur in patients with irritable bowel syndrome, but the actual mechanism of sleep dysfunction remains to be determined. Orr[122] suggested that alterations of the physiologic changes during sleep in the rectal motor contractions and anal canal pressure may be responsible for the loss of rectal continence in patients with diabetes mellitus, with autonomic neuropathy affecting the ENS.

Changes in the Urinary System in Sleep

- During sleep, urine volume decreases due to a reduction of renal blood flow and glomerular filtration rate and increased renal tubular reabsorption of water, primarily due to increased secretion of ADH, particularly in the second half of the night.[5]
- During REM sleep, there is further reduction in urine volume and increased urinary osmolality.

Changes in the Genital System During Sleep

- Sleep-related penile erections occur in all age groups, from childhood to elderly healthy men. Overall, small age-related decline is noted for total tumescence time, but there is little or no age-related decline in maximum circumference increase and number of erection episodes.[137]
- Similar tumescence occurs in the clitoris, associated with increased vaginal blood flow and uterine contractility during REM sleep in women.[5]

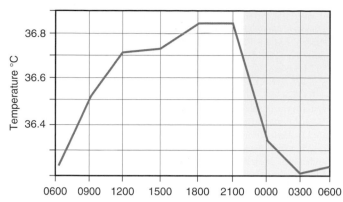

• **Figure 5.9** Body temperature follows a sinusoidal rhythm with a peak around 9 PM and a minimum (nadir) around 3 AM as a result of circadian rhythmicity.

Thermoregulation in Sleep

- While body temperature is linked to the sleep-wake cycle, it has its own distinct and independent circadian rhythm.[138–140] When sleep-wake cycles and temperature cycles are dissociated from each other, for example when environmental cues such as light are removed, the independent nature of the two becomes obvious.
- Body temperature follows a sinusoidal rhythm with a peak around 9 PM and a minimum (nadir) around 5 AM as a result of circadian rhythmicity (Fig. 5.9). Thus the core temperature nadir occurs 2–3 hours before habitual wake time, a fact that is of crucial importance in the detection and treatment of circadian rhythm disorders.
- Sedative hypnotics also have thermoregulatory effects. The somnogenic effects of melatonin[141] and the benzodiazepines[142,143] are accompanied by a decrease in core body temperature. Caffeine and amphetamines, in contrast, decrease sleep propensity and increase body temperature.
- Reduced body temperature and peripheral heat loss promote sleep onset and enhance SWS, and sleep in turn causes a further decrease in body temperature and increases heat loss, thus consolidating sleep.
- Electrical stimulation of the thermosensitive neurons located in the medial preoptic-anterior hypothalamic (POAH) region causes cutaneous vasodilation, panting, suppression of shivering, and decreased body temperature promoting heat dissipation. Lesions of the POAH cause suppression of both NREM sleep and thermoregulation.
- Since the thermoregulatory mechanism is inoperative during REM sleep, thermoregulatory homeostasis is lost. Thus thermoregulatory responses such as sweating and panting, which are noted in NREM sleep, are absent in REM sleep. As a result of complete suppression of thermoregulatory responses in REM sleep, mammals display a state of poikilothermia. Brain temperature rises during REM sleep, due to an increase in cerebral metabolic activity, and this may be one mechanism for preparing for behavioral activation during REM sleep.[144]

Clinical Relevance

- Jet lag and shift work may disrupt the linkage between thermoregulation and SWS, causing difficulty in initiating and maintaining sleep and disrupting sleep architecture and daytime function.

- Menopausal hot flashes may be a disorder of thermoregulation initiated within POAH.[138] The central thermoregulatory mechanisms underlying hot flashes may affect hypnogenic pathways inducing sleep and heat loss in these patients. It has been suggested that an impairment of thermoregulatory mechanisms in the elderly makes them susceptible to hypothermia or hyperthermia.[145]
- Finally, age-related impairment of the heat loss mechanism or phase advance in body temperature rhythm may partly explain sleep initiation or maintenance difficulty in the elderly. Thermal manipulation by adapting behavior to enhance peripheral heat loss may improve sleep. Those individuals suffering from vasospastic syndrome (e.g., cold feet) with impaired heat loss may also have a prolonged sleep onset latency.[146]

Immune Functions and Cytokines in Sleep

- Sleep is thought to act as a host defense against infection (bacterial, viral, and fungal infections enhance NREM but suppress REM sleep) and facilitates the healing process.[147,148]
- Leukocyte-produced cytokines such as interleukin (IL), interferon-alpha, and tumor necrosis factor-alpha (TNF-α) promote sleep. Other known factors enhancing sleep include delta sleep-inducing peptides, muramyl peptides, cholecystokinin, arginine vasotocin, vasoactive intestinal peptide, GHRH, somatostatin, prostaglandin D_2, nitric oxide, and adenosine.
- Adenosine in the basal forebrain inhibits cytokine release (in addition to mediating somnogenic effects of prolonged wakefulness by acting through A1 and A2a receptors).[149,150]

Glymphatic System

- A recent discovery in the CNS of mice (not yet demonstrated in humans) revealed a new metabolic waste clearing pathway (equivalent to the lymphatic system in the body), termed "the glymphatic system," because of its dependence on glial cells (astrocytes) performing a "lymphatic"-like cleansing of the brain interstitial fluid in the perivascular space between the brain blood vessels and leptomeningeal sheaths surrounding these vessels.[151–155]
- In sleep, the glial cells shrink and the extracellular pace expands, promoting clearance of interstitial waste products. Furthermore, it appears that the ability of this system to remove misfolded or aggregated proteins (demonstrated experimentally by injection of labeled beta amyloid proteins into the brains of sleeping and awake mice) is hampered.[156]

Clinical Relevance

- Sleep is essential for immunologic homeostasis and for improving immune responses; sleep deprivation leads to altered immune functions. Cytokines play an important role in the pathogenesis of excessive daytime sleepiness in a variety of sleep disorders and in sleep deprivation.[157] Increased production of the proinflammatory cytokines IL-6 and TNF-α has been noted in sleep deprivation, causing excessive sleepiness.
- Excessive sleepiness in OSA, narcolepsy, insomnia, or idiopathic hypersomnia may also be caused by such cytokines, although there have not been any valid scientific studies to prove this.
- An increased amount of circulating TNF-α may also be responsible for inflammatory disorders such as human immunodeficiency virus (HIV) infection and rheumatoid arthritis. Finally, viral or bacterial infections causing increased NREM

sleep and excessive sleepiness may have been due to the increased production of proinflammatory cytokines.

- Although the glymphatic system has yet to be replicated in humans, it is postulated that a similar mechanism may be present, and demonstration of such a system may aid in the development of drugs that promote clearance of beta amyloid and other undesirable products from the brain during sleep, thereby preventing or halting the progression of neurodegenerative diseases like Alzheimer's disease, Parkinson's disease, and so on.[158] More research is needed.

Suggested Reading

Chase MH, Morales FR. Control of motoneurons during sleep. In: Kryger MH, Roth T, Dement WC, eds. *Principles and Practice of Sleep Medicine*. 5th ed. Philadelphia, PA: Elsevier Saunders; 2005:154.

Chokroverty S. Physiologic changes in sleep. In: Chokroverty S, ed. *Sleep Disorders Medicine: Basic Science, Technical Considerations and Clinical Aspects*. 3rd ed. Philadelphia, PA: Saunders/Elsevier; 2009.

Chokroverty S, Avidan AY. Sleep and its Disorders. In: Daroff RB, Jankovic J, Mazziotta JC, Pomeroy SL, eds. *Bradley's Neurology in Clinical Practice*. 7th ed. Philadelphia, PA: Elsevier; 2015.

Peter JG, Fietze I. Physiology of the cardiovascular, endocrine and renal systems during sleep. In: Randerath WJ, Sanner BM, Somers VK, eds. *Sleep Apnea: Current Diagnosis and Treatment*. Basel: Karger; 2006:29.

White DP. Ventilation and the control of respiration during sleep: normal mechanisms, pathologic nocturnal hypoventilation, and central sleep apnea. In: Martin RJ, ed. *Cardiorespiratory Disorders During Sleep*. Mount Kisco, New York, NY: Futura; 1990:53.

6

Genetics in Sleep Medicine

NAMNI GOEL

The circadian clock interacts with the sleep homeostatic drive in humans. Chronotype and sleep parameters show substantial heritability, underscoring a genetic component to these measures. This paper reviews the genetic underpinnings of chronotype, sleep and individual differences in the context of the sleep loss as a phenotype in healthy adult sleepers, highlighting candidate gene and genome-wide association (GWA) studies.

Notably, both circadian and non-circadian genes associate with individual differences in chronotype and in sleep parameters. Furthermore, as predicted by the two-process model of sleep regulation, substantial overlap exists in the genes influencing sleep and circadian rhythms. The review concludes with a brief discussion of future research directions.

To read this chapter in its entirety, please see ExpertConsult.com.

7

Introduction to Evaluation Tools Used in Sleep Medicine

MARCEL HUNGS

Introduction

- Sleep complaints are very common in our society. Many methods are available to help determine whether a sleep complaint is truly a sleep disorder. These methods are very helpful in establishing a diagnosis but should be used thoughtfully. This chapter discusses a selection of testing tools used by sleep specialists to determine whether or not a patient has a particular sleep disorder.
- Advances in technology have truly revolutionized diagnostic opportunities in sleep medicine (Table 7.1). Over the last 2 decades, sleep testing possibilities have become far more sophisticated and user-friendly.[1] Data quality, quantity, speed of processing, and accessibility are rapidly improving with technologic advances such as the amount of data that can be easily collected and stored electronically compared with traditional paper recordings, as well as the increased mobility of testing devices.[1]

How to Approach a Patient with a Sleep Disorder

- Sleep medicine is a discipline driven foremost by clinical history and reported symptoms. The initial clinical encounter with the patient will guide the practitioner in the diagnostic approach and the assessment.
- *Initial patient encounter:* The patient reports personally experienced symptoms of sleep disturbance (Table 7.2). In some patient encounters, physicians observe an absent awareness or denial of sleep symptoms due to the lack of subjective disease burden, limiting the upfront information received in the assessment of sleep disorders. It is advantageous to have a reliable informant, such as a bed partner, roommate, parent, or caregiver, accompany the patient presenting to the office in order to give feedback about the patient's sleep. Conversation with the patient will address, among other areas, sleep perception, sleep habits, sleep environment, bedtime routine, work performance, and driving safety (see Table 7.2). To increase efficiency and accuracy of data collection during the patient encounter, physicians rely on sleep questionnaires (Table 7.3).
- *Sleep questionnaires:* Various sleep questionnaires available can help with the collection of sleep-related information (bedtime, sleep routine, checklist of symptoms) prior to the physician-patient encounter. Validated standardized sleep questionnaires complement the sleep history by providing a detailed assessment of a specific sleep symptom (see Table 7.3). Questionnaires such as the Berlin questionnaire or the STOP-BANG[3,4] can be used once upon intake (Tables 7.4 and 7.5). On each encounter, excessive daytime sleepiness (EDS) can be tracked with the Epworth Sleepiness Scale (Table 7.6).[6] The use of questionnaires streamlines the intake of patient symptoms. This approach also allows the patient to discuss sleep-related concerns such as level of snoring, witnessed apneas, parasomnias, and related events such as sleep talking and acting out dreams, to name a few, at home with spouse or family.
- *Physical examination:* The physical exam in sleep medicine will emphasize, among other factors, neck circumference,[10] Mallampati classification, airway inspection, and a neurologic and pulmonary examination (Fig. 7.1).[11,12] A careful review of the past medical history gives insights related to relevant medical conditions such as arterial hypertension, heart failure, stroke, muscle disease, and others.[12]
- *Sleep log:* A sleep log can be very helpful by providing *subjective* information regarding the patient's sleep. A sample sleep log from the American Academy of Sleep Medicine (AASM) can be seen in Fig. 7.2.[13] Using this log, patients are instructed to record details about their day, especially items that can affect

TABLE 7.1	Comparison of Available Testing Modalities					
	TYPE OF TESTING					
Features	PSG	MSLT	MWT	HSAT	Actigraphy	Oximetry
Sleep recording	Yes	Yes	Yes	No	No	No
Video recording	Yes	Optional	Optional	No	No	No
EEG recording	Yes	Yes	Yes	No	No	No
Attended	Yes	Yes	Yes	No	No	No
Ambulatory	No	No	No	Yes	Yes	Yes
Oximetry	Yes	Yes	Yes	Yes	No	Yes

EEG, Electroencephalogram; *HSAT*, home sleep apnea test; *MSLT*, multipe sleep latency test; *MWT*, maintenance of wakefullness Test; *PSG*, polysomnography.

TABLE 7.2	Suggested Topics for Questions in the Assessment of Sleep Disorders
Sleep hygiene	Bedtime, sleep-onset time, evening routine, wake time
Breathing events	Snoring, nasal congestion, tonsils, weight change, gasping, witnessed apnea, sleep position
Daytime symptoms	Naps, drowsy driving, decreased school/job performance, sleep paralysis, hypnagogic hallucinations, near car accidents
Leg, arm, body movements	Urge to move, leg discomfort, periodic limb movement, dream reenactment
Sleep maintenance	Timing, duration, frequency, associated symptoms
Symptoms upon awakening	Sleep inertia, headache, sleepiness
Nocturnal event	Timing after bedtime, sleepwalking, night terror, rhythmic movement (tonic clonic seizure-like), preservation of recall, duration of an event

TABLE 7.3	Validated Sleep Questionnaires to Supplement Sleep History
Berlin Sleep Questionnaire[2]	Estimates risk of having OSA
STOP BANG Questionnaire[3–5]	Screens patients for OSA
Epworth Sleepiness Scale[6]	Assesses general level of daytime sleepiness
International RLS Study Group Rating Scale[7]	Measures severity of Willis-Ekbom disease
Insomnia Severity Index[8]	Offers a brief screening measure for insomnia
Pittsburg Sleep Quality Index[9]	Measures sleep quality over the past month.

OSA, Obstructive sleep apnea; *RLS*, restless legs syndrome.

sleep and sleepiness, such as caffeine, alcohol, and exercise. Patients also record wake time, bedtime, naps, and other such events. In patients with insomnia, a sleep log can provide a much better assessment of their sleep in the preceding weeks than they can report on their own. Typically, patients should complete the sleep log every day for at least 2 weeks to provide adequate data for the sleep specialist, since some patients may have different sleep patterns on weekends or days off than on normal workdays.

Which Test Is Appropriate for Which Patient?

- The testing of a patient with a suspected sleep disorder is based on the discretion of the practitioner, incorporating existing guidelines and recommendations of the AASM or similar organizations. A "one-size-fits-all approach" is not appropriate for investigating a suspected sleep disorder. No single set of recommendations will suit every single patient encounter

situation, given the vast variation of possible clinical presentations and diagnostic questions. The practitioner is able to determine the appropriate testing (including possible laboratory investigation; Table 7.7) once history taking and physical examination are complete.

- Several classification systems are used to categorize available sleep testing devices (Tables 7.8 and 7.9).[21] Appropriate goal setting will require the management of patient expectations around successful treatment.
- The appropriate sleep testing selections depend on the suspected sleep disorder. For example, conditions such as psychophysiologic insomnia or Willis-Ekbom disease (WED) do not require a formal overnight polysomnography (PSG), while certain circadian misalignment conditions benefit from an actigraphy.[22]
- Patients with poorly controlled arterial hypertension, with a history of stroke or congestive heart failure, might require an overnight PSG, even in the absence of any sleep symptoms.[12]
- A patient with Parkinson's disease with suspected rapid eye movement (REM) sleep behavior disorder may need to be convinced that an overnight PSG will be of benefit, while a concerned parent of a pediatric patient with uncomplicated sleep terrors will need reassurance but not a PSG for the child.[12]

TABLE 7.4	Berlin Questionnaire[2]

Category 1
1. Do you snore?
   a. Yes
   b. No
   c. Don't know

   If you snore:
2. Your snoring is:
   a. Slightly louder than breathing
   b. As loud as talking
   c. Louder than talking
   d. Very loud—can be heard in adjacent rooms
3. How often do you snore
   a. Nearly every day
   b. Three to four times a week
   c. One to two times a week
   d. One to two times a month
   e. Never or nearly never
4. Has your snoring ever bothered other people?
   a. Yes
   b. No
   c. Don't know
5. Has anyone noticed that you quit breathing during your sleep?
   a. Nearly every day
   b. Three to four times a week
   c. One to two times a week
   d. One to two times a month
   e. Never or nearly never

Category 2
6. How often do you feel tired or fatigued after your sleep?
   a. Nearly every day
   b. Three to four times a week
   c. One to two times a week
   d. One to two times a month
   e. Never or nearly never
7. During your waking time, do you feel tired, fatigued, or not up to par?
   a. Nearly every day
   b. Three to four times a week
   c. One to two times a week
   d. One to two times a month
   e. Never or nearly never
8. Have you ever nodded off or fallen asleep while driving a vehicle?
   a. Yes
   b. No

   If yes,
9. How often does this occur?
   a. Nearly every day
   b. Three to four times a week
   c. One to two times a week
   d. One to two times a month
   e. Never or nearly never

Category 3
10. Do you have high blood pressure?
    Yes
    No
    Don't know

TABLE 7.5	STOP-BANG[3–5] Screening for Obstructive Sleep Apnea

Answer the following questions to find out if you are at risk for obstructive sleep apnea

STOP

S (snore)	Have you been told that you snore?	Yes/No
T (tired)	Are you often tired during the day?	Yes/No
O (obstruction)	Do you know if you stop breathing or has anyone witnessed you stop breathing while you are asleep?	Yes/No
P (pressure)	Do you have high blood pressure or are you on medication to control high blood pressure?	Yes/No

If you answered yes to two or more questions on the STOP portion, you are at risk for obstructive sleep apnea. It is recommended that you contact your primary care provider to discuss a possible sleep disorder.

To find out if you are at moderate to severe risk of obstructive sleep apnea, complete the following BANG questions:

BANG

B (body mass index [BMI])	Is your BMI greater than 28?	Yes/No
A (age)	Are you 50 years old or older?	Yes/No
N (neck)	Are you a male with a neck circumference greater than 17 inches or a female with a neck circumference greater than 16 inches?	Yes/No
G (gender)	Are you a male?	Yes/No

TABLE 7.6	Epworth Sleepiness Scale[6]

How likely are you to doze off or fall asleep in the following situations, in contrast to feeling just tired? This refers to your usual way of life in recent times. Even if you have not done some of these things recently, try to work out how they would have affected you. Use the following scale to choose the most appropriate number for each situation:

0 = No chance of dozing
1 = Slight chance of dozing
2 = Moderate chance of dozing
3 = High chance of dozing

Situation	Chance of Dozing
Sitting and reading	_____
Watching TV	_____
Sitting inactive in a public place (e.g., a theatre or a meeting)	_____
As a passenger in a car for an hour without a break	_____
Lying down to rest in the afternoon when circumstances permit	_____
Sitting and talking to someone	_____
Sitting quietly after a lunch without alcohol	_____
In a car while stopped for a few minutes in traffic	_____
Total score	_____

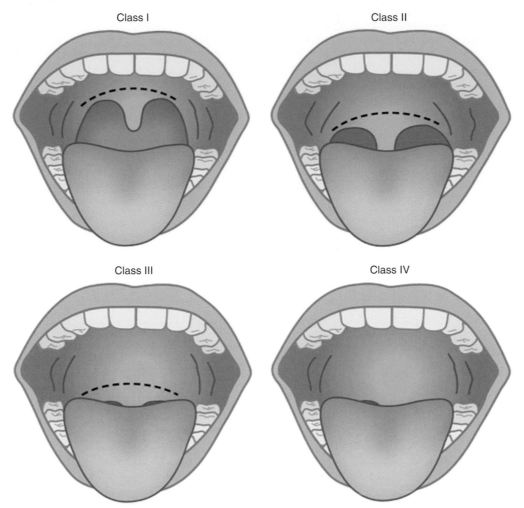

Class I   Class II

Class III   Class IV

• **Figure 7.1** Mallampati Classification. *Class I*, Soft palate, fauces, uvula, and pillars visible. *Class II*, Soft palate, fauces, and uvula visible. *Class III*, Soft palate and the base of uvula visible. *Class IV*, Soft palate not visible. (Reprinted with permission from Townsend CM, Beauchamp RD, Evers BM, eds. *Sabiston Textbook of Surgery: The Biological Basis of Modern Surgical Practice.* 18th ed. Philadelphia, PA: WB Saunders; 2007.)

TABLE 7.7	Selected Laboratory Testing Suggested in Sleep Disorders
CSF hypocretin/CSF orexin[14,15]	Narcolepsy
Ferritin/iron studies[16,17]	Willis-Ekbom disease
Complete blood count	Sleepiness
Thyroid testing	Sleepiness/insomnia
Human leukocyte antigen[18,19]	Narcolepsy
Comprehensive metabolic panel	Sleepiness/insomnia
Vitamin D levels[19]	Sleepiness

TABLE 7.8	Four AASM Categories of Sleep Monitoring Devices Are Used in the Diagnosis of Sleep Disorders[20]
Type 1	In-laboratory, technician-attended, PSG (including baseline PSG, MSLT, MWT, PAP titration study)
Type 2	Full PSG outside of laboratory, unattended
Type 3	Monitoring devices that do not record the signals to determine sleep stages. Typically channels include: • Two respiratory variables (e.g., respiratory movement and airflow) • Cardiac variable (e.g., heart rate or an electrocardiogram) • Arterial oxygen saturation Some devices may record snoring and detect light or body position.
Type 4	Continuous single or dual parameter recording (e.g., oximetry, airflow).

AASM, American Academy of Sleep Medicine; *MSLT*, multiple sleep latency test; *MWT*, maintenance of wakefulness test; *PAP*, positive airway pressure; *PSG*, polysomnography.

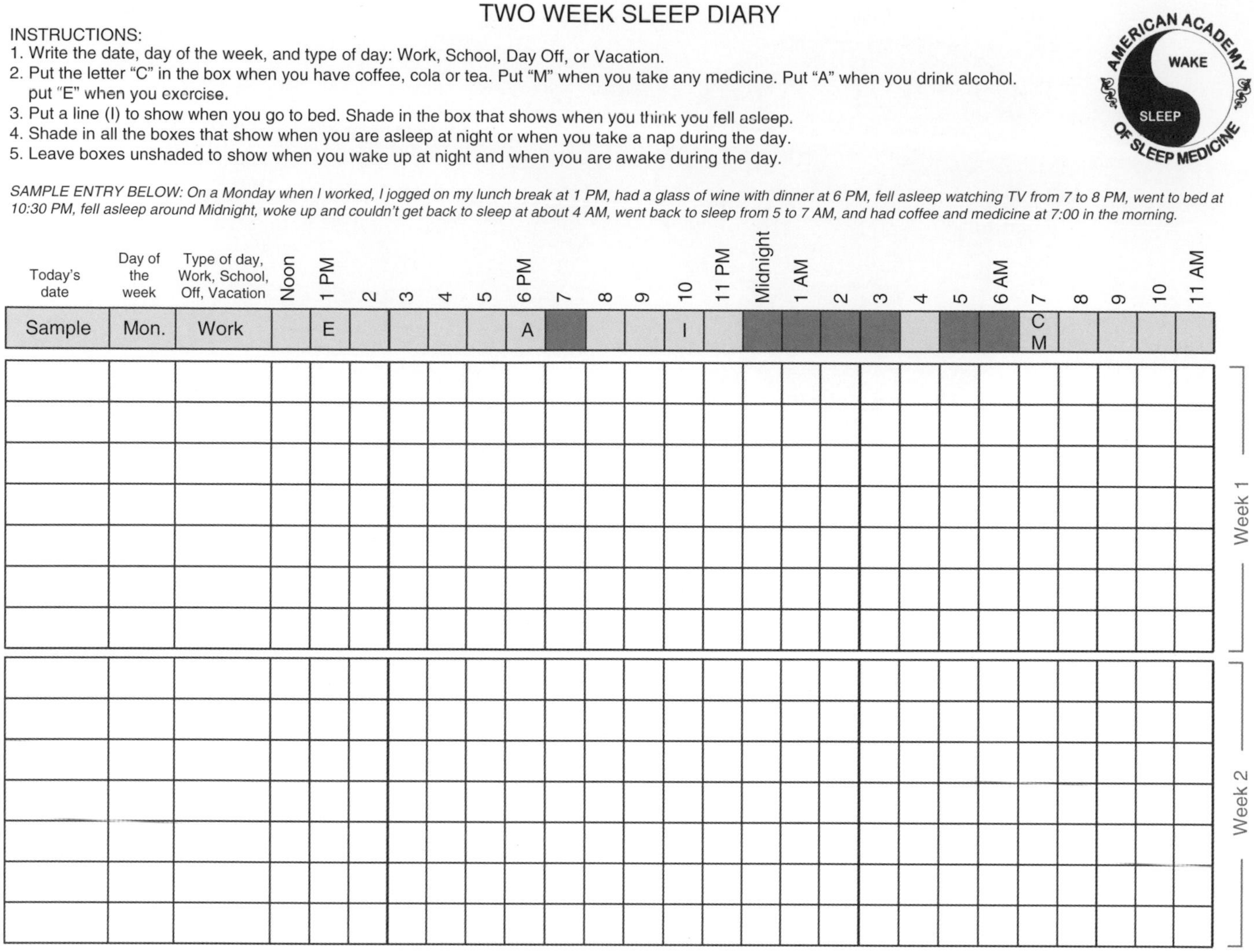

TWO WEEK SLEEP DIARY

INSTRUCTIONS:
1. Write the date, day of the week, and type of day: Work, School, Day Off, or Vacation.
2. Put the letter "C" in the box when you have coffee, cola or tea. Put "M" when you take any medicine. Put "A" when you drink alcohol. put "E" when you exercise.
3. Put a line (I) to show when you go to bed. Shade in the box that shows when you think you fell asleep.
4. Shade in all the boxes that show when you are asleep at night or when you take a nap during the day.
5. Leave boxes unshaded to show when you wake up at night and when you are awake during the day.

SAMPLE ENTRY BELOW: On a Monday when I worked, I jogged on my lunch break at 1 PM, had a glass of wine with dinner at 6 PM, fell asleep watching TV from 7 to 8 PM, went to bed at 10:30 PM, fell asleep around Midnight, woke up and couldn't get back to sleep at about 4 AM, went back to sleep from 5 to 7 AM, and had coffee and medicine at 7:00 in the morning.

Today's date	Day of the week	Type of day, Work, School, Off, Vacation	Noon	1 PM	2	3	4	5	6 PM	7	8	9	10	11 PM	Midnight	1 AM	2	3	4	5	6 AM	7	8	9	10	11 AM
Sample	Mon.	Work		E					A					I								C M				

• **Figure 7.2** A sample sleep log from the American Academy of Sleep Medicine accessed from http://sleepeducation.org/docs/default-document-library/sleep-diary.pdf.

TABLE 7.9	Categorization of Out-of-Center Devices Based on Measurements of Sleep, Cardiovascular, Oximetry, Position, Effort, and Respiratory Parameters[21]					
S1—Sleep by 3 EEG channels + with EOG and chin EMG	C1—more than 1 ECG lead—can derive events	O1—Oximetry (finger or ear) with recommended sampling	P1—Video or visual position measurement	E1—2 RIP belts	R1—Nasal pressure and thermal device
S2—Sleep by less than 3 EEG + with or without EOG or chin EMG	C2—Peripheral arterial tonometry	O1x—Oximetry (finger or ear)	P2—Nonvisual position measurement	E2—1 RIP belt	R2—Nasal pressure
S3—Sleep surrogate (e.g., actigraphy)	C3—Standard ECG measure (1 lead)	O2—Oximetry with alternative site (e.g., forehead)	—	3—Derived effort (e.g., forehead versus pressure, FVP)	R3—Thermal device
S4—Other sleep measure	C4—Derived pulse (typically from oximetry)	O3—Other oximetry	—	E4—Other effort measure (including piezo belts)	R4—End-Tidal CO$_2$ (ETCO2)
	C5—Other cardiac measure	—	—	—	R5—Other respiratory measure

ECG, Electrocardiogram; EEG, electroencephalogram; EMG, electromyogram; EOG, electrooculogram.

TABLE 7.10	Sample Polysomnography Parameters Reported

Total sleep period time (min)

Sleep efficiency index (%)

Sleep and REM sleep latency (min)

Number of awakenings

Wake after sleep onset (WASO, min)

Sleep stages and distribution, sleep fragmentation

Number and index of obstructive/mixed and central apneas

Apnea-hypopnea index (AHI)

Number and index of respiratory effort related arousals (RERAs, RDI)

Minimum oxygen saturation (%)

Presence or absence of REM sleep atonia

Abnormal electroencephalogram patterns

Amount of periodic limb movement with and without arousals

Electrocardiogram abnormalities

RDI, Respiratory disturbance index; *REM*, rapid eye movement.

TABLE 7.11	Selected Recommendations of the AASM Practice Guidelines for the Use of Polysomnography

PSG is routinely indicated for the diagnosis of SRBD.

PSG is indicated for (PAP titration in patients with SRBD.

A preoperative clinical evaluation that includes PSG or an attended cardiorespiratory (Type 3) sleep study is routinely indicated to evaluate for the presence of obstructive sleep apnea in patients before they undergo upper airway surgery for snoring or obstructive sleep apnea.

Follow-up PSG is routinely indicated for the assessment of treatment results in the following circumstances:
- After substantial weight loss (e.g., 10% of body weight) has occurred in patients on CPAP for treatment of SRBDs to ascertain whether CPAP is still needed at the previously titrated pressure
- After substantial weight gain (e.g., 10% of body weight) has occurred in patients previously treated with CPAP successfully, who are again symptomatic despite the continued use of CPAP, to ascertain whether pressure adjustments are needed
- When clinical response is insufficient or when symptoms return despite a good initial response to treatment with CPAP. In these circumstances, testing should be devised with consideration that a concurrent sleep disorder may be present (e.g., sleep apnea and narcolepsy).

Patients with systolic or diastolic heart failure should undergo PSG if they have nocturnal symptoms suggestive of SRBD (disturbed sleep, nocturnal dyspnea, snoring) or if they remain symptomatic despite optimal medical management of congestive heart failure.

Patients with coronary artery disease should be evaluated for symptoms and signs of sleep apnea. If there is suspicion of sleep apnea, the patients should undergo a sleep study.

Patients with history of stroke or transient ischemic attacks should be evaluated for symptoms and signs of sleep apnea. If there is suspicion of sleep apnea, the patients should undergo a sleep study.

Patients referred for evaluation of significant tachyarrhythmias or bradyarrhythmias should be questioned about symptoms of sleep apnea. A sleep study is indicated if questioning results in a reasonable suspicion that obstructive or central sleep apnea are present.

AASM, American Academy of Sleep Medicine; *CPAP*, continuous positive airway pressure; *PAP*, positive airway pressure; *PSG*, polysomnography; *SRBD*, sleep-related breathing disorder.

To summarize, the choice of appropriate testing is guided by the clinical questions identified in the initial patient encounter.[12]

What Are the Testing Modalities?

Polysomnography

Description

- The facility-based standard PSG provides the most reliable and complete information for the evaluation of sleep and sleep-related breathing disorders (SRBDs), including obstructive sleep apnea (OSA), central sleep apnea (CSA), and Cheyne-Stokes respiration (CSR), among others (Tables 7.10 and 7.11).[12] A PSG records central and occipital electroencephalogram (EEG), surface chin and leg electromyogram (EMG), left and right eye electrooculograms (EOGs), electrocardiogram (EKG), snoring, nasal/oral airflow, nasal pressure transducer, thoracic and abdominal effort with respiratory inductance plethysmography belts, pulse oximetry, and body position.[12] A selection of reported PSG parameters is listed in Table 7.10.
- Video is recorded throughout the night to observe the patient and preserve any behavioral episodes that may occur.[12] Video is correlated with PSG recorded sleep-related events, such as parasomnias, including REM behavior disorder (RBD) and seizures.[12]
- The standard PSG montage can be extended by additional EEG or EMG electrodes, further enhancing the detection of parasomnias (such as RBD), movement disorders of sleep, and seizure detection.[12]
- A baseline PSG allows the most accurate assessment of various sleep parameters, sleep phenomena, and sleep disorders. In the ideal setting, a patient with suspected sleep apnea attends the overnight PSG and returns the following night for a PSG with positive airway pressure (PAP) titration, also called a *full-night titration study.*[12]
- Numerous factors, such as long waits to schedule sleep studies, patient preferences, and increased economic stress on the health care system, have led to the use of so-called *split-night studies.*[12] In the first part of the study, a baseline sleep and respiratory assessment is conducted, which might identify SRBDs; if SRBD is found, the second part of the night allows for the addition of a titration of PAP to eliminate the SRBD. The use of *split-night PSG* is an AASM acceptable method for assessing and treating SRBD patients.[12] Although the benefits for the patient of *split-night PSG* include a single night test (compared with a two-night test), potentially reduced appointment wait time, and potentially a reduced economical health care cost burden,

a first night effect (when the sleep of the patient is more disrupted during their first night of recording in the sleep laboratory) may not allow for an accurate sleep recording. Shorter overnight PAP titration time during a *split-night PSG* (compared with full-night titration) may lead to unsuccessful treatment of the sleep patient, subsequently resulting in delayed OSA treatment. In the case of a patient who does not tolerate PAP easily, the time restraints of the split night study may require an additional full-night PAP titration PSG to successfully control the SRBD.

Indication

- SRBDs:
PSG is the established leading tool to evaluate sleep, and to diagnose a majority of sleep-related disorders.[12] The most common indication for a PSG is suspected SRBD, including OSA, CSA, and CSR (see Table 7.11). Although unattended portable monitoring (PM) is increasingly used in the diagnosis of sleep apnea, PSG remains the gold standard in the diagnosis and treatment of a patient with SRBD.[23]
- Hypersomnia:
PSG is also commonly used in the workup of hypersomnia. Narcolepsy, for example, is a hypersomnia of central nervous system origin, where PSG is able to address possible differential diagnoses such as nocturnal seizures, periodic limb movement disorder (PLMD), and causes of sleep fragmentation.[12] PSG will document an uneventful nocturnal sleep before a multiple sleep latency test (MSLT; discussed in detail as follows).[12] A short REM sleep latency (SOREM) on a PSG of less than 15 min can be used in combination with a second SOREM on the following MSLT to diagnose narcolepsy.[24]
- Epilepsy:
PSG is used in the evaluation of a nocturnal seizure disorder.[12] Nocturnal video PSG is the gold standard test for nocturnal frontal lobe epilepsy.[24] Patients with nocturnal movements or sleep-related events of unclear etiology benefit from a PSG to further clarify the diagnosis.[12] Detailed history and physical examination during the initial patient encounter will guide the different testing steps in patients with suspected clinical episodes at night, such as stereotypical behavior or unusual movements.[12] Additional EEG recording channels can capture abnormal electroencephalographic patterns and help with the differential diagnosis of complex nocturnal events such as seizures, RBD, PLMD, sleep talking, bruxism, and rhythmic movement disorder, to name a few.[12] PSG testing can be an important tool as part of a comprehensive epilepsy workup.[24]
- Parasomnia:
PSG is the leading tool to investigate suspected parasomnia.[12] Time-synchronized video-polysomnographic (vPSG) recording is essential to support the diagnosis of parasomnia.
  - Additional EEG channels can record postarousal EEG patterns in sleepwalking, demonstrating a partial or complete persistence of sleep, with diffuse, rhythmic delta activity; diffuse delta and theta activity; mixed delta, theta, alpha, and beta activity; or at times alpha and beta activity.[24]
  - Placing additional EMG recording channels, for example in the upper limbs, allows a more thorough evaluation of the sleep-related movement. Suspicion for a parasomnia can be raised in many situations, such as patients observing unusual circumstances upon awakening (e.g., objects moved in the house, a kitchen in disarray), or finding themselves in other parts of the house. It is of course of great help if an informant such as a bed partner or family member can

report to the sleep provider observation of the nocturnal events (see Table 7.2). However, the use of PSG depends on the clinical setting, as some parasomnias are diagnosed clinically.[12] Bed partner or family history about the sleep-related events might, at times, allow a diagnosis without the use of PSG.[12]
- Typical parasomnias such as sleep terrors, somniloquy, and nightmares may not need a PSG for evaluation, as the clinical history is often diagnostic. Other parasomnias require a PSG, especially if the presumed parasomnia is associated with snoring or apneic spells, the presumed parasomnia does not respond to conventional treatment, injuries occur at night, or atypical features are reported. The only parasomnia, however, that requires PSG for diagnostic confirmation is RBD, as it requires demonstration of REM sleep without atonia.
- Comorbid sleep disorders:
Although PSG is not indicated in the routine evaluation of insomnia, it may be useful to rule out comorbid sleep disorders (e.g., sleep-disordered breathing) among some patients who appear to meet criteria for chronic insomnia disorder.[12,22,24]

In conclusion, clinical history and the assessment of the sleep provider remain the guiding principles for determining the proper use of PSG. Used appropriately, PSG will provide a crucial host of information relevant to the successful identification and management of a sleep disorder. That said, a PSG may not provide any clinically significant information in the diagnosis of circadian rhythm disorders, WED, insomnia, and chronic lung disease, among others.[12,22]

Preparations Prior to the Polysomnography

PSG testing has to be arranged diligently:

- During the office encounter, it is helpful to educate the patient about possible sleep disorders, symptoms, specific testing plans, and implications of the results (such as the future use of a PAP). The better prepared patients are for a PSG, the more reliable their attendance during the PSG and their acceptance of the results. The detailed explanation of the PSG indication along with possible events during the PSG, such as electrodes, recording equipment, and PAP titration, will increase both compliance and success of the testing.
- A sleep log obtained prior to the office visit encounter will help identify the ideal timing of the sleep study (see Fig. 7.2). Although most patients follow a traditional sleep-wake cycle, with daytime alertness and nighttime sleep, sleep-wake cycles may in some instances differ. Some patients may have delayed sleep phase syndrome, and a sleep study should accommodate the patient's bedtime routine in order to obtain the most accurate PSG results. Other times, the patient is a shift worker and a daytime sleep study is more appropriate.
- The patient also needs to be educated about the use of medications, alcohol, and other factors prior to the study that may influence his/her experience in the sleep lab and testing results.
- A family member can accompany a child, an elderly, or a disabled patient during a sleep study in order to decrease testing anxiety, obtain a harmonious encounter, and have a more relaxed sleep lab experience.
- Depending on the clinical presentation and PSG indication, all medications are taken as usual during the day of the PSG in order to avoid any withdrawal effect on sleep and the PSG recording results. Sometimes it seems reasonable to wean medication several weeks prior to the sleep study in order to

get a PSG without medication interaction—for example, if the patient is on an antidepressant (REM suppressing agents) and is being tested for narcolepsy.[25]

- Some patients have significant anxiety around the testing, and a light sleeping aid can be prescribed as long as it's not expected to interfere with the diagnostic testing. For example, a patient with suspected sleep-disordered breathing may benefit from a low-dose short-acting nonbenzodiazepine hypnotic for the night of the testing. A CNS acting agent to induce sleep prior to PSG would be inappropriate if, for example, the patient is being tested for RBD or sleepwalking, as the agent could mask or trigger sleep-related phenomena. Patients treated for RBD with melatonin or clonazepam should also be taken off these agents several days prior to testing, as these could mask the abnormal muscle atonia or behavioral spell that the patient is evaluated for.

Polysomnography Challenges

The PSG is the gold standard for the diagnosis and treatment of numerous sleep disorders, such as sleep-disordered breathing, RBD, and PLMD, to name a few.[12,23] However, some circumstances can also lead to false positive or false negative PSG results.

- An extensive *first-night effect* (i.e., the effect of the environment and PSG recording apparatus on the quality of the patient's sleep the first night of recording) can cause sleep difficulties. The first night effect can reduce sleep efficiency and mask the true manifestation of the sleep disorder. For example, the first night effect may lead to an underestimation of sleep apnea by not reaching supine REM sleep.
- Although many sleep disorders occur on a nightly basis, some might only occur sporadically. RBD or epilepsy patients may not necessarily have typical events during the night of the recording. Repeated PSGs are sometimes necessary to capture the reported clinical event.
- Inaccurate PSG recordings are observed in patients with recent medication changes, in patients with *first-night effect*, and potentially related to lack of adaptation to a continuous positive airway pressure (CPAP) mask.

Multiple Sleep Latency Test

The MSLT is a validated, objective, in-laboratory test that measures the tendency of a patient to fall asleep in the setting of no external alerting factors.[25] This test correlates subjective excessive sleepiness with objectively shortened sleep latency.[25]

- Protocol:
The current standards for the test are five daytime naps performed at 2-hour intervals, with the first nap starting 1.5–3 hours after the end of the preceding overnight PSG.[25] Each nap allows 20 min for sleep onset (defined as the first epoch of any stage of sleep). If sleep occurs during the nap, the test continues for 15 min after sleep onset to allow the occurrence of REM sleep. If sleep does not occur, the nap is terminated at 20 min.
- Practical tips:
The patient stays awake in between naps and is not allowed any alerting agents, such as caffeine, medications, or exercise. The MSLT requires specific preparations. The MSLT is performed in immediate conjunction with a PSG. It is recommended that a patient has at least 6 hours of sleep, documented by PSG the night preceding an MSLT.[24,25] A urine toxicology screen on the day of the MSLT follows a 2-week washout period off stimulants and medication that suppress REM sleep. A general good rule

of thumb is to stop CNS agents for at least five times the half-life of the drug, which for most drugs works for at least 2 weeks before the MSLT.

- Indications:
The MSLT is used primarily for the evaluation of patients with hypersomnia, such as narcolepsy, or to help differentiate idiopathic hypersomnia from narcolepsy.[25] Patients with narcolepsy characteristically have a shortened sleep latency and sleep-onset REM periods ("SOREMPs"). The MSLT is not to be used as a single diagnostic test for narcolepsy, but rather as part of the overall evaluation. In other sleep disorders, such as OSA and PLMD, the MSLT would not be used in the initial evaluation, nor as a way to evaluate the response to treatment.[25] Rather, the MSLT can be helpful in evaluating patients with OSA or PLMD who are still sleepy despite adequate treatment.
- Suggested normal values:
A mean sleep latency on the MSLT of less than 8 min should be considered abnormal.[24] The average sleep latency in control subjects during five naps MSLT is 11.6 ± 5.2 min.[25]

Maintenance of Wakefulness Test

The maintenance of wakefulness test (MWT) measures the patient's ability to remain awake in a setting that is devoid of altering factors such as light and noise.[25]

- Protocol:
The MWT consists of four trials of 40-min duration each. Similar to the MSLT, the MWT starts the first trial period between 1.5 and 3 hours after the patient wakes up in the morning, and then subsequent trials are separated by 2 hours.[25] Sleep onset is defined as the first epoch in which there is 15 sec of cumulative sleep.
- Suggested normal values:
A mean sleep latency on the MWT of less than 8 min should be considered abnormal. A sleep latency of between 8 and 40 min on average for the test is inconclusive and needs to be considered with other factors.[25] The average sleep latency in control subjects during MWT is 30.4 ± 11.2 min.[25]
- Indications:
The MWT has two main uses in the evaluation of patients with sleep disorders.
  - MWT is used in patients with EDS from a known sleep disorder, such as narcolepsy, as a measure of the patient's response to treatment. Patients with OSA and PLMD can also be tested with the MWT for this purpose.[25] There are no defined absolute values of mean sleep latency on the MWT. Instead, the clinician needs to evaluate the decrease in mean sleep latency on the MWT in the clinical setting. As with the MSLT, the MWT should not be used alone, but provides benefit when used with other evaluation tools, such as the patient's own subjective history.
  - MWT is used to assess patients with a known sleep disorder, such as OSA or narcolepsy, for their ability to maintain wakefulness and therefore keep a job involving public or personal safety issues.[25] Although there is no documented predictive value of the MWT or MSLT thus far regarding traffic safety and accident risk, the MWT has found a use in this arena. It must be stressed again that the MWT should not be used in isolation for this purpose, but rather as part of the entire evaluation of a patient—for example, adherence to PAP therapy. In addition, it should be noted that patients'

ability to stay awake during the MWT does not guarantee that they will stay awake in the work environment. However, patients who remain awake on all four of the 40-min trials of the MWT have the best chance of maintaining wakefulness in other settings.[25]

Actigraphy

Description

Actigraphy is a measure of an individual's movement, typically using a device that looks like a wristwatch.[26] The actigraph converts mechanical motion into an electronic signal that is sampled several times a second and then displayed in a graph format (Fig. 7.3).[1,26] The actigraph data are downloaded to a computer, and a program then scores wake versus inactivity ("sleep"). Typically, the data are organized into 30- or 60-sec epochs of wake or sleep, based on the assumption that the patient moves much less during sleep than during wakefulness. Some actigraphy models can also measure noise, ambient light, and body temperature, and have event markers to provide more data to the sleep specialist. The patient wears the device on either the wrist or the ankle for several days, and thus an assessment of the 24-hour sleep-wake pattern can be obtained.

Indication

Actigraphy is useful in the assessment of specific aspects of circadian rhythm disorders and EDS.[26]

- Actigraphy can be used to study sleep in normal healthy adults, such as in a research setting.[26]
- For circadian rhythm disorders and insomnia, actigraphy can be used to more objectively assess the patient's sleep and sleep patterns, as well as response to treatment.[26]
- Actigraphy may also be helpful in the evaluation of patients with shift work sleep disorder, especially with an actigraph that can measure the amount and duration of ambient light exposure.[26]
- Actigraphy can document, in a 2-week period prior to a PSG/MSLT testing for hypersomnia, the sleep-wake cycle, reinforcing subjective reported sleep log data.[26]
- Overall, actigraphy is a very useful tool in evaluating patients with complaints of insomnia, restless sleep, insufficient sleep, circadian abnormalities, and EDS. While actigraphy alone cannot be used to make a diagnosis, using the data from actigraphy along with sleep logs, the patient's history, and other clinical data provides important input for the diagnosis of circadian rhythm disorders, among other sleep disorders.[26]

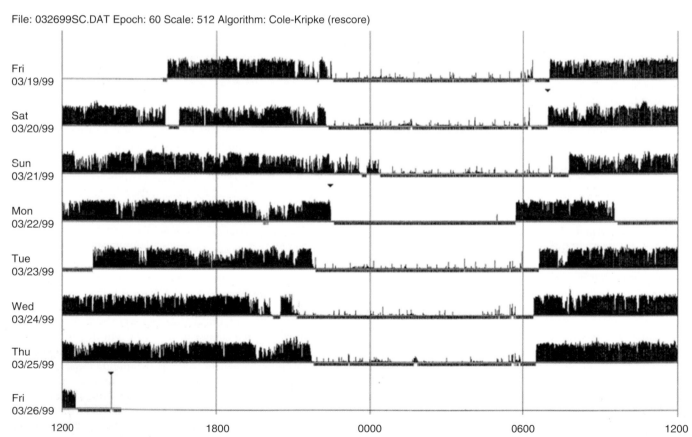

File: 032699SC.DAT Epoch: 60 Scale: 512 Algorithm: Cole-Kripke (rescore)

• **Figure 7.3** Normal sleep-wake schedule. Wrist actigraphic recording from a 55-year-old healthy woman without sleep complaints. This shows a fairly regular sleep-wake schedule, except one weekend night (third from the top). She goes to bed between 10:30 PM and 11:00 PM and wakes up around 7:00 AM, except on the third day. Physiologic body shifts and movements during sleep are indicated by a few *black bars* in the *white areas*. The waking period is indicated by *black bars*. (Reprinted with permission from Chokroverty S, Thomas R. *Atlas of Sleep Medicine*. 2nd ed. Boston: Elsevier; 2014: 255–299.)

Portable Monitoring

Description

Home sleep apnea testing (HSAT) has been considered by the AASM to be an acceptable form of testing for OSA in selected patients.[23] HSAT offers some advantages over in-laboratory PSG, such as convenience for the patient, lower cost, and speed of results. However, in the absence of sleep recording, HSAT may underestimate the severity of OSA compared with the in-laboratory PSG.[23] Portable PSG, PM, and HSAT are generic terms that encompass several different types of monitors, each with their own ability or lack of ability to detect OSA (see Tables 7.8 and 7.9).[20,21] Newer types of HSAT do not fit the AASM Type 1–4 classifications well and can instead be organized using the SCOPER system (see Table 7.9).[20,21] The most commonly used HSAT is the Type 3 or level III, with a minimum of four channels, including at least two channels of respiratory movement or airflow, heart rate or EKG, and oxygen saturation.[23] Typically a type 3 device does not measure sleep, and therefore respiratory effort–related arousals will not be scored. This means that the results will give the clinician an apnea-hypopnea index (AHI) only, but not a respiratory disturbance index (RDI), as one would obtain in a PSG. The AHI is the total number of apnea and hypopnea events per hour of sleep, and the RDI is the number of apnea, hypopnea, and respiratory effort–related arousal events per hour of sleep. In addition, since sleep is not measured, the sum of the apnea and hypopnea events is divided by the total recording time, thus lowering the AHI in comparison to what would have been obtained if sleep were measured and used as the denominator for determination of the AHI. The AASM suggest the term *respiratory event index* (REI), which is the number of respiratory events/monitoring time (in hours), as an alternative to AHI when referring to the index derived from HSAT.

Indication

HSAT may be used under the auspices of an AASM-accredited comprehensive sleep medicine program for unattended monitoring studies in the patient's home.[23]

- The AASM recommends that HSAT be used only in conjunction with a comprehensive sleep evaluation, and that a board-certified sleep specialist supervise the HSAT evaluation.[23] In the absence of a comprehensive sleep evaluation, no PM is indicated. The reasoning behind this recommendation is that a skill set for appropriate use of HSAT is required. This skill set includes an understanding of differential diagnosis of a broad array of symptoms, the ability to interpret HSAT results and sources of error, and the experience needed to use the HSAT results in the context of the individual patient's history and physical examination.[23]
- The AASM recommends that HSAT be used in place of an in-laboratory study only in patients with a high pretest probability of moderate to severe OSA, and not be used in patients with comorbid conditions, other sleep disorders, or for screening purposes.[23]
- HSAT may be indicated for patients for whom an in-laboratory study is not possible for various reasons (e.g., illness, safety concerns) and can be considered for use as a way to monitor the patient's response to non-CPAP therapies for OSA, such as dental devices, surgery, or weight loss.[23]
- HSAT is not appropriate for the diagnostic evaluation of OSA in patients suspected of having other sleep disorders, including CSA, PLMD, insomnia, parasomnia, circadian rhythm disorders, or narcolepsy.[23]

- Negative or technically inadequate HSAT tests in patients with a high pretest probability of moderate to severe OSA should prompt in-laboratory PSG.[23]

Oximetry

Pulse oximetry is part of the standard in-laboratory polysomnogram, as well as many PM studies (see Tables 7.1, 7.8, and 7.9). The pulse oximeter is a device that has a two-wavelength light and sensor and is placed on a superficial pulsating vascular bed, such as the fingertip or earlobe. Several studies have shown that overall pulse oximetry is not an adequate screening test for patients suspected of having OSA.

Imaging Studies

Imaging studies are not commonly used in the assessment of sleep disorders, but can serve an important function in select clinical questions.

Cephalometry

One way to assess the upper airway in patients who may have OSA is through cephalometry, a radiograph of the upper airway; this is often used in dental sleep medicine (Fig. 7.4). Practically, the test is performed with the patient in a sitting position and the head in a rigid structure. The radiograph is taken at end-expiration as the upper airway structures change relative to one another with the respiratory cycle. Cephalometry is two-dimensional and allows for measurements of the mandible, maxilla, and hyoid bone, and their respective angles.[27] Information about the soft tissues in the upper airway such as the tongue and soft palate can be obtained from cephalometry as well. Patients with micrognathia, retrognathia, and small mandibles are more precisely identified in the assessment of OSA. In addition, if the hyoid bone is displaced inferiorly, the patient is at increased risk for OSA. Oral surgeons may use cephalometry to evaluate the upper airway before performing surgeries for OSA in patients with craniofacial abnormalities (e.g., bimaxillary advancement and mandibular advancement).[28] In the treatment of OSA, cephalometry can also be used to assess the degree of displacement that occurs with oral appliances. The advantages of using cephalometry are that it is relatively easy to perform and less expensive than more detailed tests such as computed tomography (CT) and magnetic resonance imaging (MRI). Its disadvantages are that it exposes the patient to radiation, it provides only a two-dimensional view of the upper airway without characterization of sleep dynamic changes of airways, and it does not give information on the lateral soft tissue structures.

Computed Tomography

CT of the upper airway provides a more detailed evaluation of the soft tissue structures than cephalometry.[28] CT also allows three-dimensional volumetric reconstruction of the upper airway.[28] In patients with OSA, CT shows that the retropalatal area is narrowed, and in obese patients with OSA, it shows them to have a larger tongue volume.[28] CT of the upper airway has some predictive value in determining success after uvulopalatopharyngoplasty (UPPP)—specifically, whether or not retropalatal obstruction is present. However, routine use of CT for the evaluation of a patient with probable OSA is not practical for several reasons. CT is associated with significant radiation exposure and, except in patients undergoing UPPP, provides no additional clinical benefit. Although CT of the upper airway has been an exciting research tool and

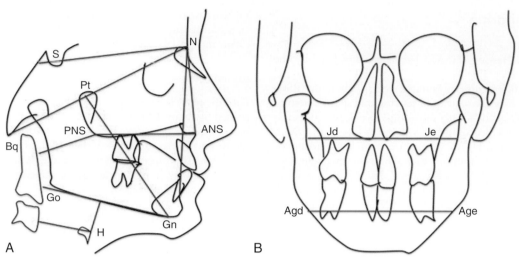

• **Figure 7.4 A,** Representative cephalometric lateral image with the evaluated measures. **B,** Representative cephalometric anteroposterior image with the evaluated measures. (Reprinted with permission from Braga A, Grechi TH, Eckeli A, et al. Predictors of uvulopalatopharyngoplasty success in the treatment of obstructive sleep apnea syndrome. *Sleep Med.* 2013;14:1266–1271.)

has helped dramatically in our understanding of upper airway anatomy and physiology in patients with OSA, it is not very useful in the clinical setting except to identify suitable surgical candidates.

Magnetic Resonance Imaging

MRI has also been used for evaluation of the upper airway structures and physiology of patients with OSA. It has resulted in great advances in our understanding of the dynamics of the upper airway in patients with OSA. Soft tissue and adipose tissue are easily seen on MRI, and the cross-sectional area of the upper airway can be determined (Fig. 7.5). Although much has been learned in research by the use of MRI in patients with OSA, clinical applications have yet to be elucidated. MRI of the brain allows a more detailed assessment of CNS structures. MRI studies are not part of the routine repertoire of evaluation of sleep disorders. Neurologic conditions are, at times, associated with sleep disorders, raising red flags for CNS pathology and the need for CNS imaging. While it is highly unusual to find an abnormal MRI in sleep disorders such as hypersomnia, sleep-disordered breathing, or parasomnias, one should consider CNS imaging when a neurologic injury is temporally associated with the evolution of the sleep disturbance (i.e., RBD following a pontine stroke, or narcolepsy symptoms in the setting of traumatic brain injury).

Selected Laboratory Testing

The clinical presentation of the patient will guide the laboratory testing in the evaluation of a sleep disorder. Thyroid stimulating hormone, complete blood count, electrolytes, creatinine, BUN, and hepatic function panel can be used to screen for numerous conditions, including thyroid dysfunction, anemia, infection, and liver or kidney disease.

Human Leukocyte Antigen

Narcolepsy/hypocretin deficiency has one of the strongest human leukocyte antigen (HLA) associations known, with more than 99% of patients carrying HLA DQB1*06:02, as well as HLA DQA1*01:02. However, 12%–38% of healthy individuals have this allele as well, making HLA typing for the sole purpose of diagnosing narcolepsy of limited value.[18,19]

Ferritin

Problems with maintaining adequate iron occur for each of the three major secondary causes of WED—end-stage renal disease, iron deficiency, and pregnancy.[17] When each of these conditions resolves, the iron status improves and so does the WED.[17] Iron studies and evaluation of hemoglobin are key in determining whether iron deficiency is present. Low ferritin levels (<50 ng/mL) are associated with symptoms of WED, even without coexisting anemia.[17]

CSF Hypocfretin/CSF Orexin

CSF hypocretin/orexin testing is one possible tool in the diagnosis of Narcolepsy type 1.[14,15,24] Narcolepsy type 1 is caused by a deficiency of hypothalamic hypocretin (orexin) signaling.[14] Patients with low or undetectable concentrations of hypocretin-1 in the CSF compose a specific disease population with a single etiology and relatively homogenous clinical and polysomnographic features.[14,24] Nevertheless, the majority of narcolepsy patients are diagnosed on clinical grounds, complemented by PSG/MSLT testing.[24] While CSF hypocretin/orexin have been studied in a large number of medical conditions, no clear consensus exists if CSF hypocretin is truly of a practical clinical significance in any other disease apart from narcolepsy.[15] Patients with Niemann-Pick disease type C, myotonic dystrophy, Coffin-Lowry syndrome, Norrie's disease, and Prader-Willi syndrome have been reported to show hypersomnia and in some cases decreased CSF hypocretin-1 concentrations, while patients with Parkinson's disease, multiple system atrophy, dementia with Lewy bodies, progressive supranuclear palsy, and corticobasal degeneration have normal CSF hypocretin-1 concentrations.[15]

Vitamin D

Some reports suggest a role for inadequate vitamin D in the development of symptoms of wake impairment commonly associated

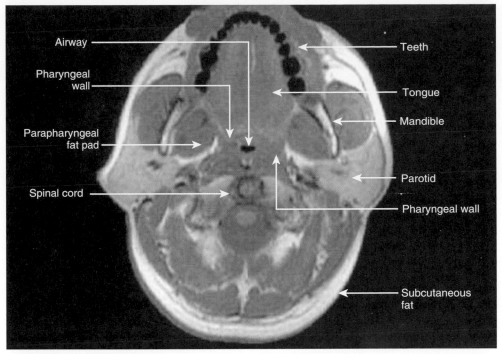

• **Figure 7.5** Axial magnetic resonance image of the retropalatal area in a normal subject. (Reprinted with permission from Schwab RJ. Upper airway imaging. *Clin Chest Med*. 1998;19[1]:33–54.)

with sleep disorders. Persistent inadequacy of vitamin D may also increase the risk for OSA via promotion of adenotonsillar hypertrophy, airway muscle myopathy, and/or chronic rhinitis.[29]

Conclusion

This chapter introduces a wide variety of sleep evaluation tools intended to familiarize the practitioner with the advantages and limits of different testing options. Some tools do not require the use of technology, such as sleep questionnaires and sleep logs. The decision to perform a facility-based or ambulatory test is driven by interactions with the patient, clinical history, and differential diagnoses of the sleep-related concern. Circadian rhythm disorders are typically evaluated with an ambulatory test—an actigraphy. RBD requires a facility-based, attended PSG. SRBDs are most commonly tested using a facility-based PSG, but can, in limited instances, also be addressed using HSAT. Laboratory test and imaging studies will complement the workup. It is critical for the practitioner to be highly familiar with different sleep evaluation options in order to advocate for the most appropriate testing of a sleep disorder in a world of increasingly managed health care.

Suggested Reading

American Academy of Sleep Medicine. *International Classification of Sleep Disorders*. 3rd ed. Darien, IL: American Academy of Sleep Medicine; 2014.

Collop NA, Anderson WM, Boehlecke B, et al. Clinical guidelines for the use of unattended portable monitors in the diagnosis of obstructive sleep apnea in adult patients. Portable Monitoring Task Force of the American Academy of Sleep Medicine. *J Clin Sleep Med*. 2007;3:737-747.

Collop NA, Tracy SL, Kapur V, et al. Obstructive sleep apnea devices for out-of-center (OOC) testing: technology evaluation. *J Clin Sleep Med*. 2011;7(5):531-548.

Horowitz SL, Hungs M. Utility of sleep studies in neurologic practice. *Neurol Clin Pract*. 2014;4:53-62.

Kushida CA, Littner MR, Morgenthaler T, et al. Practice parameters for the indications for polysomnography and related procedures: an update for 2005. *Sleep*. 2005;28:499-521.

8

An Overview of Polysomnography

SHARON A. KEENAN

Introduction

- The term polysomnography (PSG) was proposed by Holland et al.[1] to describe the recording, analysis, and interpretation of multiple simultaneous physiologic parameters during sleep.

- This 1974 publication followed long-standing efforts on the part of Dement and colleagues at Stanford to have PSG accepted as a medical test.
- This was a historic event because it created the groundwork necessary for reimbursement for this comprehensive, time-, and cost-intensive test performed on outpatients who sleep in a medical facility.
- As a tool, PSG is considered the "gold standard" for the formulation of diagnoses of sleep disorders and to enhance our understanding of both normal sleep and sleep disorders.[2-15] It is a complex procedure that should be performed by a trained technologist.[16] Today's clinical sleep laboratories continue to undergo technologic evolution,[17-21] and the collection of data outside the traditional sleep laboratory setting is common.[22] The ongoing evolution requires in-depth knowledge of equipment, protocols, and procedures.
- This chapter is a review of the technical and clinical aspects of PSG and includes standards from *The American Academy of Sleep Medicine (AASM) Manual for the Scoring of Sleep and Associated Events*,[23] the *International Classification of Sleep Disorders* (ICSD-3),[24] and other standards of practice publications.[25-35]
- PSG is used to investigate sleep-related changes in physiology, the impact of these changes on sleep, and the consequences on waking function, performance, and behavior. Issues such as shift work, time zone change, or suspected advanced or delayed sleep phase syndrome should be considered when scheduling the study. PSG should be conducted during the patient's usual major sleep period to avoid confounding circadian rhythm factors.
- Questionnaires regarding sleep-wake history and a sleep diary provide information about major sleep periods and naps. Questionnaires can be used to identify and triage patients before laboratory testing.[36-45]
  1. The prestudy/2 week/24-hour log
  2. Date
  3. Time awake
  4. Time asleep
  5. Exercise
  6. Treatment
  7. Sleep quality
  8. Medications
  9. Comments
     a. The prestudy log should be completed by the patient for a period of 2 weeks before the study. For each hour of the day, the sleep or wake time, naps, and periods of sleepiness should be indicated.

- The results of polysomnography can be influenced significantly by circadian factors. For example, sleep-onset time (latency from lights out to sleep) can be dramatically increased if a patient is asked to initiate sleep at a time much earlier than their usual bedtime.
- In addition, rapid eye movement sleep may appear in early naps of a multiple sleep latency test if the patient was awakened much earlier than his or her usual wake time. This is of greatest concern in the adolescent population where delayed sleep phase syndrome is common.

Indications for Polysomnography

According to the AASM practice parameters,[31] PSG is considered standard practice for:

1. Diagnosis of sleep-related breathing disorders (SRBDs)
2. Titration of positive airway pressure treatment
3. Preoperative assessment for snoring or obstructive sleep apnea (OSA) surgery
4. Evaluating results of the following treatments: oral appliances for moderate to severe OSA, surgical procedures for moderate to severe OSA, or surgical or dental procedures in patients with the return of symptoms of SRBD
5. Substantial weight loss or gain (10% of body weight)
6. When clinical response is insufficient or when symptoms return
7. Patients with systolic or diastolic heart failure and nocturnal symptoms of SRBD
8. Patients whose symptoms continue despite optimal management of congestive heart failure
9. Neuromuscular disorders with sleep-related symptoms
10. Narcolepsy (multiple sleep latency test [MSLT][46,47] to follow PSG; Table 8.1)
11. Periodic limb movement disorder in cases secondary to complaints by the patient or observer (movements during sleep, frequent awakenings, excessive daytime sleepiness)

PSG is not indicated for:

1. Parasomnias (except in cases of rapid eye movement [REM] sleep behavior disorder or when differentiation from nocturnal seizures is required)
2. Seizure disorders
3. Restless legs syndrome
4. Common, uncomplicated noninjurious events (arousals, nightmares, enuresis, sleep talking, bruxism)
5. Circadian rhythm disorders
6. Diagnosis by clinical evaluation alone is the standard in these cases. Standard clinical evaluation includes the history; details of behavior; age at onset; and time, frequency, regularity, and duration of events. It is useful if patients provide video documentation of the events in question, if possible, captured by a bed partner, family member, or roommate. Circadian rhythm disorders evaluation relies heavily on actigraphy. Actigraphy allows for the indexing of sleep as a function of decreased motor activity. Environmental light level is also collected. Actigraphy data are collected over a period of at least 3 days, and frequently longer.

Prestudy Questionnaires

- It is common for patients, particularly those with excessive sleepiness, to have diminished capacity to evaluate their level

TABLE 8.1 Normative Values for Multiple Sleep Latency Test and Maintenance of Wakefulness Test

	"Normal/Control Values" Mean Sleep Latency ± SD (min)
Multiple Sleep Latency Test	
4-Nap protocol	10.4 ± 4.3
5-Nap protocol	11.6 ± 5.2
Patients with narcolepsy	3.1 ± 2.9
Maintenance of Wakefulness Test	
40-minute protocol (latency to first epoch of sleep)	30.4 ± 11.20

This table summarizes normative data for the multiple sleep latency test (MSLT; four and five naps), with comparison to a group of patients with narcolepsy, and for the maintenance of wakefulness test (MWT; 40 min). Establishing normative values for both the MSLT and MWT has been complicated and challenging. Studies reporting normative data frequently lack information regarding previous sleep time and sleep quality, operational definitions for sleep onset, nap termination, number of naps, and whether caffeine was allowed. In addition, although the clinical protocol for the MSLT has been standardized, at least four different protocols have been used for the MWT. These data represent the current evidence available and may only approximate data from large, well-controlled studies across all age groups. The data reported here are for persons aged 10 years and older.
SD, Standard deviation.
Data from the American Academy of Sleep Medicine Standards of Practice Committee. Practice parameters for clinical use of the multiple sleep latency test and the maintenance of wakefulness test. *Sleep.* 2005;28(1):113–121.

of alertness. In addition, many patients with difficulty initiating and maintaining sleep often report a subjective evaluation of their total sleep time and sleep quality that is at odds with the objective data collected in the laboratory, referred to as *sleep state misperception*, an ICSD-3 diagnosis classification.[24,30] For these reasons it is recommended that subjective data be collected systematically as part of the sleep laboratory evaluation.

- The Stanford Sleepiness Scale (SSS)[37,38] is an instrument used to assess a patient's subjective evaluation of sleepiness before PSG. The SSS is presented to the patient immediately before the study. It offers a series of phrases describing states of arousal or sleepiness. Patients respond by selecting the set of adjectives that most closely corresponds to their current state of sleepiness or alertness. The scale is used extensively in both clinical and research environments; however, it has two noteworthy limitations: it is not suitable for children who have a limited vocabulary or for adults who speak English as a second language. In these situations, a linear analog scale is recommended. One end of the scale represents extreme sleepiness, and the other end represents alertness. Patients mark the scale to describe their state just before testing.

Instruments for a Quick Subjective Evaluation of Sleepiness

- Subjective evaluation of sleepiness
  - SSS[36,37]
    - Feeling active and vital; alert; wide awake.
    - Functioning at a high level, but not at peak; able to concentrate.

• BOX 8.1 Overview of the Clinical Use of the Multiple Sleep Latency Test and Maintenance of Wakefulness Test

- The multiple sleep latency test (MSLT) and the maintenance of wakefulness test (MWT) are laboratory-based clinical tools that allow characterization of excessive sleepiness (MSLT) and assessment of the ability to stay awake (MWT). Both tests require integration of a thorough history and clinical judgment for proper assessment. Both tests suffer from the lack of a large, multicenter, systematically collected repository of normative data across all age groups. The following is an overview of the indications and protocols for both tests.

Multiple Sleep Latency Test

- The MSLT provides an objective measure of sleepiness and is thought to measure the physiologic tendency to fall asleep in the absence of alerting factors. Expression of physiologic sleep tendency is demonstrated in the speed of falling asleep, given appropriate conditions and instructions. The score for the test is the mean value of individual scores collected throughout the individual's habitual time of being awake.
- The MSLT is indicated in patients suspected of having narcolepsy and to support a diagnosis of idiopathic hypersomnia.
- The MSLT is not routinely indicated for the initial evaluation of obstructive sleep apnea, assessment of treatment with continuous positive airway pressure, or the evaluation of sleepiness in patients with medical and neurologic disorders (other than in the setting of suspected narcolepsy), insomnia, or circadian rhythm disorders.
- The MSLT protocol consists of a series of four or five naps (or opportunities to fall asleep) at 2-hour intervals. The first nap is given 1.5–3 hours after final wakening from a required polysomnogram.
  - Each nap consists of a 20-min opportunity to fall asleep. Each nap is ended after 20 min if no sleep occurs or 15 min after sleep onset.

- MSLT sleep onset is defined as the first epoch of greater than 15 sec of cumulative sleep in a 30-sec epoch.
- The instructions given to the patient before the test are to "Please lie quietly, assume a comfortable position, keep your eyes closed, and try to fall asleep."
- The conventional recording montage for the MSLT includes central (C3-M2, C4-M1) and occipital (01-M2, 02-M1) electroencephalogram derivations, left and right eye electrooculograms (EOGs), vertical EOG, mental/submental electromyogram, and electrocardiogram.
- Most patients with narcolepsy have objective evidence of sleepiness associated with a mean sleep latency of 3.1 min (Table 8.1). The presence of two or more sleep-onset rapid eye movement (REM) periods, defined as REM sleep at any time during the nap, was associated with a sensitivity of 78% and a specificity of 93%. It is noted that other reasons for REM to appear (such as sleep deprivation, sleep fragmentation, medications, timing of the nap) should be considered before the final diagnosis.
- The reader should be aware that in the *International Classification of Sleep Disorders*, 3rd edition, published by the American Academy of Sleep Medicine, a mean sleep latency of less than 8 min on the MSLT is used to define pathologic sleepiness for diagnostic purposes. This value has been shown to be the best cut-off in the context of diagnosing narcolepsy, with approximately 90% of narcoleptic patients having latency below this level.

Maintenance of Wakefulness Test

- The MWT measures the ability to stay awake under nonstimulating conditions. The MWT is used primarily to assess the effectiveness of treatment of a sleep disorder, particularly in situations of patient or public safety.

- Relaxed; awake; not at full alertness; responsive.
- A little foggy; not at peak; let down.
- Fogginess; beginning to lose interest in remaining awake; slowed down.
- Sleepiness; prefer to be lying down; fighting sleep; woozy.
- Almost in reverie; on the verge of sleep onset; with a lost struggle to remain awake.
  - Linear Analog Scale
    - Just before starting the test, the technologist should ask the patient to make a mark on a straight line stretching from point 1 ("wide-awake") to point 7 ("very sleepy"). The mark they make on the line should correspond with their subjective evaluation of sleepiness or alertness at that moment. The results using the linear analog scale have shown strong correlation with results of the SSS.[36,37]
    - Another instrument for collecting subjective data, the *Epworth Sleepiness Scale*,[36] provides information about chronic sleepiness. Patients are asked to report the likelihood of falling asleep in eight conditions, such as riding as a passenger in a car or watching television, and so on.
- Also prior to the study, patients are also asked about their medication history, smoking history, any unusual events during the course of the day, their last meal before the study, alcohol intake, and a sleep history for the prior 24 hours, including naps. Involvement of the patient in providing this information usually translates into increased cooperation during the study. A technologist's complete awareness of specific patient idiosyncrasies, in the context of the questions to be addressed by the study, ensures a good foundation for the collection of high-quality data (Box 8.1).

Nap Studies

- A proposed alternative to PSG has been the nap study[26] (to be distinguished from the MSLT[46,47]). The rationale is that if a patient has a sleep disorder, it will be expressed during an afternoon nap, as well as during more extensive PSG.
- The nap study approach was used most frequently for the diagnosis of SRBDs and was proposed in an effort to reduce the cost of the sleep laboratory evaluation. The thinking is that a short study in the afternoon avoids the necessity of having a technologist present for an overnight study.
- Serious limitations in the use of nap studies include the possibility of false-negative results or misinterpretation of the severity of SRBDs, especially if the patient is sedated or deprived of sleep before the study. If a nap study is performed, it should follow the guidelines published by the American Thoracic Society.[26]
- Although minimal systematic data exist on the value of nap recordings, nap studies of 2–4 hours' duration may be used to confirm the diagnosis of sleep apnea, provided that all routine PSG variables are recorded, that both nonrapid eye movement (NREM) sleep and REM sleep are sampled, and that the patient spends at least part of the time in the supine position.
- Sleep deprivation and the use of drugs to induce a nap are contraindicated.
- Nap studies are inadequate to definitively exclude a diagnosis of sleep apnea.

Data Collection

- Data are collected by using a combination of alternating current (AC) channels and direct current (DC) channels. The most important tool in PSG is the differential amplifier. The characteristics of the differential amplifier allow display of the signal of interest (electroencephalogram [EEG], for example) and greatly diminish the display of unwanted signals (artifacts).
- Equipment for performing PSG is produced by a number of manufacturers. Each instrument may have a distinctive appearance and some idiosyncratic features, but there is remarkable similarity when the basic functioning of the instrument is examined. Proper use of the equipment calls for an understanding of how the filters and sensitivity of the amplifiers affect the data collected.[16]
- The amplifiers used to record physiologic data are very sensitive, so it is essential to eliminate unwanted signals from the recording.
- By using a combination of high- and low-frequency filters and appropriate sensitivity settings, the likelihood of recording and displaying the signals of interest is maximized, and the possibility of recording extraneous signals is decreased.
- Care must be taken when using the high- and low-frequency filters, however, to ensure that an appropriate window for recording specific frequencies is established and that the filters do not eliminate important data.
- For example, if the question for the sleep study is to rule out or capture seizure activity, the high frequency filter should be set at 70 Hz or higher. The usual setting of 35 Hz is acceptable for studies not asking a seizure question. At a setting of 35 Hz, the presentation of common muscle artifacts is reduced in the EEG channels. If, however, the interest is in displaying spikes, the filter needs to be increased to allow for the faster spike activity to be displayed. This is a logical place to mention the use of the 60 Hz filter, which in general should be avoided for all studies, but is particularly important to avoid the use of the 60 Hz (AC/line/notch) filter when recording for possible seizure activity.

Alternating Current Amplifiers

- Differential, AC amplifiers are used to record physiologic parameters of high frequency, such as the EEG, the electro-oculogram (EOG), the electromyogram (EMG), and the electrocardiogram (ECG).
- The AC amplifier has both high- and low-frequency filters. The low-frequency filter makes it possible to attenuate slow potentials not associated with the physiology of interest; such potentials include the galvanic skin response, DC electrode imbalance, and breathing reflected in an EMG, EEG, or EOG channel.
- Combinations of specific settings of the high- and low-frequency filters make it possible to focus on specific bandwidths associated with the signal of interest. For example, breathing is a very slow signal (roughly 12–18 breaths/min) when compared with the EMG signal, which has a much higher frequency (approximately 20–200 Hz or cycles/sec).

Direct Current Amplifiers

- In contrast to AC amplifiers, DC amplifiers do not have a low-frequency filter. DC amplifiers are typically used to record slower moving potentials, such as output from the oximeter or pH meter, changes in pressure in patients being treated with positive airway pressure, or output from transducers that record changes in endoesophageal pressure or body temperature. Airflow and effort of breathing can be recorded successfully with either AC or DC amplifiers, because they are very slow signals as compared with EEG or EMG.
- An understanding of the appropriate use of filters for clinical PSG is essential for proper recording technique.[48,49] Table 8.2

TABLE 8.2	Recording Montage Filter Settings and Sampling Rates			
Derivation	Low-Frequency Filter (Hz)	High-Frequency Filter (Hz)	Minimal Sampling Rate (Hz)	Desirable Sampling Rate (Hz)
• EEG	• 0.3*	• 30–35†	• 200	• 500
• EOG	• 0.3	• 30–35	• 200	• 500
• EMG	• 10*	• 100	• 200	• 500
• Breathing (airflow and effort)	• 0.1 Hz	• 15	• 25	• 100
• Oximetry	• None	• Not listed	• 10	• 25

*Low-frequency filters are related to the time constant, which is usually recorded in seconds. A low-frequency filter of 0.3 Hz equals a time constant of 0.4 sec, and a low-frequency filter of 5 Hz equals a time constant of 0.03 sec. A setting of 10 Hz is even shorter. The AASM scoring manual recommends 500 Hz as the desirable sampling rate for the EEG, EOG, EMG, and electrocardiography channels. However, recording multiple channels at this rate will result in very large files. From a practice perspective, the difference between 200- and 500-Hz sampling resolution is not discernible unless the recording is displayed on a very large screen.

†Note that if the clinical question involves the detection of seizure activity, the high-frequency filter should be set at 70 Hz. There are no specifications for individual channel sensitivities. Historically, the EEG has been recorded at 50 μV/cm. This usually needs to be translated to accommodate to the ±128-μV screen display for EEG channels.

EEG, Electroencephalography; *EMG*, electromyography; *EOG*, electro-oculography.
From AASM, American Academy of Sleep Medicine.

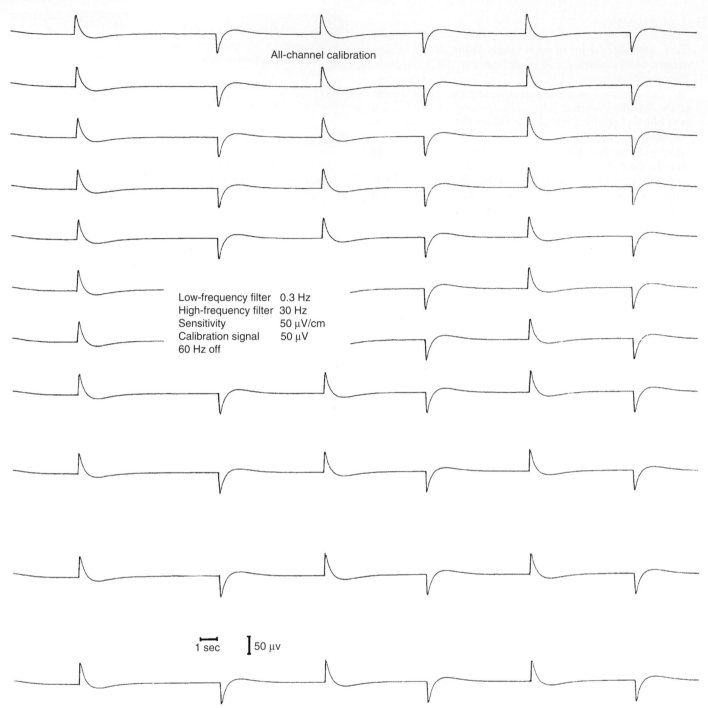

All-channel calibration

Low-frequency filter   0.3 Hz
High-frequency filter   30 Hz
Sensitivity   50 µV/cm
Calibration signal   50 µV
60 Hz off

1 sec   50 µv

• **Figure 8.1** All-channel calibration is shown. All amplifiers have the same sensitivity and high- and low-frequency filter settings. All channels should look the same.

provides recommendations for filter settings for various physiologic parameters according to the AASM.

Calibration of the Equipment

- The PSG recording instrument must be calibrated to ensure adequate functioning of the amplifiers and appropriate settings for the specific protocol.

- The first calibration is an all-channel calibration (Fig. 8.1). During this calibration, all amplifiers are set to the same sensitivity and high- and low-frequency filter settings, and a known signal (e.g., 50 µV) is sent through all amplifiers simultaneously. Proper functioning of all amplifiers is thus demonstrated, thereby ensuring that all are functioning in an identical fashion.
- A second calibration (Fig. 8.2) is performed for the specific study protocol. During this calibration the amplifiers are set

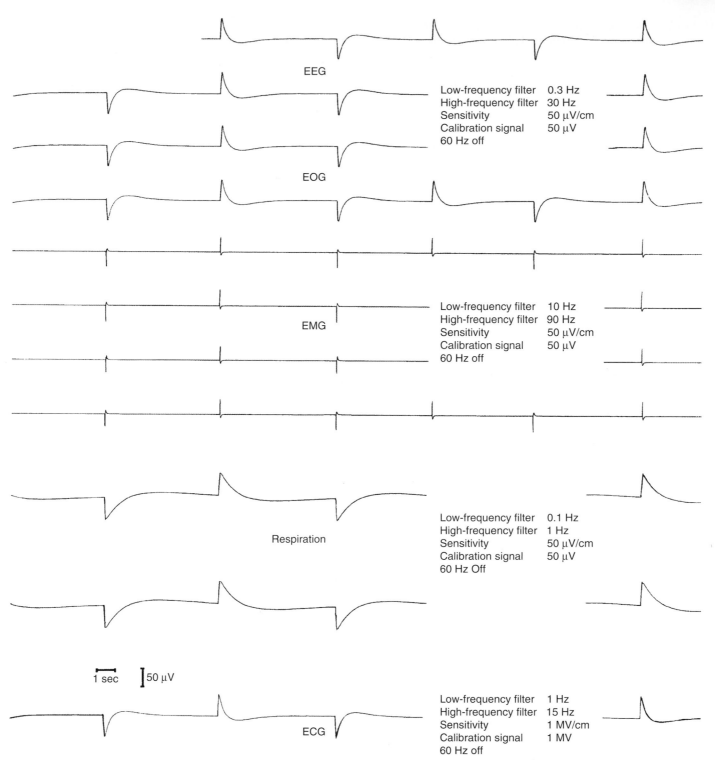

• **Figure 8.2** The montage calibration (calibration for the protocol for the study) shows changes in the high- and low-frequency filter settings from the all-channel calibration to display a variety of physiologic signals for the polysomnogram: electroencephalogram (EEG), electrooculogram (EOG), electromyogram (EMG), electrocardiogram (ECG), and breathing. Note the difference in the appearance of the signals, especially for the EMG and respiration channels. The difference is due to a difference in the settings for the filters.

with high- and low-frequency filter and sensitivity settings appropriate for each channel; the settings are dictated by the requirements of the specific physiologic parameter recorded on each channel (see Table 8.2).

- The calibration protocol ensures that all amplifiers are set to ideal conditions for recording the parameter of interest. Filter and sensitivity settings should be clearly documented for each channel.

CRITICAL POINT BOX 3

- A test of the integrity of the recording device via calibration with a known voltage ensures and documents the proper functioning of the equipment. This step is commonly missed in routine clinical practice.
- Later in this chapter a third set of calibrations will be discussed. The physiologic or patient calibrations ("bio-cals") include documentation of the patient's response to specific behaviors requested (open eyes, close eyes, etc.). This allows the opportunity to observe the data being collected and check the recording to be able to address any technical problems that may exist.

Data Display and Analysis

- The process of sleep stage scoring and analysis of abnormalities is accomplished by an epoch-by-epoch review of the data.

- Historically, a common paper speed for analog PSG was 10 mm/sec, which provides a 30-sec epoch (30 sec/page). Another widely accepted paper speed was 15 mm/sec, which produced a 20-sec epoch.
- An expanded time base may be necessary to visualize EEG data, specifically the spike activity associated with epileptic discharges. Compressed displays of greater than a 30-sec screen for the EEG should be avoided because they compromise adequate display of the EEG data. Data such as oxygen saturation and other breathing parameters can be visualized more easily when the display time is compressed to 2–5 min/screen. A major advantage of digital systems lies in the ability to manipulate the display of data after collection.

Electrode/Monitor Application Process

- The quality of the tracing generated depends on the quality of the electrode application.[48,49] Before any electrode or monitor is applied, the patient should be instructed about the procedure and given an opportunity to ask questions.
- The first step in the electrode application process involves measurement of the patient's head. The international 10–20 system[50] of electrode placement is used to localize specific electrode sites (Fig. 8.3). The following sections address the

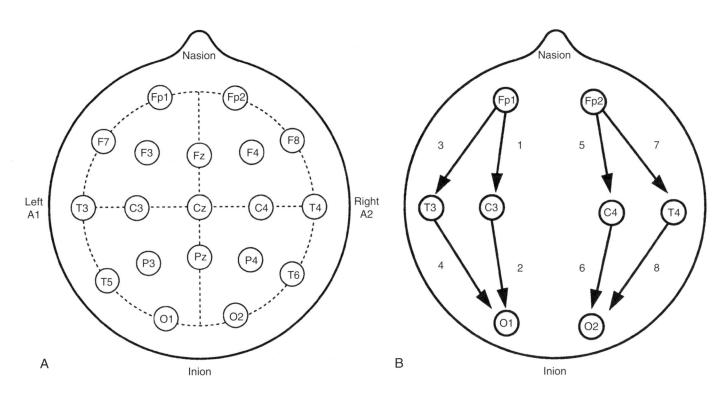

• **Figure 8.3 A,** The 10–20 system of electrode placement. Note "A1" and "A2" (left and right auricular) are in the figure. These placements are used in routine electroencephalogram (EEG). In the sleep laboratory, "M1" and "M2" are used. These electrodes are placed on the surface of the skin above the mastoid process. This placement affords a more stable surface for the electrode, helps to reduce electrocardiogram (ECG) contamination of the EEG, and avoids conflict of space for the ear oximeter. **B,** Suggested montage for recording sleep-related seizure activity for a 12-channel study: Fp1-C3; C3-O1; Fp1-T3; T3-O1; Fp2-C4; C4-O2; Fp2-T4; T4-O2; EMG-submentalis-mentalis; Right outer canthus-left outer canthus; Nasal/oral airflow; ECG. Suggested montage for recording sleep-related seizure activity for a 21-channel study: Fp1-F3; F3-C3; C3-P3; P3-O1; Fp2-F4; F4-C4; C4-P4; P4-O2; Fp1-F7; F7-T3; T3-T5; T5-O1; Fp2-F8; F8-T4; T4-T6; T6-O2; EMG-submentalis-mentalis; Right outer canthus E2/M1; Left outer canthus E1/M2; Nasal/oral airflow; ECG.

application process for EEG, EOG, EMG,[51] and ECG electrodes.

Electroencephalography

- The EEG probably reflects local changes in potential that occur on the soma and large apical dendrites of pyramidal cell neurons. The EEG is not likely to reflect action potentials of the neurons.[51]
- The cerebral cortex is believed to be the structure that generates most of the electric potential measured on the scalp. Synaptic input to neurons in the cerebral cortex consists of two types: inhibitory postsynaptic potentials (IPSPs) and excitatory postsynaptic potentials (EPSPs).
- EPSPs and IPSPs produce local changes in potential, which in turn produce the changes in the surrounding electrical field that we see reflected in the recorded EEG.
- To record the EEG, the standard electrode derivations for monitoring EEG activity during sleep are C3/M2 or C4/M1 and O1/M2 or O2/M1. (F3/M2 and F4/M1 are added to enhance detection of frontal slow activity.)
- Historically, the references have been labeled A1 and A2, and the reader should be aware that many publications prior to 2012 will show the previous terminology. The change in nomenclature has to do with the recognition that it is the mastoid reference (instead of the auricular reference) that is most commonly used in PSG. Other references, such as Cz, have been used as well.
- In PSG, our questions are most commonly answered by information about the frequency and voltage aspects of the EEG. The choice of reference and location becomes more critical in routine EEG studies when localization of activity is also important. In the sleep laboratory our most important EEG questions are: Is the patient awake or asleep? And if they are asleep, what stage of sleep (Figs. 8.4–8.10)?
- Additional EEG electrodes are necessary to rule out the possibility of epileptic seizures during sleep or the presence of any other sleep-related EEG abnormality (Figs. 8.11–8.14).
- For recording an EEG, a gold cup electrode with a hole in the center is commonly used. Silver–silver chloride electrodes are also useful to record an EEG, although they may have limitations such as increased maintenance (as evidenced by the need for repeated chloride treatments) and an inability to attach these electrodes to the scalp.
- Placement of C3, C4, O1, and O2 electrodes is determined by the international 10–20 system of electrode placement. The AASM manual also recommends the use of frontal F3 and F4 electrodes for enhancing the display of frontally predominant slow-frequency EEG activity. Reference electrodes are placed on the bony surface of the mastoid process and are labeled M2 on the right and M1 on the left (Box 8.2).
- A variety of methods are used to attach electrodes.[48–52] The collodion technique has long been an accepted and preferred method of application for EEG scalp and reference electrodes.
- This technique ensures long-term placement and allows the correction of high (>5000 Ω) impedance values after application. Other methods involving the use of electrode paste and conductive medium are acceptable and sometimes necessary in certain conditions. The goal, regardless of the application technique, is a secure placement for the duration of the study with acceptable impedance levels.

• BOX 8.2   Measuring the Head for F3, F4, C3, C4, O1, and O2 Electrodes

- Before measuring the head, it is helpful to make an initial mark at the inion, the nasion, and the two preauricular points.
- Measure the distance from the nasion to the inion along the midline through the vertex. Make a preliminary mark at the midpoint (Cz). An electrode might not be placed on this spot, but it will always be used as a landmark.
- Center this point in the transverse plane by marking the halfway point between the left and right preauricular points. The intersection of marks from steps 1 and 2 gives the precise location of Cz.
- Reposition the measuring tape at the midline through Cz and mark the points 10% up from the inion (Oz) and nasion (Fpz).
- Reposition the measuring tape in the transverse plane, through Cz, and mark 10% (T3) and 30% (C3) up from the left preauricular point, and 10% (T4) and 30% (C4) up from the right preauricular point.
- Position the tape around the head through Fpz, T3, Oz, and T4, and end at Fpz again. Ten percent of this circumference distance is the distance between Fp1 and Fp2 and between O1 and O2. Mark these four locations on either side of the midline.
- The second marks for O1 and O2 are made by continuing the horizontal mark for Oz. Do this by holding the tape at T3 and T4 through Oz, and extend the horizontal mark to intersect the previous O1 and O2 marks.
- To establish the final mark for C3, place the tape from O1 to Fp1 and make a mark at the midpoint of this line. When extended, this mark will intersect the previous C3 mark. Repeat on the right side for C4.
- F3 is midway between the distance between C3 and Fp1; F4 is midway between C4 and Fp2.

Electrooculography

- The EOG is a reflection of the movement of the electrical field associated with the cornea-retinal potential difference within the eye.[51] The retina has a relatively more negative electrical field than the cornea. Thus the eye exists as a dipole within the head, which serves as the volume conductor for that field. It is important to recognize that the EOG as described here does not measure changes in eye muscle potential (Fig. 8.15).
- EOG electrodes are typically applied to the surface of the skin with an adhesive collar.
- An electrode is typically applied at the outer canthus of the right eye. This electrode site has previously been referred to as right outer canthus (ROC) and is now called E2. E2 is offset by 1 cm above the outer canthus. Another electrode is applied to the outer canthus of the left eye, previously referred to as left outer canthus (LOC) and now called E1. The E1 electrode is offset by 1 cm below the outer canthus. The previously mentioned M1 and M2 reference electrodes can be used as follows: E2/M1 and E1/M2. In this configuration each eye is referred to the opposite reference to generate the greatest amplitude signal.
- The AASM recommends that both eyes be referred to the same reference electrode. Additional electrodes can be applied above and below for either the right or left eye. The infraorbital and supraorbital electrodes enhance the ability to detect eye movements that occur in the vertical plane and can be particularly useful in the MSLT.
- EOG electrodes allow the recording of waking eye movements, slow rolling eye movements of drowsiness, and stage N1, and

Text continued on p. 84

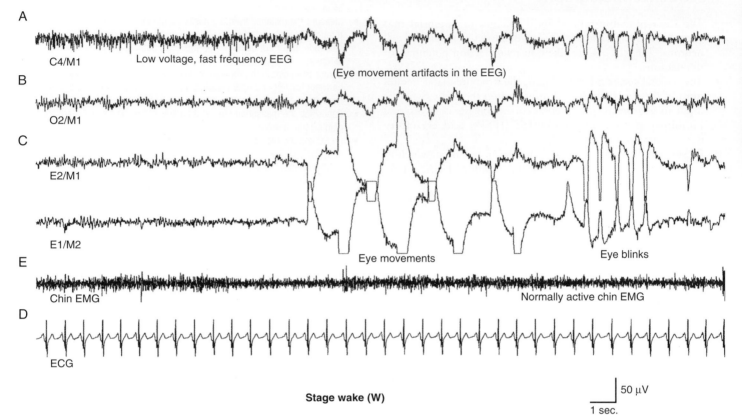

A, Low voltage, fast frequency EEG

C4/M1

(Eye movement artifacts in the EEG)

B, O2/M1

C, E2/M1

E1/M2

Eye movements

Eye blinks

E, Chin EMG

Normally active chin EMG

D, ECG

Stage wake (W)

50 µV
1 sec.

• **Figure 8.4 A,** This stage wake (W) example is an excerpt from the biocalibrations at the start of a study. It shows waking electroencephalogram (EEG), eye movements, and eye movement artifact in the EEG channels. The C4/M1 channel shows low voltage and mixed frequency EEG at the start of the epoch. This pattern changes to a mixture of the underlying EEG and a high-amplitude, slower frequency. If the reader looks down in the example, to the channels below (along the time axis), the correspondence to the eye movements can be observed. This is particularly pronounced in association with "eye blinks." **B,** The occipital EEG channel (O2/M1) also shows alpha EEG activity and a reflection of eye movements, but the amplitude of the eye movement artifact is different (as compared with the C4/M1 derivation on the first channel). This is secondary to the increased distance between the occipital electrodes and the dipole of the electrical field the eyes. The pattern of low-voltage EEG activity in the 8–13-Hz band is best seen in recordings from the occipital cortex and seen best if eyes are closed (see Fig. 8.5). **C,** When the patient is asked to look right, look left, and then blink, the channels recording eye movement document those conditions and the EEG channel (O2/M1) also shows a reflection of the movement of the electrical fields of each eye. Please note in this example the eye movement electrodes are referred to the opposite reference electrode (E2/M1 and E1/M2). This differs from the American Academy of Sleep Medicine manual, which suggests to refer both eyes to the same reference electrode. If the eye movement electrodes are referred to the same reference electrode, there are significant differences in the amplitude of the signals. This is due to the difference in the distance between the E1 and E2 electrodes from the single reference electrode. If the electrodes are referred to the opposite references, the eye movements appear more symmetrical in amplitude and sometimes easier to observe. **D,** The EEG is also reflected in the eye movement channels (E2/M1 and E1/M2). The settings for the high and low frequency filters are set to the same conditions for the EEG and electrooculogram channels. This affords the opportunity to see the reflection of EEG in the eye channels. Often this is helpful, especially when scoring slow wave sleep, or other more frontally predominant wave forms, such as K-complexes. The decisions for sleep stage scoring, however, are always made from the C3 or C4 electrodes. **E,** The chin EMG shows a normal pattern associated with relaxed wakefulness. The ECG shows normal sinus rhythm. (Reproduced with permission from Butkov N. *Atlas of Clinical Polysomnography.* 2nd ed. Medford, OR: Synapse Media; 2010.)

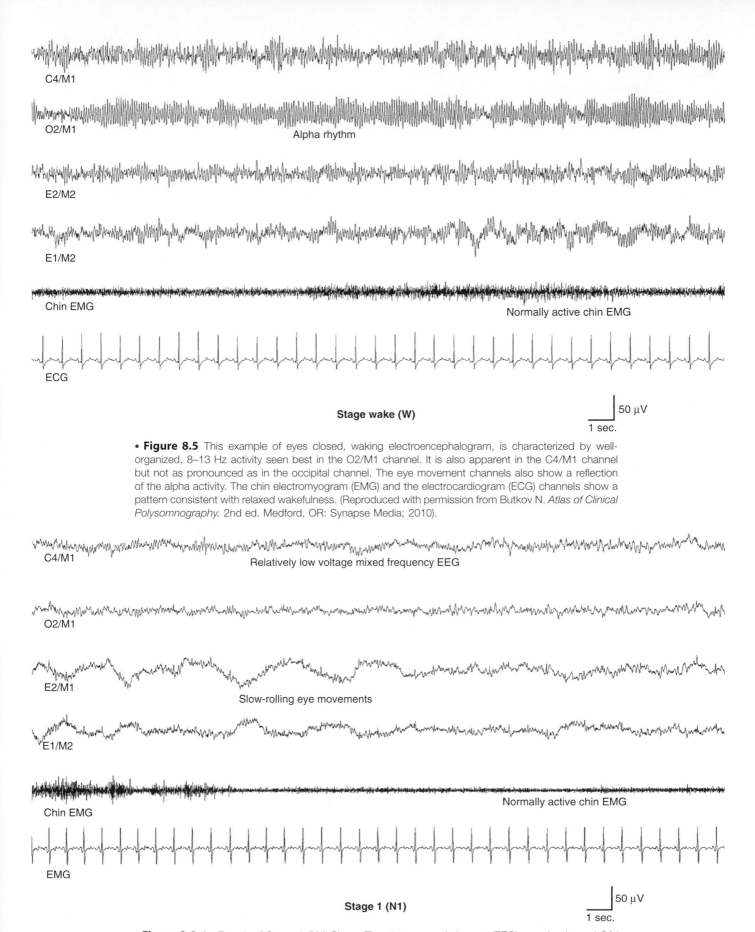

C4/M1

O2/M1 — Alpha rhythm

E2/M2

E1/M2

Chin EMG — Normally active chin EMG

ECG

Stage wake (W)

50 μV
1 sec.

• **Figure 8.5** This example of eyes closed, waking electroencephalogram, is characterized by well-organized, 8–13 Hz activity seen best in the O2/M1 channel. It is also apparent in the C4/M1 channel but not as pronounced as in the occipital channel. The eye movement channels also show a reflection of the alpha activity. The chin electromyogram (EMG) and the electrocardiogram (ECG) channels show a pattern consistent with relaxed wakefulness. (Reproduced with permission from Butkov N. *Atlas of Clinical Polysomnography.* 2nd ed. Medford, OR: Synapse Media; 2010).

C4/M1 — Relatively low voltage mixed frequency EEG

O2/M1

E2/M1 — Slow-rolling eye movements

E1/M2

Chin EMG — Normally active chin EMG

EMG

Stage 1 (N1)

50 μV
1 sec.

• **Figure 8.6** An Epoch of Stage 1 (N1) Sleep. The electroencephalogram (EEG) seen in channel O2/M1 is characterized by low voltage mixed frequency activity in the 5–7 Hz range for more than, or equal to, 50% of the epoch. The eye movement channels (E2/M1 and E1/M2) show the characteristic slow rolling eye movements often seen at the transition from wake to sleep. The electromyogram (EMG) shows a decreased, but still present EMG signal. (Reproduced with permission from Butkov N. *Atlas of Clinical Polysomnography.* 2nd ed. Medford, OR: Synapse Media; 2010.)

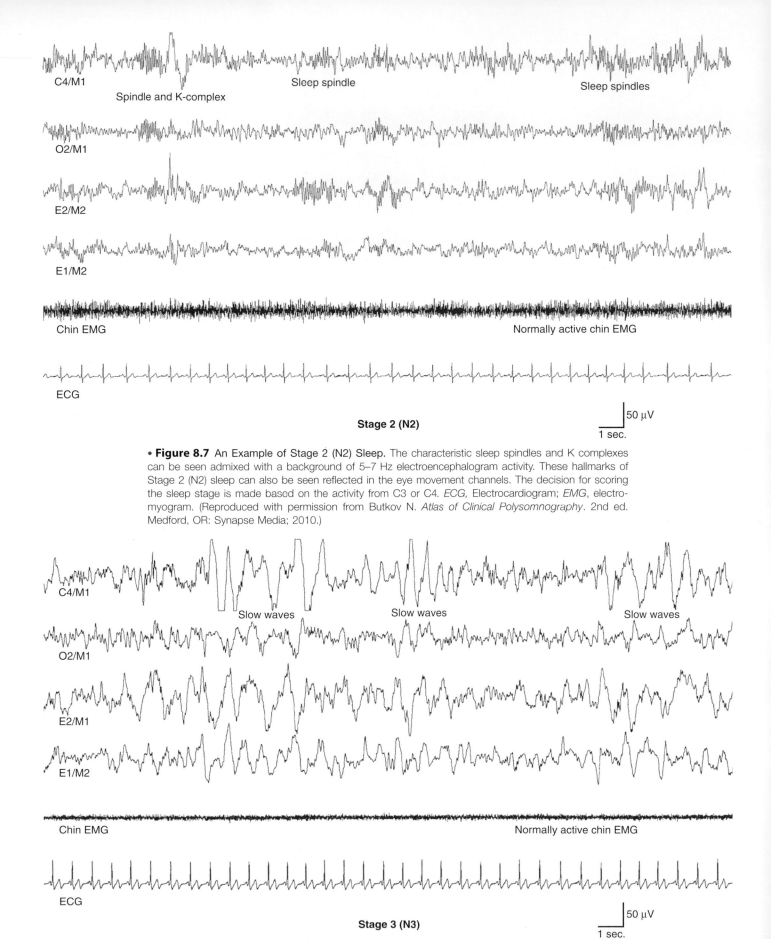

Stage 2 (N2)

50 μV

1 sec.

• **Figure 8.7** An Example of Stage 2 (N2) Sleep. The characteristic sleep spindles and K complexes can be seen admixed with a background of 5–7 Hz electroencephalogram activity. These hallmarks of Stage 2 (N2) sleep can also be seen reflected in the eye movement channels. The decision for scoring the sleep stage is made based on the activity from C3 or C4. *ECG,* Electrocardiogram; *EMG,* electromyogram. (Reproduced with permission from Butkov N. *Atlas of Clinical Polysomnography*. 2nd ed. Medford, OR: Synapse Media; 2010.)

Stage 3 (N3)

50 μV

1 sec.

• **Figure 8.8** An Example of N3 (Stage 3) Sleep. More than 20% of the epoch is characterized by high amplitude (>75 μV), slow frequency (0.5–2 Hz). The eye movement channels show a reflection of the high amplitude electroencephalogram. This is common and increases confidence about scoring slow wave sleep. The scoring decision however is made from the C3 or C4 channel. *ECG,* Electrocardiogram; *EMG,* electromyogram. (Reproduced with permission from Butkov N. *Atlas of Clinical Polysomnography*. 2nd ed. Medford, OR: Synapse Media; 2010.)

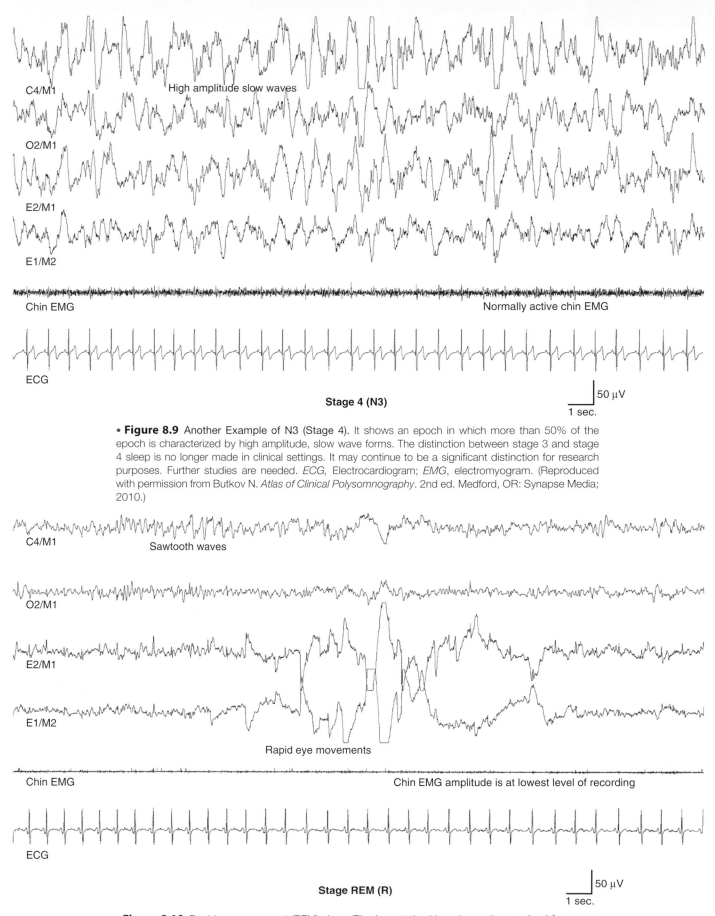

Stage 4 (N3)

50 µV

1 sec.

• **Figure 8.9** Another Example of N3 (Stage 4). It shows an epoch in which more than 50% of the epoch is characterized by high amplitude, slow wave forms. The distinction between stage 3 and stage 4 sleep is no longer made in clinical settings. It may continue to be a significant distinction for research purposes. Further studies are needed. *ECG*, Electrocardiogram; *EMG*, electromyogram. (Reproduced with permission from Butkov N. *Atlas of Clinical Polysomnography*. 2nd ed. Medford, OR: Synapse Media; 2010.)

Stage REM (R)

50 µV

1 sec.

• **Figure 8.10** Rapid eye movement (REM) sleep (R), characterized by a low voltage, mixed frequency electroencephalogram (5–7 Hz), eye movements, and a dramatic reduction in electromyogram (EMG) tone. The interesting notched wave forms appearing in the C4/M1 channel are called sawtooth waves. They appear in REM but do not need to be present to score REM sleep (R). *ECG*, Electrocardiogram. (Reproduced with permission from Butkov N. *Atlas of Clinical Polysomnography*. 2nd ed. Medford, OR: Synapse Media; 2010.)

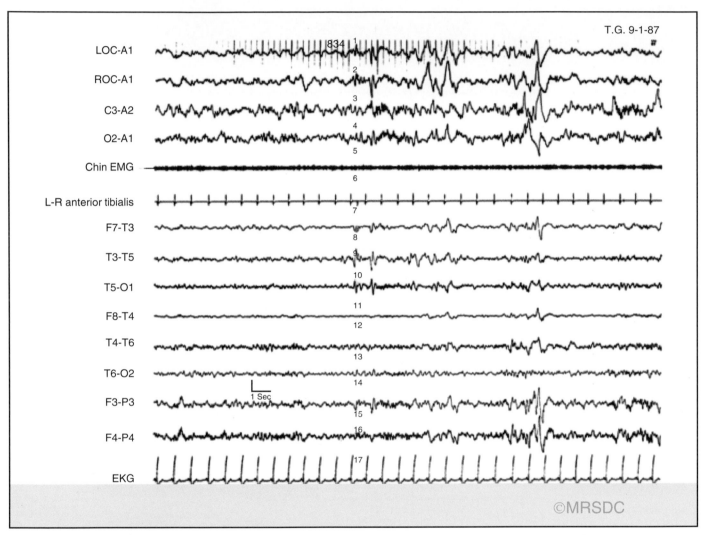

• **Figure 8.11** Shows an expanded electroencephalogram montage to be able to demonstrate the epileptogenic activity that appears in the left temporal region. Close examination of the wave forms shows a phase reversal at T5 about midway through the epoch. Notice the absence of this activity along the time axis on the right side of the brain (T6). *EKG*, Electrocardiogram; *EMG*, electromyogram. (Courtesy Dr. Mark Mahowald.)

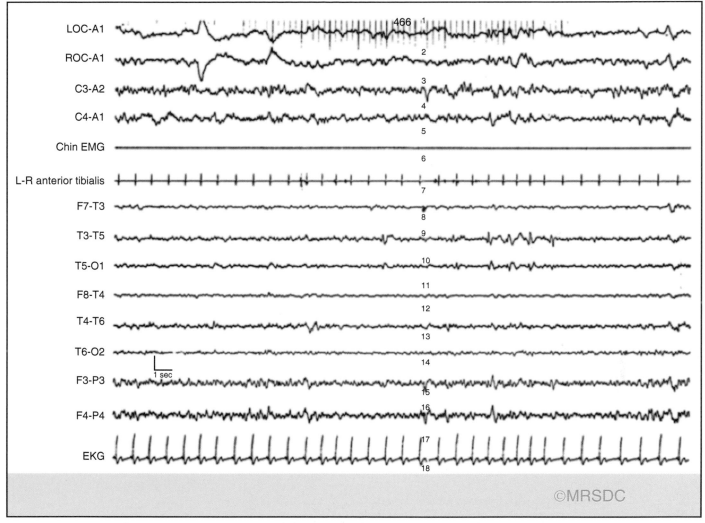

• **Figure 8.12** Shows similar sharp, spike, and wave activity at T5 during REM sleep. This activity is not present at the same time on the right side (T6). *EKG*, Electrocardiogram; *EMG*, electromyogram. (Courtesy Dr. Mark Mahowald.)

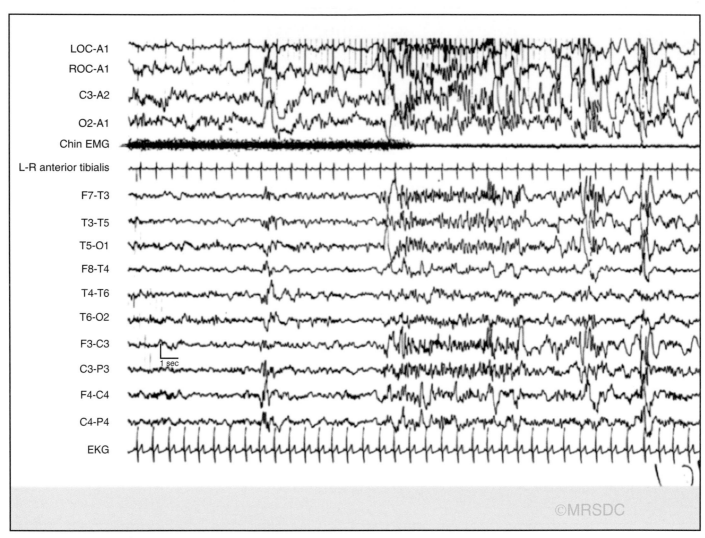

• **Figure 8.13** Shows left-sided spike and slow wave and paroxysmal rhythmic activity during apparent N2 (stage 2) sleep. *EKG,* Electrocardiogram; *EMG,* electromyogram. (Courtesy Dr. Mark Mahowald.)

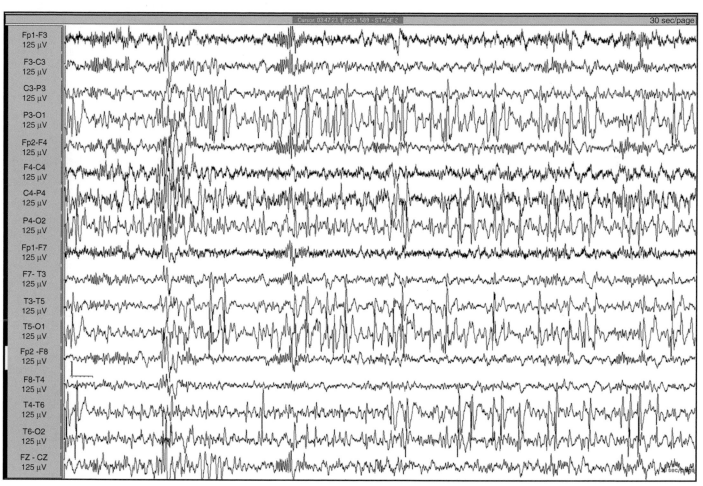

• **Figure 8.14** Is tracing showing status epilepticus during N2 (stage 2) sleep. (Courtesy Dr. Mark Mahowald.)

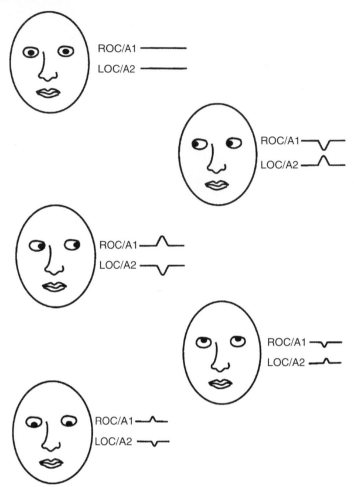

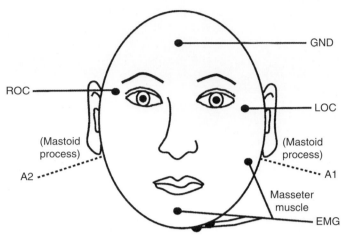

• **Figure 8.16** Schematic diagram showing placement of the electromyographic (EMG) electrodes to record activity from the mental, submental, and masseter muscles. *GND,* Ground (earth); *LOC (E1),* outer canthi of the left eye; *ROC (E2),* outer canthi of the right eye.

• **Figure 8.15** The recording montage for a two-channel electroooculogram demonstrates out-of-phase signal deflection in association with conjugate eye movements. Recall that ROC = E2 and LOC = E1. If reference electrodes are placed on the mastoid process, they are labeled M1 and M2 (previously called A1, A2). *LOC,* Left outer canthus; *ROC,* right outer canthus.

the faster eye movements of REM sleep. If the amplifiers for the EOG channels are set to the same conditions as the EEG channels, the eye movement channel data often helps answer EEG channel questions (see Figs. 8.4–8.6 and 8.10).

Electromyography

- The EMG recording represents a summation of the electrical activity of muscle fibers and nerve impulses along the nerves and neuromuscular junctions.[50]
- A gold cup or a silver–silver chloride electrode attached with an adhesive collar is used to record EMG activity from the mentalis and submentalis muscles. At least three EMG electrodes are applied. This allows the use of an alternative electrode in the event that artifact develops in one of the electrodes. The additional electrode can be placed over the masseter muscle to allow detection of bursts of EMG activity associated with bruxism (Fig. 8.16).
- Additional bipolar EMG electrodes are placed on the surface of the anterior tibialis muscles to record periodic limb movements in sleep[52–54] and on the surface of the extensor digitorum muscles if REM sleep behavior disorder[54] is suspected.

Electrocardiography

- There are a variety of approaches for recording the ECG during PSG. The simplest approach involves the use of standard gold cup electrodes; however, disposable electrodes are also available.
- ECG electrodes are applied with an adhesive collar to the surface of the skin, just beneath the right clavicle and on the left side at the level of the seventh rib. A stress loop is incorporated into the lead wire to ensure long-term placement. This represents a modified "lead II" derivation, which is commonly used in cardiopulmonary laboratories.

Monitoring Breathing During Sleep

- It is necessary to record airflow and effort to breathe, and it is with these two measures that breathing irregularities can be detected. There are many sophisticated technical advances on the horizon, but the following describes common clinical practice:
  - It is well recognized that the pneumotachograph is the "gold standard" for measuring airflow. It is customary, however, for many clinical studies to rely on qualitative methods that simply index airflow during sleep. Historically, thermistors or thermocouples were used, whereas presently a more accepted practice is to record change in pressure to monitor airflow.[32,33]
  - Respiratory inductive plethysmography is often thought of as a reliable, noninvasive measure of the work of breathing. If calibrated, it can give a measure of changes in tidal volume. There have been reports of difficulty maintaining calibration for the duration of the study.
  - Piezoelectric crystals embedded into adjustable belts worn around the chest and abdomen reflect effort to breathe and are commonly used. There are numerous ways to index breathing effort, including but not limited to intercostal or diaphragmatic EMG and impedance pneumography.
  - A quantitative measure of the work of breathing can be obtained with endoesophageal manometry.[55]
  - For greatest confidence, multiple methods of monitoring airflow and effort of breathing should be used.

- Noninvasive blood gas monitoring during sleep is essential for assessing the severity of SRBD.

CRITICAL POINT BOX 4

- It is important to understand how the signals on polysomnography are produced. For example, how are airflow and effort data being collected? Change in temperature of inhalation versus exhalation has been used to index breathing, but change in pressure is considered to be a more reliable measure. Effort of breathing is measured in many ways. Most commonly in clinical practice we rely on qualitative changes to detect sleep-related breathing disorders. Changes in endoesophageal pressure (Pes) are quantitative (but more invasive and not used routinely). Pes can give more sensitive measures of the work of breathing and allow detection of respiratory effort–related arousals, or "RERAs."[35]

Gastroesophageal Reflux Studies

- It is common for PSG to include the monitoring of endo-esophageal pH when patients complain of reflux or waking with a choking sensation.[56] Commercially available devices allow the recording of changes in pH at the distal esophageal level during sleep.
- Reflux events and the "clearing time," or the time necessary to return to normal acid levels, can be demonstrated and correlated with other physiologic events like changes in heart or breathing rates, or EEG arousals.

Impedance Check

- Before recording, the electrodes should be visually inspected to check the security of their placement, and an impedance check should be performed and documented.
- Adjustments should be made to EEG, EOG, or chin EMG electrodes with impedance greater than 5000 Ω. Higher impedance values (20 kΩ) are accepted for leg, arm, intercostal EMG, and ECG

Physiologic Calibrations

- Physiologic calibrations are performed after the electrode and monitor application is complete. This calibration allows documentation of proper functioning of the electrodes and other monitoring devices and provides baseline data for review and comparison when scoring the PSG.
- Specific instructions are given to the patient for this calibration and include the following conditions:
  1. Eyes open, look straight ahead for 30 sec.
  2. Hold head still; look to the left and right, up and down. Repeat.
  3. Hold head still; blink eyes slowly five times.
  4. Grit teeth, clench jaw, or smile.
  5. Inhale and exhale.
  6. Hold breath for 10 sec.
  7. Flex right foot; flex left foot.
  8. Flex right hand; flex left hand.
- As the patient follows these instructions, the technologist examines the tracing and documents the patient's responses.
  - When the patient stares straight ahead for 30 sec with the eyes open, the background EEG activity is examined.

- As the patient looks right and left, the tracing is examined for out-of-phase deflections of the signals associated with recording the EOG.
- Out-of-phase deflection occurs if the input to consecutive channels of the polygraph is E2/M1 (historically ROC/A1) for the first EOG channel and E1/M2 (historically LOC/A2) for the second.
- It is also important, when patients close their eyes, to observe the reactivity of the alpha rhythm seen most prominently in the occipital EEG (O1/M2 or O2/M1; historically O1/A2 and O2/A1). Usually alpha is best visualized when the patient's eyes are closed and when they are in a relaxed state.
- The patient is also asked to blink five times to observe the corresponding output on the eye movement channels and possible EOG artifact reflected in the EEG channels.
- The mentalis/submentalis EMG signal is checked by asking patients to grit their teeth, clench their jaws, or yawn.
- The technologist documents proper functioning of the electrodes and amplifiers used to monitor anterior tibialis EMG activity by asking patients to flex their right foot and left foot in turn.
- If REM sleep behavior disorder is suspected, an expanded four-limb EMG montage should be ordered, and additional electrodes should be applied to the surface of the skin above the extensor digitorum muscles of each arm. Patients are asked to flex their wrists while the technologist examines the recording for the corresponding increase in amplitude of the EMG channel.
- Inhalation and exhalation allow examination of channels monitoring airflow and effort of breathing. A suggested convention is that inhalation causes an upward deflection of the signal and exhalation causes a downward deflection.
- It is most important that the signals on all the channels monitoring breathing be in phase with each other to avoid possible confusion with paradoxical breathing, which could be observed in association with obstructive events. The technologist should observe a flattening of the trace for the duration of a voluntary apnea.
- If a 60- or 50-Hz notch filter is in use, a brief examination (2–4 sec) of portions of the tracing with the filter in the off position is essential. This allows identification of any 60- or 50-Hz interference that may be masked by the filter.
  - Care should be taken to eliminate any source of interference and to ensure that the 60- or 50-Hz notch filter is used only as a last resort.
  - This is most important when recording patients suspected of having seizure activity, because the notch filter attenuates the amplitude of the spike activity seen in association with epileptogenic activity.
  - If other monitors are used, the technologist should incorporate the necessary calibrations.
- The physiologic calibrations enable the technologist to determine the quality of data before the PSG begins.
  - If an artifact is noted during the physiologic calibrations, it is imperative that every effort be made to correct the problem, because the condition is likely to become worse through the remaining portions of the recording.
  - The functioning of alternative (spare) electrodes should also be examined during this calibration.
- When a satisfactory calibration procedure is completed and all other aspects of patient and equipment preparation are concluded, data collection can begin. This is referred to as "lights out," and the time should be noted clearly.

Monitoring, Recording, and Documentation

- Complete documentation for the PSG is essential and includes identification of the patient (patient's full name and medical record number), date of recording, and a full description of the study.
- The names of the technologists performing the recording and any technologists involved in preparation of the patient and equipment should be noted.
- The specific instrument used to generate the recording should be identified. This is particularly useful in the event that artifact is noted during the analysis portion (scoring) of the sleep study.
- Specific parameters recorded on each channel should be noted clearly, as should a full description of the sensitivity, filter, and calibration settings for each channel.
- The time of the beginning and end of the recording must be noted, as well as specific events that occur during the night.
- Usually a predetermined montage is available as a simple software selection.
- Any changes made in filter and sensitivity settings should be clearly noted.
- The technologist is also responsible for providing a clinical description of unusual events. For example, if a patient experiences an epileptic seizure during the study, the clinical manifestations of the seizure must be detailed: deviation of the eyes or head to one side or the other, movement of the extremities, presence of vomiting or incontinence, duration of the seizure, and postictal status.
- Similar information should be reported on any clinical event observed in the laboratory, such as somnambulism or clinical features of REM sleep behavior disorder. Any complaints reported by the patient are also noted.

Troubleshooting/Artifact Recognition

- In general, when difficulties arise during recording, the troubleshooting inquiry begins with the patient and follows the path of the signal to the recording device.
- More often than not, the problem can be identified as difficulty with an electrode or other monitoring device. It is less likely that artifact is the result of a problem with an amplifier.
- If the artifact is generalized (i.e., on most channels), the integrity of the ground electrode and the instrument cable should be checked.
- If the artifact is localized (i.e., on a limited number of channels), the question should be "Which channels have this artifact in common, and what is common to the channels involved?" The artifact is probably the result of a problem located in an electrode or monitoring device that is common to both channels.
- If the artifact is isolated to a single channel, the source of the artifact is limited to the input to the specific amplifier or the amplifier itself (Figs. 8.17 and 8.18).

Ending the Study

- Often clinical circumstances and laboratory protocol dictate whether the patient is awakened at a specific time or allowed to awaken spontaneously.
- It is critical to know the difference between the wake-up time for the study and to compare it with the usual wake-up time for the patient. Comparison can be made to patient reports on the sleep log.
- Ideally the patient is awakened at their usual time. If this is not the case, the difference is important clinical information and must be taken into account for proper interpretation of the study.
- After awakening, to end the study the patient should be asked to perform the physiologic calibrations to ensure that the electrodes and other monitoring devices are still functioning properly.
- The equipment should be calibrated at the settings used for the study, and finally, the amplifiers should be set to identical settings for high- and low-frequency filters and sensitivity and an all-channel calibration should be performed.
- This is essentially the reverse of the calibration procedures mentioned for the beginning of the study.
- A subjective evaluation is made by the patient. The patient is asked to estimate how long it took to fall asleep, the amount of time spent asleep, and whether there were any disruptions during the sleep period. Patients should report on the quality of their sleep and level of alertness on arousal.
- It is also worthwhile for the sleep laboratory staff to know how patients intend to leave the laboratory.
- A patient who is determined to have severe level of sleepiness should avoid driving. Support around transportation from the study is important, particularly if the patient has withdrawn from stimulant medications for the purpose of the study.

The Final Report

- Interpretation of the PSG is a process involving a review of the clinical findings and history, as well as parametric analysis of the PSG.
- The variables listed in Table 8.3 are most commonly used to assist in interpretation and create the final report. Clinical judgment is of the utmost importance when providing interpretation of the PSG.

Digital Systems

- Digital systems have made it possible to manipulate data after recording and to permit extraction of previously inaccessible information.
- Digital systems provide flexibility in the manipulation of filter settings, sensitivities, and changes in the display of montages after collection.
- The first digital EEG systems became available in the late 1980s and catalyzed a revolution in EEG and PSG technologies.[17–21]
- This revolution has been primarily in making the static format of analog system data more flexible, enhancing storage and allowing for novel ways and means for analysis.
- Significant advantages of digital systems include autocorrection of amplifier gains; self-diagnostic tests of amplifier functions; and software-controlled, in-line impedance testing.

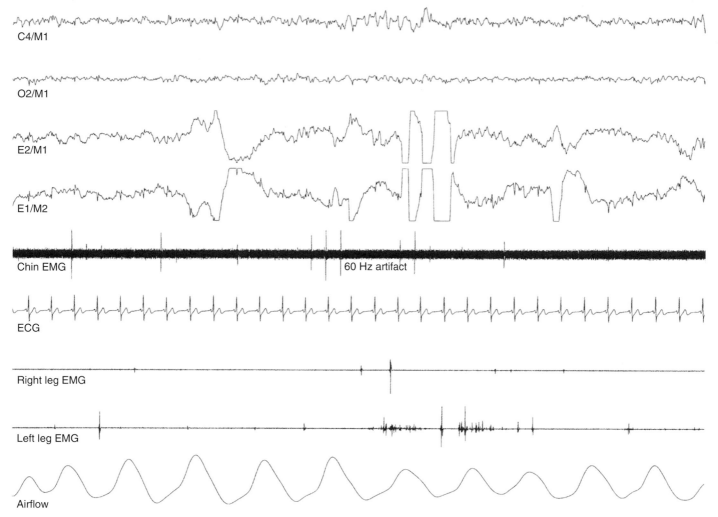

C4/M1

O2/M1

E2/M1

E1/M2

Chin EMG   60 Hz artifact

ECG

Right leg EMG

Left leg EMG

Airflow

• **Figure 8.17** The chin electromyogram (EMG) channel shows 60 Hz artifact. The electroencephalogram and electrooculogram are characteristic of stage rapid eye movement (R) sleep. This is often due to a poor electrode connection to the skin. Choosing another chin EMG electrode input to this channel will solve the problem. With most systems this kind of correction can be made during the study or during playback. (Reproduced with permission from Butkov N. *Atlas of Clinical Polysomnography*. 2nd ed. Medford, OR: Synapse Media; 2010.)

CRITICAL POINT BOX 6

- Interpretation of the polysomnography (PSG) can be challenging. Data from the PSG are always integrated in light of the history and chief complaint of the patient. Frequently, the results may be "gray" (as compared with blood gas values for example). Our goal is to diagnose and treat patients who suffer from sleep disorders and experience sleepiness during the waking hours. Ideally, the physician providing interpretation has the opportunity to review the raw data from the PSG so that impressions can be created before using the numbers provided from the scoring process.
- The clinician can answer global questions such as the following:
    1. Did the patient sleep or not?
    2. How does the waking electroencephalogram (EEG) appear?
    3. What do the stage 2 (N2) phenomena look like? That is, are well-developed K complexes or sleep spindles present?
    4. Was slow wave sleep (N3) observed?
    5. What does the patient's rapid eye movement sleep look like?
    6. Was the distribution of sleep stages within normal limits or not?
    7. Did the patient have problems with breathing during sleep or not?
    8. Did the patient have excessive movement or any unusual events or not?
    9. This global impression should be used in conjunction with the final report numbers generated by the technologist who scores the PSG. If there are great variances between the global clinical impression and the scoring report of the technologist, they should be discussed and understood before making a final interpretation. In the end (as with EEG), it is the patient not the PSG recording that is treated.
    10. Moreover, we do not "rush to treat" findings on the PSG (such as frequent leg movements) in the absence of a complaint or significant disruption of sleep.

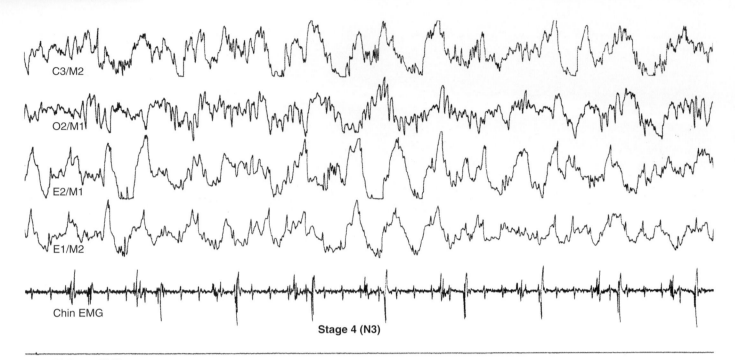

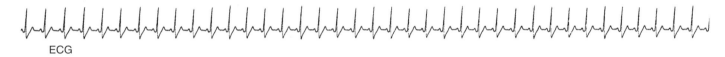

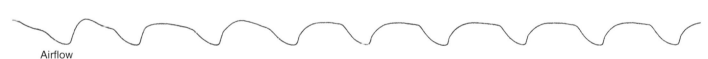

• **Figure 8.18** The chin electromyogram (EMG) channel shows electrode artifact. It is repetitive in nature and in time with breathing. Electrocardiogram (ECG) artifact is also present in this channel. The solution is to change the input for this channel to avoid the use of the faulty electrode. (Reproduced with permission from Butkov N. *Atlas of Clinical Polysomnography*. 2nd ed. Medford, OR: Synapse Media; 2010.)

- The use of computers has facilitated storage of data, manipulation of data after collection, and presentation of different views of the data.
- Both analog and digital systems require electrodes and other sensors to be applied with the greatest of care.
- Ideally, calibration procedures are performed to document and ensure the collection of high-quality data at the beginning and end of the recording.
- Knowledge of the specifics of the equipment and of the physiology of interest is important to ensure accurate signal processing.
- In digital systems it is rare to encounter breakdown of any mechanical component; the most frequently encountered problems involve cables, sensors, or electrodes. The most important problems to avoid for trouble-free operation are mechanical shock, dust, and static electricity.

- An important factor for understanding digital PSG systems is the concept of sampling rate. Sampling rate is the frequency at which the signal is reviewed (sampled) for conversion to a digital signal. The minimum acceptable sampling rate for the EEG, EOG, and EMG in PSG is 200 Hz.
- Another issue unique to digital systems is the accuracy or precision of recordings. The resolution of the signal is a function of the number of binary bits used to represent the digital values.
- Readers will recall that a bit is a value of 1 or 0. Eight bits is 2 to the 8th power, or 256. For example, if we assume an EEG voltage greater than 256 μV, from negative 128 μV to positive 127 μV, this would result in a resolution with an 8-bit system of a 1-μV difference, being represented in 1 bit of change.

TABLE 8.3 Polysomnography Variables

Variable	Units	Variable	Units
Lights out	Time	WASO	Minutes
Lights on	Time	WAFA	Minutes
Lights out to SO	Minutes	TST/TIB	Minutes
SO	Minutes	SE	%
SO to N1 (NREM stage 1)	Minutes	TST	%
SO to N2 (NREM stage 2)	Minutes	Events	
SO to N3 (NREM stages 3 and 4)	Minutes	Average O_2 saturation	%
SO to R (REM)	Minutes	Low O_2 saturations	%
TMT	Minutes	Total Events	
TN1	Minutes, %TST	OSA	#
TN2	Minutes, %TST	CSA	#
TN3	Minutes, %TST	HYP	#
TREM	Minutes, %TST	Indexes	
TRT	Minutes	AHI	#
TSWS	Minutes	RDI	#
TWT	Minutes	AI	#

AHI, Apnea-hypopnea index; *AI*, apnea index; *CSA*, central sleep apnea; *HYP*, hypopnea; *N1*, stage 1; *N2*, stage 2; *N3*, slow wave sleep; *NREM*, nonrapid eye movement; *OSA*, obstructive sleep apnea; *RDI*, respiratory disturbance index; *REM*, rapid eye movement; *SE*, sleep efficiency (TST/TIB); *SO*, sleep onset; *TMT*, total movement time; *TN1*, total N1; *TN2*, total N2; *TN3*, total N3; *TREM*, total REM; *TRT*, total recording time; *TST*, total sleep time; *TST/TIB*, total sleep time/time in bed; *TSWS*, total slow wave sleep; *TWT*, total wake time; *WAFA*, wake after final wakening; *WASO*, wake after sleep onset.

- The 8-bit system provides the least amount of precision.
- A 12-bit system (2 to the 12th power) provides a range of values between −2048 and +2047 (the number line includes "0"). The 12-bit successive digital values represent a 0.0625-µV change in the analog signal. The 12-bit representation is far more precise and reflects a smaller change in the analog signal. (It is interesting to note that the equivalent precision of paper tracings is approximately 6 bits. The decreased precision of analog systems is a function of the limitation of the amount of paper available for one channel and pen thickness.)

- Also to be considered is the display resolution, which is determined by the resolution of the monitor. The screen used for reviewing the data must be at least 20 inches in size and display a resolution of 1280 × 1024 pixels (flicker free; i.e., 75-Hz monitor scan rate).[21]

Recording Samples

- Examples of PSG data (Figs. 8.19–8.21) are from the *Atlas of Clinical Polysomnography*, used with permission of the author and publisher.[57]

Summary

- Throughout its evolution, PSG has proved to be a robust tool for enhancing our understanding of sleep and its disorders. It is an essential diagnostic procedure.
- PSG is complex and labor intensive. It requires specialized technical skills and knowledge of normal sleep and sleep disorders.
- Technologists need to be experts with equipment, competent in dealing with medically ill patients, and capable of dealing with emergencies that may be encountered in the sleep laboratory. They must also be skilled enough to work in many circumstances outside the traditional laboratory setting.
- Our field faces many challenges. Evaluation of sleep disorders must be made readily available to the millions of patients with sleep disorders who lack diagnosis and treatment.[58–61]

- Cost-effectiveness in sleep health care and maintenance of high-quality evaluation and treatment remain important challenges. Digital systems facilitate data storage, manipulation, and analysis.
- Any system works best when the user is knowledgeable about the tools and clear about the questions. Ongoing innovations in technology hold great promise for advances in knowledge about sleep.
- PSG is incomplete without the use of EEG monitoring. The EEG to date is the only parameter that allows evaluation of the person's physiologic state of sleep or wakefulness during the recording.
- Many exciting surrogates hold promise as tools for furthering insights into brain state, but to date, it is hard to match the power of the EEG in increasing our understanding of sleep and wakefulness.

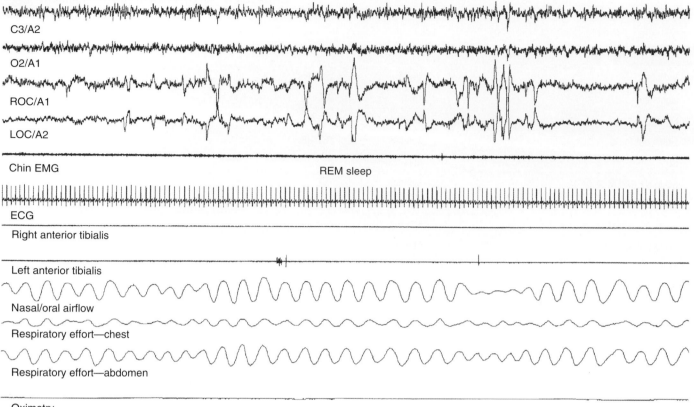

C3/A2

O2/A1

ROC/A1

LOC/A2

Chin EMG

REM sleep

ECG

Right anterior tibialis

Left anterior tibialis

Nasal/oral airflow

Respiratory effort—chest

Respiratory effort—abdomen

Oximetry

• **Figure 8.19** Digital Record Sample of Rapid Eye Movement Sleep. Though altered by time scale compression, the sleep stage pattern seen in this sample can readily be identified as rapid eye movement (REM). Note the mild respiratory irregularity, which is a normal variant of REM sleep physiology. *ECG,* Electrocardiogram; *EMG,* electromyogram; *LOC,* left outer canthus; *ROC,* right outer canthus. (Reproduced with permission from Butkov N. *Atlas of Clinical Polysomnography.* 2nd ed. Medford, OR: Synapse Media; 2010.)

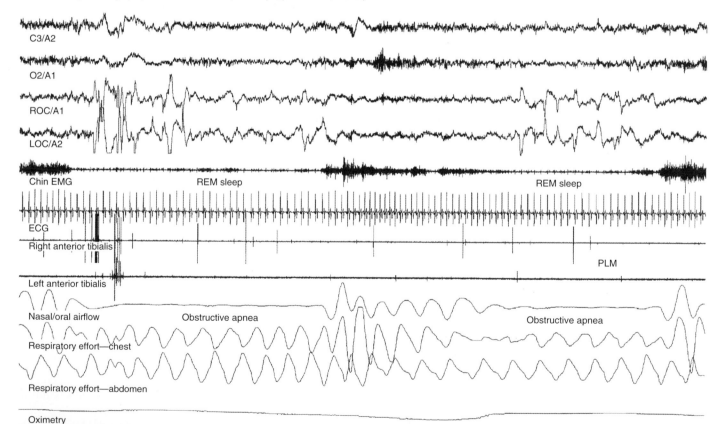

C3/A2

O2/A1

ROC/A1

LOC/A2

Chin EMG

REM sleep

REM sleep

ECG

Right anterior tibialis

PLM

Left anterior tibialis

Nasal/oral airflow

Obstructive apnea

Obstructive apnea

Respiratory effort—chest

Respiratory effort—abdomen

Oximetry

• **Figure 8.20** Digital Record Sample of Patient With Obstructive Apnea. This sample shows a compressed display of repetitive obstructive apnea occurring during rapid eye movement (REM) sleep. As noted previously, this represents the extreme end of the sleep-disordered breathing continuum. In the preceding example, all the features of classic obstructive sleep apnea are present, including distinct paradoxical (out-of-phase) respiratory effort, instances of complete cessation of airflow, subsequent electroencephalographic arousal, and cyclic O2 desaturation. *ECG,* Electrocardiogram; *EMG,* electromyogram; *LOC,* left outer canthus; *PLM,* periodic limb movement; *ROC,* right outer canthus. (Reproduced with permission from Butkov N. *Atlas of Clinical Polysomnography.* 2nd ed. Medford, OR: Synapse Media; 2010.)

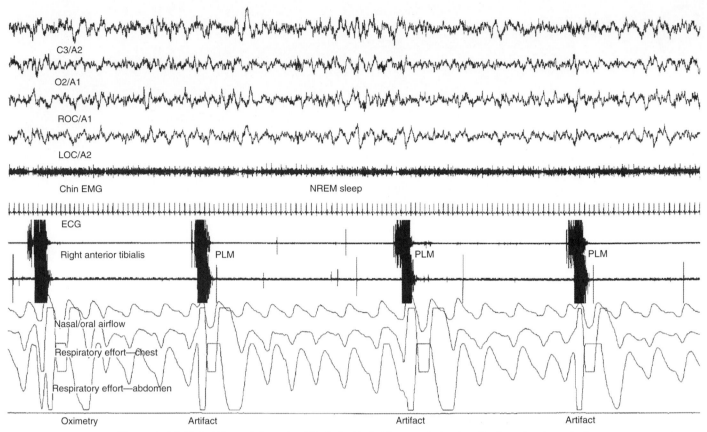

• **Figure 8.21** Digital Record Sample of Periodic Limb Movement. As described previously, periodic limb movements (PLMs) often generate artifacts in the respiratory channels that appear similar to cyclic hypopnea. This sample shows a compressed version of the characteristic pattern of PLM recorded by the right and left anterior tibialis electromyogram (EMG) channel. Note that the respiratory channel artifact appears almost identical to the cyclic hypopnea seen in the preceding sample. *ECG,* Electrocardiogram; *LOC,* left outer canthus; *ROC,* right outer canthus. (Reproduced with permission from Butkov N. *Atlas of Clinical Polysomnography.* 2nd ed. Medford, OR: Synapse Media; 2010.)

Suggested Reading

American Academy of Sleep Medicine. *International Classification of Sleep Disorders.* 3rd ed. (ICSD-3): Westchester, IL: 2014.

Butkov N. *Atlas of Clinical Polysomnography.* 2nd ed. Medford, OR: Synapse Media; 2010.

Kryger M, Roth T, Dement W, eds. *Principles and Practice of Sleep Medicine.* 6th ed. Philadelphia, PA: Elsevier; 2017.

Sheldon S, Kryger M, Ferber R, Gozal D, eds. *Principles and Practice of Pediatric Sleep Medicine.* 2nd ed. Philadelphia, PA: Elsevier; 2014.

The AASM Manual for the Scoring of Sleep and Associated Events. Westchester, IL: American Academy of Sleep Medicine; 2016.

9

Sleep Stage Scoring

NIC BUTKOV

Introduction

The standard method for identifying and scoring sleep stages was developed in 1968 by Rechtschaffen and Kales (R&K).[1] With this method, the entire polysomnogram (PSG) is divided into epochs, and each epoch is assigned a score. Each score represents one of the basic stages of sleep. These stages are identified by examining and correlating the electroencephalogram (EEG), the electrooculogram (EOG), and the chin electromyogram (EMG) tracings.

In 2007 the American Academy of Sleep Medicine (AASM) published a new scoring manual[2] and mandated its use for AASM-accredited sleep centers in 2008. Though largely based on consensus, the AASM scoring manual was concomitantly incorporated into the board-certifying examination for physicians and the registry examination for technologists. The visual rules for scoring sleep stages presented by the AASM originate from the R&K scoring system with relatively few changes; however, subsequent revisions and additions have since been made by a Scoring Manual Committee of the AASM. Since its inception, the AASM manual has been replicated in digital form and made available to subscribers online. The version cited at the time of this writing is 2.3, released April 1, 2016.[3]

This chapter provides an overview of sleep stage scoring and summarizes both the traditional R&K and the revised AASM scoring methods, along with relevant commentary. For board examination purposes, the reader needs to follow the current AASM specifications. For a more global perspective, familiarity with both scoring systems is useful. The reader should also be aware that the existing scoring rules are based on stereotypical patterns seen in normal subjects, which do not always accommodate the various abnormal findings seen on a clinical PSG. Common confounding factors that significantly alter the appearance of the PSG include coexisting pathologies, use of certain prescription medications, and recording artifacts. Consequently, the scorer must learn to combine existing rules with practice-based clinical judgment to most accurately interpret the substance of the data.

Historical Background

Recordings of electrical activity produced by the human brain during wakefulness and sleep were first performed during the 1920s by Hans Berger, a German psychiatrist who recorded the world's first EEG. Initially identifying a wave pattern of approximately 10 Hz (or cycles per second), Berger named the pattern "alpha" as the first waveforms isolated in the human EEG. Berger also discovered that the alpha pattern diminished with concentration—or when a subject's eyes were open—and that the pattern was replaced by low-voltage, mixed-frequency activity with the onset of sleep.

Early efforts to describe and classify sleep stages followed in the 1930s when Alfred Lee Loomis and colleagues began performing continuous overnight EEG recordings of sleeping patients. In the absence of other physiologic parameters, sleep staging was predominately based on the presence of stereotypical EEG features, which included alpha activity, beta activity, theta activity, sleep spindles, and slow wave activity. Although rudimentary eye movement recordings were obtained during these early studies, the discovery of rapid eye movement (REM) sleep did not occur until nearly 2 decades later. Sleep stages were initially described as stages A, B, C, D, and E. Stage A was identified by the presence of alpha rhythm and slow, rolling eye movements. Stage B consisted of low-voltage activity without alpha rhythm or spindles. Stage C was identified by the presence of spindles with a low-voltage EEG background. Stage D included both spindles and random slow waves. Stage E consisted predominately of high-amplitude slow waves.

The discovery of REM sleep was described in 1953 by Nathaniel Kleitman and Eugene Aserinsky. Later that decade, Nathaniel Kleitman and William C. Dement refined the techniques for recording and measuring the EEG and eye movement activity and charted the patterns of sleep and dreaming over the course of a night. By combining the EEG with recordings of eye movements and later with recordings of chin muscle activity, Kleitman and Dement laid the foundation for the establishment of four distinct nonrapid eye movement (NREM) sleep stages alternating with REM sleep.

Rechtschaffen and Kales Scoring Manual

Recognizing the ever-increasing need for standardization of sleep scoring, a committee was formed by members of the Sleep Research Society to develop a standardized scoring manual. The committee, chaired by Alan Rechtschaffen and Anthony Kales, developed and published *A Manual of Standardized Terminology, Techniques and Scoring Systems for Sleep Stages of Human Subjects*. Since its introduction in 1968, the R&K manual has been used extensively for both research and clinical purposes and is probably the most often quoted reference manual in sleep medicine worldwide.

One of the key stipulations of the R&K manual is that EEG criteria for scoring sleep stages be derived from central electrode placements C3 or C4, referenced to an opposite mastoid. The reason for a standardized central derivation is that most critical features, such as sleep spindles, K-complexes, vertex sharp waves, and high-amplitude slow waves, are clearly recorded from the C3 or C4 electrode sites. The manual specifies the use of an opposite ear or mastoid (A1 or A2) as a standard reference because this maximizes interelectrode distances and avoids mixing EEG activity from two different scalp areas.

Though not required by the R&K manual, most sleep centers include an occipital EEG channel (derived from O1 or O2) as part of the PSG recording montage. In most subjects, alpha activity appears most prominently in the occipital region; therefore the occipital EEG is often helpful for identifying wakefulness and for determining sleep onset when the alpha rhythm disappears.

To record eye movements, the R&K manual specifies at least two EOG channels with signals derived from electrodes placed approximately 1 cm above and slightly lateral to the outer canthus of one eye and 1 cm below and slightly lateral to the outer canthus of the other eye. The manual recommends referencing both eye electrodes to the same ear or mastoid (in actual practice, many sleep centers prefer to use a contralateral mastoid to maximize both EOG signals and to equalize the out-of-phase deflections seen with conjugate eye movements). The R&K manual discourages the use of a supranasion reference (Fpz) because vertical eye movements (appearing as in-phase deflections with this arrangement) can be confused with artifacts.

For chin EMG recordings, the R&K manual recommends the use of electrodes placed over muscle areas on and beneath the chin (mental, submental). To ensure sufficient amplitudes when recording tonic EMG activity during NREM sleep, the manual recommends the use of a high gain (sensitivity) of 20 μV/cm or higher, along with minimal high-frequency filtering.

The R&K manual provides definitions for scoring stage wake; NREM stages 1, 2, 3, and 4; stage REM; and stage movement time (MT). Each epoch is scored according to the predominance of characteristic features of a particular sleep stage, as recorded by the EEG, EOG, and chin EMG. The R&K manual also provides specific rules for identifying the boundaries between stages, particularly in the context of stage 2 sleep and REM sleep.

American Academy of Sleep Medicine Scoring Manual

The AASM manual closely follows the original R&K sleep stage scoring criteria, with a few notable exceptions. The current manual specifies a minimum of three EEG derivations, including the addition of frontal leads for scoring slow wave sleep, but reduces the traditional four stages of NREM sleep to three by combining stage 3 and 4 sleep. A few changes have also been made regarding the continuity of stage 2 sleep and REM sleep. The AASM manual has also changed some of the nomenclature, with NREM sleep stages being identified as N1, N2, and N3, and stage REM further being abbreviated as stage R. The mastoid reference sites A1 and A2 have been renamed M1 and M2.

One of the more controversial aspects of the AASM scoring manual has been the sanctioning of alternative EEG and EOG derivations. The manual allows the use of bipolar EEG derivations (Fz/Cz and Cz/Oz) in addition to the standard C4/M1 derivation. In practice, the use of bipolar EEG derivations for scoring sleep stages is incongruous because signals derived from electrodes in close proximity to each other are significantly attenuated by common mode rejection.[1]

This especially applies to the use of bipolar frontal leads in the context of scoring slow wave sleep. The use of alternative derivations defeats the goal of standardization because each of the proposed electrode combinations, including the backup options, yields different results. The current version of the AASM manual states that the "acceptable" bipolar EEG derivation of Fz/Cz should not be used for scoring slow wave sleep, but that instead slow wave activity can be measured from the left eye electrode (E1) referenced to Fpz. The manual also states that when using the *acceptable* EEG derivations along with the *recommended* EOG derivations, slow wave activity for determining slow wave sleep should be measured from C4/M1 or C3/M2 (essentially defaulting back to R&K criteria).

---

[1]Common mode rejection is a function of differential signal amplification, as used in EEG and PSG recordings, whereby signals of dissimilar voltage or polarity are amplified, while any identical, in-phase signals are rejected.

On the positive side, the AASM manual has helped clarify some of the ambiguities related to the scoring of transitions between sleep stages and has identified some of the characteristic features of shifts in stage that follow arousals. The manual also offers technical specifications for digital PSG recordings, including filter configurations, sampling rates, computer monitor resolution, on-screen calibration capabilities, impedance measurements, and other requirements. This is an important step toward setting standards for the sleep recording industry, although more work is needed in this area. Another positive development seen in the most current version of the manual is the addition of notes regarding alterations in appearance of the EEG caused by certain pathologies and by recording artifacts. Recognizing these phenomena is a critical prerequisite to accurate visual scoring. It is hoped that future versions of the manual will similarly address pharmaceutical drug effects on the PSG, a common finding in routine clinical sleep studies that significantly impacts the scoring process.

Technical Challenges

A fundamental consideration for accurately scoring and interpreting PSG data is recording quality. This in turn is determined by three factors: the integrity of the electrode and sensor application, the quality of the equipment used to produce the recording, and the maintenance of the recording for the duration of the sleep study.

The application of electrodes and sensors represents the most essential, yet most vulnerable, link in the entire chain of connections between the patient and the data output. Despite ongoing advancements in technology, the old adage "garbage in = garbage out" still stands. Without proper attention to this process, the recorded data become questionable. Readers are encouraged to establish rigorous standards within their facilities regarding the manner in which electrodes and sensors are applied to the patient, specifically paying attention to proper skin preparation techniques, electrode impedance levels, and accurate placement.

The second factor to consider is recording equipment. Historically, PSG data were recorded with high caliber paper-based analog instruments or polygraphs that were capable of yielding optimal signal quality and minimizing signal distortion, while preserving all the necessary detail for accurate data analysis. Although the advent of digital polysomnography has added tremendous flexibility and practicality to this process, it has also been associated with many flaws. The general trend in digital PSG has been software development, while downplaying the importance of a solid hardware foundation. As a result, many contemporary PSG recording systems produce marginal results, even when optimal application techniques are exercised by the attending technologists. Problems stem from fundamental defects such as loose electrode connections, excessively long electrode leads (necessitated by some contemporary headboard designs), inferior components, and overall lack of quality control. To compensate for these problems, PSG signals are often overprocessed, which makes it difficult for scorers to discern between factual data and noise-related artifacts that *resemble* physiologic data. Readers are encouraged to thoroughly research their equipment before making a purchase, bearing in mind that so-called upgrades and changes in design are not always indicative of product improvement.

The third consideration is recording maintenance, which relies on the skills and vigilance of the attending technologist. Because sleep studies are conducted over an extended period of time on patients who are unrestricted in movement, recording problems and subsequent artifacts are common. To help facilitate accurate data scoring, it is essential for the attending technologists to know how to recognize and properly address recording problems that arise during the course of the study. It is equally important for technologists to document any changes made to the recording and to convey any additional information regarding the study that might be helpful to the scorer or interpreter of the study.

Data Display

Another essential issue in scoring the PSG is the manner in which the data are displayed. In the past, analog-based PSG recordings were presented in uniform size, typically on grid paper marked with millimeter and centimeter lines. In the present day, digital recordings can be displayed and manipulated in many different ways. Although this offers greater flexibility, it also raises many practical issues. For example, if the signal display is overcrowded, overattenuated, or overfiltered, it alters the scorer's perception of the data. This is a common problem with many contemporary digital PSG recordings. To enable accurate scoring and data interpretation, PSG signals need to be free of excessive noise (but not overfiltered), and displayed with sufficient amplitudes to facilitate clear visual perception of all essential detail.

Display Calibration

Although the AASM scoring manual recommends performing a standard calibration routine with a negative 50-μV DC voltage, it does not specify how to apply this calibration to the computer screen display. If the user wants to achieve an actual calibration of 50 μV/cm (or any other desired calibration), some adjustments must be made. On many digital PSG systems, the default sensitivity settings for the individual channels are too low and must be increased to achieve adequate amplitude resolution. The signal display dimensions are further determined by the size and shape of the monitor screen, the available work space within the screen, and on some systems, the total number of channels simultaneously displayed within the work space.

To achieve a precise screen calibration, the user can hold a ruler or measuring tape against the monitor screen while applying the calibration signal. Most recording systems provide reference brackets, or threshold lines, that can be adjusted to increase or decrease individual channel sensitivity settings. Similar attention must be paid to the time scale of the display. Historically, the time scale used for sleep stage scoring has been 1 cm/sec, with 30 sec per page (epoch) being presented. When viewing a digital PSG, the actual dimensions of a 30-sec epoch are usually "stretched" to fit the width of the computer screen. In general, this does not pose a problem, as long as the time scale is not altered excessively. In some instances, PSG data are displayed on wide-screen monitors or projected onto a large screen. When doing so, it is important to maintain the correct aspect ratio (i.e., the vertical and horizontal proportions of the signals should be preserved).

Establishing a Work Space

It is important to exercise care when setting up a display work space. With ever-increasing options presented by digital recording systems, it is easy to overlook essential channel settings that might be set incorrectly and render the visual representation of the entire recording inaccurate. Incorrect filter settings, inverted polarity, wrong sensitivity adjustments, or any combination thereof can distort the data to such an extent that sleep stages and other scoring variables can be grossly misinterpreted. Once an appropriate work space is established, it is advisable to save the settings and make certain that everyone involved in the scoring and interpretation process views the data in the same manner.

Recording Artifacts

Descriptions of the various types of recording artifacts are beyond the scope of this chapter and are discussed elsewhere in this publication. However, from a scoring perspective, it is important to understand the way in which artifacts can influence the scoring and interpretation process.

PSG recording artifacts are defined as extraneous signals appearing within any of the recorded parameters of the study. Most artifacts can be readily identified by their exaggerated or distorted appearance and by their lack of correlation to adjacent channels. However, some artifacts may closely resemble physiologic activity and may lead to misinterpretation of the data. This is more likely to happen when PSG signals are over-processed to the extent that extraneous interference is reduced to narrow bandwidths that appear similar to EEG, EMG, or other PSG signals. An extreme example of this is seen with some recording systems, whereby extraneous electrical signals *resembling* the EEG or other parameters appear on the display even when the patient is disconnected from the equipment.

It is important to note that not all artifacts are undesirable. For example, artifacts in the chin EMG caused by snoring help confirm that the patient snored, while muscle-generated artifacts in the EEG, EOG, and EMG occurring with body movements help confirm that the patient moved. Even undesirable artifacts serve a purpose, because they indicate the presence of a faulty signal that needs correction.

Therefore it is a mistake to try to eliminate all artifacts, especially by attempting to "clean up" the study with filters. In particular, it should not be standard practice to rely on 50- or 60-Hz notch filters to eliminate power line frequency interference. In general, the presence of such interference indicates high electrode impedances, faulty electrode connections, faulty ground, or inferior recording equipment. A 50- or 60-Hz artifact can also occur when using extra-long unshielded electrode leads from the patient to the jack box. Unfortunately, the design of some equipment necessitates the routine use of 50- or 60-Hz filters, even when proper application techniques are performed. The problem with this practice is that the electrical noise is still there, but it may instead replicate the appearance of alpha or beta activity in the EEG or muscle activity in the EMG. In these instances, terms such as "high definition" or "high resolution" become moot, because the study essentially yields a highly detailed depiction of noise, and the reader of the study can longer be certain whether the data represent real physiologic activity, or a narrow bandwidth of artifact, or some combination of both. It is hoped that future editions of the scoring manual will address these issues, particularly with regard to PSG recording equipment design.

Recognition of Electroencephalogram Patterns

As noted earlier, the existing criteria for scoring sleep stages are based on normal subjects who expectedly exhibit normal EEG patterns. In actual practice, EEG patterns vary widely, even in normal individuals. A side-by-side comparison of recordings obtained from different subjects may reveal patterns that hold different meanings for each subject (i.e., one person's stage wake may resemble another person's stage 1 or stage REM). Consequently, to accurately interpret the data, the scorer must rely on pattern recognition skills relative to each individual subject. A biocalibration routine conducted at the beginning of the study helps provide the scorer with a baseline reference for stage wake with eyes open and with eyes closed. Additional references are gleaned from the study during the scoring process by viewing the changing patterns within the context of the recording.

In this manner, sleep stage scoring is analogous to reading handwritten script, whereby the reader learns to recognize familiar patterns within the context of preceding and succeeding epochs and interprets them accordingly. While fundamental scoring rules are necessary to form a common language and to develop some degree of consistency among scorers, an equally important element is practice-based clinical judgment.

The following list describes the basic criteria for identifying EEG patterns relative to sleep stage scoring. These patterns are described according to their frequency (cycles per second or hertz), amplitude (measure of voltage), and morphology (characteristic shape or structure).

- EEG frequencies (or bandwidths) are identified as alpha, beta, theta, and delta (Fig. 9.1).
- When the EEG pattern appears mixed without a dominant frequency, it is described as "mixed-frequency EEG." Mixed-frequency EEG can be seen during stage 1 sleep, during REM sleep, and as the background frequency during stage 2 sleep (Fig. 9.2).
- The amplitude of an EEG waveform is represented by its vertical size, measured peak to peak. The amplitude of the EEG represents the voltage of the waves, which is measured against a calibration signal of known value. (Typically a negative 50-μV direct current [DC] signal is used [Fig. 9.3].)
- EEG waves can also be described in terms of their characteristic shape or structure. Examples include vertex waves, K-complexes, sleep spindles, and sawtooth waves (Fig. 9.4).

Sleep stages are identified by correlating specific EEG patterns with other recorded parameters, including the EOG and chin EMG. In general, each epoch is scored according to the predominance of a particular sleep stage. Thus, when a characteristic pattern of a particular sleep stage begins during the first half of an epoch, the entire epoch is scored as that stage. When the pattern begins during the last half of the epoch, the score is carried over to the following epoch. An exception to this rule involves the scoring of slow wave sleep (N3). Slow wave sleep is scored according to the overall percentage of high-amplitude slow waves occupying the epoch, regardless of whether they occur during the first or the last half of the epoch.

Sleep Stage Definitions

The following sleep stage descriptions include both traditional R&K and AASM scoring definitions. The AASM manual uses abbreviations (W, N1, N2, N3, and R) to label the sleep stages.

Stage Wake (W)

Stage wake can appear in two forms. When a subject's eyes are open, the EEG usually shows a fast, mixed-frequency pattern with low amplitude. The EOG displays eye movements and eye blinks in the presence of elevated chin EMG activity (Fig. 9.5).

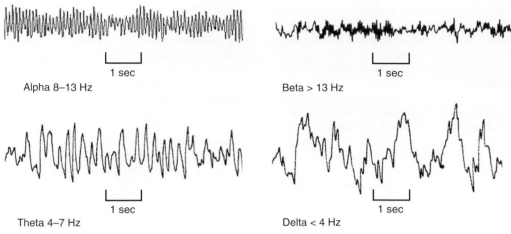

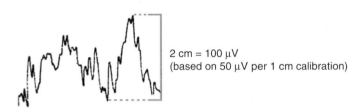

• Figure 9.1 Electroencephalographic bandwidths. (Reprinted with permission from Butkov N. *Atlas of Clinical Polysomnography.* 2nd ed. Medford, OR: Synapse Media; 2010.)

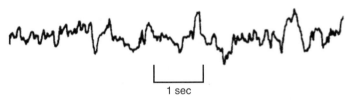

•Figure 9.2 Mixed-frequency electroencephalographic tracing. (Reprinted with permission from Butkov N. *Atlas of Clinical Polysomnography.* 2nd ed. Medford, OR: Synapse Media; 2010.)

2 cm = 100 μV
(based on 50 μV per 1 cm calibration)

• Figure 9.3 Measuring electroencephalographic wave amplitude. (Reprinted with permission from Butkov N. *Atlas of Clinical Polysomnography.* 2nd ed. Medford, OR: Synapse Media; 2010.)

When the eyes are closed, a predominance of alpha rhythm (8–13 Hz) is seen in most individuals. Alpha activity is usually more prominent in the occipital EEG, but it is also seen in the central EEG and the EOG (Fig. 9.6). Alpha activity becomes attenuated or disappears with concentration or when subjects open their eyes.

The AASM manual has added a definition for "reading eye movements," described as trains of conjugate eye movements consisting of a slow phase followed by a rapid phase in the opposite direction. However, reading patterns can vary widely, and the act of reading or any other activity during wakefulness is best confirmed by direct patient observation or video monitoring.

During stage wake, the chin EMG should show normal baseline muscle tone. Although the chin EMG is in general regarded as a qualitative signal, it is important to establish sufficient amplitude in the chin EMG during relaxed wakefulness. Overattenuated chin EMG tracings are a common finding in many digital PSG

recordings. Establishing adequate baseline chin EMG amplitude is essential for identifying subsequent changes, particularly with the onset of REM sleep.

According to both the R&K and AASM criteria, stage wake is scored when greater than 50% of an epoch shows a wake pattern. The wake pattern is identified either by the presence of alpha rhythm or by the presence of REMs associated with normal or high chin muscle tone. Stage wake is also scored during intervals when a patient is temporarily disconnected from the equipment during the course of a sleep study.

Stage 1 (N1)

Stage 1 sleep represents a transition from wakefulness to sleep. Stage 1 is identified by relatively low-voltage, mixed-frequency EEG activity, with a predominance of theta frequency (4–7 Hz). Alpha activity is expected to diminish or disappear with sleep onset (Fig. 9.7). The EOG channels often display slow rolling eye movements, especially during the initial onset of sleep. During the latter part of stage 1 sleep, vertex sharp waves may appear in the central EEG (Fig. 9.8).

Chin EMG levels are variable and may drop below those seen during relaxed wakefulness, but they continue to maintain normal tonic levels associated with NREM sleep.

According to both the R&K and AASM criteria, stage 1 sleep (N1) is scored when alpha rhythm is attenuated and replaced by relatively low-voltage, mixed-frequency EEG activity for greater than 50% of an epoch. The AASM manual recommends that in subjects who do not generate alpha rhythms, N1 can be scored by the presence of a slowing of background EEG frequencies with activity in the range of 4–7 Hz or by the presence of either vertex sharp waves or slow, rolling eye movements.

An important addition to the current version of the AASM manual is a note stating that "theta frequency (4–7 Hz) waveforms that are of pathological origin (such as those resulting from neurological impairment, encephalopathy or epilepsy) should not be considered toward the determination of Stage N1 sleep. In a person with a slow background EEG in the awake state, further non-pathological slowing of the background activity of >1 Hz from that seen in the wake state would be considered evidence of Stage N1 sleep."

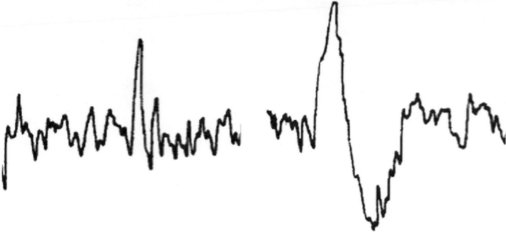

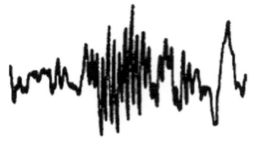

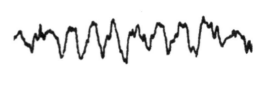

Vertex waves—sharp negative waves appearing over the vertex of the scalp, usually within the theta frequency range, typically appearing during the latter part of stage 1 sleep.

K-complex—a sharp negative wave followed by a slower positive compenent; a characteristic feature of stage 2 sleep.

• **Figure 9.4** Examples of electroencephalographic wave structures. (Reprinted with permission from Butkov N. *Atlas of Clinical Polysomnography.* 2nd ed. Medford, OR: Synapse Media; 2010.)

Sleep spindle—short rhythmic waveform clusters of 12–14 Hz, often showing a waxing and waning appearance; a characteristic feature of stage 2 sleep.

Sawtooth waves—relatively low-amplitude waves with a notched, sawtooth appearance; a common feature of REM sleep.

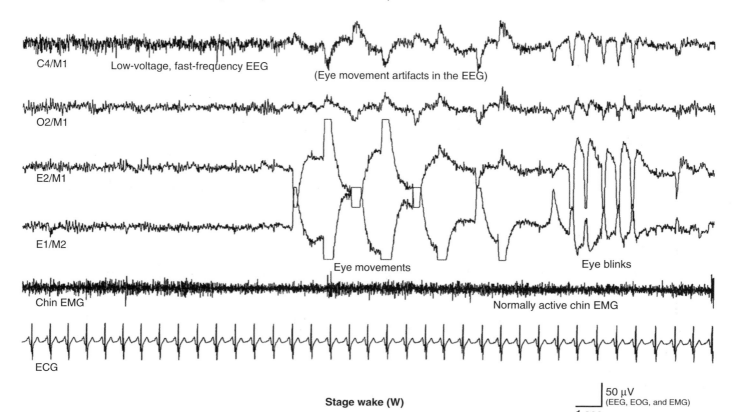

C4/M1   Low-voltage, fast-frequency EEG   (Eye movement artifacts in the EEG)

O2/M1

E2/M1

E1/M2

Eye movements   Eye blinks

Chin EMG   Normally active chin EMG

ECG

Stage wake (W)

50 μV
(EEG, EOG, and EMG)
1 sec

• **Figure 9.5** Stage wake (W), eyes open with eye movements. This is a sample obtained during a biocalibration routine. With the subject's eyes open, the electroencephalogram (EEG) is low in amplitude and relatively fast. The distinctive out-of-phase deflections in the electrooculogram (EOG) channels represent eye movements and eye blinks. The chin electromyogram (EMG) shows normal activity with variations in amplitude. (Reprinted with permission from Butkov N. *Atlas of Clinical Polysomnography.* 2nd ed. Medford, OR: Synapse Media; 2010.)

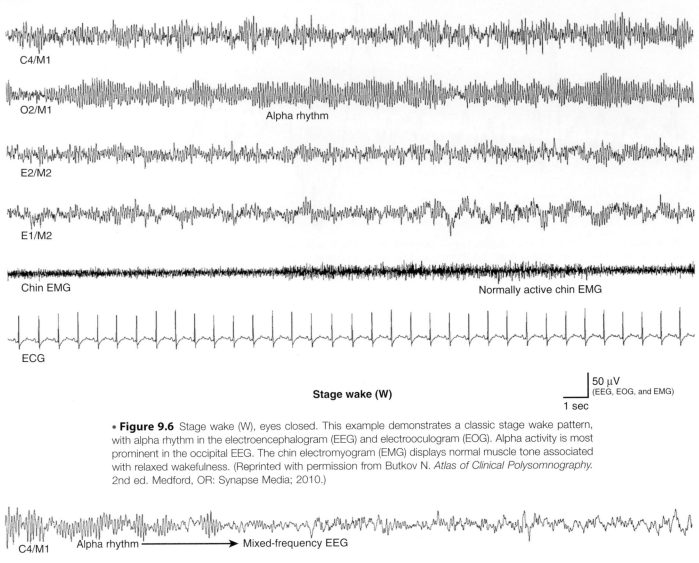

Stage wake (W)

50 µV
(EEG, EOG, and EMG)

1 sec

• **Figure 9.6** Stage wake (W), eyes closed. This example demonstrates a classic stage wake pattern, with alpha rhythm in the electroencephalogram (EEG) and electrooculogram (EOG). Alpha activity is most prominent in the occipital EEG. The chin electromyogram (EMG) displays normal muscle tone associated with relaxed wakefulness. (Reprinted with permission from Butkov N. *Atlas of Clinical Polysomnography.* 2nd ed. Medford, OR: Synapse Media; 2010.)

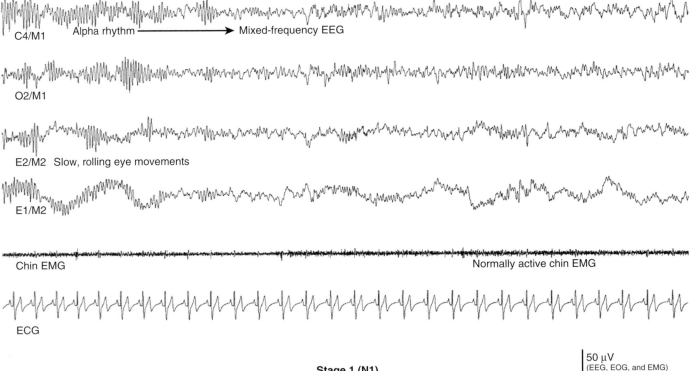

Stage 1 (N1)

50 µV
(EEG, EOG, and EMG)

1 sec

• **Figure 9.7** Stage 1 sleep (N1). In this sample, the onset of stage 1 sleep is clearly identified by the disappearance of alpha rhythm, which is replaced by a relatively low-voltage, mixed-frequency electro-encephalogram (EEG) with a predominance of theta activity. Note that the right electrooculogram (EOG; E2) electrode is referenced to M2. The slow eye movements may be detected better if the E2 electrode is referenced to the opposite mastoid (M1). (Reprinted with permission from Butkov N. *Atlas of Clinical Polysomnography.* 2nd ed. Medford, OR: Synapse Media; 2010.)

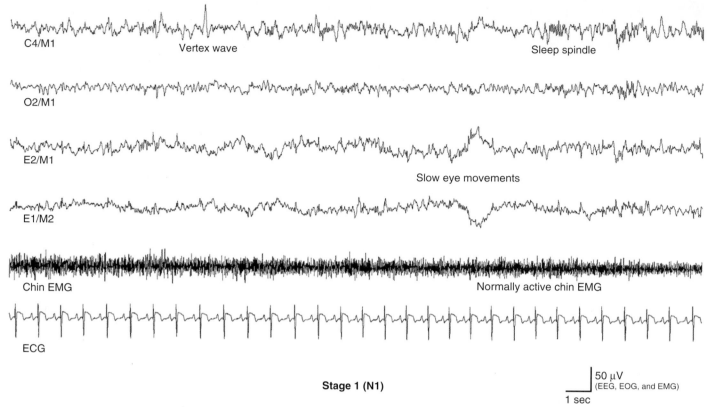

C4/M1   Vertex wave   Sleep spindle

O2/M1

E2/M1   Slow eye movements

E1/M2

Chin EMG   Normally active chin EMG

ECG

Stage 1 (N1)

50 μV
(EEG, EOG, and EMG)
1 sec

• **Figure 9.8** Stage 1 sleep (N1) transitioning to stage 2 (N2). This sample shows a continuation of stage 1 sleep, with the first prominent sleep spindle appearing in the last half of the epoch. In this example, stage 2 sleep would be scored in the following epoch. The small wave cluster appearing in the middle of the epoch could potentially be interpreted as a sleep spindle, although it is not quite as distinct as the spindles that follow. (Reprinted with permission from Butkov N. *Atlas of Clinical Polysomnography.* 2nd ed. Medford, OR: Synapse Media; 2010.)

Stage 2 (N2)

Stage 2 represents established NREM sleep. Stage 2 is identified by the presence of K-complexes or sleep spindles (or both) against a background of mixed-frequency EEG and an absence of sufficient high-amplitude slow wave activity to qualify for slow wave sleep (Fig. 9.9).

The R&K manual does not specify the exact starting point for scoring stage 2, whereas the AASM manual specifically defines the beginning of stage 2 (N2) to be when one or more K-complexes or sleep spindles appear on the first half of an epoch or on the last half of the preceding epoch.

Sleep spindles, K-complexes, or both do not need to appear on every epoch to continue scoring stage 2 sleep. The R&K manual had previously established a "three minute rule," whereby stage 2 can be scored for the duration of 3 min without K-complexes or sleep spindles. The AASM manual has discontinued this rule and recommends that stage N2 be interrupted only if the patient awakens, if an arousal occurs, or if the patient transitions to REM sleep or slow wave sleep. The AASM manual uses the term "non-arousal K-complex" to differentiate normally occurring K-complexes during stage 2 sleep from K-complexes associated with arousal.

Stages 3 and 4 (N3)

Stages 3 and 4 represent the deepest stages of sleep and are also described as slow wave sleep. The presence of high-amplitude slow waves with a frequency of 0.5–2 Hz and amplitudes greater than 75 μV identify both stages.

According to the R&K manual, stage 3 sleep is scored when at least 20% but not more than 50% of an epoch consists of slow waves meeting the aforementioned criteria (Fig. 9.10). Stage 4 sleep is scored when more than 50% of the epoch contains these high-amplitude slow waves (Fig. 9.11).

The AASM manual has combined stages 3 and 4 sleep and renamed them as stage N3. The AASM manual uses the same frequency and voltage criteria for scoring N3 as the R&K manual, but recommends using frontal EEG derivations F4/M1 or F3/M2 for measuring the slow waves.

Because of variations in slow wave morphology and the blending of faster and slower waves, which are often superimposed over one another, an *exact* measure of slow wave percentages meeting stage 3 or 4 criteria is often difficult to achieve. In many instances, scorers must use their judgment to decide how to score a particular epoch based on pattern recognition, rather than using precise measurements.

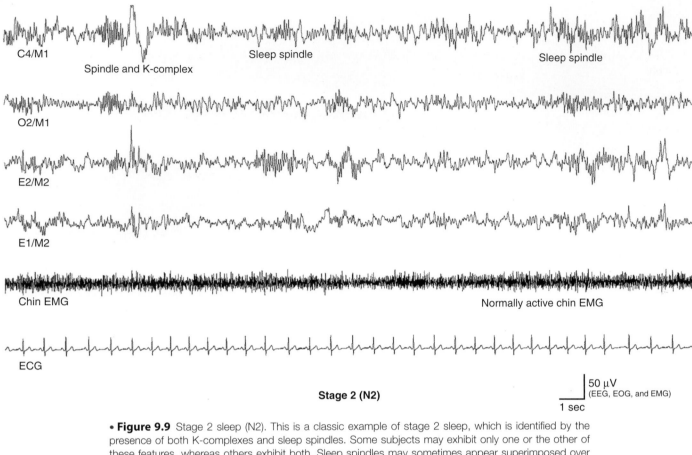

Stage 2 (N2)

50 µV
(EEG, EOG, and EMG)
1 sec

• **Figure 9.9** Stage 2 sleep (N2). This is a classic example of stage 2 sleep, which is identified by the presence of both K-complexes and sleep spindles. Some subjects may exhibit only one or the other of these features, whereas others exhibit both. Sleep spindles may sometimes appear superimposed over a K-complex or immediately precede or follow a K-complex. (Reprinted with permission from Butkov N. *Atlas of Clinical Polysomnography.* 2nd ed. Medford, OR: Synapse Media; 2010.)

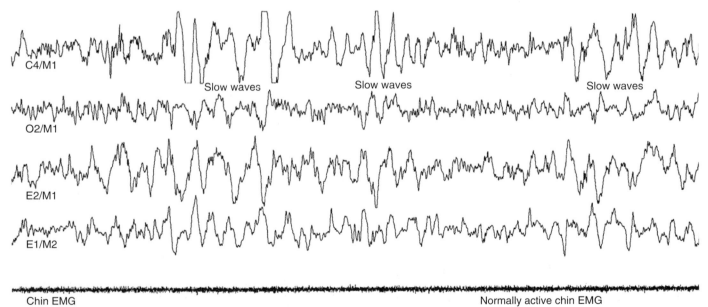

Stage 3 (N3)

50 µV
(EEG,EOG, and EMG)
1 sec

• **Figure 9.10** Stage 3 sleep (N3). The percentage of high-amplitude slow wave activity in this sample is greater than 20% of the epoch. To qualify for stage 3 (N3), the slow waves must have a frequency of 0.5–2 Hz and amplitudes greater than 75 µV. (Reprinted with permission from Butkov N. *Atlas of Clinical Polysomnography.* 2nd ed. Medford, OR: Synapse Media; 2010.)

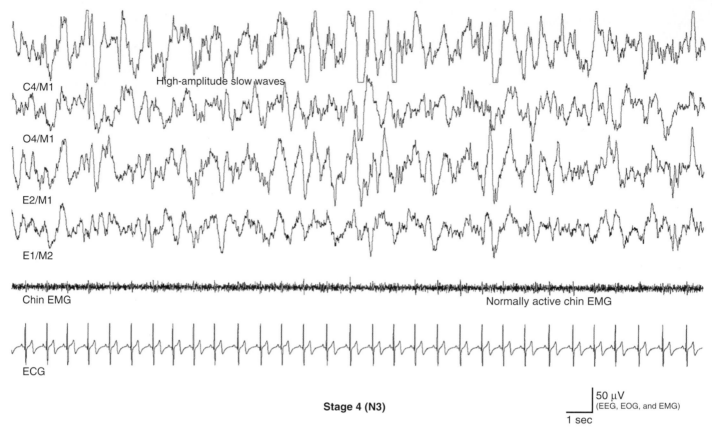

C4/M1

High-amplitude slow waves

O4/M1

E2/M1

E1/M2

Chin EMG

Normally active chin EMG

ECG

50 µV
(EEG, EOG, and EMG)

1 sec

Stage 4 (N3)

• **Figure 9.11** Stage 4 sleep (N3). In this example, high-amplitude slow waves occupy greater than 50% of the epoch and thus demonstrate deep slow wave sleep. This epoch is scored as stage 4 according to the Rechtschaffen and Kales criteria or as N3 according to the American Academy of Sleep Medicine criteria. (Reprinted with permission from Butkov N. *Atlas of Clinical Polysomnography.* 2nd ed. Medford, OR: Synapse Media; 2010.)

A recent addition to the AASM manual is a note stating that "pathological wave forms that meet the slow wave activity criteria, such as those generated by metabolic encephalopathies, epileptic, or epileptiform activity, are not counted as slow wave activity of sleep. Similarly, waveforms produced by artifact or those of non-cerebral origin should not be included in the scoring of slow waves." Readers should also note that artifacts in the EEG can stem from atypical eye movements during NREM sleep, which are more prominently seen in frontal EEG derivations.

Stage Rapid Eye Movement (R)

REM sleep is commonly described as paradoxical sleep and is characterized by a highly activated brain within a paralyzed body. According to both R&K and AASM criteria, REM sleep is identified by the combination of the following three conditions (Fig. 9.12):
1. The EEG returns to a relatively low-voltage, mixed-frequency pattern with cessation of sleep spindles, K-complexes, and high-amplitude slow waves.
2. The chin EMG falls to the lowest level of the recording.
3. The EOG channels demonstrate the presence of REMs.

Additional features of REM sleep, seen in many but not all subjects, include sawtooth EEG waves and phasic muscle twitches. Sawtooth waves are described by the AASM manual as "trains of sharply contoured or triangular, often serrated, 2–6 Hz waves maximal in amplitude over the central head regions and often, but not always, preceding a burst of rapid eye movements." Phasic muscle twitches are described as transient muscle activity consisting of "short irregular bursts of EMG activity usually with duration <0.25 seconds superimposed on low EMG tone." According to both R&K and the AASM, these additional features may be supportive, but not required, for identifying REM sleep.

Identifying the beginning and ending of stage REM is similar in both manuals. Once the requisite criteria for REM sleep (as listed previously) have been identified, the scorer can look back over the preceding epochs and begin scoring stage REM from the time when either the chin EMG falls to the lowest level or the last K-complex or sleep spindle is noted—whichever occurs last. The end of stage REM is identified when the chin EMG amplitude increases for greater than 50% of the epoch, when sleep spindles or K-complexes (or both) resume, or when the subject awakens.

The R&K and AASM manuals likewise have comparable recommendations for defining REM sleep continuity in the presence of K-complexes or sleep spindles. According to R&K, the presence

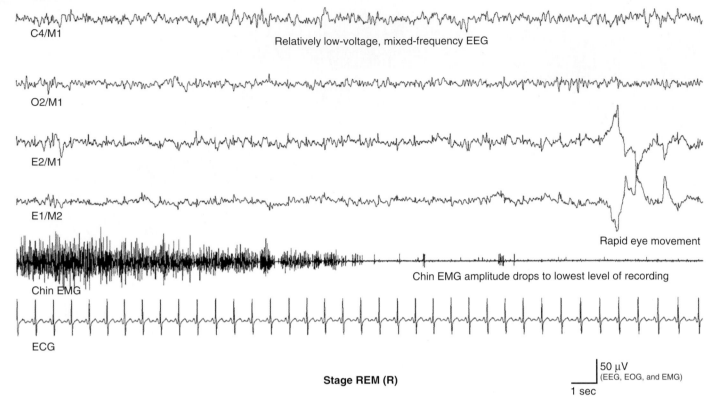

C4/M1

Relatively low-voltage, mixed-frequency EEG

O2/M1

E2/M1

E1/M2

Rapid eye movement

Chin EMG amplitude drops to lowest level of recording

Chin EMG

ECG

Stage REM (R)

50 µV
(EEG, EOG, and EMG)

1 sec

• **Figure 9.12** Stage REM (R). This sample shows a classic onset of rapid eye movement (REM) sleep with an abrupt drop in chin electromyogram (EMG) amplitude; relatively low-voltage, mixed-frequency electroencephalogram (EEG); and the appearance of rapid eye movements seen as out-of-phase deflections in the electrooculogram (EOG) channels. (Reprinted with permission from Butkov N. *Atlas of Clinical Polysomnography.* 2nd ed. Medford, OR: Synapse Media; 2010.)

of an isolated K-complex or sleep spindle does not interrupt the scoring of stage REM; however, if there are two K-complexes or sleep spindles without intervening REMs, then the interval between the K-complexes and/or sleep spindles is scored as stage 2. The AASM manual similarly recommends interrupting stage REM if an interval between two K-complexes or sleep spindles does not contain REMs, but to continue scoring uninterrupted stage REM if only one K-complex or sleep spindle occurs, followed by REMs on subsequent epochs.

The AASM manual is a bit confusing because it also states that stage REM should end if "one or more non-arousal associated K-complexes or sleep spindles are present in the first half of the epoch in the absence of rapid eye movements, even if the chin EMG tone remains low" (rule I.6e). However, this rule would presumably apply only if there were no REMs in subsequent epochs. As illustrated by the AASM figures, an isolated K-complex or sleep spindle should not interrupt stage REM, as long as the chin EMG remains low and REMs resume in subsequent epochs. This essentially reflects the original R&K recommendations of ignoring single isolated K-complexes and sleep spindles when scoring stage REM.

Commentary Regarding the Scoring of Stage Rapid Eye Movement

Identifying REM sleep is an essential part of accurately interpreting the PSG. This especially applies to scoring diagnostic and treatment studies of patients with obstructive sleep disordered breathing or sleep related hypoventilation, where in general REM sleep unveils the most severe symptoms. As noted earlier, various pathologies,

medications, and recording artifacts can significantly alter the appearance of the PSG, including the characteristic features of stage REM. Significant differences in stage REM can even be seen in normal subjects, particularly in younger individuals whose EEG patterns during REM sleep often include high amplitude slow and biphasic waves that are more typically seen during stages 2 or slow wave sleep in older individuals. In other instances, stage REM may closely resemble stage wake or stage 1 sleep. Optimal recordings of the chin EMG are especially critical in helping identify REM sleep; however, chin EMG recordings are susceptible to artifacts, and their overall integrity is greatly dependent on proper electrode application technique and high-caliber recording equipment. Other factors that may affect the scoring of REM are "pseudo-spindles" or other aberrations in the EEG as a result of medication use.

For these reasons, it is important to learn the characteristic signs of REM sleep and then apply them to uncharacteristic or abnormal sleep recordings. Both the R&K and the AASM manual attempt to cover the many contingencies encountered in scoring REM sleep; however, in actual practice, there are far more variables than can adequately be described by words or diagrams. In many instances, identifying REM sleep, and its beginning and ending, can only be adequately accomplished by viewing the patterns within the context of the recording

Movement Time

The R&K manual defines MT as an epoch that is obscured by movement artifact to such an extent that it becomes impossible to determine the sleep stage (Fig. 9.13). The MT score is used

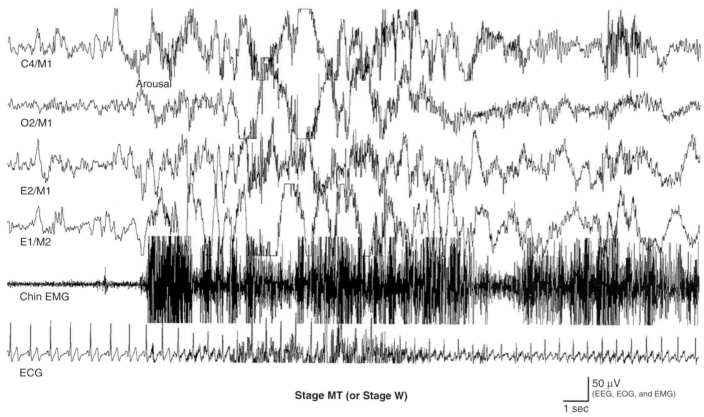

Stage MT (or Stage W)

50 μV
(EEG, EOG, and EMG)
1 sec

• **Figure 9.13** Movement time (MT). According to the Rechtschaffen and Kales scoring criteria, this epoch is scored as movement time (greater than 50% of the epoch is obscured by artifact and the epoch is preceded by sleep). According to the American Academy of Sleep Medicine manual, this epoch is scored as stage wake (W) based on the presence of alpha rhythm during the last portion of the epoch. (Reprinted with permission from Butkov N. *Atlas of Clinical Polysomnography*. 2nd ed. Medford, OR: Synapse Media; 2010.)

only when the preceding epoch is scored as sleep, and only when greater than 50% of the epoch is obscured by artifact.

The AASM manual has discontinued the use of the MT score and recommends that epochs obscured by artifact be scored the same as the succeeding epoch or as stage wake if any alpha rhythm is seen within the epoch. According to both manuals, epochs obscured by artifact that are preceded or followed by wakefulness are scored as stage wake.

Comparison of the Rechtschaffen and Kales and American Academy of Sleep Medicine Scoring Systems

As noted earlier, overall changes to the R&K manual recommended by the AASM have been relatively minor. However, a detailed comparison of the two scoring systems, published in the journal *Sleep*,[4] has suggested that some of the differences in scoring necessitate the establishment of new normative data for the AASM scoring method. According to the study, influences on total sleep time, sleep efficiency, and stage REM are minimal, but the distribution of NREM sleep stages and the calculation of wake after sleep onset (WASO) are affected by the AASM revisions.

Some of the differences are related to the use of frontal leads (Fig. 9.14), with subjects having borderline slow wave amplitudes recorded from the central EEG, potentially showing higher amplitudes when frontal EEG leads are used. However, the study notes that using frontal leads to identify K-complexes also results in scoring more NREM intrusions into REM sleep, thereby reducing total REM scores in younger subjects. The frontal lead discrepancy is further complicated by the suggestion of alternative bipolar derivations, which result in varying EEG amplitudes (Fig. 9.15). It is hoped that future revisions of the AASM scoring manual will address these concerns.

Arousal Scoring

The importance of identifying arousals and other forms of activation during sleep has gained widespread recognition since the early days of polysomnography. Elevated numbers of arousals have been linked to impaired daytime functioning, even when total sleep time appears to be unaffected.[5] The presence of frequent or cyclic arousals may be associated with increased upper airway resistance.[6] Arousals typically accompany the termination of obstructive respiratory events, but they can also be associated with other phenomena, such as periodic limb movements. Elevated numbers of arousal and other sleep-related disturbances are

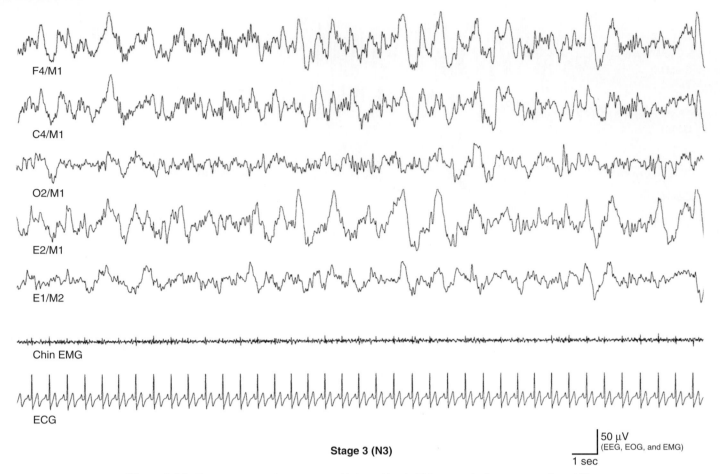

F4/M1

C4/M1

O2/M1

E2/M1

E1/M2

Chin EMG

ECG

50 μV
(EEG, EOG, and EMG)

1 sec

Stage 3 (N3)

• **Figure 9.14** Sleep stage–scoring montage with frontal leads. This example demonstrates the addition of frontal EEG as described by the American Academy of Sleep Medicine scoring manual. Scoring from frontal referential electroencephalographic derivations may increase percentages of slow wave sleep in some individuals, although overall differences between the C4/M1 and F4/M1 derivations are often minor. Note that the highest slow wave amplitudes are usually seen in the right EOG channel when referenced to the opposite mastoid. (Reprinted with permission from Butkov N. *Atlas of Clinical Polysomnography.* 2nd ed. Medford, OR: Synapse Media; 2010.)

also often seen in patients taking certain types of prescription medications. Arousals that do not appear to be associated with specific sleep-related events are commonly described as spontaneous arousals.

Although the term "arousal" implies awakening, in actuality, the subject often remains asleep during these events. In most instances the scored events are better described as partial arousals—or EEG activations—rather than awakenings. A number of different arousal-scoring definitions have been proposed, including a paper published in 1992 by the American Sleep Disorders Association (ASDA) (since renamed the American Academy of Sleep Medicine).[7]

The AASM scoring manual offers a brief definition of arousal based on the 1992 ASDA publication. The current criteria limit the definition of arousal to an abrupt shift in EEG frequency that includes alpha, theta, and/or frequencies above 16 Hz, but not spindles; lasts for at least 3 sec; and is preceded by at least 10 sec of sleep (Fig. 9.16). An arousal during REM sleep also requires a concurrent increase in the chin EMG lasting at least 1 sec (Fig. 9.17).

SLEEP STAGE DEFINITION SUMMARY

- **Stage wake (W)**—Relatively low-voltage, mixed-frequency electroencephalogram (EEG) with eye movements, eye blinks, and normally active chin electromyogram (EMG) or alpha rhythm, and normally active chin EMG.
- **Stage 1 (N1)**—Relatively low-voltage, mixed-frequency EEG (slower than during stage wake), slow rolling eye movements, and normally active chin EMG
- **Stage 2 (N2)**—The presence of K-complexes, sleep spindles, or both against a background of mixed-frequency EEG
- **Stage 3 (N3)**—Slow waves with frequencies of 0.5–2 Hz and amplitudes greater than 75 μV, occupying 20% or more of an epoch
- **Stage 4 (N3)**—Slow waves with frequencies of 0.5–2 Hz and amplitudes greater than 75 μV, occupying more than 50% of an epoch
- **Stage REM (R)**—Relatively low-voltage, mixed-frequency EEG, chin EMG falling to the lowest level of the recording, and the presence of rapid eye movements
- **Stage MT**—Greater than 50% of an epoch preceded by sleep and obscured by artifact (stage MT is not used by the AASM scoring manual)

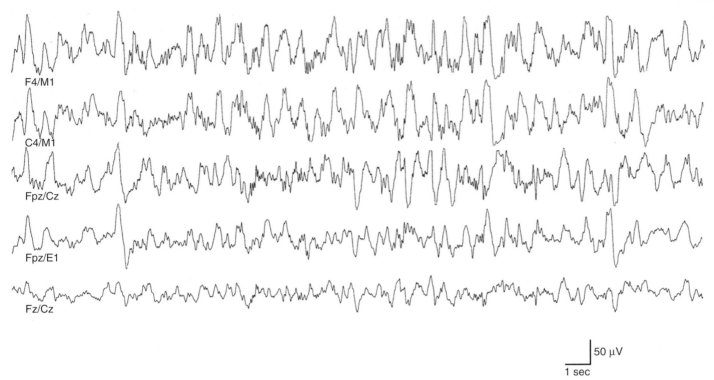

50 µV

1 sec

• **Figure 9.15** Electroencephalographic (EEG) derivation amplitude comparison. This example illustrates the problem of using alternative EEG derivations for sleep stage scoring. Each of the derivations yields different results. Note that the C4/M1 and F4/M1 referential derivations are the most similar in appearance, whereas the bipolar derivations are significantly attenuated. (Reprinted with permission from Butkov N. *Atlas of Clinical Polysomnography.* 2nd ed. Medford, OR: Synapse Media; 2010.)

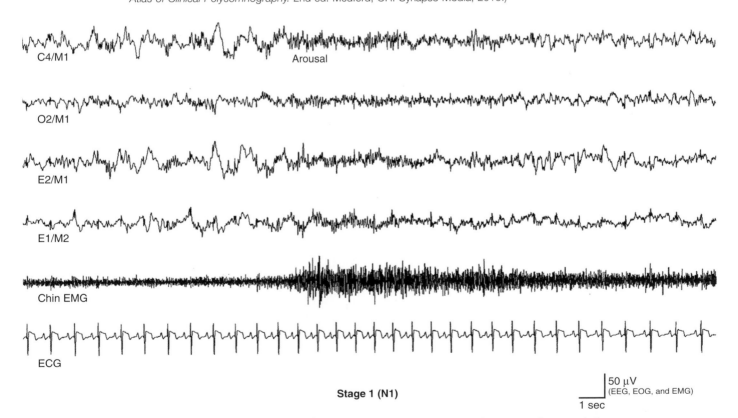

Stage 1 (N1)

50 µV
(EEG, EOG, and EMG)

1 sec

• **Figure 9.16** Arousal during nonrapid eye movement sleep. In this example an arousal occurs during the first half of the epoch, followed by a pattern that suggests return to stage 1 sleep. (Reprinted with permission from Butkov N. *Atlas of Clinical Polysomnography.* 2nd ed. Medford, OR: Synapse Media; 2010.)

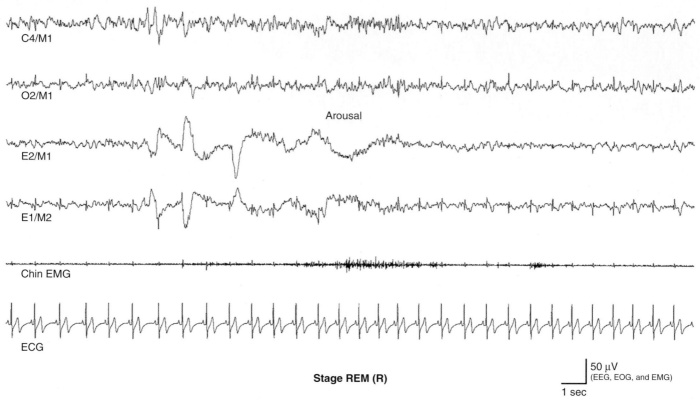

C4/M1

O2/M1

Arousal

E2/M1

E1/M2

Chin EMG

ECG

Stage REM (R)

50 µV
(EEG, EOG, and EMG)
1 sec

• **Figure 9.17** Arousal during rapid eye movement (REM) sleep. In this sample a brief arousal is seen during REM sleep. According to the American Academy of Sleep Medicine arousal-scoring criteria, an arousal during REM sleep requires an increase in chin EMG activity for at least 1 sec. (Reprinted with permission from Butkov N. *Atlas of Clinical Polysomnography.* 2nd ed. Medford, OR: Synapse Media; 2010.)

Other measures of arousal have been described, including the more intricate cyclic alternating pattern (CAP) scoring system developed by Terzano et al. in 1985,[8] which identifies a broader spectrum of EEG activations, including intermittent alpha rhythm, vertex wave or K-complex clusters, and delta bursts.

Changes in Sleep Stage with Arousals

A common question arises regarding the effects of arousals on sleep stage scoring.

The AASM manual states that if an arousal occurs during N2, the stage should be changed to N1 until a nonarousal K-complex or sleep spindle reoccurs. This differs from the 1992 ASDA recommendation, which states that an arousal can proceed to stage wake, or it can be followed by a lighter stage or by the same stage. The AASM manual applies similar guidelines to REM sleep, except that a brief arousal during stage REM does not alter the REM score unless followed by slow eye movements and other characteristics of N1 sleep.

Atypical Arousals and Other Forms of Activation

Although the AASM/ASDA criteria for scoring arousals help quantify certain types of sleep disturbances, they do not address other forms of activation commonly seen in sleep studies. For example, younger patients often exhibit abrupt shifts to *slower* frequencies as an arousal response; these shifts appear in the form of paroxysmal K-complex bursts or slow wave clusters (Fig. 9.18). The significance of these events is not yet fully understood, but their presence often helps the reader of the study establish a connection with respiratory disturbances, periodic limb movements, and other sleep-related events.

American Academy of Sleep Medicine Manual Technical Specifications

The AASM scoring manual includes technical specifications for the visual scoring of sleep and associated events. These specifications are described in the following sections, with explanation and commentary.

Impedance Measurements

The AASM scoring manual specifies that the maximum electrode impedance be 5 kΩ. The manual specifies that individual electrode impedances should be measured against a reference (the latter may be the sum of all other applied electrodes).

Impedance is defined as a combined measure of resistance and reactance (reactance can be inductive, capacitive, or a combination

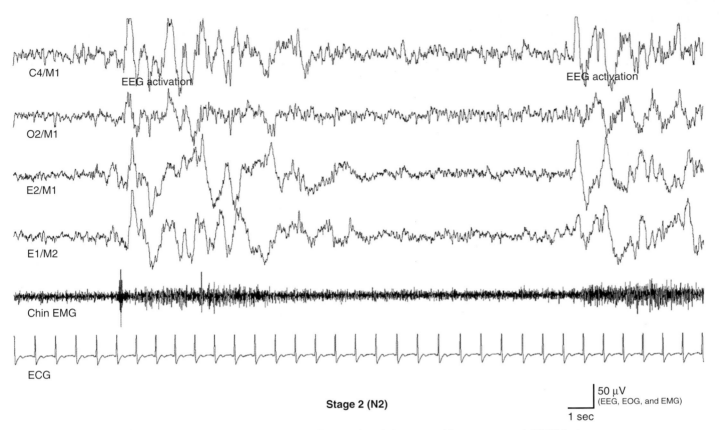

C4/M1

EEG activation

EEG activation

O2/M1

E2/M1

E1/M2

Chin EMG

ECG

Stage 2 (N2)

50 μV
(EEG, EOG, and EMG)

1 sec

• **Figure 9.18** Electroencephalogram (EEG) activation during nonrapid eye movement (NREM) sleep. This sample shows a pattern of slow wave clusters during NREM sleep accompanied by increases in chin EMG amplitude. Although these patterns do not meet the American Academy of Sleep Medicine arousal-scoring criteria, they are noteworthy because they represent a form of sleep disturbance. According to the cyclic alternating pattern definitions, these patterns are described as phase A1 delta bursts. EEG activations consisting of K-complex clusters or delta bursts are often seen in younger patients with obstructive sleep-disordered breathing instead of shifts to faster frequencies, which are more commonly seen in older patients. (Reprinted with permission from Butkov N. *Atlas of Clinical Polysomnography*. 2nd ed. Medford, OR: Synapse Media; 2010.)

of both). Electrode impedance values can be read by using a handheld alternating current (AC) impedance meter connected to the electrode jack box, or be obtained directly from the recording system. However, some recording systems provide imbalance readings only between pairs of electrodes, which are not the same as individual electrode impedance measurements.

Bit Resolution

The AASM manual specifies a minimum digital resolution of 12 bits per sample.

Bit resolution refers to the number of binary units (bits) used to represent the numeric value of each sampled interval during analog-to-digital conversion. Bit resolution determines the amplitude resolution of a digital recording. In general, contemporary digital PSG systems have the capability of 16-bit resolution; however, some systems have selectable bit resolution, which should be verified before starting a recording.

Sampling Rates

The AASM recommendations for minimal and desirable sampling rates are as follows.

Channel	Minimal Rate (Hz)	Desirable Rate (Hz)
EEG, EOG, EMG, ECG, and snoring	200	500
Respiratory airflow and effort	25	100
Oximetry	10	25
Body position	1	1

ECG, Electrocardiogram; *EEG*, electroencephalogram; *EMG*, electromyogram; *EOG*, electrooculogram.

Sampling rate refers to the number of sampled intervals obtained in the span of 1 sec by the analog-to-digital converter. The sampling rate determines the frequency resolution of a digital recording. Reconstruction of a digitized waveform follows the Nyquist theorem, which states that the sampling rate must be twice the rate of the highest frequency sampled to obtain basic frequency resolution. Higher sampling rates are necessary to obtain an adequate graphic representation of the analog signals; therefore sampling rates of 5–10 times the Nyquist rate are commonly used.

Using higher sampling rates was problematic in the past because of slow processing speeds and limited data storage capacity. Present-day computer processing and storage capabilities are better suited for faster sampling rates; however, even contemporary systems have practical limitations if excessively high sampling rates are applied to multiple channels. In clinical practice, in general, sampling rates of 200 Hz per channel are adequate for most PSG recordings.

Filter Settings

The AASM recommendations for low- and high-frequency filter settings are as follows.

Channel	Low-Frequency Filter (Hz)	High-Frequency Filter (Hz)
EEG and EOG	0.3	35
EMG and snoring	10	100
ECG	0.3	70
Nasal pressure	DC or ≤0.03	100
Positive airway pressure (PAP) Flow	DC	DC
Thermal flow and respiratory effort belt signals	0.1	15

ECG, Electrocardiogram; *EEG*, electroencephalogram; *EMG*, electromyogram; *EOG*, electrooculogram.

Low- and high-frequency filters are used to minimize signal interference by attenuating or removing undesirable frequencies outside the selected bandwidth for each channel. Contemporary digital equipment may include a broader range of filter-setting options than previously available. For example, the low-frequency filter settings for the respiratory channels may be set below 0.1 Hz on some systems. This can be advantageous for demonstrating the flattening effect of airflow waveforms seen with flow limitation.

Filter Design

The AASM recommends a filter design that functionally replicates conventional analog-style frequency-response curves.

Digital filters can be designed to replicate conventional frequency-response curves, or they can be made to produce a more radical effect on the signal by essentially removing all frequencies outside the range of the selected bandwidth. The latter design is problematic in that it can mask poor signal quality. When filters are used to eliminate the possibility of any signal interference, the operator of the system can no longer determine whether the recorded signals represent physiologic activity or a narrow bandwidth of artifact. Conventional filter frequency-response curves allow sufficient attenuation of undesirable frequencies, but if signal degradation occurs, the distinct presence of artifact alerts the operator that a problem exists.

50/60-Hz Filter Controls

The AASM recommends a separate 50/60-Hz filter control for each channel.

50- or 60-Hz filters are used to reduce or eliminate line frequency interference (60-Hz line frequency is used in the United States, Canada, and many South American countries; most European and Australasian countries use 50-Hz line frequency). Under normal circumstances, these filters should not be used because they can potentially mask a poor-quality signal. The availability of separate filter controls for each channel allows the operator to use these filters selectively and only when necessary. Most commonly, 50- or 60-Hz filters are used in leg EMG recordings, which tend to be more susceptible to line frequency interference.

Calibration

The AASM manual specifies the use of a standard negative 50-μV DC calibration signal for all channels to demonstrate polarity, amplitude, and time constant settings for each recorded parameter.

A calibration signal generated by the recording system is an essential feature for confirming and documenting the instrument settings for each channel. The AASM manual does not provide actual specifications for polarity, amplitude, and time constant values. Historically, PSGs have been recorded according to the EEG polarity convention, whereby a negative voltage produces an upward deflection. Signal amplitudes are determined by individual channel sensitivity settings. The EEG, EOG, and EMG channels are typically adjusted to produce 1-cm deflection in response to a 50-μV signal (some laboratories routinely use 70 μV/cm). For pediatric studies, a calibration of 100 μV/cm is typically used for the EEG and EOG. Time constant refers to the duration of the calibration wave, which is determined by the settings of the high- and low-frequency filters. Actual time constant values can vary depending on equipment design. The purpose of evaluating the time constant is to confirm correct filter settings and appropriate signal responses in each channel.

Polysomnogram Display

The AASM recommends that the recording system provide the capability of retaining and viewing the data in the way in which it was recorded by the attending technologist, as well as in the same manner in which it was scored by the scoring technologist.

Most contemporary digital systems provide the capability of developing a customized work space that can be replicated at each work station. In addition, any changes or annotations made by the recording or scoring technologists should be made available to the reading physician.

Computer Monitor Resolution

The AASM recommends a monitor resolution of at least 1600 × 1200 for displaying and scoring raw PSG data.

Most high-end computer monitors provide the capability of 1600 × 1200 screen resolution; however, the resolution setting must be confirmed within the system software.

Histogram

The AASM recommends the generation of a histogram that includes sleep stages, respiratory events, leg movements, O_2 saturation, and arousals.

In general, histogram options are included with digital PSG software.

Time Scales

The AASM recommends having the ability to choose time scales, ranging from 5 sec per screen to an entire study on the screen.

The standard time scale for scoring sleep stages is 30 sec per screen. The ability to compress the time scale is useful for evaluating respiratory patterns. Expanding the time scale may be useful for examining the ECG or for resolving fast-frequency EEG waves.

Video Recording

The AASM recommends the capability of recording video data synchronized with the PSG, with an accuracy of at least one video frame per second.

In general, synchronized video capabilities are provided by the equipment manufacturers.

Documentation of Scoring Mode

The AASM recommends that the recording system provide the capability of identifying whether sleep stage scoring was performed visually or computed by the system.

To date, the use of automated sleep stage scoring has not been validated.

Optional Features

The AASM scoring manual lists several additional optional features that largely pertain to screen navigation and software functions.

The use of computers in polysomnography has opened the door to many new possibilities for processing, displaying, manipulating, and tabulating physiologic data. Although some of these features are useful, many are superfluous, and some are clearly inappropriate. It is essential that sleep professionals fully understand the purpose, function, and consequence of every new option or feature presented to them.

Practical Considerations for Sleep Stage Scoring

The most important concept in scoring sleep stages (as well as sleep-related events) is to learn to see the "bigger picture." Instead of focusing on individual waveforms, the scorer must learn to visually scan the data, identify stereotypical patterns, and interpret the patterns within the context of the recording. Like any pattern recognition skill, this takes time and practice. It is essential to apply rigorous standards to the electrode and sensor application process, and to the integrity of the recording equipment, in order to ensure accurate and detailed PSG data.

As noted earlier, individual PSG patterns vary widely. The record samples shown in this chapter demonstrate classic sleep stage patterns, as typically described by textbooks and scoring manuals. In actual practice, the appearance of the EEG and other PSG parameters can be significantly altered by medications, by various pathologies, and by recording artifacts. Common aberrations include alpha sleep, absence of alpha during wakefulness, increased beta activity and pseudo-spindles, exaggerated theta activity, generalized slowing of the EEG, atypical eye movements during NREM sleep, increased motor activity during REM sleep, disorganized sleep-wake EEG, and various other forms of sleep stage dissociation. The high incidence of these phenomena emphasize the fact that PSG scoring cannot be confined to a set of rigid scoring rules but must include a certain degree of clinical judgment and common sense.

A fundamental challenge of a rule-based scoring manual is the daunting task of attempting to describe every possible deviation and confounding artifact that can be found in a clinical sleep study. In many instances, these variations cannot be adequately described by words or diagrams; they actually have to be seen to be appreciated. While a scoring manual serves well as a basic learning tool, the reader should make every attempt to further refine his or her skills through systematic practice and experience. Sleep stage scoring need not be excessively tedious or time-consuming, nor should it be done in a robotic manner that focuses on minutia but overlooks the obvious. Experienced scorers are able to recognize signature patterns indicative of pathology, atypical sleep architecture, medication effects, and so on just by visually scanning the data. Those who are less familiar with the process have often attempted to oversimplify and automate the practice, to the detriment of data accuracy and detail. Readers are encouraged to study all aspects of the recording process, correlate it with our existing knowledge of sleep physiology, and master the art of visually recognizing and interpreting the countless nuances found within the PSG.

Suggested Reading

Berry RB, Brooks R, Gamaldo CE, et al. *The AASM Manual for the Scoring of Sleep and Associated Events: Rules, Terminology and Technical Specifications, Version 2.0.* Darian, IL: American Academy of Sleep Medicine; 2014. www.aasmnet.org.

Butkov N. *Atlas of Clinical Polysomnography.* 2nd ed. Medford, OR: Synapse Media; 2010.

Iber C, Ancoli-Israel S, Chesson AL, Quan SF. *The AASM Manual for the Scoring of Sleep and Associated Events: Rules, Terminology and Technical Specifications.* Westchester, IL: American Academy of Sleep Medicine; 2007.

Rechtschaffen A, Kales A, eds. *A Manual of Standardized Terminology, Techniques and Scoring System for Sleep Stages of Human Subjects.* Bethesda, MD: U.S. National Institute of Neurological Diseases and Blindness, Neurological Information Network; 1968.

Silber MH, Ancoli-Israel S, Bonnet MH, et al. The visual scoring of sleep in adults. *J Clin Sleep Med.* 2007;3(2):121-129.

10

Sleep Deprivation

SIGRID C. VEASEY

- **Definition:** Sleep deprivation may be defined as any condition of insufficient sleep, whether acute or chronic, total, or partial.
- **Consequences:** Neurobehavioral and peripheral physiologic effects of sleep loss vary with duration and across species. In all species, however, the severity of neurobehavioral impairment following sleep deprivation varies with intensity of homeostatic drive, circadian time, and overall brain health.
- **Evidence:** Studies in both humans and laboratory animals have unveiled the importance of obtaining sufficient sleep by demonstrating important effects on brain health, immune function, and metabolic function.
  - Acute total sleep loss (1 night) results in lapses in attention, disturbed executive function, impaired newly learned skills, poor mood in healthy individuals, and temporarily improved mood in some depressed individuals.
  - Chronic partial sleep deprivation is highly prevalent, particularly in developed countries. Significantly, chronic short sleep in humans is an important risk factor for fatal motor vehicle accidents and several morbid conditions, including cardiovascular disease, obesity, diabetes, and particular cancers.

Epidemiology

- The Institute of Medicine has declared sleep deprivation from either insufficient sleep time or sleep disorders an unmet significant public health problem.
- It is estimated that 50–70 million Americans chronically suffer from inadequate sleep and that hundreds of billions of dollars are spent annually in the United States alone for health care visits and medications related to inadequate sleep and sleep disorders.
- The National Institutes of Health recommends that school-age children obtain at least 10 hours of sleep, teenagers at least 9, and adults at least 7 hours regularly. In the United States more

than 30% of adults do not obtain 7 hours of sleep regularly across the work week.[1]
- A nationwide survey performed by the Centers for Disease Control in 2009 revealed that more than a third of adults (18 years and older) reported falling asleep unintentionally at least once in the past month prior to the survey and greater than 2% of adults admitted to falling asleep while driving in the past month.
- Sleepiness and fatigue is implicated as a key risk factor in over half of all fatal crashes involving trucks.
While a majority of individuals are at risk of sleep deprivation at various times across their lives, several groups have heightened risk for chronic insufficient sleep.
- Adolescents, particularly those with computers, phones, and televisions in the bedroom and those with high school load and extracurricular activities.
- Shift workers for rotating, night, and early morning shifts.
- Individuals performing multiple jobs for greater than 40 hours/week.
- Individuals with long commutes (>1 hour each way).
- Individuals regularly using alcohol, stimulants, including caffeine, or medications and illicit drugs that interfere with sleep.
- Individuals exposed to increased environmental noise and/or light.
- Individuals with psychiatric illnesses or conditions disturbing sleep.
- Individuals with medical conditions that disrupt sleep, including chronic respiratory conditions, heart failure, sleep apnea, and restless legs syndrome.

Sleep Loss Studies in Animal Models

- Early data: A series of total sleep deprivation studies in rats across weeks was led by Alan Rechtschaffen in the 1980s. In these studies, rats were prompted to walk along a rotating platform every time the animal's electrography suggested sleep.[2]
  - Control animals were exposed to a similar environment but allowed to sleep for the majority of the experiment and effectively had almost 80% of their normal 24 hour/day sleep time, while the sleep-deprived animals had <10% sleep consecutively over days and weeks.
  - Most of the effects observed in sleep-deprived animals were related to peripheral metabolism and immune function. Remarkably, very few findings were evident in the brain. Specifically, animals lost tremendous amounts of weight,

despite eating more than control animals, and sleep-deprived rats showed skin lesions, and bacterial infections, while brains showed no evidence overall of neuron loss.

- A summary of the effects of sleep deprivation in these animal studies is presented in Table 10.1.
- More recent studies in adult animals suggest that there may be important effects of sleep deprivation on both neuron survival and memory.
  - For example, 1 week of shift work extended wake periods in the adult mouse results in a loss of locus coeruleus neurons, and long-term sleep deprivation impairs hippocampal-dependent memory in the adult rat.[3]
  - Both locus coeruleus and cognitive studies found increased tumor necrosis factor-alpha upregulated by chronic sleep loss, suggesting that sleep loss can be proinflammatory.[4]
- Sleep deprivation can also have important negative and lasting effects on brain development in young animals.
  - Several studies in both mammals and invertebrates demonstrate lasting effects of early life sleep loss. Specifically, during a critical period of development in the cat, occluding vision in one eye remodels circuits to optimize ocular dominance, but only if the animals are allowed sleep, where rapid eye movement (REM) sleep was critical for this ocular dominance.[5]
  - Kittens deprived of REM sleep across this critical time never developed plasticity and adaption for improved vision. In the fruit fly, where specific sleep stages have not been characterized, early life sleep loss has lasting effects on impairing courtship behavior.

Sleep Loss in Humans

- Sleep loss in humans is typically distinguished as partial sleep loss, total sleep loss, REM sleep, or nonrapid eye movement (NREM) sleep selective deprivation and sleep fragmentation.

TABLE 10.1	Physiologic Effects of Sleep Loss in the Rat	
Increased energy expenditure	Increased thyroxine and norepinephrine
Initially increased and then reduced body temperature	Weight loss
Infection, ultimately bacteremia and sepsis	Hair loss, ulcerative, and hyperkeratotic skin changes
Death after 11–22 days	If allowed to recover midway, a large REM sleep rebound was observed.

- Sleep homeostasis varies across these types of sleep deprivation, yet with all of these sleep loss conditions, there are important predictable findings. Across continued sleep loss, the pressure to sleep builds (sleep homeostasis), and the likelihood of temporarily shifting into sleep becomes more likely (wake state instability).
- Sustained tasks therefore are difficult to continue to do well, particularly sedentary tasks requiring little more than paying attention (e.g., driving long stretches of straight highways). Circadian timing also contributes to overall alertness, and thus the time of day across sleep loss can have significant effects on alertness.
- Consider Fig. 10.1. If an individual is regularly sleeping from 10 PM until 6 AM, homeostatic drive (process S, *red*) is greatest just at bedtime, and process S declines all across sleep and is lowest at 6 AM.[6]
- Across the daytime, process S slowly builds with daytime waking. With no sleep debt, there is a beautifully balanced circadian wakefulness (process C, *green*) and process S, so that alertness is remarkably stable across the day, even after a healthy lunch, so that there should not be a postprandial dip in alertness with adequate sleep.
- Now imagine staying up all night. Process S would continue to steadily rise, while process C would not be affected. Thus the gradient between the pressure to sleep and circadian wakefulness becomes greater and greater.
- Imagine also the condition of chronic short sleep, going to sleep at midnight but still waking at 6 AM. Process S would be far higher at 12 AM and would fall with sleep but be higher than each C below so that the next day there will be at all time points higher process S relative to C and thus sleepiness and sleep-wake instability.
- Chronic sleep restriction reduces the metabolic rate of the frontal cortices, while increasing activity in the default regions in the brain during quiet wakefulness. Intriguingly, during mental tasks relevant brain regions may show *increased* activation, possibly representing a short-term compensatory mechanism.

Effects of Sleep Loss on Attention

- The most reliable indicator of sleepiness-impaired performance is a measure of sustained attention to a simple task, called the psychomotor vigilance test.[3] This test measures an individual's reaction time and accuracy in detecting random numbers shown on a computer screen in a small box, as below in Fig. 10.2.
- Progressively across chronic partial sleep deprivation (obtaining ≤7 hours sleep/night), there is a steady decline in performance, with more lapses, more false responses, and slowed responses, especially across the duration of the test.[7]

SC   SC   SC   SC   SC   SC   Sc   Sc   Sc   Sc   Sc   SC
08 AM 10 AM 12 PM 02 PM 04 PM 06 PM 08 PM 10 PM 12 AM 02 AM 04 AM 06 AM

- **Figure 10.1** Homeostatic and circadian influences on sleep, wakefulness, and alertness behaviors. Across a 24-hour period, a balance of homeostatic sleep drive (process S, *red S*) and circadian (process C, *green C*) governs sleep and wake propensities. When well rested and regularly waking an hour or so after dawn, both circadian and homeostatic influences are low. Across the day, sleep homeostasis builds but is balanced perfectly by increases in circadian alertness. Just after sunset, circadian influences may start to wane, while sleep homeostasis continues to build as long as one is awake. The high process S and low process C are ideal for sleep. Across sleep, process S declines, as does process C, so that sleep continues until dawn and the process is repeated.

Psychomotor vigilance test:
performance across chronic short sleep

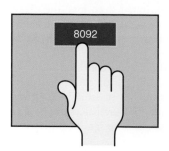

- More lapses
- More false responses
- Slower responses
- Instability of performance
- Delayed recovery (>3 days)
- Circadian variation in performance

• **Figure 10.2** The psychomotor vigilance test as an index of vigilance stability. *Left,* a schematic of the test screen in which numbers appear in the *darker blue* screen and the subject must respond simply by touching a screen or button. Sleep-deprived individuals may start out performing well with this test. However, as the test goes on, these subjects will experience more lapses, delays in response, and even more false starts. Because sleepiness is dictated by both sleep homeostatic and circadian influences, performance with this test is also very sensitive to circadian time of day.

- Remarkably, even after 3 nights of 9 hours time in bed, the reaction times in subjects that are sleep restricted do not return to normal, suggesting delayed recovery beyond sleep homeostasis.
- When vigilance fully returns is not presently known. Significantly, across chronic sleep deprivation, subjects begin to progressively underestimate their sleepiness and impairment.
- In addition to impaired attention or vigilance, numerous studies have consistently shown that mood is negatively impacted by sleep deprivation in healthy humans, while acute sleep deprivation in depressed individuals may improve mood on a short-term basis.
- Beyond mood, extended periods of sleep deprivation may also disturb the ability to integrate information and make complex decisions, and may also increase anxiety and pain thresholds, and impair motor skills, particularly if newly learned skills.[8]
- Metabolic activity in the brain declines upon long-term sleep deprivation, particularly in the cortices, as shown in Fig. 10.3.[9]
- Neurobehavioral effects of sleep deprivation in humans are summarized in Table 10.2, stratified to healthy adults and adults with psychiatric comorbidities.

Sleep Fragmentation

- It is evident that brief arousals across sleep while obtaining the same total sleep time also cause sleepiness and impaired vigilance. The frequency of arousals has important effects on sleepiness and performance.
- Arousals every 20 min have minimal effects in young adult humans, while arousals once per minute cause similar effect of total sleep deprivation for the same duration on sleepiness. Sleep fragmentation acutely in healthy humans can increase insulin resistance.

Physiologic Effects of Sleep Deprivation

- A large collection of studies in both animals and humans provides evidence of metabolic dysregulation in response to sleep loss.[5,6] Most effects are similar for both acute (1 night) and chronic

TABLE 10.2	Neurobehavioral Effects of Sleep Deprivation in Humans	
Healthy Adults	**Adults with Psychiatric Conditions or Predispositions**
Mood changes: irritability, lack of interest, decreased motivation	Acute sleep loss: improvement in depression; Chronic sleep loss: worsening
Poor motor learning of new skills	Anxiety
Cognitive inflexibility, complex reasoning	Mania
Accident prone	Paranoid delusions
Visual hallucinations (if prolonged sleep loss)	Auditory hallucinations (if schizophrenic disorder)

TABLE 10.3	Physiologic Effects of Sleep Loss in Humans	
Acute	**Chronic**
↓ growth hormone	↓ growth hormone
↑ leptin, increased hunger	↑ leptin, increased hunger
↑ cytokines: TNF-α and IL-1β	cytokines: TNF-α and IL-1β
↓ insulin sensitivity	↓ insulin sensitivity
↑ metabolic rate	↓ metabolic rate
↓ seizure threshold	—

(over at least several consecutive days), as highlighted in Table 10.3.
- Metabolic rate may increase with acute sleep loss and then decline by the second night and onward. Note this is in significant contrast with the Rechtschaffen rat studies, which found a progressive increase in metabolic rate.
- Whether this difference is species specific or related to the type of sleep deprivation is not known. *There are several hormones that are not significant in humans across sleep deprivation, including cortisol and melatonin, providing light exposures do not change.*
- Sleep deprivation is a powerful stimulus for specific types of seizures, especially in children with juvenile myoclonic epilepsy and grand mal seizures. Significantly, treating sleep disorders and increasing sleep time can reduce seizure frequency.

Conclusions

- Rat studies show substantial peripheral effects of sleep loss on metabolism, infection, and endocrinologic function.
- Circadian and homeostatic influences contribute to sleep loss effects on cognitive performance.
- Recently there has a paradigmal shift in appreciation of the neurobehavioral and metabolic consequences of chronic insufficient sleep.
- Chronic sleep loss and/or chronic sleep disruption can have lasting effects on cognition and neuronal function and survival.

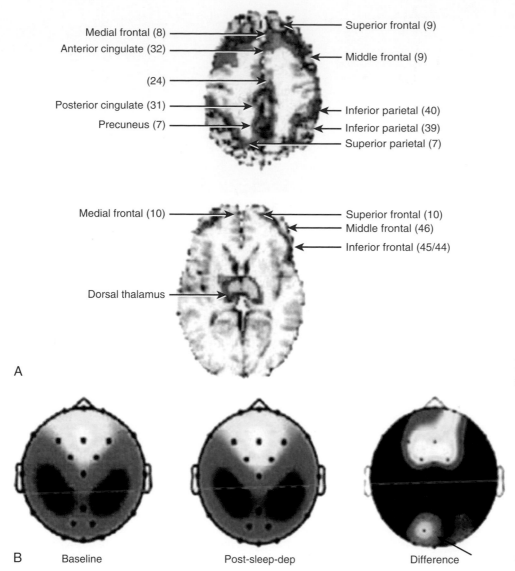

• **Figure 10.3** Metabolic and slow wave electroencephalographic responses to acute total sleep deprivation for 24 hours in healthy young adults. **A,** Images show regions identified by 18s FDG-PET scan imaging evidencing reductions in metabolic rate. Regions with color on a scale from *blue* to *yellow* show moderate to pronounced reductions in glucose uptake. Fronto-parietal cortices and thalamus show the largest reductions in glucose uptake after sleep deprivation. **B,** An electroencephalographic correlate shows increases in slow wave activity within the frontal and cingulate cortices with reductions in the occipital cortex. (From Nofzinger EA. Neuroimaging and sleep medicine. *Sleep Med Rev.* 2005;9[3]:157–172.)

• Future studies are needed in humans to determine the extent of reversibility and the extent of lasting neurobehavioral impairment.

Suggested Reading

Covassin N, Singh P. Sleep duration and cardiovascular disease risk: epidemiologic and experimental evidence. *Sleep Med Clin.* 2016;11(1):81-89.

Durmer JS, Dinges DF. Neurocognitive consequences of sleep deprivation. *Semin Neurol.* 2005;25(1):117-129.

Hirotsu C, Tufik S, Andersen ML. Interactions between sleep, stress, and metabolism: from physiological to pathological conditions. *Sleep Sci.* 2015;8(3):143-152.

McEwen BS, Karatsoreos IN. Sleep deprivation and circadian disruption: stress, allostasis, and allostatic load. *Sleep Med Clin.* 2015;10(1):1-10.

Owens J. Adolescent sleep working group; committee on adolescence. Insufficient sleep in adolescents and young adults: an update on causes and consequences. *Pediatrics.* 2014;134(3):e921-e932.

11

The Insomnias

DAVID N. NEUBAUER

Introduction and Definitions

- **Definitions**: Insomnia is a common clinical problem that for many individuals is a diagnosable disorder. Fundamentally insomnia represents dissatisfaction with sleep characterized by difficulty initiating or maintaining sleep; however, the addition of daytime distress or impairment presumably related to the sleep disturbance allows patients to meet criteria for insomnia disorders.
- **Insomnia as a public health problem**: Insomnia is a significant public health problem due to its high prevalence, chronicity, association with risks and consequences, societal economic burden, and treatment challenges. Insomnia is the most common type of sleep disorder in the general population.
- **Comorbid insomnia**: It may occur independently or exist with comorbid disorders, including psychiatric, medical, and other sleep disorders. The considerable overlap with psychiatric illness, especially mood and anxiety disorders, warrants special attention.
- This chapter addresses the evaluation and management of insomnia based on two key resources that provide comprehensive information representing current perspectives regarding insomnia disorders.
  - *International Classification of Sleep Disorders, 3rd ed*[1] (ICSD-3) published by the American Academy of Sleep Medicine (AASM) in 2014
  - "Clinical Guideline for Evaluation and Management of Chronic Insomnia in Adults"[2] (Clinical Guideline) published by the AASM in 2008

Insomnia Evaluation

- Overview
  - The AASM Clinical Guideline offers a general discussion as well as specific recommendations regarding the evaluation of patients presenting with chronic insomnia. The key elements of the evaluation of insomnia are offered in this section.
  - As with other clinical complaints, the evaluation of insomnia rests upon a careful and detailed history, along with physical and mental status examinations. While focusing on sleep-related details, the history should also assess potential comorbid conditions and the use of medications and other substances.
  - The major components of the sleep history are the primary insomnia complaint, presleep conditions, sleep-wake schedule, nocturnal symptoms, and daytime activities and function (Table 11.1). In addition, the insomnia evaluation may involve a review of subjective and objective supporting information.
- **Insomnia complaint**: The primary insomnia complaint should be characterized in terms of the pattern of sleep disturbance, duration of symptoms, frequency of sleep difficulty, severity of nighttime insomnia, daytime effects, and the course of the sleep disturbance over time.
  - The insomnia pattern may include difficulty falling asleep, remaining asleep, awakening excessively early, or a combination of these.
  - The duration of symptoms may range from days to decades.
  - The frequency may be nightly, occasional, weekly, or monthly in a predictable pattern, or unpredictably irregular.
  - The severity may be mild to extreme.
  - The daytime symptoms may include cognitive, affective, and physical complaints.
  - Attempts should be made to identify past or present precipitants and factors that may be perpetuating the insomnia.
  - In addition, the history should include past and current treatments and how the patient responded to them.
- **Presleep conditions**: The assessment of presleep conditions should consider the bedroom environment, the patient's activities and mental state in the evening as bedtime approaches, and the conditions under which the individual attempts to fall asleep or return to sleep following awakenings.
  - This information may be very helpful in the identification of factors that may perpetuate insomnia. For example, patients may be spending excessive wakeful time in bed; may be in bed reading, eating, watching television, using an electronic

TABLE 11.1	Major Components of the Sleep History[2]

- Primary insomnia complaint
- Presleep conditions
- Sleep-wake schedule
- Nocturnal symptoms
- Daytime activities and function

device with a screen, or talking on a telephone; or may be repeatedly watching a clock when they are unable to sleep.

- In the evening as bedtime approaches, insomnia sufferers may feel increasingly anxious and worried about how poorly they might sleep—anticipating another bad night followed by another bad day.
- The bedroom environment should be characterized with regard to a patient's sleeping room and surface, whether there is a bed partner or others nearby, the presence of pets, and also with regard to the temperature, noise, and light levels.

- **Sleep-wake schedule**: Considerable attention should be given to a patient's sleep-wake schedule, including routine school and workdays, weekends and vacations, and any other variations in schedule.
  - The regularity of bedtimes and wake-up times should be ascertained.
  - It is important to estimate key sleep parameters, such as the total sleep duration, time needed to fall asleep, number of awakenings, and wake time after sleep onset.
  - The presence of napping and the associated timing, frequency, and duration should be documented.
  - In the morning does the patient awaken spontaneously or typically require an alarm clock?
  - Is the patient allowing sufficient time in bed to achieve adequate sleep?

- **Nocturnal symptoms**: The sleep history should explore nocturnal symptoms that may be associated with comorbid sleep, psychiatric, neurologic, and medical conditions that may be accompanied by insomnia complaints.
  - Snoring, gasping, and coughing may suggest obstructive sleep apnea.
  - Certain behaviors or experiences may result from parasomnias.
  - Twitches or leg kicks may represent periodic limb movements or rapid eye movement (REM) sleep behavior disorder.
  - Stereotypic movements and behaviors may indicate a seizure disorder.
  - Patients may describe palpitations, pain, gastroesophageal reflux, and emotional states of sadness or a sense of anxiety associated with awakenings.

- **Daytime activities and functioning**: There is a reciprocal relationship between the activities and experiences during the daytime and the characteristics of nighttime sleep: poor sleep may result in daytime impairment, and activities during the daytime can have an impact on the quality and quantity of nighttime sleep.
  - Some degree of daytime impairment is essential for the formal diagnosis of an insomnia disorder.
  - There are multiple domains of potential daytime impairment reflected in the ICSD-3 insomnia disorder diagnostic criteria.

- The sleep history should explore the extent to which patients report fatigue and sleepiness, napping and inadvertent sleep episodes, mood disturbances and cognitive difficulties, functioning in work and school settings, aspects of decrement in quality of life, and possible changes in symptoms of comorbid conditions.
- A review of daytime and evening schedules and activities that may impact sleep is important. Relevant issues may include lifestyle choices, such as level of activity, exercise, and light exposure, as well as work and school schedules.

- **Health history**: In addition to a detailed sleep history, the insomnia evaluation should include the individual's medical and psychiatric history, review of systems, family health history, social and occupational history, and all currently used medications and substances.
  - Both physical and mental status examinations should be performed.
  - Key mental status elements should include concentration, alertness, memory, anxiety, mood, and thoughts of suicide.
  - Patients should complete a general questionnaire that includes medical and psychiatric conditions, as well as medications used; a standardized sleepiness assessment, such as the Epworth Sleepiness Scale[3]; and a sleep log covering at least 2 weeks.

- **Additional testing?** Although *polysomnography* and *actigraphy* are not part of the routine evaluation of patients with insomnia, they may be indicated for selected patients with histories or physical characteristics suggestive of comorbid sleep or medical disorders.

Diagnosis

- Overview:
  - The 2014 publication of the ICSD-3 incorporated vast changes in the approach to insomnia diagnosis.[1]
  - The authors of the ICSD-3 insomnia nosology aimed for conceptual simplicity with a system that *subsumes children and adults with just three insomnia disorder options*, based primarily on the duration of the symptoms.
  - No longer is there a differentiation between primary and secondary insomnias. It was concluded that this was not a useful distinction, since often there is considerable overlap in symptoms, insomnia can have an independent course that remains clinically significant after effective treatment of coexisting conditions, insomnia sometimes adversely affects other presumably underlying disorders, and effective insomnia treatment may benefit coexisting disorders.
  - Insomnia disorder diagnoses are made independent of the presence of comorbid disorders. The multiple specific insomnia diagnoses have been abandoned due to questionable reliability and validity; however, these previous (ICSD-2) specific insomnia diagnoses are reviewed as follows, since several remain in common usage and are included in the 2014 ICSD-3 discussion.
  - Essential and fundamental insomnia disorder diagnosis elements (Table 11.2):
    - *Persistent sleep difficulty*
    - *Adequate opportunity* for sleep
    - *Daytime dysfunction*, presumably associated with the nighttime sleep disturbance
  - The reported sleep and wake difficulties should not be better explained by another sleep disorder.

TABLE 11.2	Insomnia Disorder Essential Elements[1]

- Persistent sleep difficulty
- Adequate opportunity and circumstances for sleep
- Associated daytime dysfunction

- The duration of the sleep-related complaints differentiates chronic from short-term insomnia disorder.
- The sleep disturbance may involve *sleep initiation*, *duration of sleep*, *sleep consolidation*, and *sleep quality*.
- The sleep complaints typically include one or more of the following: *difficulty falling asleep*, *difficulty remaining asleep*, and *waking up excessively early*.
- There may be frequent nighttime awakenings or fewer but longer duration wakeful periods with difficulty returning to sleep.
- These all represent *subjective assessments*, as *the nosology does not include objective thresholds for these parameters*.
- The sleep disturbance criterion options also include resistance to going to bed on an appropriate schedule and difficulty sleeping without a parent or caregiver intervention, both typically associated with childhood insomnia but potentially relevant for older adults with dementia.
  - Sleep disturbance history may be provided by parents or care providers.
  - The childhood sleep-onset association option should be reserved for significantly delayed or disrupted sleep with frequent interventions.
- **Persistent sleep difficulty**: New to the ICSD-3 is the "A" criterion that individuals report or are observed to experience actual sleep onset or sleep maintenance difficulty. *No longer can isolated complaints of nonrestorative, unrefreshing, or poor-quality sleep satisfy this criterion.*
- **Adequate opportunity for sleep**: This criterion emphasizes that the patient complaints should not result from an insufficient time in bed allotted for sleep. In addition, the sleep opportunity should include an environment that is not adverse to comfortable sleep. The sleep environment should be regarded as safe and free of temperature extremes and disturbing light and noise.
- **Daytime dysfunction**: These options are plentiful and diverse.
  - While some people report daytime sleepiness, more commonly patients with insomnia describe an inability to nap and a lack of inadvertent sleep episodes.
  - A common description is feeling "tired and wired."
  - Complaints of *fatigue*, *lack of energy*, *reduced alertness*, *general malaise*, *irritability* or *decreased mood*, *impaired functioning*, *decreased motivation*, *behavioral problems*, and proneness for *accidents or errors* all may satisfy the "B" daytime dysfunction criterion.
  - The daytime impairment may relate to *vocational or social function* or *reduced quality of life*, or in children it may be indicated by *poor school performance*.
  - Finally, *concerns about or dissatisfaction with sleep* satisfies this diagnostic option.
  - Although not incorporated into the diagnostic criteria, patients with insomnia also frequently present with assorted physical symptoms, such as headache and muscle tension.

TABLE 11.3	ICSD-3 Insomnia Diagnoses[1]

- Chronic insomnia disorder
- Short-term insomnia disorder
- Other insomnia disorder

ICSD-3, International Classification of Sleep Disorders, 3rd ed.

TABLE 11.4	ICSD-3 Chronic Insomnia Disorder[1]

Elements from A–F must be present.
A. Patients, parents, or caregivers report or observe one or more of the following:
  1. Difficulty initiating sleep
  2. Difficulty maintaining sleep
  3. Waking up earlier than desired
  4. Resistance to going to bed on an appropriate schedule
  5. Difficulty sleeping without a parent or caregiver intervention
B. Patients, parents, or caregivers report or observe one or more of the following:
  1. Fatigue/malaise
  2. Attention, concentration, or memory impairment
  3. Impaired social, family, occupational, or academic performance
  4. Mood disturbance or irritability
  5. Daytime sleepiness
  6. Behavioral problems (such as hyperactivity, impulsivity, aggression)
  7. Reduced motivation, energy, or initiative
  8. Proneness for errors or accidents
  9. Dissatisfaction or concerns about sleep
C. The sleep- or wake-related complaints cannot be explained exclusively due to inadequate opportunity or circumstances for sleep.
D. The frequency of the sleep disturbance and associated daytime symptoms must be at least three times per week.
E. The duration of the sleep disturbance and associated daytime symptoms must be at least 3 months.
F. The difficulty with sleep and wakefulness cannot be better explained by another sleep disorder.

ICSD-3, International Classification of Sleep Disorders, 3rd ed.

- Insomnia disorders (ICSD-3)
  - There are three ICSD-3 insomnia disorder diagnoses (Table 11.3):
    - Chronic insomnia disorder
    - Short-term insomnia disorder
    - Other insomnia disorder
  - The *chronic insomnia diagnostic* criteria (Table 11.4) specify that the sleep difficulty and associated daytime symptoms should be present *at least 3 days per week* and that these disturbances must be present for *at least 3 months*. The notes accompanying the ICSD-3 diagnostic criteria state possible alternatives for these criteria.
    - Patients may be diagnosed with chronic insomnia disorder without the 3-month duration requirement if they have had recurrent episodes lasting several weeks over a period of several years.
    - Patients currently sleeping well with the use of a hypnotic medication may be diagnosed with chronic insomnia disorder, when presumably they would meet the criteria without the medication, and particularly when they express

TABLE 11.5 ICSD-3 Short-Term Insomnia Disorder[1]

Elements from A–E must be present
A. Patients, parents, or caregivers report or observe one or more of the following:
  1. Difficulty initiating sleep
  2. Difficulty maintaining sleep
  3. Waking up earlier than desired
  4. Resistance to going to bed on an appropriate schedule
  5. Difficulty sleeping without a parent or caregiver intervention
B. Patients, parents, or caregivers report or observe one or more of the following:
  1. Fatigue/malaise
  2. Attention, concentration, or memory impairment
  3. Impaired social, family, occupational, or academic performance
  4. Mood disturbance or irritability
  5. Daytime sleepiness
  6. Behavioral problems (such as, hyperactivity, impulsivity, aggression)
  7. Reduced motivation, energy, or initiative
  8. Proneness for errors or accidents
  9. Dissatisfaction or concerns about sleep
C. The sleep- or wake-related complaints cannot be explained exclusively due to an inadequate opportunity or circumstances for sleep
D. The duration of the sleep disturbance and associated daytime symptoms must be less than 3 months
E. The difficulty with sleep and wakefulness cannot be better explained by another sleep disorder

ICSD-3, International Classification of Sleep Disorders, 3rd ed.

TABLE 11.6 Other Insomnia Disorder[1]

- Diagnostic option for people with difficulty initiating and maintaining sleep without meeting full criteria for chronic or short-term insomnia disorder
- May be used on a provisional basis when further information is required to establish an alternate diagnosis
- Should be used sparingly

TABLE 11.7 Historic Specific Insomnia Diagnoses (ICSD-2)[4]

- Adjustment insomnia
- Psychophysiologic insomnia
- Paradoxic insomnia
- Idiopathic insomnia
- Insomnia caused by a mental disorder
- Inadequate sleep hygiene
- Behavioral insomnia of childhood
- Insomnia associated with a drug or substance (alcohol)
- Insomnia caused by a medical condition
- Insomnia not caused by a substance or known physiologic condition, unspecified (nonorganic)
- Physiologic (organic) insomnia, unspecified

ICSD-2, International Classification of Sleep Disorders, 2nd ed.

concern about not being able to sleep without taking a medication.
- The *short-term insomnia criteria* (Table 11.5) specify a duration of *less than 3 months*, although there is no weekly frequency requirement.
  - This diagnosis should be reserved for situations when a sleep disturbance is a focus of concern and warrants independent clinical attention.
  - Short-term insomnia should not necessarily be diagnosed when the sleep difficulty is a component of acute stress, as may occur with grief or acute pain.
- *Other insomnia disorder* (Table 11.6) is provided as option for circumstances where patients report difficulty with sleep onset or maintenance but do not meet the full criteria for short-term or chronic insomnia disorder.
  - This nonspecific diagnosis should be used sparingly.
  - It may be used on a provisional basis when further information is necessary to establish another insomnia diagnosis.
- The *ICSD-2 (2005) insomnia nosology* provided general insomnia criteria with 11 specific insomnia disorders

representing three broader categories: (1) *primary insomnia* (psychophysiologic, idiopathic, and paradoxic), (2) *insomnia due to medical or psychiatric disorders or drug/substance abuse*, and (3) *insomnia associated with other sleep disorders* (sleep-related breathing disorders, movement disorders, or circadian rhythm disorders).[4] Although ICSD-2 disorders have been replaced by the simplified ICSD-3 nosology, several of the descriptions remain useful and are included in the ICSD-3 text. The following are brief summaries of the ICSD-2 specific insomnia disorders (Table 11.7).

- **Adjustment insomnia**: The key feature of adjustment insomnia, also sometimes termed acute insomnia, is the presence of an *identifiable stressor* that is *temporally associated with a sleep disturbance* lasting *less than 3 months*. The stressor may be psychologic, psychosocial, interpersonal, environmental, or physical in nature. The insomnia symptoms are expected to improve with resolution of the acute stressor or as the individual adapts to the stressor. Adjustment insomnia may be associated with symptoms that are *psychologic* (e.g., anxiety, worry, ruminative thoughts, sadness, depression) or *physical* (e.g., muscle tension, gastrointestinal upset, headaches). Individuals with adjustment insomnia also may report fatigue, concentration difficulty, and irritability.
- **Psychophysiologic insomnia**: The essential features of psychophysiologic insomnia include evidence of *conditioned sleep difficulty* and/or *heightened arousal in bed*. At least one of the following five evidence types should be present:
  - Excessive focus on or heightened anxiety regarding sleep
  - Difficulty falling asleep in bed at one's desired bedtime or with planned naps, but not when one is not intending to sleep
  - An ability to sleep better when away from home
  - Mental arousal in bed with intrusive thoughts or a perceived inability to cease sleep-preventing mental activity
  - Heightened somatic tension in bed reflecting a perceived inability to relax the body

    Psychophysiologic insomnia patients are viewed as having *learned sleep-preventing associations*, contributing to their heightened arousal that together lead to the sleep disturbance and daytime impairment. They often describe a sense of having a "racing mind" that they "can't shut off." They may experience a conditioned arousal associated with their typical bedtime routines. While other precipitating factors may have initiated an insomnia episode, the evolution of a conditioned *hyperarousal* may lead to the long-term perpetuation of insomnia. Concern about insomnia may become a round-the-clock preoccupation.

- **Paradoxic insomnia**: Previously termed sleep state misperception, paradoxic insomnia represents the condition where individuals present complaints of severe insomnia *without objective evidence of sleep disturbance or significant daytime impairment*. The diagnostic criteria specify that one or more of the following be present:
  - Patient reports of little or no sleep most nights with rare nights of relatively normal sleep
  - Sleep log data showing very short average sleep time, often with no sleep some nights and typically no daytime napping
  - A consistent marked mismatch between the subjective sleep estimates (self-report or sleep diary) and simultaneous objective findings (polysomnography or actigraphy)

    In addition, patients should report a near constant awareness through the night of environmental stimuli or of conscious thoughts or ruminations while recumbent in bed. While paradoxic insomnia patients may report daytime impairment, they should not have evidence consistent with their reports of extreme sleep deprivation, such as intrusive daytime sleep episodes or other difficulties resulting from markedly decreased alertness or vigilance.

    Many people with insomnia overestimate their sleep latency and underestimate their total sleep time; however, these claims are greatly magnified in those with paradoxic insomnia. The severity of the sleep loss among paradoxic insomnia patients typically appears physiologically impossible and inconsistent with their daytime functioning. Paradoxic insomnia is the one specific insomnia diagnosis that may be supported by polysomnographic testing due to the relatively normal results regarding standard sleep parameters and sleep staging.

- **Idiopathic insomnia**: Idiopathic insomnia is an especially chronic form of insomnia characterized by an early insidious onset (infancy or childhood), the lack of an identifiable precipitant or cause, and an unremitting course without periods of sustained remission.

- **Insomnia due to mental disorder**: The insomnia due to a mental disorder diagnosis may be applied when a mental disorder has been diagnosed using standard criteria. There should be a temporal association between the insomnia and the mental disorder, although the sleep disturbance may predate the associated mental disorder by a few days or weeks. While insomnia may be a common symptom or even an element in the diagnostic criteria for the associated mental disorder, the additional diagnosis of insomnia due to a mental disorder should be applied when there is marked distress related to the sleep disturbance, or when it represents an independent focus of treatment. Insomnia due to a mental disorder is viewed as a symptom of the associated mental disorder and in general is expected to follow its course. While insomnia may occur with many psychiatric conditions, it is especially prominent with mood, anxiety, and trauma/stressor-related disorders.

- **Inadequate sleep hygiene**: The diagnosis inadequate sleep hygiene may be applied when insomnia has persisted and at least one type of evidence indicates the presence of inadequate sleep hygiene practice: (1) improper sleep scheduling (e.g., frequent daytime napping, highly variable bedtime and rising times, or excessive time in bed); (2) routine use of alcohol, nicotine, or caffeine (especially preceding bedtime); (3) mentally stimulating, physically activating, or emotionally upsetting activities close to bedtime; (4) excessive use of bed for nonsleep activities (e.g., television viewing, reading, studying, and eating); or (5) lack of a comfortable sleeping environment.

  Inadequate sleep hygiene practices are viewed as under the individual's voluntary control and are inconsistent with the promotion of good quality sleep and wake time alertness. These practices either directly increase arousal when sleep is desired or otherwise undermine sleep-wake cycle organization. Patients often do not recognize the degree to which their behaviors are contributing to their persistent sleep difficulties and may incorrectly believe that these practices (e.g., excessive time in bed or bedtime alcohol) might improve their sleep.

- **Behavioral insomnia of childhood**: The diagnosis of behavioral insomnia of childhood is based on parent or other caregiver reports. There are two general patterns, sleep-onset association type and limit-setting type, although a combined type also is a diagnostic option. With the *sleep-onset association type*, each of the following should be present: (1) sleep onset is a prolonged process requiring special conditions; (2) the sleep-onset associations are demanding or highly problematic; (3) without the associated conditions, sleep onset is delayed or sleep is otherwise disrupted; and (4) caregiver intervention is required during nighttime awakenings. The *limit-setting type* requires the presence of each of the following: (1) difficulty initiating or maintaining sleep, (2) stalling or refusing to go to bed or return to bed at appropriate times, and (3) insufficient or inappropriate limit setting on the part of the caregiver to establish appropriate sleeping behavior in the child.

  As the name suggests, the behavioral insomnia of childhood disorder is viewed as having an identified behavioral etiology. In the sleep-onset association type, there is the child's dependency on specific conditions in order to be able fall asleep, and in the limit-setting type there is bedtime stalling or refusal coupled with inadequate caregiver responses. With either type, the sleep disturbance should be regarded as a significant clinical problem. This diagnosis would not be appropriate for children younger than 6 months.

- **Insomnia due to drug or substance**: Insomnia due to drug or substance may be diagnosed when insomnia is temporally associated with the exposure, use or abuse, or acute withdrawal from an abused drug, medication, food, or toxin known to have sleep-disruptive properties in susceptible individuals. This diagnosis may be applicable when sleep problems are associated with prescription medication, recreational drug, caffeine, alcohol, food item,

TABLE 11.8	Insomnia General Population Prevalence[1]

- Adult chronic insomnia disorder: ~10%
- Adult short-term insomnia disorder: 15%–20%
- Adult transient insomnia symptoms: 30%–35%
- Adolescent insomnia: 3%–12%
- Childhood insomnia: 10%–30%*

*Related to limit-setting difficulties or requiring parental/caregiver presence.

TABLE 11.9	Epidemiologic Risk Factors for Insomnia Disorder Symptoms[1,2]

- Older adults
- Females
- Shift workers
- Lower socioeconomic strata
- Comorbid disorders
  - Medical
  - Psychiatric
  - Sleep
  - Substance abuse

or environmental toxin exposure. The range of drugs and other substances that may be associated with insomnia during use or discontinuation is quite broad. Although various drugs and other substances may affect sleep stages, there are no specific polysomnographic criteria for this disorder.

- **Insomnia due to medical condition**: Insomnia coexisting with a medical or physiologic condition known to disrupt sleep may be diagnosed as insomnia due to a medical condition. There should be a clear temporal association between the insomnia symptoms and the onset, resolution, or changes in severity of the associated condition. While many physical conditions may influence sleep quality, the insomnia due to medical condition diagnosis should be reserved for situations where there is marked distress or when the sleep disturbance warrants separate clinical attention. The range of medical and physiologic conditions potentially affecting sleep is very broad and may include pain, breathing problems, limited motility, and central nervous system symptoms. Pregnancy and menopause are physiologic conditions that may affect sleep quality.

Epidemiology

- Many general population epidemiologic studies have offered insomnia prevalence estimates (Table 11.8).
- The values for *insomnia symptoms* occurring at least transiently are in the range of 30%–35%.
- The prevalence of *chronic insomnia disorder* is approximately 10%, while that for *short-term insomnia disorder* is 15%–20%.
- *Adolescent insomnia* is estimated to occur in 3%–12% of individuals.
- *Childhood insomnia* that includes limit-setting difficulties or requires parental/caregiver presence has a prevalence of about 10%–30%.[1]
- The prevalence of insomnia is increased among older individuals and females. Typical risk factors for the presence of insomnia disorder symptoms are listed in Table 11.9.[2]

Pathophysiology

- **Theoretical models**: The processes underlying the pathology and pathophysiology of chronic insomnia are not well established; however, evidence has been presented to support several theoretical models of insomnia precipitation and perpetuation.[1]
  - In general, insomnia is considered to be multifactorial in origin and therefore is not likely to result from a single underlying pathologic process.
  - The etiology of insomnia may include genetic and cultural influences, personality characteristics, life circumstances,

behaviors and routines, medications and abused substances, comorbid disorders, and maladaptive thinking, attitudes, and beliefs about sleep.
- People with chronic insomnia may share certain psychologic or physiologic characteristics that make them more vulnerable for the perpetuation of their insomnia symptoms.
- Spielman's "3 Ps" model of insomnia is especially useful in highlighting the potential role of *predisposing, precipitating,* and *perpetuating factors* and how the relative influence of these elements can shift over time.[5]
- **Psychologic perspectives**: These emphasize personality characteristics, cognitive experiences, and behavioral associations.
  - Specific cognitive models of insomnia suggest that anxiety and selective attention lead to excessive monitoring of internal and external sleep-related cues and the subsequent experience of sleeplessness.[6]
- **Physiologic studies**: Insomnia models incorporate the central concept of round-the-clock hyperarousal, explaining both the nighttime and daytime insomnia symptomatology.[7]
  - Studies have demonstrated *elevated heart rate, basal skin resistance, core body temperature,* and *phasic vasoconstriction* in subjects with insomnia, compared with control individuals.
  - It has been argued that insomnia groups have abnormalities in their metabolic rate, heart rate variability, electromyographic activity, hypothalamic-pituitary-adrenal axis activity (elevated cortisol, adrenocorticotropic hormone, and corticotropin releasing factor near bedtime), immune function and cytokine levels, electroencephalogram patterns, and thermoregulation.[1]
  - Functional imaging studies have supported the argument that there is a relative increase in metabolic activity in regions associated with the regulation of the sleep-wake cycle in insomnia subjects, compared with healthy control subjects.[8,9]
  - Functional imaging data is depicted in Fig. 11.1.

Consequences and Associations

- The AASM Clinical Guideline emphasizes that insomnia causes burdens for both individuals and society, and it lists a variety of domains where chronic insomnia has been associated with negative outcomes (Table 11.10).[2]
- Daytime impairment is integral to the diagnosis of insomnia disorders.
- Worse quality of life among subjects with insomnia has been reported in numerous studies.[10]

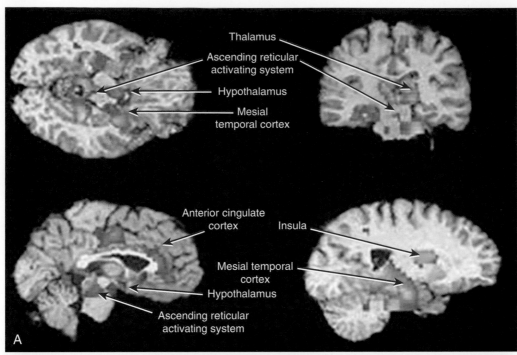

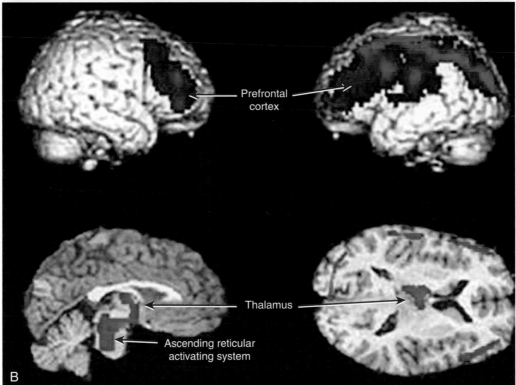

• **Figure 11.1** Functional brain changes in insomnia (^{18}F-fluorodeoxyglucose positron emission tomography). Distribution of brain glucose metabolism in patients with primary insomnia compared with healthy controls. **A,** Patients with insomnia depicted an increased global cerebral metabolic rate of glucose (CMRglu) when transitioning from waking to sleep onset, as compared with healthy subjects without insomnia, indicating that there is an overall cortical hyperarousal in insomnia. Furthermore, patients with insomnia exhibited less reduction of relative CMRglu from waking to NREM sleep in the ascending reticular activating system, hypothalamus, insular cortex, amygdala, hippocampus, anterior cingulate, and medial prefrontal cortices. **B,** Compared with insomnia patients, healthy subjects showed greater relative metabolism while awake in the prefrontal cortex, thalamus, and ascending reticular activating system. (From Dang-Vu T, Maquet P, Desseilles M. Neuroimaging techniques. In: Chokroverty S, Thomas RJ [eds]. *Atlas of Sleep Medicine.* 2nd ed. Elsevier, Inc; 2014:242–254.)

TABLE 11.10	Potential Consequences and Associations of Chronic Insomnia[2]

- Daytime impairment
  - Cognition
  - Mood
  - Performance
- Greater use of health care resources
- Greater number of physician visits
- Absenteeism
- Workplace accidents and errors
- Depression
- Suicide
- Substance abuse relapse
- Self-medication
  - Alcohol
  - Over-the-counter medications
  - Prescription medications

TABLE 11.11	Chronic Insomnia Cognitive and Behavioral Therapy Components with Recommendation Levels[2]

- Stimulus control (S)
- Relaxation training (S)
- Cognitive behavioral therapy for insomnia—CBI-I (S)
- Multicomponent therapy (without cognitive therapy; G)
- Sleep restriction (G)
- Paradoxic intention (G)
- Biofeedback therapy (G)
- Sleep hygiene therapy (N)

Recommendation levels: Standard (S), Guideline (G), and No recommendation (N).

- People with chronic insomnia have greater likelihoods of having or developing various medical and psychiatric disorders.[11,12]
- Especially prominent have been the numerous studies documenting the future risk of new-onset *depressive*, *anxiety*, and *substance use disorders*.[13]

Management

- **Overview**: Both general and specific recommendations for the treatment of insomnia are included in the AASM Clinical Guideline.[2]
  - The general items highlight the two key treatment goals:
    - Improving sleep quality and quantity
    - Improving insomnia-associated daytime impairment
  - Specific treatment goals should be reviewed with patients.
  - Management of comorbid conditions should be optimized.
  - The use of any current medications should be reviewed to determine whether dosage, timing, or other adjustments might improve the insomnia symptoms.
  - Patients should maintain sleep diaries throughout active treatment.
  - Clinical reassessment with questionnaires and survey instruments may be useful to reflect outcomes and direct treatment choices.
  - Patients should be reassessed every few weeks or monthly until the insomnia symptoms are stable or have resolved and then again every 6 months due to the high rate of relapse.
  - When particular treatment strategies have not been effective, alternate behavioral, pharmacologic, or combination approaches should be considered.
  - Further evaluation of possible comorbid disorders should be conducted in the event of treatment failure.
  - The two major evidence-based forms of treatment for chronic insomnia are[14]:
    - Psychologic and behavioral therapies
    - Pharmacotherapy
  - Although sleep hygiene recommendations often represent an important component of an insomnia patient's treatment plan, this modality alone is not considered to be an effective treatment for chronic insomnia. Accordingly, sleep hygiene

measures should be combined with other effective therapies.
- Cognitive and behavioral therapies for insomnia
  - **Overview**: The cognitive and behavioral therapy approaches to treating insomnia are consistent with theoretical models of insomnia etiology that *include cognitive hyperarousal* and problematic *behaviors that precipitate and perpetuate the insomnia symptoms*.[2]
    - Cognitive and behavioral treatment techniques for insomnia have demonstrated efficacy for patients with independent and comorbid insomnia; in adults of all ages, including older individuals; and in populations of chronic hypnotic medication users.
    - At least one behavioral intervention should be part of any initial cognitive and behavioral therapy approach.
    - Cognitive and behavioral therapy components typically are combined in a treatment program termed *cognitive behavioral therapy for insomnia (CBT-I)*. This multimodal strategy is considered most effective.
    - These approaches have been found to have *long-term efficacy* and *posttreatment durability*.[15]
    - Pharmacotherapy of insomnia may be combined with CBT-I (incorporating both cognitive and behavioral strategies); however, combined therapy has been shown to have no consistent advantage or disadvantage in comparison with CBT-I approaches without the use of medications.
  - **CBT-I components**: The major components constituting the cognitive and behavioral therapies for chronic insomnia are listed in Table 11.11. Although all may be effective, the components are supported by different levels of evidence.[2]
    - Those with the highest levels of evidence and listed as standard recommendations are stimulus control, relaxation training, and CBT-I with or without relaxation therapy.
    - Sleep restriction, paradoxic intention, biofeedback, and multicomponent therapy without cognitive therapy all have less supportive evidence and are regarded as guideline recommendations.
  - **Stimulus control therapy** attempts to help insomnia patients establish and strengthen a positive association between falling asleep and the bed and bedtime routines.
    - The underlying premise is that arousing mental states, such as frustration and worry, become conditioned responses that contribute to the perpetuation of insomnia.

TABLE 11.12 | **Insomnia Pharmacologic Treatment Approach Domains**

Prescription Required (United States)	FDA INDICATION	
	NO	**YES**
NO	Dietary supplements (Melatonin, valerian, and many others)	Over-the-counter sleep aids—all with antihistamines (Mostly diphenhydramine or doxylamine)
YES	"Off-label" for insomnia (Various antidepressants, antipsychotics, anxiolytics, antihypertensives, antiepileptics, and others)	• Benzodiazepine receptor agonists • Melatonin receptor agonist • Low-dose histamine receptor antagonist • Orexin/hypocretin receptor antagonist

FDA, US Food and Drug Administration.

- Stimulus control instructions state that patients should attempt to maintain a regular sleep-wake schedule and avoid napping, use the bed only for sleep and sexual relations, attempt to fall asleep only when sleepy, and leave the bed to pursue a relaxing activity if unable to fall asleep within about 20 min. The latter step should be repeated as necessary.
- **Relaxation training** techniques include progressive muscle relaxation, guided imagery, and abdominal breathing. These techniques may be beneficial for insomnia patients by decreasing cognitive and somatic arousal.
- **Cognitive therapy** focuses on identifying and addressing distorted beliefs and attitudes, and maladaptive behaviors related to sleep and insomnia.
- **Multicomponent therapy** (without cognitive therapy) incorporates several behavioral components for treating insomnia. Typically sleep hygiene education is a part of multicomponent therapy.
- **Sleep restriction therapy** limits the time in bed to create an increase in the sleep drive and help reduce the waking time in bed to minimize the opportunity for conditioned arousal.
  - An initial prescribed time in bed schedule is determined from a baseline sleep diary, and the schedule is modified depending on the patient's ongoing sleep efficiency.
  - Typically patients maintain a normal wakeup time, and the restriction is accomplished by delaying the bedtime. In general, the allotted time in bed would not be less than 5 hours.
- **Paradoxic intention** is a form of cognitive therapy that is intended to help decrease a patient's anxiety regarding the ability to fall asleep. Patients are instructed to try to remain awake in bed rather than trying to fall asleep, although they should not use drastic measures to maintain wakefulness.
- **Biofeedback therapy** can be achieved through a variety of modalities with the overall objective of decreasing somatic arousal, which can undermine the ability to fall asleep.
- **Sleep hygiene therapy** is typically combined with other cognitive and behavioral strategies.
  - In general, sleep hygiene recommendations include a wide range of healthy lifestyle practices that should be conducive to improved sleep.
  - Examples may include sleep-wake schedule regularity, avoidance of napping, caution regarding caffeine and alcohol use, timing of exercise, and characteristics of the bedroom environment.
- Pharmacotherapy
- **Overview**: Many different medications with varying pharmacodynamic and pharmacokinetic properties are now approved by the US Food and Drug Administration (FDA) for the treatment of insomnia.
  - In addition to those indicated for treating insomnia, several other prescription medications (e.g., antidepressants, antiepileptics, antihypertensives, and antipsychotics) are sometimes recommended on an "off-label" basis with the intention of improving sleep.
  - Insomnia sufferers may also use over-the-counter (OTC) antihistamine sleep aids or assorted unregulated dietary supplement preparations (e.g., melatonin and valerian; Table 11.12).
  - The FDA-approved insomnia medications include four broad categories: numerous *benzodiazepine receptor agonists (BZRA)*, one *selective melatonin receptor agonist*, one *selective histamine H_1 receptor antagonist*, and one *orexin/hypocretin antagonist*. Table 11.13 includes a comprehensive list of all medications available in the United States, with indications for treating insomnia with their available doses, approximate elimination half-lives, indications, common side effects, DEA classifications, and pregnancy categories.
- **BZRA hypnotics**: The broad BZRA hypnotic category includes both the *benzodiazepines*, which incorporate the characteristic benzodiazepine structure, and *nonbenzodiazepines*, which have alternate structures but share key pharmacodynamic features.
  - BZRA hypnotics are positive allosteric modulators of GABA responses at the $GABA_A$ receptor complex (Fig. 11.2).
  - Included among the BZRA, hypnotics are compounds with elimination half-lives ranging from about 1 hour to several days and products with different formulations and delivery systems.
  - All BZRA hypnotics are classed as schedule IV medications because of their identified but relatively low abuse potential.
  - The benzodiazepines are pregnancy category X, whereas the nonbenzodiazepines are pregnancy category C.
  - All of the compounds are available as immediate-release capsules or tablets, although zolpidem is also approved

TABLE 11.13 FDA-Approved Insomnia Treatment Medications

Generic (Brand) Name	Doses (mg)	Half-Life (hour)	Indications	Most Common Side Effects	DEA Class	Pregnancy Category
Benzodiazepine Immediate Release						
Flurazepam (Dalmane)	15, 30	2.3 (active metabolite 48–160)	"treatment of insomnia characterized by difficulty in falling asleep, frequent nocturnal awakenings, and/or early morning awakening"	Dizziness, drowsiness, lightheadedness, staggering, loss of coordination, falling	IV	X
Temazepam (Restoril)	7.5, 15, 22.5, 30	3.5–18.4	"short-term treatment of insomnia"	Drowsiness, dizziness, lightheadedness, difficulty with coordination	IV	X
Triazolam (Halcion)	0.125, 0.25	1.5–5.5	"short-term treatment of insomnia"	Drowsiness, headache, dizziness, lightheadedness, "pins and needles" feeling on your skin, difficulty with coordination	IV	X
Quazepam (Doral)	7.5, 15	39 (active metabolite 73)	"treatment of insomnia characterized by difficulty in falling asleep, frequent nocturnal awakenings, and/or early morning awakenings"	Drowsiness, headache	IV	X
Estazolam (ProSom)	1, 2	10–24	"short-term management of insomnia characterized by difficulty in falling asleep, frequent nocturnal awakenings, and/or early morning awakenings … administered at bedtime improved sleep induction and sleep maintenance"	Somnolence, hypokinesia, dizziness, abnormal coordination	IV	X
Nonbenzodiazepine Immediate Release						
Zolpidem (Ambien)	5, 10	~2.5	"short-term treatment of insomnia characterized by difficulties with sleep initiation"	Drowsiness, dizziness, diarrhea, drugged feelings	IV	C
Zaleplon (Sonata)	5, 10	1	"short-term treatment of insomnia … shown to decrease the time to sleep onset"	Drowsiness, lightheadedness, dizziness, "pins and needles" feeling on your skin, difficulty with coordination	IV	C
Eszopiclone (Lunesta)	1, 2, 3	~6 (~9 in elderly)	"treatment of insomnia … decrease sleep latency and improve sleep maintenance"	Unpleasant taste, headache, somnolence, respiratory infection, dizziness, dry mouth, rash, anxiety, hallucinations, viral infections	IV	C
Nonbenzodiazepine Extended Release						
Zolpidem ER (Ambien CR)	6.25, 12.5	2.8 (males)	"treatment of insomnia characterized by difficulties with sleep onset and/or sleep maintenance"	Headache, next-day somnolence, dizziness	IV	C
Nonbenzodiazepine Alternate Delivery						
Zolpidem Oral spray (ZolpiMist)	5, 10	2.7–3.0	"short-term treatment of insomnia characterized by difficulties with sleep initiation"	Drowsiness, dizziness, diarrhea, drugged feelings	IV	C
Zolpidem Sublingual (Edluar)	5, 10	~2.5	"short-term treatment of insomnia characterized by difficulties with sleep initiation"	Drowsiness, dizziness, diarrhea, drugged feelings	IV	C
Zolpidem Sublingual (Intermezzo)	1.75, 3.5	~2.5	"for use as needed for the treatment of insomnia when a middle-of-the-night awakening is followed by difficulty returning to sleep" (when the patient has at least 4 hours of bedtime remaining before the planned time of waking)	Headache, nausea, fatigue	IV	C

Continued

TABLE 11.13	**FDA-Approved Insomnia Treatment Medications—cont'd**						

Generic (Brand) Name	Doses (mg)	Half-Life (hour)	Indications	Most Common Side Effects	DEA Class	Pregnancy Category
Selective Melatonin Receptor Agonist						
Ramelteon (Rozerem)	8	1–2.6	"treatment of insomnia characterized by difficulty with sleep onset"	Somnolence, dizziness, fatigue, nausea, exacerbated insomnia	None	C
Selective Histamine H₁ Receptor Antagonist						
Doxepin (Silenor)	3, 6	15.3	"treatment of insomnia characterized by difficulties with sleep maintenance"	Somnolence/sedation, nausea, upper respiratory tract infection	None	C
Dual Orexin/Hypocretin Receptor Antagonist						
Suvorexant (Belsomra)	5, 10, 15, 20	12	"treatment of insomnia, characterized by difficulties with sleep onset and/or sleep maintenance"	Somnolence, depression (See text regarding risk of REM intrusion phenomena)	IV	C

FDA, US Food and Drug Administration; *REM*, rapid eye movement.

GABA$_A$ RECEPTOR COMPLEX

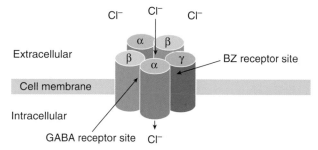

• **Figure 11.2** Representation of the GABA$_A$ transmembrane receptor complex with labeled subunits, central chloride ion channel, and GABA and benzodiazepine (BZ) agonist receptor sites. When GABA interacts with the receptor, complex chloride ions (Cl⁻) are able to enter the cell increasing the polarization and decreasing the likelihood of an action potential. The presence of a BZ agonist enhances this chloride ion entry process with greater polarization with results that may include sedation.

in extended-release, sublingual dissolvable, and oral spray formulations.
  • All BZRA hypnotics should be beneficial for sleep onset, but their efficacy for sleep maintenance depends on their duration of action. In some cases the FDA indications specify efficacy for sleep onset or sleep maintenance.
• **Melatonin receptor agonist**: The single melatonin receptor agonist is *ramelteon*, which has high affinity for the MT$_1$ and MT$_2$ melatonin receptors.
  • Ramelteon is indicated for the treatment of insomnia characterized by difficulty with sleep onset.
  • This melatonin agonist is thought to have a mechanism of action promoting sleep through effects on the endogenous circadian system, which strongly influences the sleep-wake cycle.
  • Ramelteon is a nonscheduled agent and is classed as pregnancy category C.
• **Histamine receptor antagonist**: The *low-dose doxepin* formulation is the selective histamine H$_1$ receptor antagonist

that is indicated for the treatment of insomnia characterized by difficulties with sleep maintenance.
  • Doxepin has very high selectivity for the H$_1$ receptor, and at very low doses the antihistamine sedating effect is the predominant action of the medication.
  • Low-dose doxepin for the treatment of insomnia is a nonscheduled agent and is classed as pregnancy category C.
• **Orexin/Hypocretin receptor antagonist**: *Suvorexant* so far is the only orexin/hypocretin antagonist medication approved by the FDA.
  • The specific indication is for difficulty with sleep onset and/or sleep maintenance.
  • The medication is a dual receptor antagonist.
  • The orexin/hypocretin system promotes arousal and helps stabilize wakefulness; therefore antagonist activity at these receptors should facilitate sleep.
  • One concern with the orexin/hypocretin antagonist approach to treating insomnia is the theoretical possibility of the intrusion of REM phenomena into wakefulness. These might include sleep paralysis, hypnagogic/hypnopompic hallucinations, and cataplexy-like symptoms.
  • Suvorexant is schedule IV and is pregnancy category C.
• **Clinical treatment guidelines**: The AASM Clinical Guideline document offers recommendations regarding the pharmacologic treatment of insomnia.[2] One key point is that behavioral and cognitive therapies should supplement short-term hypnotic use whenever possible. Table 11.14 lists the multiple issues that should be considered when selecting a medication to treat insomnia.
• The typical chronic insomnia medication trial sequence recommendation:
  • Begin with the use of a medication approved by the FDA for treating insomnia.
  • If the initial approach is unsuccessful, then an alternate FDA-approved insomnia medication should be tried.
  • A next step would be a trial on a sedating antidepressant, particularly when the patient has symptoms of depression or anxiety.

TABLE 11.14	Considerations in Selecting Medications to Treat Insomnia[2]

- Pattern of symptoms
- Treatment goals
- Past responses to treatment
- Patient preference
- Cost
- Availability of other treatments
- Comorbid conditions
- Contraindications
- Concurrent medication interactions
- Side effects

- A subsequent approach would combine a sedating antidepressant with an approved medication.
- Finally, additional alternate medications used on an off-label basis may be used, particularly when patients have symptoms consistent with the indications for these medications.
- The AASM Clinical Guideline does not recommend treating chronic insomnia with OTC antihistamine sleep aids, dietary supplements, and other unregulated products because of either inadequate efficacy data or safety concerns. Similarly, older insomnia medications, such as chloral hydrate and barbiturates and related drugs, are not recommended.
- General insomnia pharmacotherapy prescribing recommendations:
  - Use the lowest effective dose and tapering of the dose when appropriate.
  - Patients prescribed medications for insomnia should be educated about the *treatment goals, initial and future dosages, potential safety issues, possible drug interactions,* and *rebound insomnia on discontinuation* of the drug.
  - Chronic use of hypnotics may be appropriate for patients with severe or refractory insomnia symptoms, including those with chronic comorbid conditions.[2]
  - Whenever possible, CBT-I approaches should also be incorporated.
  - When patients are prescribed hypnotics on a short- or long-term basis, they should be evaluated regularly and assessed for continued efficacy, need for ongoing medication, adverse effects, and new symptoms or worsening of comorbid disorders.
  - Long-term hypnotic use may include *nightly, intermittent,* or *as-needed* administration.
  - No insomnia treatment medications are indicated for individuals below the age of 18 years.
  - A lower initial dose typically is appropriate in the treatment of older adults. With the exception of ramelteon, all FDA-approved insomnia medications are available in multiple doses. The FDA also has reduced the initial zolpidem dose recommendations in women, since they tend to metabolize the medication more slowly than men.
- The general AASM Clinical Guideline insomnia treatment recommendations are applicable to patients with isolated insomnia, as well as those with comorbid conditions.[2] Additional considerations may be necessary for patients with particular comorbidities, especially in the context of polypharmacy.

Insomnia and Psychiatric Comorbidities

- Both clinical experience and epidemiologic studies (cross-sectional and longitudinal) highlight the considerable overlap and bidirectionality in the relationship between sleep and psychiatric disorders.
- People with psychiatric disorders, especially during acute episodes, often report sleep disturbances—mostly insomnia, but sometimes excessive sleepiness.
- People with chronic insomnia, or even a history of persistent insomnia, are at increased risk for developing certain mental disorders— primarily depressive, anxiety, and substance abuse disorders, although *suicide also is independently associated with chronic insomnia.*[12,16,17]
- Population studies with adults and adolescents suggest that insomnia often precedes or occurs at the same time as depressive episodes, while in general insomnia occurs with or following the onset of anxiety disorders.[13,18]
- A sleep disturbance may be the first symptom signaling an acute episode of a mental disorder, and insomnia may persist as a residual symptom following the recovery from the episode.
- Among the DSM-5 anxiety disorders and trauma and stressor-related disorders, *generalized anxiety disorder (GAD), posttraumatic stress disorder (PTSD),* and *acute stress disorder* all include disturbed sleep as a diagnostic symptom option defining the disorders.[19]
  - Insomnia has increased prevalence rates in other anxiety disorders (e.g., panic disorder, obsessive-compulsive disorder, and social phobia) that do not include it as a formal diagnostic feature.
  - Insomnia and parasomnias, especially nightmares, are common occurrences in patients with PTSD and acute stress disorder.
  - It has been argued that PTSD incorporates a fundamental abnormality of REM sleep and that prazosin may be uniquely beneficial for the sleep-related symptoms (though without FDA approval for this indication).[20]
  - The majority of panic disorder patients report insomnia, and distressing panic attacks may occur during nonrapid eye movement (NREM) sleep in these individuals.
- Sleep disturbances are prominent symptoms in patients with *mood disorders.* Sleep-related symptoms are diagnostic feature options for the DSM-5 *major depressive* and *manic episode* criteria.[19]
  - Patients experiencing depressive episodes very frequently report insomnia, which may be manifest by difficulty falling asleep, difficulty remaining asleep, early morning awakening, or a combination of these.
  - A small percentage of depressed patients describe hypersomnolence.
  - Bipolar disorder patients experiencing manic episodes may report decreased need for sleep.
  - Extensive polysomnographic research has been performed comparing depressed patients with normal subjects.
    - During major depressive episodes, patients typically demonstrate sleep continuity disturbances, decreased slow wave sleep, and REM sleep abnormalities, including a shorter REM latency, longer first REM period, and increased density of REMs.[21]
  - Appropriately timed partial or complete sleep deprivation can have a transient therapeutic effect for depressed patients,

while sleep loss may precipitate manic episodes in bipolar disorder patients.[22,23]

- Patients in whom *schizophrenia* is diagnosed commonly have sleep disturbances that may include insomnia symptoms and abnormalities in the timing of their sleep-wake cycles.
  - Pronounced insomnia may represent a prodromal symptom related to the onset of the illness or acute exacerbations.
  - Reductions in total sleep time and sleep efficiency have been reported.

- Polysomnographic studies of schizophrenic patients have not revealed consistent findings, although many have found reductions in slow wave sleep.[24]
- An important treatment consideration with psychiatric disorders is the possible effects of medications on sleep characteristics. *Most psychotropic medications have the potential to influence sleep by causing insomnia, excessive sleepiness, parasomnias, or sleep architecture changes.*

Summary

- Insomnia is the most common sleep disturbance and is in general the most common type of sleep disorder.
- Insomnia typically is multifactorial in etiology and requires a broad-based evaluation to identify issues that need to be addressed in treatment.

- Considerable evidence supports the use of CBT-I and pharmacotherapeutic strategies in patients with insomnia disorders.
- The ICSD-3 insomnia nosology and the AASM Clinical Guideline provide excellent information on the range of insomnia disorders, as well as appropriate evaluation and treatment options.

Suggested Reading

Buysse DJ. Insomnia. *JAMA.* 2013;309(7):706-716.

Levenson JC, Kay DB, Buysse DJ. The pathophysiology of insomnia. *Chest.* 2015;147(4):1179-1192.

Molen YF, Carvalho LB, Prado LB, Prado GF. Insomnia: psychological and neurobiological aspects and non-pharmacological treatments. *Arq Neuropsiquiatr.* 2014;72(1):63-71.

Riemann D, Nissen C, Palagini L, et al. The neurobiology, investigation, and treatment of chronic insomnia. *Lancet Neurol.* 2015;14(5):547-558.

Winkelman JW. Clinical practice. Insomnia disorder. *N Engl J Med.* 2015;373(15):1437-1444.

12

Central Nervous System Hypersomnia: Diagnosis, Evaluation, and Treatment

EMMANUEL H. DURING, SHANNON S. SULLIVAN, EMMANUEL MIGNOT

Introduction

Definitions

- Central disorders of hypersomnolence, formerly known as "hypersomnias of central origin," refer to a group of disorders for which excessive daytime sleepiness (EDS) is a central feature, but this symptom is not due to disturbed nocturnal sleep, circadian rhythm, or sleep-related breathing disorders.[1]

- More completely understood, *hypersomnolence* (or *hypersomnia*) is a term that has been used to refer to either an excessive quantity of sleep, high sleep propensity during wakefulness,[2] or both.

Prevalence of Hypersomnia

- Hypersomnia is a common clinical complaint. EDS occurring at least 3 days per week has been reported in 4%–20% of the population, with severe EDS in 5%.[2] The estimated prevalence rate of daytime sleepiness has been estimated by questionnaire to be 4%–6.6% in children,[3,4] with prevalence increasing in adolescence to a reported 19.9%.[5]

- The occupational health and public health safety risks associated with daytime sleepiness, as well as the psychosocial and economic toll on affected individuals, are significant, thus making careful evaluation, correct diagnosis, and adequate treatment subjects of salient concern.

- This chapter focuses on the evaluation, causes, and management of hypersomnias as defined in the *International Classification of Sleep Disorders, 3rd ed* (ICSD-3; Tables 12.1 and 12.2).[1]

The Complaint of Sleepiness

Classification of Excessive Daytime Sleepiness

- According to the ICSD-3,[1] EDS is the central feature of distinct entities that include narcolepsy, idiopathic hypersomnia, Kleine-Levin syndrome (KLS, formerly known as "recurrent hypersomnia"), insufficient sleep, and hypersomnia secondary to drugs, and medical or psychiatric conditions.

- Sleepiness, or somnolence, is determined by multiple factors, including the quantity and quality of prior sleep, circadian time, substances or medications, behavioral factors such as attention, motivation, environmental stimuli, and various medical, neurologic, and psychiatric disorders.[6,7]

- The severity, timing, and duration of sleepiness are important clues to understand the underpinnings of sleepiness as a symptom; in the context of an ICSD-3–defined sleep disorder, sleepiness must have occurred daily for at least 3 months.

- A notable exception is KLS, a rare condition in which hypersomnia is episodic and the patient functions normally between episodes.

TABLE 12.1   International Classification of Sleep Disorders (ICSD-3): Diagnosis Criteria Pertaining to Commonly Encountered Central Disorders of Hypersomnolence

Disorder	Symptoms	Diagnostic Tests/Additional Criteria	Other Diagnostic Features
Narcolepsy type 1 (with cataplexy or hypocretin deficiency)	Daily periods of irrepressible need to sleep or daytime lapses into sleep occurring for at least 3 months *Note: In young children, it may present as excessively long night sleep or as resumption of previously discontinued daytime napping* A definite history of cataplexy (this criterion is not required in case of low CSF hypocretin-1)	PSG/MSLT (MSL ≤ 8 min; ≥2 SOREMPs, which can include SOREMP ≤15 min on nocturnal PSG) OR Low CSF hypocretin-1 (≤ 110 pg/mL or 1/3 of mean normal control values) *Note: In case of low CSF hypocretin-1, cataplexy is not required for the diagnosis*	Disruption of nocturnal sleep, refreshing daytime naps, frequent hypnagogic or hypnopompic multisensory hallucinations, sleep paralysis, automatic behavior, RBD, NREM parasomnias, weight gain around onset of illness Almost all patients are positive for HLA-DQB1*06:02 and predicted to have hypocretin deficiency as the cause of the pathology
Narcolepsy type 2 (without cataplexy)	Same as narcolepsy type 1 (cataplexy is absent or atypical)	Same PSG/MSLT criteria as narcolepsy type 1 Not better explained by insufficient sleep, OSA, DSP, or the effect of medication or substances or their withdrawal	Same as in narcolepsy type 1 HLA-DQB1*06:02 positive in 45% of cases only; etiologically heterogeneous
Idiopathic hypersomnia	Same as narcolepsy (cataplexy is absent)	PSG/MSLT (MSL ≤ 8 min; ≤1 SOREMP, including SOREMP ≤ 15 min on nocturnal PSG) OR Total 24-hour sleep time ≥ 11 hours (typically 12–14 hours) on 24-hour PSG monitoring (performed after correction of chronic sleep deprivation), or by wrist actigraphy in association with a sleep log (averaged over at least seven days with unrestricted sleep) *Note: These test findings may not be fulfilled if other criteria are met* Insufficient sleep syndrome is ruled out Symptoms and MSLT findings are not better explained by another sleep disorder, other medical or psychiatric disorder, or use of drugs or medications	Sleep efficiency >90% on PSG Sleep inertia (irritability, confusion, automatic behaviors), long (over an hour) unrefreshing naps, autonomic symptoms (orthostatic symptoms, temperature dysregulation, Raynaud-type peripheral vascular complaints, headaches)
Kleine-Levin syndrome	≥2 recurrent episodes of EDS and sleep duration, each persisting for 2 days–5 weeks Episodes recur at least once every 18 months (usually more than once a year) During episodes, at least one of the following: 1. Cognitive dysfunction 2. Altered perception 3. Eating disorder (anorexia or hyperphagia) 4. Disinhibited behavior (such as hypersexuality) Between episodes: normal alertness, cognitive function, behavior, and mood	No test is necessary Not better explained by another sleep, medical, neurologic, or psychiatric disorder (especially bipolar disorder), or use of drugs or medications	First episode often triggered by an infection or alcohol intake During episodes: May sleep up to 16–20 hours/day, irritability, exhaustion, apathy, confusion, slow speech, anterograde amnesia, dream-like, altered perception of the environment (derealization), may eat ravenously or eat less, may be hypersexual (usually men), childish, depressed (predominantly women), anxious, experience hallucinations and delusions. Social and occupational impairment during attacks is often severe, with teenagers bedridden for days. Termination of an episode: May be signaled by amnesia, transient dysphoria, or elation with insomnia

CSF, Lumbar sac cerebrospinal fluid; *DSP*, delayed sleep phase; *EDS*, excessive daytime sleepiness; *MSLT*, multiple sleep latency test; *OSA*, obstructive sleep apnea; *PSG*, polysomnography; *SOREMP*, sleep-onset rapid eye movement period; *TST*, total sleep time.

TABLE 12.2	**Secondary Hypersomnias**	
Condition	**Diagnostic Criteria**	
Insufficient sleep syndrome	Daily periods of irrepressible need to sleep or daytime lapses into sleep *Note: In the case of prepubertal children, there is instead a complaint of behavioral abnormalities attributable to sleepiness* Patient's sleep time is usually shorter than expected for age Curtailed sleep pattern present most days for at least 3 months Patient curtails sleep time by such measures as an alarm clock or being awakened by another person and in general sleeps longer when such measures are not used, such as on weekends or vacations Extension of total sleep time results in resolution of EDS	Not better explained by another untreated sleep disorder, the effects of medications or drugs, or other medical, neurologic, or mental disorder *Note 1: If there is doubt about the accuracy of personal history or sleep logs, actigraphy should be performed* *Note 2: In the case of long sleepers, reported habitual sleep periods may be normal based on age; however, these sleep periods may be insufficient for these patients*
Hypersomnia due to a medical condition	Daily periods of irrepressible need to sleep or daytime lapses into sleep occurring for at least 3 months EDS is a consequence of a significant underlying medical or neurologic condition	Not better explained by another untreated sleep or mental disorder, or the effects of medications or drugs If MSLT is performed (not required), MSL ≤ 8 min and ≤ 1 SOREMP are observed *Note 1: If ≥2 SOREMPs, narcolepsy type 1 or type 2 due to a medical condition should be used rather than hypersomnia due to a medical condition* *Note 2: In the subtype of residual hypersomnolence after treatment of OSA, the MSL may be >8 min*
Hypersomnia due to a medication or substance	Daily periods of irrepressible need to sleep or daytime lapses into sleep EDS is a consequence of current medication or substance use or withdrawal from a wake-promoting medication or substance	Not better explained by another untreated sleep, medical, neurologic, or mental disorder *Note 1: This diagnosis also includes hypersomnolence associated with withdrawal from amphetamines and other drugs* *Note 2: If narcolepsy or hypersomnolence existed prior to stimulant abuse, the diagnosis of hypersomnia due to a medication or substance should not be used*
Hypersomnia associated with a psychiatric disorder	Daily periods of irrepressible need to sleep or daytime lapses into sleep occurring for at least 3 months Occurs in association with a concurrent psychiatric disorder	Not better explained by another untreated sleep, medical or neurologic disorder, or the effects of medications or drugs May report excessive nocturnal sleep, daytime sleepiness, or excessive napping Patients often feel their sleep is of poor quality and nonrestorative, and often intensely focused on their hypersomnolence Psychiatric symptoms may become apparent only after prolonged interviews or psychometric testing Associated psychiatric conditions include mood disorders, conversion or undifferentiated somatoform disorder, and less frequently other mental disorders such as schizoaffective disorder, adjustment disorder, or personality disorders

EDS, Excessive daytime sleepiness; *MSLT*, multiple sleep latency test; *OSA*, obstructive sleep apnea; *SOREMP*, sleep-onset rapid eye movement period.

- The severity of sleepiness is typically greater in patients with narcolepsy, and KLS (during episodes), versus idiopathic hypersomnia (IH).

"Sleepiness" or "Fatigue"?

At times, patients with EDS do not use the word "sleepiness" to describe their symptoms. They may use vague words, such as "tired," "fatigued," "decreased energy," or similar terminology. These alternative terms may reflect either genuine sleepiness or fatigue.[8]

- Fatigue: Fatigue implies a feeling of tiredness that may have physical and psychologic components; it may occur, for example, in conditions such as depression and in other conditions such as fibromyalgia and multiple sclerosis.[8] Pure fatigue is not associated with sleepiness[9]; unfortunately, the terms are often used interchangeably, causing confusion.
- Sleepiness: In contrast to fatigue, those with bona fide sleepiness tend to fall asleep in situations that are conducive to sleep and, when severe enough, even during situations that are not soporific, even if sleeping is undesired or dangerous.[9] Furthermore, a complaint of sleepiness suggests a sleep disorder, whereas a complaint of fatigue may suggest a possible underlying medical or psychiatric disorder that is not producing any specific sleep disruption.[9]

Some conditions may involve overlapping symptoms of fatigue and sleepiness, such as multiple sclerosis, myotonic dystrophy, and Parkinson's disease.

Manifestations of Sleepiness

- Sleepiness: A condition manifested by an ability to fall asleep easily when given the opportunity, a general feeling of "decreased subjective alertness,"[6] an inability to function normally while awake that is marked by errors and suboptimal performance.[10,11]
- Sleep attacks: Defined by occurrences of sudden irresistible sleep that lead to unintentional sleep episodes during wakefulness or to frequent naps if circumstances permit.[12]
- Automatic behaviors: When severe, sleepiness may also be manifested as "automatic behavior," in which sleep attacks and microsleep episodes occur in the middle of a purposeful activity and lead to impaired performance and no memory of the event. In a typical event, a sleepy patient on the phone may continue to talk but in an unintelligible way.
- Benefit of naps: It is held that in the hypersomnia of narcolepsy, sleepiness is typically reversed temporarily by short naps,[13] whereas in the hypersomnia associated with sleep-disordered breathing (SDB) or IH, sleepiness is less likely to be relieved by napping.[14] However, there is significant clinical overlap in the way that these conditions are manifested.[15]

Physiology of Sleep and Wake

- To understand, evaluate, and treat patients with the complaint of sleepiness, it behooves one to understand basic sleep- and wake-promoting mechanisms.
- Circadian influences are critical to sleep-wake cycling, which in turn is modified by exogenous circadian cues, the most powerful being light exposure. Understanding developmental changes in circadian rhythms, such as the tendency for adolescents to have a relatively delayed sleep phase, may be critical in assessing the complaint of EDS.
- Physiologic sustenance of alertness involves a complex interaction of central nervous system (CNS) pathways and neurotransmitters influenced by extrinsic factors; these pathways are reviewed in detail elsewhere in this book.[16–18]

Neurotransmitters

- Acetylcholine
  - Location: Lateral pontine/pedunculopontine tegmentum, basal forebrain.
  - Activity: Cholinergic influences are active during wakefulness and rapid eye movement (REM) sleep.
- Norepinephrine
  - Location: Noradrenergic neurons located in the locus coeruleus project to the cortex.
  - Activity: Mainly active during wakefulness.
- Serotonin
  - Location: Raphe nuclei (mostly dorsal raphe nuclei).
  - Activity: Serotonergic activity is high during wakefulness, but absent during REM sleep.
- Histamine
  - Location: Tuberomammillary nucleus.
  - Activity: Histaminergic neurons fire most readily during wake, with gradual decrements in firing in nonrapid eye movement (NREM) and even less in REM sleep.
- Dopamine
  - Location: Produced in the ventral tegmental areas and ventral periaqueductal gray matter.
  - Activity: Not fully elucidated, involved in promoting wakefulness and volitional awake activity, likely through a connection to reward systems.
- Hypocretin-1 and hypocretin-2 (Fig. 12.1)
  - Location: Synthesized in the dorsolateral hypothalamus.
  - Activity: Key promoters of wakefulness. Involved in stabilization of wakefulness during the day and sleep during the night.

Pharmacology

- Drugs that counteract neurotransmitters that mediate alertness produce a net sedative effect. These include H_1 histaminergic antagonists, α_1-adrenergic antagonists, and hypocretin/orexin receptor 1 and 2 antagonists.
- Conversely, drugs that increase or facilitate release of these neurotransmitters in general are stimulants (acetylcholine esterase

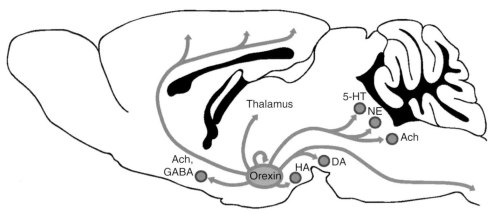

- **Figure 12.1** Orexin/Hypocretin Neurons Project Throughout the Brain to Promote and Maintain Wakefulness. Orexin/hypocretin neurons in the lateral hypothalamus project to the major arousal-promoting nuclei, including neurons producing histamine (HA; tuberomammillary nucleus), norepinephrine (NE; e.g., locus coeruleus), serotonin (5-HT; e.g., dorsal raphe), dopamine (DA; e.g., ventral tegmental area), and acetylocholine (Ach; e.g., basal forebrain, pedunculopontine and laterodorsal tegmental nuclei). The orexin/hypocretin neurons provide direct, excitatory inputs to the cortex, thalamus, and spinal cord. In addition, these neurons may be autoexcitatory. *GABA,* γ-Aminobutyric acid. (From Burgess CR, Scammell. Narcolepsy: neural mechanisms of sleepiness and cataplexy. *J Neurosci.* 2012;32[36]:12305–12311.)

inhibitors, amphetamines, monoamine reuptake inhibitors, presynaptic aminergic receptor blockers such as H_3 histamine antagonists).

- Sleep-promoting factors include γ-aminobutyric acid (GABA) and adenosine. Most sleep-inducing agents are sedatives that promote GABAergic transmission (e.g., benzodiazepine modulators, sodium oxybate).
- GABA$_A$ receptor antagonists or benzodiazepine antagonists/inverse agonists (e.g., flumazenil and clarithromycin) promote wakefulness.
- Caffeine is a well-known antagonist of adenosine, which may temporarily blunt the symptom of excessive sleepiness.
- The best example of a perturbation in an alerting pathway is narcolepsy-cataplexy phenotype, in which the loss of hypocretin neurons leads to EDS (Fig. 12.2), as well as intrusion of REM sleep-related phenomena at abnormal times, such as cataplexy, sleep paralysis, and hypnagogic hallucinations.
- Some experiments have suggested that decreased histamine or increased GABAergic transmission could be involved in the cause of some cases of hypersomnia; nonetheless, this is still speculative, and it is likely that many other contributors or biochemical causes of hypersomnia will be discovered in the future.

Making the Diagnosis

The American Academy of Sleep Medicine (AASM) practice parameters for the treatment of narcolepsy and other hypersomnias specify the importance of establishing an accurate diagnosis.[19] Given that eight subtypes of hypersomnia of central origin are identified in ICSD-3, a thorough evaluation of possible causes of EDS is required before committing to long-term therapy for hypersomnia.

Clinical History

- Mimickers and comorbid conditions: Many conditions can cause sleepiness that might imitate or coexist with central hypersomnias, including behaviorally induced insufficient sleep syndrome, obstructive sleep apnea (OSA), disorders in circadian rhythm timing, psychiatric disorders such as depression and the use of certain medications such as antidepressants, antiseizure medications. These conditions should be identified and treated, apart from using alerting medications.
- Natural evolution: The natural evolution of the symptoms should also be explored. Symptoms are stable in most primary disorders of EDS, except for periodic hypersomnia and in some psychiatric hypersomnia cases.
- Features of disease onset: Weight gain, prodromal viral illness, insomnia, timing, and the nature of the sleepiness are all important when evaluating for other diagnoses.
- Circadian rhythm pattern:
  - Advanced sleep phase disorder is associated with severe sleepiness in the evening and early morning awakening with insomnia.
  - Conversely, those with delayed sleep phase disorder experience nighttime insomnia, morning sleepiness, and sleep inertia (defined as excessive difficulty to arouse from sleep, or "sleep drunkenness").
  - A rapid onset of daytime sleepiness in the right clinical context may suggest narcolepsy.
- Cataplexy: Because of its importance to the diagnosis, questions regarding cataplexy should be asked carefully to avoid leading the patient. Cataplexy is a sudden involuntary loss of muscle tone classically triggered by humor (making a witty remark, finding something funny) involving different muscle groups, commonly orofacial and cervical muscles resulting in face sagging, jaw dropping, protrusion of the tongue particularly in children (Fig. 12.3), or lower extremity muscles resulting in knee buckling or gait unsteadiness, and in some instances the entire musculature causing individuals to slowly fall to the ground.
- Information of these events, including their triggers and various patterns of weakness, should be sought during the clinical interview.

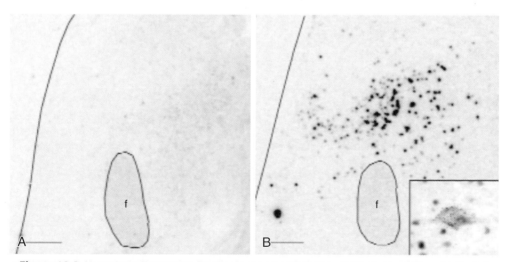

• **Figure 12.2** Hypocretin Expression Studies in the Hypothalamus of Control and Narcoleptic Subjects. Preprohypocretin transcripts are detected in the hypothalamus of control **(B)** but not narcoleptic **(A)** subjects. (From Peyron C, Faraco J, Rogers W. A mutation in a case of early onset narcolepsy and a generalized absence of hypocretin peptides in human narcoleptic brains. *Nat Med*. 2000;6[9]: 991–997).

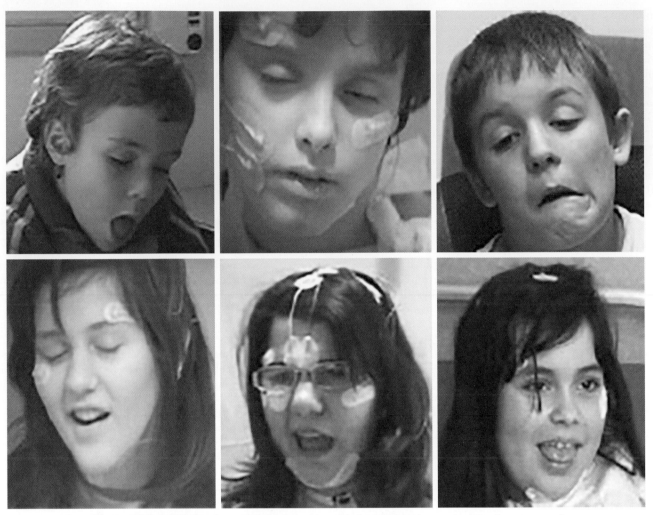

• **Figure 12.3** Facial muscle weakness, dropped eyelids (and facial grimaces keeping the eyes open), facial slackening, mouth opening and/or tongue protrusion, and a sort of "drunken/droopy look" characterize the "cataplectic facies." (From Serra L, Montagna P, Mignot E, Lugaresi E, Plazzi G. Cataplexy features in childhood narcolepsy. *Mov Disord*. 2008;23[6]:858–865.)

- Other associated symptoms:
  - Nocturnal sleep disruption or symptoms suggestive of REM sleep behavior disorder (RBD),[20] periodic limb movements (PLMs), nightmares, or other parasomnias may be associated with several sleep disorders, including narcolepsy; there may also be an association with SDB.[21]
  - EDS associated with vivid dreaming and weight gain in a child is suggestive of narcolepsy.
  - Although not specific of narcolepsy, the presence and severity of sleep paralysis and hypnagogic hallucinations should be noted. Likewise, questions about automatic behavior should be asked.
  - A particularly long nocturnal sleep duration (≥10 hours) may suggest IH (or simply a long sleeper based on reversibility of EDS with increased amount of sleep; Table 12.3).
- Social history is helpful to understand the sleep and living environment, as well as possible substance use, should be elicited. The social history may provide clues to the impact of chronic sleepiness, such as heightened risk for accidents at home or at work, poor performance at the workplace or academically, and social and marital problems.[22] Sleepiness while driving should also be thoroughly investigated and discussed.

- Family history may also reveal others with sleep disorders; disorders with a strong familial component, such as circadian rhythm disorders and OSA, may be seen in family members.[23]

Diagnostic Tests

A number of instruments have been developed to assess daytime sleepiness and cataplexy; the most frequently used in clinical practice are discussed in the following sections.

Epworth Sleepiness Scale

- The Epworth Sleepiness Scale (ESS) is a commonly used eight-item inventory for assessing the patient's likelihood of falling asleep during the course of a typical day. The total ESS score ranges from 0–24, with higher scores reflecting a greater propensity for sleep.[24]
- A total score of 10 or higher suggests pathologic sleepiness, which requires further evaluation and treatment.[25,26] Most patients with a complaint of EDS have scores of 12 or higher (e.g., >90% of narcoleptic subjects, personal data involving more than 1000 narcoleptic subjects).

TABLE 12.3	Differential Diagnosis of Central Disorders of Hypersomnolence: Normal Variants, Sleep-Related Breathing Disorders, Parasomnia, and Circadian Rhythms Sleep Disorders That May Be Confused with Hypersomnia Diagnoses		
Condition	**Diagnostic Criteria**		
Sleep-related breathing disorder	See chapter on sleep-related breathing disorder Most typically OSA syndromes	The major differential diagnosis for hypersomnia Not uncommonly, in association with a central disorder of hypersomnolence	Requires in-lab PSG confirmation May contribute only partially to overall daytime sleepiness Must be treated first before a diagnosis of hypersomnia or narcolepsy without cataplexy can be made (except if cataplexy is present)
Long sleeper	The daily total sleep time is ≥10 hours on average EDS only occurs if the patient does not obtain that amount of sleep	The sleep pattern typically has been present since childhood	Not explained by sleep-related breathing disorder, narcolepsy, idiopathic hypersomnia or medical causes of hypersomnolence As opposed to idiopathic hypersomnia, sleeping long hours is refreshing, and EDS disappears when long hours of nocturnal sleep are enforced
Circadian rhythm sleep-wake disorders	A chronic or recurrent pattern of sleep-wake rhythm disruption primarily due to alteration of the endogenous circadian timing system, or misalignment between the endogenous circadian rhythm and the sleep-wake schedule desired or required by an individual's physical environment or social/work schedules	Must lead to insomnia, sleepiness or both Cause clinically significant distress or impairment in mental, physical, social, occupational, educational, or other important areas of functioning	May be only one of the components contributing to daytime sleepiness With sleepiness, most commonly involve delayed or advanced sleep-wake phase disorder and shift work disorders More rarely: irregular sleep-wake rhythm disorder, non-24-hour sleep-wake rhythm disorder, jet lag type and secondary to a medical or psychiatric condition
Recurrent isolated sleep paralysis	Inability to move at sleep onset or upon waking up (a few seconds to a few minutes)	A parasomnia not explained by narcolepsy, hypersomnia (with sleepiness and abnormal MSLT), or another medical condition	Sleepiness is not the key associated feature, otherwise a hypersomnia diagnosis should be considered Should be considered as a normal variant if mild or infrequent May be familial
Nightmare disorder REM sleep behavior disorders	See chapter on parasomnia	When not explained by narcolepsy, hypersomnia or another condition	Sleepiness is not the key associated feature, otherwise a hypersomnia diagnosis should be considered

EDS, Excessive daytime sleepiness; *MSLT*, multiple sleep latency test; *OSA*, obstructive sleep apnea; *PSG*, polysomnography.

- However, many control subjects, approximately 25% in a general population sample, score high (≥12) on this scale.
- High scores on the ESS do not necessarily correlate well with mean sleep-onset latency (MSL), as determined by the multiple sleep latency test (MSLT).[27–29]

The Stanford Sleepiness Scale

- The Stanford Sleepiness Scale, unlike the ESS, measures a feeling of sleepiness on a 7-point scale at a particular moment in the day (Table 12.4).[30] It is used as a point-in-time estimation of the level of daytime sleepiness.
- Although sensitive to sleep deprivation,[31] it also correlates poorly with the MSLT and maintenance of wakefulness test (MWT).

Sleep Logs and Actigraphy

- Sleep logs should document sleep-onset and wake-up times, awakenings during the night, and daytime naps during a period of approximately 2 weeks. It can readily be seen whether patients suffer significant sleep restriction or circadian disruption in their sleep pattern, as well as the

TABLE 12.4	The Stanford Sleepiness Scale
Degree of Sleepiness	**Scale Rating**
Feeling active, vital, alert, or wide awake	1
Functioning at high levels, but not fully alert	2
Awake, but relaxed; responsive but not fully alert	3
Somewhat foggy, let down	4
Foggy; losing interest in remaining awake; slowed down	5
Sleepy, woozy, fighting sleep; prefer to lie down	6
No longer fighting sleep, sleep onset soon; having dream-like thoughts	7
Asleep	X

frequency and timing of nocturnal events (motor activity or parasomnias).

- Sleep logs may be used to document typical amounts of sleep over a 24-hour period and should be examined before performing the MSLT. Alternatively, actigraphy can be used to approximate sleep duration,[32,33] although it is most accurate in measuring sleep amounts in subjects without disturbed sleep or a sleep disorder.

Polysomnographic Investigations

- Most typically, an overnight sleep study, followed by the MSLT, is required, although if a coexisting sleep disorder is uncovered during polysomnography (PSG), it may be best to treat this disorder before proceeding to the MSLT.
- The MSLT should be conducted in subjects free of stimulants, stimulant-like medications, and REM-suppressing medications (listed in Table 12.5) for an adequate washout period equal to five half-lives (approximately 2–3 weeks).
- Some medications with particularly long half-lives, such as fluoxetine (and its metabolite norfluoxetine), should therefore be discontinued up to 1 month before the test.
- A good rule of thumb is to discontinue these medications for at least five times the half-life of the drug and longer-acting metabolite, confirmed by a urine drug screen.

TABLE 12.5 **Multiple Sleep Latency Testing for Narcolepsy**

1. The MSLT consists of five nap opportunities performed at 2-hour intervals. The initial nap opportunity begins 1.5–3 hours after termination of the nocturnal recording. The conventional recording montage for the MSLT includes central EEG and occipital derivations, left and right eye EOGs, mental/submental EMG, and EKG.

2. The MSLT must be performed immediately following polysomnography recorded during the patient's major sleep period. The use of MSLT to support a diagnosis of narcolepsy is suspect if total sleep time on the prior night is less than 6 hours, or if significant sleep disordered breathing is noted. The test should not be performed after a split-night sleep study and is not valid if conducted in a patient out of his normal circadian phase (shift worker), or in clearly sleep deprived subjects as documented through sleep logs.

3. Have the patient maintain a sleep diary for 2 weeks prior to sleep testing, including the following recommended questions:
   - What time did you go to bed last night?
   - What time did you turn off the light intending to sleep last night?
   - How long did it take you to fall asleep?
   - What time did you plan to wake up?
   - What time did you actually wake up?
   - Rate how rested/refreshed you feel now: 1 = very rested, … , 10 = not at all.
   - Rate the quality of your sleep last night: 1 = excellent, … , 10 = very poor.
   - How many times did you wake up during the night?
   - Estimate the amount of time you spent awake after you fell asleep (in minutes).
   - How long did you nap yesterday? (in minutes)

4. Obtain a current medication list, including OTC and illicit drugs, particularly stimulants, stimulant-like medications, and REM–suppressing medications. Medications that may suppress REM include carbamazepine, phenytoin, most antidepressant medications (serotonergic and/or noradrenergic medications), lithium, chlorpromazine, haloperidol, progesterone, beta-blockers, clonidine, diphenhydramine, loratadine, promethazine, barbiturates, and benzodiazepines.

5. Ensure that patients are drug-free for at least 15 days before sleep testing; the ideal length of time off drugs is at least five half-lives of the drug or longer-acting metabolite. Urine toxicology screening may be needed to verify the absence of medications and/or illicit drugs on the night of the sleep study or the morning after (morning of the MSLT).

6. Ensure that the patient's use of usual medications, such as antihypertensives, is planned by the sleep clinician before the MSLT so that undesired influences by the stimulating or sedating properties of the medications are minimized.

7. Prior to each nap opportunity, patients should be asked if they need to go to the bathroom or need other adjustments for comfort. Standard instructions for biocalibration prior to each nap include:
   - Lie quietly with your eyes open for 30 sec;
   - Close both eyes for 30 sec;
   - Without moving your head, look to the right, then left, right and then left;
   - Blink eyes slowly for five times;
   - Clench or grit your teeth tightly together.

8. With each nap opportunity, the subject should be given the same instructions: "Please lie quietly, assume a comfortable position, keep your eyes closed, and try to fall asleep." Immediately after these instructions are given, the lights are turned off, signaling the beginning of the test.

9. Between naps, the patient should be out of the bed and prevented from sleeping. The patient should also be advised to:
   - Stop smoking at least 30 min before each nap opportunity.
   - Avoid vigorous physical activity during the day and stop any stimulating activities by at least 15 min before each nap opportunity.
   - Abstain from all caffeine and avoid any unusual exposure to bright sunlight.
   - A light breakfast is recommended at least 1 hour prior to the first trial, and a light lunch is recommended after the termination of the second noon trial.

10. A nap session is terminated after 20 min if sleep does not occur. Sleep onset for the clinical MSLT is determined by the time from lights out to the first epoch of any stage of sleep, including stage 1 sleep. Sleep onset is defined as the first epoch of greater than 15 sec of cumulative sleep in a 30-sec epoch. The absence of sleep on a nap opportunity is recorded as a sleep latency of 20 min. This latency is included in the calculation of MSL. In order to assess for the occurrence of REM sleep, in the clinical MSLT the test continues for 15 min after the first epoch of sleep.

11. The MSLT report should include the start and end times of each nap opportunity, latency from lights out to the first epoch of sleep, mean sleep latency, and number of sleep-onset REM periods (defined as greater than 15 sec of REM sleep in a 30-sec epoch).

EKG, Electrocardiogram; *EMG*, electromyogram; *EOGs*, electrooculograms; *MSL*, mean sleep latency; *MSLT*, multiple sleep latency test; *REM*, rapid eye movement.

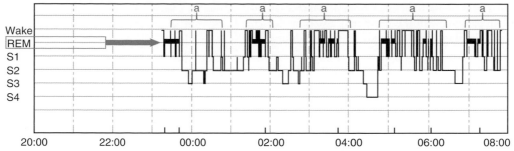

• **Figure 12.4** Typical Hypnogram Based on Nocturnal Polysomnography in a Patient with Narcolepsy. Note a highly fragmented sleep pattern with numerous awakenings *(a)* and frequent shifts between sleep states. In addition a sleep-onset REM period is present *(red arrow)*. *MT*, Movement time; *REM*, rapid eye movement sleep; *S1*, N1 sleep stage; *S2*, N2 sleep stage; *S3, S4*, N3 sleep stage (slow wave sleep). (From Overeem S, Reading P, Bassetti CL. Narcolepsy. *Sleep Med Clin.* 2012;7[2]:263–281.)

Multiple Sleep Latency Test (MSLT)

General Considerations

- The MSLT is designed to provide an objective measure of sleepiness and to estimate REM sleep onsets, the hallmark of narcolepsy.[34]
- However, caution should be taken to avoid making a diagnosis based on the MSLT alone; an understanding of the fundamental sources of error in the practical conduct of this test is critical and reviewed elsewhere. The MSLT is performed during the main period of wakefulness by using a specified protocol and is designed to determine a patient's tendency to fall asleep.[34]
- The MSL is determined from five naps. Normal subjects take more than 10 min, on average, to fall asleep; those with severe sleepiness take less than 5 min. An MSL of 8 min or less is used in the ICSD-3 classification as an indication of sleepiness.[1]
- It should, however, be noted that about 25% of the general population may have an MSL of 8 min or less.[34] Sleep deprivation, delayed sleep phase syndrome, sleep opportunities at an individual's typical sleep time, and sleep apnea are a few examples of conditions that may lead to short MSLs. Of note, the MSLT is not a validated test for children younger than 8 years (see Table 12.5).

Interpretation of MSLT

- The finding of multiple sleep-onset REM periods (SOREMPs, defined as a latency to REM sleep ≤15 min following sleep onset) during the MSLT is more predictive of pathology than a short sleep latency is.
- However, this finding is not specific of narcolepsy, as it can be seen in other situations including shift work disorder, sleep deprivation,[35] and delayed sleep phase disorder, which is particularly common in adolescents; SOREMPs in the latter case may be seen during the first two naps. Multiple SOREMPs can also be related to SDB, although the data are conflicting in this area.[36,37]
- Current ICSD-3 criteria for narcolepsy include an MSL of 8 min or less, and at least two SOREMPs, which may include a SOREMP from the preceding nocturnal PSG. Recent large studies have shown that between 4% and 9% of the general population may have multiple SOREMPs on routine clinical

MSLTs,[38–40] with about half (2%–4%) reporting daytime sleepiness and meeting the MSLT criteria for narcolepsy.
- The test-retest reliability (kappa coefficient) of the MSLT is poor, particularly in patients with type 2 narcolepsy or IH.[35,41]

SOREMP on PSG

- In contrast, although not very sensitive (~50%), finding a SOREM on a routine nocturnal PSG in patients with suspected narcolepsy (i.e., patients with hypersomnia not explained by OSA) has high specificity (96%) and an estimated positive predictive value of 92% for narcolepsy (Fig. 12.4).[42]
- Based on these findings, defining criteria for narcolepsy have been recently revised. According to the DSM-V,[43] a SOREMP on nocturnal PSG is sufficient for making the diagnosis in the correct clinical setting, regardless of the MSLT result.
- Other than narcolepsy, SOREMP on nocturnal PSG was shown to be associated with night and/or shift work (OR 4.4) and African American race (OR 4.15).[44]

Maintenance of Wakefulness Test

- The MWT is a 40-min protocol (four trials separated by 2-hour intervals) used to assess an individual's ability to stay awake. Interestingly, coefficient of correlation between the MSLT and the MWT is only partial ($r = 0.41$), accounting for less than 17% of the variability between the two tests and suggesting differences between the ability to fall asleep versus stay awake.[45]
- The MWT is not used for the diagnosis of narcolepsy and other hypersomnias, but rather, it is performed to assess the efficacy of pharmacotherapy for hypersomnia.[29,34]
- The MWT may also be helpful when there is a need to document that the patient is alert and adequately treated; for example, in cases of professional, occupational, or medicolegal inquiry. It does not, however, constitute foolproof evidence of constant alertness and can be used only as supporting data.

Continuous 24-Hour Sleep Recording

- Twenty-four-hour ambulatory or in-house PSG with electroencephalographic monitoring may be useful in the documentation of cataplexy/SOREMPs in the evaluation of narcolepsy,[46,47] documentation of a long sleep time (≥11 hours), which may replace the MSLT in patients with IH,[48] and may also be useful to detect the distribution of interictal epileptiform activity during the sleep-wake cycle.

- Standard daytime 16–20-channel electroencephalography can also be performed (with partial or total sleep deprivation the night before) to document seizures if clinically indicated. In some cases, this can be useful to distinguish atonic seizures from cataplexy.

Laboratory Tests

Routine Blood Tests. The referring physician has typically already performed these investigations before a sleep consultation, but the patient should be asked whether certain tests have recently been performed.

- Electrolytes, thyroid-stimulating hormone, and blood cell counts are helpful to exclude endocrinologic abnormalities and anemia, especially when the clinical picture suggests a component of fatigue.
- Ferritin: Patients with features suggestive of restless legs syndrome (RLS) should have ferritin measured. A ferritin less than 50 μg/L indicates a state of iron deficiency in the setting of RLS.
- Vitamin D level: Low level of vitamin D can be associated with excessive sleepiness and chronic fatigue.
- Urine drugs of abuse: Testing for selected drugs of abuse in urine samples is indicated if malingering is suspected.

Human Leukocyte Antigen (HLA) Typing

- The test is useful only when narcolepsy type 1 (hypocretin deficiency syndrome) is suspected, because almost all patients with this disorder—particularly those cases that are not caused by a central lesion or an underlying neurologic condition—carry a particular subtype of HLA-DQB1 called DQB1*06:02.[49] The association is probably close to 98% in patients in whom hypocretin deficiency has been documented inasmuch as only 10 exceptions have been documented worldwide.[50]
- It should, however, be kept in mind that 12%–35% of the general population (depending on the specific ethnic group) carry the exact same HLA subtype, DQB1*06:02.
- Since HLA "negativity" has a high negative predictive value for hypocretin-1 deficiency, HLA typing is most helpful in selecting patients prior to measurement of cerebrospinal fluid (CSF) hypocretin-1 level; in more than 300 patients with narcolepsy tested to date by multiple groups, all but four with low CSF hypocretin-1 levels have been shown to be DQB1*06:02 positive (Fig. 12.5).[51]

Cerebrospinal Fluid Hypocretin-1

- *CSF Hypocretin-1 level:* Decreased brain hypocretin neurotransmission is known to cause most cases of narcolepsy with cataplexy (see Fig. 12.2). Hypocretin cannot yet be reliably measured in blood for diagnostic purposes, but one of the two known hypocretin peptides, hypocretin-1, can easily be measured in CSF.
  - In the absence of any severe brain pathology, values below 110 pg/mL or a third of mean normal control values is the biologic defining feature of narcolepsy type 1. Although this test is highly specific and sensitive for patients with cataplexy, it is also found to be low in 5%–20% of patients without cataplexy (see Fig. 12.5).

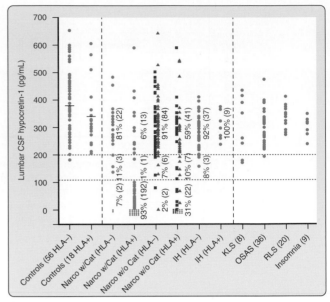

• Figure 12.5 Lumbar cerebrospinal fluid (CSF) hypocretin-1 concentrations in controls versus subjects with narcolepsy and other sleep disorders (from the Stanford Center for Narcolepsy Research database). Each point represents the concentration of hypocretin-1 as measured in unextracted lumbar CSF of a single individual. Subjects are differentiated according to HLA-DQB1*06:02 status and include controls (samples taken during both night and day). Patients are classified as having narcolepsy with or without cataplexy, and individuals without cataplexy are subdivided into those with atypical (triangle) and no (squares) cataplexy. Clinical subgroups include narcolepsy patients (Narco) with (w) and without (w/o) cataplexy (Cat), idiopathic hypersomnia (IH), Kleine-Levin syndrome (KLS), obstructive sleep apnea syndrome (OSAS), restless legs syndrome (RLS), and insomnia. Individuals with secondary narcolepsy/hypersomnia are not included. The dashed lines indicate hypocretin levels that are low (<110 pg/mL), intermediate (111–200 pg/mL), or normal (>200 pg/ml). Note that these pg/mL values are largely artificial and are meant to represent approximately 30% of mean control value as tested in a given center using direct radioimmunoassay and a set of healthy controls.13 Mean CSF hypocretin-1 concentration was not significantly different between HLADQB1*06:02 positive and negative controls. The percentage and number of subjects are specified for each group of subjects according to the two CSF hypocretin thresholds. (From Mignot E. Narcolepsy: Genetics, Immunology, and Pathophysiology. In: Kryger MH, Roth T, Dement WC, eds. *Principles and Practice of Sleep Medicine.* 6th Ed. Philadelphia: Elsevier; 2017:855–872.)

- The absence of cataplexy despite low hypocretin-1 may depend on several factors, including race, as shown in nearly one-third of African American patients.[52]
- Indication: In view of the difficulty of performing lumbar punctures, the use of CSF hypocretin-1 levels for the diagnosis of narcolepsy is typically reserved for complex cases with diagnostic challenges.[40,51]
- Such cases mostly include patients in whom the MSLT cannot be properly interpreted or with persistent clinical suspicion despite a negative or inconclusive MSLT: young children, patients with both narcolepsy and severe sleep apnea or with very disturbed nocturnal sleep, patients in whom instructions for taking an MSLT are difficult (mental retardation, psychiatric condition), and cases of secondary narcolepsy.

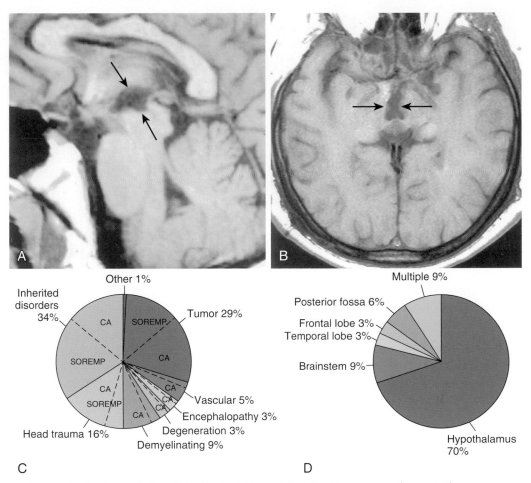

• **Figure 12.6** T1 weighted sagittal **(A)** and axial **(B)** magnetic resonance images demonstrating ex vacuo changes (between *arrows*) in the posterior hypothalamus and rostral midbrain of a patient with narcolepsy with cataplexy caused by a periprocedural stroke after removal of a craniopharyngioma. **(C)** Neurologic diseases are shown by category reported as secondary narcolepsy. Reported here are tumors, inherited disorders, and head trauma, which are the three most frequent causes. The percentage of cataplexy (CA) or sleep-onset REM periods (SOREMP) is denoted in each category with a dashed line. **(D)** Location of brain lesions in symptomatic patients with narcolepsy associated with brain tumor; the hypothalamus and adjacent structures are the most common location. Included are 113 symptomatic cases of narcolepsy. (AB, Modified from Scammell TE, Nishino S, Mignot E, Saper CB. Narcolepsy and low CSF orexin [hypocretin] concentration after a diencephalic stroke. *Neurology*. 2001;56[12]:1751–1753. CD, Modified from Kanbayashi T, Sagawa T, Takemura F, et al. The pathophysiologic basis of secondary narcolepsy and hypersomnia. *Curr Neurol Neurosci Rep*. 2011;11[2]:235–241).

• It may also be useful in patients in whom the cataplexy is atypical, when treatment response has been suboptimal, and in patients in whom more forceful treatment is needed (e.g., high-dose amphetamine or sodium oxybate). In rare instances, cost of the MSLT or inability to stop an existing essential treatment (e.g., co-occurring depression with suicidality) may also be an issue.

Imaging Studies–Magnetic Resonance Imaging of the Brain, and Other Diagnostic Tests

• These tests are indicated if a secondary medical or neurologic cause is suspected and is temporally associated with the onset of hypersomnia, or if the clinical picture or therapeutic response is atypical.

• In narcolepsy with and without cataplexy, examples include all subjects with abnormal neurologic findings on physical examination, HLA-negative subjects with isolated cataplexy, and subjects with narcolepsy plus other neurologic or endocrine symptoms, suggesting that it is part of a more complex syndrome.

• Secondary narcolepsy cases are more frequent in children than in adults (Fig. 12.6).[53,54] In children, narcolepsy-like features may occur in the context of complex genetic disorders, often with dysmorphic features.

- Specific examples include:
  - Prader–Willi syndrome: hypotonia, short stature, obesity, mental retardation, and sleep apnea.
  - Myotonic dystrophy: characteristic grip myotonia, facial and distal extremity weakness, sleep apnea, cataract, and male-pattern baldness.
  - Niemann-Pick disease type C: profound mental retardation, seizures, vertical supranuclear gaze palsy, ataxia, hepatosplenomegaly, and early death.
  - Coffin–Lowry syndrome: mental retardation with seizures.
  - Norrie's disease: ocular atrophy, deafness.
  - Late-onset congenital hypoventilation syndrome with hypothalamic abnormality.[40,55,56]
- Cataplexy may at times be difficult to differentiate from other mimics such as atonic seizures, vasovagal syncope, basilar migraines, and vertebrobasillar insufficiency.
- In both adults and children, narcolepsy with cataplexy may also be caused by a diencephalic (particularly hypothalamic) or brainstem tumor,[57–59] strokes (Fig. 12.6),[60] immune-mediated conditions including demyelinating disorders (acute disseminated encephalomyelitis, multiple sclerosis, neuromyelitis optica, Guillain–Barré syndrome),[61] and paraneoplastic syndromes, particularly when associated with anti-Ma2 antibodies[62] or in the setting of neuroblastoma.[63]
- Finally, it should be mentioned that hypersomnia is a common symptom and is associated with many neurologic disorders, including Parkinson's disease and posttraumatic brain injury.

Psychiatric Evaluation and Psychologic Testing

Sleepiness and other sleep-related symptoms can be seen in a variety of psychiatric conditions. For instance, there is an important overlap between depression and complaints of chronic fatigue or EDS. Atypical cataplexy (caused by unusual triggers such as negative emotions or stress) or sleep paralysis (with altered mental status or abnormally long in duration) can be experienced by patients with conversion or somatization disorder. Finally, hallucinations associated with a delusional theme (persecution, control) or not criticized by the individual should raise concern for an underlying psychotic disorder.

Specific Disorders

Narcolepsy

Epidemiology
- The prevalence of narcolepsy is estimated to be 1 per 2000 individuals in the general population.[64]
- Age at onset varies from early childhood to the fifth decade, with a peak in the second decade.
- Though considered a disease of adulthood, most cases are associated with onset in childhood or early adolescence.[65] Earlier reports observed that about half the patients had an onset before 15 years of age, with less than 10% having an onset before the age of 5 years.[66,67]
- More recently, it has been reported that of 1219 narcolepsy cases in one narcolepsy center database, 40% reported the onset of symptoms before the age of 15 (2.1% before the age of 5 years), although only 10% were younger than 18 years at the time of evaluation; 1.1% had cataplexy before the age of 5 years.[68]

- The delay from symptom onset to diagnosis is long in this disorder, with early work indicating that the median delay between onset and diagnosis is greater than 10 years.[69]
- However, with increased attention to narcolepsy, cases are being diagnosed with less delay, in less than 2 years from symptom onset in one series of children with narcolepsy-cataplexy.[68]

Classification
Following the discoveries of hypocretin involvement in narcolepsy with cataplexy, the ICSD-3 now differentiates:
- Type 1 narcolepsy, with either definite hypocretin deficiency—proven by CSF measurement, or probable hypocretin deficiency—in the presence of clear cataplexy and a positive MSLT
- Type 2 narcolepsy, a subtype not likely to be associated with hypocretin deficiency (i.e., cases without cataplexy but with a positive MSLT)

Clinical Presentation
Cataplexy
- Cataplexy is an abrupt and reversible bilateral decrease or loss of muscle tone, most frequently provoked by a strong emotion such as laughter or humor. It can occur multiple times daily, depending on the circumstances.
- This symptom is almost pathognomonic for narcolepsy type 1 and represents the intrusion of REM-related atonia during wakefulness (Fig. 12.7).[12,65,70]
- Importantly, as opposed to sleep attacks, consciousness remains intact and is unaffected during the episodes, which last from a few seconds to several minutes.
- Cataplexy may involve only certain muscle groups, such as orofacial and cervical muscles causing face sagging and jaw dropping with a characteristic protrusion of the tongue, particularly seen in children indicative of "cataplexy facies" (see Fig. 12.3); lower extremity muscles, resulting in knee buckling or gait unsteadiness; and in some instances the entire voluntary musculature, which may lead to a slow-motion fall typically not causing any injury.
- Cataplexy is a pure skeletal motor phenomenon devoid of any sensory component. For example, when laughing hard, non-narcoleptic patients might also feel "rubber knees" or partially experience unbuckling of the knees.
- In bone fide cataplexy, the muscle weakness is obvious and must occur more than a few times in a lifetime.
- Deep tendon reflexes (such as the "H-Reflex") are abolished during an episode,[71,72] which is particularly useful in distinguishing true cataplexy from cataplexy-like phenomena, including syncope, sleep attacks, atonic seizures, as well as conversion ("pseudocataplexy").
- The existence of a typical trigger is crucial for the recognition of genuine cataplexy. It is most commonly induced by "positive" emotional phenomena such as humor or laughter, for example, when the patient is hearing or telling a joke or funny story, or making a witty remark.[65,73]
- Less commonly, surprise, elation, or playful excitement is involved. Occasionally, emotions such as stress, startle, embarrassment, or related to sexual activity may be involved, but should not be the sole trigger. Startle is not a typical trigger.
- "Negative" emotional phenomena such as anger and fear are uncommon triggers of cataplexy.
- Cataplexy classically follows the onset of sleepiness in the natural history of narcolepsy, occurring within 5 years of the onset of

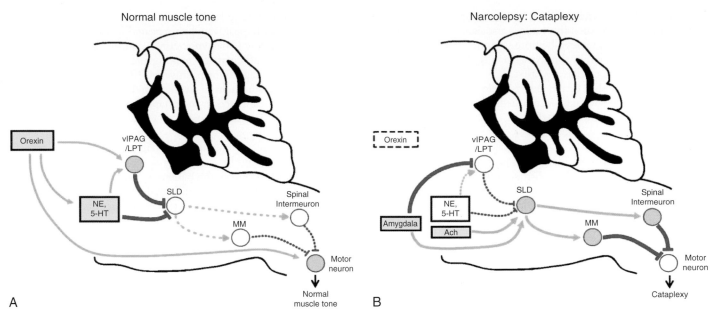

• **Figure 12.7** Atonia Pathways Triggering Cataplexy. **A,** Several pathways suppress atonia during normal wakefulness. Atonia is driven by neurons in the sublaterodorsal nucleus in the pons (SLD) that activate neurons in the spinal cord and medial medulla (MM) that inhibit motor neurons using γ-aminobutyric acid and glycine. During wakefulness, this atonia system is inhibited by neurons in the ventrolateral periaqueductal gray/lateral pontine tegmentum (vlPAG/LPT) and by monoaminergic neurons (e.g., NE and 5-HT). The orexin/hypocretin neurons are active during wake, and they help maintain normal muscle tone by exciting neurons in the vlPAG/LPT, monoamine neurons, and motor neurons. **B,** In narcolepsy, loss of the orexin/hypocretin neurons plus strong, positive emotions can trigger cataplexy. Positive emotions may activate neurons in the amygdala that excite the SLD and inhibit the vlPAG/LPT. The SLD may also be activated by cholinergic inputs and a sudden withdrawal of monoamine tone. The SLD then excites neurons in the medial medulla and spinal cord that strongly hyperpolarize motor neurons, resulting in cataplexy. Normally, the many effects of the orexin/hypocretin system and a continued monoaminergic drive to the pons and directly to motor neurons would counter this triggering of atonia, but in the absence of orexins, these excitatory drives are lost and cataplexy occurs. Solid pathways from filled nuclei are active; dashed pathways from unfilled nuclei are inactive. Green pathways are excitatory; red pathways are inhibitory. *NE,* Norepinephrine. (From Burgess CR, Scammell TE. Narcolepsy: neural mechanisms of sleepiness and cataplexy. *J Neurosci.* 2012;32[36]:12305–12311.)

EDS in two-thirds of cases.[13] In a recent analysis of 51 cases of pediatric narcolepsy with cataplexy, cataplexy occurred within 2 months of the onset of EDS 82% of the time, with similar data for prepubertal, peripubertal, and postpubertal subgroups.[68]

• In exceptional cases, in general young children, cataplexy can occur independently of daytime sleepiness in association with a complex syndrome secondary to other neurologic conditions such as Möbius syndrome, Niemann-Pick disease type C, Prader–Willi syndrome, and midbrain lesions.[40,55,56,58] In these cases, episodes of cataplexy may typically be triggered by laughing or may be difficult to distinguish from atonic seizures, especially when other seizures are also present (e.g., Coffin–Lowry syndrome).

Other Symptoms Associated with Narcolepsy

• Prodromal viral infection: If questioned closely about symptom onset in children, it may be possible to obtain a history of viral infection or streptococcal throat infection before onset, which has been reported.[74]

• Sleep paralysis is an inability to move for seconds to minutes that occurs most commonly on awakening and occasionally at sleep onset.

• Hypnagogic and hypnopompic hallucinations are dream-like visual or auditory perceptions that occur at sleep onset and on awakening, respectively.[12,65,75] These symptoms can be found in normal individuals and those with IH and OSA[75-77]; however, they can be severe in patients with narcolepsy and may require specific clinical attention.

• Weight gain and metabolic syndrome: Excessive weight gain at symptom onset. (In 51 children at Stanford University, 86% gained at least 4 kg within 6 months of symptom onset.)[68]

• Behavioral automatisms: Gestural, ambulatory, and speech automatisms; disturbed nighttime sleep, PLMs, or RBD, present in half of the cases.[78,79]

• Decreased performance in school, work, or impaired social function can also be observed, as a result of decreased attention and intrusion of sleep during academic, professional, or leisure activities.

• Disturbed and fragmented nocturnal sleep is present in approximately 50% of patients with narcolepsy-cataplexy and can be very disabling.[6,12,70] Narcolepsy is not characterized by difficulty falling asleep, but typically recurrent nighttime awakenings and a feeling of restlessness during the night are prominent.

- Nightmares and increased PLMs are often seen.[80,81] The situation becomes complex when insomnia is associated with a complaint of EDS without cataplexy, because sleepiness could be the result of insufficient sleep. In these cases it is typically recommended that the insomnia be treated first. It is also recommended in general that the SDB be treated first before diagnosing centrally mediated hypersomnias, while keeping in mind that these conditions may be associated.

Diagnosis

- Although very specific for type 1 narcolepsy, the presence of definite cataplexy together with sleepiness is not sufficient to diagnose the disorder based on ICSD-3 criteria, as it requires a positive MSLT to be consistent with the diagnosis (see Table 12.1 and Fig. 12.8).
- The advantage of requiring a positive MSLT is the exclusion of conversion disorder.
- In the event of a negative MSLT in the setting of a high pretest clinical suspicion and probability for the diagnosis, it is recommended to repeat the MSLT, as it has been shown to be consistently positive when repeated in these cases.
- In contrast, low CSF hypocretin-1 concentration, in addition to EDS, is sufficient for making the diagnosis, even in the absence of cataplexy or positive MSLT (Fig. 12.8).
- As CSF measurement of hypocretin-1 level is not available in routine clinical practice, the cataplexy should be corroborated to be definitive and typical to make a diagnosis of type 1 narcolepsy-cataplexy.
- If the cataplexy has atypical triggers, or is very rare or mild (cataplexy-like events), it is best to consider cataplexy absent and to classify the patient as having narcolepsy type 2, until the spells can be confirmed to be more definitive. It is not clear to what extent narcolepsy type 1 and type 2 have similar or overlapping pathophysiologic underpinnings of disease.
- Approximately 5%–20% of narcolepsy patients without cataplexy have low CSF hypocretin levels (<110 pg/mL), all of whom are HLA-DQB1*06:02 positive (see Fig. 12.5).

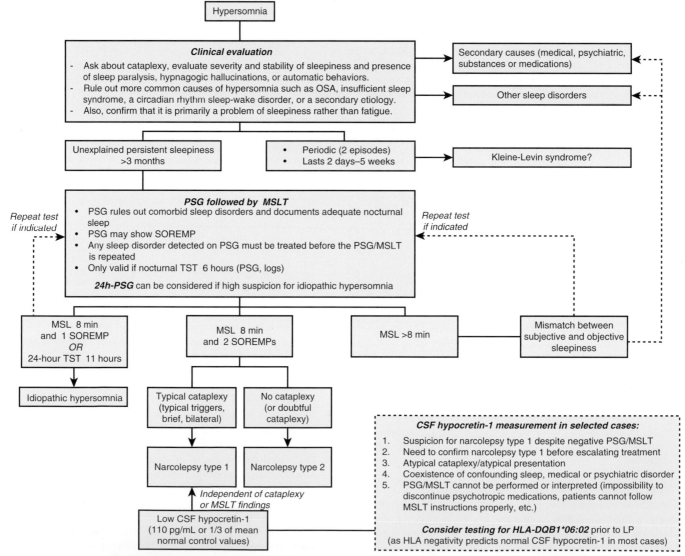

- **Figure 12.8** Diagnostic flow chart for the most commonly encountered types of hypersomnia. *CSF,* Cerebrospinal fluid; *MSL,* mean sleep latency; *MSLT,* multiple sleep latency test; *OSA,* obstructive sleep apnea; *PSG,* polysomnography; *SOREMP,* sleep-onset rapid eye movement period; *TST,* total sleep time.

- Conversely, HLA-DQB1*06:02 negative patients without cataplexy almost always have normal hypocretin levels. Patients with narcolepsy due to central lesions represent an exception to this rule, since in these cases the pathophysiology is not related to autoimmunity.

Pathophysiology

- As mentioned previously, most cases of cataplexy and a small fraction of cases without cataplexy are caused by hypocretin deficiency (see Fig. 12.7).
- Epidemiologic evidence and genetic studies in patients with narcolepsy-cataplexy suggest that, in genetically predisposed individuals, an autoimmune reaction triggered by an infection may result in the targeted destruction of hypocretin-secreting cells, likely through a process of molecular mimicry.[82]
- Almost all patients with narcolepsy type 1 are HLA-DQB1*06:02[83,84] and HLA-DQA1*01:02 positive, the gene products of which form a heterodimer that presents antigens to T-cell receptors on CD4 T cells.[85]
- Additional genetic predisposing factors include other HLA alleles and polymorphisms in T-cell receptor α (TCRα)[86] and purinergic (adenosine triphosphate) P2RY11 receptors.[87]
- DQB1*06:02 homozygotes or those with DQB1*06:02/DQB1*03:01 are at increased risk, whereas those with DQB1*06:02 and DQ1 are at decreased risk.
- The association with DQ and the TCR loci suggests that the specific HLA-DQα/β molecule B1*06:02 and DQA1*01:02 can present a specific antigen to one or a few specific TCRα/β–specific T-cell lines, with subsequent effects leading to an autoimmune reaction against hypocretin cells.
- Genetic susceptibility, although necessary in the vast majority of cases, is not sufficient for the development of narcolepsy. Indeed, identical twins are most commonly discordant.[88] Substantial stochastic effects may be necessary; for example, some individuals may or may not generate certain TCR combinations that may or may not escape negative selection by the thymus.
- Environmental factors, particularly streptococcal or influenza virus infection or vaccine, are involved in many cases through molecular mimicry. Support for the molecular mimicry theory is based on the presence of structural similarities between antigenic determinants of a pathogen (H1N1 infection) and the host hypocretin neuron autoantigens, as illustrated in Fig. 12.9.
- The onset of narcolepsy in children is often seasonal (late winter to spring), and patients close to onset have been shown to have increase antistreptolysin O (ASO) antibodies, a marker of infection with *Streptococcus pyogenes*. This finding, replicated twice in Caucasian populations,[89,90] was also confirmed in population-based studies, in which patients with narcolepsy were reported to have a fivefold increased risk when reporting a history of past streptococcal throat infection before the age of 21.[91]
- More recently, influenza infection and vaccine have also shown to be associated with increased risk for the disease.
  - In 2010 surges in incidence of narcolepsy-cataplexy were observed in different areas of the globe concomitantly affected by the H1N1 swine influenza pandemic that occurred in the winter of 2009–2010.
  - Similarly, incidence of narcolepsy increased by a factor of 12 in Europe, where onset of the disease often followed by

1–2 months the administration of a particular vaccine, Pandemrix® vaccine. This vaccine, containing a particularly potent adjuvant, may have triggered an autoimmune reaction in children and teenagers, but only in those carrying the HLA-DQB1*06:02 gene (Fig. 12.10).[82,92]
- Interestingly, increased ASO was also found in the context of patients in whom narcolepsy-cataplexy developed precipitously after adjuvant vaccination against H1N1.
- How could these infections or immune system stimulations be involved in the triggering of narcolepsy (see Fig. 12.10)?
  - In one case, a specific infection may generate peptides or molecules bridging specific DQ with specific TCR molecules and lead to cross-recognition of self-peptides in hypocretin-producing cells (molecular mimicry).
  - Alternatively, these infections could engage the immune system less specifically. For example, *S. pyogenes* is known to secrete superantigens, molecules that can stimulate a large number of T-cell clones by directly bridging the TCR and the HLA molecules and bypassing antigen presentation.
  - Similarly, the AS03 adjuvant implicated in narcolepsy after H1N1 vaccination could have such an effect. These non-specific immune stimulations could reactivate preexisting but dormant pathogenic T-cell clones, increase permeability of the blood-brain barrier to T cells, or induce an autoimmune process.
- Much less is known about the pathophysiology of narcolepsy type 2. This subtype may represent a mixed group, composed of individuals in whom cataplexy is less prominent or atypical (indicated by incidental finding of low hypocretin levels in some of them), patients suffering from other central disorders of hypersomnolence, as well as other sleep disorders and medical or psychiatric conditions, such as masked or atypical depression.

Evolution and Prognosis

- When associated with hypocretin deficiency, narcolepsy is considered irreversible and a lifelong disorder.
- The severity of the disease is often the greatest the first year around the onset, when symptoms are often evolving and cataplexy is establishing itself. In general, spontaneous amelioration has thus ensued, although the severity is greatly mitigated by aggressive therapy.
- Little is known regarding the evolution of narcolepsy without cataplexy. In some cases the cataplexy may develop years after disease onset. In other cases, the disease may regress or disappear. For this reason, it is wise to avoid aggressive therapies and a lifelong diagnosis when hypocretin deficiency has not been established.

Kleine-Levin Syndrome

In KLS (formerly called recurrent or periodic hypersomnias), the somnolence or increased sleep lasts 2 days–5 weeks, usually recurs more than once a year, and is separated by periods with normal alertness and cognitive functioning (see Table 12.1). Most episodes resolve in 30 days or less, and the periodicity of episodes is rarely more than 12–15 months.

Epidemiology

- KLS is an exceptionally rare condition; diagnosis is based primarily on clinical findings.

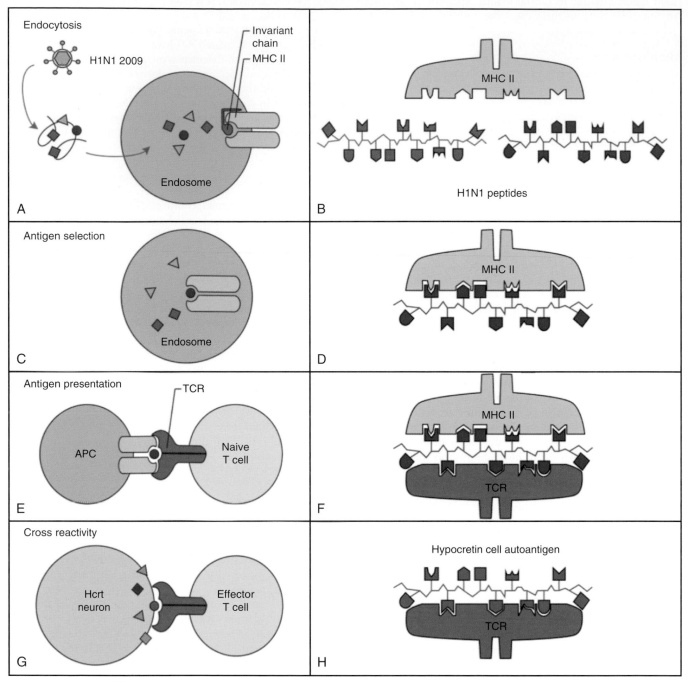

• **Figure 12.9** Molecular Mimicry Between H1n1 Peptides and Hypocretin Neuron Autoantigens. Sequence and structural homology between foreign and self-peptides are required for molecular mimicry to occur. **A,** The H1N1 virus is engulfed by an antigen presenting cell and the foreign antigenic material is digested into peptide fragments in the endosome/lysosome. **B,** The invariant chain is digested and the MHC groove is ready for occupancy by the antigenic fragment. **C** and **D,** The MHC binding groove selects the H1N1 fragment with a specific amino acid sequence in the context of DQA1*01:02-DQB1*06:02. **E,** The vesicles move to the plasma membrane and the complex is displayed at the cell surface for TCR recognition. **F,** The TCR recognizes a presented peptide with a specific amino acid sequence. **G** and **H,** Activated CD4+ T cells cross-react and recognize hypocretin neuron autoantigens as foreign molecules, prompting an autoimmune response against hypocretin neurons. *MHC,* Major histocompatibility complex; *TCR,* T-cell receptor. (From Mahlios J, De la Herrán-Arita AK, Mignot E. The Autoimmune Basis of Narcolepsy. *Curr Opin Neurobiol.* 2013;23[5]:767–773.)

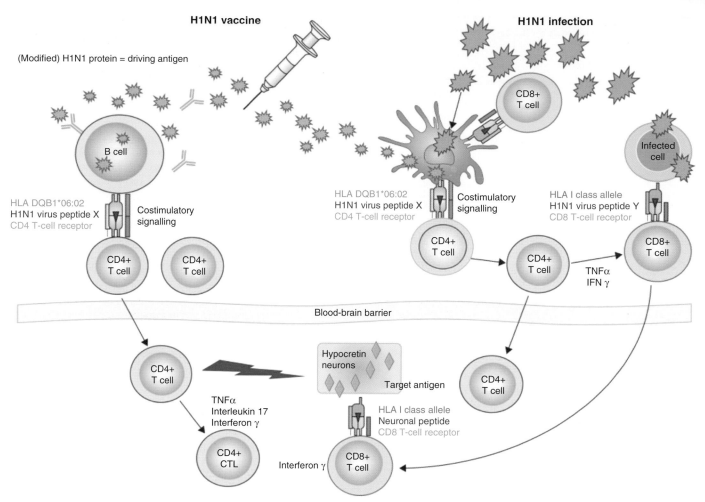

• **Figure 12.10** The role of H1N1 virus proteins and the HLA DQB1*06:02 allele in the development of type 1 narcolepsy is supported by epidemiologic studies showing increased incidence of narcolepsy after H1N1 vaccination (Pandemrix) in individuals with HLA DQB1*06:02 genotype, and by the possible cross-reactivity of hypocretin-specific CD4+ T cells with H1N1 virus protein in patients with narcolepsy. Increase in narcolepsy incidence has also been reported after H1N1 infection. In our model an H1N1 peptide X is presented in the complex of HLA DQB1*06:02 molecule to CD4+ T cells by antigen-presenting cells, such as dendritic cells or B cells. Because the risk of narcolepsy is seemingly associated only with Pandemrix and not with other adjuvanted or unadjuvanted H1N1 vaccines, an H1N1 viral antigen modified in the manufacturing process of Pandemrix might be presented as peptide X. Viral peptide X-specific CD4 T cells further activate CD8 cells, which recognize H1N1 viral peptide Y. Activated CD4 and CD8 cells cross the blood–brain barrier and infiltrate the hypothalamus, where hypocretin neurons are located. The destruction of hypocretin neurons can be mediated by inflammatory cytokines (e.g., TNFα, interferon γ, and interleukin 17) secreted by CD4 cells or DC4 cells, which acquire cytotoxic phenotype, or by cytotoxic CD8 cells. The neuronal autoantigen might show molecular mimicry with the H1N1 viral peptides X or Y, or the role of viral peptide X might be that of driving antigen of the narcolepsy-related autoimmunity. *APC*, antigen presenting cell; *CTL*, cytotoxic T lymphocyte; *TNFα*, Tumor necrosis factor α. (From Partinen M, Kornum BR, Plazzi G, Jennum P, Julkunen I, Vaarala O. Narcolepsy as an autoimmune disease: The role of H1N1 infection and vaccination. *Lancet Neurol.* 2014;13[6]:600–613.)

- This disorder frequently affects adolescent males, with the male-to-female ratio being 2 : 1, with a prevalence of one case per 1 million individuals.[93]
- Although the Ashkenazi Jewish population has been reported to be disproportionately affected, no genetic link has clearly been demonstrated. A third of patients with KLS report birth or developmental problems.[94]

Clinical Presentation

- Triggers: In more than 90% of patients with KLS, the initial episode is preceded by a prodromal event such as infection or high fever. Alcohol use, sleep deprivation, and stress have also been reported.[93] Nonetheless, less than 15% of recurrent episodes have an identified trigger.
- Onset and offset mode: In general, onset of an episode occurs over a few hours to 1 or 2 days, rarely longer, as well as offset.
- Hypersomnia: The hypersomnia associated with KLS is dramatic, with reported daily sleep durations close to 20 hours.
- Gender differences: Even though the rate of symptoms is the same in both sexes, it is reported that males exhibit more hypersexuality and females express more depressed mood.[94]

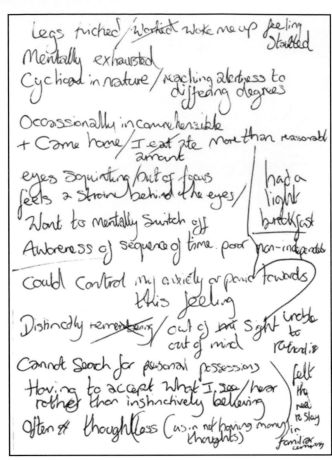

• **Figure 12.11** Symptoms as described by a 19-year-old boy during a Kleine-Levin syndrome episode. Note the incoherent and occasional wrong writing. (From Arnulf I. Kleine-Levin syndrome. *Sleep Med Clin.* 2015;10[2]:151–161.)

- Cognitive symptoms: May include cognitive impairment (cognitive slowing, impaired executive function, impaired language, slurred speech), abnormal behavior, and personality changes (apathy, regressive behaviors, "baby talk," disinhibition, irritability, aggressiveness).
- Psychiatric symptoms: These include repetitive behaviors and compulsions, altered sensorium, dissociative symptoms (derealization, depersonalization), delusion and hallucinations, as well as depressed affect, particularly in women. Fig. 12.11 illustrates the disorganization of thought and cognitive impairment in a 19-year-old boy during an episode of KLS.[95]
- Classic triad: Although the classic triad of KLS has been known as hypersomnia, hyperphagia, and behavioral changes, hyperphagia and hypersexuality may often be absent.[94,96] In fact, many patients report decreased appetite. Hypersexuality affects less than half of patients.
- Amnesia patients often display at least partial amnesia of their episodes.
- The diagnostic criteria set forth in ICSD-3 are summarized in Table 12.1.

Diagnostic Tests

- *PSG* has been conducted during and between episodes, with no clear differences noted between and during episodes.[97] However, in a recent report of 19 KLS patients who underwent PSG, when PSG was performed early (before the end of the

first half of the symptomatic period), an important reduction in slow wave sleep was always present with a progressive return to normal during the second half of the period. Conversely, REM sleep remained normal in the first half of the episode but decreased in the second half.[97]
- *MSLT* data have not been consistent in patients with KLS, but SOREMPs may be observed.[96,98]
- Imaging studies: A few functional imaging studies during the episodes, using 18F-fluorodeoxyglucose-PET single-photon emission computed tomography techniques, have shown patterns of decreased perfusion or metabolism more consistently affecting the hypothalamus, thalamus, frontal and temporal cortices, and occasionally other cortices and basal ganglia.[99–102] In a minority of patients, some of these findings persist at a lower level during asymptomatic periods.

Differential Diagnosis

- The major differential diagnoses are medical conditions, bipolar disorder, seasonal affective disorder, or other recurrent psychiatric conditions.
  - If the hypersomnia occurs in association with menstruation, a diagnosis of menstrual-related KLS may be made.[103,104]
  - This extremely rare condition is typically responsive to hormonal therapy.

Treatment

- KLS is a difficult disorder to treat, with a limited number of therapeutic options and limited data on their efficacy.
- Improvement has been reported with lithium[94,96] and anecdotally with valproic acid,[105] but stimulants have not been shown to be of great benefit.[94]
- Recent AASM practice parameters have supported the possible effectiveness of lithium carbonate for treatment of recurrent hypersomnia and behavioral symptoms associated with KLS.[19] Interestingly, lithium is a well-established and effective therapy in mood disorders, particularly bipolar disorder, a condition that has some similarities with KLS.
- One report showed that the antiviral agent amantadine given on the very first day of symptom relapse may abort the episode in as many as 42% of patients.[94]

Evolution and Prognosis

- The natural history of episodes is that they typically become less frequent, less severe, and shorter; persistent remissions can occur.
- The median duration of KLS was 8 years in a meta-analysis of 186 cases and 13 years in another.[94,96]
- Most adults are unaffected after 35 years of age.

Idiopathic Hypersomnia

Definition

- IH is a disorder of unknown etiology characterized by nonrefreshing sleep with difficulty waking from nocturnal sleep or daytime naps (or both).
- This disorder and its underpinnings are poorly understood, and exclusion of other causes of EDS—such as narcolepsy, sleep deprivation, circadian rhythm disorders, OSA, mood disorders, chronic fatigue syndrome, and others—is mandatory.[1]
- The ICSD-3 no longer differentiates between those with a long sleep time and those without a long sleep time (> or <10 hours, respectively).

Epidemiology

Although its prevalence is unknown, IH has been reported to occur 10%–60% as frequently as narcolepsy.[106,107] Symptoms typically start in adolescence or young adulthood, and there may be a familial pattern.[14,107]

Clinical Presentation

- IH is manifested as EDS despite adequate total sleep time and normal overnight sleep architecture typically associated with a high sleep efficiency (>90%), in contrast to patients with narcolepsy.
- Typically, patients report difficulty arising at wake time. Sleep inertia is a common, though not essential feature.
- In general, naps are not refreshing, in contrast to narcolepsy.
- Hypnagogic or hypnopompic hallucinations, sleep paralyses, or automatic behaviors may be present, and therefore do not distinguish IH from narcolepsy.
- Although depressive symptoms might be present, the diagnostic criteria for mood disorder must not be met.

Diagnosis

- The ICSD-3 has set forth criteria for establishing the diagnosis of IH (see Table 12.1); subjective measures of sleepiness obtained by using the scales described earlier, along with the MSLT, are important for this diagnosis.
- Alternative to the MSLT testing, the diagnosis can be made if total 24-hour sleep time exceeds 11 hours on 24-hour PSG.
- PSG was demonstrated to reveal more slow wave sleep after 6 AM in one series of patients with IH than in controls.[107]
- Actigraphy and sleep diaries can help document the 24-hour sleep-wake schedule,[108] and ascertain that the individual's EDS is not caused by insufficient opportunities to sleep. Both latter methods provide an alternative measurement of increased TST in these individuals with unexplained hypersomnia.
- Despite the ICSD-3 new criteria, the diagnosis is challenging due to the lack of a positive definition. IH presents with suggestive but variable symptoms, and may in fact represent a heterogeneous disorder. Furthermore, it is often clinically indistinguishable from narcolepsy without cataplexy, and the test-retest reliability of the MSLT has shown to be low, resulting in misclassifications for both these disorders.[41]
- Until causative mechanisms are found, IH and narcolepsy without cataplexy may be placed on a continuum of disease for which the etiology is still unclear.

Evolution and Prognosis

The evolution of IH is variable and unknown, and thus therapy is based on symptoms and should be conservative.

Pathophysiology

- As mentioned previously, this section also probably applies to most cases of narcolepsy without cataplexy (narcolepsy type 2). Identifying the cause of daytime sleepiness in these patients without cataplexy is difficult.
- These disorders are probably heterogeneous and in many cases multifactorial, and they also involve sleepiness caused by factors other than brain abnormalities.
- Consequently the diagnosis should primarily be one of exclusion (see Fig. 12.8), although this does not necessarily mean that these patients should be dismissed and left untreated.

- Factors contributing to the clinical picture may include genuine brain pathology resulting from infectious, metabolic, or autoimmune causes (yet to be discovered); sleepiness secondary to depression or anxiety (in these cases, subjective sleepiness is higher than objective, MSLT-based sleepiness); and sleep insufficiency as a result of sleep deprivation, abnormalities in circadian rhythm, irregular sleep/wake habits, or other factors.
- The disorder may also coexist with SDB or insomnia, and in such cases, participation of SDB or insomnia in the clinical picture is often difficult to assess without a therapeutic trial (e.g., continuous positive airway pressure for SDB).
- In complex cases it is suspected that the disorder is intractable because it is the result of multiple factors, some of which are psychiatric in origin.
- HLA linkage has not been definitely established,[109,110] and CSF hypocretin levels are normal.[93,111]
- A recent study found enhancement of GABA$_A$ signaling in the CSF of patients with IH or narcolepsy without cataplexy,[112] enhancement reversed after addition of flumazenil, a GABA$_A$ receptor antagonist. The authors concluded that flumazenil may act on a naturally occurring CSF constituent, present in IH patients, acting as a positive allosteric modulator of synaptic GABA$_A$ receptors. This hypothesis is supported by another study showing decreased EDS after a 14-day course of clarithromycin, another GABA$_A$ negative allosteric modulator.[113]
- Studies have shown that patients with IH and narcolepsy without cataplexy but with normal CSF hypocretin levels have decreased CSF histamine content.[114,115]
- Pitolisant, a histamine 3 receptor (H3R) antagonist, has been used in France for treating EDS in patients with narcolepsy[116] and IH[117]; however, it showed minimal efficacy in IH patients. Whether low CSF histamine is causative of sleepiness in some cases or simply reflects decreased histamine release when patients are sleepy is unknown. Unfortunately, lumbar punctures are unattractive as a diagnostic test, and this measure does not have clear clinical application at this time.
- A study by Sforza et al. demonstrated decreased slow wave activity (delta power) on spectral analysis in patients with IH.[118] This could in part explain the relative efficacy of sodium oxybate in some patients.[119]

Treatment Strategies for Central Nervous System Hypersomnia

- Treatment strategies for hypersomnias of central origin should always start with behavioral therapies but usually require pharmacologic approaches (Fig. 12.12).
- Regularizing the sleep-wake cycle with strict bed and wake-up times and scheduled napping is almost always recommended.
- Caution should be exercised with the use of amphetamine-like stimulants when the clinical picture is unclear or the sleepiness could have multiple causes (i.e., in patients without cataplexy).

Behavioral Treatments

- Good sleep hygiene, education, and compliance with treatment are important in the management of both narcolepsy and hypersomnia.[120]
- Fixed bed- and wake-up times and a regular sleep schedule are recommended. Napping every day at regular times, but not

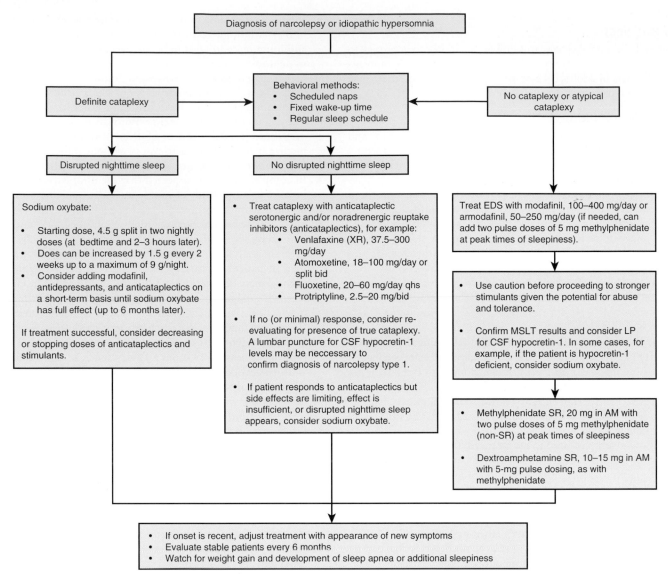

• Figure 12.12 Suggested Treatment Strategy for Narcolepsy and Idiopathic Hypersomnia. Note that other strategies for treatment are possible on a case-by-case basis. *CSF,* Cerebrospinal fluid; *EDS,* excessive daytime sleepiness; *LP,* lumbar puncture; *MSLT,* multiple sleep latency test; *SR/XR,* slow- or extended-release formula. Of note, modafinil, amphetamine, or methylphenidate may be available as single isomers or as a racemic mixture with different properties (see text). Doses indicated are for racemic mixtures except when specified (*d*-amphetamine).

excessively (one to two times per day for 15–20 min), is also beneficial.[121,122] This is especially the case for patients with hypocretin deficiency, for whom brief naps are refreshing.
- Avoidance of alcohol and some foods such as those particularly rich in proteins (tryptophan causes sleepiness) and carbohydrates (increasing cerebral utilization of tryptophan) may be helpful.[123]
- In addition, strategic timing and content of meals (incorporating snacks in between overall lower caloric meals) allow for the minimization of postprandial early afternoon dip.
- In some cases of IH, a long period of "sleep" may be reported, but the sleep periods may be distributed all through the night and day and largely occur at the wrong circadian phase. A depressive component may also be present in these cases. Light therapy, sleep restriction, and limiting napping can paradoxically be helpful in some of these cases.[124]

- Obesity may develop in patients with narcolepsy, especially in young children when onset of the disease is abrupt.[68] In these cases it is useful to restrict the diet, encourage exercise, and treat sleepiness aggressively around onset of the disease with medication.
- Given the duration from symptom onset to diagnosis, quality of life, social relationships, and function at school or work may have suffered. Patients with hypersomnias should be screened for the development of depression and substance use, and these conditions should be treated appropriately.
- Information about patient-oriented support groups such as the Narcolepsy Network (http://www.narcolepsynetwork.org/) may be provided as appropriate.
- The risk associated with driving while sleepy, especially before adequate therapy, must be discussed and, if appropriate, regulatory agencies notified.[125]

- Patients with narcolepsy or severe hypersomnia should receive counseling regarding school scheduling and avoid jobs that put others in danger (commercial driver, airline pilot). Activities that are less sedentary and involve physical work outside are often beneficial.[126] Jobs that involve repetitive tasks or sitting down and looking at a computer all day can be difficult. Employers or teachers may need to be asked to accommodate scheduled naps.

Wake-Promoting Agents

Modafinil, Armodafinil

Today, modafinil, either as a racemic mixture (*S*-modafinil) or as *R*-modafinil (armodafinil), is considered first-line therapy for EDS associated with narcolepsy[19] and may be effective for EDS in patients with IH.[19,107,127]

- Modafinil is a relatively older compound that was first made available in France in the 1980s and approved in the United States in the late 1990s. Although the mode of action of modafinil is not fully elucidated, inhibition of dopamine reuptake is likely to be involved in its wake-promoting effects.[128–130]
- The results of several multicenter trials have demonstrated improvements in objective measures of sleepiness and improved wakefulness in narcoleptic patients, and additive effects have been demonstrated when used in conjunction with sodium oxybate.[131–133]
- Armodafinil, which was approved in 2007 for the treatment of EDS in narcolepsy, has been shown to improve EDS throughout the day in randomized double-blind, placebo-controlled trials, and improve MSLT results at doses of 150–250 mg.
- Like modafinil, armodafinil is metabolized via the hepatic CYP3A4 enzyme, which can lead to induction of this enzyme pathway and effectively reduce the effectiveness of low dose oral contraceptives, so appropriate counseling about additional contraceptive options is necessary.
- The typical doses of modafinil are 100–400 mg, and those of armodafinil are 50–250 mg, with morning or morning plus noon hour administration (for modafinil). Of note, however, the 150 mg dose of armodafinil is more efficacious than 200 mg of racemic modafinil; equipotency is more likely around 125 mg.
- The elimination half-life is about 4–6 hours for *S*-modafinil and 15 hours for the *R*-enantiomer armodafinil; thus during chronic treatment with the racemic mixture, most of the effect is mediated by a stable concentration of *R*-modafinil.
- Headache can be a problematic side effect, but it usually resolves and can often be avoided by increasing the dose slowly.
- Importantly, modafinil can reduce the effectiveness of oral contraceptives, and therefore patients should be advised to use additional forms of contraception.
- The potential for abuse of this medication is low, and discontinuation of modafinil is not associated with rebound hypersomnolence, nor is there strong evidence of tolerance.

Amphetamine-Like Stimulants

Methylphenidate, dextroamphetamine, racemic amphetamine mixture, and methylamphetamine can also be used and are often stronger stimulants but have a number of disadvantages.[40,134–136]

- They are potentially addictive and should be reserved for patients with a well-established diagnosis.

- In addition, side effects such as palpitations, hypertension, and nervousness may occur because of their action on the autonomic nervous system.
- The mode of action of amphetamine-like stimulants on wakefulness is thought to involve increase dopaminergic transmission (blocking of reuptake and stimulation of release).
- Amphetamine (especially methamphetamine) should be used more cautiously than methylphenidate in as much as animal experiments have shown cytotoxicity on monoaminergic neurons with amphetamine,[137] a compound that depletes dopamine stores by interfering with the vesicular monoamine transporter.[135]
- Atomoxetine is unique in being the only medication approved by the US Food and Drug Administration (FDA; and only approved for attention-deficit/hyperactivity disorder) that selectively blocks reuptake of norepinephrine. It is also a mild stimulant and can sometimes be used to treat mild daytime sleepiness in some patients with IH. Interestingly, some patients who do not respond well to modafinil (probably a dopaminergic reuptake inhibitor) may have a favorable wake-promoting response with atomoxetine.[135]

Treatment of narcolepsy or other disorders of hypersomnolence during pregnancy represents a particular case since all CNS stimulants are category C (studies in animals show adverse effects and toxicity on fetus). In addition, modafinil has shown to decrease the efficacy of low-dose contraceptive pills, increasing the risk of undesired pregnancy. Sodium oxybate is also considered category C, and is associated with decreased Apgar scores in neonates when administered systemically during labor and delivery. It should only be used during pregnancy if the potential benefit for the mother outweighs the risk for the fetus.

Pharmacologic Management

- The most important concept when using stimulants for treating daytime sleepiness is timing. A typical scenario is to use modafinil or an extended-release methylphenidate or amphetamine formulation in the morning with pulse dosing of a short-acting medication at appropriate times throughout the day. For example, a student who still has problems with sleepiness after lunch might take 5–15 mg of short-acting methylphenidate at that time in addition to morning modafinil.
- Although stimulants are used primarily for daytime sleepiness, amphetamines (but not modafinil/armodafinil) also have some effect on cataplexy at high doses.
- Of note, short- and fast-acting stimulants are more likely to be abused, and their administration may be more difficult to control.
- In the use of stimulant medications, the specific formulation,[138] isomer,[134,139] packaging, and brand can make a tremendous difference in optimizing efficacy. More than 20 different formulations of amphetamine and methylphenidate are available, all distinguishable by their isomer content, conjugated salt, and releasing formulation.
- Selegiline, a monoamine oxidase B inhibitor that is metabolized to amphetamine, may be considered for the treatment of EDS according to practice parameters, though with reservations.[19]

Anticataplectic Agents: Antidepressants

Antidepressants may be effective in treating cataplexy, as well as sleep paralysis and hypnagogic hallucinations, which can sometimes be disabling symptoms.

- Selective norepinephrine and serotonin reuptake inhibitor medications such as venlafaxine and duloxetine are most effective.[135,140,141] Venlafaxine, a dual serotoninergic and noradrenergic reuptake inhibitor, is now typically used for the treatment of cataplexy (37.5–300 mg/day). Use of an extended-release formulation is critical, or multiple daily doses should be used.
- Tricyclic antidepressants (such as protriptyline, 2.5–20 mg/day, or clomipramine, 25–200 mg/day) are very effective in treating cataplexy, but have anticholinergic side effects and can be life-threatening in case of overdose.
- Selective serotonin reuptake inhibitors are included in the AASM practice parameters[19] for the treatment of cataplexy, sleep paralysis, and hypnagogic hallucinations, but they are only marginally effective when very specific for serotonin. Among them, fluoxetine (20–60 mg/day) has shown to be effective in some cases.
- Atomoxetine: Due to its norepinephrine reuptake blockage action, it can be used and effective at doses ranging 18–100 mg/day or split twice daily.
- All anticataplectic drugs including sodium oxybate are category C (risk cannot be ruled out) during pregnancy.
- Patients should be forewarned that rebound cataplexy almost always occurs when antidepressant medications are discontinued, changed, or skipped. Compliance is key to therapeutic efficacy as anticataplectic agents. It is occasionally difficult to wean patients from these medications because of rebound cataplexy, which may last weeks.

Sodium Oxybate

- Sodium oxybate (also called γ-hydroxybutyrate, GHB[19,131,142]) is approved by the FDA for the treatment of both cataplexy and EDS associated with narcolepsy-cataplexy.[19,131,142–145] It is the treatment of choice for narcolepsy with cataplexy because it is efficacious in alleviating multiple symptoms (EDS, cataplexy, disrupted nocturnal sleep).
- It is a strong sedative that has been used as an anesthetic agent since the 1960s and is now first-line therapy in patients with narcolepsy/hypocretin deficiency. GHB is given at night to consolidate sleep. It is thought that consolidation of nocturnal sleep with promotion of slow wave, and REM sleep leads to decreased daytime symptoms the following day.
- Recent studies have shown that sodium oxybate can be used successfully in young children with narcolepsy-cataplexy, including prepubertal children.[68]
- Although recent evidence suggests that GHB may be beneficial in patients with IH,[119] as with amphetamine stimulants, the drug should be used cautiously in patients without a clear diagnosis of narcolepsy with cataplexy.

Mechanism of Action

GHB is an endogenous CNS metabolite of GABA, with highest concentrations in the hypothalamus and basal ganglia. It is considered a neuromodulator/neurotransmitter affecting dopamine, serotonin, GABA, and endogenous opioids; it also considered to be a $GABA_B$ receptor agonist.[131,144,146–148] As a therapeutic agent for narcolepsy-cataplexy, its mechanism of action is poorly understood.

Clinical Benefit

- Clinically, it has been shown to dramatically reduce cataplexy, as well as treat daytime sleepiness and improve the sleep fragmentation/disturbed sleep typical of narcolepsy-cataplexy.[19,131,142–145,149]
- The improvement in cataplexy is much more rapid than its effect on daytime sleepiness, which may take up to 6–8 weeks, an important concept since titrating upward too quickly in an attempt to control daytime sleepiness is a common mistake.

Dosing

- In adults, the starting dose should not be higher than 4.5 g per night divided into two nightly doses (before bedtime and a second dose typically about 3 hours later, once the first dose has metabolized).
- Dosing may be gradually increased over a period of 8 weeks or longer, with a typical adult dose goal of 6–9 g, which has been shown to be effective for improvement in EDS and nocturnal sleep.[1]
- A limitation of GHB is that its efficacy is short, frequently no longer than 2 hours.[150] In these cases, varying the administration schedule may be helpful in optimizing total sleep time while keeping the dose at the therapeutic range. Variations in the schedule include letting the patient sleep during first cycle without drugs, followed by two administrations separated by 2 hours or occasionally use of three lower doses. Until the full alerting effects of GHB become manifested, other alerting agents may be used.

Adverse Effects

- Side effects include nausea, especially at initiation and with higher doses, disorientation in the middle of the night, grogginess on awakening, and enuresis.
- Occasionally, use of this medication results in dramatic weight loss, often a good outcome in an obese patient. In rare cases, however, decreased appetite and nausea can be severe and lead to excessive weight loss, thereby mandating interruption of therapy.
- Unusual parasomnia-like behavior (sleep walking, night terrors) are reversible on decreasing the total dose.
- In rare cases, sodium oxybate may induce psychologic changes such as increased anxiety, depression, or other daytime effects.
- Use of this medication also confers a significant sodium load, which may be limiting for those with fluid retention, congestive heart failure, or hypertension.
- Sodium oxybate should not be taken with alcohol or other CNS depressants.
- Experiments have also shown no acute rebound of cataplexy or other symptoms on withdrawal.[151]
- It should also be noted that the drug can be prescribed in the presence of sleep apnea if OSA is treated properly (i.e., in conjunction with positive airway pressure).
- A limitation with the use of sodium oxybate is its potential for abuse, toxicity at high doses, and illicit use.[152,153]
- As mentioned previously, sodium oxybate is considered category C in pregnant women. Despite the absence of adequate studies in pregnant women, it has shown to result in transient sleepiness in neonates when used as an anesthetic agent during labor or delivery.

Treatment of Ancillary and Associated Conditions

In the special case of narcolepsy or hypersomnia caused by another medical or neurologic condition, optimal therapy for the associated condition should be achieved first, with special attention to gaining adequate control of nocturnal sleep disturbances, which could partially or entirely be causing the daytime sleepiness.

- Depression: This is particularly important in the case of co-occurring depression or anxiety, which will often complicate compliance and response to therapy. When underlying depression is suspected, bupropion may be an agent of choice due to its dopaminergic and noradrenergic properties.
- OSA: Primary narcolepsy is also frequently associated with other sleep disorders; OSA is common and must be treated, especially if sodium oxybate is to be used, since this drug can worsen the severity of OSA.
- PLMs and REM sleep without atonia are also common, but very rarely need treatment unless associated with RLS.
  - Empiric treatment of PLMs may also be considered when these are associated with arousals that are not related to SDB.
  - PLMs in narcolepsy are more common during REM sleep than in nonnarcoleptics.

Narcolepsy-Cataplexy: Novel Approaches

- Given the emerging evidence of an autoimmune cause of narcolepsy-cataplexy, there has been increased interest in the early diagnosis of narcolepsy-cataplexy to allow the possibility of using immunomodulators, which may reduce the destruction of hypocretin-producing hypothalamic neurons and reduce or eliminate the burden of this disease.[135]
- Case reports and series of steroids, plasmapheresis, and intravenous immunoglobulin therapy have shown limited or no success, although cataplexy or improved sleepiness has been reported with the latter treatment in some cases.[154–161]

Investigational Agents

- Several novel approaches for treating narcolepsy have been proposed, including hypocretin replacement, hypocretin gene therapy, stem cell transplantation, and new pharmaceutical agents active on the thyrotropin (thyrotropin-releasing hormone), $GABA_A$ transmission, and histamine (H_3) systems to promote alertness. Among these agents, pitolisant has recently gained a particular place since two recent randomized control studies in Europe showed that this H3 receptor inverse agonist has efficacy both on symptoms of EDS[162] and cataplexy[163] in patients with narcolepsy. Although long term data is needed, this makes pitolisant a promising alternative pharmacological treatment to GHB for narcolepsy with or without cataplexy.
- Since the vast majority of narcolepsy-cataplexy patients are deficient in CNS hypocretin ("ligand deficient"), hypocretin replacement therapy is an attractive approach to treat both the sleep problems and cataplexy. Intranasal administration of hypocretin-1 in a small group of patients has shown promising results.[164] Early reports of gene therapy in murine models also demonstrate some promise.[165–166]

- Efforts to date in the pharmaceutical sector have focused on hypocretin/orexin receptor 1 and 2 antagonists as a treatment of insomnia, most notably drugs commonly referred as DORA (dual orexin receptor antagonists, such as suvorexant). Agonist molecules have been found in vitro,[167] but none have been developed as drugs. It is likely that selective and dual hypocretin receptor agonists will be found in the future and, if able to penetrate the CNS, will offer effective therapies for the treatment of narcolepsy.

Conclusion and Perspectives

- Although the diagnosis and treatment of type 1 narcolepsy have been codified and much of its pathophysiology is well understood, much less is known about narcolepsy without cataplexy, IH, KLS, and other central disorders of hypersomnolence.
- Hypersomnia disorders are increasingly being diagnosed on the basis of the MSLT alone, yet the MSLT was developed primarily as a diagnostic test for narcolepsy-cataplexy, and its diagnostic reliability for other disorders is limited. This is especially true in the context of IH, a condition most often diagnosed on the basis of a short MSL (<8 min) alone.
- With the growth of sleep medicine, patients with hypersomnia symptoms are increasingly being identified in the context of other sleep-like symptoms (fatigue) or disorders—mostly insomnia, depression, circadian abnormalities, sleep deprivation, and OSA.
- Because clear therapeutic guidelines are lacking for these conditions, in general, it is recommended that one exercise caution in the use of potentially abusable substances such as amphetamine and sodium oxybate.
- Diagnosis and management of these complex cases remain challenging but may be the next frontier in optimizing diagnosis and clinical care in the field of hypersomnia.
- New treatments of narcolepsy-cataplexy, as well as studies on the treatment of other central disorders of hypersomnolence, are needed, as are studies in special populations such as children, pregnant women, and older adults.

Suggested Reading

Bassetti C, Billiard M, Mignot E. In: Lenfant C, ed. *Narcolepsy and Hypersomnia*. New York: Informa Health Care USA Inc.; 2007:697.

Bourgin P, Zeitzer JM, Mignot E. CSF hypocretin-1 assessment in sleep and neurological disorders. *Lancet Neurol.* 2008;7(7):649-662.

Dauvilliers Y, Arnulf I, Mignot E. Narcolepsy with cataplexy. *Lancet.* 2007;369(9560):499-511.

Mignot E. Narcolepsy: genetic, immunology, and pathophysiology. In: Kryger MH, Roth T, Dement WC, eds. *Principles and Practice of Sleep Medicine*. 6th ed. Elsevier; 2017:938-956.

Mignot EJ. A practical guide to the therapy of narcolepsy and hypersomnia syndromes. *Neurotherapeutics.* 2012;9(4):739-752.

Scammell TE. Narcolepsy. *N Engl J Med.* 2015;373(27):2654-2662. doi:10.1056/NEJMra1500587.

13

Sleep-Related Breathing Disorders: Clinical Features and Evaluation

BENJAMIN H. HUGHES, CHARLES A. POLNITSKY, TEOFILO LEE-CHIONG

Introduction

A snoring person has historically been portrayed as one peacefully at rest in deepest sleep, perhaps disturbing his companions, but usually regarded with humor. The past several decades have produced an entirely new picture in which sleep-disordered breathing (SDB), ranging from snoring and mild increases in upper airway resistance to apnea with profound hypoxemia, actually causes significant physiologic reactions and contributes to multiorgan pathology. Furthermore, these conditions are now recognized in both genders and across all ages.

- The incidence of SDB appears to be increasing beyond what would be expected from newfound awareness alone.
- Obesity, allergic upper airway conditions, and other influences, including survival advantages conferred by better health care, have combined to make SDB one of the new epidemics of this millennium.

Obstructive Sleep Apnea

The terminology pertaining to obstructive sleep apnea (OSA) continues to evolve.

- Obstructive apnea (OA) occurs when there is complete or nearly complete cessation of airflow, accompanied by preservation of respiratory drive manifested as persistent respiratory muscle activity (Fig. 13.1).
- If there is a partial reduction in airflow with preservation of respiratory effort, the event is defined as obstructive hypopnea (OH; Fig. 13.2).
- Although OA and OH have different specific definitions, their pathophysiology and physiologic consequences are similar, and in clinical polysomnography (PSG) they are combined into a single measure—the apnea-hypopnea index (AHI).[1]

In general, the magnitude of AHI reflects the severity of OSA syndrome (OSAS) sequelae:

- Excessive daytime sleepiness (EDS)
- Cardiovascular risk
- Neurocognitive impairment
- Metabolic consequences

The AHI also provides objective thresholds for diagnosis and treatment reimbursement. When respiratory effort–related arousals (RERAs, see later) are included in the total number of events

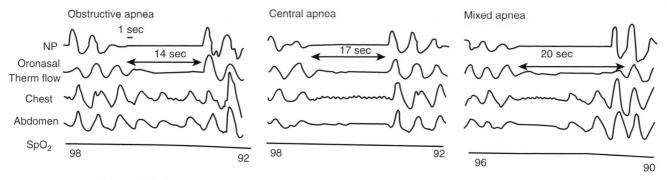

• **Figure 13.1** Comparison of Obstructive Apnea, Central Apnea, and Mixed Apnea. Note the cessation of nasal pressure (NP) and oronasal flow for at least 10 sec in all cases. In obstructive apnea, respiratory effort persists. In central apnea, respiratory effort is absent. In mixed apnea, absence of respiratory effort in the initial portion is followed by resumption of respiratory effort while absence of airflow persists. (Modified from Berry RB. *Fundamentals of Sleep Medicine*. 1st ed. Philadelphia, PA: Saunders; 2012:124.)

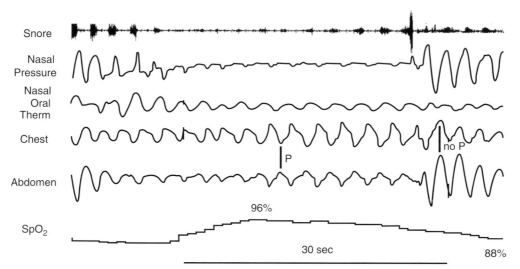

• **Figure 13.2** Obstructive Hypopnea. Note the decrease in nasal pressure signal amplitude by greater than 30% with associated oxygen desaturation. A 3% desaturation or arousal is required to score a central hypopnea if using the recommended American Academy of Sleep Medicine (AASM) criteria; a 4% desaturation is required if using the acceptable AASM criteria. To qualify as *obstructive,* the event must be accompanied by evidence of respiratory effort, such as snoring, thoracoabdominal paradox (P), and/or flattening of the inspiratory phase of the nasal pressure signal (Modified from Berry RB. *Fundamentals of Sleep Medicine*. 1st ed. Philadelphia, PA: Saunders, 2012:130.)

determined by standard PSG, the convention is to report the sum as the respiratory disturbance index (RDI).
• The term *OSA* is properly reserved to describe the objective documentation of OA and OH events.
• When psychologic or physiologic manifestations of OSA are diagnosed in an individual, that person is considered to have OSAS.

Epidemiology

• OSA was historically thought to affect approximately 3%–7% adults[2] and 1%–4% of children[3] in the United States.
• Recent data indicate that OSA can be demonstrated on PSG in up to 34% of men and 17% of women.[4] Overall, OSAS is estimated to have a prevalence of 14% in men and 5% in women.[5]

Factors That Increase Prevalence

Age, gender, body mass index (BMI), and race have important impacts on prevalence in various cohorts, with advancing age, male gender, higher BMI, and Asian or African American race all conferring increased risk for OSA at a population level.[2,6]

Comorbid Associations

In addition, there are many disease-specific associations with OSA.
• In one study, apnea was present in 60% or more of individuals who experienced a stroke.[7]
• Likelihood of OSA is also increased in the context of other chronic conditions, such as congestive heart failure (CHF),[8] polycystic ovary syndrome (PCOS),[9] and asthma.[10]
• The disease occurs in association with various neuromuscular disorders, such as myotonic dystrophy, and craniofacial disorders, such as Pierre Robin sequence and Down syndrome.

Effect of Body Mass Index, Gender, and Age

- Although OSA is more common in obese and overweight individuals, it is also found in individuals of normal weight, in whom the prevalence may be markedly underestimated because of a failure to consider this diagnosis in this population group.[11]
- A similar concern has been raised for the female gender.[12]
- OSA is not uncommon in children, for whom age-specific diagnostic criteria have been established.[13–16]

Definitions

Definitions of events vary considerably in the sleep literature, which results in potential confusion for readers and gives rise to difficulty making meaningful comparisons. The American Academy of Sleep Medicine (AASM) standards, revised in 2012, provide the most commonly used reporting system.[16]

Obstructive Apnea in Adults

- Ninety percent or greater drop in the oronasal or alternative diagnostic sensor or positive airway pressure (PAP) device flow signal for 10 or more seconds.
- Ongoing inspiratory effort must be evident to qualify as an OA.
- In the absence of inspiratory effort, the event is scored as a central apnea (CA; see later).

Scoring of Hypopnea Is Less Straightforward

The AASM recommended criteria require the following:
- The flow signal, preferably generated by a nasal pressure sensor, must drop by 30% of baseline or greater.
- The duration must be 10 sec or longer.
- A drop in oxygen saturation (SaO_2) of 3% or greater from the pre-event baseline must occur, *or* there must be an associated EEG arousal.

The AASM also presents an alternative "acceptable" definition for scoring hypopnea that calls for the same depth and duration of flow reduction plus a 4% or greater oxygen desaturation; arousals are not included in this definition. In the United States, Medicare and an increasing number of private insurers require a 4% or greater desaturation in the scoring of OH for the purposes of treatment reimbursement.

Distinguishing Obstructive Versus Central Hypopnea

OH requires evidence of respiratory effort, which may include any of the following:
- Snoring
- Inspiratory flattening in the nasal pressure signal
- Thoracoabdominal paradox

In addition, an event may occur as a mixed apnea or mixed hypopnea if it meets the aforementioned criteria but demonstrates absence of respiratory effort in its initial phase, followed by resumption of effort in the latter portion of the same event.

Pediatric Criteria

Guidelines for scoring events in children under 18 years of age have also been formulated. They contain some variations from the adult criteria. One challenge with their application is identifying the appropriate age cutoff. It has been suggested that the decision to use pediatric or adult criteria may be flexible, especially for those aged 13–18 years.[16]

Pathophysiology

OSA can develop in any given individual as a result of a combination of a variety of predisposing anatomic and physiologic aberrations in the maintenance of upper airway patency during sleep; these changes have recently been categorized into four principle variables that govern the balance between airway patency and collapse.[17]
- Critical closing pressure (P_{crit})
- Loop gain
- Upper airway dilator recruitment threshold
- Arousal threshold

Critical Closing Pressure

Critical closing pressure, the pressure at which the upper airway collapses, is higher in subjects with OSA, reflecting increased inherent collapsibility. Factors affecting P_{crit} include airway luminal diameter, external compression (for instance, by adipose tissue), and upper airway muscle function.[18,19] Therefore P_{crit} increases in the setting of obesity, craniofacial abnormalities, neuromuscular disease, and tonsillar hypertrophy. P_{crit} is a marker of upper airway collapsibility but does not independently predict OSA severity. The other physiologic determinants, described later, interact with P_{crit} to cause OA and OH.

Loop Gain

Loop gain describes the ratio of ventilatory response to derangements in oxygenation and ventilation. Subjects with OSA often have increased loop gain, or an exaggerated response to episodes of hypoxemia and/or hypercapnia; this causes transient hyperventilation and subsequent loss of respiratory drive and upper airway dilator muscle tone, resulting in repetitive obstruction and apneas.[20,21]

Upper Airway Recruitment Threshold

Upper airway recruitment threshold is a measure of the amplitude of stimuli (hypercapnia, hypoxemia, and negative intraesophageal pressure) required for activation of the upper airway dilator muscles; it is increased in OSA patients. Patients with a high recruitment threshold do not readily activate the upper airway musculature (especially genioglossus) to maintain airway patency, particularly during phasic inspiration when negative intrathoracic pressure is transmitted to the upper airway.[22]

Arousal Threshold

Arousal threshold is the negative intraesophageal pressure required to cause an arousal. Individuals with low arousal threshold develop increased sleep fragmentation and sympathetic activation. In the setting of frequent arousals, brief periods of wakefulness cause relative hyperventilation that, with return to sleep, leads to decreased respiratory drive and diminished upper airway dilator muscle tone, thereby predisposing to recurrent airway collapse.[23,24]

Interaction of Variables

All of these determinants of airway patency are dynamic in a given individual. For instance, factors such as body position, sleep deprivation, altitude, and alcohol or medication consumption have been shown to alter one or more of these variables. Therefore OSA itself is a dynamic process in which severity and pathology can change on a nightly basis.

Obesity Is a Major Risk Factor

There are various mechanisms by which increased BMI predisposes to OSA.[25]

- The simple reduction in upper airway diameter by retropharyngeal fat deposition has been seen in imaging studies.[26]
- The inspiratory resistive loading associated with increased thoracic and abdominal mass plays a role in effort-related airway collapse.
- Autonomic dysfunction, such as seen in patients with diabetes, may have a contributory role.[27]
- Weight reduction, including that which is achieved by bariatric surgery in morbidly obese individuals, can eliminate OSA or reduce its severity.[28–30] However, in many obese individuals, the need for PAP therapy remains even after weight loss.[31]

Influence of Sex Hormones

There is an overall male preponderance of OSA, but the association goes beyond simple gender influence.

- Testosterone replacement therapy in men has been reported to induce or worsen OSA.[32,33] Variation in OSA severity in women has been demonstrated through the menstrual cycle and during pregnancy.[34]
- OSA is also seen in women with PCOS in excess of the prevalence that would be expected if caused by obesity alone.[35]
- The prevalence of OSA in females is approximately tripled after menopause, which is thought to result from a drop in female hormone levels and a relative increase in androgen. This observation holds even with correction for age and BMI.[36,37]

Predisposing Factors in Childhood

- Hyperplasia of the tonsils and adenoids is responsible for most cases of OSA, and therefore adenotonsillectomy (AT) is often recommended. However, residual OSA following AT has been increasingly described, particularly in older children and those with severe baseline disease and comorbid obesity or craniofacial abnormalities.[38]
- In one recent study, less than 25% of all children and 10% of obese children experienced a cure following surgery.[39]
- In a small but significant number of children successfully treated by surgery, OSA returns in puberty or adulthood, once again calling attention to its multifactorial etiology.[40]
- Nasal obstruction in young children with allergy or congenital nasopharyngeal abnormalities can play a role.[41] Mouth breathing predisposes to snoring and increases the risk for apnea. Over time, it also results in mandibular developmental insufficiency.
- Micrognathia, retrognathia, and macroglossia, both acquired and congenital, result in pharyngeal narrowing and consequently predispose to OSA.
- Neuromuscular disorders and syndromes associated with hypotonia, most notably Down syndrome.
- Increasing BMI compounds the effects of even relatively subtle upper airway structural and functional abnormalities.
Table 13.1 presents a list of predisposing conditions.

Physiologic Consequences

Cardiac Effects

With each OA or OH event, as upper airway resistance increases, tidal volume falls, SaO_2 drops, and the carbon dioxide (CO_2) level rises. Increased sympathetic activity causes vasoconstriction and frequently tachycardia, producing an increase in blood pressure. As respiratory efforts against a narrowed or occluded airway increase, reflex bradycardia and atrioventricular block may occur. Once the

TABLE 13.1	Factors Associated with the Development of Obstructive Sleep Apnea

Ear, Nose, and Throat

Seasonal allergic rhinitis
Perennial rhinitis/sinusitis
Nasal septal deviation
Hyperplasia of the tonsils/adenoids
Retrognathia
Micrognathia
Incisor overjet
Dental mandibular crowding
Macroglossia
High arched hard palate
Extended soft palate
Enlarged/elongated uvula
Vocal cord paralysis
Reduced pharyngeal cross-sectional area
Increased pharyngeal length
Congenital and Heredofamilial Craniofacial Syndromes
    Down syndrome
    Prader-Willi syndrome
    Treacher Collins syndrome
    Pierre Robin syndrome

Metabolic/Endocrine

Obesity
Testosterone predominance:
    Male gender
    Iatrogenic androgen supplementation
    Female postmenopausal state
Pregnancy
Hypothyroidism
Mucopolysaccharidoses

Medical/Constitutional Conditions

Stroke
CHF
Autonomic dysfunction
Familial predisposition—multiple
Neuromuscular disease:
    Charcot-Marie-Tooth syndrome
    Myotonic dystrophy
    Multiple system atrophy
    Duchenne muscular dystrophy
Cervical spine injury
Sedative use
Alcohol consumption
Tobacco smoking

CHF, Congestive heart failure.

apnea has terminated, tachycardia may develop, and supraventricular and ventricular ectopy can occur in susceptible individuals.

A combination of increased preload, leftward shift of the intraventricular septum, reduction in left ventricular compliance, and increased afterload occurs. As a result, there may be a worsening of preexisting CHF.[42,43]

Systemic Consequences

The physiologic stress imposed by each event causes a number of pathologic responses:

- Release of inflammatory mediators[44–48]
- Elevation of leptin levels[49]
- Increases in platelet adhesiveness[50] and fibrinogen levels

- Reduced fibrinolytic activity.[51] Insulin resistance and the prevalence of type 2 diabetes are also increased in proportion to OSA severity.[52–54]

Hormonal Responses

In females, hyperinsulinemia shifts the androgen-estrogen balance of ovarian hormone synthesis more toward the androgen side, thereby exacerbating PCOS.[35] Secretion of atrial natriuretic peptide is augmented by a false volume overload signal, and nocturia results.[55]

Atherosclerotic Cardiovascular Disease

Cyclic elevation of microvascular resistance[56] and generalized persistent endothelial dysfunction also occur.[57,58] Sympathetic responses to the stress of apnea can lead to diurnal persistence of hypertension[59–63] and exacerbation of CHF.[64,65]

Multiple Other Consequences

- An increased propensity toward the development of atrial fibrillation and a 50% reduction in successful postcardioversion maintenance of normal sinus rhythm if the OSA is not corrected.[66]
- Pulmonary artery pressure may become transiently elevated, and in a small percentage of individuals, fixed pulmonary hypertension occurs.[67] During periods of intense apnea and hypoxia, elevated right-sided cardiac pressure can lead to opening of a patent foramen ovale, and thereby exacerbate systemic hypoxia and increase the risk for embolic stroke.[68]
- Long-term intermittent hypoxia results in oxidative stress.[46,69,70] Hypoxia may further worsen pharyngeal muscle dilator function.[71] Repetitive mechanical trauma to the pharyngeal muscles can lead to inflammation and denervation, which yields a similar effect.[72]
- The final common pathway of the multiple responses to OSA is increased atherogenesis.[73] There is evidence of acceleration of coronary artery disease,[74] the appearance of new clinical cardiovascular morbidity (recurrent atrial fibrillation, fatal and nonfatal myocardial infarction, and pulmonary hypertension), and an association with stroke.[75,76] Furthermore, studies have also shown that progression of cardiovascular disease is retarded when OSA is corrected.[77–80]

Consequences of Sleep Fragmentation

Repetitive EEG arousals result in sleep fragmentation and in some cases suppression of normal progress through deeper sleep, especially rapid eye movement (REM) sleep.

- Failure to achieve restorative sleep and the effects of oxidative stress are thought to be responsible for excessive daytime somnolence and affective complaints such as increased irritability, depression, and cognitive dysfunction, including deterioration of memory and concentration.
- Whether by intermittent hypoxia and oxidative stress or fragmentation of sleep, OSA can contribute to cognitive decline in the elderly and appears to have a link with dementia.[81,82]
- Finally, the combined influences of sleep fragmentation and intermittent hypoxia are being investigated as etiologic factors in carcinogenesis.[83]

Clinical Evaluation

The often-cited medical maxim—"unless a specific condition is considered as a possibility, timely identification of it is unlikely"—is especially true for OSA. An obese middle-aged man who snores profoundly at night and falls asleep readily during the day does not pose a diagnostic challenge. In this circumstance, EDS should always raise the possibility of OSA. A score of greater than 10 on the Epworth Sleepiness Scale (ESS) is considered abnormal, but the ESS lacks sufficient specificity and sensitivity to be relied on exclusively.

The Body Mass Index Varies Significantly

An elevated BMI in either gender and at any age increases the likelihood of a positive diagnosis; however, OSA can affect individuals with BMI in the normal or minimally elevated range.[11] Table 13.2 summarizes the clinical findings that may suggest consideration of a diagnosis of OSA.

Variable Presentations

- The typical male with OSA will report feeling groggy in the morning (despite the perception of having had a good night's sleep) and may indicate nodding off while sitting quietly or driving.
- Women are more likely to complain of insomnia, generalized daytime fatigue, and a variety of psychologic and somatic complaints, such as depression and headache.[12,84]
- Sleep fragmentation is sometimes accompanied by paroxysmal nocturnal dyspnea, palpitations, anxiety attacks, or dreams of physical exertion.
- Children may respond to sleep fragmentation from SDB with hyperactivity, behavioral difficulties, or attention-deficit/hyperactivity disorder, any of which should prompt a consideration of OSA.[85]
- Hypertension, especially when refractory to conventional treatment, has been linked to OSA.[86] It should be noted, however, that there remains some degree of controversy about the magnitude of the risk for hypertension from OSA, as well as the benefits from treatment of OSA.[87,88]
- Unexpected nocturia in both genders occurs when apnea results in alterations in circulatory dynamics and causes inappropriate nocturnal secretion of atrial natriuretic peptide.
- Gastroesophageal reflux symptoms, especially nocturnal regurgitation, may be caused or exacerbated by OSA. The recurrent microaspiration of nasopharyngeal secretions or gastric contents (or both) associated with the inspiratory gasps following airway closure can lead to persistent hoarseness, tickle in the throat, and chronic cough.
- Male erectile dysfunction can be caused by OSA, as well as by the many comorbid conditions that apnea sufferers may also have, such as hypertension and diabetes.

The presence of several specific endocrine abnormalities should raise suspicion for OSA:

- There is an association with hypothyroidism,[89] probably multifactorial and based on a reduction in the metabolic rate, macroglossia, mucosal abnormalities, obesity, and other influences.
- Women with PCOS have an increased prevalence of OSA in excess of that expected in the context of obesity alone.[35]
- There is also an increased incidence of OSA during pregnancy.

Diabetes and Metabolic Syndrome

The diagnosis of diabetes or unexpected difficulty with glycemic control may be a marker for OSA.[90] Most individuals with the metabolic syndrome (MetS) should at least be queried about

TABLE 13.2 Initial Complaints and Physical Findings Suggesting a Diagnosis of Obstructive Sleep Apnea

Sleep Related

Excessive sleep need
Snoring
Restless sleep
Insomnia
Bruxism
Nonrestorative sleep
Gasping arousals
Nocturnal gastroesophageal reflux
Nocturnal panic attacks
Nocturia
Parasomnias
Dreams of exertion or suffocation
Daytime complaints
Morning somnolence
Morning headache
Morning dry mouth
Excessive daytime somnolence
Impaired job or school performance
Generalized fatigue
Drowsy driving
Cognitive impairment
Mood disorders
Intense menopausal complaints
Reduced libido/erectile dysfunction
Somatic symptoms:
  Fibromyalgia
  Chronic fatigue syndrome
  Irritable bowel syndrome
  Headache
Refractory asthma
Difficult intubation or anesthesia recovery

Conditions

Attention deficit disorder
Dysglycemia
MetS
Polycystic ovary syndrome
Refractory systemic hypertension
Angiotensin-converting enzyme polymorphism
Chronic renal failure
Stroke
Recurrent or unexpected atrial fibrillation
Unexplained pulmonary hypertension
CHF
Acromegaly
Parkinson's disease

CHF, Congestive heart failure; *MetS,* metabolic syndrome.

symptoms and signs that might raise suspicion for OSA, especially because of the cardiovascular risks associated with MetS. After controlling for BMI and age, one study found OSA in 1 of 6 men with MetS as compared with 1 of 40 without MetS.[91]

Hypotonia Predisposes to Obstructive Sleep Apnea

- Approximately two-thirds of children with Down syndrome will be found to have OSA by PSG, with this prevalence likely increasing in adulthood.[92]

- There is also a significantly increased incidence in persons with neuromuscular diseases.[93]

Perioperative Complications

Perioperative complications, including a history of difficult endotracheal intubation, slow postoperative recovery from anesthesia, unexplained postoperative hypoxemia, or need for reintubation after anesthesia should raise suspicion for underlying OSA.[94]

Reports from Family Members or Bed Partner

Reports from family members or bed partner should also be elicited. Witnesses often report persistent nodding off, especially under inappropriate social circumstances. Bed partners may have taken to sleeping in another room or have banished the patient from the bedroom because of disruptive snoring.

Physical Examination Clues

- A neck circumference greater than 17 inches
- Craniofacial features (discussed previously)
- Nasal obstruction
- A high-arched palate
- Tonsillar hyperplasia
- Engorgement of pharyngeal tissues, and uvular prominence

Diagnosis

Attended in-laboratory PSG remains the reference standard for diagnosis.[95]

- OAs and hypopneas are detected by the various sensors of oronasal airflow and thoracic and abdominal excursion. Current AASM rules recommend the use of an oronasal thermal sensor for optimal detection of apnea, plus a nasal air pressure transducer to detect hypopnea.[16,96] The nasal device also provides information about more subtle events such as RERAs (discussed later).[97]
- Respiratory effort is preferably documented through the use of inductance plethysmography, which has replaced older measures, such as strain gauges and piezoelectric belts. Esophageal manometry continues to be used in research settings.
- In general, a body position sensor is used, but its accuracy can be suboptimal, and visual confirmation by a technician is often necessary.
- Pulse oximetry provides data on the depth and duration of apnea-associated hypoxia and response to treatment. An oximeter with appropriate sensitivity and response time is necessary to avoid over- or under-diagnosis of oxygen desaturation events.[95,98]
- Three or four EEG channels are commonly used to identify sleep stages and document arousals.
- Electrooculography and chin electromyography assist in identifying stage REM sleep.

Pediatric Sleep Laboratories

Pediatric sleep laboratories also frequently monitor transcutaneous CO_2, because identification of OSA is significantly more challenging and less well defined in children than in adults.[14]

Diagnostic Criteria

- An AHI of less than 5 is considered normal in adults, although there is strong evidence that persistent snoring and upper airway resistance syndrome (UARS, described later) confer adverse health consequences.

- An AHI of 5–14 is arbitrarily ranked as mild, 15–30 as moderate, and higher than 30 as severe disease, but the designations vary among laboratories.

A case can be made for identifying an AHI of greater than 15–20 as having increased physiologic significance, because it is at this approximate level that some of the adverse consequences (such as increased blood coagulability and platelet adhesion) appear. Additional parameters (average desaturation, event length, and frequency of events) in the context of AHI may be utilized to better define severity.[99]

In general, medicare guidelines for treatment reimbursement, adapted by most commercial insurance providers, include:

- An AHI of 5 or greater in the context of at least one of the following:
  - Hypertension
  - Ischemic heart disease
  - History of stroke
  - Insomnia or EDS
  - Depression or cognitive dysfunction
- An AHI of 15 or greater even in the absence of associated comorbid conditions.[100]

Obstructive Sleep Apnea Diagnosis in Children Is Less Precise

- The current AASM diagnostic criteria for children require at least one clinical manifestation (such as snoring, excessive somnolence, or hyperactivity) in the context of an AHI ≥1 or a $PaCO_2$ >50 for >25% of sleep time with observed evidence of SDB in the sleep lab.[101]
- However, controversy exists both with regard to AHI cutoff and AHI validity as a sole determinant of OSA in children. For instance, recent publications use an obstructive AHI cutoff of two events per hour,[102] and many pediatric sleep providers integrate other parameters, such as oxygenation, ventilation, and work of breathing when determining OSA severity.
- The sleep specialist interpreting the PSG should also use clinical discretion in both scoring criteria and diagnostic criteria in children 13 years and older.[16]

Alternative Diagnostic Approaches

Numerous alternative diagnostic approaches are available. They range from snoring recorders[89] and recording oximetry to multi-channel home PSG systems. As a screening technique, overnight oximetry has adequate sensitivity but lacks specificity and is not recommended.[95,103] Various multichannel data collectors have been used in both attended and unattended settings in an attempt to substitute for formal PSG, but the data are difficult to compare, and the accuracy of the testing continues to be evaluated.[104] In addition, smartphone applications and other novel recording techniques have recently been studied.[105,106]

The AASM guidelines continue to call for attended, in-laboratory PSG in most circumstances,[107–109] emphasizing that simple problems such as loss of electrode contact can easily be repaired; sleep staging is provided. Diagnosis of other significant conditions such as limb movement disorders, parasomnias, seizure activity, and cardiac arrhythmias is facilitated. In-laboratory PSG also affords an opportunity for PAP titration in the second half of the night. Studies have demonstrated equivalence of the split-night study to full-night PSG, followed by a second night devoted to continuous positive airway pressure (CPAP) titration alone.[110]

Unattended Portable Monitoring

Portable monitoring (PM) is endorsed by the AASM in circumstances in which PSG is unavailable or contraindicated for a variety of financial, clinical, and social reasons.[111] Data acquisition capability spans a wide range.

- Type 2 devices: seven or more channels
- Type 3 devices: four to seven channels (Fig. 13.3)
- Type 4 devices: one or two channels

If the clinician has adequate clinical patient information and a full understanding of the instrumentation and algorithms of the particular PM system being used, meaningful results can be obtained.[112,113] It is important to note that studies reporting noninferiority of PM compared with PSG have usually limited patient selection to those with a high pretest probability of OSA, and have excluded those with medical comorbidities and morbid

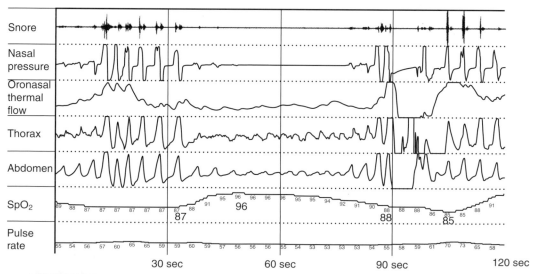

• **Figure 13.3** Representative 120-sec epoch from a type III portable monitoring device depicting an obstructive apnea. Note the suboptimal oronasal thermal flow signal; the inability to correct faulty signals is a disadvantage of unattended studies. (Modified from Berry RB. Uses and limitations of portable monitoring for diagnosis and management of obstructive sleep apnea. *Sleep Med Clin.* 2011;6[3]:311.)

obesity.[5] Medicare, the Veterans Affairs medical system, and most private insurers currently accept an OSA diagnosis and will pay for CPAP treatment based on PM.[114]

- Indications for PM[111] may include:
  - High pretest probability for OSA
  - In-laboratory PSG not possible due to immobility, safety, or critical illness
  - Monitoring response to non-CPAP treatment in patients previously diagnosed with OSA
- Contraindications for PM[111] include:
  - Low pretest probability for OSA
  - Significant medical comorbidities, including severe pulmonary disease, neuromuscular disease, or CHF
  - Clinical suspicion for alternative sleep disorders, including CA, periodic limb movement disorder, insomnia, parasomnia, circadian rhythm disorder, or narcolepsy
  - Screening of asymptomatic patients in high risk populations, including heart failure (HF), commercial truck drivers, or patients undergoing bariatric surgery
- Since most PM montages do not include staging capabilities, sleep quality and quantity may be overestimated, resulting in false negative results.[115] Therefore any patient with a high pretest probability of OSA who has a negative PM study should undergo laboratory PSG.
- Laboratory PSG may also be necessary in circumstances such as poor response to treatment of OSA or persistence of complaints, despite documented patient compliance. Underlying issues ranging from suboptimal OSA therapy to the presence of comorbid conditions (seizures, limb movement disorders, parasomnias, etc.) might thus be revealed.
- Accounting for these limitations, the AASM has proposed an algorithm for choosing in-laboratory PSG versus PM (Fig. 13.4).[111]
- Whereas in-laboratory PSG is typically accompanied by in-lab titration to determine optimal CPAP settings, in general PM requires the use of auto-titrating PAP (Fig. 13.5); in-lab titration may also be performed once the diagnosis of OSA is established by PM.

Central Apnea

- CA results from instability of controller mechanisms in the central nervous system. In contrast to OSA, in CA, there is a temporary cessation of signaling to the inspiratory muscles. Airway collapse may also occur,[116] but is not the pivotal event. Rather, gradual or abrupt cessation of airflow results from a lapse in controller signaling. Thus no inspiratory efforts accompany CA (see Fig. 13.1).
- CA frequently causes oxygen desaturation and is usually terminated by the increased partial pressure of arterial carbon dioxide ($PaCO_2$) that results from the apnea. As with OSA, sleep fragmentation is common. Because CA may occur under a diverse set of pathologic conditions, a unifying underlying mechanism is often difficult to determine.

Pathophysiology

CA occurs in a number of distinct patterns. Because instability of ventilatory control is thought to underlie all forms of apnea, it has been proposed that there is an overlap in the mechanisms responsible for CA and OA.[117]

PORTABLE MONITORING DECISION TREE

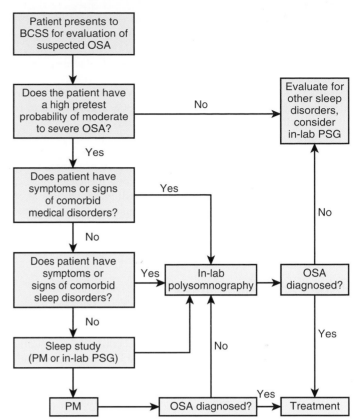

• **Figure 13.4** Diagnostic algorithm proposed by the American Academy of Sleep Medicine task force to guide the decision to perform in-laboratory polysomnography (PSG) versus portable monitoring (PM) in the diagnosis of obstructive sleep apnea (OSA). A board-certified sleep specialist (BCSS) should first evaluate the patient to determine pretest probability for OSA and determine if contraindications for PM are present. (Modified from Collop NA, Anderson WM, Boehlecke B, et al. Clinical guidelines for the use of unattended portable monitors in the diagnosis of obstructive sleep apnea in adult patients. Portable Monitoring Task Force of the American Academy of Sleep Medicine. *J Clin Sleep Med.* 2007;3[7]:741.)

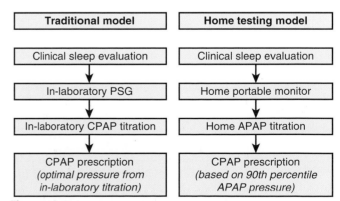

• **Figure 13.5** Comparison of strategies to determine optimal continuous positive airway pressure (CPAP) setting. In the traditional model, in-lab diagnostic polysomnography (PSG) is accompanied by in-laboratory titration. With portable monitoring, home sleep testing is accompanied by home auto-titrating positive airway pressure (APAP) titration. (Modified from Cooksey JA, Balachandran JS. Portable monitoring for the diagnosis of OSA. *Chest.* 2016;149[4]:1074–1081.)

- In sleep, most of the modulating influence originates from changes in $PaCO_2$ and PaO_2.
- Hypoxic and hypercapnic responses in general are blunted in sleep, especially in stage REM, although some gender-specific differences have been described.[118]
- Changes in PaO_2 within the normal physiologic range do not cause a large respiratory variation. Relatively small changes in $PaCO_2$, however, result in brisk, inversely proportional responses in minute ventilation. Variation in $PaCO_2$ is considered to be the dominant respiratory controller in sleep.[117]
- Because CO_2 responsiveness falls during sleep, sleep-onset CAs are commonly seen.

CAs have been described following tracheotomy for OSA, thus illustrating the overlap between the two forms of apnea.[119] Occasionally mixed apneas are encountered, in which there is an apparent initial CA event with return of respiratory effort observed during the terminal portion, giving the appearance of OA (see Fig. 13.1). The specific underlying mechanism has not been fully resolved.[120,121]

History and Examination

The manifestations of CA vary in the context of the specific form and underlying cause, as outlined in the sections that follow.[117] Patients with idiopathic CA have a variety of complaints, including fatigue and other problems found with OSA, but also insomnia or sleep fragmentation. They are often not obese. Because CA also results in hypoxic periods, as with OSA, it can cause pulmonary and systemic hypertension.

Diagnosis

PSG is the primary diagnostic tool for CA of any etiology. In general, the current standards vary somewhat but call for an AHI of greater than 5 in pure CA or for more than 80% of apneas to be central in cases of mixed disease. Central hypopnea is scored if the event meets the hypopnea criteria (discussed previously), including a 30%–90% drop in airflow, but with *decreased* respiratory effort and absence of snoring, inspiratory flattening, or paradox (Fig. 13.6).[16] Refinements in diagnosis are based on the clinical

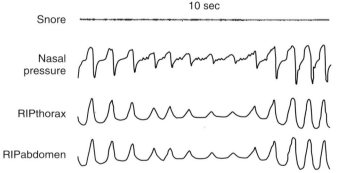

- **Figure 13.6** Central Hypopnea. In contrast to obstructive hypopnea (OH), central hypopnea (CH) is not accompanied by snoring, flattening of the inspiratory phase of the nasal pressure signature, or thoracoabdominal paradox. As with OH, a 3% desaturation or arousal is required to score a CH if using the recommended American Academy of Sleep Medicine (AASM) criteria; a 4% desaturation is required if using the acceptable AASM criteria. (Modified from Berry RB, Wagner MH. Sleep medicine pearls. 3rd ed. Philadelphia, PA: Saunders, 2014:128.)

context and patterns of frequency, such as seen in Cheyne-Stokes respiration (CSR). Specific pathologic forms of CA are outlined next.

Cheyne-Stokes Respiration

- When an alternating hyperventilation/hypoventilation cycle is evident, the term *periodic breathing* (PB) is applied. The most commonly recognized form of PB in adults is CSR, which is typically seen in the context of HF.
- The AASM has defined CSR as the presence of three or more consecutive cycles of crescendo-decrescendo amplitude in respiration with cycle length of at least 40 sec *plus* five or more CAs/hypopneas per hour of sleep (Fig. 13.7).[16]

Pathophysiology

- In general, individuals with HF-linked CSR have a reduced baseline $PaCO_2$ secondary to hyperventilation because of increased controller responsiveness to CO_2 associated with heightened sympathetic activity and pulmonary vagal stimulation.[122]
- In sleep, as the apneic threshold increases, $PaCO_2$ rises slightly to a new steady state. Sleep state transition during N1 and N2 is associated with a sudden increase in CO_2 sensitivity which triggers a ventilatory response.
- Diminished loop gain in HF, however, sets the stage for overcompensation. Minute ventilation at an increased level drives $PaCO_2$ below the apneic threshold before chemoreceptors detect the drop. Ventilation then ceases, sleep stabilizes, and $PaCO_2$ rises, once again significantly above the apneic threshold before the response fires.
- This process continues in a cyclic fashion primarily during N1 and N2 sleep.[123]
- The prolonged circulation time in patients with HF results in an overshoot of the hyperpnea and an extension of the PB cycle to yield the characteristic cyclic crescendo-decrescendo pattern of CSR with periodicity.[124]
- Thus a rhythmic oscillation between hyperpnea and hypopnea/apnea around the apneic threshold occurs.
- CSR is usually seen in non-REM (NREM) sleep. A more subtle but similar pattern can be seen during wakefulness in some HF-afflicted individuals.

Associated Conditions

- CSR has also been described in patients with stroke, but in most cases it might merely be a manifestation of coexisting occult or subclinical left ventricular dysfunction.[125]
- The hyperpneic phase of CSR may also give rise to ventricular ectopy that persists even if the associated hypoxia is corrected.[126]
- The presence of CSR in patients with HF increases their risk for mortality. Cardiac transplant lessens CSR.[127]
- However, recent data suggest that therapeutic modalities aimed at treating CSA and CSR—namely, adaptive servo-ventilation (ASV)—may increase cardiovascular mortality in patients with symptomatic HF, reduced ejection fraction less than 45%, and predominantly CA at baseline.[128] Of note, significant controversy exists regarding this finding and its application to modern ASV devices.[129]

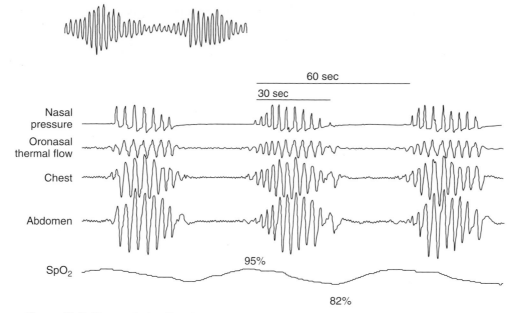

• **Figure 13.7** Cheyne-Stokes Respiration. Note the periodic crescendo-decrescendo pattern in amplitude of the respiratory effort and oronasal flow signals separated by periods of apnea, with cycle length exceeding 40 sec. Cheyne-Stokes breathing may be associated with central hypopneas, as illustrated in the upper left corner. (Modified from Berry RB. *Fundamentals of Sleep Medicine.* 1st ed. Philadelphia, PA: Saunders; 2012:133.)

High-Altitude Periodic Breathing

- Hypoxic drive is augmented by the reduced barometric pressure at high altitude, and hyperpnea and subsequent hypocapnia results. As in CSR, the hyperpnea ceases only when $PaCO_2$ falls sufficiently to trigger alkalosis-induced apnea. Increasing hypoxia will propagate the cycle, which is more pronounced in sleep.
- High-altitude PB is very common in early infancy, typically resolving within the first year of life.[130] PB at sea level, a similar disorder of respiratory control, can also infrequently occur.[131]

Idiopathic Central Sleep Apnea

- Idiopathic central sleep apnea is a relatively uncommon condition afflicting individuals with an inherently high chemoreceptor responsiveness that drives ventilation and results in hypocapnia, even at sea level.
- As with high-altitude PB, the cycling is exaggerated during sleep; in general, the smooth crescendo-decrescendo pattern of CRS and PB, however, is absent, and apneas may terminate abruptly.

Central Apnea Associated with Baseline Hypercapnia

- A wide variety of conditions with different causes come under this heading. The most common is obesity hypoventilation syndrome (OHS). Other neuromuscular diseases compromising mechanical gas exchange and leading to chronic hypercapnia can result in CA, but upper airway instability may also play a role in these instances.

TABLE 13.3	Central Apnea Classification
Nonhypercapnic	
Central sleep apnea/Cheyne-Stokes respiration	
Idiopathic central sleep apnea	
High-altitude central apnea	
Periodic breathing at sea level	
Incidental (e.g., at sleep onset)	
Hypercapnic	
Obesity-hypoventilation syndrome	
Neuromuscular diseases	
CCHS	

CCHS, Congenital central hypoventilation syndrome.

- Central alveolar hypoventilation secondary to various acquired neurologic abnormalities or lesions, especially in the brainstem (including Chiari malformation), may be accompanied by CA.[132]
- Finally, in context of the national epidemic of opioid abuse, there is increasing importance that clinicians remain aware of the possibility of CA induced by use of prescription or illicit narcotics and methadone.[133] Both ataxic and rhythmic central apneic patterns occur.[134] Table 13.3 summarizes the classification of CA.

Mixed Central and Obstructive Apnea

- Some individuals show combined OSA and CA. As control of airway stability is established with CPAP, intractable CA develops, especially during NREM sleep. This is thought to result from reflex controller inhibition as partial pharyngeal closure occurs.

This phenomenon, termed treatment-emergent CA or complex sleep apnea, reflects a common underlying pathophysiology[135] and is more common in OSA patients under conditions predisposing to CA such as high altitude dwelling.[136] Importantly, CPAP-emergent CA has been noted to resolve spontaneously in 30% or more of patients.[137]

Snoring

During sleep, vibration of upper airway structures, including the soft palate, uvula, and lateral walls of the pharynx, causes snoring. The character and timbre of the audible sound produced are influenced by the site or sites of vibration. Although snoring is often noted during inspiration, it can also occur during exhalation.

Pathophysiology: The upper airway, from the nares to the larynx, is a flexible collapsible tube that performs various functions in respiration, swallowing, and phonation.

- Airway patency is maintained by a balance of collapsing and distending forces that vary with changes in airflow and muscle tone.
- In anatomically susceptible upper airways, snoring is produced when the inspiratory luminal negative pressure exceeds the distending activity of the upper airway muscles.[138]
- Collapsibility increases during sleep as a result of a reduction in upper airway muscle tone.
- Differences in collapsibility of the upper airway, defined by its P_{crit}, determine whether snoring, hypopnea, or apnea will result.[139]
- Snoring can also stem from or be made worse by nasal obstruction. Nasal congestion may give rise to oronasal breathing, which further compromises the upper airway.[140]

Risk Factors

- Overweight and obesity
- Supine sleep position
- Male sex
- Pregnancy
- Nasal congestion
- Ingestion of alcohol, muscle relaxants, opioid analgesics, and sedative-hypnotic agents before sleep
- Smoking
- Family history of snoring or SDB
- Sleep deprivation
  Data from the Wisconsin Sleep Cohort Study revealed that habitual snorers tend to have a higher prevalence of OSA with AHI of 15 or higher.[141] Nonetheless, snoring by itself lacks specificity for OSAS.

History

Snorers may seek evaluation and management when snoring is causing significant disruption of the bed partner's or roommate's sleep or when there is concern that snoring is associated with OSA.

- The bed partner should be asked about the duration, frequency, and intensity of snoring.
- Snoring should be differentiated from stridor resulting from laryngeal narrowing, incoherent sleep talking, and expiratory groaning during sleep (catathrenia), in which the groaning usually occurs during the second part of the night during stage R and N2 sleep. Findings on otorhinolaryngologic

and neurologic evaluation are normal in patients with catathrenia.[142]

Examination

- Snorers share many of the upper airway features of patients with OSA.
- Examination may demonstrate swollen nasal mucosa; enlargement of the tonsils, uvula, and tongue; narrowing of the airway by the lateral pharyngeal walls; a low palate; and retrognathia.
- Referral to an otorhinolaryngologist for fiberoptic pharyngoscopy may provide additional information that might be useful for patients with an incomplete response to medical therapy or those who are considering surgery for their snoring. However, pharyngoscopic features do not reliably predict responses to surgical interventions for snoring.

Complications

In general, complications of snoring relate to symptoms and disruption of either the patient's or the bed partner's quality of life.

- However, snoring even in the absence of OSA is associated with carotid artery atherosclerosis,[143] with the proposed mechanism being tissue vibration and localized endothelial dysfunction.[144]
- Snoring in children, even in the absence of OSA, is associated with neurocognitive impairment.[69]

Diagnosis

Snoring is typically a clinical diagnosis. PSG is not routinely indicated in the evaluation of snorers in the absence of additional features suggestive of OSA such as witnessed apneas or daytime sleepiness. Snoring is identified during PSG either by using microphones or by sound/vibration sensors placed on the neck or near the oronasal opening or from reports of audible snoring by the sleep technologist.

Upper Airway Resistance Syndrome

As its name implies, UARS is characterized by repetitive episodes of increased resistance to airflow in the upper airways associated with arousals from sleep, resulting in sleep fragmentation and daytime hypersomnolence.[145]

History and Examination

Clinical presentation and risk factors associated with UARS largely overlaps other forms of SDB including OSAS and snoring. In addition,

- Snoring may or may not be present.
- Patients may also have less specific somatic complaints, including headaches, irritable bowel syndrome, and sleep-onset insomnia.[146]
- Other associated features include fatigue and a higher prevalence of systemic hypertension.[147]

Diagnosis

Proper identification of UARS is particularly important in patients with a presumptive diagnosis of idiopathic hypersomnia.[148] UARS

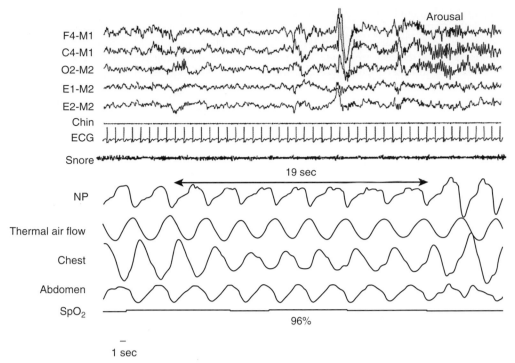

• **Figure 13.8** Respiratory effort-related arousal. Note the flattening of the nasal pressure (NP) signal, with the event terminated by arousal (A). As the decrease in NP signal is less than 30% and there is no significant desaturation, this event does not qualify as hypopnea by recommended or acceptable American Academy of Sleep Medicine criteria. (Modified from Berry RB. *Fundamentals of Sleep Medicine.* 1st ed. Philadelphia, PA: Saunders, 2012:126.)

may be distinguished from other forms of SDB by PSG. However, accurate identification of UARS is hampered by the lack of standardized diagnostic criteria. Respiratory effort-related arousal (RERA) is frequently noted (Fig. 13.8). The AASM defines RERA as follows:

- In adult patients: An arousal is preceded by a discrete episode of increased respiratory effort and/or flattening of the nasal pressure waveform lasting at least 10 sec and not meeting the criteria for either apnea or hypopnea.
- In children younger than 18 years: An arousal is preceded by an episode lasting at least the duration of two breaths and any of the following: increased respiratory effort, flattening of the inspiratory pressure signal, snoring, or elevation of end-tidal $PaCO_2$.[16]

Other PSG findings and patterns in patients with UARS may include:

- Respiratory events accompanied by increases in heart rate and systolic and diastolic pressure and changes in electrocardiographic R-R intervals.[149]
- A crescendo pattern, seen commonly during stage N1 and N2 sleep, consisting of a more negative peak end-inspiratory P_{es}, with more regular and continuous high respiratory efforts seen during stage N3 sleep.[150]
- Nasal pressure transducers capturing a pattern of airflow limitation consisting of an inspiratory "plateauing" or flattened contour of the tracing corresponding to the increasingly negative pleural pressure excursions, followed by a rounded contour during arousals.[151] Of note, although more accurate than thermistors, nasal pressure transducers may nonetheless fail to detect all abnormal breathing episodes during sleep.[150]

- PSG often demonstrates a greater total time of wakefulness after sleep onset (WASO) and a decreased duration of slow wave sleep.[146]

Obesity-Hypoventilation Syndrome

OHS is characterized by the presence of obesity (typically morbid) and hypercapnia during wakefulness. Hypercapnia develops as a result of the increased production of carbon dioxide because of greater work of breathing and lack of sufficient compensatory increases in ventilation.[152]

- Although weight is a significant factor in the pathogenesis of OHS, even among obese persons, OHS is uncommon.
- In one study of hospitalized patients with severe obesity, hypoventilation was present in 31% of subjects who did not have other reasons for hypercapnia. These patients required greater duration of intensive care, long-term care at discharge, and mechanical ventilation, and had higher mortality at 18 months after hospital discharge than did patients with simple obesity without OHS.[153]

History and Examination

Patients with OHS may have complaints of

- Hypersomnolence
- Decreased objective attention or concentration
- Peripheral edema
- Cyanosis

Evaluation may disclose the presence of periodic respiration, hypoxemia, pulmonary hypertension, and polycythemia. Severe obesity can be associated with mild to moderate degrees of restrictive ventilatory impairment.

- OSA is present in most, but not all, patients with OHS.
- Diurnal arterial blood gas measurements are worse, and pulmonary artery hypertension is more frequent in patients with OHS than in those with OSA alone.[154]
- Other causes of chronic hypoventilation, such as severe chronic obstructive pulmonary disease, neuromuscular disorders, or diaphragmatic paralysis, should be excluded.[155]

Diagnosis

According to the AASM guidelines, hypoventilation during sleep is present if the following criteria are met[16]:

- In adults: A measure of $PaCO_2$ exceeds 55 mm Hg *or* increases by at least 10 mm Hg above an awake supine baseline to a value above 50 mm Hg for a duration of at least 10 min.
- In children: A measure of $PaCO_2$ is greater than 50 mm Hg more than 25% of the total sleep time.

Congenital Central Hypoventilation Syndrome

In congenital central hypoventilation syndrome (CCHS), hypoventilation and failure of autonomic respiratory control are present from birth, and therefore CCHS most commonly presents as respiratory failure during the perinatal period or early infancy. However, late onset cases are increasingly reported.[156,157]

- Ventilatory responses to hypoxia and hypercapnia are impaired because of a disorder in central chemoreceptor responsiveness.[158]
- Hypoventilation during sleep can be severe with lack of ventilatory or arousal responses.
- Hypoventilation is characteristically most prominent during NREM sleep but in severe cases can be present even during wakefulness.[159]
- Activity and exercise can result in worsening gas exchange, with greater hypoxemia and hypercapnia and a lesser increase in heart rate.[160]
- Affected patients lack subjective sensation of dyspnea.[161]
- Despite the absence of chemoreceptor function, however, hyperpnea can occur during exercise, with increasing respiratory frequency rather than an augmentation of tidal volume being responsible for the increase in minute ventilation.[162]

Pathophysiology

Abnormalities in neural structure and autonomic function are increasingly recognized as underlying mechanisms of the disease.[163] This is supported by the association with neural crest disorders such as Hirschsprung disease and tumors of neural crest origin. Recently, paired-like homeobox 2B (*PHOX2B*) has been identified as the gene underlying CCHS.[164,165]

- The normal genotype at the disease-causing locus consists of 20 polyalanine repeats.

- Ninety percent of patients with CCHS are heterozygous for a polyalanine repeat expansion mutation, typically consisting of 24–33 polyalanine repeats.[166]
- The remaining 10% may express various polymorphisms of the *PHOX2B* gene, including missense, nonsense, and frameshift mutations.[167]
- An association between repeat mutation length and severity of the CCHS phenotype has been described.[165]

Epidemiology

- Worldwide, there have been approximately 1000 cases of CCHS with confirmed *PHOX2B* disease-causing mutations.[166]
- Although rare overall, this prevalence is thought to represent a substantial underestimate due to lack of awareness about this disease.

Presentation

The classic presentation for CCHS is respiratory failure in the neonatal period. However, given the complex autonomic manifestations and variable expressivity of the disease, CCHS has diverse clinical presentations. A careful review for the following elements may help elucidate a diagnosis of CCHS:

- Subtle dysmorphisms, including "box-shaped" short and flat face and inferior inflection of the lateral aspect of the superior vermilion border.[168]
- Tachycardia, diaphoresis, cyanosis, witnessed apnea, feeding difficulties, apparent life-threatening events, respiratory arrest, and pulmonary hypertension.
- Arrhythmias (most notably transient asystole), seizures, syncope, heat intolerance, esophageal dysmotility, and ophthalmologic abnormalities such as pupillary dysfunction.[169]
- Dysfunctional control of the heart by the autonomic nervous system and decreased heart rate variability.[170]
- Hirschsprung's disease and tumors of neural crest derivation (i.e., ganglioneuromas and neuroblastomas).[171]
- Growth impairment, hypotonia, major motor delays, and neurocognitive impairment.[158,172]

Diagnosis

- CCHS should be distinguished from other congenital syndromes associated with abnormalities in respiratory control, such as Prader-Willi syndrome and familial dysautonomia.
- Other causes of chronic hypoventilation, such as cardiopulmonary, neuromuscular, central nervous system, and metabolic disorders, should also be excluded.
- A mutation in the *PHOX2B* gene confirms the diagnosis of CCHS.[166]
  - Approximately 95% of mutations may be identified using the polyacrylamide gel electrophoresis *PHOX2B* screening test.[166]
  - If *PHOX2B* screening test is negative but a high suspicion for CCHS persists, full *PHOX2B* sequencing test may be performed.[166]

Summary

In conclusion, SDB is a highly variable condition that can be seen in all genders and ages from birth to old age. All clinicians should be aware of the possibility for overt or subtle manifestations of the problem and apply appropriate history, physical examination, and diagnostic tools. In nearly all cases, sleep laboratory evaluation is necessary to confirm a specific diagnosis, and often to assure response to treatment.

Suggested Reading

Deacon NL, Jen R, Li Y, Malhotra A. Treatment of obstructive sleep apnea. Prospects for personalized combined modality therapy. *Ann Am Thorac Soc*. 2016;13(1):101-108.

Marcus CL, Moore RH, Rosen CL, et al. A randomized trial of adenotonsillectomy for childhood sleep apnea. *N Engl J Med*. 2013;368(25): 2366-2376.

Naughton MT. Cheyne-Stokes respiration. *Sleep Med Clin*. 2014;9:13-25.

Peppard PE, Young T, Barnet JH, et al. Increased prevalence of sleep-disorder breathing in adults. *Am J Epidemiol*. 2013;177(9):1006-1014.

Selim BJ, Mithri RJ. Central sleep apnea. The complex sleep apnea syndrome. *Sleep Med Clin*. 2014;9:37-47.

14

Sleep-Related Breathing Disorders: Treatment

JOYCE K. LEE-IANNOTTI, DENNIS AUCKLEY

Introduction

- **Terminology**: The term *sleep-disordered breathing (SDB)* encompasses a wide array of breathing disturbances that occur exclusively or predominantly during sleep. SDB can be categorized into obstructive sleep apnea (OSA) disorders, central sleep apnea (CSA) syndromes, sleep-related hypoventilation syndromes, sleep-related hypoxemia disorder, snoring, and catathrenia.[1]

- **Objectives:**
  - This chapter covers the treatment of the first three of these conditions (OSA, CSA, sleep-related hypoventilation syndromes) in an evidence-based manner.
  - When applicable, the authors refer to the most recent American Academy of Sleep Medicine (AASM) systematic reviews, practice parameters, and clinical guidelines for recommendations on treatment options. These documents, which establish standards of practice for sleep medicine, use specific terminology to grade the level of each recommendation—standard, guideline, and option[2]—although the definition of these recommendation levels has evolved over time.

- **AASM Level of Evidence and Standard Recommendations**: Older reviews define a *Standard* recommendation as being supported by high- or moderate-quality evidence—either randomized controlled trials (RCTs) with low alpha and beta levels (level I studies) or a sufficient number of randomized trials with high alpha and beta levels (level II studies). Standard recommendations were meant to represent a "high degree of clinical certainty" and a "generally accepted patient-care strategy."[2] A *Guideline* recommendation was supported by moderate- to low-quality evidence—either level II evidence or general agreement among nonrandomized concurrently controlled studies (level III studies).

- **AASM Guideline Recommendations**: Guideline recommendations were meant to reflect "a moderate degree of clinical certainty."[2] An *Option* recommendation was offered when there is "either inconclusive or conflicting evidence or conflicting expert opinion" and represents "a patient-care strategy that reflects uncertain clinical use."[2]

- **AASM Grading System**: More recently the AASM has switched to a new grading scheme, known as the Grading of Recommendation Assessment, Development and Evaluation (GRADE) system.[3] This grading system has still been using the level of recommendations of Standard, Guideline, or Option, although this now considers an assessment of benefit/harm/burden along with the quality of the evidence to determine the final recommendation. This change primarily affects the most recent practice guideline on the use of oral appliances (OA) for treatment of OSA.[4]

- Future GRADE reviews and practice parameters from the AASM will use a new recommendation scheme that will include the following categories: Strong for, Weak for, Weak against, and Strong against.[5] However, this does not apply to the reviews discussed in this chapter.

Upper Airway Resistance Syndrome and Obstructive Sleep Apnea

Introduction

- SDB resulting from narrowing or collapse of the upper airway runs the spectrum from primary snoring and upper airway resistance syndrome (UARS, also known as respiratory effort–related arousals [RERAs]) to frank OSA. While isolated snoring can have an impact on the quality of life of patients and their bed partners, other medical consequences resulting from this condition are less certain, and thus it has largely been considered a cosmetic problem. In contrast, UARS and OSA have both been associated with numerous functional, physiologic, and medical consequences, and these are discussed in the preceding chapter. For the purposes of this chapter, UARS will be considered as part of OSA.
  - In adults, clinically significant OSA is defined as an *apnea-hypopnea index* (AHI: number of apneas and hypopneas per hour of sleep) ≥5 events per hour in the setting of symptoms or significant comorbid conditions, or when the AHI is ≥15 events per hour.[1]
  - Some authors also use the term *respiratory disturbance index* (RDI) when reporting OSA parameters, and this refers to the number of apneas and hypopneas and RERAs per hour of sleep.[6]

- Grading the severity of OSA depends on the result of objective testing and the severity of the daytime symptoms. However, for most clinical purposes, AHI or RDI thresholds derived from polysomnography (PSG) are used to grade severity. The standard classification recommended by the AASM and used in practice is as follows: an AHI or RDI between 5 and less than 15 events per hour indicates mild OSA, an AHI or RDI between 15 and 30 events per hour is considered moderate OSA, and an AHI or RDI of more than 30 events per hour represents severe OSA.[7] Although these thresholds are somewhat arbitrary, there is data linking worse outcomes with moderate to severe OSA (AHI ≥ 15) and growing evidence suggesting that treatment may improve these outcomes.[8,9] In children, the threshold AHI for treatment is typically 1 event per hour (or 25% of the total sleep time associated with obstructive hypoventilation),[1] although this is not universally accepted, and the threshold may vary according to the child's age.

- This chapter reviews the treatment options for OSA in adults. Pediatric OSA and its management are covered in the chapter on pediatric sleep medicine. The therapeutic options are organized into the following categories: positive airway pressure (PAP) treatment options, oxygen therapy, OA, surgical treatment options, hypoglossal nerve stimulators (HNS), nasal resistive valves, pharmacologic therapies, behavioral treatments, and miscellaneous therapies (positional therapy, negative oral pressure therapy [OPT], high flow nasal cannula therapy). An overview of an algorithmic approach to the treatment of OSA is provided in Fig. 14.1.

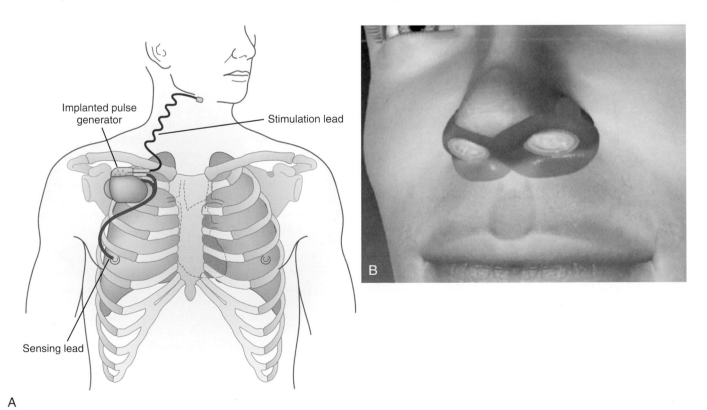

- **Figure 14.1** **A,** Hypoglossal nerve stimulator. This is one (Inspire II; Inspire Medical Systems, Inc.) of several models currently being tested. **B,** Nasal expiratory positive airway pressure device. (From Park JG, Morgenthaler TM, Gay PC. Novel and emerging nonpositive airway pressure therapies for sleep apnea. *Chest.* 2013;144[6]:1946–1952.)

Positive Airway Pressure

- PAP is considered first-line therapy for the management of OSA due to the significant body of evidence supporting its impact on clinical outcomes. A wide variety of PAP modalities have been used in the treatment of OSA, including continuous positive airway pressure *(CPAP)*, auto-adjusting CPAP *(ACPAP)*, CPAP with expiratory relief *(CPAPexp)*, bilevel PAP *(BPAP)*, adaptive servo-ventilation *(ASV)*, and volume assured pressure support *(VAPS)*. As ASV and VAPS are primarily indicated in the setting of CSA (ASV) and significant hypoventilation (VAPS), these modalities will be discussed in later sections of this chapter.

Positive Airway Pressure Modalities

- *CPAP* was the first developed and clinically implemented PAP modality[10] and is the standard therapy to which all other therapies are compared.
  - CPAP delivers a predetermined fixed pressure during both inspiration and expiration to keep the upper airway patent.
  - ACPAP differs from CPAP in that the pressure fluctuates over time between preset minimum and maximum pressure limits. The pressure fluctuations are driven by brand-specific algorithmic responses to machine-sensed snoring and/or flow limitations (i.e., by analyzing breathing waveforms) to either increase the pressure in response to perceived respiratory disturbances or decrease the pressure in response to a stable breathing pattern over a predefined period.[11]
  - CPAPexp is similar to traditional CPAP, with the exception of allowing a transient decrease in pressure during early expiration, followed by ramping of the pressure back to the fixed pressure setting by the end of expiration.[11] The patient sets the level of drop in expiratory pressure by choosing one of three settings that somewhat, although variably, correlates with a decrease in expiratory pressure of 1, 2, and 3 cm H_2O. This technology is available with both ACPAP and BPAP in some models.
  - BPAP differs from CPAP modalities by delivering a separately adjusted inspiratory pressure setting (IPAP) and expiratory pressure setting (EPAP).[11] The EPAP setting is usually slightly lower than or approximates the fixed CPAP setting need to prevent apneas, whereas the IPAP setting is a minimum of 4 cm H_2O higher, although the gradient between IPAP and EPAP may reach 10 cm H_2O or higher.
  - Auto-adjusting BPAP devices have independently fluctuating IPAP and EPAP that respond to machine-sensed breathing disturbances.[11] These are also commercially available.

Continuous Positive Airway Pressure and Other Positive Airway Pressure Modalities

- CPAP is highly effective at controlling OSA, and as a result, numerous positive outcomes have been reported with CPAP treatment of OSA. The main limitation to the efficacy of CPAP therapy is the willingness of patients to accept CPAP therapy up front and, in those who do, remaining adherent to therapy over time.
  - By creating positive pressure within the upper airway, CPAP counteracts the subatmospheric collapsing pharyngeal pressure produced during an obstructive event. Interestingly, imaging studies reveal that the greatest change in the upper airway occurs in the lateral dimension.[12] Other theories to explain the effects of CPAP on OSA have been put forth, although supportive data are largely lacking. These theories have

included rebreathing CO_2 to stimulate ventilation, increasing airway patency by creating a traction force on the trachea, and increasing airway patency by augmenting end-expiratory lung volumes.[13]

- Impact on symptoms, cognition, and mental health
  - Multiple RCTs with placebo in the forms of pills or sham CPAP have demonstrated that CPAP improves both objective and subjective sleepiness.[14] By enhancing the continuity of nighttime sleep, CPAP also improves vigilance and concentration in OSA patients during the daytime.
    - Observational studies consistently show that the higher rate of motor vehicle accidents seen in OSA patients (as compared with the general population) decreases with CPAP therapy.[15]
    - CPAP appears to improve quality of life in patients with OSA, both in short-term and in longer-term studies.[16–18] CPAP has also been shown to improve the quality of life of bed partners of patients with OSA.[14]
  - The reversal of neurocognitive deficits attributed to untreated OSA has been suggested to result from CPAP therapy but has been difficult to conclusively prove. The largest RCT to date, the Apnea Positive Pressure Long-term Efficacy Study (APPLES), failed to show an improvement in neurocognitive function following 6 months of CPAP therapy.[19] However, this study enrolled patients with normal baseline cognitive function and did not address whether or not CPAP may prevent or reverse cognitive impairment in those with reduced baseline function. A recent small RCT of elderly patients with severe OSA and baseline cognitive deficits found 3 months of treatment with CPAP improved memory and executive function as compared with the control group, and this was felt to be mediated through neuroimaging-confirmed increased connectivity in the brain and reduced cortical thinning.[20] Further work in this area is warranted.
  - CPAP therapy in OSA patients with comorbid psychiatric symptoms, such as depression and anxiety, has been studied sufficiently enough that a recent meta-analysis of this body of literature was performed.[21] Interestingly, CPAP appears to improve symptoms of both depression and anxiety in preCPAP versus postCPAP studies (moderate effect size) and when CPAP is compared with oral placebo (low effect size), but not when CPAP is compared with sham CPAP.[21] The authors hypothesized that the reduction in symptoms may have been the result of patient expectations and ongoing contact with their health care provider, and not the CPAP itself.

- Impact on cardiovascular outcomes
  - Multiple controlled trials have examined the effect of CPAP on blood pressure (BP), and at least eight meta-analyses have been performed.[22] The results have been fairly consistent across studies, showing that CPAP treatment in OSA patients has a mild effect on BP, with decreases in the systolic BP in the range of 1.5–2.5 mm Hg and in the diastolic BP of 1.5–2.0 mm Hg. The two most recent meta-analyses only included studies in subjects on CPAP for more than 4–6 weeks, and noted that the magnitude of effect on BP is greater on nighttime BP (as compared with daytime BP) and in patients with poorly controlled hypertension.[23,24] Other factors that appear to impact the BP response to CPAP include how symptomatic the patients are at baseline (e.g., level of sleepiness) and their compliance with CPAP therapy.[22] An additional meta-analysis of four studies of

patients with resistant hypertension demonstrated a more substantial effect of CPAP on BP (systolic BP decreased by 6.7 mm Hg and diastolic BP by 5.9 mm Hg).[25]

- There are considerably fewer randomized controlled data evaluating the efficacy of CPAP on other cardiovascular outcomes. Many studies have included control groups that refuse to use or are nonadherent with CPAP, thus introducing potential selection bias. Nonetheless, a number of observational studies have found that treatment with CPAP reduces detrimental composite cardiovascular outcomes.[8,26,27] Most recently, a single-center RCT of ACPAP versus usual care ($n = 122$ per arm) in nonsleepy patients with at least moderate OSA (AHI $\geq$ 15) and newly revascularized coronary artery disease failed to find a difference in the composite cardiovascular outcome at 57 months of follow-up.[28] However, when adherence to CPAP was taken into account, there was a significant risk reduction in cardiovascular outcomes (hazard ratio 0.29, confidence intervals [CI] 0.10–0.86) in those who used CPAP $\geq$4 hours per night compared with those who used it <4 hours per night.

- Data has begun to emerge examining specific cardiovascular outcomes.
  - A recent meta-analysis of atrial fibrillation in OSA patients included eight studies (only one RCT) and reported a 44% decreased risk of the recurrence of atrial fibrillation following catheter ablation in patients treated with CPAP.[29]
  - In patients with coexistent OSA and congestive heart failure (CHF), three small RCTs have demonstrated improvements in left ventricular ejection fraction (LVEF) in as short as 1–3 months after initiating treatment with fixed pressure CPAP.[30–32] Additional small studies have found significant reductions in muscle sympathetic nerve activity, heart rate variability, and baroreflex sensitivity with CPAP treatment in OSA patients with CHF.[33] However, data regarding other clinically relevant outcomes for CPAP treatment of OSA in CHF patients are lacking, and this is also the case for patients with heart failure with a preserved ejection fraction.
  - Limited observational and retrospective data suggests better cardiovascular outcomes in patients with preexisting coronary artery disease.[33] As noted earlier, a single-center RCT study failed to find superior cardiovascular outcomes in nonsleepy patients with coronary artery disease and OSA who were treated with CPAP in the intention-to-treat analysis, although subanalysis did show improvements in those who were adherent to CPAP therapy.[28] It is hoped that ongoing multicenter prospective RCTs will provide additional answers.[34,35]

- OSA has been linked to increased risk of cerebrovascular accidents (CVAs), and thus treatment of OSA with CPAP has been evaluated in terms of risk reduction for CVA as an outcome. A recent systematic review and meta-analysis found lower rates of incident CVA (relative risk 0.27, CI 0.14–0.53) with CPAP treatment of OSA in five prospective cohort studies.[36] However, this finding was not replicated in a single RCT and two administrative database studies.[36] In a series of small RCTs, survivors of CVA subsequently found to have OSA appear to have better short-term neurologic recovery following their CVA with CPAP treatment.[37–40] And in those with moderate to severe OSA who remain adherent to therapy, CPAP use leads to reduced long-term mortality.[8,41]

- Other potential cardiovascular benefits with CPAP therapy include reductions in pulmonary artery pressure, and a recent meta-analysis suggests this effect may be significant.[42]

- The positive effects of CPAP therapy on cardiovascular outcomes are probably multifactorial and mediated through CPAP-induced reductions in sympathetic activity, modulators of inflammation and coagulation, and improvements in endothelial function, all of which are found to be deranged in patients with OSA and thought to be part of the underlying pathophysiology of many cardiac diseases.[14,33]

- Impact on other outcomes
  - In addition to hypertension, OSA has been associated with other components of the metabolic syndrome, including impaired glucose tolerance and dyslipidemia.
  - The data regarding CPAP therapy and its effect on glucose control have been inconsistent[43] and may depend on the severity of the OSA, CPAP adherence, and presence or absence of obesity.[43,44]
  - Before-and-after CPAP studies suggest a significant improvement in lipid profiles with CPAP therapy,[45] although this has not been verified when only RCTs are considered (with the possible exception of improved total cholesterol).[46,47]

- *Titration and initiation of CPAP therapy*
  - Once the decision is made to initiate CPAP, the optimal pressure setting needs to be determined. Traditionally, this is determined by in-laboratory PSG with attended manual titration of CPAP by a sleep technician. While in practice a "split-night" protocol (the first half of the PSG is a diagnostic study followed by titration of CPAP) is often used, a full-night CPAP titration has been the preferred method according to the 2006 AASM practice parameters for the use of CPAP and BPAP (Guideline).[2] Recently, alternative methods for determining the optimal fixed CPAP setting have been evaluated, and these approaches will be discussed shortly.
  - Before titration or initiation of CPAP therapy, standard care should include education about CPAP (including indications, rationale, and potential side effects), a hands-on demonstration of CPAP, careful mask selection and fitting, and a short period of acclimatization (Standard).[48] In 2008 the AASM published evidence-based clinical guidelines (consensus in the absence of high-level evidence) for the manual titration of CPAP for patients with OSA.[48] These recommendations have not been updated since that time and thus are reviewed here.
  - Titration of CPAP should be targeted to eliminate apneas, hypopneas, RERAs, and snoring (Consensus).[48] In the absence of clear respiratory events, CPAP should not be titrated for hypoxia. The starting CPAP setting should be 4 cm H_2O, although higher pressure can be considered in morbidly obese patients and for retitration studies, with a maximum pressure of 15 cm H_2O in patients younger than 12 years and 20 cm H_2O in patients older than 12 years (Consensus).[48] Table 14.1 provides details of the recommended titration algorithm for patients older than 12 years. (The reader is referred to the referenced article for details on those younger than 12 years.)[48] The titration algorithm is recommended for both split-night and full-night titrations. A grading system for the adequacy of the titration is also provided and includes the following categories: optimal, good, adequate, and unacceptable (shown in Table 14.2). Figs. 14.2–14.6 provide examples of the grading system for CPAP and BPAP titrations.

TABLE 14.1	American Academy of Sleep Medicine Continuous Positive Airway Pressure Titration Algorithm for Patients >12 Years Old[48]

1. Initiate CPAP at 4 cm H_2O*.
2. Increase CPAP by ≥1 cm H_2O no less than every 5 min for the following number of events per 5 min: ≥2 obstructive apneas, ≥3 hypopneas, ≥5 RERAs, or ≥3 min of loud or unambiguous snoring.
3. Maximum pressure of 20 cm H_2O.
4. Consider "exploration" of CPAP settings up to 5 cm H_2O above pressure that eliminated the respiratory events.
5. Consider "down titration" of CPAP if ≥30 min of sleep without breathing events noted. CPAP should be decreased by ≥1 cm H_2O every 10 min.
6. Consider transitioning to BPAP if respiratory events persist on CPAP at >15 cm H_2O.

*Higher pressures may be indicated for morbidly obese patients or retitration studies.
BPAP, Bilevel PAP; *CPAP*, continuous positive airway pressure; *RERA*, respiratory effort–related arousals.
Modified from Kushida CA, Chediak A, Berry RB, et al. Clinical guidelines for the manual titration of positive airway pressure in patients with obstructive sleep apnea. *J Clin Sleep Med.* 2008;4(2):157–171.

TABLE 14.2	American Academy of Sleep Medicine Positive Airway Pressure Titration Grading System[48]

Optimal Titration: RDI <5 per hour for at least 15 min and should include supine REM sleep at the select pressure that is not continually interrupted by spontaneous arousals or awakenings.

Good Titration: RDI ≤10 per hour, or a 50% decrease if the baseline RDI is <15 per hour, and should include supine REM sleep at the select pressure that is not continually interrupted by spontaneous arousals or awakenings.

Adequate Titration: RDI not reduced to ≤10 per hour but is reduced by 75% from the baseline, or the criteria for a good or optimal titration are met except for the lack of supine REM sleep at the selected pressure.

Unacceptable Titration: Does not achieve any of the grades listed previously.

RDI, Respiratory disturbance index; *REM*, rapid eye movement.

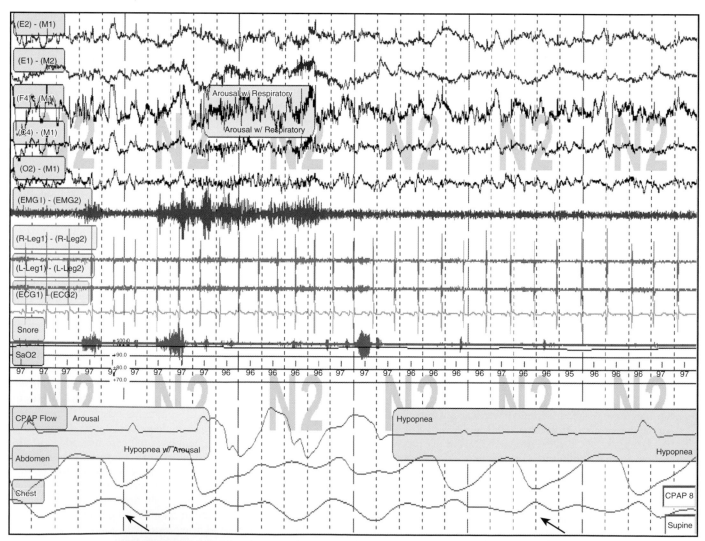

• **Figure 14.2** "Unacceptable" continuous positive airway pressure (CPAP) titration. This 30-sec epoch shows a patient maintained on CPAP at 8 cm H_2O with ongoing hypopneas associated with arousals during N2 sleep in the supine position. Paradoxical breathing is also noted *(arrows)*.

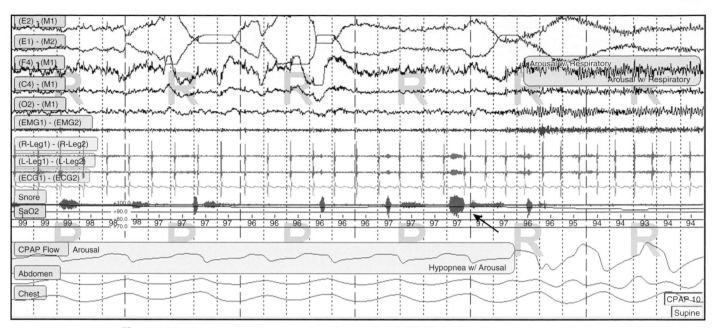

• **Figure 14.3** "Adequate" continuous positive airway pressure (CPAP) titration. This 30-sec epoch shows a patient maintained on CPAP at 10 cm H_2O with ongoing hypopneas associated with arousals during supine rapid eye movement sleep. The titration would be considered "adequate" if the respiratory disturbance index remains higher than 10 events per hour but less than 75% of the baseline RDI on the best CPAP setting. Note the snoring is still present as well *(arrow)*. (Please see also Table 14.2 and reference 48.)

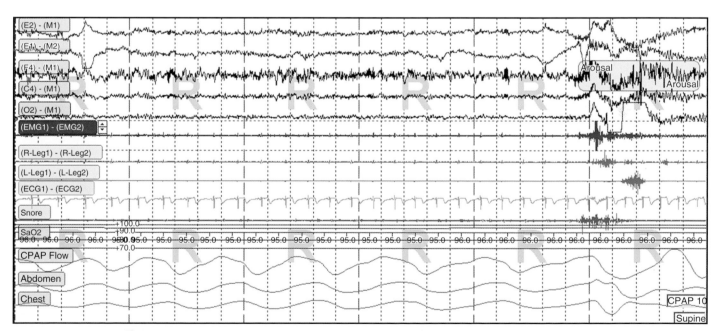

• **Figure 14.4** "Good" continuous positive airway pressure (CPAP) titration. This 30-sec epoch shows a patient maintained on CPAP at 10 cm H_2O with no clear abnormal respiratory events during supine rapid eye movement (REM) sleep but occasional arousals. The titration would be considered "good" if the respiratory disturbance index (RDI) is 10 or fewer events per hour (or a 50% or greater reduction if the baseline RDI is fewer than 15 events per hour) on the best CPAP setting. Supine REM sleep is required on the best CPAP setting. (Please see also Table 14.2 and reference 48.)

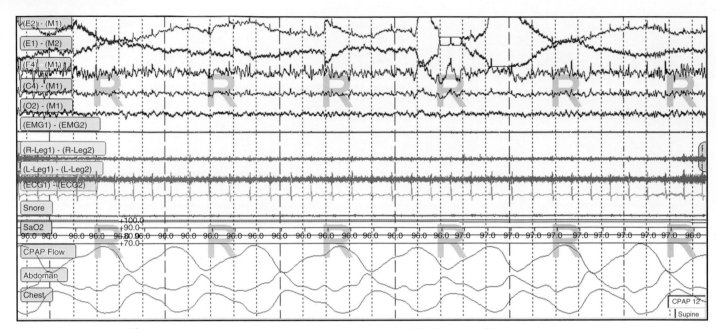

• **Figure 14.5** "Optimal" continuous positive airway pressure (CPAP) titration. This 30-sec epoch shows a patient maintained on CPAP at 12 cm H_2O with no abnormal respiratory events or arousals during supine rapid eye movement (REM) sleep. The titration would be considered "optimal" if the respiratory disturbance index (RDI) is 5 or fewer events per hour without arousals on the best CPAP setting. Fifteen minutes of supine REM sleep on the best CPAP setting is required. (Please see also Table 14.2 and reference 48.)

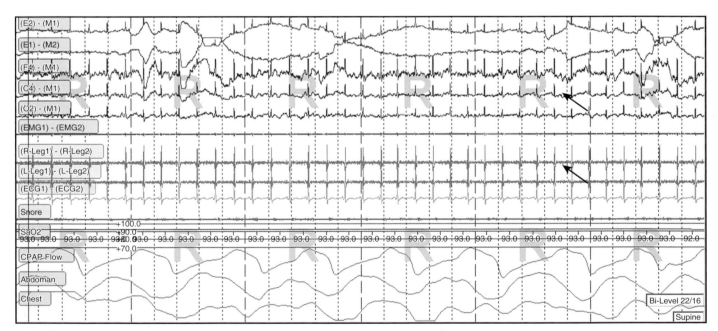

• **Figure 14.6** "Optimal" bilevel positive airway pressure (BPAP) titration. This 30-sec epoch shows a patient maintained on BPAP at 22/16 cm H_2O with no abnormal respiratory events during supine rapid eye movement (REM) sleep. The titration would be considered "optimal" if the respiratory disturbance index (RDI) is 5 or fewer events per hour without arousals on the best BPAP setting. Fifteen minutes of supine REM sleep on the best BPAP setting is required. This patient required BPAP because of reaching a continuous positive airway pressure (CPAP) of 20 cm H_2O with suboptimal control of the sleep apnea. Note the excessive electrocardiographic artifact in the leg electromyogram and all electroencephalographic leads *(arrows)*. (Please see also Table 14.2 and reference 48.)

A repeat titration study should be considered if the titration grade is not optimal or good.[48]

- Manual CPAP titration offers the benefit of an attendant sleep technician for educating the patient; troubleshooting patient complaints, mask leaks, and mask intolerance; and intervening in cases of hypoxemia. However, alternative approaches to initiation of CPAP have been suggested and evaluated.
- One such approach is the use of an *ACPAP* device for a defined period with determination of the optimal fixed pressure setting based on inspection of the machine's download.[49] In selected patient populations (diagnosed OSA, free of significant comorbid conditions), the strategy of using ACPAP to determine a fixed CPAP setting has been shown in numerous controlled trials to be equivalent to PSG-derived settings in terms of short-term (4–12 weeks) outcomes: subjective and objective sleepiness, quality-of-life measures, and CPAP adherence.[50-54] Nonetheless, many issues remain to be addressed with this approach, including the optimal duration of an ACPAP trial, how best to determine the optimal CPAP setting off the download (i.e., from the machine detected 90th or 95th percentile pressure?), and specifics regarding the algorithm of each ACPAP brand. ACPAP devices use significantly different algorithms to respond to machine-detected respiratory events.[11] The 2007 AASM practice parameters on ACPAP devices graded this approach as an option because of clinical uncertainity,[55] although based on accumulated data since that time this would be considered a reasonable treatment strategy for some patients.
- Other methods of initiating CPAP therapy have been described and include the use of pressure prediction equations,[56,57] empirical CPAP trials,[58] and patient/bed partner–driven pressure adjustments based on perceived comfort, efficacy, or observation.[59,60] These approaches were found to lack sufficient evidence for support in the 2008 AASM clinical guidelines for CPAP titration,[48] and in general, with advancements in technology, are no longer relevant.

- *Improving CPAP adherence*
  - Approximately 8%–15% of patients offered CPAP therapy will decline it up front[61] (and even up to 60% in certain populations),[62] leading to a search for alternative OSA therapies for these individuals. In those who agree to CPAP therapy, adherence is paramount to realize the benefits mentioned earlier.
  - The AASM considers objective monitoring of CPAP use to be the standard of care,[2] and devices come equipped with "time-on" pressure-monitoring capabilities. "Time-on" pressure monitoring allows the physician to review a download from the CPAP machine that shows the actual number of hours or minutes per 24-hour period that the machine is turned on and pressurized at the preset CPAP setting. Although good adherence has in general been considered to be the use of CPAP for at least 4 hours on 70% of nights, the more time patients use their CPAP while sleeping, the better their subjective and objective outcomes with regard to sleepiness and daily functioning.[63] In a multicenter study of 149 patients with moderate to severe OSA (AHI >15 by PSG) who were evaluated at baseline and after 3 months of CPAP therapy, there appeared to be a "dose-response" relationship between the hours of CPAP use and improvements in sleepiness (as measured by both the Epworth Sleepiness Scale [ESS] and the multiple sleep latency test [MSLT]) and quality

of life (as measured by the Functional Outcomes associated with Sleepiness Questionnaire [FOSQ]).[63] Nonetheless, reports of CPAP compliance suggest that only 40%–80% of patients use their CPAP for more than 4 hours on 70% of nights.[14,64]

- While studies have been inconsistent in their findings, factors reported to be associated with improved adherence include greater severity of OSA, the presence of daytime sleepiness, a higher education level of the patient, and a greater perceived benefit of therapy. Factors negatively associated with CPAP adherence include lack of daytime sleepiness, lack of a perceived benefit from therapy, previous uvulopalatopharyngoplasty (UPPP), nasal obstruction, claustrophobia, and side effects from CPAP. Because early adherence to therapy appears to predict long-term adherence, the AASM recommends that patients initiating CPAP therapy be monitored closely by a health care provider trained in sleep medicine (Standard).[2,7]
- Maneuvers to improve adherence to CPAP therapy can be broadly placed into the categories of behavioral interventions, management of CPAP-related side effects and technologic adjustments (the latter two are addressed in later sections).[65] An additional category of adjunctive sedative/hypnotic use can also be considered.
  - *Behavioral approaches* include educational interventions, supportive actions, and behavioral therapy.
    - Educational interventions reported in the literature vary from written and video instruction to group and one-on-one educational sessions lasting anywhere from 15 min to up to 4 hours.
    - Educational interventions, in low to moderate quality studies, have been shown to improve PAP adherence by about 0.60 hours per night, resulting in 13% more patients using PAP for longer than 4 hours per night. Both of these findings were statistically significant in a recent meta-analysis.[61]
    - Supportive interventions may range from a follow-up phone call by qualified personnel to computer-assisted monitoring and troubleshooting to comprehensive follow-up home visits. Early follow-up with a sleep practitioner, including review of PAP usage data, is also considered a supportive action. Supportive interventions, in low quality studies, may increase PAP adherence by 0.83 hours per night, as well as increase those crossing the 4 hours of use threshold by 16%.[61]
    - Cognitive behavioral therapy and motivational enhancement therapy are the most common behavioral therapies utilized. Training in these techniques is required prior to implementing them in practice. These modalities have been found to increase PAP use by up to 1.4 hours per night and result in a 19% increase in the number of patients exceeding the 4 hour of use standard.[61] As for these later maneuvers, the quality of these studies is low, and there is significant variability in the individual study findings.[61]
  - *Side effects* related to CPAP use are minor in general, although they may be significant enough to limit use or lead to discontinuation of therapy and thus should be aggressively managed. CPAP-related side effects can be broadly categorized into mask-related and pressure-related side effects. These side effects are listed in Table 14.3, along with possible interventions to address the problems.

TABLE 14.3	Side Effects of Positive Airway Pressure and Potential Interventions
Side Effect	**Intervention**
Mask-Related	
Discomfort	Interface change to different type or brand.
Rash	Interface change to type or brand made of different materials.
Skin breakdown	Avoid excessive tightening. Interface change (consider nasal pillows). Protective barrier for skin.
Claustrophobia	Change to nasal pillow interface. Trial of desensitization therapy.
Eye irritation	Interface assessment. Lower pressure or trial ACPAP or BPAP.
Pressure-Related	
Nasal congestion	Heated humidification. Change to full face mask. Nasal topical sprays (i.e., steroids, antihistamines). Avoid long-term decongestant use.
Sinus pain	Heated humidification. Lower pressure or trial ACPAP or BPAP. Nasal topical sprays (i.e., steroids, antihistamines).
Nasal/oral dryness	Heated humidification. Saline nasal spray or gel. Interface change. Lower pressure or trial. ACPAP or BPAP.
Epistaxis	Heated humidification. Saline nasal spray or gel. Interface change.
Rhinorrhea	Nasal ipratroprium.
Pressure intolerance	Lower pressure or trial ACPAP, CPAPexp or BPAP.
Aerophagia	Lower pressure or trial ACPAP or BPAP. Avoid full face mask. Trial of treatment for reflux.

ACPAP, Autoadjusting continuous positive airway pressure; *BPAP*, bilevel positive airway pressure; *CPAPexp*, expiratory relief continuous positive airway pressure.

A wide array of interface options is available, including nasal masks, nasal pillows, full face masks, oral interfaces, and a number of hybrids. Sleep practitioners should familiarize themselves with these options, as individualization of care will improve adherence.

- *Technologic adjustments,* including alternative PAP therapies, have included the use of ACPAP, *CPAPexp,* and *BPAP* devices. These devices were introduced, in part, with the hope of improving PAP adherence in patients with OSA. Unfortunately, these PAP alternatives have not been found to consistently improve adherence to PAP therapy, although they may be of benefit for certain individuals.
  - ACPAP has been shown to reduce the average pressure at night[66] and has the ability to respond to changes in OSA severity brought on by body position, sleep stage, or other factors. In three recent meta-analysis comparing ACPAP to CPAP, ACPAP increased PAP use by 0.18, 0.21, and 0.23 hours per night, findings that were statistically significantly in all three analyses,

but of questionable clinical significance.[67–69] For some individuals with strongly positional or sleep stage–dependent OSA or in those with some of the side effects listed in Table 14.3, ACPAP may still be a reasonable consideration. In general, ACPAP should not be used in patients at risk for central apnea (e.g., heart failure, narcotic users) or hypoventilation (e.g., neuromuscular disease, chronic obstructive pulmonary disease [COPD] such as emphysema).

- CPAPexp, by offering expiratory pressure relief, was hoped to enhance adherence by improving patient comfort. A meta-analysis of six studies examining CPAPexp found this not to be the case.[67] However, CPAPexp may play a role as "salvage" therapy for some who are struggling with fixed-pressure CPAP.
- BPAP may also play a role as salvage therapy, as it has not been found to improve PAP adherence in head-to-head trials with fixed-pressure CPAP,[67] although it allows some patients to continue PAP therapy who otherwise would abandon fixed-pressure CPAP. BPAP may be particularly useful in patients with pressure intolerance, patients with severe OSA, those requiring high treatment pressures, and when hypoventilation is also present.[70] The AASM practice parameters on CPAP and BPAP stated that BPAP could be considered in patients requiring high CPAP pressures who have difficulty exhaling against fixed-pressure CPAP or in whom coexisting central hypoventilation is present (Guideline).[2] The 2008 PAP titration guidelines supported these recommendations (see Table 14.1).[48]
- Heated humidification is another technologic adjustment hoped to improve adherence with CPAP, although data have been equivocal.[67] Despite this, the AASM recommends heated humidification be used with PAP therapy as Standard.[2,7]
- Constantly evolving interface technology may also play role in maximizing adherence. While interface choice needs to be individualized to a given patient's needs, limited head-to-head data suggests nasal pillows may improve overall patient satisfaction with fewer side effects compared with a nasal mask, and that nasal masks may be preferred and enhance PAP usage when compared with full face masks.[71]
- *Adjunctive sedative / hypnotic use,* primarily in the form of *benzodiazepine receptor agonists* used short-term, has garnered some interest as an intervention to improve adherence to CPAP when patients are initiating therapy. A retrospective study suggested that the use of a sedative/hypnotic (zolpidem or eszopiclone) just on the night of the titration sleep study could improve early CPAP adherence.[72] Two subsequent RCTs of either a single dose of ezopiclone[73] or zaleplon[74] on the night of the CPAP titration study yielded conflicting results regarding adherence at 1 month. Likewise, there is inconsistent data regarding the use of benzodiazepine receptor agonists during the first 2 weeks of CPAP initiation on short-term CPAP adherence.[75,76] Some of the differences in the study outcomes likely reflect variability in protocols, including the medication provided (eszopiclone versus zolpidem versus zaleplon). Additional data regarding this tactic appears warranted.

Oxygen Therapy

- *Oxygen therapy* has been studied for the treatment of OSA, although the data are limited.
  - Compared with no therapy, oxygen will improve the hypoxemia seen in OSA, reduce the AHI (though not normalize it) in some subjects, and can improve daytime sleepiness.[77,78] However, when compared with CPAP, oxygen is far inferior for reducing the AHI[78] and thus should not be considered as a first-line therapy. Furthermore, the use of oxygen may prolong the duration of apneas[78] and runs the risk of worsening hypoventilation in some patients.[79]
  - In contrast, oxygen may be used as a supplement to PAP therapy in some cases when patients remain hypoxic on PAP; the 2008 AASM clinical guideline on manual PAP titration considers this a Consensus recommendation.[48] In addition, oxygen therapy may be appropriate for individuals who fail or refuse all other OSA treatments and have significant nocturnal hypoxia associated with their sleep apnea, although this should be determined on a case by case basis.

Oral Appliance Therapy

- According to the 2015 AASM practice parameter update regarding the use of OA, such therapy is indicated, rather than no treatment, for patients with OSA who are intolerant of CPAP therapy or prefer alternate therapy (Standard).[4] OAs can also be used in patients with primary snoring who fail conservative measures such as weight loss, sleep position therapy, and avoidance of alcohol (Standard).[4]
  - The presence or absence of OSA must be determined before initiating treatment with OA. This is necessary to identify patients at risk for complications of sleep apnea, as well as to provide a baseline to measure the severity of the OSA and establish the effectiveness of subsequent treatment. Before fitting of an OA, an evaluation should be conducted by a qualified dental professional who has the technical skills, knowledge, and judgment regarding the outcomes and risks of OA therapy.[4] The assessment should include a dental history, a complete intraoral examination, and dental radiographs or a Panorex survey to look for underlying dental pathology.[80] Dental personnel will determine the candidacy for OA therapy and the type of device needed to improve upper airway patency.[80]
  - There are two main types of OAs:
    1. *mandibular-repositioning appliances (MRAs)*, which cover the upper and lower teeth and advance the mandible forward in relation to the resting tongue, and
    2. *tongue-retaining devices (TRDs)*, which hold the tongue forward without affecting the resting mandibular position.
       - Both devices improve upper airway patency during sleep by enlarging the upper airway or decreasing airway collapsibility, or both.[80] MRA therapy requires an adequate number of healthy teeth to anchor the OA (the exact number of teeth necessary for adequate support of an MRA has not been identified, but consensus holds that the presence of at least 6–10 teeth in the upper and lower dental arches is desirable), absence of significant TMJ disorder, adequate jaw range of motion, and sufficient manual dexterity and motivation to insert and remove the device.[80] Custom

titratable devices are recommended over noncustom devices (Guideline).[4]
       - When patients are deemed to be unsuitable for MRA therapy or if they have a large tongue, a TRD may be used as an alternative, although data regarding TRDs and their impact on outcomes is significantly more limited than MRAs.[81] TRDs do not require dentition to keep them in place and may be an alternative for edentulous patients.[80]
  - The goals of OA therapy are to resolve the clinical symptoms and signs of OSA and to normalize the AHI and oxyhemoglobin saturation. To ensure adequate therapeutic benefit with OA therapy, the patient with OSA should undergo repeat sleep testing with the appliance in place after final adjustments and fit have been performed (Guideline).[4] It should be noted that about one-third of patients will not respond to OA therapy, and factors predicting success are not agreed upon.[82] A single night OA titration during PSG is being evaluated as a possible strategy to differentiate responders from nonresponders.[82]
- OAs have been compared with placebo and CPAP therapy in controlled trials.
  - In these trials, OA therapy has been shown to improve the AHI, reduce the arousal index, and improve oxygen saturation, although they do not have a significant effect on sleep architecture or efficiency.[4] These changes have led to improved daytime function and quality of life when studied.[82] In general, however, CPAP appears superior to OAs for improving parameters measured by PSG, although the two therapies appear similar in terms of quality of life outcomes.[4,82] Controlled trials have demonstrated that OA therapy improves BP and may be as effective as CPAP therapy in select patient populations for this outcome.[4,82] A single observational study reported no difference in cardiovascular mortality in OSA patients treated with CPAP or OA at a median follow-up of 6.6 years,[83] although no randomized control trials have addressed other cardiovascular endpoints with OA therapy for OSA.
  - Acceptance and preference of OAs versus CPAP varies by individual. Adherence to OA therapy is considered to be superior to CPAP, with reports of usage at 76% at 1 year and 62% at 4 years, although these are self-reports which may be overestimating use.[82] Recent technologic advances have led to the development of temperature sensing OA devices to allow for measurement of objective compliance.[82] A study utilizing this technology demonstrated relatively high adherence rates at 3 and 12 months of OA therapy.[84]
- Once a patient has been started on OA therapy, it is recommended that periodic office visits with both the sleep physician and qualified dentist occur to ensure ongoing efficacy and to monitor for dental-related side effects (Guideline).[4]
  - The purpose of each visit is to reassess the patient's signs and symptoms, confirm compliance in use of the OA device, and provide repair and readjustment as needed.[7] Although OAs are well tolerated in general, there are a number of potential side effects of which patients should be made aware. Most of them are considered minor and temporary, including transient TMJ pain, myofascial pain, tooth pain, excessive salivation or dry mouth, and gum irritation. However, these symptoms can be severe or continuous (or both), thus prompting the need to adjust or discontinue therapy. In addition, the potential for tooth movement, skeletal changes,

and alterations in occlusion with the long-term use of OA, although not common, warrants monitoring by a dental specialist with an understanding of these issues.

Surgical Therapies

- Before the advent of CPAP therapy for OSA in the early 1980s, surgery was the primary treatment option for patients with OSA, typically in the form of tracheostomy, although limited use of pharyngeal surgery and mandibular advancement surgery had been reported.[85] Since that time, a wide array of surgical procedures have been developed to address OSA, but most have met with limited or varied success, thus hampering their widespread applicability.
  - The definition of successful treatment of OSA in most surgical studies is considered to be the combination of a decrease in the AHI to less than 20 and an overall reduction of the AHI by 50% of the presurgical value.
  - As an example, "successful" surgical treatment of OSA might be considered a postsurgical AHI of 18 in a patient with a presurgical AHI of 50. This definition may result in patients with "successful" surgery being left with what would otherwise be considered clinically significant OSA. In addition, limited long-term follow-up data and a paucity of RCTs leave the surgical literature deficient, particularly when comparing the efficacy of surgical intervention with that of other treatment options.
  - Despite the lack of high-level evidence to support surgical procedures for the management of OSA, a wide variety of surgeries are currently used in practice and the most common surgical options for OSA are listed in Table 14.4.
- The AASM last performed a review and published a practice parameter on surgical treatment options for adult OSA patients in October 2010.[86]
  - This practice parameter on the surgical treatment of OSA reviewed the literature regarding the following specific surgical procedures: *tracheostomy, maxillomandibular advancement (MMA), laser-assisted uvulopalatoplasty (LAUP), UPPP, radiofrequency ablation (RFA), and palatal implants.*

TABLE 14.4 Surgical Approaches for the Management of Obstructive Sleep Apnea

Anatomic Site of Surgery	Surgery
Nasopharynx	Septoplasty Turbinate reduction Adenoidectomy/Polypectomy
Oropharynx	Tonsillectomy Uvulopalatopharyngoplasty (and variants)
Hypopharynx	Midline glossectomy Base of tongue reduction Genioglossus advancement Hyoid suspension Mandibular advancement
Trachea	Tracheostomy
Multiple sites	Maxillomandibular advancement
Weight loss	Bariatric surgery

- In addition, specific recommendations regarding the role of surgery, outcomes with which to measure success, and follow-up after surgery were commented on. These recommendations, with their level of evidence grade, are summarized here and supplemented as warranted by more recent literature. Additional surgeries (e.g., nasal surgery, tonsillectomy) not addressed in the practice parameter will be commented on as well.
- Establishing a diagnosis of OSA and its severity by PSG before any surgical intervention was recommended (Standard).[86] Furthermore, so that patients can make an informed decision regarding therapy, it was recommended that all patients be advised of the potential success rates, as well as complications, related to surgical intervention, as compared with the alternative treatment options for their OSA (namely, PAP therapy and OA therapy; Standard).[86] If patients chose to undergo surgery, clinical follow-up to include PSG was recommended to document resolution of the signs and symptoms of OSA, as well as, and perhaps most importantly, to document normalization of the AHI, oxygen saturation, and sleep architecture (Standard).[86] Long-term follow-up to monitor for recurrence of OSA was also recommended (Standard).[86]
- Regarding the specific procedures, as of 2010 none had received more than a recommendation of option as an intervention for the management of OSA.[86] The only exception was a recommendation *against* using *LAUP* as a treatment of OSA (Standard).[86] This was in line with a 2009 systematic review that found two RCTs of LAUP that showed no benefit.[87] A synopsis of comments from the practice parameter on the specific surgical procedures follows.[86]
  - *Tracheostomy* is still considered an option for the treatment of OSA, but it was recommended that it be reserved for patients who fail all other therapies, have refused all other therapies, or have no other therapeutic options left. In occasional instances (e.g., profound respiratory failure related to severe OSA unable to be controlled with PAP therapy), the clinical situation may dictate tracheostomy as an immediate and necessary treatment. A 2014 meta-analysis of tracheostomy for OSA management that was based primarily on case series demonstrated a reduced AHI, improved quality of life, and apparent reductions in overall and cardiovascular mortality (compared with historic controls) following tracheostomy.[88] There are both short-term and long-term risks and complications associated with this procedure (including stomal complications and psychologic trauma) that limit its use.
  - *MMA* (Fig. 14.7)[89] can be considered for severe OSA when the patient has failed or refuses PAP therapy or when OA therapy is unacceptable (fails or refuses). A recent meta-analysis of before and after studies of MMA surgery found marked improvements in AHI, oxygenation, and sleepiness following surgery, with 85.5% "success" rates (as defined earlier) and a 38.5% cure rate (AHI < 5).[90] Risks with MMA surgery include malocclusion, facial numbness, cosmetic changes, and prolonged recovery times.[91] In general, patients undergoing this surgery are highly selected based on craniofacial anatomy, and a multidisciplinary approach is recommended to identify appropriate patients for this surgery.
  - *UPPP* (Fig. 14.8),[89] alone or in combination with tonsillectomy, was not recommended as first-line therapy for patients with moderate to severe OSA, and further

research regarding outcomes with this procedure has been suggested.

- Success rates for UPPP vary from 16%–33% when performed alone, to as high as 60% when combined with other procedures.[44,91] Persistent side effects may occur with palatal procedures, including difficulty swallowing, globus sensation, velopharyngeal insufficiency, and impairment of future CPAP use (due to leak and pressure intolerance).[44,87] Furthermore, recurrence of OSA over time has been reported.[92]
- *RFA* of the soft palate was also given an Option recommendation by the AASM as a surgical procedure for patients with mild to moderate OSA who fail or refuse PAP or when OA therapy is unacceptable, although careful selection of patients is recommended. Likewise, soft palatal implants can be considered in patients with mild OSA who fail or refuse PAP or when OA therapy is unacceptable, although data on their efficacy is limited and somewhat inconclusive.[93]

- Multilevel or stepwise surgery was given an Option recommendation as an alternative in patients with OSA and documentation of multiple sites of upper airway narrowing.
- *Nasal surgery* as a standalone intervention for patients with OSA and nasal obstruction was not addressed by the 2010 AASM practice parameter though has been subject to study. Interestingly, a 2015 meta-analysis of nasal surgery (two RCTs, seven prospective studies, and one retrospective study) found significant improvements in the ESS and the RDI but not the AHI.[94]
- *Tonsillectomy,* considered a first-line procedure for childhood OSA, may be of some use in adults with significant tonsillar hypertrophy though careful patient selection is required.[81,95]
- And finally, a myriad of tongue-related procedures, including RFA to the base of the tongue, posterior midline glossectomy, and tongue-repositioning procedures, are available.[91] These are most commonly performed as part of multilevel surgeries, and their efficacy as isolated interventions has not been well-studied.

- Even though surgery is not considered first-line therapy for OSA in the majority of patients, there are some patients for whom surgery is appropriate.
  - For example, patients with mild to moderate OSA who are not obese and have clear anatomic abnormalities in their upper airway are likely to benefit the most from surgical intervention. Careful patient selection is key in making these judgments, and additional data on selection strategies will be helpful to guide treatment decisions.
  - Surgery may also play a role in certain cases as adjunctive therapy to other long-term OSA treatment options. For instance, surgical intervention to remove the tonsils in a morbidly obese patient may reduce the severity of the OSA and thereby lead to lower CPAP requirements and improved compliance with CPAP therapy.[96] A recent review found that a variety of nasal, oral and multilevel procedures improve the AHI enough to lead to a reduction in CPAP pressure settings and better compliance with CPAP following surgery, although the overall quality of the data is low.[97]
  - Aside from airway surgery, gastric bypass surgery (GBS), a surgical intervention that leads to dramatic weight loss in the morbidly obese, can significantly improve OSA without directly operating on the upper airway. GBS is discussed later in the section on weight loss.

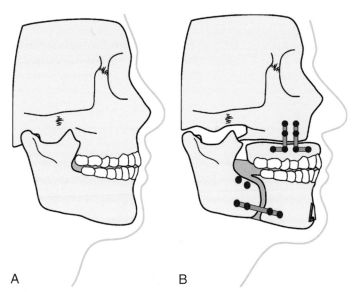

- **Figure 14.7** Before **(A)** and after **(B)** maxillomandibular advancement surgery. (From Holty JC, Guilleminault C. Maxillomandibular expansion and advancement for the treatment of sleep-disordered breathing in children and adults. *Semin Orthod.* 2012;18[2]:162–170.)

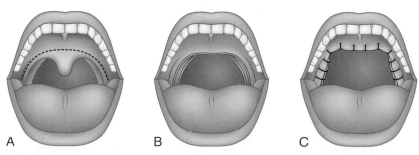

- **Figure 14.8** Technique of Uvulopalatopharyngoplasty. **A,** Redundant soft palate and tonsillar pillar mucosa are outlined. **B,** Tonsils, tonsil pillar mucosa, and posterior soft palate are excised. **C,** Mucosal flaps of the lateral pharyngeal wall and nasal palatal muscle are advanced to the anterior pillar and/or mucosa of the soft palate. (Modified from Berry RB, Wagner MH. Surgical treatment for obstructive sleep apnea. In *Sleep Medicine Pearls*. 3rd ed. 2015;341–348.)

- With all surgical interventions, follow-up testing is recommended to assess the impact of the surgery on the OSA. In addition, long-term follow-up is indicated as the efficacy of many surgical interventions decreases with weight gain and aging. Overall, there remains a need for larger, well-controlled trials of surgical interventions in the management of OSA to determine how best to use these treatment options in clinical practice.

Hypoglossal Nerve Stimulators

- Stimulation of the hypoglossal nerve leading to activation of the genioglossus muscle has been a treatment concept under investigation for some time,[98] although only recently has it been shown to be a safely tolerated and effective therapy for select patients with OSA.[99]
  - *HNS* are placed surgically with a sensing electrode on an intercostal muscle to synchronize pacing to inspiration and a pacing electrode on the hypoglossal nerve to stimulate the genioglossus muscle, increasing upper airway motor tone and thus upper airway patency (Fig. 14.9).[100]
- In a large multicenter study of 126 patients with moderate to severe OSA intolerant of CPAP therapy, HNS therapy resulted in a 68% reduction in the AHI at 1 year, as well as improvements in the ESS and quality-of-life measures.[99] A meta-analysis of HNS treatment found five prospective case series and one case report, reporting that the AHI decreased by 50%–57% at 3–12-month intervals, with significant improvements in the oxygen desaturation index and the ESS.[101] Adherence to therapy appears to be high (85% of nights with 5.4–7.5 hours of use), and the devices appear to be well-tolerated.[101]
- In general, complications are mild and transient and include tongue weakness/soreness, neck pain/swelling, fever, and lack of tongue response to stimulation, although approximately 4.5% of patients had serious complications requiring removal of the device.[101]
- It should be noted that the eligibility criteria for receiving a HNS implantation in these studies has been fairly narrow and limit generalizability. Most patients studied have failed or refused CPAP therapy, have a body mass index (BMI) <32 kg/m^2, an AHI between 20 and 60 events per hour, and a lack of concentric collapse at the level of the soft palate during drug-induced sleep endoscopy. And finally, this therapy is expensive relative to other treatment options for OSA, and comparative cost-effectiveness studies are needed.

Nasal Expiratory Positive Airway Pressure

- The use of one-way valves at the nose to create positive pressure on expiration (EPAP) was developed as an alternative to CPAP therapy for the management of OSA.[102] *Nasal EPAP* devices are disposable adhesives placed over the nostrils that increase airflow resistance on expiration, creating increased end-expiratory

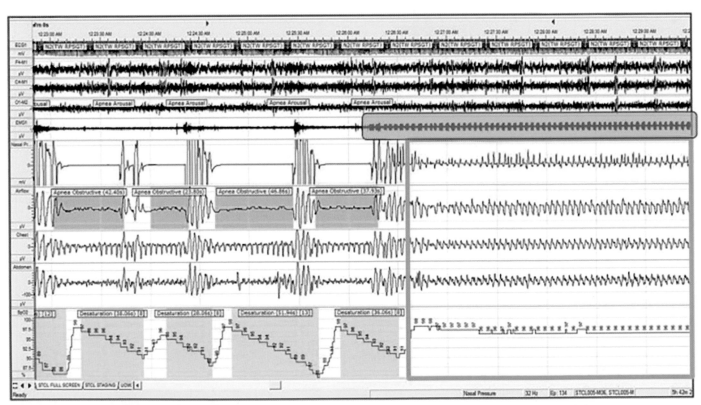

- **Figure 14.9** Titration of Hypoglossal Nerve Stimulators Therapy During Polysomnography. Polysomnography snapshot showing an approximately 6-min respiratory window. The left side of the image shows periodic airflow limitation, fluctuating respiratory effort, and associated oxygen desaturations consistent with obstructive sleep apnea. Device activation is illustrated by the green box. After the device synchronizes with ventilatory effort, immediate improvement in control of breathing and oximetry is observed. (From Soose RJ. Novel surgical approaches for the treatment of obstructive sleep apnea. *Sleep Med Clin.* 2016;11[2]:189–202.)

pressure leading to upper airway dilation and making the upper airway more resistant to collapse with the next inspiration.[103]

- The majority of studies suggest nasal EPAP may be effective at improving the AHI and the ESS in patients with mild to moderate OSA, although some concern has been raised about their utility in patients with more severe OSA, particularly following withdrawal of CPAP.[103,104] A 2015 systematic review and meta-analysis, which included conference abstracts as 10 of the 18 studies, found that nasal EPAP reduced the AHI by 53% and improved the lowest oxygen saturation by 3%, as well as reduced the ESS by 2.5 units.[103]
- However, there are some caveats regarding nasal EPAP worth mentioning.
  - First, many of the studies included select patient populations free of major comorbidities and without significant nasal congestion.
  - Second, individual patient response is variable (suggesting a need for follow-up testing to verify adequacy of therapy), and patient characteristics that might be predictive of a favorable treatment response have not been identified.
  - Third, while self-reported adherence appears high (80%–99%), objective measures of adherence have not been reported.
  - Fourth and finally, long-term data on control of OSA, and particularly cardiovascular outcomes, are lacking.
- Given these limitations, nasal EPAP devices might be considered in select patients where close clinical follow-up is available.

Pharmacologic Therapies

- In the context of a growing array of available treatment options for OSA, all of which possess some shortcomings, extensive research into potential pharmacotherapies for the management of OSA has been an active area of investigation.
- All the drugs evaluated have reasonable physiologic underpinnings with regard to why they might work to alleviate OSA, but to date there is no single pharmacologic agent that can be recommended for the primary treatment of OSA. This body of literature was reviewed in an AASM practice parameter published in 2006, but has not been updated since.[105] The findings from this document are highlighted when appropriate, although the more recent 2013 Cochrane review of drug therapy for adult OSA will also be discussed.[106] A few medications can play an adjunctive role in managing select patients with OSA, and these are reviewed as well. It should also be noted that studies regarding medications as therapies for OSA have primarily focused on the AHI as the main outcome, with little data on other relevant outcomes.
- Medications affecting airway neuromechanical properties
- The neurotransmitter serotonin (also known as 5-hydroxytryptamine [5-HT]) plays an integral role in maintaining patency of the upper airway by activating the upper airway dilator muscles. However, at least 14 different serotonin receptor subtypes have been identified, and some of them, when stimulated, exhibit inhibitory effects on upper airway motor tone. It is likely that mixed serotonin receptor agonist-antagonist medications are needed to produce clinically significant changes.
  - Unfortunately, human studies with *mirtazapine,* a 5-HT$_1$ receptor agonist and 5-HT$_2$ and 5-HT$_3$ receptor antagonists, have failed to show a benefit (despite promising earlier results in animal models).[107]

- A more recent small single-center trial demonstrated a 40% reduction in the AHI in the group randomized to the higher dose *ondansetron* (5-HT3 antagonist) combined with *fluoxetine* (selective serotonin re-uptake inhibitor), although there was considerable variability in individual responses and only 30% achieved an AHI less than 10.[108]
- *Protriptyline* is a nonsedating tricyclic antidepressant with rapid eye movement (REM) sleep–suppressing properties that also stimulates the hypoglossal motor neurons to increase upper airway muscle activity. Older studies have not shown clinically significant improvements in OSA (two studies found statistically significant reductions in the AHI, although moderate to severe OSA persisted). There is also a high frequency of intolerable anticholinergic side effects. The 2006 AASM practice parameters concluded that protriptyline should not be used as primary treatment of OSA (Guideline).[105]
- Other medications proposed to act on upper airway motor tone include *paroxetine* (selective serotonin re-uptake inhibitor), *buspirone* (azaprione anxiolytic acting on serotonin receptors), and *salmeterol* (long acting beta-agonist). These medications have been evaluated in small studies with limited to no significant benefit on controlling OSA.[106] More recently, there has been interest in the use of cannabinoids to improve upper airway motor tone, although only pilot data are available.[109]
- Nasal airflow resistance may contribute significantly to the development of OSA. OSA is more common in individuals with chronic nasal congestion than in those without. Only one placebo-controlled study has examined the impact of *nasal steroids* on parameters of OSA in adults with concomitant allergic rhinitis.[110] This small study (23 patients total) showed an improvement in the AHI in treated patients, and of the five individuals in whom the AHI decreased to less than 5, three had an AHI of between 5 and 10 with placebo. These data suggest that in select patients with mild OSA and allergic rhinitis, nasal steroid therapy could potentially play a role in treatment. In the 2006 AASM practice parameters, nasal steroids were recommended as a possible adjunct to other primary therapies for OSA (Guideline), whereas nasal decongestants were not thought to be indicated as treatment of OSA (Option).[105] Small studies examining nasal decongestants and topical airway lubricants have failed to show much benefit.[106]
- Medications affecting control of breathing in general
  - *Medroxyprogesterone (MPA)* is a recognized ventilatory stimulant, although it may exert some stimulatory effects on the upper airway motor neurons as well. An early small uncontrolled study found that MPA improved OSA in a subset of patients with baseline hypercapnia, although a subsequent small controlled trial found no benefit.[106] Its role in treating patients with OSA and obesity-hypoventilation syndrome (OHS) is uncertain and discussed in the section on hypoventilation syndromes. Estrogen has effects on the upper airway musculature, in addition to possible centrally mediated effects on respiration. In postmenopausal women receiving hormone replacement therapy (HRT), the incidence of OSA remains low. In 2003 two small pilot studies also suggested improvement in the AHI with estrogen therapy.[111,112] Despite these findings, no large RCTs of HRT in postmenopausal women with OSA have been reported, and the risks of HRT would need to be weighed against any possible

benefits. The AASM practice parameter did not recommend estrogen therapy as treatment of OSA (Standard).[105]

- *Theophylline* is a methylxanthine that inhibits adenosine, a centrally acting ventilatory depressant, as well as enhances the ventilatory response to hypoxia and hypercapnia. However, OSA has failed to improve following therapeutic-range dosing of theophylline in a number of controlled trials. The AASM practice parameter concluded that methylxanthine derivatives should not be used as treatment of OSA (Standard).[105]

- *Acetazolamide,* a carbonic anhydrase inhibitor, produces metabolic acidosis and thus stimulates respiration. This drug has traditionally been considered in the treatment of CSA as opposed to OSA. Older studies found that in patients with OSA, the AHI variably improved following treatment, but that clinically significant OSA often persisted. There has been renewed interest in this medication, as it is being investigated as a potential treatment for patients with OSA who have high loop gain (an unstable ventilatory pattern).[113,114] However, side effects, including intolerable paresthesias and severe metabolic acidosis seen at higher doses, may restrict its clinical utility. Acetazolamide is not currently recommended for the treatment of OSA.

- Hypothyroidism depresses the ventilatory drive, can impair upper airway muscle function as a result of myopathy, and may narrow the upper airway secondary to deposition of mucopolysaccharide. A number of small case series of *thyroid replacement therapy* have yielded conflicting results, with some showing dramatic decreases in the AHI and others showing no effect. It is unclear whether those failing to respond have irreversible changes from hypothyroidism or whether other factors contributing to risk for OSA (such as obesity or craniofacial abnormalities) may be playing a role. No RCTs addressing thyroid replacement in hypothyroid patients with OSA have been reported. Based on the data available, it is reasonable to use thyroid replacement therapy with close clinical follow-up as monotherapy for hypothyroid patients with mild OSA, but adjunctive conventional treatments should be considered for those with significant OSA-related symptoms or more severe OSA. All patients should undergo repeat evaluation of their sleep apnea once euthyroid status is achieved. Of note, the 2006 AASM practice parameter thought that there was insufficient evidence to support the formulation of a practice parameter on thyroid replacement therapy.[105]

- Additional agents that were studied in hopes that they would aid in the treatment of OSA by affecting control of breathing have included *naloxone, naltrexone, doxapram,* and *almitrine,* although none have proven to be effective therapies.[106]

- Medications that minimize symptoms
  - Despite optimal treatment of OSA, subjective daytime sleepiness may persist in as much as 22% of patients.[63] The reason for this is not entirely clear, but these ongoing symptoms can have an adverse impact on quality of life and potentially increase the risk for accidents. Therefore therapies to further reduce daytime symptoms of OSA in those already undergoing conventional treatment have been studied.
  - *Modafinil* and its R-isomer, armodafinil, are centrally acting wake-promoting agents that have no effect on respiratory events in sleep. Since the original randomized

placebo-controlled trials of these agents for residual sleepiness in OSA patients on PAP therapy,[115,116] a sufficient number of controlled trials have been reported that no less than 3 meta-analysis have recently been performed.[117–119] These analyses included 6, 10, and 16 studies and found remarkably consistent improvements in both subjective and objective measures of sleepiness. Subjective sleepiness, as measured by the ESS, has been shown to improve by 2.2–3 units, while objective sleepiness, as measured by the maintenance of wakefulness test, improved by 2.5–3 min.[117–119] There was little difference in outcomes between the modafinil and armodafinil in these meta-analysis that compared them.[118] Individual studies have also demonstrated improvements in tests of vigilance and measures of quality of life. A trend toward a decrease in CPAP use (0.12 hours less) was noted with stimulant use in one of the meta-analyses, although this was not statistically significant.[117] However, this remains a potential concern outside of a clinical trial setting.

- Based on the available data at the time, the 2006 AASM practice parameter concluded that modafinil could be considered as an adjunct to effective PAP therapy for patients with residual OSA-related daytime sleepiness in the absence of other known causes of their sleepiness (Standard).[105]

- Close monitoring of CPAP use is encouraged. Other stimulants have not been tested in this setting.

- Serum *tumor necrosis factor-α (TNF-α)* and interleukin-6 levels are elevated in individuals with OSA and have been proposed as mediators of the excessive daytime sleepiness that accompanies OSA. Etanercept neutralizes TNF-α and thus was tested in a small placebo-controlled pilot study of patients with OSA to assess its effects on OSA and OSA-related symptoms.[120] Though having a marginal impact on AHI (decreased from 53 to 44, statistically but not clinically significant), substantial improvement in an objective measure of sleepiness was seen (3.1 min on the MSLT). No subjective ratings of sleepiness or other quality-of-life measures were reported. There have been no additional studies of etanercept as an adjunctive therapy for persistent daytime symptoms in patients with treated OSA.

- Other medications
  - There has been interest in *proton pump inhibitor* treatment of gastroesophageal reflux as a potential OSA therapy, although this has not been shown to be effective in reducing the AHI.[121]

  - The 2006 AASM practice parameters did not find enough support to develop a practice parameter recommendation regarding the following additional medications: *nicotine, bromocriptine* in acromegalics, and *androgen blockade.*[105]

  - Other categories of medications studied for the treatment of OSA, but for which there are insufficient data (and were not addressed in the 2006 AASM practice parameter), include cholinesterase inhibitors (*physostigmine, donepezil), fenofibrate, clonidine,* and *eszopiclone,* which were all discussed in the 2013 Cochrane review.[106] Of interest, the single study of eszopiclone noted that eszopiclone had the greatest impact on the AHI in patients with a low arousal threshold at baseline, presumably by increasing the arousal threshold resulting in more stable breathing.[122] This is noteworthy when one considers the growing interest in a more "tailored" individual approach to OSA therapy, which will be addressed at the end of the section on OSA.

Weight Loss Therapies

- Because most but not all patients with OSA are obese, weight loss is usually recommended as part of the treatment program. The literature on weight loss as treatment of OSA has been extensively reviewed.[123,124]
- Weight loss
  - Successful *dietary-induced weight loss* can result in a decrease in the AHI, and there appears to be a correlation between the amount of weight lost and the degree of improvement in the OSA.[123] A 2014 systematic review and meta-analysis that included four RCTs of intensive lifestyle changes, typically requiring very-low-calorie diets (ranging from 450 to 800 kcal/day), reported significant reductions in the AHI with complete resolution of OSA in some patients.[123] The most substantial changes were seen in those who lost the most weight, and the outcomes were maintained at 12 months.[123] The severity of the caloric restriction in these studies may limit their utility in clinical practice, and the benefits beyond 1 year require additional study.
  - Surgical intervention via *GBS* can lead to dramatic weight loss that should improve OSA in obese subjects. Generally accepted guidelines for GBS include a BMI >40 kg/m^2 or a BMI >35 kg/m^2 associated with 1 or more significant comorbidities (e.g., hypertension, diabetes, OSA, etc.), and the absence of comorbid conditions that would preclude surgery (including pregnancy).[125] GBS involves a Roux-en-Y procedure, which can be performed laparoscopically. There are a variety of surgical techniques to accomplish this, and these include open or laparoscopic Roux-en-Y, sleeve gastrectomy, adjustable gastric banding, and biliopancreatic diversion with duodenal switch gastric bypass (BDDS). Limited data suggests similar outcomes for all techniques except for gastric banding, which had the least favorable outcome.[126]
    - For patients with severe obesity, BDDS may lead to the most weight loss, although the data is quite limited.[126] Bariatric patients typically lose 45%–70% of excess body weight within the first year following surgery, which is often sufficient to improve or resolve their OSA.[127] A 2009 meta-analysis of 12 studies (342 patients) that had data on before and after GBS reported that on average the AHI improved from 54.7 to 15.8, while the BMI decreased from 55.3 kg/m^2 to 37.7 kg/m^2.[128] However, only a minority of patients successfully resolve their OSA to the point where additional therapy is no longer needed, highlighting the need for postoperative sleep evaluation and management.[129] There are also reports of recurrence of OSA years after GBS, particularly if weight is regained.
    - Complications associated with GBS also have to be considered as well when assessing GBS as a treatment option. Nonetheless, when compared with nonsurgical weight loss interventions, GBS has been shown to lead to greater improvements in BMI and AHI.[124,125]
  - *Medications to induce weight loss* have also been evaluated in obese OSA patients and have met with limited success. When compared with CPAP therapy, medication-induced weight loss as a treatment of OSA is far inferior.[130–132] This therapy can only be recommended as a possible adjunct to other primary therapies in patients failing to lose weight by other measures.
- In general, other behavioral maneuvers recommended for patients with OSA include minimizing or eliminating alcohol consumption, avoiding benzodiazepine use, ceasing tobacco use, and avoiding sleep deprivation. These recommendations are based on limited data, suggesting that each of these factors may exacerbate underlying OSA. No controlled trials on their effectiveness as interventions are available.

Miscellaneous Therapies

- A number of additional therapeutic options for the treatment of OSA have been investigated, although most are lacking sufficient data on which to make solid recommendations. These will briefly be reviewed here.
- Positional therapy
  - Of the alternative miscellaneous therapies in this section, positional therapy appears to have the most data supporting its use.
  - Position-dependent OSA is usually defined as an AHI that is at least twofold higher when sleeping supine than when sleeping nonsupine. Depending on the study population and the definition used, position-dependent OSA is found in anywhere from 30%–69% of OSA patients.[133,134]
  - *Positional therapy* maintains the patient in the nonsupine position during sleep and avoids supine sleep. A variety of devices have been used to maintain nonsupine sleep, ranging from verbal instruction and positional alarms to tennis balls attached to the back and vests/pillow positioners.[135] The latter of these are likely the most effective, and a number of small single-night studies have suggested reasonably good control of OSA, similar to that achieved with CPAP, although CPAP tends to be slightly more effective.[135] In the 2006 AASM practice parameter on medical therapies for OSA, positional therapy was considered a viable treatment as a secondary therapy or an adjunct to primary therapy in patients with mild OSA (Guideline).[105]
  - If positional therapy is prescribed for a patient with position-dependent OSA, control of the respiratory events should be objectively documented while the patient is sleeping with the device. And while short-term self-reported adherence to positional therapy appears equal or superior to CPAP adherence, long-term adherence appears to be very poor (19%–29% at 14–30 months), limiting enthusiasm for this modality as a durable treatment option.[136,137] Patients report nonadherence for a variety reasons, including discomfort from the device, backaches, a sense of ineffectiveness, and no improvement in sleep quality or alertness.[135]
- *Negative OPT*
  - As opposed to using positive pressure to splint the upper airway, negative OPT creates negative intraoral pressure, pulling the tongue and soft palate forward to create space in the posterior upper airway. The negative pressure is generated by a vacuum pump that is connected to a mouthpiece and requires a good seal to be effective.
  - After an initial feasibility study demonstrated a reduction in the AHI from 38.7 to 24.6 with 38% of patients achieving an AHI ≤ 10,[138] a prospective multicenter randomized crossover trial was performed.[139] This study included 63 patients with a wide spectrum of OSA severity, and found a decrease in the AHI from 27.5 to 14.8 at day 28 of OPT. Other outcomes included improved sleep quality, a decrease

in the ESS and good compliance with the OPT (average 6 hours per night). However, only 32% of the patients achieved an AHI ≤ 10 associated with a greater than 50% decrease in the AHI from baseline. In addition, the group was highly selected, with 43% of potential enrollees excluded due to poor mouthpiece fit, inability to get a good vacuum seal, or device intolerability.[139] Further study of this therapy is needed.

- *Upper airway exercises (myofunctional therapy)*
  - After two trials of upper airway exercises[139,140] suggested that these maneuvers can improve SDB in patients with mild to moderate OSA, a series of studies have evaluated the effect of myofunctional therapy on OSA.
  - A systematic review and meta-analysis found that this therapy could improve the AHI by about 50% in adults with additional benefits of improved oxygenation and a reduced ESS.[141] However, the overall effect is somewhat modest, and it is currently recommended only as an adjunct to other therapies.[141]
- *High flow nasal cannula therapy*
  - Nasal insufflation of high-flow warm humidified air has been reported to improve OSA in both adults and children in small trials.[142–144] Additional work on this therapeutic option appears warranted.

Individualized Therapy

- Recent work has begun to better elucidate the underlying pathophysiologic mechanisms contributing to OSA, demonstrating considerable interindividual variability in OSA phenotypes.[145]
  - The primary areas of focus include anatomic abnormalities, impairment of upper airway dilator muscles, unstable ventilatory control due to increased loop gain, and a decreased arousal threshold.[145]
  - Patients may exhibit problems in one or more of these pathophysiologic traits, and thus it stands to reason that therapies could be targeted to address the specific OSA phenotype.[146] For example, while a patient with reduced upper airway motor tone may benefit from hypoglossal nerve stimulation, another patient with high loop gain as their primary pathophysiologic risk factor may be better treated with oxygen or medications to reduce loop gain.[146] This novel approach to the management of OSA appears to hold promise, and further data on this therapeutic strategy is anticipated.

Central Sleep Apnea

- CSA is characterized by a lack of drive to breathe during sleep, which results in repetitive periods of insufficient ventilation and gas exchange. CSA is diagnosed by PSG, when more than five central apneas occur per hour of sleep, each lasting 10 sec or longer, and more than 50% of the events are determined to be central rather than obstructive in nature.[1] This nocturnal breathing disturbance can lead to significant comorbidity and increased risk for adverse cardiovascular outcomes.
  - The International Classification of Sleep Disorders (ICSD)-3[1] identifies eight different forms of CSA: (1) CSA with Cheyne-Stokes breathing (CSB), (2) CSA due to a medical disorder without CSB, (3) CSA due to high altitude periodic breathing, (4) CSA due to a medication or substance, (5) Primary CSA,

(6) Treatment-emergent CSA, (7) Primary CSA of infancy, and (8) Primary CSA of prematurity.
- An alternative classification system is based on etiology, where CSA can be idiopathic (e.g., primary CSA) or secondary. Secondary CSA includes CSB (usually attributable to heart failure or stroke), CSA caused by drug or substance abuse, apnea from high-altitude breathing, or CSA caused by a medical condition (e.g., thyroid disease, atrial fibrillation, renal failure). Please refer to the previous chapter for a discussion of the pathophysiology related to CSA. This section reviews the various therapeutic options currently available.
- At present there are no clear guidelines stating when or whether to treat CSA in the absence of symptoms, particularly when CSA is discovered after PSG is performed for unrelated symptoms.
  - Up to 20% of cases of CSA have been suggested to resolve spontaneously. If the patient is asymptomatic, observation may be the appropriate initial step. This is typically seen in patients who have CSA during sleep-wake transition patterns (i.e., postarousal central events), in patients without significant oxygen desaturation, or in those who experience CSA during CPAP treatment for OSA (treatment-emergent CSA or treatment-emergent central sleep apnea [TECSA]).
  - However, when symptoms are present, treatment is warranted. Individuals with CSA tend to complain less of excessive daytime sleepiness but may note poor sleep with sleep fragmentation, sleep maintenance insomnia, and daytime fatigue. Morning headaches and snoring may be present as well. Initial treatment should be directed at any condition that may be causing or perpetuating the CSA. If symptoms are still present despite optimization of such therapy (e.g., inotropic support in those with heart failure), other therapeutic measures should be undertaken.
  - Several different treatments that have been used for CSA include PAP therapy in the form of CPAP, BPAP, or ASV; supplemental oxygen; inhalation of carbon dioxide; overdrive atrial pacing (OAP); and implantation of cardiac devices. In addition, several pharmacologic agents have been studied for the treatment of CSA.

Positive Airway Pressure Therapy

- PAP is the most common and best studied intervention for treating CSA. The 2012 AASM practice parameters on the treatment of CSA syndromes in adults graded PAP therapy (CPAP, BPAP-ST, ASV) as an Option due to clinical uncertainty.[147] The consensus stated that the literature on the use of PAP therapy for the treatment of primary CSA is very limited but has potential to ameliorate central respiratory events without significant risks.
- *CPAP*
  - CPAP for treatment of CSA appears to be most beneficial in patients who have some form of nasal obstruction or pharyngeal airway collapse, are obese in body habitus, have idiopathic CSA, or have CSB-CSA. CPAP therapy is thought to prevent airway closure and increase arterial carbon dioxide levels (PCO_2), which results in PCO_2 levels being maintained above the apnea threshold.[147,148]
    - The apnea threshold is defined as the PCO_2 level below which ventilation will stop. Normal ventilation is closely regulated to maintain normal arterial PCO_2 levels within a narrow range and above the apnea threshold via feedback

loops that involve peripheral and central chemoreceptors, the vagal receptors within the pulmonary system, the brainstem respiratory control centers, and the respiratory muscles. Although during wakefulness conscious cortical stimulation can influence respiration, termed behavioral control of ventilation, the main underlying control mechanism is heavily dependent on chemical control (termed *metabolic control of ventilation*), with PCO_2 levels being the primary driving force. Thus, in the absence of behavioral override of the metabolic control system (e.g., during sleep), a reduction in PCO_2 levels of just a few mm Hg below the apneic threshold will result in cessation of ventilation (leading to central apnea) until the PCO_2 rises above this threshold.

- The majority of studies evaluating CPAP involve patients with CSA related to heart failure. In this patient population, CPAP therapy has been shown to be most effective in improving cardiac function by reducing cardiac transmural pressure and substantially reducing the frequency of apneas with chronic CPAP use.[149,150]
- A study published in 2000 suggested that CPAP may reduce the combined rate of mortality and cardiac transplantation in heart failure patients with CSA-CSB.[151] This prompted a large prospective RCT, the Canadian Prospective Continuous Positive Airway Pressure (CANPAP) study for CSA in patients with CHF, which revealed that treatment with CPAP resulted in attenuation of CSA, improvement in nocturnal oxygenation, lowering of plasma norepinephrine levels, improvement in LVEF, and an increase in 6-min walk distance. Despite these changes, the study failed to show a mortality benefit.[152] Suboptimal treatment of the CSA (the AHI during CPAP therapy was close to 20) and an unexpected improvement in CHF-specific mortality during enrollment, resulting in an underpowered study, were the major limitations of the study.
  - Subsequent post hoc analysis found that in the subset of patients undergoing CPAP treatment whose sleep apnea was controlled (AHI < 15, about 57% of the CPAP-treated arm), lower mortality rate and cardiac transplantation rates were seen compared with those in the control arm or those suboptimally treated with CPAP (33% event rate in the effectively treated CPAP group versus 56% in the control group; relative risk reduction, 67%, $P = .059$).[153] Therefore CPAP therapy, as long as it is documented to control the central events, remains a viable treatment option in patients with CHF and CSA.
  - Of interest, in an extension of the CANPAP trial, spontaneous conversion of central events to obstructive events over time in the control cohort was associated with a significant improvement in cardiac function (3.5% increase in LVEF, 8.2 sec decrease in lung-to-ear circulation time) compared with the nonconversion group.[154]
- As mentioned earlier, there is limited data for the use CPAP in patients with opioid-related CSA or idiopathic CSA, and many patients will not respond to this therapy, although a subset will and an attempt at control of the CSA with CPAP is reasonable.[147,155]

- *BPAP*
  - With BPAP, IPAP is higher than EPAP, and a high IPAP-to-EPAP gradient provides breath-by-breath pressure support to facilitate ventilation.[11] As a result, BPAP is effective in treating CSA associated with hypoventilation and ventilatory

failure, as in patients with neuromuscular disorders, chest wall–related disorders, and central nervous system disease (e.g., amyotrophic lateral sclerosis).
  - Some patients with nonhypercapnic CSA, such as CSB-CSA and primary CSA, have been shown to benefit from BPAP as well.[156] A small RCT compared BPAP-S (spontaneous mode) ($n = 10$) to standard medical therapy ($n = 11$) and found a substantial improvement in the LVEF at 3 months (20.3%) in the BPAP-S group only. There was also a suggestion of improved survival with BPAP-S (100%) versus standard care (63%), although survival was not a primary outcome of the study.[157]
    - However, BPAP, especially when used with a high IPAP-to-EPAP differential, has the potential to worsen CSA by lowering PCO_2 below the apnea threshold. Further studies are needed to better assess the role of BPAP treatment in this group of patients.
  - Pressure-cycled BPAP is preferred over volume-cycled ventilation because of cost-effectiveness and the ability to adjust for high leaks and humidification.
  - Adjunctive measures to improve breathing include elevating the head of the bed to 45–60 degrees, which dramatically decreases pressure requirements, and using a backup rate, particularly for central apneas that are longer in duration.
  - BPAP in the spontaneous timed (ST) mode is a mode similar to the traditional spontaneous mode (BPAP-S), but initiates a breath and controls the duration of IPAP and lowering of the EPAP within a set time period. BPAP-ST has been shown to have similar effects to CPAP with regard to improving the EF and lowering the AHI.[156] According to the 2012 AASM practice parameters,[147] BPAP-ST therapy can be considered for treatment of CSA related to CHF, only if there is no response to adequate trials of CPAP, ASV (although this is controversial now, as discussed in the following section), and oxygen therapies. It received an Option grading due to the paucity of data and considerable increase in cost compared with CPAP (two to four times more).
- *ASV*
- ASV is a form of closed-loop mechanical ventilation that effectively attenuates hyperventilation by delivering a target minute ventilation or target peak flow (which depends on the brand of the device) for the treatment of CSA.
- ASV provides EPAP that can be either manually or automatically titrated starting at 4–5 cm H_2O and a variable IPAP that allows pressure swings between 5 and 25 cm H_2O through a high-gain integral controller system.[158] In older models, EPAP was adjusted manually to eliminate obstructive apneas, and the IPAP pressure limits are set to resolve hypopneas and central events. Recent technology allows for auto-adjusting of the EPAP. When ASV is used at its starting support settings, there is a minimum EPAP of 4–5 cm H_2O (ASV machine brand specific) and a maximum support of 9–10 cm H_2O. If the patient's breathing decreases, the servo-controlled mechanism increases the pressure swings to achieve a target ventilation or peak flow of 90%–95% of the patient's baseline ventilation over a 3–4-min window to minimize hypo- or hyperventilation.[158] With adjustments of the IPAP pressure limit, a maximum pressure swing of 25 cm H_2O (i.e., a maximum pressure of 25 cm H_2O and a minimum of 5 cm H_2O) can be achieved with some ASV devices.
- Studies have shown that ASV is superior to conventional PAP therapy for controlling the number of CSAs, upgrading sleep architecture, and improving daytime hypersomnolence,

particularly for CSB-CSA, primary CSA syndrome, and TECSA.[159,160]

- In patients with CHF,
  - Studies have found that ASV improves LVEF by 6% (CI 4%–8%) and decreases the AHI by 31 (CI –25 to –36) compared with baseline, and decreases the AHI by 12–23 more than CPAP.[147] In addition, adherence with ASV has been reported to be significantly higher than with CPAP, roughly around 1–1.5 more hours per night.[159,161] Based on these and other studies, the 2012 AASM practice parameters considered ASV as a Standard treatment for CSA related to CHF.[147]
  - However, a recent landmark study, the Treatment of SDB with Predominant CSA by ASV in Patients with Heart Failure (*SERVE-HF*) trial published in September 2015, has raised concerns about the use of ASV in patients with impaired left ventricular function.[162]
    - This RCT showed that in symptomatic CHF patients (LVEF ≤ 45%) with moderate to severe predominant CSA, ASV had no significant effect on the composite primary end point of time to all-cause mortality, lifesaving cardiovascular intervention, or unplanned hospitalization for worsening heart failure (HR 1.14, CI 0.974, 1.325, $P = .104$).[162]
    - Unexpectedly, there was an increase in both all-cause mortality and cardiovascular-specific mortality (2.5% absolute increased risk of cardiovascular-specific mortality) for those patients who received ASV therapy compared with those in the control group.[162]
    - Based on these findings, the manufacturer of the device used in the study, ResMed, released a safety notice stating that patients with symptomatic CHF (NYHA II-IV) with reduced LVEF (≤45%) on ASV therapy for treatment of moderate to severe CSA should be informed that there is a increased risk of cardiovascular death and that alternative therapies should be considered.[163]
  - Speculation regarding a possible cause-and-effect explanation of the findings from the SERVE-HF trial by the investigators included (1) that CSA may be a compensatory mechanism with protective cardiac effects in CHF patients and/or (2) that ASV may cause increased intrathoracic pressures that lead to adverse cardiovascular complications.[162]
  - Recent commentaries suggest that multiple confounding factors call the study's findings into question.[164,165] Issues raised include the use of outdated, previous-generation ASV devices (with fixed EPAP) that could lead to uncontrolled sleep apnea and hypoxemia, poor patient selection (including some patients with LVEF greater than 45%, with an LVEF in the range of 9%–71% in the control arm and 10%–54% in the ASV arm), patient crossover between arms of the study, incomplete data collection (missing data points and significant dropout rates), and overall poor treatment adherence (average adherence of 3.7 hours/night, approximately 40% of patients with a total of ≤3 hours of use per night).[164,165]
  - Further post hoc analyses of the SERVE-HF study are forthcoming. In addition, ongoing trials, including ADVENT-HF, which investigates the use of ASV (with automatic end-expiratory titration) in patients with CHF and either OSA or CSA, are hoped to add further insight into the long-term effects and consequences of ASV therapy in patients with CSA related to CHF.[166]

- For subjects with CSA related to opioid use, a small study demonstrated that ASV was more effective in reducing central apneas and the overall AHI in patients taking opiates long-term,[167] although a companion study failed to find much benefit of ASV in patients with opioid-associated SDB.[168] Subsequent work has suggested that some but not all patients with opioid-related CSA can be controlled with ASV.[155,169] More studies in this CSA subtype are needed.

Oxygen Therapy

- Several studies suggest that *oxygen* may be a useful form of therapy for CSA.
  - A small case series observed complete resolution of central apneas in two patients with primary CSA.[170] Another study found a significant reduction in the number of central apneic events in patients with central alveolar hypoventilation syndrome treated with oxygen.[171]
  - In addition, supplemental oxygen may be effective in some patients with CSB-CSA and has also been shown to improve the ejection fraction.[172] In a cohort of 55 patients with CHF (NYHA class II-III and LVEF ≤ 45%) and CSB-CSA, home oxygen therapy over a 12-week period improved SDB (AHI reduced from 21.0 to 10.0 event per hour, $P < .001$), LVEF (EF 34.7%–38.2%, $P = .022$), and quality of life.[172] In a follow-up study, the efficacy of oxygen therapy was sustained over a 52-week monitoring period.[173]
    - The mechanism of its effectiveness is still unclear but thought to involve a rise in PCO_2 (thus widening the difference between eucapnic PCO_2 and apneic PCO_2 levels), a reduction in the ventilatory response to CO_2, and increasing pulmonary alveolar concentrations of oxygen.[174]
    - The 2012 AASM practice parameters graded nocturnal oxygen therapy as a Standard for treatment of CSA in CHF patients based on the abundance of literature supporting the benefits of use, relatively low cost, and wide availability.[147]
  - Oxygen is also effective in treating CSA caused by high-altitude periodic breathing. Any patient with CSA and significant hypoxemia is a potential candidate for a trial with supplemental oxygen. The optimal flow rate can be titrated during PSG.

Carbon Dioxide Inhalation

- Increasing CO_2 levels during inspiration has been shown to be effective against both primary CSA and CSB-CSA in reducing the overall AHI.
  - This can be achieved by *rebreathing devices* (e.g., enhanced expiratory rebreathing space or EERS) or by directly adding supplemental CO_2 (0.5%–5%) through a sealed interface with close monitoring of CO_2 levels. These techniques can increase CO_2 reserves above the apneic threshold. The increase in PCO_2 is usually minimal (approximately 2–4 mm Hg) but is enough to be effective in stabilizing the breathing pattern.[175]
  - CO_2 therapy is not currently commercially available because of safety concerns regarding CO_2 rebreathing in an unmonitored setting, and the failure of this therapy to reduce arousals in sleep.[176] And arousals from sleep in patients with CSB-CSA can lead to fluctuations in BP and sympathetic nervous

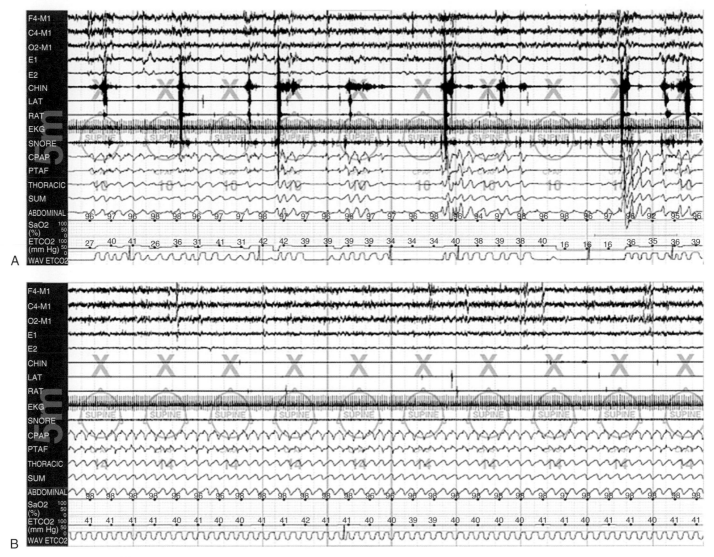

• **Figure 14.10** Potential Effects of Treatment with Acetazolamide for Central Sleep Apnea. **Panel A,** Before acetazolamide treatment of resistant sleep apnea. At the start of this PSG, the patient was failing CPAP, 150 mL enhanced expiratory rebreathing space (EERS), and supplemental O_2. **Panel B,** Postacetazolamide effects, 1 hour later. The patient received a single dose of 250 mg acetazolamide about 2 hours before this snapshot. Note the complete resolution of CSA, which was maintained for the rest of the night. 50 mL of EERS was continued. (From Thomas RJ. Alternative approaches to treatment of central sleep apnea. *Sleep Med Clin.* 2014;9[1]:87–104.)

system activation, potential contributors to the poor prognosis of heart failure patients with CSA.

Pharmacologic Therapy

- The role of pharmacologic agents in the treatment of CSA is modest and limited by the lack of controlled clinical trials to investigate their effectiveness. Therefore current evidence is insufficient to justify the standard use of pharmacologic agents for the treatment of CSA.
    - Several proposed medications aimed at improving CSA have been studied and include respiratory stimulants, such as acetazolamide and theophylline, and sedative-hypnotic agents.
    - *Acetazolamide* is a carbonic anhydrase inhibitor that causes metabolic acidosis, which stimulates respiration and presumably shifts the apneic threshold of PCO_2 to a lower level

(Fig. 14.10).[175] In a study involving six patients with CSA, administration of 250 mg of acetazolamide four times daily resulted in a substantial decrease in central apnea over a 1- to 2-week period.[177] In a study of 14 patients with CSA, acetazolamide led to improvement in daytime hypersomnolence.[178] Acetazolamide has been shown to be effective therapy for primary CSA and CSA caused by high-altitude periodic breathing, with some beneficial effects in CHF-CSB.[179] However, several studies have reported the emergence of OSA after acetazolamide use, although to be related to the respiratory-stimulating activity of the medication. When little ventilatory effort is present, the apneas appear to be central; however, when respiration is stimulated, obstructive events develop.[180] In addition, intolerable side effects (e.g., paresthesias, severe metabolic acidosis, gastrointestinal symptoms, tinnitus, drowsiness), particularly at higher doses, limit its utility. The 2012 AASM practice parameters on treatment of CSA graded azetazolamide use as an Option due to limited supporting evidence for efficacy.[147]

- *Theophylline* has been studied in patients with CSA in the setting of heart failure, as well as in patients with brainstem lesions, and was found to be effective in attenuating CSB.[181,182] However, it is rarely used because it tends to fragment sleep, has interaction with other medications, and carries a risk for toxicity—particularly cardiac arrhythmias that could potentially lead to sudden death. Furthermore, since this class of medications does fragment sleep, patients often experience a persistence of daytime symptoms, thus hampering compliance.

- *Sedative-hypnotic agents* have been used successfully in treating nonhypercapnic CSA.[175] Triazolam and zolpidem, in particular, are believed to work by suppressing arousals and consolidating sleep, minimizing the instability in ventilation induced by sleep-wake transitions. In a small case series, triazolam was found to decrease the overall AHI (borderline statistical significance, $P = .05$) and significantly decrease the central AHI in five patients with primary CSA.[183] In a nonrandomized open label treatment trial, zolpidem decreased the overall AHI from 30 to 13.5 ($P = .001$) and the central AHI from 26 to 7.1 ($P < .001$) in 20 patients with idiopathic CSA over a 9-week treatment period.[184] This study also reported decreases in the arousal frequency with improved subjective scores of sleep quality and daytime sleepiness.[184] More controlled studies are needed to verify these findings. The 2012 AASM practice parameters zolpidem and triazolam may be considered for the treatment of CSA in patients without underlying respiratory depression (Option).[147]

Overdrive Atrial Pacing

- *OAP* paces the atria at a higher rate, typically 15–20 beats above the baseline heart rate. Data suggests that it may be effective in reducing SDB, primarily CSA, in some patients with a dual-chambered pacemaker in place.

- An early study reported a reduction in AHI of approximately 60% in patients who had pacemakers implanted for symptomatic sinus bradycardia.[185] Obstructive apneas fell from 6 to 3 apneas per hour, central apneas from 13 to 6 per hour, and the overall AHI from 28 to 11 events per hour.[185]

- Since that report, multiple other studies have been published on the use of OAP for sleep apnea with mixed results. Two meta-analyses examined the role of OAP for the treatment of sleep apnea.
  - The first found that the overall AHI was reduced by only 4.7 events per hour and thus did not recommend OAP for the treatment of sleep apnea.[186] This study did not differentiate central and obstructive disease.
  - The second meta-analysis reported that the AHI in patients with CSA decreased by an average of 17 events per hour, whereas the AHI in patients with OSA decreased by an average of only three events per hour.[187] It was concluded that this therapy may be appropriate for patients with central-predominant SDB.

- The exact mechanism of OAP in sleep apnea is not fully understood. However, some have proposed that atrial pacing might stabilize respiration by preventing nocturnal vagotonia and heart rate variability seen with parasympathetic activation in sleep apnea. Another possibility is that improvements in

cardiac output with OAP may lead to reduction in lung to chemoreceptor circulation times and left ventricular filling pressures, thereby reducing loop gain and preventing the hyperventilation that initiates CSA. This theory would better explain the greater effect on CSA rather than OSA, where the instability of the respiratory control system plays less of a pathophysiologic role.[187]

Miscellaneous

- *Heart transplantation* has also been reported to either resolve CSB-CSA or decrease the cycle length of CSB in patients with heart failure.
  - In an RCT comparing 13 heart transplant patients with CHF and CSA and nine transplant subjects with CHF but no CSA, LVEF improved in both groups, but the CHF subjects with CSA pretransplant had a variable response regarding their sleep apnea: six were cured of CSA, three had persistent CSA, and four developed OSA.[188]
- Additional case reports have noted that implantation of *left ventricular or biventricular assist devices* in heart failure patients can significantly improve or resolve CSA, thus supporting the assertion that CSA-CSB in patients with CHF is a result of the heart failure.

Conclusions

- Treatment of CSA must be individualized and aimed towards treating the underlying etiology, if determined. Only after such therapy has been optimized and the CSA persists should additional treatment be considered.
- For patients with CSA, a trial of CPAP should be considered, although oxygen therapy may be acceptable for some patients with heart failure and CSA. Further data is awaited regarding the role of ASV in patients with CHF and CSA, although this may be a viable option for some patients with opioid-related CSA.
- Conversely, for patients with CSA associated with hypoventilation, BPAP should be used. Alternative therapies, including pharmacologic agents and overdrive pacing, can be considered in select patients but lack sufficient data to support their routine use in the management of CSA. The inhalation of CO_2 is promising but not ready for clinical use at this time.

Treatment-Emergent Central Sleep Apnea

- The term TECSA, previously called "complex sleep apnea," was adopted by ICSD-3 nosology and should be used when discussing this specific entity. It describes the occurrence of central apneas during titration of CPAP therapy for previously documented OSA.[189]
  - More specifically, the diagnosis of TECSA requires demonstration of predominately OSA (five or more obstructive respiratory events per hour of sleep) on the diagnostic portion of a PSG, followed by significant resolution of the obstructive apnea and emergence or persistence of CSA (not caused by another identifiable comorbidity such as CSB or substance) during the PAP titration (Fig. 14.11).
  - The clinical significance of these events is controversial.[190,191] Although some data suggest that the central apneas persist with CPAP treatment and thus alternative therapies, such as ASV, are required to eliminate the SDB,[192] others have

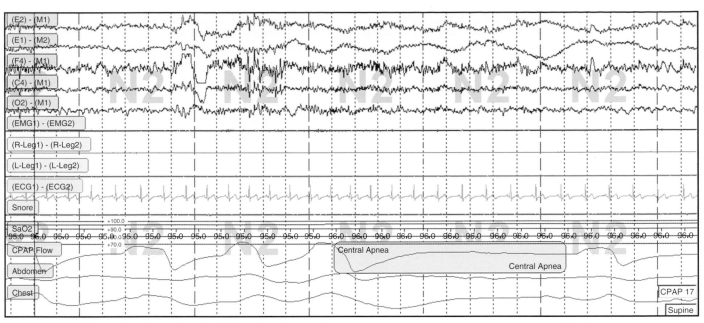

• **Figure 14.11** Treatment of emerging central apneas during continuous positive airway pressure (CPAP) titration. This 30-sec epoch shows the emergence of central apneas during supine N2 sleep in a patient titrated to CPAP at 17 cm H_2O. This may suggest over-titration of CPAP, and reducing CPAP may resolve the problem.

suggested that the central apneas tend to resolve in the majority of patients following 2–3 months of CPAP therapy (set at the pressure that eliminates the obstructive events).[193–195] In patients in whom resolution does not occur, ASV therapy may be a consideration.[160]

• Additional data examining the natural course and treatment strategies for this particular form of sleep apnea are needed.

Hypoventilation Syndromes

• According to the ICSD-3,[1] sleep-related hypoventilation disorders are categorized as follows:
  • OHS,
  • congenital central alveolar hypoventilation syndrome,
  • late-onset central hypoventilation with hypothalamic dysfunction,
  • idiopathic central alveolar hypoventilation,
  • sleep-related hypoventilation due to a medical or substance, and
  • sleep-related hypoventilation due to a medical disorder.

• The criteria for sleep-related hypoventilation syndromes requires demonstration of elevated PCO_2 levels during sleep, either by direct determination with arterial blood gases or, more commonly, by proxy measures such as end-tidal or transcutaneous CO_2 measurements. Daytime hypoventilation may or may not be present.

Congenital Central Hypoventilation Syndrome

• Congenital central hypoventilation syndrome (CCHS) is a respiratory disorder that is fatal if untreated. Persons afflicted with CCHS classically suffer from a serious form of CSA involving failure of autonomic control of breathing.
  • In general, patients require *tracheotomies* and *lifetime mechanical ventilation* to survive.

• In some patients, noninvasive negative pressure ventilation may be an option, thus avoiding tracheostomy. *Biphasic cuirass ventilation (BCV)* is a method of ventilation in which the patient wears an upper body shell or cuirass attached to a pump that actively controls both the inspiratory and expiratory phases of the respiratory cycle. In a study of nine patients with central hypoventilation syndrome who were treated with BCV, the authors concluded that it was an effective means of respiratory support in infants with CCHS.[196]

• An alternative to a mechanical ventilator is *phrenic nerve pacing (PNP)*.[197] PNP, or diaphragm pacing, is the rhythmic application of electrical impulses to the diaphragm to induce respiration in patients who would otherwise be dependent on a mechanical ventilator. Studies are limited to individual case reports, however.

Obesity-Hypoventilation Syndrome

• OHS has historically been defined as obesity associated with alveolar hypoventilation that occurs in the absence of any other condition known to cause hypoventilation.[198] The current definition entails more specific identifying features, including obesity (BMI $\geq$ 30 kg/m^2), chronic alveolar hypoventilation resulting in daytime hypercapnia and hypoxia ($PCO_2 \geq$ 45 mm Hg and $PO_2 <$ 70 mm Hg), and some form of SDB.[199]

• To make the diagnosis, other causes of alveolar hypoventilation (e.g., severe obstructive or restrictive pulmonary disease, significant kyphoscoliosis, severe hypothyroidism, neuromuscular diseases, or other central hypoventilation syndromes) must be excluded.

• Patients with OHS have symptoms similar to those with OSA, including excessive daytime sleepiness and fatigue, although this is accompanied by daytime hypercapnia and hypoxemia.

- This syndrome has been associated with pulmonary hypertension, right-sided CHF (cor pulmonale), and high mortality rates. Therefore prompt diagnosis and treatment are important.
- In general, therapeutic goals for patients with hypoventilation are aimed toward achieving an improved PCO_2 level, maintaining adequate ventilation, improving daytime oxygenation, preventing significant oxygen desaturation during sleep, and limiting sleep fragmentation.[200] It should be noted that attempting to normalize PCO_2 in patients with OHS who are in acute respiratory failure is contraindicated because it may precipitate significant life-threatening alkalosis. A gradual reduction in PCO_2 over a period of days will allow time for the kidneys to eliminate bicarbonate and prevent dangerous alkalosis from developing. In most patients with chronic OHS, complete normalization of PCO_2 during the daytime is not achieved, even with adequate nocturnal ventilation.[199]
- *CPAP*
  - In patients with both OHS and OSA, CPAP therapy is frequently effective.[201] CPAP maintains upper airway patency, eliminates obstructive apneas and hypopneas, and improves daytime hypercapnia.[199–203] Only a couple of RCTs have compared CPAP to BPAP for control of OHS and found that, in general, BPAP offers no significant benefit over CPAP alone, although the longest trial was only 3 months in duration.[204,205] In the largest of the RCTs ($n = 221$), CPAP was equivalent BPAP in all sleep-related outcomes, although some daytime parameters (6-min walk and spirometry) were better in the BPAP group at 2 months.[205] There is also a subset of patients with OHS who will remain hypoxic on CPAP and thus may require therapy with BPAP (Fig. 14.12).[206,207]

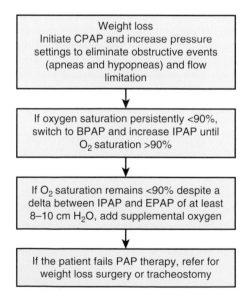

Weight loss
Initiate CPAP and increase pressure settings to eliminate obstructive events (apneas and hypopneas) and flow limitation

If oxygen saturation persistently <90%, switch to BPAP and increase IPAP until O_2 saturation >90%

If O_2 saturation remains <90% despite a delta between IPAP and EPAP of at least 8–10 cm H_2O, add supplemental oxygen

If the patient fails PAP therapy, refer for weight loss surgery or tracheostomy

IPAP = Inspiratory positive airway pressure
EPAP = Expiratory positive airway pressure

- **Figure 14.12.** Treatment algorithm for obesity-hypoventilation syndrome. *BPAP,* Bilevel positive airway pressure; *CPAP,* continuous positive airway pressure; *PAP,* positive airway pressure. (Modified from Mokhlesi B, Tulaimat A. Recent advances in obesity hypoventilation syndrome. *Chest.* 2007;132[4]:1322–1336.)

- *Noninvasive mechanical ventilation*
  - Noninvasive mechanical ventilation is effective for almost all patients with OHS. It involves the use of either a fixed pressure BPAP device or volume-targeted ventilators. BPAP devices and volume-targeted systems allow independent adjustment of inspiratory and expiratory pressure, which assists lung inflation, permits effective ventilation, and maintains upper airway patency. Volume ventilators have the added advantage of allowing higher peak inspiratory pressure and, by targeting a predetermined tidal volume, can guarantee adequate support over time.[206]
  - In recent studies, *VAPS* has been introduced as a new mode for bilevel pressure ventilation in OHS. VAPS differs from traditional BPAP in its ability to ensure a more consistent minute ventilation by automatically adjusting inspiratory positive airway pressure (IPAP) to achieve a predetermined tidal volume.[11] In short, it is a cross between the volume and pressure-assisted modes of ventilation. Studies to date show that VAPS may more efficiently decrease PCO_2 levels compared with BPAP, although it has not been demonstrated to improve other important outcomes regarding sleep quality, adherence to therapy and quality of life measures in short-term studies (up to 3 months).[208,209]
  - If severe hypoxia or hypercapnia persist despite optimal therapy with CPAP, BPAP, BPAP-ST or VAPS, or if patients are intolerant of PAP therapy, tracheostomy should be considered.[206]
- *Tracheostomy*
  - Creation of a surgical opening in the trachea is a treatment of last resort for people with OHS.[206] A tracheostomy is performed at the area of the sternal notch. Since this area lies below the upper airway, a tracheostomy bypasses the upper airway obstruction seen in OSA, thereby maintaining airflow. This treatment may improve OHS by permitting uninterrupted respiration and, if indicated, by allowing supported ventilation. As persistent hypoventilation and hypoxemia may occur, some patients will require additional PAP therapy and/or oxygen even after tracheostomy.[206,210]
  - In general, there is a lack of quality long-term data on outcomes and quality of life for tracheostomy in OHS/OSA.[210] In addition, this procedure is invasive and is often difficult to perform and manage in morbidly obese patients. Tracheostomy in this patient population may lead to complications, including granuloma formation within the airways, narrowing or collapse of the airway above the tube's location, obstruction of the tube by soft tissue or mucous plugs, accidental dislodgement of the tube, tracheoesophageal fistula formation leading to recurrent pneumonias, and psychologic trauma.[206]
- Pharmacologic therapy
  - *Progesterone,* which acts as a respiratory stimulant, has shown benefit in the treatment of OHS. In a older small case series, progestin therapy was associated with improvement in hypoxemia and hypercapnia while awake.[211] A recent 6-week RCT confirmed these effects with MPA, although the subjects also had an increase in their AHI compared with when on CPAP, and their sleep quality worsened on MPA.[212] The data are very limited regarding long-term outcomes, and the potential for adverse effects (e.g., alopecia, decreased libido, and increased risk for venous thromboembolism) prevents more common use in clinical practice. Experts do

not currently recommend progesterone therapy as standard therapy for OHS.[206]

- Other medications, including *acetazolamide, theophylline,* and *protriptyline,* have been evaluated in small clinical trials and been shown to be of no benefit in patients with OHS.[213,214]
- *Weight loss*
  - Weight loss is imperative in the treatment of patients with OHS and is considered, in the long-term, the best solution for treatment of OHS.[206] Weight loss of at least 10 kg has been shown to significantly improve vital capacity and voluntary ventilation with a marked reduction in daytime PCO_2.[215]
  - A reduction in the BMI can be achieved through lifestyle modification (including dietary restriction, exercise, and behavioral modification), GBS, and medications. These treatment approaches are all reviewed under the treatment of OSA section, though a few caveats are warranted. First, these patients are at increased risk for perioperative morbidity and mortality, primarily due to respiratory failure and risk of pulmonary embolism.[216] Therefore the use of perioperative PAP therapy is advocated.[206] Second, long-term monitoring is warranted following GBS due to the risk of potential weight gain 3.5–7 years out from surgery and thus recurrence of disease.[217] Finally, the medications for weight loss have yielded variable findings, and they often result in insufficient total weight loss in the face of concerns about side effects.
- *Medications to avoid in patients with OHS*
  - Agents that reduce the ventilatory drive or cause disruption of upper airway patency should be avoided. Such agents include alcohol, benzodiazepines, opiates, and barbiturates.

Hypoventilation Caused by Lung Disease

- Hypoventilation is not uncommon in patients with severe COPD.
  - Alveolar hypoventilation in patients with COPD does not usually occur unless the forced expiratory volume in 1 sec (FEV_1) is less than 1 L or roughly 35% of the predicted value.
  - When hypoventilation leads to significant hypoxemia, the mainstay of treatment typically entails the use of supplemental oxygen. Older studies have shown amelioration of pulmonary hypertension, better quality of life, and improved overall survival in patients treated with supplemental oxygen.[218]
  - However, oxygen therapy does not treat the underlying hypoventilation, and may actually worsen hypercapnia during sleep.[219,220] As such, *BPAP* has been studied for the treatment of hypoventilation in COPD patients.[221] While earlier trials were disappointing, more recent studies have suggested that BPAP can improve diurnal PCO_2 values.[221] Most recently, a reasonable large ($n = 195$) RCT of stable GOLD stage IV COPD patients with daytime PCO_2 values ≥52 mm Hg found improved survival at 1 year with treatment with BPAP compared with standard care.[222] In addition, high intensity BPAP using the highest possible inspiratory pressures tolerated has appeared promising in improving physiologic parameters and tolerance.[223] However, there is often a lack of subjective improvement in symptoms in many patients, and this hampers adherence and can lead to rejection of this therapy long-term. Conversely, based on multiple systematic meta-analyses,

noninvasive positive pressure ventilation (NPPV) has assumed a role as standard treatment of acute ventilatory failure associated with COPD.

- Recent data suggest that *VAPS* may be another treatment option for nocturnal support. However, preliminary studies comparing VAPS to BPAP have not shown significant differences in parameters of ventilation (daytime PCO_2, mean oxygen saturation, mean minute ventilation), adherence to therapy, or subjective measures.[224–226]

Hypoventilation Caused by Neuromuscular Disease

- Neuromuscular diseases that can cause alveolar hypoventilation include myasthenia gravis, amyotrophic lateral sclerosis, Guillain-Barré syndrome, and muscular dystrophy. These patients have rapid, shallow breathing because of severe muscle weakness or abnormal motor neuron function, which leads to hypoventilation. The central respiratory drive is typically maintained in patients with neuromuscular disorders.
  - NPPV, usually in the form of *BPAP*, is indicated for use in patients with neuromuscular disorders who exhibit morning headaches, daytime hypersomnolence, sleep difficulties, or cognitive dysfunction. If the patient is asymptomatic, NPPV is recommended when PCO_2 is greater than 45 mm Hg or when PO_2 is less than 60 mm Hg on morning arterial blood gas analysis.[227]
  - NPPV has been shown to improve quality of life and enhance survival in patients with neuromuscular disorders,[228–232] although survival may be disease specific.[233]
  - The 2010 AASM Task Force for NPPV for hypoventilation syndromes recommended that titration of NPPV in patients with neuromuscular disease be performed during an attended PSG.[234]
  - Daytime ventilation should be used when these patients have a PCO_2 greater than 50 mm Hg or oxygen saturation of less than 92%.[235]
  - *VAPS* has shown benefit in patients with neuromuscular disease. The major benefit of VAPS over BPAP is that it guarantees a delivered tidal volume despite variability in the patient's effort, changes in airway resistance, and worsening lung or chest compliance as the disease progresses. Data suggests VAPS may improve ventilation better than BPAP,[236] improves compliance,[237] and can be well-tolerated out to 1 year of use.[238] Further data on other outcomes is awaited.
  - *Tracheostomy* and *mechanical ventilation* can be considered if attempts at noninvasive ventilation fail to benefit the patient, although this needs to be placed in the context of the patient's overall disease prognosis and goals of care.

Conclusions

- The treatment options for OSA have greatly expanded in the last decade, and now include a variety of PAP therapies, OA; a number of surgical treatment options, HNS; nasal resistive valves; select pharmacologic therapies; behavioral treatments; positional therapy; negative OPT; and potentially even high flow nasal cannula therapy. However, the quality of data supporting the routine use of the majority of these interventions is quite limited and PAP therapy remains the first-line treatment option for most patients. Oral appliance therapy may also be considered as an initial treatment option for patients with mild to moderate OSA, and select patients may be candidates for other specific interventions depending on the characteristics of their OSA (e.g., anatomy, positional dependence, etc.). There is growing interest in targeted OSA therapy based on the patient's OSA phenotype, and future work on this treatment approach is anticipated.

- The therapeutic armamentarium for CSA and TECSA has also grown and now includes PAP therapy in the form of CPAP, BPAP, or ASV, oxygen therapy, OAP, implantation of cardiac devices, and pharmacologic agents. The type of therapy chosen for a given patient should be tailored to the underlying etiology of their CSA. Currently, there is controversy regarding the role of ASV in patients with CSA and reduced ejection fraction heart failure. Ongoing research is hoped to provide additional guidance in this area. Carbon dioxide inhalation appears to hold promise as a treatment option for CSA, although safety concerns remain and it is not ready for use in clinical practice at this time.

- The mainstay of treatment for hypoventilation syndromes remains ventilatory support. Technologic advances with interfaces and ventilator modalities have improved how this therapy can be delivered, although it is not clear if these innovations result in better outcomes for all hypoventilation syndromes. For example, VAPS appears superior to traditional BPAP for neuromuscular disease-related hypoventilation, but the role of VAPS in the management of OHS and hypoventilation related to underlying lung disease remains to be defined.

Suggested Reading

Aurora RN, Casey KR, Kristo D, et al. Practice parameters for the surgical modifications of the upper airway for obstructive sleep apnea in adults. *Sleep*. 2010;33(10):1408-1413.

Aurora RN, Chowdhuri S, Ramar K, et al. The treatment of central sleep apnea syndromes in adults: practice parameters with an evidence-based literature review and meta-analyses. *Sleep*. 2012;35(1):17-40.

Berry RB, Chediak A, Brown LK, et al. Best clinical practices for the sleep center adjustment of noninvasive positive pressure ventilation (NPPV) in stable chronic alveolar hypoventilation syndromes. *J Clin Sleep Med*. 2010;6(5):491-509.

Epstein L, Kristo D, Strollo P, et al. Clinical Guideline for the evaluation, management and long-term care of obstructive sleep apnea in adults. *J Clin Sleep Med*. 2009;5(3):263-275.

Kushida CA, Chediak A, Berry RB, et al. Clinical guidelines for the manual titration of positive airway pressure in patients with obstructive sleep apnea. *J Clin Sleep Med*. 2008;4(2):157-171.

Ramar K, Dort LC, Katz SG, et al. Clinical practice guideline for the treatment of obstructive sleep apnea and snoring with oral appliance therapy: an update for 2015. *J Clin Sleep Med*. 2015;11(7):773-827.

15

Circadian Rhythm Sleep-Wake Disorders

SABRA M. ABBOTT, KATHRYN J. REID

Introduction

Disorders of sleep-wake timing include what the *International Classification of Sleep Disorders*, 3rd Edition (ICSD-3)[1] terms circadian rhythm sleep-wake disorders (CRSWD). There are seven CRSWD classified in the ICSD: delayed sleep-wake phase disorder (DSWPD), advanced sleep-wake phase disorder (ASWPD), irregular sleep-wake rhythm disorder (ISWRD), non-24-hour sleep-wake rhythm disorder (N24SWD), jet lag disorder, shift work disorder (SWD), and CRSWD not otherwise specified (NOS).

Basic Information

- General criteria for CRSWD include:
  - A persistent or recurrent pattern of sleep disturbance due to either alterations of the circadian timekeeping system, or a misalignment between the endogenous circadian clock

and exogenous factors that influence the timing and duration of sleep
  - The circadian disruption leads to insomnia and or excessive sleepiness.
  - The disruption results in impairment of social, occupational, or other areas of functioning.[1]
- Most disorders of sleep-wake timing result from a complex interaction between physiology, social, environmental, and behavioral factors.
- Even though disruption of the sleep-wake cycle is often associated with insomnia and/or excessive sleepiness, CRSWD are often underrecognized clinically.
- In a clinical setting, CRSWD should be considered in the differential diagnosis of any patient presenting with insomnia and/or hypersomnia. In the following sections each of the CRSWD will be described along with their pathophysiology, epidemiology, diagnosis, and management.

The Two Process Model

- The sleep-wake cycle is regulated by a complex interaction of circadian and homeostatic processes.[2,3]
- The circadian clock is located in the suprachiasmatic nucleus (SCN) of the hypothalamus.
- The SCN acts as a central pacemaker to control the regulation of many physiologic processes including sleep-wake, blood pressure, core body temperature, melatonin, and cortisol.[4]
- Each of these physiologic functions has a temporal relationship with each other that is controlled via the SCN.
- Circadian misalignment can result in symptoms ranging from insomnia and sleepiness to gastrointestinal upset.
- SCN neurons generate and maintain a self-sustaining circadian rhythm via an autoregulatory feedback loop.
- Oscillating circadian gene products regulate their own expression through a complex system of transcription, translation, and posttranslational processes (Fig. 15.1).[5]

- The SCN produces an alerting signal that promotes wakefulness during the day (Process C).[2,3]
- This opposes the homeostatic drive for sleep that increases across the waking day (Process S).
- The combined effects of Process C and Process S are to maintain sustained wakefulness during the day, and sustained sleep at night (Fig. 15.2).
- Sleep timing and duration are also influenced by behavioral (e.g., work, family, social activities, etc.) and environmental factors (e.g., ambient light, noise, etc.).

Circadian Regulation

Light

- The light-dark cycle is an important *Zeitgeber* (German for "time giver") for regulating the timing of the circadian clock.
- Light reaches the SCN via afferent projections from the retina via the retinohypothalamic tract (Fig. 15.3).[4]

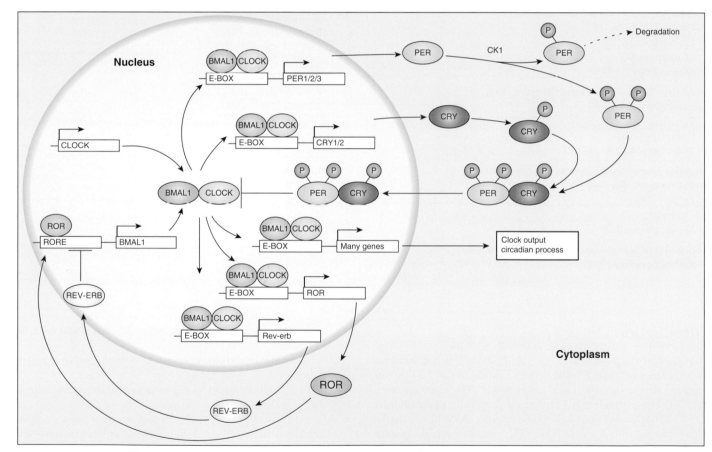

• **Figure 15.1** A Schematic of the Molecular Transcription/Translation Feedback Loop. Two genes, brain and muscle arnt-like protein 1 *(Bmal1)* and circadian locomotor output clock kaput *(CLOCK)*, are transcribed and translated. BMAL1 and CLOCK proteins then form heterodimers, which promote the transcription of Perid *(Per)* and Cryptochrome *(Cry)*. PER and CRY proteins in turn dimerize and are translocated back into the nucleus, where they inhibit transcription of *Bmal1* and *Cry*. The rate of translocation of PER/CRY heterodimers is regulated through phosphorylation by casein kinase 1 (CK1). Retinoic acid receptor-related orphan nuclear receptor (ROR) and reverse viral erythroblastic oncogene product (REV-ERB) provide additional regulation of this process through activation and repression of *Bmal1* transcription respectively. Overall each cycle takes ~24 hours to complete.

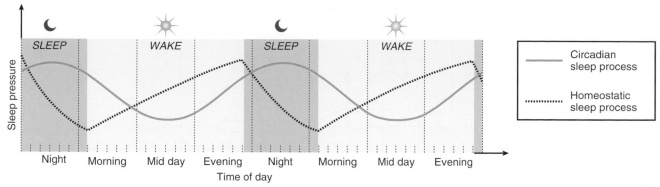

• **Figure 15.2** The Two-Process Model for Regulation of Sleep-Wake State. The homeostatic drive for sleep rises with increasing wakefulness, while the circadian system provides an alerting signal during the day, and creates a permissive state for sleep at night.

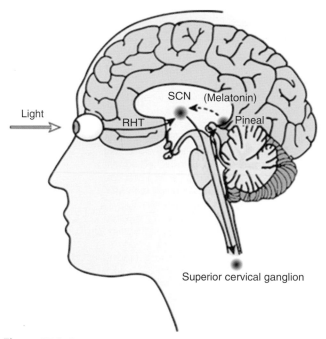

• **Figure 15.3** Schematic representation of the neural pathways for light input to the circadian system. Light information from the eyes travels to the suprachiasmatic nucleus (SCN) via the retinohypothalamic tract (RHT). The SCN then signals the pineal gland via the superior cervical ganglion to inhibit the production of melatonin. In the absence of light, this inhibition is removed. (From Reid KJ, Zee PC. Circadian rhythm disorders. *Semin Neurol.* 2009;29:393–405.)

• Timing, duration, intensity, and wavelength of light all play a role in the influence of light on the circadian clock and can be expressed as a phase response curve (PRC) to light (Fig. 15.4).[6–9]
• Bright light exposure prior to the core body temperature minimum (CBTmin; a phase marker of the circadian clock) phase delays (shifts the circadian clock later).
• Bright light exposure after the CBTmin results in a phase advance (shifts the circadian clock earlier).[6,7,10]

• Light exposure at an inappropriate circadian time can exacerbate and perpetuate circadian disruption, while exposure at the right circadian time can be used as a treatment for many CRSWD.[10,11]

Melatonin

• Melatonin is also an important modulator of circadian rhythms,[12] and can be used to phase shift the circadian clock.
• The timing of melatonin production and release is controlled by the SCN via an indirect pathway, a noradrenergic synapse from the superior cervical ganglion to the pineal gland.[13]
• Melatonin also has soporific effects, particularly when given at time when its production is low.[14,15]
• The PRC to melatonin is about 12 hours out of phase with the light PRC (see Fig. 15.4).[16]
• Melatonin (0.3–5 mg) given prior to the CBTmin will phase advance the circadian clock and melatonin administered after the CBTmin will phase delay the circadian clock.[16–19]
• Melatonin is not approved by the US Federal Drug Administration (FDA) for treatment of any disorder, and there is limited data available for the optimal dose required to treat CRSWD.

Circadian Rhythm Sleep-Wake Disorders

Delayed Sleep-Wake Phase Disorder

• DSWPD is a CRSWD characterized by a stable delay in the timing of the sleep-wake cycle of several hours compared with desired times.
• Sleep onset is typically between 1 and 6 AM, and wake time ranges from 10 AM–1 PM (Fig. 15.5).[20,21]
• Complaints include sleep onset insomnia and/or difficulty waking at the desired time.
• With work/social/school commitments, the long sleep latency and early wake time result in sleep loss, which can impact daytime functioning.
• Physiologically the circadian rhythm of other physiologic functions including CBTmin[22,23] and dim-light melatonin onset[24–26] are delayed.

HUMAN PHASE RESPONSE CURVES TO BRIGHT LIGHT AND MELATONIN

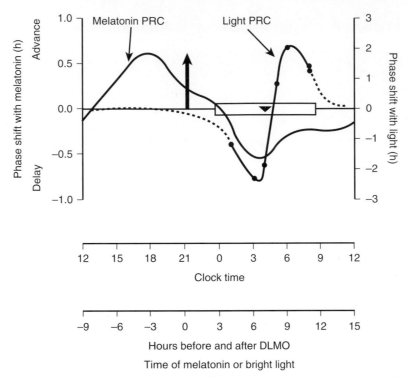

• **Figure 15.4** The light phase response curve (PRC) was generated from seven subjects who free-ran through about 3 days (73.5 hours) of an ultradian LD cycle (2.5 hours wake in dim light <100 lux alternating with 1.5 hour sleep in dark; Eastman and Burgess, unpublished data). Subjects lived on the ultradian schedule on two different occasions, once with bright light pulses, about 3500 lux, for 2 hours at the same time each day, and once without bright light pulses, counterbalanced. Phase shifts of the midpoint of the melatonin rhythm collected in dim light (<5 lux) before and after the 3 days were plotted against the time of the light pulse relative to each subject's baseline dim-light melatonin onset (DLMO) and corrected for the free run when the bright light was not applied. Upward *arrow*: average baseline DLMO, rectangle: average baseline sleep schedule, triangle: estimated time of body temperature minimum (DLMO + 7 hours). The solid line is a smoothed curve fit to the seven points. The melatonin PRC was calculated from the data of Lewy et al. (1998). Subjects (*n* = 6), living at home, took 0.5 mg melatonin at the same time each day for 4 days. Phase shifts of the DLMO were plotted against the time of melatonin administration relative to each subject's baseline DLMO. A smoothed curve was fit to the data after averaging the 70 data points into 3-hour bins. (Reprinted with permission from Revell VL, Eastman CI. How to trick mother nature into letting you fly around or stay up all night. *J Biol Rhythms.* 2005;20:353–365.)

• The prevalence of mood and personality disorders is high in DSWPD.[27–29]

Pathophysiology

• The pathophysiology of DSWPD is unknown, but there are several proposed causes.
  • A longer circadian period may make it difficult for the circadian system to make the small adjustments each day to maintain a 24-hour cycle at the desired time[30,31] and has been demonstrated in both melatonin and temperature rhythms in patients with DSWPD.[32]
  • DSWPD patients may have alterations in the response to circadian synchronizing agents such as light. In a study of melatonin suppression using 1000 lux broad spectrum light at night, those with DSWPD had greater suppression of melatonin compared with controls.[33]
  • Those with DSWPD may also have an abnormally small response to the phase advancing portion of the PRC to light.

People with an evening circadian preference have a reduced electroretinogram response to morning light.[34]
• Alternatively since those with DSWPD are going to bed and waking later than desired, the combination of more light exposure during the phase delaying portion of the light PRC (evening), and less light exposure during the phase advance portion of the light PRC (morning) may maintain or perpetuate the delay in the circadian clock and sleep. There is evidence that even relatively low levels of light (100 lux) in the late evening can impact the circadian clock.[35]
• Patterns of melatonin release differ in DSWPD, with a later dim-light melatonin onset (DLMO) and decreased melatonin surge following DLMO.[36]
• DSWPD may also have a genetic basis with an autosomal dominant mode of inheritance. There have been a number of potential genes identified, including polymorphisms in *hPer3*, Arylalkylamine N-acetyltransferase, HLA, and *CLOCK*.[37–40]

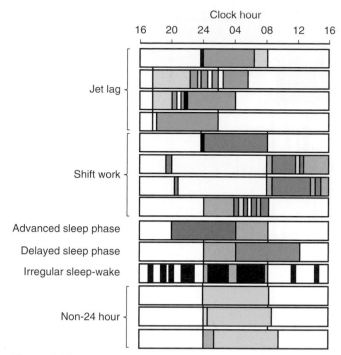

Clock hour

Jet lag

Shift work

Advanced sleep phase

Delayed sleep phase

Irregular sleep-wake

Non-24 hour

• **Figure 15.5** Schematic Representation of the Four Major Circadian Rhythm Sleep Disorders. The *black bars* indicate sleep and the white bars indicate wake; the gray bar indicates a "normal" sleep time. (Reprinted with permission from Reid KJ, Chang AM, Zee PC. Circadian rhythm sleep disorders. *Med Clin North Am.* 2004;88:631–651, viii.)

- Finally, there may be alterations in homeostatic processes. Following 24 hours of sleep deprivation, DSWPD subjects had a decreased ability to compensate for sleep loss during the subjective day and the first hours of subjective night when compared with controls.[41,42]

Epidemiology

- Prevalence ranges from 0.17%–8.9% in community-dwelling adults,[43,44] to 3%–16% in adolescents[45–47] and 5%–10% in patients treated for clinical insomnia.[21]

Diagnosis

- ICSD criteria[1] require a stable delay in sleep-wake period relative to desired sleep times, and a complaint of insomnia and excessive daytime sleepiness that impairs daily function.
- Confirmatory tests include sleep logs and/or wrist activity monitoring for at least 7 days and preferably 14 days (Fig. 15.6).
- The sleep complaint should not be better explained by any other medical, neurologic, or medication use disorder.
- Polysomnography (PSG) is only required to rule out other sleep disorders if suspected when appropriate.
- Assessment of circadian phase using DLMO or urinary 6-sulfatoxymelatonin can be useful.

Management

- For a summary of treatment options for DSWPD, see Table 15.1.
- Behavioral interventions are the first line of treatment for all CRSWD, although there is insufficient evidence that this is

effective as a standalone treatment,[48] working best in combination with other interventions (e.g., bright light or melatonin).
- Good sleep hygiene is essential, including a quiet, cool, and dark place to sleep; keeping a stable sleep/wake schedule; avoiding caffeine close to desired sleep times; and reducing alcohol consumption.
- Avoiding light in the evening and seeking light in the morning is recommended, although caution must be maintained to avoid light prior to the CBTmin (phase delay portion of the light PRC), as this may perpetuate the delay.[49]
- Chronotherapy, involving deliberate delay of the sleep-wake period by several hours each day until the desired sleep time is reached, has been met with limited success.[30] For some individuals it can be difficult to maintain the new sleep-wake time due to a natural tendency to delay or social/occupational factors that do not permit keeping a consistent schedule.[50]
- Melatonin administered in doses between 0.3 and 5 mg, between 1.5 and 6 hours prior to bedtime has been reported to improve sleep latency, phase shift the circadian clock, and improve daytime function,[51–58] and the most recent clinical practice guidelines for CRSWDs report weak evidence for the use of timed melatonin in adults and children. For treatment of DSWPD, we will typically give 0.5 mg, approximately 5 hours prior to habitual bedtime.
- Bright light exposure upon natural wake time for 1–2 hours has been shown to improve daytime alertness and reduce sleep onset.[56,59–62]
- There is insufficient evidence to support the use of bright light as monotherapy. However, in children and adolescents there is weak evidence to support the use of light in conjunction with behavioral treatments,[48] while in adults, combined therapy with light and melatonin results in an advance in sleep-wake patterns and DLMO,[63] and improved daytime sleepiness and cognitive performance (Fig. 15.7).[64]

Advanced Sleep-Wake Phase Disorder

- ASWPD is a CRSWD characterized by a stable advance in the sleep-wake period relative to desired times (see Fig. 15.5).
- Complaints include early morning wakening insomnia, sleep maintenance insomnia, and sleepiness in the late afternoon and/or early evening.
- Sleep onset is typically between 6 and 9 PM, and wake time is between 2 and 5 AM (see Fig. 15.5).
- Early evening sleepiness makes it difficult to participate in activities at this time, and sleep is often truncated, resulting in impairments in daily functioning.
- Physiologic functions including CBTmin and dim-light melatonin onset are also advanced.[65,66]

Pathophysiology

- There are several proposed mechanisms for ASWPD based on our current knowledge of circadian and sleep regulatory systems, including:
  - A shorter than normal endogenous circadian period, reported two individuals.[11,65]
  - Alterations in the response to light including a reduced ability to phase delay or a stronger than normal phase advance to light. Or simply having less light in the evening due to the early bedtime (phase delay region of the light PRC) and more light in the morning (phase advance region of the

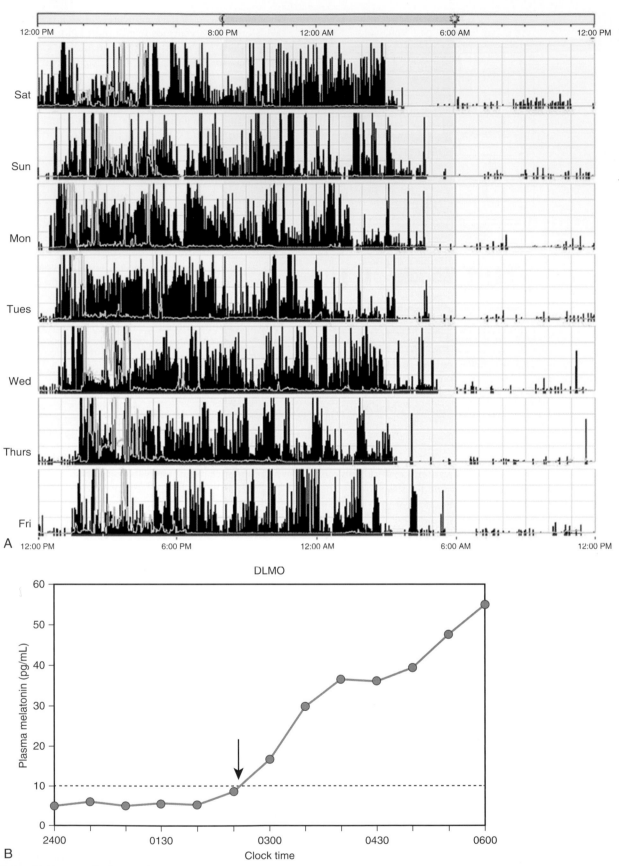

• **Figure 15.6 A,** An example of rest-activity cycle from a patient with delayed sleep phase disorder using wrist actigraphy monitoring. The *black bars* indicate activity level, and *yellow lines* indicate ambient light exposure at the nondominant wrist. This individual had a typical bedtime of 3–5 AM and wake time of 12–2 PM. **B,** An example of plasma dim-light melatonin onset (DLMO) of the same individual. In plasma, DLMO is defined as the time at which the melatonin level reaches 10 pg/mL. The DLMO typically occurs about 2 hours before sleep onset. In this individual the DLMO was at about 2:30 AM *(arrow)* and sleep time was at 4:30 AM. (From Malkani R, Zee PC. Basic circadian rhythms and circadian sleep disorders. In Chokroverty S, Thomas R, eds. *Atlas of Sleep Medicine.* 2nd ed. 2014:119–126.)

TABLE 15.1 Summary of the Possible Treatment Options for Circadian Rhythm Sleep-Wake Disorders

Circadian Rhythm Sleep-Wake Disorder	Clinical Presentation	Population	Preferred Sleep Times	Treatment Options
DSWPD	Difficulty falling asleep at night and difficulty waking up in the morning	Adolescents > Older adults	Bedtime: 2–6 AM Waketime: 10 AM–1 PM	• Good sleep hygiene • Avoid bright light in the evening prior to bed • Seek bright light in the morning (2 hours, at least 5000 lux) • Melatonin (0.5 mg) 5–7 hours prior to habitual sleep onset
ASWPD	Difficulty staying awake at night and early morning awakenings	Older adults > adolescents	Bedtime: 6–9 PM Waketime: 2–5 AM	• Good sleep hygiene • Avoid bright light in the morning • Seek bright light in the evening 7–9 PM (2 hours, at least 4000 lux)
ISWRD	≥3 sleep bouts in 24 hours, total sleep time normal for age	Institutionalized and patients with neurodegenerative disorders	Variable, lack of consolidated sleep	Older adults • Multimodal approaches using a combination of treatments • Increase exposure to circadian entraining agents such as light and activity • Good sleep hygiene and environment Children with mental retardation • Melatonin (2–20 mg) administration prior to bed
N24SWD	Progressive delay of the sleep-wake cycle resulting in daytime sleepiness and insomnia	Blind individuals	Later each day	Blind • 0.5 mg of melatonin ~9 PM (or 2 hours before bedtime) once the sleep period has drifted to desired/conventional time • Tasimelteon 20 mg prior to bedtime Sighted • Morning bright light exposure • ~3 mg of melatonin at bedtime
SWD	Insomnia and sleepiness associated with rotating shift work	Shift workers	—	• Good sleep hygiene • Avoid light on the way home (dark glasses) • Bright light exposure during the first half of the night shift • Napping prior to work or during work • Stimulants including caffeine (avoid too close to bedtime) • Wake promoting agents: modafinil and armodafinil • Melatonin (0.5–3 mg) prior to sleep during the day
Jet lag disorder	Insomnia and sleepiness associated with travel across ≥2 time zones	Travelers	—	Eastward travel (phase advance) Prior to travel • 3 days prior to travel move the sleep period 1 hour earlier each day • Bright light exposure in the morning upon waking for 1 hour • Exogenous melatonin 5 hours prior to habitual bedtime Upon arrival at destination • Avoid light in the morning (dark sunglasses or remain indoors) • Seek light in the afternoon (go outdoors, or light box) • Exogenous melatonin 5 hours prior to habitual bedtime (when at home) • Hypnotics at bedtime • Caffeine during waking hours but not too close to bedtime • Short nap (no longer than 30 min) • Good sleep hygiene Westward travel (phase delay) Prior to travel • No adaptation usually necessary, but can seek bright light in the evening 1–2 days prior to travel Upon arrival at destination • Avoid light in the early morning (dark sunglasses or remain indoors) • Seek light in the evening (outdoors, or light box) • Hypnotics at bedtime • Caffeine during wake, not too close to bedtime • Short nap (no longer than 30 min) • Good sleep hygiene

ASWPD, Advanced sleep-wake phase disorder; *DSWPD*, delayed sleep-wake phase disorder; *ISWRD*, irregular sleep-wake rhythm disorder; *N24SWD*, non-24-hour sleep-wake rhythm disorder; *SWD*, shift work disorder.

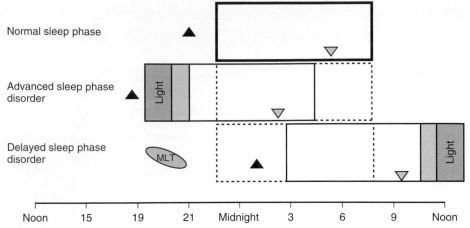

• **Figure 15.7** Schematic Representation of Treatment Strategies for Advanced Sleep Phase Disorder and Delayed Sleep Phase Disorder. In this example, the primary sleep period is indicated by the solid lines and the desired sleep phase following treatment is indicated by the *dashed line*. The estimated core body temperature rhythm minimum (CBTmin) and the dim-light melatonin onset, both common markers of circadian phase, are indicated by triangles. The CBTmin occurs ~2–3 hours prior to habitual wake time *(gray triangles)* and dim-light melatonin onset occurs ~2 hours prior to habitual sleep onset *(black triangles)*. When light is administered prior to the CBTmin, it results in a phase delay of the circadian clock (moves it later), and when light is given after the CBTmin, it results in a phase advance of the circadian clock (moves it earlier). To phase delay the sleep period of an individual with advanced sleep-wake phase disorder, bright light should be administered during the first half of the evening; in this example, light is given from 7–9 PM (indicated by the *gray box*). To phase advance the sleep period of an individual with delayed sleep-wake phase disorder (DSWPD), bright light should be administered in the morning after the estimated CBTmin; in this example, light is administered between 11:00 AM and 1:00 PM (indicated by the gray box). The current examples try to minimize the amount of sleep lost to maximize the phase shifting effects of the light. Melatonin (MLT) given in the evening is also used to phase advance circadian rhythms in DSWPD. Melatonin administered relative to the dim-light melatonin onset has shown the most consistent phase advances in DSWPD, and administration 5 hours prior to dim-light melatonin onset or 7 hours prior to habitual sleep onset gives consistent phase advances. In this example, melatonin would be administered at 8:00 PM. (Reprinted with permission from Reid KJ, Zee PC. Circadian rhythm disorders. *Semin Neurol.* 2009;29:393–405.)

light PRC) due to the early morning awakening may exacerbate and perpetuate the disorder.
• In older adults, altered exposure to entraining agents such as light and physical activity[67–69] may result in a phase advance.
• Several familial cases of ASWPD have been reported with an autosomal dominant mode of inheritance.[65,66,70] There have also been links to circadian clock gene polymorphisms associated with ASWPD, including a phosphorylation site mutation in the circadian clock gene in *hPer2*[71] and in another family, a CKI-Δ mutation.[72]

Epidemiology

• The prevalence of ASWPD in the general population is unknown, but it is believed to be quite low, around 1% in middle aged adults, and more common in older adults.[43,73]

Diagnosis

• ASWPD is diagnosed by detailed history, with the ICSD criteria[1] requiring the following:
  • A stable advance in sleep-wake period relative to desired sleep times
  • A complaint of difficulty sleeping as long as desired and excessive sleepiness in the evening that impairs daily function

• Diagnosis is confirmed with at least 7 days but preferably 14 days of sleep log and/or wrist activity monitoring.
• Additional confirmation of the advance of the circadian clock with circadian phase markers such as the DLMO or CBTmin can be useful.
• The sleep complaint should not be better explained by any other medical, neurologic, or medication use disorder.
• Fig. 15.8 depicts an actogram of rest-activity, recorded using wrist activity monitoring, from an individual with ASPS.

Management

• There is limited data available on the treatment of ASWPD. For a summary of treatment options for ASWPD, see Table 15.1.
• The practice parameters as outlined by the American Academy of Sleep Medicine recommend appropriately timed bright light as a treatment option for ASWPD.[48]
  • Studies of early morning awakening insomniacs have successfully used bright light (2500 lux) exposure in the evening between 8 PM and 12 AM to phase delay the circadian clock and improve sleep duration.[74,75]
  • In sleep maintenance insomniacs bright light exposure (>4000 lux) from 9–11 PM did not improve sleep,[76] but an earlier study by the same group reported a similar protocol with

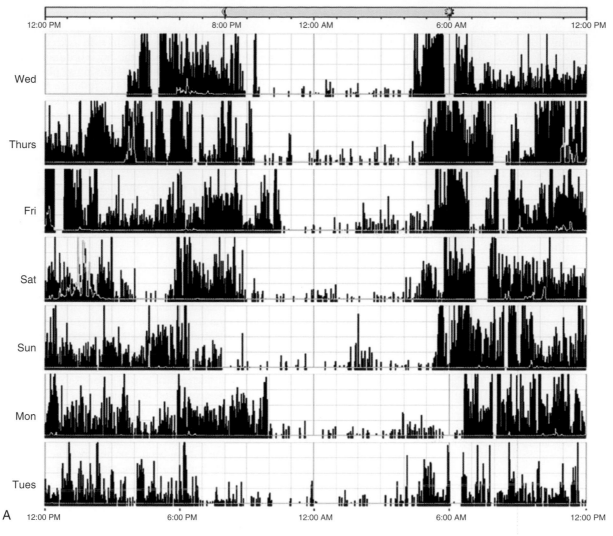

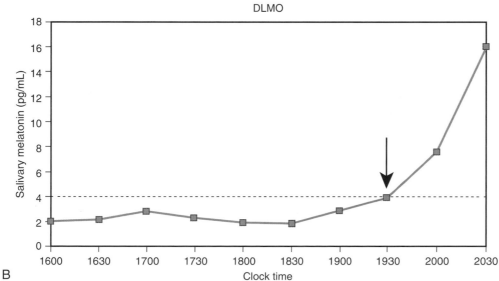

• **Figure 15.8 A,** An example of rest-activity cycle from a patient with advanced sleep phase disorder using wrist actigraphy monitoring. The *black bars* indicate activity level, and *yellow lines* indicate ambient light exposure at the nondominant wrist. This individual had a typical bedtime of 9 PM and wake time of 4 AM. **B,** An example of salivary dim-light melatonin onset (DLMO). In saliva the DLMO time is determined when the melatonin level reaches 3–4 pg/mL, which corresponds to a plasma melatonin level of 10 pg/mL. In this case the DLMO is at approximately 7 PM *(arrow)*, which corresponds to a circadian sleep onset of 9 PM. (From Malkani R, Zee PC. Basic circadian rhythms and circadian sleep disorders. In Chokroverty S, Thomas R, eds. *Atlas of Sleep Medicine.* 2nd ed. 2014:119–126.)

improvement in sleep duration, sleep efficiency, and wake after sleep onset (see Fig. 15.7).[77]

- Timed melatonin on awakening could theoretically provide treatment benefit by delaying the circadian clock; however there are no published studies in ASWPD as to the effectiveness of this therapy.[78]

Irregular Sleep-Wake Rhythm Disorder

- ISWRD is a CRSWD that is characterized by a lack of a single distinct sleep period; rather there are three or more sleep episodes in a 24-hour period (see Fig. 15.5).
- Sleep episodes vary in length, and napping may be common. The total sleep duration during the 24-hour period is typically normal for the patient's age.[1]
- This disorder is often seen in neurodegenerative disorders, including institutionalized elderly and persons with dementia, and in children with neurodevelopmental disorders.[79]

Pathophysiology

- ISWRD is thought to be the result of impairments either in the circadian clock itself[80,81] or to alterations in the exposure to circadian Zeitgebers such as light and physical and social activity,[82–84] often encountered in institutionalized care.

Epidemiology

- The prevalence of ISWRD is unknown; however, it is believed to be rare.

Diagnosis

- ISWRD is diagnosed by detailed history. The ICSD criteria[1] require a chronic complaint of insomnia and or excessive sleepiness present for at least 3 months.
- The disruption to the sleep-wake period should be confirmed with at least 7 days and preferably 14 days of sleep logs and/or wrist activity monitoring, demonstrating several (≥3) sleep periods during the 24-hour day.
- The sleep complaint should not be better explained by any other medical, neurologic, or medication use disorder. Poor sleep hygiene and voluntary irregular sleep schedule should be ruled out.

Management

- The treatment of ISWRD is aimed at consolidating the sleep period. Due to cognitive and physical limitations in the population, the effectiveness of many of these treatments is often variable and difficult to maintain for long periods of time. For a summary of treatment options for ISWRD, see Table 15.1.
- Increasing the exposure to circadian timing agents such bright light and physical activity has been successful in consolidating the sleep-wake cycle.
- In the elderly, bright light therapy (typically 2 hours in the morning) is recommended in the practice parameters created by the American Academy of Sleep Medicine.[48]
- In children/adolescents with neurologic disorders, melatonin (2–10 mg) 1 hour prior to bedtime can improve sleep[85–87]; however, using melatonin alone in elderly patients with dementia may be harmful and should be avoided.[48]

- Combination therapy may be effective, including bright light exposure (≥2500 lux in the morning), exogenous melatonin (5 mg), behavioral interventions such as keeping nursing home residents out of bed during the day, a bedtime routine, reducing light and noise at night, and structured physical activity,[88–92] although recent recommendations from the American Academy of Sleep Medicine advise against the use of combination therapy that includes melatonin in elderly demented patients.[48]
- Fig. 15.9A depicts an actogram of rest activity, recorded using wrist activity monitoring, from an individual with ISWRD.
- Fig. 15.9B illustrates a sleep log from a patient with ISWRD.

Non-24-Hour Sleep-Wake Rhythm Disorder

- N24SWD is a CRSWD characterized by a daily delay in the sleep-wake period by about 1–2 hours per day (see Fig. 15.5).

Pathophysiology

- N24SWD is believed to be the result of a lack of photic entrainment, decreased sensitivity of the circadian clock to light, or an alteration in entrainment pathways that result in weakened or lack of entrainment of the endogenous circadian clock.[93]
- For many blind people the most likely cause of N24SWD is a lack of photic entrainment. However, there are some blind people whose circadian clock responds to photic input despite no visual perception of light,[94] as well as others who most likely entrain to nonphotic inputs such as social or work schedules.
- Sighted individuals can also develop N24SWD, but the cause is unclear.
  - A few cases have been reported after head injury, and it is assumed that the injury resulted in some sort of damage to the circadian entrainment pathways.[95,96]
  - In the other cases, a longer than normal endogenous circadian period that is beyond the range of entrainment to the 24-hour day is believed to be the cause.[97]
  - It has also been suggested that N24SWD is a severe form of DSWPD, since some patients with DSWPD have developed N24SWD following treatment with chronotherapy.[98]

Epidemiology

- The prevalence of N24SWD in the general population is unknown, but it does tend to be more common in blind individuals. Estimates are that up to 50% of totally blind individuals have N24SWD[99] and that 70% of blind individuals report sleep complaints.[100,101]
- The disorder has also been reported in sighted individuals[93,102–104] and following head injury.[95,96]

Diagnosis

- N24SWD is diagnosed by a detailed history. The ICSD-3[1] criteria require a complaint of insomnia or excessive sleepiness related to attempting to sleep at an inappropriate circadian time.
- The daily drift (usually a delay of 1–2 hours) in the sleep-wake period should be confirmed with at least 14 days of sleep logs and/or wrist activity monitoring (Fig. 15.10).
- The sleep complaint should not be better explained by any other medical, neurologic, or medication use disorder.

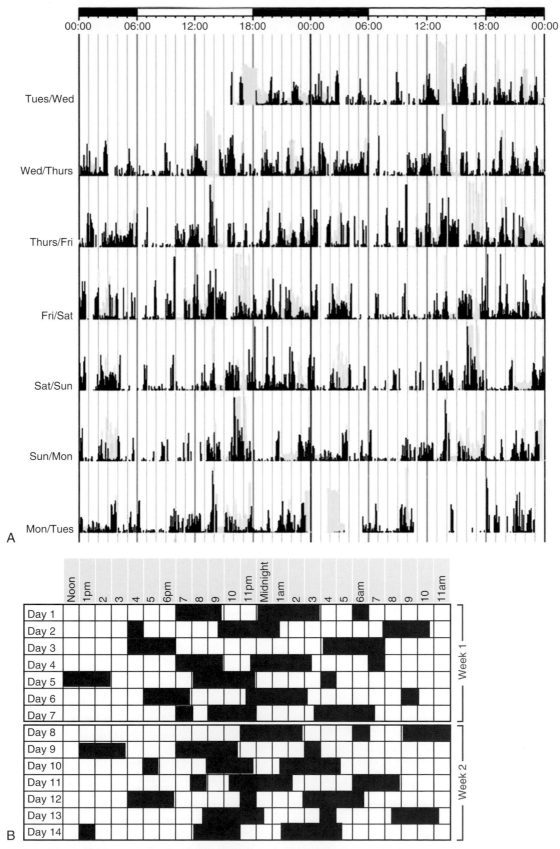

• **Figure 15.9 A,** Rest-activity recorded with wrist actigraphy monitoring of an older adult with irregular sleep-wake disorder. The *black bars* indicate activity levels, and the *yellow bars* indicate the level of ambient light exposure recorded at the nondominant wrist. There is a lack of discernible circadian sleep-wake rhythm. Sleep is characterized by nocturnal fragmentation and multiple short periods of sleep and wake across the entire 24-hour day. **B,** Example sleep log data from an individual with irregular sleep-wake type. Each line represents 24 hours, with block boxes indicating the sleep period. Note that the individual has multiple sleep bouts throughout the 24-hour period, but total sleep time is within normal limits. (**A,** From Malkani R, Zee PC. Basic circadian rhythms and circadian sleep disorders. In Chokroverty S, Thomas R, eds. *Atlas of Sleep Medicine.* 2nd ed. 2014:119–126; **B,** From Abbott SM, Reid KJ, Zee PC. Circadian rhythm sleep-wake disorders. *Psychiatr Clin North Am.* 2015;38[4]:805–823.)

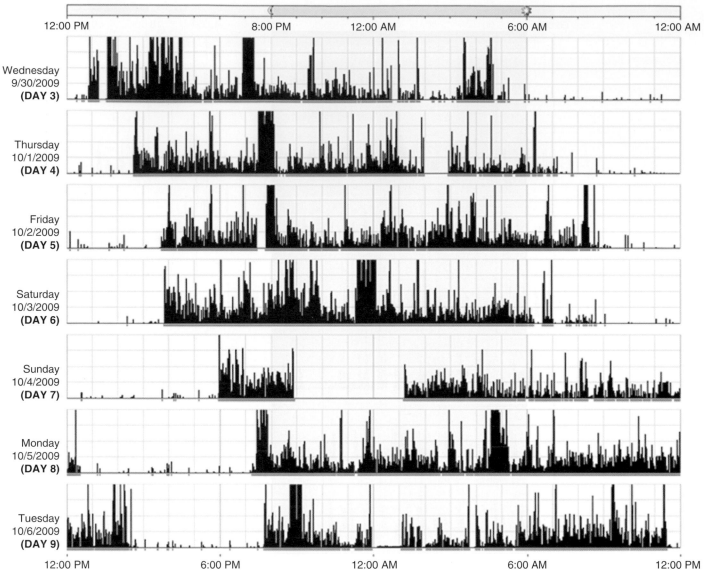

• **Figure 15.10** An actogram of rest-activity, recorded using wrist activity monitoring, from an individual with free running disorder (non-24-hour sleep-wake rhythm disorder). This individual has a progressively delaying sleep period. On day 3 they go to bed at approximately 5 AM, on day 4 at 7 AM, and on day 5 at 8 AM, and wake up between 1:00 and 3:00 PM on these days.

Management

- Treatment of N24SWD is dependent on whether the patient has circadian light perception or not.
- Melatonin is recommended for blind individuals according to the practice parameters outlined by the American Academy of Sleep Medicine,[48] while the evidence is less strong for the use of melatonin and/or bright light therapy in sighted patients with N24SWD. For a summary of treatment options for N24SWD, see Table 15.1.
- In general, for blind and sighted patients, exogenous melatonin administration of between 0.5 and 10 mg has been successful in entraining the circadian clock.
  - Typically treatment with melatonin is started when the sleep period has drifted to the desired or conventional times. Melatonin as low as 0.5 mg about 1–2 hours prior to desired sleep time has been shown to entrain rhythms and also to then maintain entrainment with continue daily use.[8,105–112]

- More recently tasimelteon, a melatonin agonist, has been approved for the treatment of blind individuals with N24SWD.[113]
- For sighted patients or blind individuals with circadian light perception, bright light (2 hours at 2500 lux upon waking) is also an option for treatment.[48,114]

Shift Work Disorder

- SWD is a CRSWD characterized by excessive sleepiness and/or insomnia associated with a work schedule that occurs primarily during the sleep period.
- Insomnia results from sleeping when the circadian alerting signal is high, while excessive sleepiness results from a combination of both sleep loss and being awake when the circadian alerting signal is low.
- Night work and early morning start times (before 6 AM) are associated with the greatest impairment in sleep, with between

1 and 4 hours less sleep reported in shift workers compared with day workers.[115–117]

Pathophysiology

- SWD results from a misalignment between the sleep-wake period and the circadian clock due to the work schedule.
- Not all shift workers experience the CRSWD SWD, even though they may experience many of the symptoms at some point in their shift working life. Factors influencing the ability to cope with shift work include:
  - Age[118]
  - Domestic responsibilities[119]
  - Commute times
  - Diurnal preference
  - Presence of comorbid sleep disorders
- The symptoms of SWD can persist into days off, since most shift workers revert back to a "normal" sleep-wake schedule at this time in order to participate in social and family responsibilities.
  - Those with SWD may experience insomnia due to sleeping at a circadian time when they would normally be awake, and the circadian alerting signal is high, even though they may have accumulated a significant homeostatic sleep load.
  - Symptoms may also vary depending on how many consecutive shifts are worked. As the circadian clock adjusts to the new schedule, some symptoms may lessen, although the sleep loss experienced earlier in the work cycle may mean that the worker still experiences excessive sleepiness when awake.

Epidemiology

- Data from the United States estimates that 1% of the general population and up to 10% of night and rotating shift workers have the CRSWD SWD.[120]
- Since it is estimated that about 20% of the workforce in industrialized countries is used in some kind of shift work, then the overall prevalence could be quite high.[121]

Diagnosis

- SWD is diagnosed by detailed history.
- ICSD criteria[1] require a complaint of insomnia or excessive sleepiness associated with a work schedule occurring during the normal sleep time for at least 1 month.
- A sleep log and/or actigraphy monitoring for at least 7 days should be used to confirm the misalignment between the sleep period and normal circadian timing. The sleep complaint should not be better explained by any other medical, neurologic, or medication use disorder.

Management

- There are two basic strategies for the treatment of SWD:
  - Realigning the endogenous circadian clock with the sleep-wake cycle, and/or
  - Treating the symptoms (i.e., insomnia and excessive sleepiness)
- For a summary of treatment options for SWD, see Table 15.1.
- Treatment needs to be tailored to each person:
  - For example, a patient may be a permanent night worker, but they may work as few as 1 or 14 or more consecutive

nights in a row. Since the circadian clock will only phase shift about an hour a day, if the shift worker is only working, say, 2 consecutive nights before a day off, or rotating to another schedule then realigning, the circadian clock is not very feasible, and treating the symptoms of insomnia (hypnotics) and or sleepiness (caffeine, bright light, naps, modafinil, or armodafinol) may be preferred.[122,123]

- In contrast, if the person works 5 consecutive night shifts, then using bright light and/or melatonin may be a more practical solution to aid in realigning the circadian clock with the sleep-wake cycle.
- The practice parameters outlined by the American Academy of Sleep Medicine for the treatment of SWD indicate that timed light exposure, melatonin administration, hypnotics, and alerting agents are guidelines, and that caffeine is an option.[124]
- In general, treatment involves the realignment of the endogenous circadian clock with the sleep-wake cycle in combination with good sleep hygiene.
  - Bright light exposure during the first half of the work period and avoiding bright light in the morning on the way home after a night shift will aid the circadian clock in adjusting to the new schedule.
  - Napping either before or during work to combat sleepiness can be useful.[125–127]
  - Caffeine taken during the work period may also help, but not for the last few hours of the shift, since it may interfere with later sleep.[128–131]
  - Modafinil and armodafinil are both approved for the treatment of excessive sleepiness associated with SWD.[122,123]
    - Modafinil (200 mg) and armodafinil (150 mg) taken 30–60 prior to each night shift significantly reduced nighttime sleepiness, although for modafinil the levels of sleepiness were still quite high.[122,123]
    - Armodafinil was also associated with significant improvements in measures of clinical condition, long-term memory, and attention compared with placebo.[123]
  - When at home make sure the sleep environment is conducive to sleep. This may require blackout blinds on the windows and instructing friends and family not to make noise or call during the sleep period.
  - Melatonin administration to phase shift the circadian clock has not been as successful as avoiding bright light in the morning, or using bright light during the night shift. However, there are a few studies both simulated and in shift workers that indicate that melatonin (1.8–6 mg) taken prior to sleep results in improved daytime sleep durations.[132–135]
- For the permanent night worker, an experimental paradigm aimed at achieving a compromise phase position has shown some promise as a way to manage or minimize the symptoms of SWD, both during work and on days off.
  - In a simulated shift work study, participants underwent 2 consecutive night shifts followed by 2 days off and then another 4 night shifts.[136–138]
  - During the night shift the experimental group was exposed to intermittent bright light in 15 min sessions (for 75 or 120 min). They wore dark sunglasses when outside and slept in a dark bedroom at scheduled times after night shifts and on days off. (Sleep was scheduled from 08:30 to 15:30 [7 hours] after the first 2 night shifts, from 08:30 to 13:30 [5 hours] after the third night shifts, from 03:00 to 12:00 [9 hours] on the 2 weekend days off, and again from 08:30

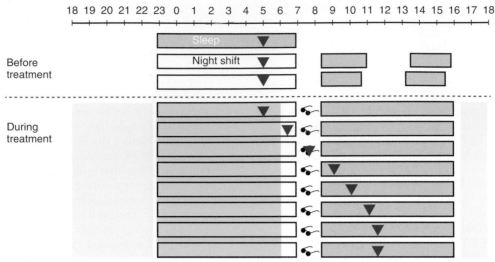

• **Figure 15.11** Schematic representation of a strategy using timed light exposure and avoidance to attain circadian realignment in shift work disorder. The *triangles* represent the core body temperature (CBT) nadir. *Dark shaded boxes* represent the sleep period; *empty boxes* represent work during the night shift. Before treatment, night shift workers work when the circadian alerting signals are low, resulting in excessive sleepiness during the shift; they sleep during the day when circadian alerting signals are high and have disturbed and shortened sleep during the day. Treatment is aimed at realignment of the circadian rhythm. During treatment, bright light therapy *(dark yellow)* during the night shift can delay the circadian phase and improve alertness. Bright light therapy should be stopped 1–2 hours before the end of the night shift. In the morning before sleep, such as during the commute home, light should be avoided *(sunglasses)* to prevent phase advance. When home and sleeping, the sleep environment should be kept dark. The CBT nadir will gradually shift to the daytime, which will improve daytime sleep. Upon awakening, individuals may be exposed to regular light (e.g., sunlight or ambient light, *light yellow*), which may help to prevent overshooting the intended phase delay. (From Malkani R, Zee PC. Basic circadian rhythms and circadian sleep disorders. In Chokroverty S, Thomas R, eds. *Atlas of Sleep Medicine.* 2nd ed. 2014:119–126.)

to 15:30 after the final 4 night shifts.) They received outdoor light exposure upon awakening from sleep.
- The control group remained in dim room light during night shifts, wore lighter sunglasses, and had unrestricted sleep and outdoor light exposure.
- This complicated regime resulted in an average phase shift of the circadian clock to a position that was a compromise for work days and days off (4:30 AM).
- The participants in the experimental condition were able to sleep most of the time allotted for sleep both after night shifts and on days off, and they performed better than control subjects during the simulated night shifts.[136]
- A schematic highlighting the strategy using timed light exposure and avoidance to attain circadian realignment in SWD is illustrated in Fig. 15.11.
- Fig. 15.12 summarizes treatment options for the management of SWD utilizing melatonin, light exposure/avoidance, and wake promoting agents.

Jet Lag Disorder

- Jet lag disorder is a CRSWD as a result of circadian misalignment between the internal circadian clock and the external environment following transmeridian travel over at least two time zones.[1]

Pathophysiology

- Jet lag disorder results from the mismatch between the endogenous circadian clock and the external environment due to transmeridian travel over at least two time zones.[1]
- Not all travelers experience jet lag disorder. Factors that may influence jet lag disorder are age, number of time zones crossed, and circadian preference.

Epidemiology

- The prevalence of jet lag disorder is unknown; however, one study of 500 travelers reported a high prevalence of symptoms, including disturbed sleep (78%), daytime fatigue (49%), impaired mental performance (26%), gastrointestinal complaints (24%), and irritability (18%).[139]
- Given the prevalence of these complaints and high prevalence of jet travel (over 30 million international travelers crossing three or more times zones departing the United States in 2009[140]), the occurrence of jet lag disorder is suspected to be high.

Diagnosis

- Jet lag disorder is diagnosed by detailed history and physical examination.

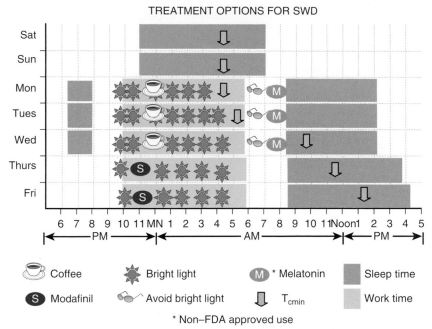

TREATMENT OPTIONS FOR SWD

	Coffee		Bright light		* Melatonin		Sleep time
S	Modafinil		Avoid bright light		T$_{cmin}$		Work time

* Non–FDA approved use

• Figure 15.12 Treatment Options for the Management of Shift Work Disorder. This example illustrates the timing of light exposure and the use of pharmacologic agents, either alone or in combination, for the management of shift work disorder (SWD). The habitual preshift sleep time of this 42-year-old man is 11 PM–7 AM. The new work shift requires that he work from 10 PM–6 AM for 4–5 days per week. Circadian alignment can be achieved by manipulating light and dark exposure. To delay his circadian rhythm, bright-light exposure (continuous or intermittent) should start early in the shift and stop about 1–2 hours before the shift ends, with sunglasses worn to avoid advancing circadian rhythms in the morning. If needed, melatonin taken before bedtime may help improve sleep quality. To address the issue of excessive sleepiness, a scheduled 1- to 2-hour nap before the shift work, if possible a short 30-min nap in the middle of the shift, and/or caffeine can help decrease sleepiness at work. If sleepiness persists, modafinil, 200 mg, and armodafinil, 150 mg, have been shown to improve alertness during work and are approved by the US Federal Drug Administration (FDA) for the treatment of excessive sleepiness in patients with SWD. (From Zhu L, Zee PC. Circadian rhythm sleep disorders. *Neurol Clin.* 2012;30[4]:1167–1191.)

- The ICSD-3 criteria[1] requires a complaint of insomnia and/or excessive sleepiness after transmeridian travel across at least two time zones.
- These complaints are associated with impaired daytime function, and the sleep disturbance or other symptoms should not be better explained by any other medical, neurologic, or medication use disorder.
- Other causes for some of the symptoms of jet lag disorder should be ruled out—for example, gastrointestinal upset may be the result of a preexisting condition.
- PSG is not required unless another sleep disorder such as sleep apnea is suspected. If the complaints continue for more than 2 weeks following travel, psychophysiologic insomnia may be the cause, particularly if poor sleep habits are present.

Management

- There are two basic strategies for the treatment of jet lag disorder:
  - Realigning the circadian clock to the new time zone as quickly as possible
  - Treating the symptoms
- Timed melatonin administration is a "standard" treatment, and timed and dosed bright light is a treatment "option" for jet lag

disorder according to the practice parameters laid out by the American Academy of Sleep Medicine.[124]
- For a summary of treatment options for jet lag disorder, see Table 15.1.
- Realigning the circadian clock to the new time zone can be started prior to travel or upon arrival at the new destination, with the timing of these interventions dependent on the direction of travel.
- Symptoms of jet lag tend to be worse following eastward travel compared with westward travel,[141] because eastward travel requires a phase advance of the circadian clock and westward travel requires a phase delay.
  - It is usually easier to phase delay the circadian clock than it is to phase advance, since the circadian period of humans tends to be slightly longer than 24 hours.[142]

Eastward Travel

- When traveling east, people usually experience difficulty initiating and maintaining sleep because they are attempting to sleep at a time when the circadian alerting signal is high. They are also likely to still be sleepy when they wake up, because the circadian alerting signal will be low at this time.
- When travelling east, phase advancing the circadian clock prior to travel by approximately 2.5 hours requires shifting the sleep

period by 1 hour earlier each day starting 3 days prior to departure, in combination with melatonin administration (0.5 mg or 3 mg) 5 hours prior to habitual bedtime along with morning bright light (four 30 min pulses of 5000 lux).[143]
  - A similar protocol without the addition of melatonin resulted in about a 2-hour phase advance.[144]
- When at the new destination, it is recommended to avoid light (by wearing dark sunglasses or remaining indoors) during the morning to avoid inducing phase delays.
- It is also recommended to seek light exposure (by going outside or using a light box) in the afternoon in order to further phase advance the circadian clock.[145,146]
- Melatonin could be taken prior to bedtime to aid with the phase advance,[147] but again if light exposure occurs at the wrong time, exogenous melatonin administration will not be as successful.[148]
- Melatonin agonists tasimelteon (10–100 mg) and ramelteon (1–8 mg) have also been studied as a treatment for phase advancing the circadian clock following a 5-hour phase advance either due to real[149] or simulated[150] travel.
- Ramelteon 1 mg taken just prior to bedtime (~5 min) improved latency to persistent sleep at the 1 mg dose on night 2-to-4 after travel,[149] while tasimelteon 30 min prior to bedtime increased sleep efficiency and total sleep time and decreased latency to persistent sleep.[150]
- These treatment options remain investigational, and at the time of writing this manuscript are not approved by the FDA.

Westward Travel

- When travelling west, people may experience sleepiness prior to bedtime, which may make falling asleep easier, but they may have difficulty maintaining sleep for as long as desired since the internal circadian alerting signal will be rising during the sleep period.
- In general, since it is easier to travel west, preflight adjustment may not be necessary. However, if desired, 2 hours of bright light exposure (~4000 lux) prior to bed and a 4-hour delay of bedtime will phase delay the circadian clock by about 1.5 hours.[151]
  - If a similar protocol is followed for several days with a 2-hour (rather than 4 hours) delay of the sleep period, along with a bright light pulse of ~5000 lux, there may be up to a 4.4-hour delay.[152]
- Upon arrival in the new destination, avoid light in the early morning and get as much light as possible in the evening for the first few days.[146]
- Some studies suggest that melatonin administration (5 mg) may be useful, at least subjectively, for treating the symptoms of jet lag following westward travel.[153,154]
  - In these two studies 5 mg of melatonin was taken prior to departure (~10 AM–12 PM) and upon arrival in the new destination (~10 PM–12 AM).
- Fig. 15.13 summarizes innovative strategies to accelerate circadian adaption to jet lag when traveling eastward and westward.

Other Circadian Rhythm Sleep-Wake Disorders

- There are also CRSWD that are either due to medical, neurologic, or psychiatric disorders, or NOS. There is less information about these disorders compared with the other CRSWD.[1]

Pathophysiology

- Several medical and neurologic conditions are associated with disruption of circadian rhythms, including dementia, movement disorders (such as Parkinson's), blindness, and hepatic encephalopathy.
- The type of circadian rhythm sleep disturbance reported in dementia (see ISWRD and blindness) and blindness (see N24SWD) has been mentioned in other sections of this chapter.
- For those with Parkinson's disease, there are various types of circadian disruption and sleep disturbance.[155–157]
- Hepatic encephalopathy can be associated with a delayed sleep phase.[158]

Epidemiology

- The specific prevalence of these disorders is unknown; however, it is dependent on the prevalence of the underlying medical disorder involved.

Diagnosis

- The CRSWD NOS is diagnosed by a detailed history.
- ICSD criteria[1] require a complaint of insomnia, excessive sleepiness related to alterations in the circadian timing system, or misalignment between the endogenous circadian clock and exogenous factors that influence the timing of sleep.
- Sleep log and/or actigraphy for at least 7 days and preferably 14 days confirms a disturbed or low amplitude circadian rhythm.
- The sleep complaint should not be better explained by any other sleep, mental, medication, or substance use disorder and does not meet criteria for any other CRSWD classified in the ICSD.

Management

- Treatment of these disorders is dependent on the cause, but there is no specific data available for the treatment of any of these disorders.

Conclusions

- As the field gains a greater knowledge about the regulation of sleep and the circadian system, the understanding of the pathophysiology and treatment options for circadian rhythm sleep disorders improves.
- There is still a lack of well-designed placebo-controlled clinical trials for many of the treatments currently available, even for the most common circadian rhythm sleep disorders.
  - For example, there is not a clear understanding of the dose of melatonin to be used for phase shifting sleep-wake in the various disorders.
  - Furthermore, while melatonin is widely used, it is not approved by the FDA for any use. There are limited studies of melatonin agonist drugs, and as yet none are FDA approved for CRSWD.
  - It is similar to studies using bright light treatment that report various durations, wavelength, and intensity of light.
  - Combination therapies appear in a few preliminary studies to be successful for treating some CRSWD, but again there is limited data available to determine the best dose or combinations.

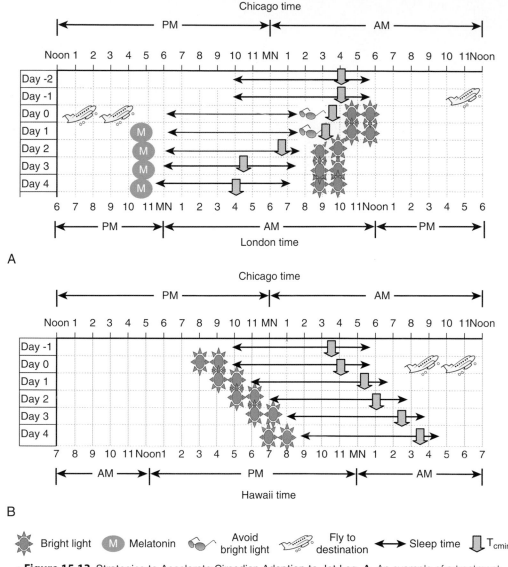

Chicago time

London time

A

Chicago time

Hawaii time

B

☀ Bright light Ⓜ Melatonin 👓 Avoid bright light ✈ Fly to destination ↔ Sleep time ⬇ T$_{cmin}$

• **Figure 15.13** Strategies to Accelerate Circadian Adaption to Jet Lag. **A,** An example of a treatment strategy for jet lag associated with an eastward flight over six time zones (from Chicago to London). Adjustment requires an equal number of hours of phase advance. On arrival, the traveler should avoid bright light in the early-morning hours (before 9 AM) for the first 2 days so that light does not decrease before nadir of the core body temperature (which will induce a phase delay), and exposure to bright light after 9 AM to induce phase advances. In addition, melatonin, 1–5 mg taken at 18:00 local time on the departure day and at local bedtime (22:00–23:00) on arrival for 4 days has been shown to be effective. **B,** Treatment strategy for jet lag associated with a westward flight over five time zones (from Chicago to Hawaii). The subject should be exposed to as much as light as possible in the late afternoon and early evening at the destination, which will result in the required phase delay. (**A,** From Morgenthaler TI, Lee-Chiong T, Alessi C, et al. Practice parameters for the clinical evaluation and treatment of circadian rhythm sleep disorders. An American Academy of Sleep Medicine report. *Sleep.* 2007;30:1445–1459; **B,** From Zhu L, Zee PC. Circadian rhythm sleep disorders. *Neurol Clin.* 2012;30[4]:1167–1191.)

• Therefore, in summary, there is still much to discover about the prevalence, pathophysiology, and management of the CRSWD.

Suggested Reading

American Academy of Sleep Medicine. *The International Classification of Sleep Disorders: Diagnostic and Coding Manual.* 3rd ed. Westchester, IL.: American Academy of Sleep Medicine; 2014.

Auger RR, Burgess HJ, Emens JS, et al. Clinical practice guideline for the treatment of intrinsic circadian rhythm sleep-wake disorders:

advanced sleep-wake phase disorder (ASWPD), delayed sleep-wake phase disorder (DSWPD), non-24-hour sleep-wake rhythm disorder (N24SWD), and irregular sleep-wake rhythm disorder (ISWRD). An update for 2015: an American Academy of Sleep Medicine Clinical Practice Guideline. *J Clin Sleep Med.* 2015;11:1199-1236.

Burgess HJ, Revell VL, Eastman CI. A three pulse phase response curve to three milligrams of melatonin in humans. *J Physiol.* 2008;586:639-647.

Dunlap JC. Molecular bases for circadian clocks. *Cell.* 1999;96:271-290.

Khalsa SB, Jewett ME, Cajochen C, Czeisler CA. A phase response curve to single bright light pulses in human subjects. *J Physiol.* 2003;549:945-952.

16

Diagnosis and Treatment of Parasomnias

SHELBY F. HARRIS, MICHAEL J. THORPY

Introduction

- **Definition**:
  - The parasomnias include some of the most fascinating and heterogeneous of all sleep disorders and are undesirable physical events or experiences that occur at entry into sleep, during sleep, or during arousals from sleep.[1,2]
  - They are characterized by abnormal behavioral or physiologic events that accompany particular sleep stages or transitions associated with activation of the central nervous system, changes in the autonomic nervous system, and increases in skeletal muscle activity.
  - Parasomnias often involve complex, seemingly purposeful, goal-directed behavior that is outside the awareness of the individual. Therefore they are automatisms, which are a nonreflex act without conscious volition.
- **Etiology and pathophysiology**: The cause of most parasomnias is unknown; however, psychopathology can influence some disorders such as nightmares, and neurologic disorders can be associated with others such as rapid eye movement (REM) sleep behavior disorder (RBD). It is suspected that underlying genetic mechanisms affect the pathophysiology of some parasomnias, since they often tend to run in families.[3]
- **Consequences**: Many parasomnias are benign, especially when they occur in childhood. However, the consequences of chronic parasomnias may include disruption of sleep, poor health, increased stress, and physical harm. Some can be associated with violence to a bed partner, whereas others, such as sleep terrors or sleepwalking, can lead to injury from leaving the bed.
- **Management**: Management involves pharmacologic, psychologic, and behavioral interventions. Because no large-scale controlled trials have been conducted, in general, treatment is guided by small clinical trials and anecdotal evidence. This chapter presents an overview of parasomnias, as well as the current pharmacologic and behavioral treatments.

Clinical Diagnosis and Evaluation

- The clinical evaluation of parasomnias requires a complete clinical history from the patient and family.
- Overnight polysomnography (PSG) may be required to accurately establish the diagnosis, particularly when the behavior is violent or extreme, and a detailed montage is often required to rule

TABLE 16.1 Listing of Parasomnias[2]

Disorders of Arousal (From NREM Sleep)

Confusional arousals
Sleepwalking
Sleep terrors
Sleep-related eating disorder

REM-Related Parasomnias

REM sleep behavior disorder
Recurrent isolated sleep paralysis
Nightmare disorder

Other Parasomnias

Exploding head syndrome
Sleep enuresis
Parasomnia due to a medical disorder
Parasomnia due to a medication or substance
Parasomnia, unspecified

Isolated Symptoms and Normal Variants

Sleep talking

NREM, Nonrapid eye movement; *REM*, rapid eye movement.

out alternative diagnoses, such as nocturnal seizures, obstructive sleep apnea syndrome, and others.

- Sleep deprivation and forced arousals during slow wave sleep (SWS) have been shown to induce a sleepwalking episode in predisposed adults.[4] Performance of this procedure during video-PSG can help establish the diagnosis. Neuroimaging is not usually helpful in the evaluation of parasomnias, unless the patient has RBD or a neurologic basis for the parasomnia is suspected.
- Parasomnias are categorized by the sleep stage in which they occur. REM sleep, nonrapid eye movement (NREM) sleep, as well as the category "other parasomnias."
- Table 16.1 presents a list of the parasomnias as defined by the International Classification of Sleep Disorders-3.

Disorders of Arousal

- Disorders of arousal are arousals that occur during NREM sleep, most often sleep stage N3 (SWS).
- The majority of NREM SWS occurs in the first third of the night, and disorders of arousal are most commonly seen in the beginning of the nocturnal sleep period.
  - Such disorders include confusional arousals, sleepwalking, and sleep terrors.
  - Dreaming is often absent during these episodes, although the patient may occasionally report vague and fragmented dreams.
- Arousal disorders are believed to be a continuum of behaviors involving the re-establishment of full alertness, self-control, and rapid alternation between sleeping and waking states.[5] Furthermore, all three arousal disorders can coexist, making them difficult to distinguish from one another.
- NREM disorders of arousal have been found to have a genetic basis. A person whose first-degree relative has a disorder of arousal is 10 times more likely to have a similar disorder than a person who does not have an affected relative.[6] The HLA

gene *DQB1* is reported to be present in 35% of sleepwalkers versus 26% of normal controls.

- The diagnosis is primarily guided by the patient's clinical history. Although PSG is useful to rule out other sleep disorders (e.g., RBD or nocturnal seizures), behavioral events rarely occur in the sleep laboratory.[7,8] If events do occur during PSG, they are usually less intricate than events that patients report having at home.
- Nocturnal seizures may be differentiated from disorders of arousal, since the latter show a pattern of episodes that occur out of stage N3 sleep during the first third of the night, are not stereotyped, and have a sustained autonomic component. They also tend to disappear or decrease after adolescence. PSG with expanded electromyogram (EMG) and electroencephalographic (EEG) montages is extremely useful for proper diagnosis and differentiation between parasomnias and seizures.

Confusional Arousals

- Related to both sleepwalking and sleep terrors, confusional arousals are brief and incomplete arousals typically starting in N3 sleep.
- The aroused individual appears confused in general. Patients who experience confusional arousals usually do not leave the bed, thus differing from sleepwalking.
- As with sleep terrors, confusional arousals most commonly occur during the first third of the night, but they can also take place in other NREM stages or during the later part of the night.
- Common examples include picking at clothing and sitting up in bed, making uncomplicated vocalizations.
- The terms "sleep drunkenness" and "sleep inertia" are also used to describe these events since the episodes (particularly those following arousal in the morning) are often accompanied by disorientation, behavioral disturbance, and impaired cognition.
- Confusional arousals are seen in children during both nocturnal sleep and daytime naps.
- About 10%–20% of children and 2%–5% of adults experience confusional arousals at some point in their lives.
- Anxiety, sleep deprivation, fever, and endocrine factors (e.g., pregnancy) can increase the frequency of episodes. In adults, primary sleep disorders (e.g., obstructive sleep apnea, periodic leg movement disorder) can also aggravate such conditions. Other precipitating factors include the consumption of alcohol, hypnotics, lithium, antihistamines, and potentially other medications that tend to elevate the arousal threshold.

Sleepwalking

- Sleepwalking (somnambulism) is initiated during SWS and in general occurs within the first third of the sleep period.
- Sleepwalking involves a series of complex motor behaviors and results in walking during altered consciousness.
- About 10%–20% of children and 1%–4% of adults experience sleepwalking, and it is most prevalent in children between 5 and 10 years of age.[9]
- Sleepwalking events range from simple to complex, such as walking, unlocking doors, putting on makeup, and even driving.
  - Episodes usually last from a few seconds to half an hour, and in general patient recall of these events is vague or absent the following morning.

- There is a lack of dreaming in the sleepwalking state; the individual's eyes are open, and if awakened, a sleepwalker may respond with simple phrases and non sequiturs.
- Frequent sleepwalking in adults may be associated with dangerous or violent activity, thus warranting treatment.
- Patients evaluated for sleepwalking most often have normal findings on neurologic examination, but the presence of another contributing medical disorder or medication should be investigated before a definitive diagnosis is made.
- Sleepwalking is linked to NREM sleep instability, particularly an abnormality in regulation of SWS.[10,11] Although frequent arousals from SWS, decreased slow wave activity, and the presence of hypersynchronous delta waves have all been linked to sleepwalking, these findings lack specificity and sensitivity.[12]
- Episodes may be precipitated in predisposed people by the consumption of alcohol, hypnotics, lithium, antihistamines, and other medications that can elevate the arousal threshold. Sleepwalking can occur in association with other sleep disorders, such as obstructive sleep apnea syndrome.

Sleep Terrors

- Similar to sleepwalking, sleep terrors (night terrors, pavor nocturnus) are characterized by arousal from N3 sleep.
- Sleep terrors begin with incomplete arousal from SWS and are associated with activation of the autonomic nervous system and reports of frightening imagery.
  - Events may terrify the patient, who often abruptly screams and exhibits autonomic and behavioral manifestations of intense fear.
  - Sleep terrors are associated with agitation, hyperpnea, tachycardia, and sweating.
- Differentiation between sleep terrors and other parasomnias is presented in Table 16.2.

- In general, episodes occur in the first third of the night.
- Patients have very little, if any, recall of the event the following morning, with witnesses often being more distressed by the events than the patients themselves.
- Sleep terrors occur in 5% of children and 1%–2% of adults.[13]
  - Fortunately, children with sleep terrors tend to grow out of them.
  - Events in adults may be brought on by stressors such as psychologic pressure, sleep deprivation, alcohol use, and shift work.
  - Adults with sleep terrors should be thoroughly assessed for comorbid psychiatric disorders.
  - Fig. 16.1 displays a postarousal EEG pattern during a behavioral arousal from stage 4 sleep in a 19-year-old man.

Sleep-Related Eating Disorder

- Sleep-related eating disorder (SRED) involves partial arousals from sleep where patients involuntarily eat and drink.
  - Patients have little to no memory of these events.
  - Foods consumed may comprise peculiar combinations or even inedible and toxic substances such as coffee grounds, frozen food, and cleaning materials.
  - Some patients have unexplained weight gain and a lack of appetite in the morning.
- Patients should be evaluated thoroughly for any comorbid disorders. SRED is more often seen in those with a history of sleepwalking or eating disorders, but is also seen as comorbid with restless legs syndrome, periodic limb movements, and SRBD.
- Medications such as zolpidem, anticholinergics, and lithium have been reported to alleviate SRED.[14,15] Both topiramate and dopaminergic medications have been effective for some patients with SRED.[16,17]

TABLE 16.2	**Differential Diagnosis of Parasomnias**					
	Confusional Arousals	**Sleep Terrors**	**Sleepwalking**	**Nightmares**	**REM Sleep Behavior Disorder**	**Nocturnal Seizures**
Time of night	Early	Early	Early–mid	Late	Late	Any/first half
Sleep stage	SWA	SWA	SWA	REM	REM	Any
EEG discharges	–	–	–	–	–	±
Scream	–	++++	–	++	+	+
CNS activation	+	++++	+	+	+	+
Motor activity	–	+	+++	+	++++	++++
Awakens	–	–	–	+	+	+
Duration (min)	0.5–10	1–10	2–30	3–20	1–10	0.5–15
Postevent confusion	+	+	+	–	–	+
Age	Child	Child	Child	Child/adult	Older adult	Young adult
Genetics	+	+	+	–	–	±
Organic CNS lesion	–	–	–	–	++	++++

+, Usually present; –, not usually present; ±, occasionally present. *CNS*, Central nervous system; *EEG*, electroencephalographic; *REM*, rapid eye movement; *SWA*, slow wave activity.
Modified from Avidan AY, Kaplish N. The parasomnias: epidemiology, clinical features, and diagnostic approach. *Clin Chest Med*. 2010;31:353–370.

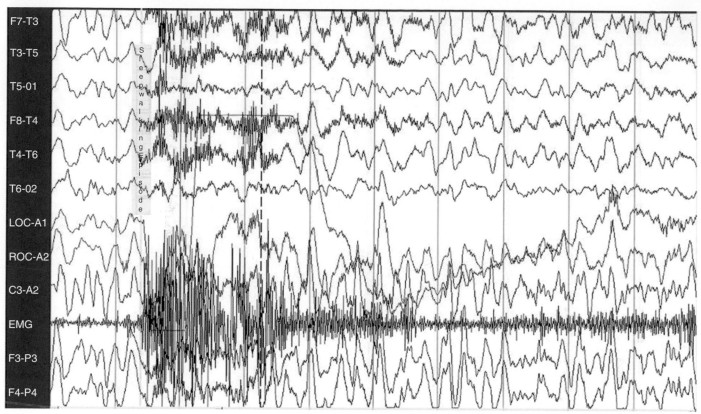

• **Figure 16.1** Postarousal Electroencephalographic (EEG) Pattern During a Behavioral Arousal from Stage 4 Sleep in a 19-Year-Old Man. The EEG shows diffuse and rhythmic delta activity and is most predominant in the anterior regions. *EMG*, Electromyogram; *LOC*, left outer canthus; *ROC*, right outer canthus. (Reprinted with permission from Zadra A, Montplaisir J. Sleepwalking. In: Thorpy MJ, Plazzi G, eds. *The Parasomnias.* Cambridge, UK: Cambridge University Press; 2010.)

Treatment of Arousal Disorders

Pharmacologic and behavioral treatments of arousal disorders overlap significantly and will be addressed with the disorder-specific treatment recommendations.

- When an arousal disorder is diagnosed, a treatment plan must account for the nature of the symptoms.
- Most arousal disorders in the general population are mild, occur in childhood, and resolve over time.
- Overnight PSG should be restricted to those whose behavior is violent or bothersome to others or when an underlying sleep disorder is suspected, such as obstructive sleep apnea.
- In determining a course of treatment, one must consider the frequency and severity of the episodes because arousal disorders are mild and therefore pharmacologic intervention is not usually indicated. Other treatment may be necessary for any concurrent sleep disorders (e.g., sleep apnea, periodic limb movements) that may trigger arousals.

Education

- Proper education is key to addressing arousal disorders.
- Patients should be informed of their diagnosis and taught about the pathophysiology, which may increase the possibility of recurrence.
- It should be explained to patients and family that many arousal disorders require no intervention, and that these events often diminish or disappear over time.

- It is particularly important to educate parents about the diagnosis in children, because parents may erroneously believe that these events indicate underlying medical or psychologic illness or trauma. Stress may be a factor in arousal disorders, but this should not be the clinician's immediate conclusion, particularly in children.

Safety

- Safety is critical when treating patients with arousal disorders.
- There is no "one size fits all" solution for all patients, and each patient's safety must be individually tailored. For example, one may reduce the risk for injury by placing the mattress on the floor or installing gates at the top of staircases and in doorways. Safety suggestions are listed in Table 16.3.
- Table 16.4 lists various indications for a PSG to diagnose parasomnia.

Sleep Hygiene and Sleep-Wake Scheduling

- Good sleep hygiene may help reduce arousals.
  - Regularly scheduled sleep-wake times and adequate sleep durations are important because sleep deprivation may trigger SWS episodes.
  - Sources of arousal such as noise or light should be limited. For example, earplugs to block noise and light-blocking shades are both common suggestions.

TABLE 16.3	Suggestions to Ensure Safety in Patients with Arousal Disorders

Place the mattress on the floor.
Light outside hallways.
Install alarm systems to alert when someone has left the room or house.
Place gates at the top of staircases and in doorways.
Remove and/or lock away dangerous objects.
Cover windows and glass doors with thick drapes.
Remove coat hooks from doors.
Remove obstructions from rooms.
Sleep in a separate bed from the bed partner.
Lock doors with a double lock.
Place bells on the outside of doors.

TABLE 16.4	When to Conduct a PSG for Suspected Parasomnia

Uncommon age of onset for presenting symptoms
Medical and legal consequences
Associated excessive daytime sleepiness
High frequency of episodes
Injury to self or others during events
Safety risks such as leaving the house

- Exercise, drugs, and alcohol should all be avoided within 3 hours of bedtime.

Avoid Restraint

- Refrain from engaging the patient in the middle of an episode. Confronting patients during events is to be avoided; instead, the patient must be quietly guided back to bed without awakening. Confrontation can prolong the event and may even worsen a patient's behavior and possibly lead to dangerous or violent situations.

Scheduled Awakenings

- Several case studies have found that scheduled awakenings can reduce nighttime events.[18]
- They may diminish the overall duration of SWS, although the exact mechanism of action remains unclear.[19,20]
- Awaken the patient 15 min before the time of the usual first arousal. A nightly sleep diary should be kept to record the time of each event. Patients must be stimulated enough to open their eyes and speak a few words. The observer must wake the patient in this fashion nightly before each arousal until the events subside.
- If the arousal events reoccur, treatment is reinstated.
- Caution must be exercised with this treatment because it may worsen the arousals.

Stress Management

- Because psychologic strain can precipitate arousals, stress management treatments are commonly recommended.
- Practicing progressive muscle relaxation (PMR) before bedtime may be helpful, as reported in case studies involving both adults and children.[21]

- Although the data are sparse, some support the proposition that muscle relaxation helps alleviate arousal disorders.[22]

Psychotherapy

- If underlying psychologic issues are present (e.g., anxiety, trauma, depression), psychotherapy may be useful in treating arousal disorders.
- Psychopathology may occur more frequently in adults with arousal disorders, and such adults should be evaluated for psychiatric comorbid conditions.
- Limited data exist on the efficacy of psychotherapy in treating parasomnias, but its success has been demonstrated in case studies. In addition, a number of different approaches to psychotherapy exist (e.g., cognitive behavior therapy, dynamic therapies, psychoanalysis), but no study has evaluated the efficaciousness of one type over another.
- Kales et al. reported case studies of three adult male patients, each of whom was married and educated and had lengthy arousal disorders.[23]
  - Through the use of psychodynamic therapy, patients with sleep terrors were better able to understand how they internalized their emotional states.
  - They were taught ways to effectively cope with stress.
  - As self-esteem and coping abilities increased, the patients gradually worked through their emotional conflicts and, as Kales and associates suggested, reduced the internalized aggression and conflict that were manifested as sleep terrors.

Hypnosis

- Single case studies and small case series that have been reported in the literature document the value of hypnosis in treating arousal disorders, specifically night terrors and sleepwalking.[24–26]
- A decrease in tonic levels as a result of hypnosis may help decrease events.[27]
- Hauri et al. noted that although hypnosis was helpful in most parasomnias, it was least beneficial for sleep terrors.[28]
- Further studies may clarify the role that hypnosis can play in treating arousal disorders.

Medications

- Pharmacologic treatment is necessary when events become frequent, put the family and patient at risk for harm, or disrupt overall family life.
- Benzodiazepines (e.g., clonazepam, diazepam) have successfully reduced both arousals and SWS. Benzodiazepines may be used continuously or when great risk for harm is suspected.
- Even though patients have responded well to desipramine, paroxetine, and imipramine, few cases have been reported.
- Table 16.5 summarizes the most commonly used medications for parasomnias.

Treatment Summary

Since the arousal disorder episodes occur during NREM sleep, it is challenging to try to awaken patients; however, if awakened, patients can be confused or aggressive. Despite reports of many medications being effective in isolated cases, there is no good evidence that any one medication is superior. Ensuring the safety of the environment is essential for some patients.

TABLE 16.5	Typical Pharmacologic Interventions for Parasomnias		
Medication	Effective Dose Range (mg)	Appropriate Patient Population	Possible Side Effects
NREM Parasomnias			
Diazepam	5–10	Can be effective for ST	Rebound insomnia on discontinuation
Clonazepam	0.5–2.0	Can be effective for SW, ST, CA	Daytime somnolence, cognitive dysfunction
Imipramine	10–300	Can be effective for ST, CA	Anticholinergic effects
Paroxetine	20–40	Can be effective for SW, ST	Nausea
Melatonin	3–15	Can be effective for SW, ST	Not FDA approved or regulated in the United States; daytime somnolence
Trazodone	25–150	May be effective for ST	Nausea, daytime somnolence, dizziness
REM-Related Parasomnias			
Clonazepam	0.5–2.0	First-line treatment of RBD	Daytime somnolence, cognitive dysfunction
Melatonin	3–12	Has been effective for RBD	Not FDA approved or regulated in the United States, daytime somnolence
Pramipexole	0.5–1.5	May help RBD	Nausea, daytime somnolence
Tricyclic antidepressants	Variable	May suppress NM	Anticholinergic side effects
Prazosin	1.0–5.0	Effective for NM	Worsens cataplexy in narcoleptics
Gabapentin	300–3600	May reduce NM	Dizziness, daytime somnolence, nausea
Olanzapine	10–20	May reduce NM	Dizziness, daytime somnolence, weight gain
Topiramate	75	May reduce NM	Paresthesias, cognitive dysfunction
Other Parasomnias			
Venlafaxine	37.5	May be useful for RISP	May exacerbate RLS

CA, Confusional arousals; *FDA*, US Food and Drug Administration; *NM*, nightmares; *NREM*, nonrapid eye movement; *RBD*, REM sleep behavior disorder; *REM*, rapid eye movement; *RISP*, recurrent isolated sleep paralysis; *RLS*, restless legs syndrome; *ST*, sleep terrors; *SW*, sleepwalking.

Parasomnias Usually Associated with Rapid Eye Movement Sleep

Rapid Eye Movement Sleep Behavior Disorder

- The hallmark of RBD is vigorous motor activity, typically occurring in REM sleep and thus in the absence of muscle atonia (commonly referred to as REM sleep without atonia [RSWA]).
- The prevalence of RBD in the general population is unknown but estimated to be 0.5%.[29] RBD usually consists of injurious dream enactment activity from vivid, often unpleasant dreaming.
- RBD is symptomatically complex and may involve behavior that is dangerous to the patient and those nearby.
- Although most RBD diagnoses are made in middle-aged and older adult men, it can be seen in patients of either gender or age group.
- Patients experiencing RBD should consult a sleep specialist for a thorough evaluation.
- Since RBD can be idiopathic or related to underlying neurologic conditions (secondary RBD), patients should undergo a thorough physical examination to identify any comorbid disorders that may disrupt REM sleep.
- Acute RBD can be induced by medications (including monamine oxidase inhibitors [MAOIs], tricyclic antidepressants [TCAs], and serotonin reuptake inhibitors), benzodiazepine withdrawal, and alcohol.

- Table 16.6 describes the various RSWA and RBD subtypes and terminology.
- Figure 16.2 presents a 30-sec PSG epoch for a patient with RBD. The polysomnogram shows RSWA, manifest by increased muscle activity in REM sleep, with or without an arousal from REM sleep with increased motor activity.
- The exact pathophysiology of RBD is currently unknown, but recent animal models of RBD suggest an interruption in REM muscle atonia and disinhibition of brainstem motor pattern generators, particularly in the pontine tegmentum.[31,32]
  - Neuroimaging in adults with RBD has shown evidence of structural lesions in the brainstem, thus implicating the pons and dorsal midbrain.
- RBD is thought to be a prodrome of neurodegenerative disease[33]—in particular, diffuse Lewy body dementia, Parkinson's disease, and multiple system atrophy[34]—and has been linked with α-synuclein-mediated degeneration of sleep-regulating nuclei in the brainstem, with a focus on the pontine tegmentum.
  - Upwards of 81% of men with RBD over the age of 50 evidence a delayed emergence of Parkinson's disease or dementia (over a decade after the initial RBD diagnosis).[35,36]
- Clinical and pathophysiologic subtypes of RBD
  - Parasomnia overlap disorder occurs when a patient has both RBD and a disorder of arousal, rhythmic movement disorder, sexsomnia, or SRED. Although it can occur at any age,

TABLE 16.6	Definitions for REM Sleep without Atonia and REM Sleep Behavior Disorder[30]

REM Sleep without Atonia

- Electrographic finding of EMG augmentation during REM sleep

Dream Enactment Behavior

- Recurrent nocturnal behavior that is interpreted by the observer as acting out dreams, often with associated injuries or potential for injury
- The dreams are typically (though not always) associated with chasing or attacking themes
- Not specific for RBD

REM Sleep Behavior Disorder

- Presence of RSWA and DEB
- Absence of any linked seizure activity during events

Subclinical REM Sleep Behavior Disorder

- PSG finding of RSWA

Clinically Probable RBD/Probable RBD

- Recurrent DEB (especially when access to PSG is limited)

Idiopathic/Cryptogenic REM Sleep Behavior Disorder

- RSWA with DEB
- RBD occurring in the absence of any associated neurologic disorder

Secondary or Symptomatic REM Sleep Behavior Disorder

- RBD plus another neurologic/neurodegenerative disease

DEB, Dream enactment behavior; *EMG*, electromyogram; *PSG*, polysomnography; *REM*, rapid eye movement; *RBD*, REM sleep behavior disorder; *RSWA*, REM sleep without atonia.

many cases begin during childhood or adolescence and predominantly in males. In some cases, it may be idiopathic, whereas in others it may be a symptom of another disorder such as narcolepsy, brain tumor, brain trauma, psychiatric disorders, substance abuse, and multiple sclerosis.

- Status dissociatus is a subtype of RBD that is an extreme form of state dissociation without typical identifiable sleep stages, but does have sleep and dream enactment behaviors. Patients have no obvious PSG markers for REM sleep, NREM sleep, and wakefulness. Oftentimes, the patient believes he is awake, yet observers assume he is asleep and engaging in dream enactment behaviors (or vice versa). Confusion as to whether the patient is awake, asleep, or dreaming tends to be the hallmark observable issue. In almost all cases, an underlying neurologic or medical condition is the root cause.
- Level B (suggested) treatments for RBD include clonazepam (0.5–2.0 mg) and melatonin.
- Level C (may be considered) interventions include pramipexole, paroxetine, L-DOPA, and acetylcholinesterase inhibitors.
- Other Level C interventions may be considered, although limited data exist. These medications include zopiclone, temazepam, triazolam, alprazolam, carbamazepine, desipramine, clozapine, yi-gan san (an herbal medication), and sodium oxybate.[37–40]
- In general, RBD can be managed with medication, but behavioral interventions are also helpful.

- Successful and comprehensive treatment of RBD must emphasize the patient's safety. Safety is paramount, and the measures discussed previously in treating arousal disorders should be taken to keep the room safe (see Table 16.3). Patients should sleep alone in a different bed from their partner until the episodes are controlled. Patient and family education is critical because violent episodes may strain relationships.

Recurrent Isolated Sleep Paralysis

- Sleep paralysis occurs when REM muscle atonia persists into wakefulness.
- Eye movements and respiratory activity remain intact, but somatic movements are not possible.
- Episodes may accompany a dream-related fear or anxiety when the patient realizes that movement is impossible.
- Each episode may last as long as a few minutes and may be terminated by an external stimulus (e.g., noise or touch).
- Sleep deprivation and alcohol can induce these episodes, and those with infrequent sleep paralysis in general do not require treatment.
- For recurring episodes, depression and other psychiatric conditions should be evaluated because they have the potential to produce sleep disturbances.
- With severe, frequent cases, pharmacologic intervention with antidepressants may help.[41–43]

Nightmares

- Nightmares are frightening dreams that can wake the sleeper from REM sleep.
- Although nightmares may occur at any time during the night, they take place mostly during the final third of the night when REM sleep is prominent.
- In general, the memory of a nightmare is detailed and vivid.
- Nightmares are often associated with the emotions of fear and anxiety, but anger, embarrassment, and sadness may also be present.
- Table 16.2 further differentiates nightmares from night terrors.
- Nearly 75% of children report experiencing a nightmare at least once, with 40% of children aged 6–10 years experiencing chronic nightmares.
  - The peak age for nightmares is between 6 and 10 years of age, and boys and girls are affected equally.
  - After 12 years of age, females appear to have more nightmares.[44,45]
- Occasional nightmares are common in the adult population, with 85% reporting at least 1 within a 12-month period. Between 2% and 6% of adults have chronic, weekly nightmares.[46]
- Stress and antidepressant or antihypertensive medications can be precipitating factors.
- Nightmare disorder—experiencing recurrent nightmares—can be idiopathic or related to an underlying psychologic trauma or psychopathology (e.g., depression, anxiety, posttraumatic stress disorder [PTSD]).
- Recurrent or frequent nightmares can result in diminished quality of life.
- Despite the prevalence of nightmares in the general population, many clinicians are still unaware of the psychiatric and medical toll that nightmares take on patients. Effective behavioral and

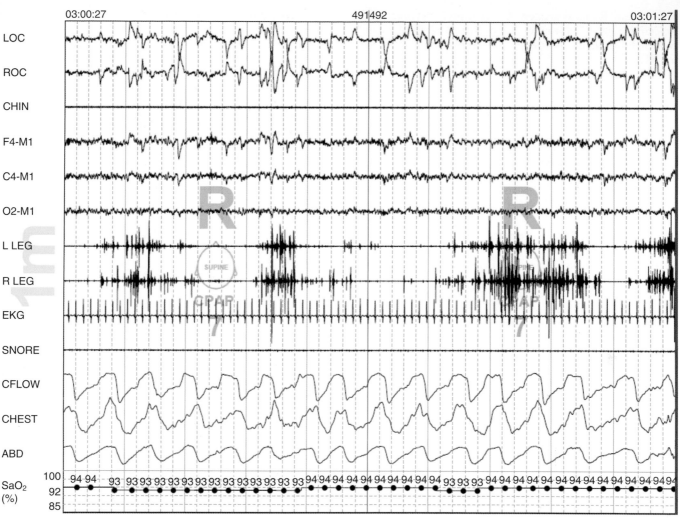

• **Figure 16.2** A 30-Sec Polysomnography Epoch for a Patient with Rbd. The polysomnogram shows rapid eye movement (REM) sleep without atonia, manifest by increased muscle activity in REM sleep, with or without an arousal from REM sleep with increased motor activity. Channels are as follows: electro-oculogram (left, left outer canthus [LOC]-A2; right, right outer canthus [ROC]-A1), chin electromyogram (EMG), electroencephalogram (left central, right central, left occipital, right occipital), two electrocardiogram (EKG) channels, limb EMG (LAT), snore channel, nasal-oral airflow, respiratory effort (THOR: thoracic, abdominal), and oxygen saturation (SaO2). *ABD*, Abdominal. (Copyright Alon Y. Avidan, M.D., MPH.)

pharmacologic treatments exist to treat nightmares, and careful evaluation can help lead to successful outcomes.

- Due to the increase in treatment studies (both pharmacologic and psychologic) in the past decade, the American Academy of Sleep Medicine's Standards of Practice Committee published guidelines for the treatment of nightmare disorder in adults.[47]
  - Both pharmacologic and psychologic treatments (especially imagery rehearsal therapy [IRT] and prazosin) for nightmares have been shown to have a moderate effect, reducing intensity, distress, and frequency.[48]
  - Studies have demonstrated that improvements in sleep quality and quality of life result from successful treatment of nightmares, thus suggesting that nightmares are a primary disorder or comorbid condition, rather than simply a symptom of a primary psychiatric disorder.[49,50]
  - This places less weight on nightmares as a symptom and highlights nightmares as an individual diagnostic entity.

Pharmacologic Treatment of Nightmares

- Despite the availability of some promising pharmacologic treatments, some commonly used medications can instead cause or increase the frequency of nightmares.
- Medications that can exacerbate nightmares include antidepressants (especially those that react with dopamine, norepinephrine, and serotonin), β-blockers, amphetamines, and sedatives.[51] Synthetic cannabinoid may lead to improvements in nightmares.[52]

Prazosin

- Prazosin is the only pharmacotherapy currently recommended as a treatment for PTSD-related nightmares, and has been demonstrated to have significant improvements posttreatment.[47,48,53]
- Prazosin blocks central α_1-adrenoceptors and has been used safely in general medicine to treat hypertension.

- Taylor and Raskind suggested that central nervous system α_1-adrenergic receptor stimulation disrupts sleep physiology, which leads to the heightened reactivity seen as the basis of PTSD.[54]
  - The pharmacologic blockade of postsynaptic α_1-receptors may actually provide symptomatic relief from nightmares related to trauma, sleep disturbance, and other PTSD symptoms.
- Prazosin has shown very promising results in the effort to diminish nightmares.[55–57]
- Prazosin must be taken continuously to consistently reduce nightmare frequency, or they can reappear on cessation of prazosin.

Antidepressants

- Early research on the use of antidepressants to treat idiopathic nightmares was unsuccessful, but their application to PTSD-related recurrent nightmares has been inconclusive and thus warrants more investigation.[58]
  - Certain selective serotonin reuptake inhibitors (SSRIs; e.g., sertraline) have been associated with insomnia.
  - More research is necessary to understand this side effect and its impact on insomnia and nightmares.
- A number of medications that may be considered for PTSD-related nightmares, but caution that studies backing up their use are sparse and they should be judiciously used.[47]
  - Fluvoxamine has been shown helpful in treating nightmares,[59] with trazodone and cyproheptadine—medications that potentiate serotonin while also acting as serotonin 5-HT$_2$ receptor agonists—also reducing PTSD-related nightmares.
  - Trazodone is indicated solely for the treatment of depression but is commonly used in psychiatry for its hypnotic side effects as a treatment for insomnia.[60] Research on the use of trazodone to treat nightmares is limited, although two studies have shown it to be successful when used for the treatment for patients with PTSD, insomnia, and nightmares.[61,62]
  - Nefazodone is not recommended as a first-line treatment for nightmares because of an increased risk of hepatoxicity.[47]
  - Results from limited datasets have been reported for the use of TCAs and MAOIs in the treatment of nightmares.
    - Studies investigating the use of phenelzine in patients with PTSD have shown the best results.[63]
    - Poor patient compliance and the adverse effects associated with TCAs and MAOIs suggest that these medications will probably not be studied in further detail.

Psychotherapeutic Approaches to the Treatment of Nightmares

Imagery Rehearsal Therapy

- Cognitive behavioral treatment (CBT) of nightmares has the largest body of empirical support for the treatment of nightmares[64]; IRT is the most researched of all such interventions.
  - Accordingly, IRT is often recommended as a first-line (or adjunctive) therapy for treating nightmares.[47,65,66]
  - Many studies combine various psychologic interventions, but sole IRT is considered the best available treatment for idiopathic nightmares, with solid outcomes for PTSD-related nightmares as well.[48]
- Chronic nightmare sufferers may feel as though they have no control over their nightmares. IRT allows patients to have control.
- IRT was originally developed to treat idiopathic nightmares and is now used to treat both the idiopathic and PTSD-related varieties.
- The IRT intervention is actually fairly simple. IRT consists of (1) writing down a nightmare, (2) changing it any way that the patient wishes, (3) writing down the changed dream, and finally (4) imaginal rehearsal of the newly changed dream for 5–20 min daily.[67]
  - Patients need to be able to clearly visualize, in their mind's eye, images that they would like to see.
  - IRT is less likely to be successful if a patient has difficulty painting a mental picture.
  - Participants are encouraged to start with minimally distressing nightmares and not an exact replication of any actual trauma.
  - Since IRT is a rather straightforward and simple technique, many research protocols test this treatment in a group setting.[50,68]
- Krakow and associates developed sleep dynamic therapy (SDT) in an attempt to expand IRT and incorporate interventions for both insomnia and nightmares.[69]
  - This program was composed of CBT for insomnia, IRT, and emotional processing. Patients are taught to compare their sleep habits with those of normal sleepers to help them recognize the indicators of poor sleep quality and to help identify sleep movement disorders or sleep-disordered breathing.
  - SDT was administered in 2-hour weekly group sessions for 6 weeks to fire evacuees who were experiencing PTSD, nightmare disorder, and insomnia.
  - The results showed moderate increases in sleep quality, total sleep time, and sleep efficiency, with small effects noted at the 3-month follow-up.
  - These modest improvements may be due to the large number of patients with sleep-disordered breathing in the population, or there may be difficulties inherent in dealing with personal and emotional information in a large group of patients.[70]
  - As no control group was included in this study, the overall effects of SDT are not fully known.
- IRT is reported to be successful in reducing nightmares in as many as 90% or more of the individuals who use it.[71]
- Despite the high success rate, there are limitations to IRT.
  - Some patients find imagery to be too difficult or may instead be flooded with negative imagery. These patients may require structured guidance in positive imagery practice and specific cognitive behavioral interventions at the beginning to help moderate the negative imagery.
  - Most of the research on IRT has been conducted by one single research group.[64] More studies are warranted to compare IRT with other techniques, such as exposure and pharmacologic treatment, and larger patient populations should also be used.

Lucid Dreaming Therapy

- In lucid dreaming therapy (LDT), patients learn to change a nightmare within and during the nightmare itself.

- Because higher rates of lucid dreaming have been reported in patients with greater nightmare frequencies, it is suggested that nightmares may elicit lucid dreaming.[72]
- Few case studies have investigated the effects of LDT on nightmares, and each has shown reductions in overall nightmare frequency.[73–76]
- Given the lack of research conducted on LDT, any conclusions regarding its efficacy should be made with caution and it is not considered a first-line treatment for nightmares.[47]

Psychodynamic Psychotherapy

- Traditional models of psychotherapy viewed nightmares as a symptom of a larger primary psychiatric illness.[77]
- These therapies work on the belief that successful treatment of a "primary" psychiatric disorder (e.g., depression, anxiety, PTSD) will ultimately resolve the nightmares.
- No empirical support has demonstrated that the use of traditional psychotherapeutic models is efficacious in treating nightmares.[47,78]

Prolonged Exposure

- Nightmares are frequently seen in patients with PTSD.[79]
- Prolonged exposure (PE) is a highly effective treatment of PTSD that has been researched in numerous controlled trials across a wide cross section of trauma survivors.[80]
- Even though PE is recommended as a first-line treatment of PTSD,[58] most studies have not investigated the impact of PE on sleep disturbance, although it is very common complaint reported in patients with PTSD.
- Two studies evaluated the effect of PE on nightmares, but the results are inconclusive.[81,82]
  - In each study, CBT reduced recurrent nightmares, but in one study, nearly half of patients reported continued insomnia.
  - Additional research is warranted in this field, with an emphasis on sleep outcomes. Such research will help in modifying overall treatment plans for those with PTSD by aiding in the understanding of which treatments help patients with particular symptoms.[47]

Exposure and Systematic Desensitization

- Exposure therapy for nightmares consists of the patient writing down a nightmare and then "reliving" the nightmare in the patient's imagination until the patient's anxiety decreases by at least half.
  - The patient is instructed to engage in daily practice of this nightmare imagining.
  - Anxiety from the nightmare practice peaks and is recorded on a homework sheet.
  - The patient continues the exercise until the anxiety has subsided by at least half of the peak.
  - The goal is to expose the patient to the anxiety so that the patient eventually acclimates to the anxiety.
  - Patients must avoid distractions during the exercise because diversions will prevent the anxiety from properly habituating.
  - Relaxation and other coping techniques may be taught before or after the exercise, but their use during the exercise is discouraged.
- Little research exists to draw any conclusions regarding exposure therapy for the treatment of nightmares, although guidelines suggest it may be considered for treatment of PTSD-related nightmares.[47,83] Burgess et al. reported the only straight exposure studies comparing exposure with relaxation.[84]
- Systematic desensitization (SD) is a different form of exposure therapy that uses coping strategies such as relaxation.[85]
  - SD for the treatment of nightmares starts with the patient first being taught relaxation skills and given education that these skills will help counteract fear and anxiety.
  - The clinician works with the patient to create a hierarchy of nightmares based on the intensity of fear.
  - Once the patient learns relaxation techniques, the patient then applies them while imagining nightmares.
  - The patient can also be taught coping strategies such as positive self-statements (e.g., "I can get through this") or given cognitive therapy for catastrophizing during the exposure practice.
  - SD is suggested as a possible treatment for idiopathic nightmares.[47]
- Traditional exposure is favored over SD in most CBT protocols for the management of anxiety.
  - This maximizes habituation by denying coping strategies only during the exposure exercise.
  - Still, in nightmare treatment there is little research to draw any conclusions that SD has been shown to be effective.
  - Adequately powered studies should be devised to compare SD with IRT and exposure.

Relaxation

- Few studies have investigated relaxation strategies for the treatment of nightmare disorder.
- Miller and DiPilato[86] compared PMR, SD, and waitlist control in patients with nightmares.
  - The results indicated that both relaxation and SD produced a reduction in nightmare intensity, with an 80% reduction in nightmares in 63% of patients.
  - More favorable outcomes were noted for SD at the 25-week follow-up, with clients noting significantly reduced nightmares.
- Burgess et al. researched PMR, self-exposure, and wait list control in 170 adults with nightmares.[84]
  - At the 1- and 6-month follow-up, the exposure group reported a lower frequency of nightmares than the other groups did.

Nightmare Recording

- Recording of nightmare content inconsistently reduces the frequency of nightmares and has not been shown to successfully reduce associated complaints such as anxiety, depression, and diminished quality of life.
- Neidhardt et al. compared IRT with nightmare recording.[87]
  - All participants were instructed to write down their nightmares for 1 month. The recording group received no additional treatment, whereas the IRT participants received instructions for IRT.
  - The results indicated a significant decrease in nightmare frequency in both treatment groups.

Hypnosis

- Hypnosis is reported to help in the treatment of nightmares.[88]
- A patient under hypnosis can control the nightmare by changing a part of the dream or creating a less frightening ending, much like in LDT.

- Hauri et al. reported on a 5-year follow-up study of hypnosis in 36 patients.[28]
  - The results showed that hypnosis was effective in both short- and long-term follow-up of the nightmares, with 67% of patients being either free of symptoms or greatly improved at the 5-year follow-up.

Other Parasomnias

Sleep Enuresis

- Sleep enuresis is characterized by recurrent and involuntary urination during sleep.
- Although bed-wetting may be normal for some ages, it becomes pathologic when it occurs twice weekly or more during sleep in patients who are at least 5 years old.
- Patients with primary enuresis (those who are never consistently dry during sleep) may have a neurologic impairment or deficient release of vasopressin.
- Patients with secondary enuresis have had periods of remaining dry during sleep for at least 6 months in duration.
- Enuresis has been linked to urinary tract infection, diabetes mellitus, epilepsy, obstructive sleep apnea, and psychologic stress.
- In general, treatment includes reassurance and, in children, positive reinforcement for achieving goals.
  - Patients should refrain from drinking fluids during the evening.
  - Behavioral conditioning treatment (such as bell and pad alarms) may be useful.[89-91]
  - Desmopressin has most commonly been used to reduce urine production, and TCAs have been found to be helpful for short-term management of enuresis.[89]

Exploding Head Syndrome

- Patients suffering from "exploding head syndrome" report waking up because of a sensation of a loud, explosion-like sound inside their head that is described as being a nonobjective auditory experience ranging from a subtle sound to a loud bang.
- These noises typically occur just as the patient is falling asleep.
- Although the experience is usually painless, some patients note pain with the sound.
- The "explosions" are often exacerbated by sleep deprivation and stress.
- Treatment emphasizes reassuring the patient that these events are benign.
- If symptoms are disabling to the point that the patient loses sleep, case studies suggest the use of clomipramine (50 mg), flunarizine (10 mg), and nifedipine (90 mg).[92,93]

Sleep-Related Hallucinations

- Arguably the least studied of the parasomnias, sleep-related hallucinations (SRHs) are hallucinations that occur either at sleep onset (hypnagogic) or on awakening (hypnopompic).
- Most often visual in nature, SRHs can also include auditory, tactile, or kinetic sensations. SRHs range in description from very simple (such as vague colors or shapes) to complex images and sensations of falling or flying.

- Hypnagogic hallucinations are difficult to distinguish from sleep-onset dreaming, whereas hypnopompic hallucinations may be confused with early morning REM sleep.
- Events tend to be brief in duration, but they can occasionally last for a few minutes.
- Increasing ambient light tends to terminate the hallucination.
- Some patients are upset and frightened by SRHs because they initially perceive them to be real.
- Although SRH is in itself a distinct diagnosis, it is also seen during episodes of sleep paralysis and narcolepsy.
- Some patients may also experience separate, non-SRHs during the daytime.
- Little is known about the differences between hypnagogic and hypnopompic hallucinations.
- Proper assessment of SRHs should include asking the patient, "When you fall asleep or wake up, do you see, hear, or feel things that are not actually there?"
- SRHs are worsened by cigarette smoking, sleep deprivation, sedative-hypnotics, and certain antidepressants.[94]
- Various treatments have been used with overall poor results, including TCAs, benzodiazepines, olanzapine, hypnosis, and psychotherapy.[95,96]

Isolated Symptoms and Normal Variants

Sleep Talking

- Sleep talking (somniloquy) refers to speaking words or sounds during sleep without any awareness of the event as it happens.
- Occurring during stage 2, SWS or REM, sleep talking is most often seen during the first half of the night.
- Episodes may be worsened by acute medical illness, stress, a comorbid sleep disorder, or new medications.
- Sleep talking does not usually require intervention unless another sleep disorder is present.
- If treatment is required, patients are instructed to follow good sleep hygiene and reduce exacerbating factors such as alcohol.
- Sleep talking, rhythmic movement disorders, and bruxism are all differentiated from nocturnal seizures by taking a detailed history and completing a PSG.

Other Disorders in the Differential Diagnosis of Parasomnias

- Many other disorders that can occur during sleep, many of which are related to medical or psychiatric dysfunctions (or both), have been described in the literature.
- Some need specific medical intervention, whereas others require only reassurance.

Forensic Implications of Parasomnias

- Violent and other undesired behavior may take place during sleep and can occur without the affected individual being aware of the behavior.
- Such sleep-related behavior has been reported in 2% of the population and can occasionally have significant forensic implications.[97]

- A few prominent legal cases involving murder, apparent suicide, and assault have been linked to disorders of arousal, psychogenic states, sleep-related seizures, or RBD.
- It is in the clinician's professional interest to become informed of the medical and legal implications if the law assumes intentionality when aberrant behavior is present.
- Further investigation is needed to understand the prevalence of these disorders, how to diagnose and treat them, and how to protect those affected by the patient.

Conclusion

- Parasomnias may be considered some of the most fascinating of all the sleep disorders.
- They are common nocturnal events that can occur at any stage of sleep and have been well described behaviorally but remain poorly understood in terms of their underlying mechanisms.
- A full or extended EEG montage during PSG is often necessary to differentiate parasomnias from a seizure disorder.
- Genetic studies reveal that parasomnias commonly run in families, but although genetic susceptibility to parasomnias has been confirmed, not all variants of the disorder demonstrate a clear linkage.

- Further investigation of gene-environment interactions and other possible causes should be conducted to understand the precise nature of such disorders.
- The patient and clinician must work in tandem to tailor the treatment to the patient to reduce the patient's risk for injury, increase the safety of family members, and enhance the patient's overall quality of life.

Suggested Reading

Augedal AW, Hansen KS, Kronhaug CR, et al. Randomized controlled trials of psychological and pharmacological treatments for nightmares: a meta-analysis. *Sleep Med Rev.* 2013;17:143-152.

Aurora RN, Zak RS, Casey KR, et al. Best practice guide for the treatment of nightmare disorder in adults. *J Clin Sleep Med.* 2010;15:389-401.

Aurora RN, Zak RS, Maganti RK, et al. Best practice guide for the treatment of REM sleep behavior disorder (RBD). *J Clin Sleep Med.* 2010;6:85-95.

Iranzo A, Santamaria J, Tolosa E. The clinical and pathophysiological relevance of REM sleep behavior disorder in neurodegenerative diseases. *Sleep Med Rev.* 2009;13:385-401.

Schenck CH, Boeve BF, Mahowald MW. Delayed emergence of a parkinsonian disorder or dementia in 81% of older males initially diagnosed with idiopathic REM sleep behavior disorder (RBD): 16 year update on a previously reported series. *Sleep Med.* 2013;14:744-748.

17

Sleep-Related Movement Disorders

RICHARD P. ALLEN

Introduction

- Chapter emphasis on restless legs syndrome (RLS)/periodic leg movements in sleep (PLMS): Though few, the sleep-related movement disorders are perhaps the most common of the sleep disorders and, particularly for RLS with the closely related PLMS, represent a major public health problem that has yet to be adequately addressed and treated.
- Most of this chapter focuses on RLS and PLMS in recognition of their relative importance and common occurrence in the clinical practice of sleep medicine, but the other major disorders are also covered.
- Overview of the sleep-related movement disorders:
  - The definition of what a sleep-related movement disorder is involves somewhat arbitrary distinctions.
  - Parasomnias are not included here since they are viewed as indicating a pathology that is disrupting sleep maintenance mechanisms, such as occurs with rapid eye movement (REM) sleep behavior disorder (RBD), or sleepwalking/sleep terrors.
- Similarly, the usual daytime movement disorders with elements of disordered movement persisting in sleep, such as occurs with Parkinson's disease or some tremors, are usually considered features secondary to the daytime symptoms of the disease and are not primary sleep-related movement disorders. Sleep-related epilepsy (e.g., sleep-related hypermotor epilepsy[1]) produces abnormal movements sometimes only in sleep that are considered part of epilepsy rather than a movement disorder.
- This leaves us with a small collection of seven primary sleep-related disorders identified in *International Classification of Sleep Disorders*, 3rd edition (ICSD-3)[2]: RLS, periodic limb movement disorder (PLMD), sleep-related leg cramps, sleep-related bruxism, sleep-related rhythmic movement disorder, benign sleep myoclonus of infancy, and propriospinal

myoclonus at sleep onset. The last two of these will not be covered in this chapter, aside from listing the diagnostic criteria in the tables. Benign sleep myoclonus has little clinical significance, and propriospinal myoclonus at sleep onset is both rare and closely related if not the same as daytime propriospinal myoclonus, except for its more frequent expression with drowsiness. It neither occurs in sleep nor has any related features occurring in sleep.

- The ICSD-3 also recognizes some minor sleep-related phenomena of uncertain status, possibly atypical variants of another condition, or variants of normal physiology with uncertain clinical significance, such as excessive fragmentary myoclonus, hypnagogic foot tremor, alternating leg muscle activity, or sleep starts (hypnic jerks). Given the uncertain status of these conditions, they will not be covered in this chapter, except for a brief note about alternating leg muscle activation (ALMA) in relation to the issue of scoring the bilateral movements. Finally, the ICSD-3 notes that if the diagnosed movement disorder in sleep results from a medical disorder, medication, or substance, the diagnosis is not changed but should note this association. Table 17.1 lists the ICSD-3 classifications and codes for sleep-related movement disorders.

Restless Legs Syndrome

- Significance: RLS is the most significant of the movement disorders of sleep and, after sleep-disordered breathing (SDB), is perhaps the most clinically significant common sleep disorder. It produces significant health and personal morbidity, including the most profound chronic loss of sleep of any sleep-related disorder, yet it is not commonly recognized, diagnosed, and treated. Thus it is a significant and underrecognized public health problem in North America and Europe.[3]

History

- First medical description: Though indirectly described in several early literary texts, the eminent 17th century English physician Tomas Willis provided the first known medical description. He reported a case of extreme motor activity during resting and sleep that was successfully treated with an opioid.[4] He aptly describes the torture experienced by those with what we recognize today as severe RLS (Fig. 17.1).
- Diagnosis development: Despite occasional references in the medical literature indicating some recognition of the disorder,

TABLE 17.1	ICSD-3 Diagnosis (Codes) for Sleep-Related Movement Disorders

Primary Sleep-Related Movement Disorders (ICD-9-CM, ICD-10-CM codes)

- Restless legs syndrome (RLS) (333.99, G25.81)
- Periodic limb movement disorder (PLMD) (327.51, G47.61)
- Sleep-related leg cramps (327.52, G47.62)
- Sleep-related bruxism (327.53, G47.63)
- Sleep-related rhythmic movement disorder (327.59, G47.69)
- Benign sleep myoclonus of infancy (327.59, G47.69)
- Propriospinal myoclonus at sleep onset (327.59, G47.69)

Isolated Symptoms, Apparently Normal Variants and Unresolved Issues

- Sleep starts (hypnic jerks)
- Hypnagogic foot tremor and alternating leg muscle activation (ALMA) during sleep
- Excessive fragmentary myoclonus (not covered in this chapter)

ICSD-3, International Classification of Sleep Disorders, 3rd edition.

1692:
1st medical description

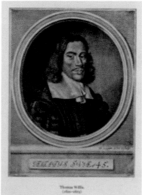

Wherefore to fome, when being a Bed they betake themfelves to fleep, prefently in the Arms and Legs, Leapings and Contractions of the Tendons, and fo great a Reftleffnefs and Toffings of their Members enfue, that the difeafed are no more able to fleep, than if they were in a Place of the greateft Torture.

1945:
1st systematic study

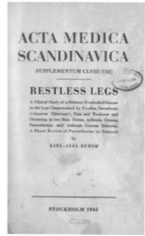

- **Figure 17.1** Significant historic identification of restless legs syndrome. (Copyright Richard P. Allen.)

it was another 300 years before careful medical analysis for diagnosis of this condition was performed. This was provided in 1945 by the thorough and thoughtful monograph of the noted Swedish neurologist Karl Ekbom. He gave various names to the disorder, including classical Latin ones, but titled his monograph "Restless Legs" (see Fig. 17.1)[5] and, in a latter manuscript, "Restless Legs Syndrome."[6] Willis emphasized the movements, whereas Ekbom emphasized the sensory disturbance associated with RLS. These were combined in the currently accepted medical definition of the disorder developed by the International RLS Study Group (IRLSSG; Table 17.2).[7] The updated diagnosis criteria emphasize differential diagnosis, excluding conditions that produce symptoms that at times mimic those of RLS. The updated diagnosis also adds two significant specifiers for the diagnosis—that is, clinical course (chronic, persistent vs. intermittent) and clinical significance.

- Recognition increases: The major boost for recognition and treatment of RLS comes from the serendipitous discovery in 1982 by Dr. Akpinar in Ankara, Turkey, of the dramatically effective treatment provided by levodopa and dopamine agonists.[8,9] Levodopa was later shown to be more effective than what was at that time a commonly used opioid propoxyphene.[10] Just as continuous positive airway pressure restored wakefulness in patients with sleep apnea, so dopamine restored sleep for

patients with RLS. It provided relief to thousands suffering with this sleep disorder. Like sleep apnea, RLS was recognized as a common disorder with significant morbidity[11] that could be effectively treated in many patients. Unfortunately, the long-term complications of the dopaminergic treatments have limited the potential benefits, thus raising new challenges for the future development of treatments (e.g., alpha-2-delta [$\alpha2\delta$] drugs as alternate first-line treatment[12] and possible modification of the course of the disease.

Diagnosis

RLS is defined by sensory symptoms, not movements, based on four essential features of the sensory symptom.

- The primary sensory symptom:
  - Sensory symptom location and descriptions: The four essential diagnostic criteria for RLS start with the primary symptom of akathisia, or an urge to move focused on the legs. Akathisia involving the legs is required to make the diagnosis. Other body parts may also be included, such as the arms and even the trunk, but rarely the feet or hands and even less commonly the face. Both or only one leg may be affected, and the usual distal to proximal pattern observed for peripheral neuropathies does not occur. The urge to move is often accompanied by strange, unpleasant sensations that patients have trouble describing. Both the urge to move and the sensations are unique to RLS patients and in general rarely, if ever, experienced by others; there is, therefore, no common shared experience and thus no language to describe these sensory phenomena. The choice of words suggests a somewhat dynamic feeling not on the surface but deeper in the leg and sometimes involving the joints but very rarely limited to the joints (Table 17.3). The sensations usually affect both legs but not necessarily equally or at the same time; when exclusively limited to one leg, the clinician should be concerned that a radiculopathy or some other unilateral physical factor may be present that is contributing to the disorder. The sensations appear to be on a dimension associated with

TABLE 17.2	Essential Diagnostic Criteria for Restless Legs Syndrome

Essential diagnostic criteria (all must be met):
1. An urge to move the legs usually but not always accompanied by, or felt to be caused by, uncomfortable and unpleasant sensations in the legs.
2. The urge to move the legs and any accompanying unpleasant sensations begin or worsen during periods of rest or inactivity such as lying down or sitting.
3. The urge to move the legs and any accompanying unpleasant sensations are partially or totally relieved by movement, such as walking or stretching, at least as long as the activity continues.
4. The urge to move the legs and any accompanying unpleasant sensations during rest or inactivity only occur or are worse in the evening or night than during the day.
5. The occurrence of the above features is not solely accounted for as symptoms primary to another medical or a behavioral condition (e.g., myalgia, venous stasis, leg edema, arthritis, leg cramps, positional discomfort, habitual foot tapping).

Specifiers for Clinical Course of Restless Legs Syndrome/ Willis-Ekbom Disease (RLS/WED)

A. Chronic-persistent RLS/WED: symptoms when not treated would occur on average at least twice weekly for the past year.
B. Intermittent RLS/WED: symptoms when not treated would occur on average <2/week for the past year, with at least five lifetime events.

Specifier for Clinical Significance of RLS/WED

The symptoms of RLS/WED cause significant distress or impairment in social, occupational, educational, or other important areas of functioning by their impact on sleep, energy/vitality, daily activities, behavior, cognition, or mood.

Modified from Allen RP, Picchietti D, Garcia-Borreguero, et al. Restless legs syndrome/ Willis–Ekbom disease diagnostic criteria: updated International Restless Legs Syndrome Study Group (IRLSSG) consensus criteria—history, rationale, description, and significance. *Sleep Med.* 2014;15:860–873.

TABLE 17.3	Words Commonly Used by Patients with Restless Legs Syndrome to Describe Their Leg Sensations

Creepy-crawly
Ants crawling
Jittery
Worms moving
Soda bubbling in the veins
Electric current, shock-like feelings
Pain
Burning
Jimmy legs/Elvis legs
Throbbing
Grabbing sensation
Itching bones
Crazy legs
Just need to move

Modified slightly from Allen RP, Picchietti D, Hening WA, et al. Restless legs syndrome: diagnostic criteria, special considerations, and epidemiology. A report from the restless legs syndrome diagnosis and epidemiology workshop at the National Institutes of Health. *Sleep Med.* 2003;4(2):101–119.

pain and are often reported as painful.[13] The words describing the sensation, however, differ from those used for peripheral neuropathy[14] and are more consistent with the studies indicating that they involve the central or emotional pain pathways in the brain.[15]

- Movements without sensory symptoms do not define RLS: It is important to note that the urge to move the legs is a strong sensory phenomenon and not something that happens unconsciously. Thus patients reporting surprise that others tell them they are moving their legs all the time do not meet this diagnostic criterion unless they are themselves sometimes aware of the urge to move. Habitual foot tapping or involuntary leg movements (LMs) may commonly occur with RLS, but do not suffice to make the diagnosis. This important distinction is often lost when making the diagnosis.
- RLS sensations are episodic during waking: The sensations are rarely always present; instead, they come and go, frequently with a rather abrupt onset. They persist for at least a few minutes and sometimes hours if the patient does nothing to relieve them. Factors affecting when the symptoms occur and how they can be relieved serve to further define the disease.
- Three critical factors must affect expression of the primary RLS sensations: (1) onset associated with rest, usually sitting or lying down; (2) at least partial or complete relief with movement; and (3) a circadian pattern with symptoms worse in the evening and night for a normally entrained 24-hour cycle.
  - In general, onset with rest occurs in relation to the duration of rest and requires resting of both the body and mind. Since not all rest induces the symptoms, the critical question is whether the sensory symptoms ever start when active. This should essentially never occur in patients with RLS, unless the disorder is so severe that it occurs most of the time.
  - Relief with movement may be partial or complete, and the severity of the symptoms often returns when the movement stops. When the symptoms become severe, the movements may need to be strenuous, such as fast walking, to experience appreciable relief. Other activities also reduce the symptoms, particularly any activity that increases alertness and decreases sleepiness, but significant movement should always have some effect. Shifting the leg to a new position and not continuing with any movement should provide minimal and short-lived benefit, if any at all. If this suffices for prolonged benefit, the diagnosis should be reconsidered.
  - Circadian pattern—worse at night: Symptoms are worse or may be present only in the evening or nighttime in patients with a normal circadian cycle. This must be carefully separated from the role of inactivity producing symptoms. Studies involving maintained rest or periods of rest throughout the day have demonstrated that this circadian pattern of symptoms occurs independent of either the level of activity or sleep loss.[16,17] These studies demonstrate a somewhat protected period in the morning, usually 8–12 AM, when symptoms are mild if they occur at all. As the disease becomes worse, symptoms spread to earlier in the evening and then into the afternoon but rarely occur during this protected morning period. The critical issue is not that the symptoms are worse in the evening or night, but rather whether the patient can remain at rest longer in the morning than in the evening or at night.

- Features of RLS supporting the diagnosis: Four clinical features of RLS that support the diagnosis should be noted: periodic limb movements (PLMs), family history, therapeutic response to dopamine treatment, and lack of profound daytime sleepiness despite significant sleep loss (Table 17.4).
  - PLMS occur in about 80%–90% of patients with RLS, especially when evaluated over more than 1 night.[18] The LMs during sleep and also frequently during resting wakefulness provide a sensitive but not specific indication of RLS.[19] Patients with RLS who do not have these movements should be reviewed carefully to ensure that the diagnosis is correct. RLS often runs in families, particularly if the RLS symptoms start before the age of 45. Thus another first-degree relative with RLS provides supportive evidence for the diagnosis in uncertain cases.
  - Dopaminergic treatment (levodopa and presumably any D_2/D_3 dopamine agonist) benefit almost all patients with RLS, and symptoms severe enough to be treated respond well to this treatment.[20] Failure to respond at least initially to these dopaminergic treatments should raise serious concerns about the diagnosis, but placebo responses also occur in patients who have leg symptoms but not RLS. Thus this feature, like PLMS, is very sensitive but may not be very specific.
  - Lack of significant sleepiness occurs for RLS despite low levels of significant sleep. RLS patients report sleepiness on the Epworth Sleepiness Scale (ESS) that ranges in general over the normal range, except for some younger RLS patients with less distressing RLS symptoms.[13] There is one report of a relatively small group of RLS patients with high ESS

TABLE 17.4	Features Supporting the Diagnosis of Restless Legs Syndrome

Family History

The prevalence of RLS in the first-degree relatives of a person with RLS that starts early in life (before the age of 45) is about seven times greater than for relatives of a person without RLS.

Response to Dopaminergic Therapy

Nearly all people with RLS show at least an initial positive therapeutic response to either levodopa or a D2/D3 dopamine receptor agonist at appropriate doses. This initial response may not persist.

Periodic Limb Movements (During Wakefulness or Sleep)

PLMS occur in most but not all patients with RLS. PLMS also commonly occur in other disorders and in healthy elderly individuals. Children rarely have significant PLMS unless RLS or a related disorder is present.

Lack of Profound Daytime Sleepiness

RLS patients may have chronic short sleep times but do not usually have the level of sleepiness expected for the degree of sleep loss and very rarely have profound daytime sleepiness. Thus patient alertness when evaluated in the day despite reporting sleep loss supports the diagnosis. Conversely, when profound daytime sleepiness is present, possible causes other than RLS should be evaluated.

PLMS, Periodic limb movements during sleep; *RLS*, restless legs syndrome.
Modified from Allen RP, Picchietti D, Garcia-Borreguero, et al. Restless legs syndrome/Willis-Ekbom Disease diagnostic criteria: updated international restless legs syndrome study group (IRLSSG) consensus criteria—history, rationale, description and significance. *Sleep Med.* 2014;15:860–873.

values, but these patients had on average only about 6 hours of sleep a night, which for some is inadequate to maintain daytime alertness.[21] Overall, sleepiness when present is in general significantly less than would be expected for the degree of sleep loss.[22] Thus when RLS patients present in a medical office, they may not be sleepy despite chronic severe sleep loss. Profound sleepiness may indicate a disorder other than RLS or effects of RLS treatment.[21]

Differential Diagnosis

- The differential diagnosis must be done carefully to exclude conditions that produce symptoms mimicking at least some of the characteristics of RLS. The most common but also easily discerned in a clinical setting are positional discomfort, leg cramps, positional ischemia (numbness), arthritis, leg shaking, jitters, and generalized nervousness.[23] In general, careful questioning differentiates the symptoms resulting from these conditions from those of RLS. Particularly critical considerations in the differential diagnosis are onset only when inactive, intermittent periods of symptoms and sometimes with an abrupt onset or worsening, some relief with movement soon after the movement starts, minimal involvement of joints, degree of awareness of the movements, efforts to resist making the movements indicating awareness of the movements, and a strong circadian pattern with relief in the morning. The differential diagnosis of neuropathies, myopathies, and venous stasis can be particularly difficult, and any indication of these problems should lead to careful evaluation to separate any RLS symptoms to be treated from those of the other medical conditions (Table 17.5).

Restless Legs Syndrome Phenotypes

- There are four dimensions defining clinically significant RLS phenotypes that should be considered when making the diagnosis: chronicity-persistence (clinical course), age at onset, family history, and indications for major secondary causes.
- Chronicity-persistence relates to the severity of the symptoms and is considered the most important clinical phenotype, since

TABLE 17.5	Common Considerations in the Differential Diagnosis of Restless Legs Syndrome

Nocturnal leg cramps
Positional discomfort
Local leg injury/arthritis
Positional ischemia (numbness)
Nerve damage (neuropathy, radiculopathy)
Sleep transition phenomena (e.g., hypnic jerks)
Leg shaking, jitters
Generalized nervousness
Myopathies
Venous stasis
Peripheral neuropathy
Akathisia
Claudication

Modified from Hening WA, Allen RP, Washburn M, et al. The four diagnostic criteria for the restless legs syndrome are unable to exclude confounding conditions ("mimics"). *Sleep Med.* 2009;10(9):976–981.

it signifies the potential need for treatment. RLS has a wide range of severity and when very mild may be intermittent, sometimes occurring only a few times a year. Most cases deserving treatment, however, are chronic and reasonably frequent. Thus phenotypes can be identified as either a chronic and persistent pattern that if not treated would have occurred on average at least twice a week for the past year versus an intermittent pattern with symptoms that occur less often or for a shorter period. Some consider only the chronic-persistent phenotype as RLS. This unfortunately confounds the need to treat with diagnosis. It fails to appreciate RLS is a neurologic disease with a sensory-motor abnormality producing symptoms that are not an extension of normal experience. Frequency, persistence, and clinical significance, while important for treatment, are not relevant for diagnosis, aside from having enough episodes to evaluate symptoms and circadian timing. Clinical specifiers for these phenotypes are included in the diagnostic criteria (see Table 17.2).

- The age at onset and family history phenotypes are closely associated. The risk for RLS is only about two times greater for relatives of RLS patients whose symptoms started after the age of 45.[24,25] Thus both the age at onset and the family history define this interesting population of familial RLS. Age at onset is the preferred measure, since the family history is distorted by a varying number of first-degree relatives, which is often very small.
- Secondary RLS produced by another medical condition: RLS starts with development of the other condition and in general improves with a reduction in the effects of this other condition. Three medical conditions produce RLS: (1) *end-stage renal disease,*[26] (2) *pregnancy,*[27] and (3) *iron deficiency anemia.*[28] RLS occurs in 30%–40% of patients with any one of these medical conditions, and in most cases the symptoms of RLS stop when the associated medical condition is resolved. These conditions all involve compromised iron status, and in general, any condition reducing the availability of iron to the brain will increase the risk for RLS.[29] Thus medical conditions producing iron deficiency, such as frequent blood donations[30] and major surgery,[31,32] have been associated with increased occurrence of RLS.
- RLS produced or exacerbated by medications: Some medications, particularly serotonin and norepinephrine reuptake inhibitors, may also produce or exacerbate RLS, although the supporting documentation has relied on a few clinical reports and some evidence linking increased PLMS to use of the medications. Use of levodopa has also converted patients with only PLMS into ones with clear RLS.[33] This effect of levodopa may explain the high prevalence of RLS with Parkinson's disease.[34]

Epidemiology

- Flawed methods overestimated prevalence at 10%–20%: Many of the studies on the epidemiology of RLS have used one to five questions answered by the subject that covered the four diagnostic criteria for RLS. These questions have rarely been validated against a clinical diagnosis of RLS, and there has been little effort to even remove the more common RLS mimics. When these questionnaires were validated against clinical diagnoses, they have been found to have a specificity of about 50%–60%,[35,36] and the early reports of an RLS prevalence of 10%–20% or higher should not be considered valid.

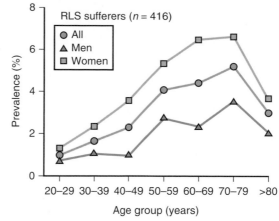

Overall prevalence: 3%–7%
- Lower in some Asian populations
- Higher in women over age 30
- Prevalence increases with age

REST studies
- Prevalence in childhood
  - 1.9%–2.0% any RLS
  - 0.5%–1.0% RLS sufferer

• **Figure 17.2** Graph for prevalence of sufferers of restless legs syndrome (RLS) in Western Europe and the United States by gender and age from the REST study. RLS sufferer defined by RLS symptoms occurring ≥2/week with moderate or extreme distress.[40,41] (Modified from Allen RP, Walter AS, Montplaisir J, et al. Restless legs syndrome prevalence and impact: REST general population study. *Arch Intern Med.* 2005;165:1286–1292.)

- Better validated methods, questionnaires—RLS prevalence 5%–7%. Three methods can be used to reduce the inaccuracies of self-reported questionnaire ascertainment of RLS.
  - First, some studies have focused on more severe illness and defined RLS "sufferers" as those with symptoms occurring at least twice a week for the past year with at least moderate distress when present, thereby removing the less certain, milder cases.[11]
  - Second, questionnaires have added items designed to exclude those with the more common mimics such as leg cramps, positional discomfort, and habitual responses.[23] Currently, there is one such validated questionnaire[37] that has been used successfully to exclude mimics in one study on work productivity and RLS. As expected, it showed that about 50% of those reporting the usual RLS symptoms had one of the major mimics producing the RLS symptoms.[35]
  - Third, studies have used a screening questionnaire followed by physician diagnosis.[36] The results from these more careful studies have tended to converge and indicate an overall prevalence in Western Europe and the United States for current (past year) RLS of about 5%–7% and for current RLS sufferers of 2%–4%.[11,36]
- Age and prior pregnancy increase RLS prevalence: In general, the prevalence of RLS increases with age up to about 60 years and may then decrease somewhat in the oldest age group. After about age 35, RLS is about twice as common in women than in men, but childhood and young adult life do not show a significant gender difference. Moreover, nulliparous women show the same risk of RLS as men,[38,39] indicating the gender difference may be mostly if not entirely due to delayed effects of pregnancy. The prevalence in children ages 8–17 is about 1%–2%, with no gender difference (Fig. 17.2).[40]
- RLS is common, clinically significant, yet not diagnosed: Despite its common occurrence and significant adverse effect on health, it remains underdiagnosed and undertreated. In one study, physicians indicated that in about 1% of all patients seen in their primary care, RLS severely decreased their health and well-being. These patients with severe RLS had on average 5.2 hours of sleep per night. Yet in that study RLS had not been previously diagnosed or treated in 71% of those with this severe RLS.[36]
- General population risk of developing RLS may be about 33%: Although primary RLS occurs in only about 5% of the population, this does not reflect the actual population risk for developing RLS. RLS, as noted previously, develops with medication conditions, particularly iron deficiency. However, about two-thirds of the population with iron deficiency do not get RLS, regardless of the severity of the iron deprivation (ID).[28] There appear to be genetic or epigenetic factors that strongly moderate risk of RLS with ID and presumably also the other conditions that produce RLS. This suggests that the risk of developing RLS, given the appropriate environmental factors, is present in about a third of the general population, at least for Europe and America.
- Prevalence summary: Overall, epidemiologic studies indicate that RLS is a common disease that increases in prevalence with age and affects adult women, particularly those who have been pregnant, more than men. It remains largely undiagnosed and untreated.

Neurobiology/Pathophysiology

- Research has identified more about the biology of RLS than we know about many similarly common chronic conditions such as depression, essential tremor, and fibromyalgia. The clinical features of RLS point to four major areas, with each demonstrating significant biologic abnormalities: dopamine, given the excellent treatment response to dopamine agonists and levodopa[19]; iron, given the clear indication that any condition compromising iron status increases the risk for and severity of RLS[27]; sleep disruption, producing a primary morbidity of RLS; and PLMS, the only motor sign of the disorder.[18]
- Iron: altered iron regulation with low brain iron
  - Low brain iron: It has long been known since the seminal studies by Ekbom and the more recent careful studies by O'Keeffe[42,43] and Allen[44] that lower peripheral iron status increases risk for the development and severity of symptoms. The presumed mechanism involves decreased availability of brain iron for metabolic activity, particularly in support of oxidative metabolism. Nordlander first proposed body tissue

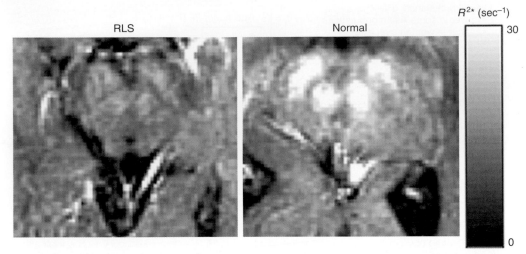

• **Figure 17.3** Magnetic resonance image showing the reduced iron content in the substantia nigra and red nucleus of a patient with restless legs syndrome (RLS) with respect to an age- and gender-matched control. The higher *(brighter)* R^{2*} relaxation rate indicates more iron concentration. (From Allen RP, Barker PB, Wehrl F, et al. MRI measurement of brain iron in patients with restless legs syndrome. *Neurology*. 2001;56[2]:263–265.)

iron deficiency as a primary cause of RLS and reported, in a small group of patients, successful treatment with intravenously administered iron.[45] More recent imaging work with both magnetic resonance imaging[46–48] and ultrasound[49] has documented brain iron deficiency in the substantia nigra of patients with RLS (Fig. 17.3). Decreased brain iron status has been further supported by decreased ferritin and increased transferrin in the cerebrospinal fluid (CSF) of RLS patients, despite normal peripheral iron levels.[50] Earlier age at onset of RLS appears to reflect a more significant brain iron abnormality,[51] although even patients with late-onset RLS have been found to have decreased brain iron.[48]

• Abnormal central and peripheral iron regulation in RLS: Autopsy studies have documented that the nigral iron deficiency occurs in the cytosol but not in the mitochondria, which in contrast to the cytosol have increased ferritin, a finding indicative of increased iron acquisition and storage.[52] Thus the iron metabolism disorder of RLS probably involves mitochondrial metabolic changes with increased iron demand producing cytosolic iron deficiency, possibly problems with iron-sulfur complexes and activation of the hypoxic pathway. This metabolic abnormality with hypoxic activation may to some extent involve tissue other than that from the brain. Lymphocytes in women with early-onset RLS have been found to show a pattern of abnormal iron regulatory proteins consistent with increased iron turnover (increased transferrin and also ferroportin), possibly related to mitochondrial iron increases.[53] The leg muscles of patients with RLS also show signs of activation of the hypoxic pathway expected for the iron metabolic problem of RLS.[54,55] In agreement with these findings was the leg weakness noted by Ekbom to be common in RLS patients.[5]

• Animal models—low brain iron and dopamine: The lower brain iron content provides a basis for an animal model of RLS involving dietary iron deficiency. Several studies have found that dietary ID, either starting with the fetus or after weaning, decreases rat and mouse brain iron levels. These models have found that lower brain iron decreases striatal

dopamine-2 receptor (D_2R) proportional to the amount of iron loss[56] and increases tyrosine hydroxylase (TH)[57] and extracellular dopamine, along with increases in the amplitude of the circadian changes in extracellular dopamine.[58] These ID animals also showed decreased dopamine transporter (DAT) that mostly involved membrane-bound DAT, thus indicating reduced trafficking of DAT to the cell surface, producing decreased functional DAT.[59]

• Iron—animal models for treatment evaluations: The problem with these models has been that they produce significant iron deficiency in both peripheral tissue and the brain, whereas RLS is associated with significant brain iron loss without significant peripheral iron deficiency and with normal hemoglobin.[50] The peripheral iron loss complicates evaluating efficacy of treatment. What is needed is a genetically identified mouse strain that responds to dietary iron deficiency with decreased brain iron, while maintaining normal hemoglobin. Such a strain has been identified (BXD strain 40[60]) and has been used to evaluate effects of IV iron treatment on brain iron.[61] It potentially provides a better behavioral model for the effects of brain iron deficiency characteristic of RLS and can be particularly useful for evaluating treatments of RLS, such as the IV iron study noted previously.

• Dopamine, increased in RLS: Despite the dramatic reduction in RLS symptoms produced by levodopa, the initial efforts failed to define a dopamine abnormality in patients with RLS.

  • Positron emission tomography (PET) studies found striatal D_2R upregulated, down-regulated, and not changed.[62–64] Single-proton emission computed tomography (SPECT) studies found no differences in striatal DAT between RLS patients and controls.[65–68]

  • CSF studies found no dopamine-related abnormalities in patients with RLS.[69,70] Fortunately, the ID animal studies demonstrated where to look for dopamine abnormalities in individuals with RLS. The animal studies indicated that DAT would be much more abnormal for membrane-bound DAT than for the total cellular DAT measured by most SPECT studies.

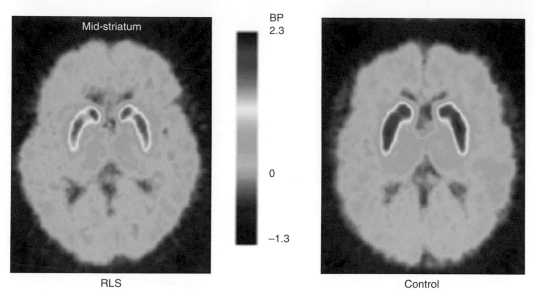

• **Figure 17.4** Examples of DAT binding in the striatum of a patient with RLS *(left)* when off any RLS treatment for at least 12 day and a matched control subject *(right)*. *BP,* Binding potential for dopamine site; *DAT,* dopamine transporter; *RLS,* restless legs syndrome. (Reprinted with permission from Earley C, Kuwabara H, Wong D, et al. The dopamine transporter is decreased in the striatum of subjects with restless legs syndrome. *Sleep.* 2011;34[3]:341–347.)

• Two recent PET studies involving ligand binding to the dopamine site of the dopamine transporter (DAT) that were more sensitive to membrane-bound DAT found the expected decrease in DAT in RLS patients in comparison to controls,[71] as shown in Fig. 17.4. Autopsy studies confirmed for RLS the decrease in striatal D_2R seen in the animal models but discovered that this was limited to more severe cases of RLS. This decrease was not present in milder cases of RLS, similar to those used in recent studies failing to find the decrease in D_2R.[57]

• Finally, autopsy studies also found the increased TH expected from the ID animal studies.[57] A closer look at the CSF found increased 3-*O*-methyldopa (3-OMD) in those with RLS that related to severity and also correlated with homovanillic acid levels,[72] consistent with increased TH activity. Thus, as expected from the animal studies, RLS in humans is characterized by a hyperdopaminergic state with increased dopamine production, decreased D_2R, and decreased DAT. The circadian expression of symptoms appears to reflect problems in the balance between postsynaptic receptors and the increased amplitude of the circadian variation in dopamine.

• Sleep-hyperarousal in RLS: Although reduced sleep time is the primary morbidity in RLS, dopaminergic treatments, despite reducing PLMS and RLS symptoms, in general fail to significantly increase sleep times.[73,74] A recent study reported magnetic resonance spectroscopy data showing that a measure of thalamic glutamate levels was increased in individuals with RLS, thus suggesting increased thalamic activity and, accordingly, reduced inhibitory activity required to maintain sleep.[75] Thus in addition to dopaminergic there may be some glutamatergic abnormality in RLS producing the sleep loss. This abnormality may have limited response to dopaminergic treatment.

• PLMS: The primary motor sign of RLS. See the section on PLMD.

Genetics of Restless Legs Syndrome

• Although several linkage studies have identified probable association of RLS within some families to regions on several chromosomes, they have failed to identify any specific gene associated with the occurrence of RLS.

• Genome-wide association studies, however, have identified increased relative risk for RLS to be significantly associated with 10 allelic variations (for homozygous carriers) in five different genomic regions: *MEIS1* on chromosome 2p, *BDBT9* on 6p, *MAP2K4/LBXCOR1* on 15q, and *PTPRD* on 9p.[76–79]

• The allelic variations are on introns, indicating probable regulation of expression rather than alteration of the proteins. *MEIS1*, one of the genes associated with a larger relative increase in risk for RLS, has, in one study, decreased expression with decreased protein in the brains of subjects with RLS.[80] Possible biologic pathways relating these genes to RLS pathology are being studied.

• Some promising studies have related these genes to PLMS[79,81,82] and iron metabolism[83] in humans. They have also been related to iron metabolism in *Caenorhabditis elegans*[84] and to both dopamine and iron status in drosophila.[85]

Restless Legs Syndrome Evaluation

• The IRLS scale: Subjective evaluation of the severity of RLS relies mostly on the IRLSSG's RLS severity scale, the IRLS (http://www.rls.org.au/pdf/PKGD6.pdf). Its 10 items are scored 0–4, with 4 indicating more severity. The 0–40 range has been somewhat arbitrarily divided into 0–10 for minimal/mild symptoms, 10–20 for moderate RLS, 20–30 for severe, and 30–40 for very severe.[86]

- The scale has been well validated and shows good interrater reliability, stability, good internal consistency, and good convergent validity.[87]
- It somewhat distorts mild ratings, so even very mild symptoms occurring for less than an hour a day only 1 day per week might produce a score of close to 10; consequently, patients with IRLS scores of 10 or less after treatment are often called remitters, whereas those with scores of zero are called symptom-free.[88]
- The scale has two subscales, one consisting of five items related to basic RLS symptoms and the other consisting of three items related to the impact of these symptoms on functioning.[89]
- Clinical history: As noted in the earlier section on epidemiology, the subjective frequency of symptoms in terms of days per week that symptoms occur is also used as a marker of severity. This is sometimes combined with an evaluation of the degree of distress caused by the symptoms when present.[11]
- Sleep studies: PLMS and sleep quality—objective evaluation of RLS severity has relied primarily on the rate of PLMs per hour of sleep. This has been found to correlate with the IRLS,[90,91] but this assessment is complicated by the increase in PLMS observed with age.[92] The benefits of treatment are sometimes evaluated in terms of decreases in PLMS and, less commonly, improvements in sleep on a polysomnogram. Various sleep studies at home or in the lab are useful for differential diagnosis and in some cases for treatment evaluations. While sleep studies are not required for diagnosis, improved multiple night at-home recordings would be very helpful for differential diagnosis, assessment, and treatment evaluation. Improving technology may make these available and practical in the near future.

Restless Legs Syndrome Morbidity

- Quality of life: As RLS becomes more severe, it profoundly affects the patient's ability to rest and relax, with reduced resting times in the afternoon and evening and significantly reduced sleep. It also appears to be associated with discomfort and pain, and in some cases with leg muscle weakness.[5,54]
- Patients with moderate to severe RLS (RLS sufferers with symptoms at least twice per week that are at least moderately distressing when present) are found to have reduced quality of life on most standard quality-of-life scales, such as the short-form health survey (SF-36).[11]
- RLS reduces mostly the subscales on the SF-36 related to energy/vitality and physical symptoms impairing normal daily functioning. RLS has been associated with an increased incidence of depression and anxiety disorders, particularly panic disorders,[93,94] but curiously, the quality-of-life scales indicate that the physical distress and decreased energy in patients with RLS affect their quality of life more than the mental health effects of the disease (Fig. 17.5).
- Daytime function/work productivity: Moderate to severe RLS significantly impairs daytime function[95] and produces 20%–50% loss of work productivity[35]
- Sleep disturbance: Patients with moderate to severe RLS have sleep times of less than 5.5 hours on most nights, and many sleep less than 5 hours per night most nights.[36] This degree of chronic sleep loss is greater than seen with most other disorders, yet RLS patients do not report the expected level of severe daytime sleepiness. Thus RLS patients, even with severe symptoms and short sleep at night, do not sleep late in the morning and show at most only moderate degrees of daytime sleepiness, much less than expected for the amount of sleep loss.[96] Overall,

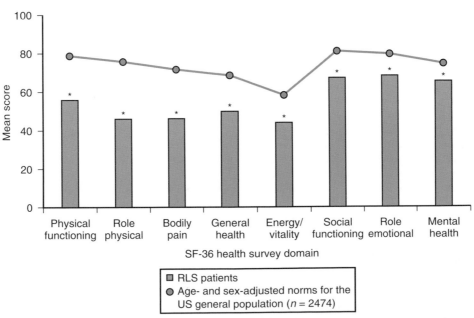

- **Figure 17.5** Short-form health survey (SF-36) scores for a population-based sample of untreated patients with restless legs syndrome (RLS) who reported that symptoms occur two or more times per week and cause moderate to severe distress (RLS sufferers, n = 375) versus US normative values. *Stars* above the *bars* indicate statistically significant differences. (From Allen RP, Walters AS, Montplaisir J, et al. Restless legs syndrome prevalence and impact: REST general population study. *Arch Intern Med.* 2005;165[11]:1286–1292.)

then, RLS produces a hyperarousal that disrupts and decreases sleep at night and reduces the expected daytime sleepiness from the shortened sleep at night.

- Cardiovascular disease (CVD): Possible association of RLS with either CVD or high blood pressure (HBP) has been evaluated in several population studies, but unfortunately using inadequate and unvalidated questionnaires for ascertainment of RLS producing mixed results, as might be expected given the limitations of the methods (see the section on epidemiology).
  - One study using a validated diagnostic interview has, however, reported an association with CVD,[97] and another prospective study of women using physician diagnosed RLS reported an increased risk for myocardial infarction and fatal CVD for those who had RLS for more than 3 years.[98]
  - Another study using physician diagnoses reported a significant increase in risk of CVD only for RLS, occurring secondary to another medical condition not for primary RLS. In contrast, primary RLS was associated with increased risk of HBP.[99] Possible mechanisms for these deficits include the chronic effects of frequent PLMS and sleep disruption associated with autonomic arousals and episodic transient blood pressure increases (see the "Periodic Leg Movements/Periodic Limb Movement Disorder of Sleep" section).[100]

Treatment

See Fig. 17.6 for overview and Table 17.6 for more details.

Medical Evaluation

- Medical history: In all cases of RLS, the medical history should be reviewed for indications of possible medical or medication factors contributing to the RLS. Treatment of associated medical problems such as iron deficiency may reduce the RLS symptoms. Medications known to cause problems with RLS (Table 17.7) should be reviewed to see whether they can be discontinued or if the dose can be decreased.
- Iron status: Patients should always be evaluated with at least a serum ferritin level from a morning blood sample. Those with a serum ferritin concentration of less than 75 μg/L should be considered for oral iron treatment, such as ferrous sulfate taken with a small dose of vitamin C (200 mg) to increase absorption. In some patients intolerant to oral iron or refractory to their RLS treatment, intravenous iron can be considered as described later in this chapter.
- Vitamin D deficiency: Low vitamin D may be related to increase risk of RLS.[101] In some studies, replacement treatment for vitamin D deficiency has been reported to reduce RLS symptoms.[102] Vitamin D levels should be considered, particularly for older patients and for those with limited exposure to sunlight. Excessive oral supplements can, however, produce vitamin D toxicity.

Nonmedication/Behavioral Treatment

- RLS symptoms, particularly when mild and intermittent, can often be adequately managed with behavioral adjustments, such as avoiding longer periods of inactivity, increasing alertness, and maintaining good sleep hygiene with slightly late bed and waking times.

TABLE 17.6	Details of Treatment Algorithm for Restless Legs Syndrome

All RLS

Behavioral management:
  Sleep hygiene, delayed sleep, regular activity, reduction of situations prolonging inactivity
Avoid medications that exacerbate RLS
Treat medical problems exacerbating or causing RLS as appropriate
Check iron status:
  Serum ferritin <50 μg/L, consider oral iron
  Ferrous sulfate with 200 mg vitamin C 2–3×/day as tolerated
  Stop iron treatment if percent saturation of transferrin ≤50% or serum ferritin >75 μg/L
  (Note intravenous iron treatment of refractory cases below)
Check vitamin D and supplement as needed; avoid overdose.

Intermittent RLS (<2/week)

PRN medications:
  Levodopa
  Milder opioids (hydrocodone, oxycodone)
  GABA-active hypnotics
  Ropinirole, pramipexole (low dose if tolerated)

Frequent Chronic RLS (>2/week, Persisting for Past Few Months)

First choice daily:
  Dopaminergic medications:
  Pramipexole, ropinirole, rotigotine
  α2δ Anticonvulsants
  Gabapentin, enacarbil, pregabalin
  Lower-potency opioids
  Hydrocodone, oxycodone
  (GABA-active hypnotics added/used PRN for sleep problems)

Refractory RLS (Not Responding to Initial 1st Choice Treatment—or Augmented)

Tailor treatment to specific need:
  Rotigotine 24-hour patch
    Provides response when other medications fail
  Combine treatment:
    Dopamine agonist + other type of drug
  Methadone (or other long-acting high-potency opioid)—for very severe cases, especially augmentation
  Consider 250–1000 mg iron intravenously when
    Iron deficiency persists despite adequate duration/dose of oral iron AND
    Serum transferrin percent saturation is low (<20%) and serum ferritin also remains low
    Avoid high-molecular-weight dextran

GABA, γ-aminobutyric acid; *PRN*, as needed; *RLS*, restless legs syndrome.
From Ondo WG. Intravenous iron dextran for severe refractory restless legs syndrome. *Sleep Med.* 2010;11(5):494–496.

- Behavioral interventions may also be used with more severe RLS to keep the medication dose lower. Nonmedical management also includes avoiding medications that may exacerbate or trigger RLS symptoms—particularly antihistamines that produce drowsiness.

Medication Treatment Guidelines

- Table 17.8 lists the current, commonly used pharmacologic treatments of moderate to severe RLS. Treatment with

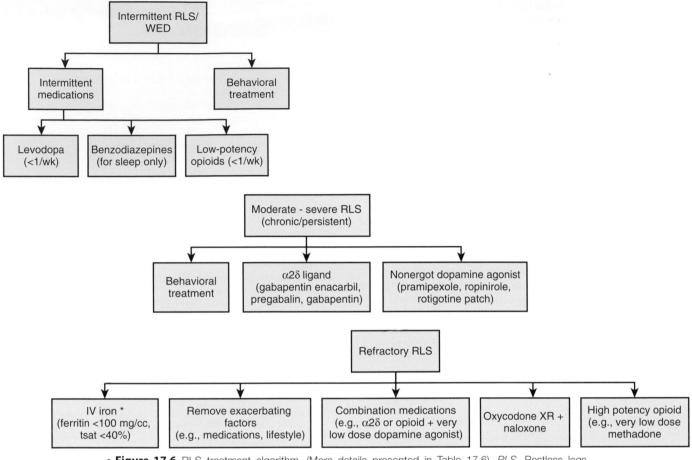

• **Figure 17.6** RLS treatment algorithm. (More details presented in Table 17.6). *RLS*, Restless legs syndrome; *WED*, Willis-Ekbom disease. (Adapted from Silber M, Becker P, Farley C, el al. Willis-Ekbom disease foundation revised consensus statement on the management of restless legs syndrome. *Mayo Clinic Proc.* 2013;88[9]:977–986.)

TABLE 17.7	Medications and Other Factors That Exacerbate Restless Legs Syndrome

To Be Avoided in Most Cases

Dopamine agonists (antiemetics, antipsychotics)
Antihistamines that are centrally active

To Be Used with Caution

SSRIs (e.g., fluoxetine, paroxetine, sertraline)
SNRIs (e.g., venlafaxine)
Tricyclic antidepressants (e.g., amitriptyline)
Tetracyclic antidepressants (e.g., mianserin, mirtazapine)
Lithium
Alcohol (especially lower doses)

SNRIs, Serotonin-norepinephrine reuptake inhibitors; *SSRIs*, selective serotonin reuptake inhibitors.

medications depends largely on the severity, timing, and morbidity of the RLS.

Infrequent or mild RLS can often be treated with behavioral adjustments, such as avoiding longer periods of inactivity, increasing alertness, and maintaining good sleep hygiene with slightly late bed and waking times. Behavioral interventions may also be used with more severe RLS to keep the medication dose lower.

Medication Treatment Considerations

- Table 17.8 lists the current, commonly used pharmacologic treatments of moderate to severe RLS. Treatment with medications depends largely on the severity, timing, and morbidity of the RLS.
- Mild or intermittent RLS symptoms (<2/week):
  - Mild RLS rarely needs medication treatment beyond oral iron and intermittent treatment for occasional situations where the RLS becomes a problem.
  - Intermittent RLS can be managed with very low doses of short-acting dopaminergic medications, particularly levodopa (100 mg with a drug to prevent peripheral uptake of levodopa; e.g., carbidopa or benserazide). Very low dose dopamine agonists can also be used if tolerated. These medications should not be given more than on average once a week. This approach requires early recognition of the start of the symptoms, so that the medication can be taken while the patient can still move about to manage the symptoms until the medication becomes effective. Behavioral management is particularly important for the management of intermittent RLS.
- Persistent moderate to severe RLS (≥2/week on average for past year): RLS occurring on average at least twice a week with moderate to severe distress usually requires medication to allow a satisfactory and functioning life.

TABLE 17.8 Commonly Used Pharmacologic Treatments of Restless Legs Syndrome with Total Daily Doses

Dopaminergic Drugs (Usual First-Line Treatment)

Drug	Receptor Affinity	Half-Life (h)	Starting Dose	Usual Dose	Usual Max Dose	Dose Schedule	Aug 1–3 year	Cautions	Comments
Levodopa	All D1–D5	1–2	50 mg	100 mg	200 mg	PRN, 1–2×/day	80%	Morning rebound. Use mainly PRN	Daily use is associated with severe augmentation and should in general be avoided.
Pramipexole	D1–D3	8–12	0.125 mg	≤0.5 mg	1 mg	1–2×/day	30%	FDA approved; max, 0.5 mg	
Ropinirole	D2–D3	6	0.25–0.5 mg	≤2 mg	4 mg	1–2×/day	7%–20%	FDA approved; max, 4 mg	
Rotigotine patch	D1–D3	N/A	0.5 mg/ 24 hours	1–2 mg/ 24 hours	3 mg/ 24 hours	1/day	2%–5%	Occasional skin rash	Rotigotine is available and approved in Europe. It is not available in the United States but is expected to be available in 2011–2012.
Cabergoline	D2–D3	60	0.5 mg	≤2 mg	7 mg	1/day	4%–9%	Rare fibrosis High cost in United States	Cabergoline is an ergot derivative and produces some significant fibrosis with valvular heart disease, so regular cardiac evaluation is recommended. It is not approved for the treatment of restless legs syndrome by any regulatory authority.

α2δ Anticonvulsants (First- or Second-Line Treatment)

Drug	Half-Life (h)	Starting Dose (mg)	Usual Dose (mg)	Usual Max Dose	Dose Schedule	Cautions	Comments
Gabapentin	5–7 (variable)	300	600–1200	2400	1–3×/day	Uptake may vary over time	
Enacarbil (gabapentin pro)	6–10	300–600	600	1200	1/day	FDA approved; 600 mg	Enacarbil has been approved in Japan and the United States. 300 mg dose should be adjusted in patients with renal impairment. Not recommended in RLS patients with a creatinine clearance less than 15 on hemodialysis.
Pregabalin		50–100	150–300	300–450	1/day	Approved for pain but not RLS	Pregabalin, though studied for RLS, has not at the time of writing this chapter been submitted anywhere for approval for use in patients with RLS.

Opioids (Second-Line Treatment, Particularly for More Severe RLS or Augmented RLS)

Drug	Half-Life (h)	Starting Dose (mg)	Usual Daily Dose (mg)	Usual Max Daily Dose	Dose Schedule	Cautions	Comments
Oxycodone-naloxone	12	5/2.5 mg	20/10 mg	40/20 mg	2×/day	EMA approved for RLS	Prolonged release oxycodone with naloxone. The doses are shown for oxycodone/ naloxone. Currently available only in the European Union. Biphasic fast followed by slow release of oxycodone.
Tramadol	6–7	50	50–200	200	1–2×/day	May produce augmentation	
Hydrocodone	3–4.5	5	5–15	20–25	1–2×/day		
Oxycodone	3–4	2.5–5	5–15	20–25	1–2×/day		
Methadone	15–30	2.5–5	10	20–30	1–2×/day		Methadone dose is lower than that for chronic pain or drug dependence Opioid use should be at the lowest possible dose and the patient monitored for dependence, respiratory suppression, sleep apnea, and depression.

Continued

TABLE 17.8   Commonly Used Pharmacologic Treatments of Restless Legs Syndrome with Total Daily Doses—cont'd

Oral and IV Iron Treatments Used with RLS

Oral Iron	Usual Dose	Method	Dose Schedule	Usual Max Daily Dose	Dose Schedule	Cautions	Comment
Ferrous sulfate		325 mg (65 mg iron)	325 mg	650 mg	1/day	Increases hepcidin, so once daily is preferred	All oral iron dosing should be adjusted to reduce adverse effects.
IV iron	Usual dose	Method	Initial dose	Initial schedule of doses	Iron available	Cautions	
Low–molecular-weight dextran	500–1000 mg	Slow infusion diluted (1 hour) or slow IV push	1000 mg	One treatment	2–4 weeks		
Ferric carboxy maltose	750 mg	Slow push	1500 mg	2 treatments 5 days apart Max dose	2–4 weeks		
Iron-sucrose	100–200 mg	Slow injection over 2–5 min	1000 mg	5–10 treatments 2×/week	About 6 hours	Rapid iron release—more immediate AE	
Iron-gluconate	125 mg	1 hour infusion diluted or slow injection over 10 min	1000 mg	8 treatments 2×/week	About 6 hours	Rapid iron release-more immediate AE	

GABA-Active Hypnotics (Improve Sleep for RLS patients, but Have No Significant Effect on RLS)

Drug	Half-Life (h)	Starting Dose (mg)	Usual Daily Dose (mg)	Usual Max Daily Dose	Dose Schedule	Cautions	Comment
Clonazepam	30–40	0.5	0.5–1	2	1/day	Reported to be very hard to stop	GABA-active hypnotics are not approved for long-term use, and dependence may be a problem. For a more complete listing and description, the reader is referred to Hening, Allen, Chokroverty, Earley, eds. *Restless Legs Syndrome*. Philadelphia: WB Saunders; 2009:238–278.
Zolpidem	2.5	5	5–10	10	1/day		

This table gives only the currently used medications. For some of these medications, there are limited reports indicating the usual clinical doses. Many other medications have been used with restless legs syndrome with varying degree of success. These other medications include most of the dopamine agonists, opioids, and γ-aminobutyric acid (GABA)-active hypnotics. *FDA*, US Food and Drug Administration; *N/A*, not available; *RLS*, restless legs syndrome.

- The first drugs approved by the US Food and Drug Administration (FDA) and EMA were the short acting nonergotamine dopamine agonists (ropinirole and pramipexole) given in doses considerably lower than that used for Parkinson's disease. When these were used over several months and years, they were found to commonly produce significant problems with tolerance and increased severity or augmentation of the RLS symptoms—worse than before starting treatment (see discussion later in this chapter).
- To avoid this significant problem, initial treatment of RLS has now shifted more to the ($\alpha2\delta$) ligands. The $\alpha2\delta$ ligand pregabalin (Lyrica) in a 1-year blinded controlled clinical trial was found to be as effective without the high rate of augmentation of pramipexole (Fig. 17.7).[12] This appears to be a drug class affect. Thus the $\alpha2\delta$ agents are considered an alternate and, for many, the preferred first line treatment of RLS.
- Refractory (nonresponsive) RLS:
  - Except for one opioid medication (oxycodone ER and naloxone, available in Europe), there are no blinded controlled clinical trials on the treatment of RLS patients who fail to have adequate response to the first-line medications noted previously.
  - Opioids including high potency opioids (e.g., methadone)[103] and IV iron[104] have been reported to be useful in this population. Drug combinations such as opioids with lower doses of dopamine agonists may have clinical appeal, but they have not been evaluated for RLS treatment.
- RLS augmentation: A common and a major problem producing severe RLS symptoms with long-term dopaminergic treatment. This often presents complicated treatment problems.
  - Identification and rates of occurrence: The major problem with long-term dopaminergic treatment of RLS is the development of an augmentation of the RLS symptoms. In this condition, all of the symptoms of RLS become worse and they spread both in time of day and body parts involved.
    - The most common characteristic is an advance in the first time of the day that the symptoms usually occur from the evening into the afternoon and even morning.[33] Augmentation seems to be related to the dose and specific medication.

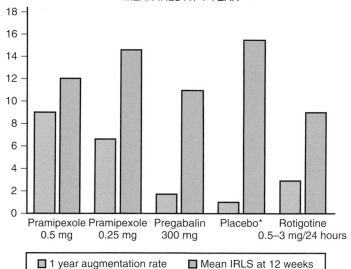

AUGMENTATION RATE % PER YEAR VERSUS EFFICACY-MEAN IRLS AT 1 YEAR

Legend:
□ 1 year augmentation rate   ■ Mean IRLS at 12 weeks

x-axis categories: Pramipexole 0.5 mg, Pramipexole 0.25 mg, Pregabalin 300 mg, Placebo*, Rotigotine 0.5–3 mg/24 hours

• **Figure 17.7** α2δ agent compared with dopamine agonists for efficacy and augmentation. Lower bars indicate better outcome for: IRLS efficacy *(red bars)* and percent with restless legs syndrome augmentation *(blue bars)* for dopamine agonist pramipexole (low and highest approved dose), compared with the α2δ agent pregabalin at 300 mg, placebo, and rotigotine patch (dose titrated for efficacy). Efficacy is from the double blind period for the 12 weeks. Augmentation is the rate over 1 year blinded study, with rates for placebo and rotigotine pro-rated from a 6-month blinded study for clinically relevant augmentation. *IRLS,* International restless legs syndrome study. (Copyright Richard P. Allen; Data are taken from Allen R, Chen C, Garcia-Borreguero D, et al. Comparison of pregabalin with pramipexole for restless legs syndrome. *N Engl J Med.* 2014;370:621–632; and Benes H, Garcia-Borreguero D, Ferini-Strambi L, et al. Augmentation in the treatment of restless legs syndrome with transdermal rotigotine. *Sleep Med.* [2012] 13:589–597.)

- Augmentation has been reported for all dopaminergic medications evaluated[105,106] and for tramadol,[107,108] but not for other opioids and not for α2δ anticonvulsants (see Fig. 17.7).
- Levodopa appears to produce augmentation in 30%–80% of patients within the first year of treatment.[33]
- Pramipexole has been reported to produce augmentation in about 30% of patients during the first 2–3 years of treatment.[109,110] A case series reported that augmentation in patients continuing with pramipexole treatment developed at a steady rate of about 7% per year for 9 years.[111]
- Very-long-acting dopaminergic medications such as cabergoline or transdermal rotigotine have been reported to have less augmentation.[112–114]
- Augmentation treatment:
  - Augmentation can sometimes be managed by advancing the time of treatment to cover the earlier onset of symptoms.
  - Keeping the dopamine agonist dose low and within the FDA-approved guidelines may also reduce the risk for significant augmentation.
  - When present, augmentation often eventually causes significant treatment problems that usually eventually

require a switch to alternative medications, either by a gradual decrease in the dopaminergic while introducing the new medication or by a gradual tapering of the dopaminergic with a few days free from medication before starting a new medication.[115] Fig. 17.8 presents the treatment options recommended by the IRLSSG to avoid or to manage RLS augmentation.

Commonly Used Medications for Restless Legs Syndrome Treatment

- α2δ ligands: As a class these are considered to be effective treatment for epilepsy (add-on for partial seizures), neuropathic pain, migraine, and generalized anxiety in addition to RLS. In general, these show efficacy for RLS within 1–7 days after starting treatment without long-term treatment problems of tolerance or augmentation. Slow titration to the therapeutic dose with increases weekly is advised.
  - Gabapentin (typically 300–2400 mg daily; two to three times a day): In general, this oldest α2δ ligand is available in generic form at lower prices than the other α2δ ligands. It has been found to be effective compared with placebo in several small double-blinded clinical trials, but has not been evaluated adequately in a large clinical trial. It has a major problem of variable and limited uptake into the blood that reduces efficacy and essentially prevents obtaining adequate therapeutic blood levels in some patients. This complicates dose adjustment and long-term treatment.
  - Gabapentin enacarbil (horizant; usual dose: 300–1200 mg, once daily): This prodrug of gabapentin resolves the uptake problem of gabapentin, providing reliable effective treatment usually lasting about 14 to almost 24 hours depending on dose. This has been shown to be effective compared with placebo for RLS in several large clinical trials.[116–118]
    - This is the only α2δ that has been approved by the FDA for use with RLS.
    - Starting and maintenance doses of 600 mg are standard but 300 mg is recommended for patients with compromised renal function, and dosed based on creatinine clearance (CrCl). No generic versions are available.
  - Pregabalin (Lyrica; usual doses of 150–450 mg, once daily): This drug has been evaluated compared with placebo in two reasonably large clinical trials,[119] including a trial with a blinded 1-year extension showing, if anything, better treatment outcome than the dopamine agonist pramipexole (see Fig. 17.7).[12] In general, this drug is effective for about 10–15 hours so that for most patients once daily dosing suffices, but twice daily may be required for more severe RLS. Generic versions of this drug are available in Canada and the United Kingdom and are expected to be available after 2018 in the United States.
  - α2δ agents common adverse effects: Sleepiness, dizziness, confusion, and weight gain may occur at least initially in treatment with these drugs. Dizziness may be a problem to watch, particularly for older RLS patients. More serious adverse effects of suicidal ideation, angioedema, and drug dependency have been reported for pregabalin. Pregabalin has also been listed as a schedule V drug, owing to the abuse potential. These more serious adverse effects have not been adequately documented to occur more than in the general population with the other α2δ ligands, but caution is advised

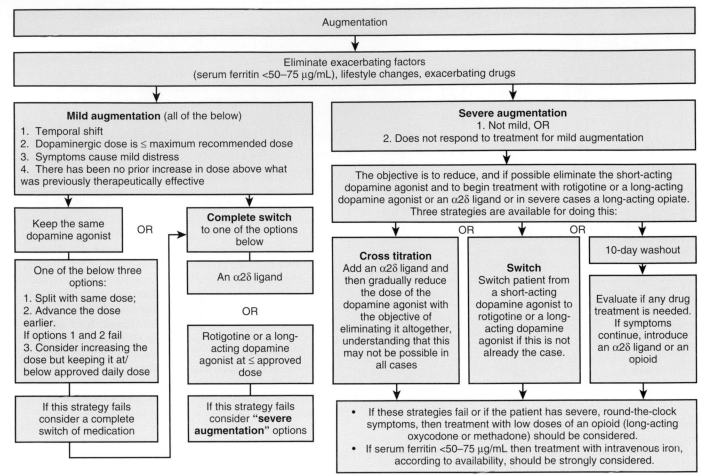

- **Figure 17.8** Treatment options for restless legs syndrome augmentation on dopaminergic drugs. (Reproduced with permission from the International Restless Legs Syndrome Study Group Foundation from Garcia Borreguero D, Silber M, Winkelman J, et al. Guidelines for the first-line treatment of RLS/ WED, prevention and treatment of dopaminergic augmentation. *Sleep Med.* 2016;21:1–11.)

about rare occurrences of these, especially for suicidal ideation.

- Dopaminergic medications: These are the most commonly used drugs for RLS. They are immediately effective the day they are taken but show long-term problems with tolerance and augmentation, particularly at higher doses. It is strongly recommended that for RLS the dose of these drugs is kept low and does not exceed the recommended maximum. Generic versions are available for all of these drugs except the long-acting dopamine agonists.
  - Levodopa (Sinemet, Madopar, Prolopa). Usual doses of 100–200 mg are given two to three times daily. This was the first dopamine drug found to be effective in treatment of RLS.[8] Levodopa is associated with a high risk of rapid development of worsening of RLS (augmentation)[33,120] and is not recommended, except for limited PRN use no more than once or twice weekly. It is strongly recommended not to exceed 200 mg daily dose for treatment of RLS.
  - Dopamine agonists—intermediate duration of action (Pramipexole: Mirapex, Sifrol. Ropinirole: Requip). Usual doses of pramipexole are 0.125–0.5 mg and ropinirole are 0.5–2 mg, both given one to two times a day. These are currently the most commonly used first-line medications for RLS and are available as generics. Their efficacy compared

with placebo for RLS has been supported by several large clinical trials,[121] but they both have a high risk of developing augmentation.[106,111,122] Both the FDA and the EMA have approved these for treatment of RLS. It is strongly recommended not to exceed the maximum daily dose of 0.5 mg for pramipexole and 4 mg of ropinirole.

- Long-acting dopamine agonists. (Rotigotine patch: Nupro. Extended release pramipexole: Mirapex ER. Ropinirole extended release: Requip Modutab). Usual given as once daily doses. For the rotigotine patch, use 1–3 mg/2 hours. ER pramipexole and ropinirole ER doses are not established, but consider the same range as shorter acting forms.
  - Rotigotine has been demonstrated effective compared with placebo for treatment of RLS in several large clinical trials[88,113,123] and is approved by both the FDA and EMA. This is the first medication for which treatment is reported to produce a large percentage of remitters (50%–60%), as well as patients symptom free (23%) for months.[88] The extended release versions of pramipexole and ropinirole have not been evaluated for efficacy treating RLS in clinical trials and have not been used in general for treatment of RLS.
- Common dopaminergic adverse effects: Dopaminergic treatment of RLS is associated with the usual short-term

problems seen with the treatment of Parkinson's disease, particularly nausea, insomnia, and peripheral edema. Orthostatic hypotension, hallucinations, and dyskinesia occur with dopaminergic treatment of Parkinson's disease but have only very rarely if ever been associated with treatment of RLS.

- Three more serious dopaminergic adverse effects: augmentation, sleepiness, and impulsive behavior:
  - Augmentation unlike the other adverse effects of dopaminergic treatment is unique to RLS. It is common, often severe, and hard to manage.
  - Increased impulsive behavior such as inappropriate shopping, gambling, and sexual activity has been reported to occur in about 9% of RLS patients undergoing dopaminergic treatment.[124] Patients may not be aware that these problems have developed, so it is important for the clinician to always warn and ask about these potential problems. They appear to be dose related.[124] Reducing the dose or switching to a different medication may be needed to correct these problems.
  - Significant daytime sleepiness with sleep attacks while driving have also been reported for RLS patients on higher doses of dopamine agonists.[125]
- Opioid medications: Almost all opioids have been reported to benefit RLS, but opioid treatment of RLS has been studied very little. A small double-blind placebo-controlled study showed oxycodone compared with placebo provided effective RLS treatment.[126] One large clinical trial demonstrated that prolonged-release oxycodone combined with naloxone (Targin) was more effective than placebo for treatment of RLS patients who had failed to have adequate treatment with a dopaminergic drug.[127] The EMA approved this drug for this second-line treatment of RLS. Table 17.8 lists the more commonly used opioids.
  - High potency opioids (e.g., methadone): Very severe RLS, particularly those with severe RLS augmentation, have been reported to respond well to treatment with long-acting higher-potency opioids such as methadone at doses lower than usual for chronic pain.[94,95]
  - Major opioid adverse effects: Aside from the usual opioid adverse effects (e.g., constipation, sleepiness), RLS patients treated with opioids need to be carefully monitored for problems of dependence, depression, and decreased respiratory drive.

Special Note on IV Iron Treatment of Restless Legs Syndrome

- Treats RLS biology: IV iron treatment has an obvious appeal of one treatment, potentially providing fairly long-term correction of a primary pathophysiology of RLS (i.e., low brain iron). It has several small to medium studies indicating efficacy and safety that differs by IV iron formulation.
- Preclinical efficacy and safety: One preclinical study with a dietary iron-deficient murine RLS model used iron isomaltoside at an IV dose of equivalent to the 1000 mg dose commonly used in humans. The evaluations at 3 and 10 days after treatment showed significant increases in brain iron only for the areas that had low iron resulting from the diet (ventral midbrain, nucleus accumbens). The results indicated regional brain iron regulation takes up the iron only where there is an iron deficiency. There was no indication for iron overload and in particular no

change in regions that were not iron deficient.[61] This study, while supportive of safety and efficacy of IV iron treatment, only evaluated a limited number of brain regions.

- Clinical efficacy and safety indicate the preferred choice of iron formulation:
  - The three controlled trials of IV iron treatment using 1000 mg iron sucrose showed mixed results in RLS patients with normal or low-normal serum ferritin.[128,129]
  - A clinical case series showed benefits for IV iron sucrose treatment of pediatric RLS/PLMS with reduced low serum ferritin.[130] One controlled clinical trial using 1000 mg ferric carboxymaltose showed significant treatment benefit compared with placebo for RLS patients not screened to exclude iron deficiency.[131]
  - Four open-label clinical trials have reported effective treatment for about 50%–60% of RLS patients with 1000 mg IV iron dextran.[132–134] No significant safety or adverse effects have been reported in these clinical trials, aside from the possible anaphylaxis response to high-molecular-weight iron dextran, an iron formulation that should not be used with RLS patients. The other formulations have very low risk of this significant reaction.
  - The clinical data further indicate that in general iron formulations that release the iron quickly (e.g., iron sucrose) have less benefit for RLS than the formulations that release the iron more slowly (e.g., ferric carboxymaltose, low-molecular-weight iron dextran). Table 17.8 provides the currently available IV iron formulations that have been tested in RLS patients.
- IV iron treatment guidelines:
  - No formal guidelines have been developed for IV iron treatment of RLS. At this point, IV iron treatment has not been adequately validated in placebo-controlled trials to be considered an effective initial treatment for RLS. Its use, therefore, is limited in general to those cases with low iron status, particularly iron-deficient anemia,[135] but it has found increasing use with patients who are not responding well to other treatments.
  - Care must be taken to avoid high-molecular-weight dextran and to ensure availability of adequate response to potential adverse effects, including the very unlikely but possible anaphylaxis. A few repeated doses can be considered for some patients who respond well initially to IV iron treatment but had a return of symptoms. Repeat IV iron can be considered with transferrin saturation less than 45% and serum ferritin less than 300 mcg/L.

Periodic Leg Movements/Periodic Limb Movement Disorder of Sleep

History

- Earliest identification—myoclonic to periodic events: When Symonds discovered the periodic leg muscle jerking in sleep, he saw it as a myoclonic type of activity modulated by the sleep state and gave it the name used in much of the early literature: sleep-related myoclonus.[136] However, the report by Lugaresi and colleagues of these movements in RLS patients[137] served to redefine these as periodic events of sleep that do not in either form or pattern relate to myoclonus. They were then somewhat more appropriately referred to as PLMs of sleep. These movements were associated with arousals and, particularly in RLS patients, appeared to be part of their sleep problem.

- Development of recording methods:
  - Electromyographic (EMG) studies using surface electrodes to record activation of various muscles in the legs found that in these periodic events the anterior tibialis was the primary and most commonly activated muscle. It produces dorsiflexion of the foot at the ankle.
  - Extension of the large toe is often also seen with these movements reflecting contraction of the hallucis longus. Neither of these muscles actually produces a LM; nonetheless, recording of the anterior tibialis alone is the standard for defining PLMS.
  - Some early studies identified somewhat similar periodic movements in the arms that unfortunately led to the current use of the term "periodic limb movements" of sleep. But this resulted from a very loose definition of periodicity that counted all the movements that occurred within 5–90 sec of each other. Recent studies have demonstrated that these arm movements during sleep in general do not show the periodicity defining PLMS.[138] Thus PLMS in this chapter refers only to LMs, not limb movements.
- Recognition and limits as a sleep disorder:
  - When recorded as part of a routine sleep evaluation, it was discovered that PLMS are common in adults. Their appearance in patients with sleep complaints led to the concept that these movements either caused some of the sleep problems or marked a process disrupting sleep.
  - Early efforts to classify PLMS as significant led to establishing a criterion of greater than 5 per hour of sleep, as indicating a possible sleep disorder. Since they occurred in patients without any indication of RLS or other sleep disorder, they were considered to reflect a new sleep disorder referred to as "periodic limb movement disorder." It was only with the increasing attention to sleep recordings in adults without any sleep complaints that PLMS was appreciated to commonly occur without any significant sleep-related symptoms. The movements increase to high rates in older adults, without association with any sleep complaints.[92]
  - PLMS have been documented to occur with many sleep disorders, particularly those involving dopamine pathology, but in small case series they have not been related to the insomnia or hypersomnia sleep complaints.[139,140] A large population-based study, however, found them related to poor sleep quality in older men.[141]
  - PLMS unrelated to RLS are now considered to have uncertain significance for sleep disturbance, but they may be significant for the associated transitory increases in heart rate and blood pressure or indicators of autonomic arousal (see the section on PLMS morbidity that follows).[142,143] The prevalence of PLMD is currently unknown.

Current Limitations and Development of New Periodic Limb Movements in Sleep Standards

- A basic problem with the extensive literature on PLMS is the failure to evaluate the periodicity of the movements.
- The criteria used to define PLMS effectively included all anterior tibialis contractions (foot dorsiflexions) that occurred within 5–90 sec of each other. There was no requirement that these showed a periodic process with a reasonably well-defined mean period and modest variance about the period, as observed in

the early work by Symonds and common for RLS patients. New standards emphasizing periodicity have been developed, as discussed later. These may significantly alter the issues of relation of PLMS to sleep, age, and medical conditions. It may be that these better defined PLMS mark a basic periodic process reflecting varying degrees of autonomic if not EEG arousal activity in sleep. These PLMS with a clear periodicity, pronounced frequency, and magnitude, as they tend to be in RLS, may therefore identify a process disturbing health and sleep. If so, their measurement becomes an important aspect of sleep evaluation.

Measurement of Periodic Leg Movements

- Criteria defining LMs and PLM: The updated standards of the International Restless Legs Study Group/World Association of Sleep Medicine for scoring PLM emphasize the periodic process more than in prior standards.[144]
  - An LM is defined as an increase in anterior tibialis EMG activity of 8 μV above the resting baseline that persists as a movement until the EMG activity drops below 2 μV above resting level and stays below that level for at least 0.5 sec. The LM must be at least 0.5 sec long and have a morphology that includes a burst of persistent activity lasting at least 0.5 sec with the median EMG, exceeding 2 μv above the resting level.
  - A candidate leg movement (CLM) for a PLM must be a LM with duration <10 sec (Fig. 17.9).
  - Bilateral LMs are counted as one LM, even if they overlap within 0.5 sec; otherwise each monolateral movement is evaluated as a separate LM.
    - A bilateral CLM for a PLM cannot contain more than four separate overlapping monolateral LMs. This often excludes alternating LMs, as noted later.
  - PLM must occur in a consecutive series of at least 4 CLM that each have an intermovement interval (IMI, time between consecutive movements) of 10–90 sec.
    - This series must not include any LM that is not a CLM or any CLM with an IMI less than 10 sec. In general, the CLM with IMI less than 10 sec have a distribution pattern that differs from those with IMI greater than 10 (Fig. 17.10).
- A LM–associated arousal is an EEG arousal occurring within 0.5 sec before or after the LM.
- Respiratory associated LM are defined as LM that occur within (before or after) 0.5 sec of the end of the SDB event. Some studies have indicated that for moderate to severe obstructive sleep apnea, the LM that start between 1.5 sec before to 2.5 sec after the sleep apnea should be excluded for the PLMS, excluding SDB LM.
- PLM are first calculated for all LM, and then if there are significant SDB events, the PLM are recalculated excluding all SDB-associated LM. This gives two PLMS rates—one including and one excluding the LM associated with SDB.
- Conditions for assessing PLM. PLM have been found to occur during both sleep and resting waking. Here the pattern suggests that the sleep-related movements intrude into wakeful resting rather than the reverse, as seen for most other movement disorders such as tics. Thus PLM are disordered movements of sleep and wakeful resting, and not full awakening. PLM during sleep are referred to as PLMS, whereas during waking they are called periodic leg movements during wakefulness (PLMW).

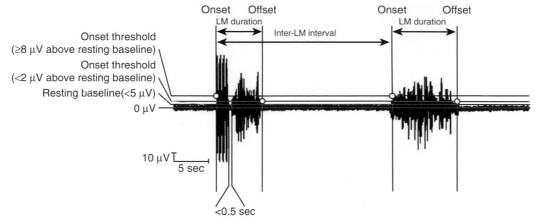

• **Figure 17.9** Overview of criteria for scoring periodic leg movement (PLM). Candidate PLMs are defined by electromyographic (EMG) onset of 8 µV or greater above the resting level with offset criteria being 0.5 sec or longer at an EMG value of less than 2 µV above the resting level. The duration of leg movement must be 0.5–10 sec. PLMs are defined as four or more consecutive leg movements with intervals of 5–90 sec between movements. Movement events that do not meet the criteria for PLM stop the run of PLM. *LM*, Leg movement. (From Zucconi M, Ferri R, Allen R, et al. The official World Association of Sleep Medicine [WASM] standards for recording and scoring periodic leg movements in sleep [PLMS] and wakefulness [PLMW] developed in collaboration with a task force from the International Restless Legs Syndrome Study Group [IRLSSG]. *Sleep Med*. 2006;7[2]:175–183.)

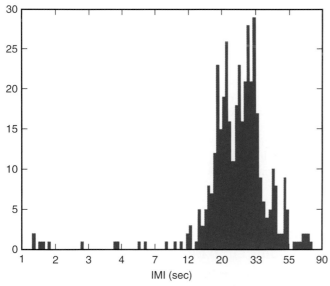

• **Figure 17.10** Histogram of the occurrence of candidate leg movements (CLM) of a restless legs syndrome patient by intermovement interval (seconds shown on natural log scale). There is an approximate log-normal distribution for intermovement interval (IMI) ≥ 10 sec. These represent the periodic process for periodic leg movements in sleep. For IMI < 10 sec the CLM appear randomly distributed and not periodic. (Data provided by Dr. Richard P Allen, Neurology, Johns Hopkins University; Copyright Richard P. Allen.)

PLMW occur in wake time during the night sleep period and during resting while awake in the daytime. The suggested immobilization test (SIT) involves sitting up in bed relaxed and awake with the legs stretched out for an hour. The SIT demonstrates high rates of PLMW (>40/hour) in RLS patients[145] that occur much more frequently in the evening and during night awakenings than in the daytime. PLMW tend to be provoked by a longer duration of resting and thus are more

pronounced after 40 min than during the first 20 min of resting in a SIT.[146]

Periodic Limb Movements in Sleep Biology

- PLMS are a consequence and sign but not a cause of autonomic arousal. Several studies have identified a pattern of autonomic activation in which an increased heart rate and delta EEG activity precede the PLMs.[147–149] Thus PLMs represent the consequences and not the cause of episodic autonomic arousal events during sleep. These arousal events have been found to include increases in blood pressure averaging 22 mm Hg for systolic and 11 for diastolic. The increases were larger for PLMS with more cortical EEG arousal, such as those more commonly seen in patients with RLS.[142,143] The arousal events are not usually recognized by the sleeper. They suggest a progression of central nervous system activation from brainstem to cortical levels. The medical significance of frequent episodic autonomic arousal and increases in blood pressure remains uncertain, but it has been suggested that they could contribute to the increased risk for CVD reported for RLS patients.[150]
- Spinal mechanisms for PLMS: The autonomic arousals with PLMS appear to occur with some disinhibition of spinal mechanisms. Thus there is evidence of increased spinal motor excitability in patients with RLS and PLMS.[151,152] It has been suggested that the disinhibited spinal system produces in part the periodicity. Consequently, PLM will be seen in patients with high cord lesions.[151,152] PLM may represent a complicated interaction of brainstem and cortical arousal disinhibiting spinal motor mechanisms, which in turn contribute to periodic reoccurrence of the related CNS and autonomic events.
- Genetics and iron—PLMS: Genetics and iron relate to occurrence of PLMS (Fig. 17.11). The very first study on RLS genetics noted the relation of BTBD9 to both serum ferritin and PLMS.[79]
  - Two recent studies have reported that the major genetic allelic variations increasing the risk of RLS are also associated with more PLMS. This occurs in a general population

- Genetics: Shares risk alleles with RLS
  - Stefansson, H 2007: BTBD9
    - Moore, 2014 : BTBD9, MEIS1, Tox3/BC034767, PTPRD(A)
    - Winkelman, 2015: BTBD9 (2), MEIS1(1), MAP2K5/SKOR1(1)
- Iron: Low ferritin in a general population (not selected for RLS
  - PLMS/hour <15 predicted by low ferritin (<50 mcg/L)
    - OR 1.55 (1.18, 1.91) $P <.020$
      (Li, J et al Sleep Med. (2015) 16(11): 1413–8)
- Iron: Substantia Nigra brain iron ppm
  versus PLMS/hour
  RLS patients
  r = 0.54 (p <0.01)
  PLMS- reflects brain iron status
  (Xu, L et al Sleep Med [2016] in press)

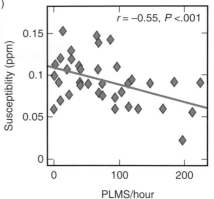

- **Figure 17.11** Genetics and iron both relate to PLMS following the same pattern that they relate to restless legs syndrome (RLS). *PLMS/hour,* Periodic leg movements in sleep per hour of sleep; *OR,* odds ratio with 95% confidence limits. (Figure reproduced from Xu L, Allen RP, Earley CJ, et al. Brain iron deficiency in idiopathic restless legs syndrome measured by quantitative magnetic susceptibility at 7 Tesla. *Sleep Med.* 2016;22:75–82; Other References: Stefansson H, Rye DB, Hicks A, et al. A genetic risk factor for periodic limb movements in sleep. *N Engl J Med.* 2007;357[7]:639–647; Moore H 4th, Winkelmann J, Lin L, Finn L, Peppard P, Mignot E. Periodic leg movements during sleep are associated with polymorphisms in BTBD9, TOX3/BC034767, MEIS1, MAP2K5/SKOR1, and PTPRD. *Sleep.* 2014;37[9]:1535–1542; Winkelman J, Finn L, Young T. *Sleep Med.* 2006;7[7]:545–552; and Li J, Moore H, Lin L. Association of low ferritin with PLM in the Wisconsin Sleep Cohort. *Sleep Med.* 2015;16[11]:1413–1418.)

not selected to include only those with RLS. In particular these studies identified significant association with the RLS risk alleles on BTBD9, TOX3/BC034767, MEIS1, MAP2K5/SKOR1, and PTPRD, but not for the intergenic region rs6747972(A). The association with MAP2K5/SKOR1 was somewhat marginal.[81,82] Despite considerable overlap, it appeared the relative importance of the alleles and genes differed somewhat for PLMS compared with that for RLS.

- A general population study has confirmed the association of low serum ferritin with high PLMS/hour (>15). An MRI study has confirmed the expected relation between substantia nigra iron and the PLMS/hour in RLS patients. It is noteworthy that recent studies with children who have PLMS and sleep disturbance have reported oral and IV iron provide significant relief.[130,153,154]

Epidemiology of Periodic Leg Movements

- Age effects differ for PLMS and PLMW: In general, PLMS are low in childhood and into young adult life. They may be somewhat higher in younger children than in young adults, but the major increase occurs after the age of 40. The average PLMs per hour of sleep for normal adults is about 15 for those 50–59 and about 20 for those older than 60 years, but there is a large variance, even among healthy adults.[92] PLMS have IMI peaks of around 15–35 sec in adults older than 40 years, but not in younger adults or children, thus suggesting a lack of structured periodicity of LMs in those younger than 40 without any sleep disorder. PLMW during nighttime sleep were, in contrast to PLMS, higher in younger than older subjects.[92]

- PLMS occur more in families with RLS. PLMS appear to be increased more than expected for age in patients with RLS and in many individuals with other dopamine-related disorders such as Parkinson's disease and narcolepsy. The commonly occurring age-related increase in PLMS has been reported to not occur in subjects who were selected as first-degree relatives of healthy adults experiencing PLMS at a rate lower than 10/hour.[155] This is consistent with the shared genetics of RLS and PLMS.

Morbidity of Periodic Leg Movements of Sleep and Periodic Limb Movement Disorder

- Limited relation of PLMS per se to sleep disruption: Despite the striking appearance of multiple PLMS on the polysomnogram, there has been very limited evidence relating the PLMS per se to any significant sleep-related morbidity in small studies.[156–158] A large general population study, however, found PLMS related to poor quality sleep in older men.[141] Moreover, dopaminergic medications reduce PLMS in RLS patients but do not significantly improve total sleep times.[73,74,159] The γ-aminobutyric acid (GABA)–active hypnotics, in contrast, improve sleep times and reduce arousals, but have relatively little effect on PLMS.[160,161] It should be noted, however, that these prior studies did not evaluate actual periodicity, nor did they evaluate the degree of actual LMs versus foot dorsiflexion.

- PLMS and cardiovascular morbidity: PLMS are clearly related to significant transitory effects on blood pressure and heart rate noted earlier, and reflect significant autonomic arousal. Studies of the clinical significance have suggested some increased risks for poorer outcomes for cardiac patients.[162] Children with PLMS may have increased nocturnal blood pressure.[163] Overall, except for children and patients with cardiac disease, health-related morbidity of PLMS remains unclear, as does the relation to sleep quality. A recent study, however, found that dopamine agonist treatment of RLS patients significantly reduced their frequent transitory increases in blood pressure and heart rate,[164] raising the question of whether these have enough consequences to warrant dopamine treatment, at least for RLS patients.

Periodic Limb Movement Disorder as a Significant Sleep Disorder

- Despite the limited published clinical data, there remains a clear awareness among sleep medicine specialists that some of their patients with sleep-related complaints and very high rates of PLMS with associated arousals benefit from the diagnosis of PLMD and appropriate treatment.[160,165] Lacking more large clinical studies of PLMD and PLMS, the consensus among clinicians is to maintain the status of PLMD as a clinically significant sleep-related movement disorder.

Diagnosis of Periodic Limb Movement Disorder

- PLMD diagnostic criteria for adults and children: PLMD requires an overnight sleep study documenting the number of PLMS, along with clinical evidence linking the PLMS to a sleep-wake complaint (Table 17.9 for the diagnostic criteria for PLMD). The initial definition of PLMD required five PLMs per hour, but recognition of the high rate of PLMS in healthy normal sleepers has changed this standard. The adult diagnostic criterion is now ≥15 PLMS per hour, and clinical judgment is needed to recognize the relevance of PLMS for sleep-wake complaints. The requirement of clinical judgment recognizes the wide individual differences in the sleep-related effects of PLMS. Children, in contrast to adults, have low rates of PLMS, so the

TABLE 17.9	**Diagnosis of PLMD (Slightly Modified from ICSD-3)**

A. Polysomnogram-demonstrated PLMS
B. PLMS >15/h for adults and >5/h for children
C. PLMS must be seen as causing significant sleep disturbance or impaired functioning (mental, physical, social, occupational, educational, behavior, or other significant area).
D. The PLMS is not better explained by another current sleep disorder, medical, or neurologic disorder, mental disorder, medication use, or substance use disorder (note that leg movements occurring with apneas are not counted as PLMS for the diagnosis of PLMD).
E. Diagnosis requires all of the above.

If PLMS are present without clinical sleep disturbance or daytime impairment, the PLMS can be noted as a polysomnographic finding, but criteria are not met for diagnosis of PLMS. The presence of insomnia or hypersomnia with PLMS does not suffice for the diagnosis; the PLMS must be seen as having a causal relation to the sleep complaint. Other possible causes of the sleep complaint need to be explored before assuming the PLMS are the cause. PLMS occur commonly with RLS, REM behavior disorder, and narcolepsy, and care should be taken to ensure the sleep compliant is not better explained by the other disorder. RLS in particular removes the option for a diagnosis of PLMD, and the PLMS should be noted as part of the RLS. PLMS secondary to medication should be specifically noted as such (i.e., not PLMD but sleep-related movement disorder due to a medication or substance).

AASM, American Academy of Sleep Medicine; *ICSD-3, International Classification of Sleep Disorders*, 3rd edition; *PLMD*, periodic limb movement disorder; *PLMS*, periodic leg movements of sleep.

standard of ≥5 PLMS per hour defines an abnormality of potential clinical significance. In all cases, possible medical or medication causes of the PLMS should be excluded before making the PLMD diagnosis.

- Night-to-night variability and at-home leg meters. The major problem with determining rates of PLMS is the large night-to-night variation. An excellent study by Trotti and colleagues using at-home leg meters showed that determining a stable rate of PLMS per hour required 5 nights of repeated recording for RLS patients.[166] There is no reason to think the same would not be true for all patients with PLMS. Use of ambulatory leg meters for multiple nights might be preferred instead of a 1-night sleep evaluation, provided, of course, that PLMS associated with SDB are known to not be a significant issue. Such devices have been reasonably well validated for adults,[167] though not for children.[168]

Treatment of Periodic Limb Movement Disorder

- PLMD medication treatments:
  - No treatments of PLMD have been approved by the FDA, nor are there any large clinical trials evaluating treatment.
  - Levodopa and dopamine agonists produce a dramatic reduction in PLMS,[169] but unfortunately they can also engender for the first time symptoms of RLS in patients with PLMS without RLS.[33,170] Thus these medications should be used with caution.
  - Most studies have shown that the GABA-active hypnotics produce improved sleep for patients with PLMD, although they have little effect on PLMS. These drugs are usually considered the primary treatments with the usual caution about dependence and increase in doses with continued use. They should be used in their usual clinical doses for insomnia.
- PLMD medical management: Avoid or reduce medications that may exacerbate or even produce PLMS (e.g., most antidepressants), particularly the selective serotonin reuptake inhibitors (SSRIs) and serotonin-norepinephrine reuptake inhibitors (SNRIs). The exceptions are trazodone[171] and bupropion.[172] Iron status should be checked and oral iron treatment considered, as for individuals with RLS, particularly children with PLMD.[154,173]

Sleep-Related Leg Cramps

Diagnosis

- Clinical features:
  - Sleep-related leg cramps involve sudden, involuntary, and usually very painful, mostly unilateral, contractions in the muscle or muscle groups of the legs or feet during the sleep period.
  - They occur most commonly in the calf but can also involve the foot or thigh.[174] They may occur while lying awake in bed or may arise during sleep and result in awakening.
  - In some cases a prodrome of strange feelings in the affected muscles precedes the leg cramp by a few seconds. The affected muscle contraction includes the usual physical characteristics of hardening and bulging of the muscle.
  - The contraction is usually relieved by forceful stretching of the affected muscles, which leads to relaxation of the contraction.

- Soreness in the affected muscle after the contraction ends may persist for up to 30 min and longer in very extreme cases.
- The muscle contractions are associated with intense high-frequency EMG activity that exceeds the range observed for normal movements or voluntary contractions.
- These events mostly occur only once or possibly twice per night and in general have a variable duration that lasts a few minutes (an average of about 9 min for adults), but they may rarely continue much longer.
- Diagnosis method: The diagnosis is almost always made easily from the clinical description of the events. It is further supported by the lack of any wake time consequences, aside from some muscle soreness and fatigue from lack of sleep in extreme cases. The official diagnostic criteria are listed in Table 17.10.
- Differential diagnosis: The major diagnostic problem is excluding the many metabolic diseases that are associated with increased risk for leg cramps (Table 17.11).

Epidemiology

- Sleep-related leg cramps may occur at any age but are more common in older adults. They have been reported to occur in 7% of children, starting at 8 years of age, and increase in frequency to peak levels in children at the age of 16–18. Most pediatric cases report one to four episodes per year.[175] In one survey, 16% of college students complained of awakening with nocturnal leg cramps twice a month or more.[176] In older adults the occurrence is even higher. Nocturnal leg cramps were reported by 56% of veterans in one medical center. A survey from a general adult practice register found the overall prevalence of "rest cramps" to be 37% with an age-related increase.[177] About

---

TABLE 17.10   Diagnosis of Sleep-Related Leg Cramps

A. A painful sensation in the leg or foot is associated with sudden involuntary muscle hardness or tightness indicative of a strong muscle contraction.

B. The painful muscle contraction in the legs or feet occurs during the time in bed for sleep, although they may arise during either wakefulness or sleep.

C. The pain is relieved by forceful stretching of the affected muscle to release the contraction.

TABLE 17.11   Conditions Associated with Increased Risk for Sleep-Related Leg Cramps

Endocrine: Thyroid disorder, Addison's disease, diabetes
Metabolic: Hyperkalemia or hypokalemia, hypocalcemia, hypoglycemia, dialysis, diarrhea
Neurologic: Neuropathy, dystonia, Parkinson's disease, multiple sclerosis, nerve root compression
Drugs: Contraceptives, diuretics, nifedipine, alcohol, steroids, lithium, statins, fibrates, phenothiazines, penicillamine, terbutaline, cimetidine, morphine withdrawal
Toxins: Lead toxicity, strychnine poisoning, tetanus
Congenital: Familial cramping disease, McArdle's disease

Modified with changes from Monderer RS, Wu WP, Thorpy MJ. Nocturnal leg cramps. *Curr Neurol Neurosci Rep.* 2010;10(1):53–59.

40% of the patients reporting cramps during rest had them three times a week or more often, and 6% (about 2% of the total practice population) reported daily occurrence.[178] The natural course of the disorder has not been studied, but there appears to be episodes of repeated events that resolve spontaneously, although they may reoccur some time later. No gender difference has been reported.
- The prevalence is thought to be high during pregnancy (about 30%),[178] when taking oral contraceptives, and also in patients with diabetes, end stage renal disease, and conditions causing limited mobility (e.g., Parkinson's disease or arthritis).

Pathophysiology

- Little is known about the pathophysiology of these very painful events. The nocturnal cramps occur in any stage of sleep, as well as during waking, and thus do not appear to be related to sleep physiology.
  - The association with various metabolic diseases suggests possible problems with hypocalcemia, but it may be that any basic chemical imbalance could contribute to this condition.
  - Patients with peripheral vascular disease and neuropathy also have a high prevalence of nocturnal leg cramps, which supports the concept that any loss of enervation, nutrient supply, or chemical balance contributes to this condition. It may be that these medical conditions produce muscle hypersensitivity and an extreme response to stimulation. Thus it has been reported that decreasing stimulation by avoiding plantar flexor or other flexor activity may reduce leg cramps.
  - It has also been suggested that the cramping results from failure to maintain adequate muscle length and that regular stretching exercises could possibly reduce this problem.[176,179] The so-called squatting hypothesis advances the concept that the modern Western lifestyle of not squatting permits tendon shortening and leads to the physiologic conditions known to produce the leg cramps.[176]
  - Strenuous muscle activation, however, can also induce cramping. A recent study noted indications for a strong seasonal prevalence increase to be as much as double in the summer compared with the winter.[180] There is no clear explanation for this seasonality of leg cramps.

Treatment

- This condition, although extremely painful, resolves spontaneously and has an overall benign course. Strenuous stretching almost always suffices to resolve the cramping.
- Regular exercise with mild stretching of the muscle is the preferred treatment to reduce the occurrence of nocturnal leg cramps.[179] In the past, quinine and vitamin E (4000 IU) have each also been recommended to reduce the frequency of leg cramps.
- The therapeutic value of these treatments remains uncertain, with the best evidence, though limited, supporting some benefit for longer-term, relatively high doses of quinine.[181] Quinine has several significant adverse effects, however, including ocular toxicity, rare thrombocytopenia, and fatal hypersensitivity reactions.[182] Given its limited benefit, it is not recommended for the treatment of leg cramps, and in 1995 the FDA stopped the marketing of quinine for the treatment of nocturnal leg

TABLE 17.12	Treatments Reported to Benefit Nocturnal Leg Cramps	
Medication	**Dose**	**Problems**
Behavioral		
Stretching the affected muscle to lengthen the tendon		
Reasonable Indication for Efficacy		
Botulinum toxin	80–400 U	Very limited data, appears effective
Quinine sulfate	200–550 mg	Potential serious ocular toxicity, rare thrombocytopenia and fatal hypersensitivity reactions. The FDA has published a strong advisory against this use.*
Possible Efficacy		
Verapamil	120 mg	Limited data, possibly effective
Diltiazem	30 mg	Limited data, possibly effective
Vitamin B complex	Unknown	Very limited data, possibly effective
Orphenadrine citrate	100 mg	Very limited data, possibly effective
Naftidrofuryl oxalate	30 mg	Not available in the United States
Probably Not Effective		
Magnesium sulfate	300–900 mg	Not effective in clinical trial
Vitamin E	400–800 IU	Clinical reports of efficacy. Not supported by studies. Appears to not be effective.

*See US Food and Drug Administration (FDA) advisory at http://www.fda.gov/Drugs/DrugSafety/PostmarketDrugSafetyInformationforPatientsandProviders/ucm218202.htm.

cramps. Vitamin E appears to have little benefit in patients with leg cramps.
- Medications that have been reported to have some possible benefit for more severe cases include verapamil (120 mg)[183] and diltiazem,[184] but other calcium channel blockers that do not directly inhibit neurotransmitter release, such as nifedipine, may increase leg cramps.[184] Both injection of lidocaine into the gastrocnemius "trigger point"[185] and injection of botulinum toxin into the affected calf muscle have been reported to be effective.[186] Magnesium failed to provide any benefit in one well-controlled clinical trial.[187] Table 17.12 lists possible treatments, but data supporting the efficacy of any medication are limited overall. The best treatment recommendation appears to be exclusion of medical causes and stretching exercises designed to lengthen leg tendons.[179]

Sleep-Related Bruxism

Diagnosis

- This condition involves frequent and either sustained jaw clenching or repetitive masticator muscle enervation, which when marked produces grinding of the teeth. Fig. 17.12 provides a polysomnogram recording of sleep-related bruxism. The tooth grinding, with its often loud and irritating sound, is considered classic sleep bruxism and is particularly common in children. Both the clenching and bruxism qualify for the diagnosis. The diagnosis is based on the patient's report of teeth clenching or grinding during sleep, plus verification by wear on the teeth, jaw muscle problems related to excessive intense activity, or masticator muscle hypertrophy during strong forced clenching. The patient's report often comes from the bed partner, since

TABLE 17.13	Diagnosis of Sleep-Related Bruxism

A. The presence of regular or frequent tooth grinding sounds during sleep
B. One or more of the following are present:
  i. Abnormal wear of the teeth consistent with the reports of tooth grinding during sleep.
  ii. Transient morning jaw muscle fatigue or pain; and/or temporal headache; and jaw locking on awakening consistent with the reports of tooth grinding during sleep.

Note the diagnosis does not require a polysomnogram but when considered for this disorder the masseter muscle activity should be recorded with audio-visual signal to improve diagnosis.
Modified slightly from the *International Classification of Sleep Disorders*, 3rd edition.

most patients with this problem are unaware of this behavior during sleep.
- Table 17.13 provides the basic diagnostic criteria for sleep-related bruxism.

Pathophysiology

- Little is known about the processes producing bruxism. Rhythmic masticatory muscle activity commonly occurs during sleep without any teeth grinding. Bruxism occurs at apparently greater intensity with a higher rate of these rhythmic activities[188] and may represent an extreme or exaggerated expression of a normal physiologic process in sleep. There are no indications of dopamine deficiency or any neurochemical abnormality in bruxism, although levodopa and propranolol treatments have been

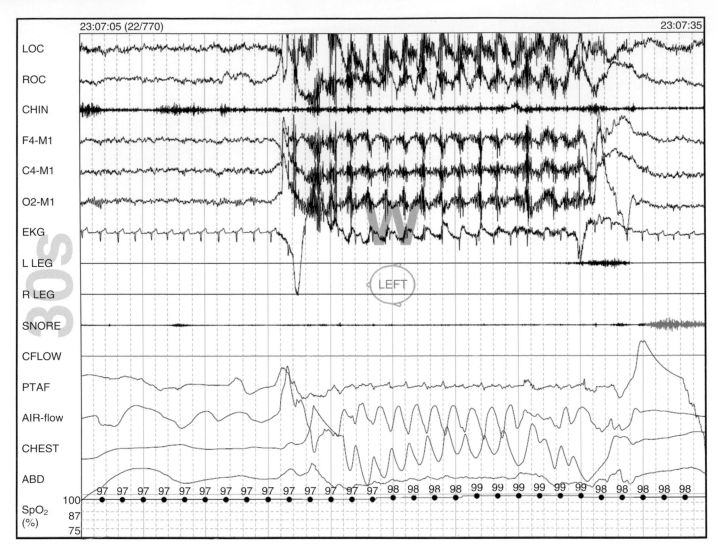

• **Figure 17.12** Channel key: 30 sec epoch. The standard polysomnogram montage was used and included: LOC and ROC left and respectively right outer cantus electrooculography; CHIN1-CHIN2, submental electromyography (EMG) signal; Electroencephalogram (EEG) = (F4/C4/O2-M1), right frontal/central/occipital, references to left mastoid. Limb EMG (left leg, right leg); EKG, electrocardiogram; SNORE, snore sensor sound; CFLOW, mark flow (inactive); AIR-flow, nasal-oral airflow; PTAF, nasal pressure transducer channel; CHEST and ABD, chest and abdominal walls motion effort; SpO2, percent oxygen saturation by pulse oximetry by finger probe. Bruxism. 29-year-old female with subvalvular stenosis was noted to have several episodes of prolonged 1–2 Hz disturbance in EEG and chin EMG. Prominent gritting sounds were heard on video replay. (Copyright Alon Y. Avidan, MD, MPH.)

associated with a reduction in bruxism in some patients. This may, however, have more to do with nonspecific effects on sleep. Bruxism appears to be related to the cyclical alternating pattern (CAP) of sleep associated with microarousal activity.[189] Physiologic recordings suggest that the bruxism occurs with microarousal events in sleep.[190]

Treatment

• Certain medications and conditions can exacerbate or even produce sleep-related bruxism, such as SSRIs[191] and antidopaminergic medications.[192] Appropriate adjustment of such drugs may help. Most management of bruxism focuses on reducing both the complaints of sleep disruption and the risk for damage to orofacial structures. Sleep can be improved with behavioral treatments appropriate for insomnia. Dental treatments consisting of soft mouth guards or hard occlusal splints reduce damage to the teeth. Medications reported to reduce bruxism have not been adequately evaluated and apparently have not gained any general clinical acceptance.[193] More severe bruxism has, however, been treated successfully with injections of botulinum toxin type A.[194]

Rhythmic Movement Disorder

Diagnosis

• This primarily pediatric disorder covers a wide range of large individually stereotyped muscle rhythmic movements that usually occur in drowsy wakefulness before the first onset of sleep. They can continue in light sleep but only very rarely arise during deep slow wave or active REM sleep. The rhythmic pattern occurs at a frequency of 0.5–2 Hz, much slower than tremors that may occur during sleep or at sleep onset. They may also take place at times of drowsiness while awake during the day. The movements occur as a cluster that persists for a few minutes up to half an hour or sometimes longer. Humming or inarticulate vocalizations may accompany the movements. Patients are often amnestic for the events and may have limited response to external stimulation during an event. Since the behavior usually involves movement of the head and neck, in 1905 Zappert originally called this condition *jactatio capitis nocturna*.[195] Fig. 17.13 gives an example of a polysomnogram recording of a head-banging episode of rhythmic movement disorder. Variations of similar specific stereotyped behaviors have been identified by other diagnostic terms, such as head banging, head rolling, body rocking, and body rolling. All share the common pattern of expression described earlier and, despite the differences in the involved body parts or movement characteristics, are considered to be examples of this one sleep-related disorder.

- Diagnosis requires both the movements and some significant problem caused by these movements, such as sleep disruption, impaired daytime functioning, bodily injury, or the likelihood of injury without protective methods. The diagnosis is usually easily made from a medical history describing these movements, when they occur, and their consequences (Table 17.14 presents the ICSD-3 diagnostic criteria). Occasionally, the history may not provide enough detail to exclude epilepsy or an arousal parasomnia, in which case a detailed video polysomnogram should be considered to confirm the diagnosis.

Epidemiology

- The prevalence of sleep-related rhythmic movement disorder is not known, but it is certainly not a rare disorder. It usually starts in infancy and only very rarely persists beyond the age of four. In very rare cases it has been described in adolescents and adults. This disorder is more common in mentally retarded

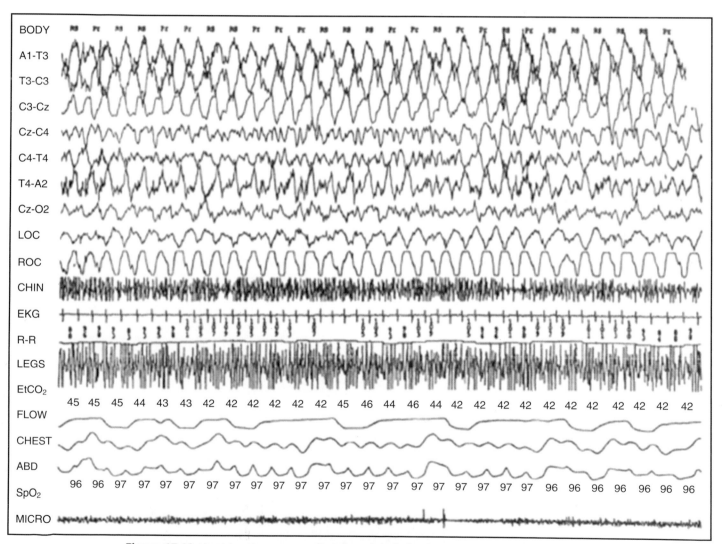

- **Figure 17.13** Head banging as a manifestation of rhythmic movement disorder is demonstrated. Repetitive artifact is noted in the electroencephalogram (channels 2–8) and in the eye lead channels (LOC and ROC). *ABD*, Abdominal; *EKG*, electrocardiogram; *LOC*, left outer cantus; *ROC*, right outer cantus. (From Walters A. Simple sleep-related movement disorders of childhood including benign sleep myoclonus of infancy, rhythmic movement disorder, and childhood restless legs syndrome and periodic limb movements in sleep. *Sleep Med Clin.* 2007;2[3]:419–432.)

TABLE 17.14	Diagnosis of Sleep-Related Rhythmic Movement Disorder

A. The patient exhibits repetitive, stereotyped, and rhythmic motor behavior involving large muscle groups.

B. The movements are predominately sleep related and occur near nap time or bedtime or when the patient appears drowsy or asleep.

C. The movements result in a significant complaint meeting one of the following:
  i. Interference with normal sleep
  ii. Significant impairment in daytime function
  iii. Self-inflicted body injury or likelihood of injury without preventive methods

D. The rhythmic movements are not better explained by another movement disorder or epilepsy.

When sleep-related rhythmic movement disorder occurs without clinical consequences, it should be noted, but the term "disorder" is not used.
Modified slightly from the International Classification of Sleep Disorders, 3rd edition.

individuals and has sometimes been seen, particularly when the movements are less violent, as a soothing motion used to promote sleep.

Pathophysiology

- The cause of these movements has not been established. They have been described after head injury,[196] and mental retardation and autism are associated with this disorder when it persists into later childhood or adult life. A basal ganglia abnormality has been suggested,[197] but there has been no evidence of any pathophysiologic abnormality associated with the disorder.

Treatment

- This condition commonly has a short benign course, especially in infants, and remits spontaneously. Treatment, if any, in general focuses on environmental protection to reduce the risk for physical harm. Behavioral management, when required, focuses

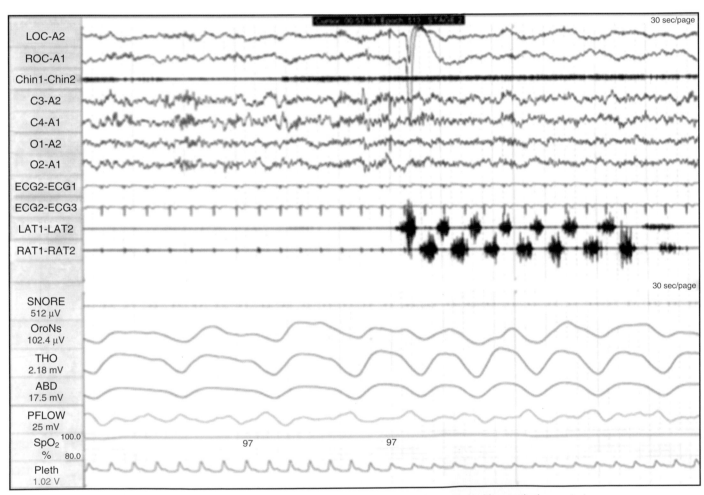

• **Figure 17.14** Alternating leg muscle activation. This 30-sec polysomnographic epoch demonstrates alternating leg movements on limb electromyogram (LAT1-LAT2, RAT1-RAT2) arising from light nonrapid eye movement sleep in a 16-year-old boy. *ABD*, Abdominal; *Chin1-Chin2*, submental electromyography (EMG) signal; *ECG*, electrocardiogram; *LOC*, left outer cantus; *ROC*, right outer cantus. (Reproduced from Hoban TF. Pediatric polysomnography. In: Kryger MH. *Atlas of Sleep Medicine*. 2nd ed. Philadelphia: Saunders; 2014:331–359.)

on avoiding emotional stress and reducing arousing activities or stimuli during the presleep period. Medical treatment of older patients or more severe cases includes short-acting GABA-active hypnotic[198] and clonazepam.[199] Imipramine has been reported to help in one adult case when hypnotics did not suffice.[200]

Alternating Leg Muscle Activation

- An interesting pattern of quickly alternating anterior tibialis activation was described in sections of polysomnograms in 16 patients who were being evaluated for SDB.[201] Fig. 17.14 provides an example of ALMA. These movements met the criteria for PLMs occurring at a somewhat fast rate of one to two events per second, but with regular alternation of one leg and then the other. A subsequent case report showed that these movements responded to pramipexole treatment much like any other case of PLMS.[202] It has been suggested that these events represent triggering or release of a spinal generator pattern for walking, but this remains to be further evaluated. At this point, these movements are considered a variant of PLMS and not classical PLMS. Their clinical significance is unclear.

Suggested Reading

Allen RP, Chen C, Garcia-Borreguero D, et al. Comparison of pregabalin with pramipexole for restless legs syndrome. *N Engl J Med*. 2014;370:621-631.

Allen RP, Picchietti DL, Garcia-Borreguero D, et al. Restless legs syndrome/Willis-Ekbom disease diagnostic criteria: updated International Restless Legs Syndrome Study Group (IRLSSG) consensus criteria—history, rationale, description, and significance. *Sleep Med*. 2014;15:860-873.

Connor JR, Wang X, Allen RP, et al. Altered Dopaminergic Profile in the Putamen and Substantia Nigra in Restless Leg Syndrome. *Brain*. 2009;132:2403-2412.

Earley CJ, Silber MH. Restless legs syndrome: understanding its consequences and the need for better treatment. *Sleep Med*. 2010;11:807-815.

Garcia-Borreguero D, Silber M, Winkelman J, et al. Guidelines for the first-line treatment of RLS/WED, prevention and treatment of dopaminergic augmentation. *Sleep Med*. 2016;21:1-11.

18

Overview of Electroencephalography and Epilepsy

DEREK J. CHONG, CARL W. BAZIL

Basics of Electroencephalography

Electroencephalography

- Compares the difference in electrical activity (also known as electrical potential) between two regions on the surface of the brain over time.
- Records microvoltages derived from the cortex through electrodes attached directly to the scalp. The signal is then filtered considerably in order to eliminate electrical noise and amplify.
- Is derived from *extracellular* currents generated from excitatory and inhibitory postsynaptic potentials (EPSPs and IPSPs, respectively), primarily from pyramidal neurons of the cerebral cortex, and an aggregate of an estimated 10 neurons contribute to the electrical field at a given electrode.[1,2]

Setup for Electroencephalography

The International 10-20 system is the standard electroencephalogram (EEG) lead placement system in North America.[3]
- For detection of epileptiform activity, a minimum of 21 electrodes are placed on the head.
- Naming conventions are listed in Figs. 18.1 and 18.2. Sagittal electrodes are given a suffix of "z," left-sided electrodes are odd numbered, and those on the right are even numbered. Electrodes on the mandibular angle (M) can substitute for auricular electrodes. There is a subtle change with the modified international 10-20 system, as T3 and T4 were renamed T7 and T8, while T5 and T6 were renamed P7 and T7 to allow for further electrodes to be placed, including inferior temporal electrodes (Fig. 18.1).
- The distance from the nasion to the inion is measured, and the first electrodes are 10%; the remaining are 20% of the distances (Fig. 18.2). Similar measurements are made from both preauricular areas to determine the placements of the remaining electrodes. This allows standardization of placement across a wide variety of head sizes, from premature infants to individuals with hydrocephalus.

Electrodes
- Are made of silver chloride or similar electrically conductive discs that are cup-shaped to hold conducting paste or glue

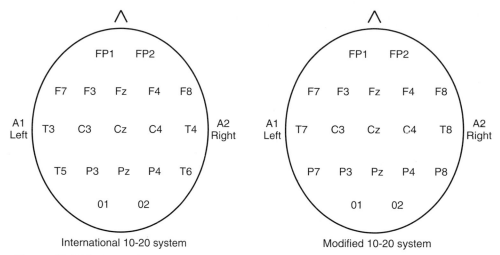

International 10-20 system   Modified 10-20 system

• **Figure 18.1** The International 10-20 System of Electrocardiogram Electrode Placement. By convention, left-sided electrodes are odd numbered, whereas those on the right are even numbered, and midline electrodes are given the subscript "z." The letters of the 10-20 system refer to the frontopolar (Fp), frontal (F), temporal (T), central (C), parietal (P), and occipital (O) regions, in addition to the auricle (A), for which the mastoid (M) may be substituted. Eye channels are often added, although they are technically not part of this nomenclature, with electrodes being placed at the left lower canthus and right upper canthus. In the modified 10-20 system, the system was refined to ensure that the larger the number, the farther away the electrode placement is from midline, with T3/T4 being changed to T7/T8 and T5/T6 to P7/P8 (see Fig. 18.2).

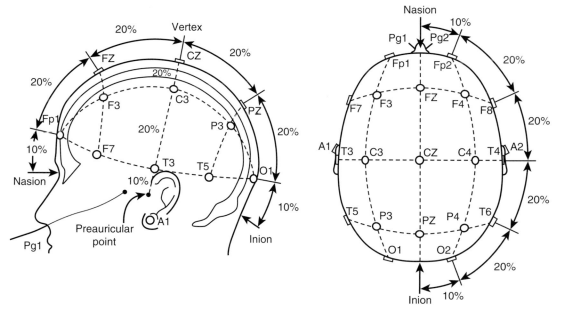

• **Figure 18.2** The 10-20 system is named for the distances of electrodes from each other. The distance from the nasion to the inion is measured, and 10% and 20% of the distance is calculated. The most inferior electrodes are placed along a circumference above from the nasion and inion that is 10% of the total distance, and the remainder of electrodes are placed 20% of that distance away from each other. (From Jasper HH. Report of the committee on methods of clinical examination in electroencephalography. *Electroencephogr Clin Neurophysiol.* 1958;10:370–371.)

Fp	Frontopolar	z	Midline/sagittal
F	Frontal	Odd	Left side
C	Central	Even	Ride side
P	Parietal	Small numbers	Close to midline/anterior
T	Temporal	Larger	Further from z
0	Occipital	—	—

• Shorter recordings can employ conductive paste between the scalp and electrodes, acting as the adhesive itself (our lab prefers 10-20 paste). A headwrap keeps the electrodes in place for moving patients and are recommended for overnight recordings, including polysomnograms (PSGs).

• Collodian is a type of biologic glue used for extended monitoring or for very active or sweaty patients.

	10-20 Paste	EC-2	Collodion
Time	Easiest of methods. Can use head wrap for overnight recordings	Medium effort	Significant time and effort to hook up: releases fumes (requires exhaust) while drying (requires blown air to expedite). Disconnection requires use of a solvent.
Maintenance issues	Easy quick fixes	Medium efforts	More stable connection for longer recordings and sweating patients
Pregnancy issues	None known	None known	Contraindicated
Storage	—	—	Flammable

Technical Basics of Electroencephalography

Each EEG channel is derived from the difference in the electrical input recorded from two different regions.

- Channels are displayed in order—for instance, Fp1-F3 means that Fp1 is input 1 and F3 is input 2.
- By convention, an upward deflection on the EEG tracing indicates that input 1 is relatively negative compared with input 2, which could mean either a negative discharge at input 1 or a positive discharge at input 2 (Fig. 18.3). Using montages (see the next section), it can be surmised whether the discharge is positive or negative.
- Signals that are identical throughout are likely to be either artifact (electrical activity is present constantly around us) or inconsequential, and are thus rejected and termed "common mode rejection." Only the difference between two sites is amplified.

The Electroencephalogram Amplifier Utilizes

Differential Amplification: Amplify *dislike* signals while eliminating *like* signals.

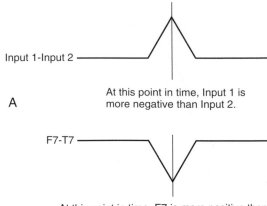

Input 1-Input 2

A

At this point in time, Input 1 is more negative than Input 2.

F7-T7

At this point in time, F7 is more positive than T7. To cause this downward deflection, there is either a relative positivity at F7 or relative negativity at T7.

B

- **Figure 18.3** Polarity on the Electroencephalogram. Each line, or channel, on the electroencephalogram is a comparison of the two inputs. A single channel does not provide information about whether the underlying discharge is positive or negative. When the input 1 is more negative than input 2, an upward deflection will result **(A)**, whereas if input 1 is more positive than input 2, a downward deflection will result. An example is provided in **B**, in which F7 (left frontotemporal) is compared with T7 (left midtemporal), as would be seen in a long bipolar montage. With this single channel, the downward deflection indicates that F7 is relatively more negative than T7, and there are two equally possible hypotheses: there is either negativity underlying F7 or positivity underlying T7. The size of the deflection reflects the magnitude of the difference. If there is no difference in the two inputs being compared, no deflection will take place. A very large region of negativity can be recorded equally below two adjacent electrodes and result in zero deflection in that channel.

Bipolar Montages
- Advantages: Best at identifying relatively focal discharges and abnormalities
- Disadvantages: Can miss large regional changes, as each electrode is compared with its neighbor, if both have the same amount of negativity the tracing will appear flat, and the entire chain can appear flat if the chain is picking up similar activity. Broad low amplitude δ slowing can be missed.

Montages

EEG represents the difference in electrical potential over time, with the first electrode compared to the second. (The math is slightly different due to differential amplification.)

- Comparisons between the electrodes are modifiable and set up in relatively standard arrangements, called "montages." Just as a lung lesion can be better visualized when comparing different views on a chest x-ray, different montages are utilized to better detect, isolate, or otherwise "visualize" various types of cerebral potentials.
  Bipolar montages: Compares one electrode with another electrode, often adjacent, typically arranged in straight lines, frequently referred to as "chains."
    - Longitudinal bipolar (Fig. 18.4A): Also known as the "double banana." The electrode comparisons are configured to create a parasagittal and a temporal "chain." For instance, Fp1-F3, F3-C3, C3-P3, and P3-O1 are

four sequential electrode pair comparisons that make up the left parasagittal chain. The temporal chain actually lies over the perisylvian fissure, just superior to the temporal lobe. An inferior temporal chain, with the use of additional electrodes (T9, T10, P9, and P10), can be added when temporal lobe epilepsy (TLE) is being evaluated.
    - Transverse bipolar (see Fig. 18.4B): Arranged in a coronal fashion, with left to right slices taken from an anterior to posterior direction. One chain would consist of T3-C3, C3-Cz, Cz-C4, and C4-T4. This montage accentuates activity at the midline, and thus sleep transients are well visualized.
  Referential montages: Each electrode compared with the identical "reference." Examples include:
    - A common point (e.g., common reference montage), such as referential Cz, which is good for determining

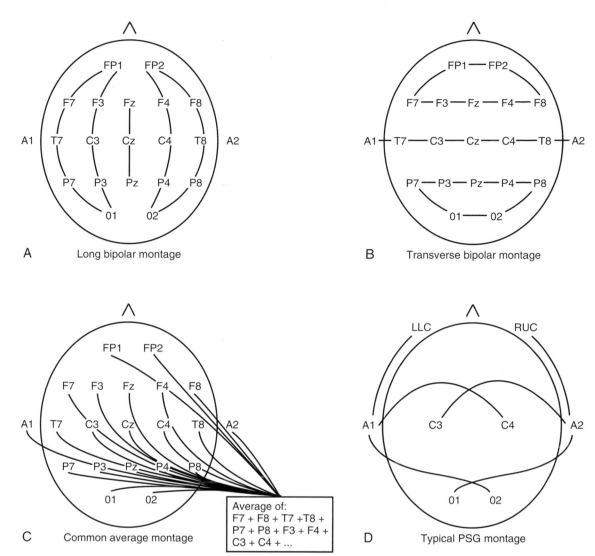

• **Figure 18.4** Frequently Used Electroencephalographic Montages. **A,** Long bipolar or "double banana." **B,** Transverse. **C,** A common average montage. **D,** Typical polysomnographic (PSG) montage. The common average montage will compare each electrode with the mean of a large group of other electrodes, often 12, 15, or 17, with Fp electrodes being omitted from the average, for instance, because these electrodes are typically affected by noncerebral artifact. The letters of the 10-20 system refer to the frontopolar (Fp), frontal (F), temporal (T), central (C), parietal (P), and occipital (O) regions. On the lateral margins of the eyes are two other electrodes: LLC, left lower canthus; RUC, right upper canthus. Some may use the auricle (A) or alternatively the mastoid (M).

Referential Montage Advantages and Disadvantages

Advantages: Identifies regional changes better, as it will be seen in multiple channels.

Disadvantages: The reference can become "contaminated" when one or more electrodes used in the reference have a waveform or artifact that is significant. For example, if the discharge is occurring at Cz itself, it will show up in every electrode comparison. It may also be difficult to identify small amplitude abnormalities.

Sleep activity will also be seen in all channels with Cz as a reference.

• An average of all or many electrode potentials (e.g., common average montage; see Fig. 18.4C).
  • The common average determines how much that electrode stands out from its peers.

An example of a large focus of negativity (an epileptiform spike) is displayed in a long bipolar and an average montage (Fig. 18.5).

Typical Montages for Limited Polysomnogram-Electroencephalogram

• Contralateral referential montage (see Fig. 18.4D) is typical.
• Large distances make for large amplitudes.
• Ear/mastoid references can be contaminated by activity of the temporal regions.

symmetry and limits muscle artifact (no muscle under Cz). But the greater distance from Cz to the temporal chain than to the parasagittal chain will make it more likely temporal derivations will show larger amplitudes.

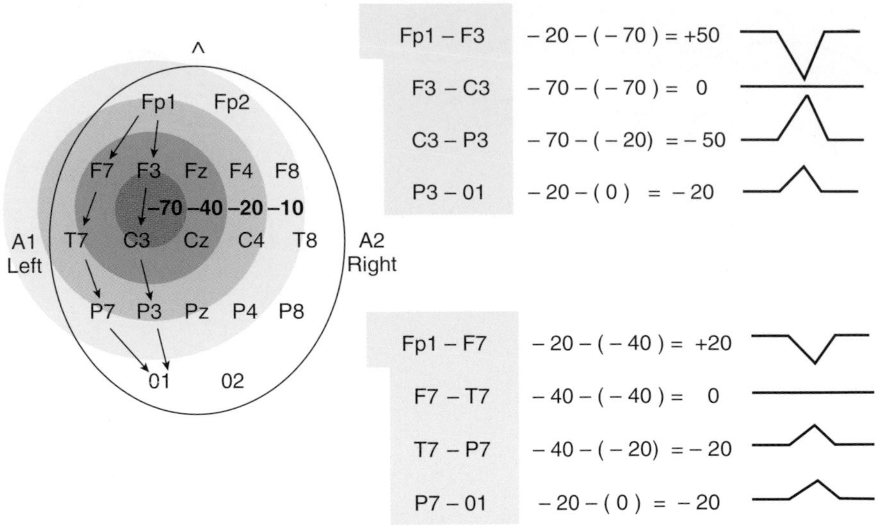

Fp1 – F3	– 20 – (– 70) = +50	
F3 – C3	– 70 – (– 70) = 0	
C3 – P3	– 70 – (– 20) = – 50	
P3 – 01	– 20 – (0) = – 20	

Fp1 – F7	– 20 – (– 40) = +20	
F7 – T7	– 40 – (– 40) = 0	
T7 – P7	– 40 – (– 20) = – 20	
P7 – 01	– 20 – (0) = – 20	

• **Figure 18.5** A diagram of a spike discharge arising from the left fronto-central region, with maximal negativity between F3 and C3, the darkest shaded area being –70 μV, and a drop-off in field in concentric circles, depicted with lighter gray shading. *Arrows* depict the left hemisphere electrode connections to create the longitudinal bipolar montage shown on the right. The Fp1 electrode would read –20 μV, while the F3 electrode would read –70 μV. Simplifying the mathematics of electroencephalogram (EEG), the channel Fp1-F3 would be –20 – (–70) = +50. By convention, negative is upward, so the EEG would deflect downward significantly. Building the remainder of the channels through similar mathematics, the typical spike seen on EEG can be derived. For simplicity, the mathematics of the differential amplifier used in EEG was left out of this example. The EEG electrode labels are from the modified 10-20 system (see Fig. 18.1).

Electroencephalography Parameters

Waveform Frequencies (Fig. 18.6)

- Waveforms are measured in cycles per second, or hertz (see Fig. 18.6).
- Refers to how many turns of a wave actually occurred in 1 sec or how many of a single, nonrepeating wave would fit into 1 sec.

A standard definition of frequencies is as follows[4]:
- δ: <4 Hz
- θ: 4 to <8 Hz
- α: 8–13 Hz
- β: >13–40 Hz
- γ: >40 Hz

Amplitude

- Measured in microvolts from the low to the high, peak to peak (not from the baseline) of waveforms
- Is the product of signal voltage × display sensitivity (or pen writer if using paper EEG)
- The voltage is the potential difference between two points and is not directly related to the power of cerebral activity.
- Interelectrode distance alters amplitude: The greater the distance between electrodes (up to 8 cm), the greater the disparity in the underlying potentials and greater amplitudes will be displayed. (This presumes the voltages of the brain differ more, the further away they are from each other.)
- Asymmetries in voltage need to be corroborated either by using another bipolar montage perpendicular to the first or by using a referential montage.

- If all points of the brain have the same potential, it is termed *isoelectric* and indicates a lack of perceptible cortical activity.

Electroencephalogram Amplitude Is Dependent on Several Factors

- The distance between the two points of measurement
- The volume of functioning brain generating the activity under each point
- The amount of absorption causing attenuation of the signal above the two areas (i.e., skull thickness, subdural fluid accumulations)

Sensitivity

- The ratio of input voltage to the degree of signal displayed (or deflection), measured in microvolts per millimeter (μV/mm)
- A standard setting for EEG is 7 μV/mm with a range of normal being 5–10 μV/mm
- Amplitudes of waveforms can be calculated as the product of the sensitivity and the height of the waveform.
- Waves with very small voltages require lower valued sensitivity settings to avoid overlooking subtleties.

Filters

- EEG signal can be "framed" by a series of filters so that only frequencies of interest are displayed. Filters modify the signal to attenuate frequencies based on a user-defined frequency cutoff point.

  Low-frequency filters (LFFs), also known as high-pass filters, exert their effect on slower waves (lower frequencies).
- When LFF is 1 Hz, waves of 1 cycle/sec will be slightly attenuated (20%–30%, depending on the machine's algorithm), while increasingly slower waves will be increasingly attenuated.

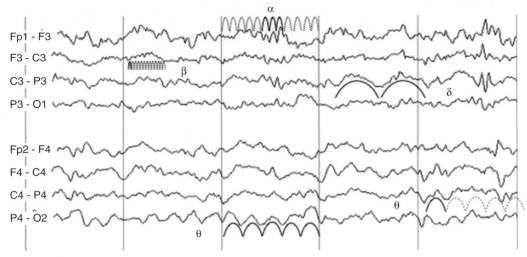

• **Figure 18.6** The electroencephalogram (EEG) of this patient has examples of β, α, θ, and δ frequencies, often with multiple frequencies simultaneously, with fast activity overriding slower waveforms. There are two examples of θ waves shown, one in a series of rhythmic θ, and also as a single waveform, for which if imagined to repeat (in *dotted lines*) would be 5/sec. Similar to the α example shown, it does not need to continue for the entire second and can be estimated. The EEG electrode labels are from the modified 10-20 system (see Fig. 18.1).

• Setting LFF to 1 Hz still affects frequencies higher than 1 Hz, but to a much lesser degree with the effect, becoming negligible as frequencies increase.
• An LFF set incorrectly can completely mask pathologic slowing, or slow waves seen during normal sleep.

High-frequency filters (HFFs), known also as low-pass filters: When HFF is 70 Hz, waves of 70 cycles/sec and faster will be attenuated.

• As the frequency of the wave increases, so does the attenuation.
• Setting the HFF too low can make muscle artifact appear as normal brain waves (α or β frequency) or as epileptiform activity (described later).
• HFF typically have even less effects below the cutoff point than the LFF has above its cutoff point.

Notch filter: Excises an artifact produced by power line activity (60 Hz in North America) using sharp cutoffs.

Polysomnography Electroencephalogram

The notch filter should be used with caution, since 60 Hz artifact in isolated leads may denote poor electrode contact (see Fig. 18.32), or poor ground or reference connection to the scalp. Data from poorly connected leads can be extremely misleading, so this artifact is a warning.

• LFF: Set low enough to view clearly slow waves of 1 Hz (typically between 0.1 and 1 Hz).
• Setting LFF above the respiratory rate can eliminate respiratory artifact.
• HFF: Should include faster waveforms (typically 70 Hz is sufficient) to avoid the filtering of fast noncerebral frequencies to appear as possibly cerebral.
Electromyogram (EMG): Muscle activity produces fast waveforms.

• LFF: As high as 10 Hz can provide a view of all of the desired muscle activity while attenuating slow artifact such as body movement.
• HFF: Can be set as high as 100 Hz or turned off.

Paper Speed

• Standard EEG: The scrolling of the "paper" is 30 mm/sec, such that typically 10–15 sec are now viewed on a digital page.
• PSG: 10 mm/sec used for scoring (30 sec/page) compresses the waveforms, but is a "virtual setting" in digital systems, which allows for both staging sleep and detecting epileptiform abnormalities.

The Normal Electroencephalogram

Electroencephalogram Concepts

• An electrical discharge from a region of the brain should be paralleled by a *sensible field*, meaning that the highest amplitude and clearest morphology are seen in one or a few adjacent electrodes, with gradual dropoff in surrounding electrodes.
  • Electrical activity from the cerebral cortex is often compared with "ripples in a pond," growing fainter with distance from the center of the source. This is true of most normal and abnormal discharges, whereas most artifacts (e.g., faulty electrode) will have no affect on surrounding electrodes and thus no sensible field.
  • "What and where": The "what" are descriptions of the frequencies and amplitudes, and the "where" is their location. The "what" was described in the preceding section.

The "Where": Location of Waveforms

See Fig. 18.7.
• Frequencies and amplitudes vary from region to region in a normal brain.

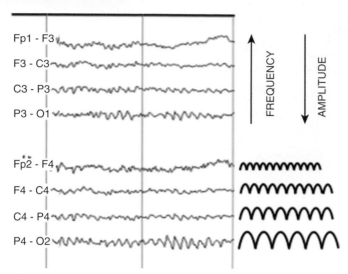

• **Figure 18.7** The electroencephalogram (EEG) of an awake and relaxed patient is shown, with a good example of an anterior to posterior gradient. The more anterior channels, Fp1-F4 and Fp1-F3, show low amplitude but faster β activity, while the posterior channels P3-O1 and P4-O2 show higher amplitude but slower α frequencies. This "organization" of the background is necessary in order to classify posterior rhythms as a posterior dominant rhythm or α rhythm, which in this case is measured at approximately 11 Hz. The EEG electrode labels are from the modified 10-20 system (see Fig. 18.1).

• Awake rhythms should be "organized" in an "anterior to posterior" gradient
  • Lower amplitude but faster frequencies at the front of the head
  • Higher-amplitude rhythms at the back with lower frequency
  • The posterior waveforms thus appear more prominent and are termed the posterior dominant rhythm (PDR), sometimes referred to as the α *rhythm* (not α frequency) or simply the "alpha."

The Posterior Dominant Rhythm

• Must be stereotyped and should become obliterated reliably ("blocking") with eye opening or when the mind is occupied (i.e., concentrating on math questions).
• Is best appreciated in relaxed, awake patients with their eyes closed
• Is typically occipital but can be temporal or parietal

> Posterior dominant rhythm (PDR) with age: On average, the PDR reaches 3 Hz by the age of 1 year, 8 Hz by the age of 3 years, and 8.5–12 Hz in adolescence and adulthood.

Normal Awake Adult Electroencephalogram Characteristics

• Low-voltage fast activity with few or no frequencies slower than 8 Hz
• Voltages most commonly seen are between 30 and 250 μV.
• Frequent eye movement artifact and EMG

• The patient is fully aware of the environment, and muscle tone is high.
• The background is relatively symmetrical with respect to the amplitudes, frequencies, and morphologies of activity over analogous regions on both sides of the head.

Benign Waveforms of Wakefulness

Mu

• μ Waves are arch-shaped, 7–11-Hz trains of moderate voltage seen best in the central regions. They are blocked when moving the contralateral limb or even planning the movement. They can be asynchronous and asymmetrical.

Lambda

• λ Waves are posterior, sharply contoured waveforms seen during visual scanning, particularly during reading (Fig. 18.8). They are positive discharges at 01 and 02.

Excess Beta

• When diffuse, β activity can be a sign of drowsiness or be seen during sleep, especially in the pediatric population. It is also a normal EEG reaction following the administration of certain medications—namely benzodiazepines and barbiturates. Excess diffuse β activity can obscure details of the normal background.

Normal Adult Sleep

Sleep staging is covered extensively in Chapter 5 and will be only briefly discussed here.
• Each sleep phase has the potential for alterations, which can be normal phenomena, may represent a sleep disorder, or could be confused with epilepsy.
• Sleep is divided into two general classes: rapid eye movement (REM) sleep and non-REM (NREM) sleep.[5] Each stage is defined by a combination of electrophysiologic parameters, including the EEG (Fig. 18.9), respiration, eye movements, and EMG.
• NREM sleep is divided into three stages, N1–N3, each with a further, progressive decrease in muscle tone.
• Stage N1: Onset of low-voltage, intermixed pattern of frequencies on EEG and interruption of the PDR. Vertex waves (Fig. 18.10) may be present during late N1, as may positive occipital sharp transients of sleep (POSTS; Fig. 18.11). Bursts of high-amplitude, diffuse, rhythmic δ-θ activity can occur, particularly in children and adolescents (hypnagogic hypersynchrony, Fig. 18.12), although it is rarely seen outside 6 months to 12 years of age. Eye movements may be present, but these movements are slow and rolling, as opposed to the sharp, predominantly vertical movements occurring with wakeful blinking. There is a slight relaxation in the musculature. Physiologically, this stage is "drowsiness." Patients may have some continued awareness of their surroundings and can easily be aroused.
• Stage N2, the low-voltage intermixed pattern along with sleep spindles (bursts of 14–16-Hz vertex activity lasting at least 0.5 sec) or K-complexes (high-amplitude biphasic discharges at the vertex), or both, must be present. Arousal is slightly more difficult from stage N2 than stage N1.
• Stage N3, also called slow wave sleep (SWS), consists of high voltage δ activity, are the most difficult to arouse from, and can be associated with transient confusion on awakening.

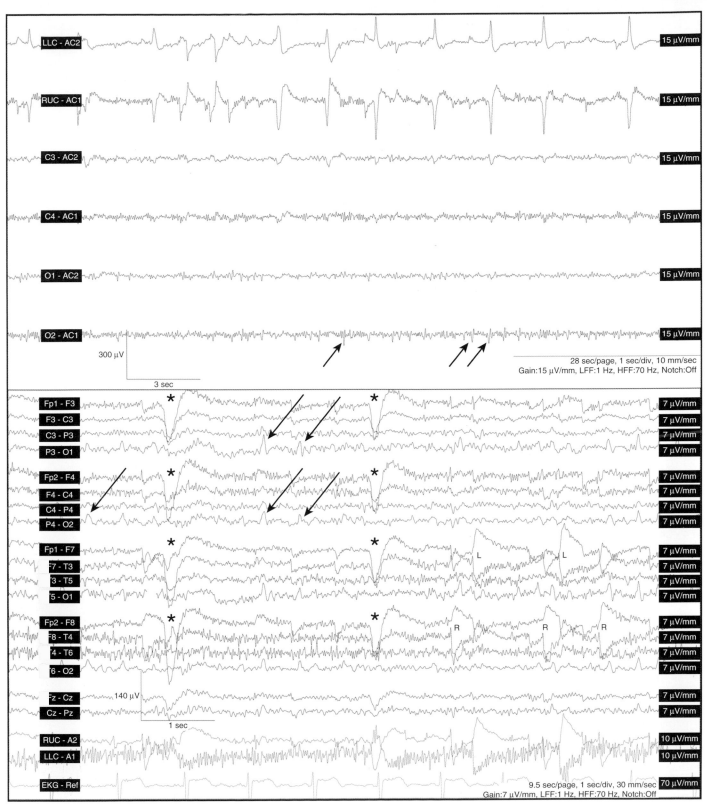

• **Figure 18.8** λ Waves *(arrows)*, or positive potentials in the occipital leads that are associated with saccadic pursuit, are often seen during reading. Note the vertical eye movements *(asterisks)*, probably related to blinks. Right (R) and left (L) lateral eye movements can be identified by ipsilateral lateral rectus muscle artifacts followed by positivity from the cornea moving toward F8 or F7, respectively. A typical polysomnographic montage has 10-mm/sec reading speed (above) and 30-mm/sec electroencephalographic reading speed in the long bipolar montage (below). A1 and AC1, left auricle; A2 and AC2, right auricle. Please refer to Fig. 18.1 for other EEG electrode definitions. *EKG,* Electrocardiogram; *LLC,* left lower canthus; *RUC,* right upper canthus.

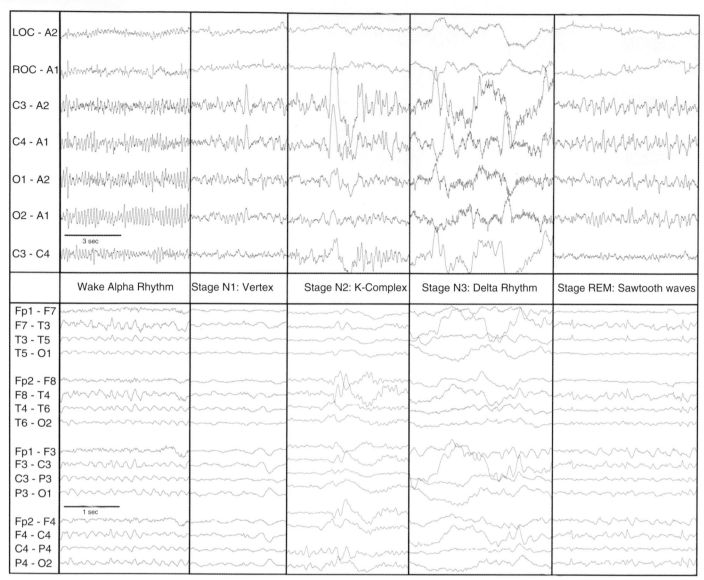

• **Figure 18.9** Comparison of normal awake and asleep patterns on a typical polysomnogram (PSG) and long bipolar electroencephalogram (EEG) montages. Note differing paper speeds: EEG at 30 mm/sec and PSG at 10 mm/sec. The EEG electrode labels are from the modified 10-20 system (see Fig. 18.1). *REM,* Rapid eye movement.

• REM sleep is a physiologic return to a low-voltage intermixed pattern. It differs from stage N1 by a profound reduction in muscle tone, the presence of REMs, irregular respiration, and occasionally sawtooth waves on the PSG EEG. The most vivid dreams occur in this state.

• In normal patients, nocturnal sleep consists of a fairly stereotyped pattern of cycling through the various sleep stages. Patients will descend through stages N1, N2, and N3, followed by REM sleep, in a cycle lasting about 90 min. The cycle then repeats over the night, with progressively less time spent in SWS and more in REM sleep. In a normal young adult, stage N1 is less than 10% of the recording, stage N2 is about 50%, and slow wave and REM sleep represent about 25% each. Sleep efficiency (the time spent asleep divided by the total time in bed) should be well in excess of 90%.

The Older Adult

• Mild temporal slowing can be seen shifting between sides in individuals older than 60 years, particularly as drowsiness ensues, and though not technically normal, such slowing occurs in asymptomatic individuals.[6]

Neonatal Recordings (The Very Basics)

• EEG channels can differ, using fewer electrodes, and differing placement (including Fp3/Fp4, which are halfway between Fp1/Fp2 and F3/F4).

• Similar to PSG, the "paper speed" is often slowed to 15 mm/sec, as δ is the predominant waveform and the compression allows trends and symmetry to be better evaluated.

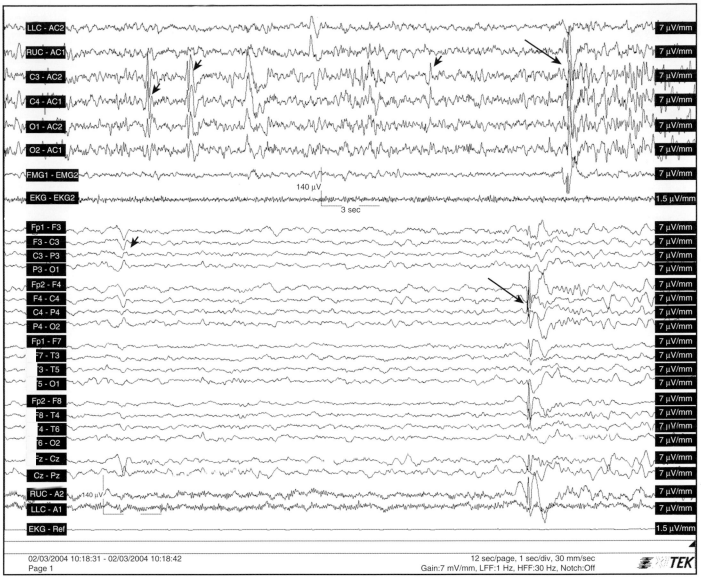

• **Figure 18.10** Vertex waves *(arrow heads)* and focal spike-wave complexes *(longer arrows)* during the same recording on both polysomnographic (at 10 mm/sec above) and electroencephalographic (EEG) long bipolar (at 30 mm/sec, below) montages. Epileptiform activity is often activated during sleep, thus making differentiation of spikes from normal sleep transients difficult but important. Identification is easier with a full EEG montage. The EEG electrode labels are from the modified 10-20 system (see Fig. 18.1). *EKG,* Electrocardiogram; *EMG,* electromyogram.

- Noncerebral channels (electro-oculogram [EOM], electrocardiogram [EKG], respiratory, submental EMG) help identify state changes, and help identify noncerebral artifacts such as hiccough.
- The main features to note on neonatal EEG evolve over the weeks of gestational age; the reader tracks continuity (periods of EEG attenuation), symmetry of the background (amplitude differences between sides), synchrony (waveforms occurring within 1 sec of each other), and the patterns and paroxysms, such as:
  - δ Brushes: A combination of a δ wave with superimposed faster "buzz" of 8–20 Hz activity, seen both in awake and sleep states, and can be in any location (though less frequently frontal), typically asynchronous but symmetric overall. Peak

abundance at 32–34 weeks chronological age (CA), they may still be present at term during trace alternant (TA), and should disappear by 44 weeks CA.
- Sharp electrographic transients (SETs) are sharply contoured and a brief duration that stand out from the background and may not be pathologic.
  - Sharp wave 100–500 msec
  - Spikes less than 100 msec
  - Encoche frontal: Greater than 150 µV biphasic transients maximal in the frontal region—typically bilateral synchronous and symmetric, most abundant during active sleep to quiet sleep transition, and considered normal during these states up to 44 weeks CA. When seen during wakefulness, they may indicate dysfunction or a structural problem,

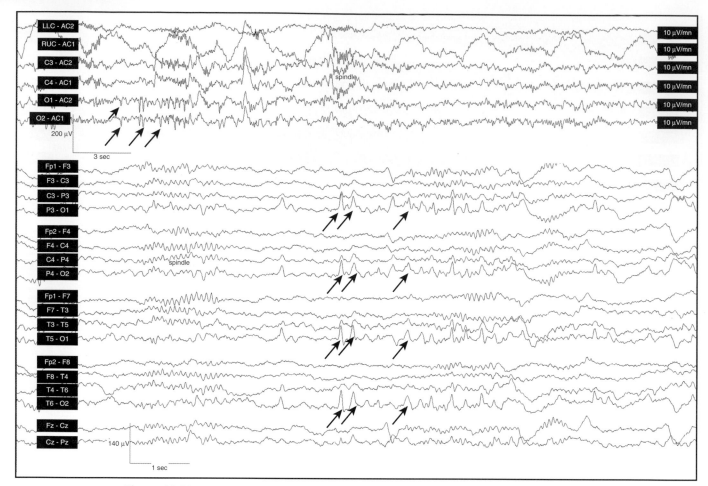

• **Figure 18.11.** Positive occipital sharp transients of sleep *(arrows)* during stage 2 sleep (note the spindles) can also occur in late stage 1 sleep and are maximal over the posterior regions. They can be determined to be positive by using a referential montage as the downward deflection in O1/O2-AC (polysomnogram, above). The large-amplitude upward deflection at P3-O1/P4-O2 (electroencephalogram, below) without clear phase reversal anteriorly is also supportive that the discharge is positive and situated more posteriorly (the other half of the deflection cannot be seen because it is at the end of the chain). Other electroencephalogram electrode labels are from the modified 10-20 system (see Fig. 18.1). *AC1,* Left auricle; *AC2,* right auricle; *LLC,* left lower canthus; *RUC,* right upper canthus.

and if markedly asymmetric with spike-morphology, they may denote a true epileptogenic potential.

- Negative-polarity SETs tend to be more commonly seen in the temporal (T3/T4) and central parasagittal (C3/C4) region, and can be normal when symmetric and occurring ≤1/min. Spike-morphology, runs, and lateralization to one hemisphere over the other may be associated with seizures. Occipital and midline predominance has been seen with diffuse encephalopathies.
- Positive sharp waves (PSW), less than 500 msec with predominant surface-positive-polarity, are often rolandic (PRS), vertex (PVS), or temporal (PTS). PRSs and PVSs are associated with structural abnormalities, often deep white matter lesions, such as intraventricular hemorrhages (IVH). PTSs may also occur with lesions, but can be seen in normal neonates disappearing by term, and should be symmetric and broad.
- Neonatal seizures can be surface negative or positive, and can be so focal as to be restricted to a single electrode, but should

show evolution, with a discernable beginning, middle, and end. Many morphologies and frequencies are possible, sometimes appearing bizarre. Two seizures in different locations with different frequencies can occur simultaneously.

- Rhythmic patterns less than 10 sec in duration are termed brief ictal rhythmic discharges (BIRDs).

Ontogeny of Sleep Patterns

See Fig. 18.13.
- Active sleep is the equivalent of REM sleep.
  - EEG is continuous and consists mainly of θ and δ activity.
  - As in older children and adults, this is characterized by active eye movements and decreased EMG.
  - At term, this state occupies about half of sleep.
- Quiet sleep is the equivalent of NREM sleep.
  - EEG has predominantly slower-frequency δ activity with some intermixed faster frequencies.

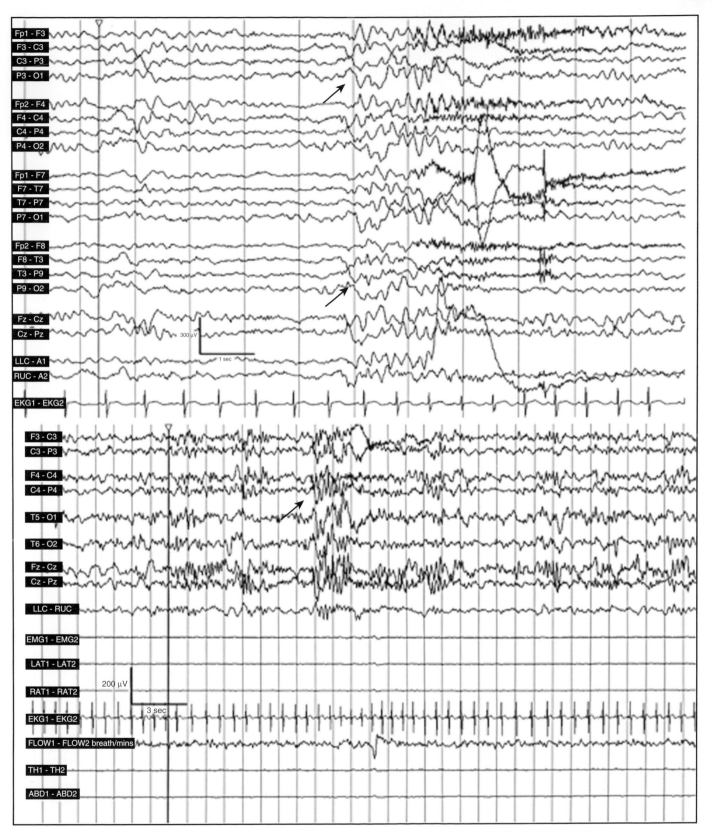

• **Figure 18.12** Hypnogogic hypersynchrony in a 4-year-old seen on a standard electroencephalographic (EEG) long bipolar montage at 30 mm/sec and on a polysomnographic montage at 10 mm/sec. *Arrows* show the onset of a short burst of high-amplitude rhythmic δ-θ activity synchronized between the hemispheres. These bursts can be more prolonged and frequently last 10 sec. EEG electrode labels are from the modified and international 10-20 systems (see Fig. 18.1). Other channels are as follows: Chin (EMG1-EMG2), limb electromyogram (EMG; LAT1-LAT2 and RAT1-RAT2), electrocardiogram (EKG), nasal-oral airflow (FLOW), and respiratory effort channels (TH, thoracic; ABD, abdominal).

EGA   EEG evolution

8   ⟶ First appearance of EEG signal across cortex
<24   ⟶ Discontinuous EEG; no state cycling
24   ⟶ Some continuous EEG; mostly discontinuous EEG; early state cycling
30–32   ⟶ Definite state cycling—early appearance of cycling
32–34   ⟶ Consolidation of behavioral states; definite cycling between discontinuous
                and continuous EEG
40   ⟶ Predictable cycles of "active" and "quiet" sleep
44–46   ⟶ First appearance of sleep spindles during quiet sleep

4 months
postterm   ⟶ Sleep-onset quiet sleep and emergence of mature sleep architecture

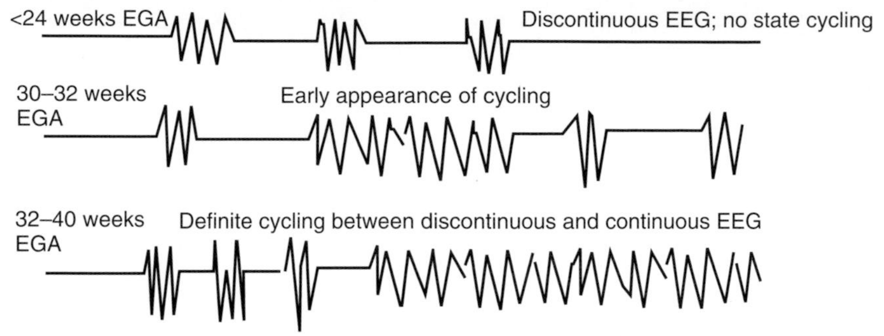

<24 weeks EGA ⟩⟩⟩ ... ⟩⟩⟩ ... ⟩⟩ Discontinuous EEG; no state cycling

30–32 weeks
EGA   Early appearance of cycling

32–40 weeks   Definite cycling between discontinuous and continuous EEG
EGA

• **Figure 18.13** Evolution of the electroencephalogram (EEG) over time during the neonatal period to early childhood. *EGA*, Estimated gestational age. (Modified from Kellway P, Crawley JW. *A Primer of Electroencephalography of Infants, Section II and I: Methodology and Criteria of Normality*. Houston, TX: Baylor University College of Medicine; 1964.)

- Regular respiration, absent eye movements, and relatively preserved EMG
- Tracé discontinu (TD): Present between 30 and 34 weeks CA, bursts of high-amplitude θ-δ (≤200 μV) activity separated by less than 25 μV periods, known as the interburst interval (IBI). Clinical correlate of quiet sleep, whereas awake and active sleep appear the same at this age.
- TA seen at 35–36 weeks CA, similar to TD but less than the periods of relative attenuation in the IBI, are now 25–50 μV, shortening to 2–4 sec by full term, and bursts consist of δ admixed with faster frequencies.
- Continuous slow-wave sleep (CWSW): δ/θ (50–300 μV) resembling adult SWS, without IBI. This can be seen from 35 weeks CA, slowly taking over the percentage of quiet sleep/TA.
- Sleep spindles: 12–14 Hz activity maximal Cz appear at 44–49 weeks CA, and should be well-developed by 3 months of age, symmetric in amplitude, but typically are asynchronous until age 2 years. Duration before this age can be prolonged, up to 8 sec (extreme spindles). Morphology may be arciform.
- Vertex waves and K-complexes are reliably present at 5–6 months of age but can appear earlier.
  - Vertex waves in 3–5 year olds can be very sharply contoured and repetitive, and be misinterpreted as epileptiform activity.
- Hypnogogic hypersynchrony (see Fig. 18.12): From age 1 to 2 months, infants should transition from wakefulness into quiet sleep, rather than active sleep. This drowsy state may show an abrupt increase in amplitude that is highly synchronous and rhythmic in the low θ range. It can be confused with 3–4 Hz spike-wave activity.

- In early childhood both hypnogogic and hypnopompic hypersynchrony can be seen, again typically 3–5 Hz, high amplitude, and rhythmic, but should not be seen in any other circumstances other than arousals and drowsiness, and becomes rare to absent before adolescence.
- Posterior slow waves of youth: 1.5–3 Hz occipitally predominant waves intermixed with α should block with eye-opening, similar to the PDR. This begins at age 3 and can persist into early adulthood.
- POSTS (see Fig. 18.11) can be seen from 6 years of age.

Abnormalities of Background

Frequency

- Slowing:
  - Slowing is generally considered to be due to regional subcortical dysfunction.
  - Continuous slowing has been associated with underlying structural lesions (tumor, stroke, abscess), although intermittent slowing can be due to similar causes (Fig. 18.14).
  - In specific contexts (history of seizures), regional slowing can also be associated with an elevated risk for seizure activity[7] (see Fig. 18.14).
  - On PSG, continuous or intermittent slowing can make accurate sleep staging more difficult.
- Focal β activity:
  - Diffuse β activity is associated with medication effect or drowsiness/sleep.
  - Focal β activity has been associated with structural or otherwise epileptogenic regions. Areas of dysplastic cerebral cortex

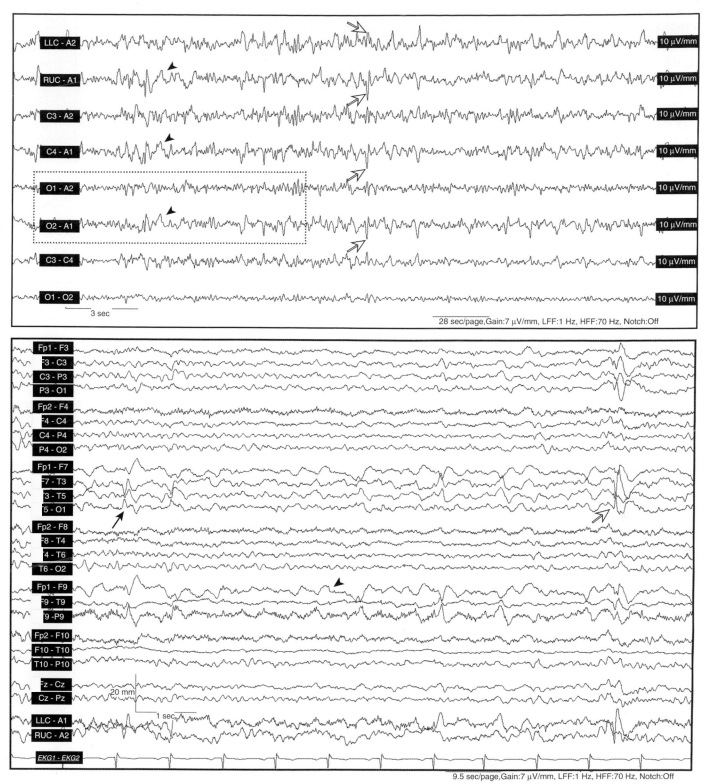

• Figure 18.14 The *arrowhead* shows left inferior temporal intermittent rhythmic δ activity (TIRDA), sharp waves *(barbed arrows)*, and spikes *(open arrows)*, all markers of temporal lobe epilepsy. On a basic polysomnographic montage at 10 mm/sec (above), the temporal activity is well recorded by the left lower canthus (LLC) and the A1 reference, but it is also broadly distributed over the left frontocentral regions. Thus the major asymmetry in channels (see the *dotted box*) is between O2 and A1 (in which O2 is inert but the A1 reference is involved) and O1 and A2 (neither lead is involved, thus showing a normal posterior dominant rhythm). All other leads are involved to some extent. On the long bipolar montage at 10 mm/sec with extra electrodes (inferior temporal leads), the TIRDA is easily localized to the left inferior temporal region. Interspersed with the TIRDA are frequent spikes, maximal in the left temporal region. Electroencephalographic electrode labels are from the modified 10-20 system. The F9, T9, and P9 and F10, T10, and P10 electrodes represent the left and right inferior temporal electrodes, respectively. *RUC*, Right upper canthus.

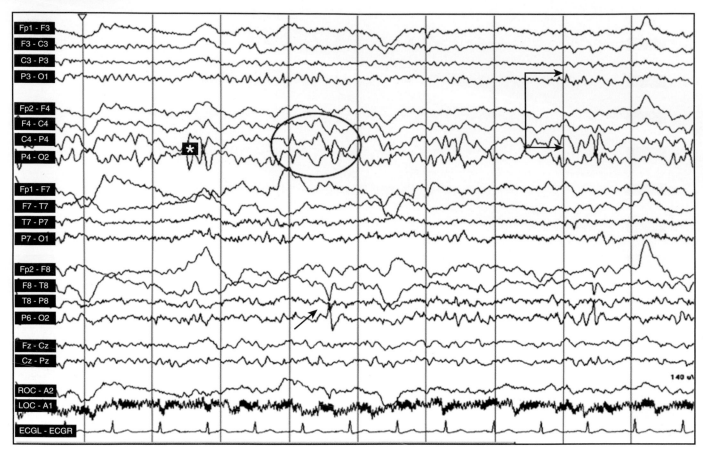

• **Figure 18.15** Breach rhythm and focal δ slowing in a 55-year-old patient after right hemispheric brain surgery to remove an arteriovenous malformation. The electroencephalogram (EEG) can be difficult to interpret in such patients. Breach rhythm refers to increased amplitude of the faster frequencies through a skull defect and is demonstrated when comparing the left and right posterior regions *(double-headed arrow)*. There is less resistance for electrical activity to escape through the skull defect; this gives a sharper appearance to the underlying background activity *(asterisk)*, which can be difficult to differentiate from epileptiform activity. In this example there is a true sharp wave *(arrow)*, electromaximal at T8–P8 (involving both the T8 and P8 electrodes equally). There is also continuous δ slowing in the same right posterior region *(oval)*. The long bipolar montage was recorded at 30 mm/sec, with EEG electrode labels from the modified 10-20 system.

have been implicated, although the sensitivity and specificity of the association have not been well documented.[7]

Voltage

- Attenuation (decreased voltage)
  - Determined relative to the background voltage.
  - Low (<20 μV), medium (20–40 μV), and high (>50 μV) are used loosely to describe voltage.
  - Cortical damage (as a result of anoxic injury or stroke, for example) is associated with focal attenuation, particularly of faster-frequency activity.
  - Can also be seen when additional substances absorb the electrical activity of the brain before it reaches the electrodes (such as blood in a subdural hematoma).
  - Voltages often normalize with time following cerebral injuries.
  - Focal or regional attenuation can also be artifactual, caused by small differences in electrode distances, or can be presumed

to be due to increased voltage on the opposite side as a result of a "*breach artifact*" (Fig. 18.15), which in essence is a skull abnormality characterized by increased amplitude (because of decreased resistance).

- Increased voltage:
  - Focal high-voltage activity is unusual and often due to a "*breach artifact*" (see Fig. 18.15) caused by cranial defect, such as prior craniotomies, and also minor skull fractures or thinning.

Basics of Clinical Epilepsy

- Epilepsy affects an estimated 0.4%–1.0% of the population, with a lifetime prevalence of 1.8%–2.6%.[8] The prevalence of definite epilepsy (recurrent, unprovoked seizures) is estimated to be 6.5 per 1000 in the United States.[1]
- Most cases of epilepsy have an unknown etiology (Fig. 18.16), with other various causes being vascular, congenital, or secondary to neoplasm. The head trauma must be severe enough to cause

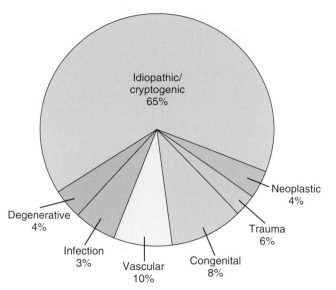

• **Figure 18.16** Etiology of newly diagnosed epilepsy in Rochester, Minnesota, 1935–1984. (Data extracted from Hauser WA, Annegers JF, Kurland LT. Incidence of epilepsy and unprovoked seizures in Rochester, Minnesota: 1935–1984. *Epilepsia.* 1993;34[3]:453–468.)

loss of consciousness to carry an appreciable risk for subsequent epilepsy.

• Epileptic conditions can be classified by seizure type or by etiology. With a history of probable epilepsy, documentation of an unprovoked seizure during an EEG recording would make the diagnosis definite.

• A history of "paroxysmal episodes" or spells, along with epileptiform activity, would be very suspicious for an epileptic condition.

Epileptiform Abnormalities and Seizures

• Interictal (meaning "between seizures") epileptiform activity classically includes spikes and sharp waves, and can be either focal or generalized.

• Sleep and sleep deprivation are known to increase the occurrence of all of these discharges.[9,10]
  • For focal discharges, the greatest frequency occurs during SWS, whereas REM sleep has the opposite effect, a dramatic decrease in all discharges.[11]

Focal Spike

See Figs. 18.10 and 18.14.

• Transient potential stands out from the background; duration of the base is 20–70 msec.

• Typically negative in polarity with a sensible electrical field (a region of maximal amplitude with lesser amplitudes in neighboring electrodes as a result of the discharge originating from a discrete region of the cerebral cortex). Can be positive in neonates.

• Often followed by a slow wave of negative polarity that disrupts the background.

Sharp Wave

See Figs. 18.10 and 18.14.

• Similar to a spike but 70–200 msec in duration.

Multifocal Epileptiform Discharges

• Spikes or sharp waves (or both) with a discrete origin occur in at least two locations on one hemisphere and in one on the contralateral hemisphere. For example, although F7 may denote one anterotemporal focality, a second focus at P7 and any on the right side would together denote multifocality, thus implying a more refractory epilepsy syndrome.

Generalized Epileptiform Discharges

See Fig. 18.17.

• Generalized spike-wave and polyspike-wave discharges can occur in runs and trains.

• Discharges typical of absence epilepsy repeat at frequencies of nearly exactly 3 Hz (Fig. 18.18), with faster frequencies being related to juvenile myoclonic epilepsy and slower frequencies being related to other generalized epilepsies.

Seizures

• Classically electrographic seizures are defined as rhythmic discharges or rhythms that evolve in the frequency of the rhythmic pattern (speed up, then slow down, and end abruptly), with spread of the electrical field, usually increase in amplitude during the seizure, with attenuation or slowing following immediately. Significant artifact often obscures the EEG if there is a convulsive component (Fig. 18.19).

• There is wide variability in seizures—in terms of location, frequency, and evolution pattern.

• Most seizures have both a clinical and EEG correlate.

• Others, such as frontal lobe seizures, can be diagnosed on clinical grounds with no clear correlate on EEG.

• Nocturnal seizures: Both generalized and partial epilepsy syndromes can have a diurnal pattern. Many nocturnal paroxysmal events are not epileptic, and EEG on overnight PSG can be helpful in the diagnosis. In addition, specific features can be elicited during a brief clinical evaluation, with the differential diagnosis of events and disorders being listed in Tables 18.1 and 18.2, respectively.

Generalized Epilepsy and Electroencephalography

• Generalized epilepsy is conceptualized to have seizures generated from both hemispheres essentially simultaneously.

• Idiopathic generalized epilepsy (IGE), also known as primary generalized epilepsy or PGE in the past, includes multiple syndromes in people of normal intellect, each of which may have different seizure types, including generalized tonic-clonic (GTC) seizures.

• Juvenile myoclonic epilepsy and absence epilepsy are the most common IGE syndromes.

Generalized Tonic-Clonic Seizures

• Can be either primary generalized (no known or suspected cause or location of onset) or secondarily generalized from an epileptogenic focus (see the section on localization-related epilepsy and Fig. 18.16).

• Can occur day or night. If exclusively nocturnal, the seizures are more likely to be idiopathic[12] and tend to occur during the onset or at end of sleep, and rarely out of REM sleep.

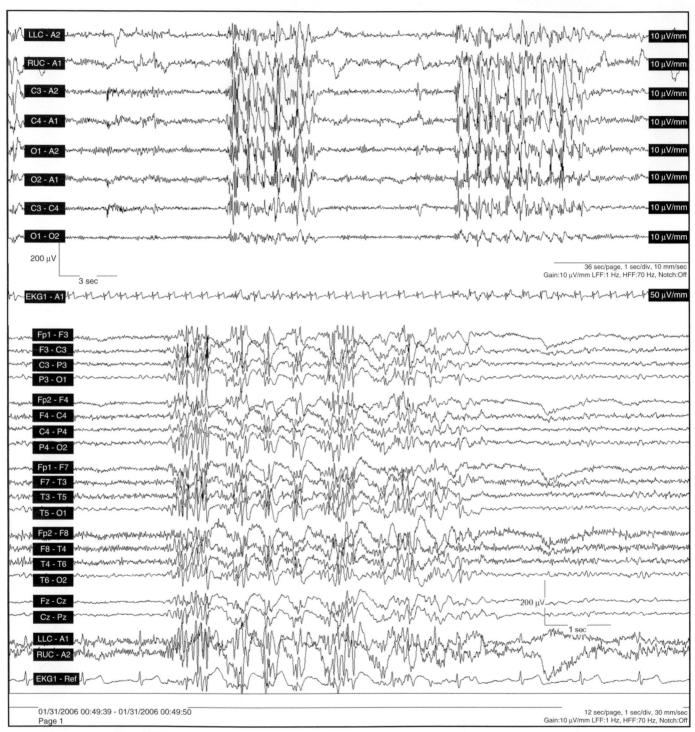

• **Figure 18.17** Burst of generalized epileptiform activity consisting of polyspikes and polyspike-wave complexes seen with a typical polysomnographic montage and reading speed (above) and electroencephalographic (EEG) reading speed in a long bipolar montage (below). Polyspike-wave complexes are typical of a generalized epilepsy syndrome, including juvenile myoclonic epilepsy. The EEG electrode labels are from the modified 10-20 system (see Fig. 18.1). *EKG,* Electrocardiogram; *LLC,* left lower canthus; *RUC,* right upper canthus.

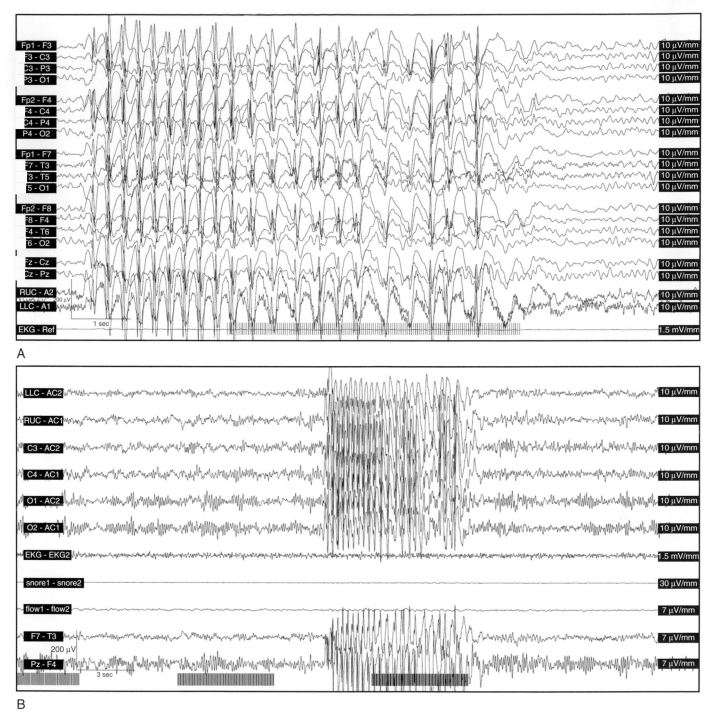

• **Figure 18.18** Absence seizure featuring classic 3-Hz spike and wave activity shown at a standard electroencephalographic (EEG) reading speed of 30 mm/sec **(A)** and compressed at a standard polysomnographic scoring speed of 10 mm/sec. **B,** The EEG electrodes are as per Fig. 18.1; other electrodes include the left auricle (AC1), right auricle (AC2), electrocardiogram (EKG), snore (snore 1–snore 2) and nasal-oral flow (flow 1–flow 2). *LLC,* Left lower canthus; *RUC,* right upper canthus.

• In IGE onset should be bisynchronous, typically maximal in the anterior regions, although a shifting asymmetry is sometimes seen.
• EEG may only show an arousal and a typical pattern of muscle artifact, which obscures the EEG tracing but parallels the tonic (sustained contraction) and then clonic (rhythmic brief contractions) components of the seizure.

• Diffuse background slowing in the δ range is seen in the postictal phase.

Juvenile Myoclonic Epilepsy
• The most benign of the many myoclonic epileptic disorders, although it is still a lifelong condition (see Fig. 18.17)[12]

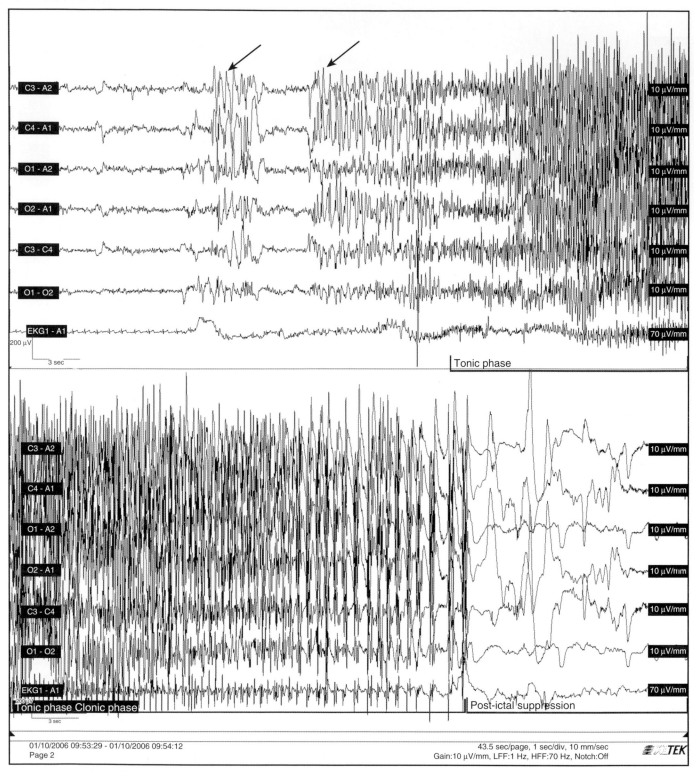

43.5 sec/page, 1 sec/div, 10 mm/sec
Gain:10 µV/mm, LFF:1 Hz, HFF:70 Hz, Notch:Off

• **Figure 18.19** Relatively short generalized tonic-clonic seizure on a typical polysomnographic montage at 10 mm/sec. Rapid clinical onset caused a muscle artifact to obscure electroencephalographic (EEG) evidence of the seizure, but the pattern of muscle artifact matches the clinical phenomena. The densest muscle artifact occurs during the tonic phase of the seizure, with a progressively relenting on-off muscle pattern matching each clonic movement. The actual onset of the seizure may have been heralded by myoclonic activity *(arrows)*. This rapid onset may be due to either a primary generalized epilepsy syndrome or a rapidly secondarily generalized partial-onset seizure. These seizures can be overlooked as simple arousal and muscle artifact, with the only EEG correlate being postictal slowing and attenuation, which is diffuse in this case, but if focal it may suggest partial onset. EEG scalp electrodes are as per the modified 10-20 system (see Fig. 18.1). *EKG,* Electrocardiogram.

TABLE 18.1	Nocturnal Events: Differential Diagnosis						
	Incontinence	Tongue Biting	Confusion	Tonic-Clonic Movement	Drooling	Amnesia	Occur While Awake
Seizure	+	+	+	+	+	+	+
Sleep drunkenness	–	–	+	–	–	+	–
Sleep terror	–	–	+	–	–	–	–
Somnambulism	–	–	+	–	–	+	–
Somniloquy	–	–	+	–	–	+	–
Sleep enuresis	+	–	–	–	–	–	–
PLMS/RLS	–	–	–	–	–	–	+
Nightmare	–	–	–	–	–	–	–
Cataplexy	–	–	–	–	–	–	+
Sleep paralysis	–	–	–	–	–	–	+
Hypnic hallucination	–	–	–	–	–	–	+
REM behavior disorder	–	–	+	–	–	–	—

PLMS, Periodic limb movements during sleep; *REM*, rapid eye movement; *RLS*, restless legs syndrome.

TABLE 18.2	Effects of Antiepileptic Drugs on Sleep and Sleep Disorders				
	EFFECTS ON SLEEP			EFFECTS ON SLEEP DISORDERS	
Antiepileptic Drug	Positive	Negative		Improves/Treats	Worsens
Barbiturates	Decreased latency	Decreased REM		Sleep-onset insomnia	OSA
Benzodiazepines	Decreased latency	Decreased REM, SWS		Sleep-onset insomnia	OSA
Carbamazepine	—	Decreased REM?		RLS	—
Phenytoin	Decreased latency	Increased arousals and stage 1; decreased REM		—	—
Valproic acid	—	Increased stage 1		—	OSA*
Felbamate	?	?		OSA*	Insomnia
Gabapentin	Increased SWS, decreased arousals	None		RLS	—
Lacosamide	?	?		—	—
Lamotrigine	None	Decreased SWS?		—	—
Levetiracetam	Increased SWS	None		—	—
Pregabalin	Increased SWS, decreased arousals	None		RLS	OSA*
Tiagabine	Increased SWS	None		—	—
Topiramate	?	?		OSA*	—
Zonisamide	?	?		OSA*	—

*Indirectly through weight change.
OSA, Obstructive sleep apnea; *REM*, rapid eye movement; *RLS*, restless legs syndrome; *SWS*, slow wave sleep; ?, unknown.

- Onset between 0 and 18 years of age, although it can present much later
- Familial tendency; typically occurs in otherwise healthy individuals
- Myoclonic jerks or GTC seizures early or first thing in the morning, especially with sleep deprivation
- Myoclonic jerks can be very mild and relatively asymptomatic, but they can also consist of whole-body myoclonic activity.
- EEG spike-wave and polyspike-wave activity, sometimes repetitive but irregular 4–6 Hz. Photic stimulation can activate EEG abnormalities and seizures. Most commonly seen during early sleep and upon awakening.

Absence Epilepsy

- Childhood form is more benign: onset is 3–12 years, with a peak at 6–7 years (see Fig. 18.18).
- The juvenile form starts later and is more likely to be associated with GTC seizures and be refractory to treatment.[12]
- Typical absence seizures occur in neurologically normal individuals and consist of a brief (usually <15 sec but up to 30 sec) behavioral arrest with rapid onset and offset.
- 3-Hz generalized spike and wave complex (often appearing with maximal amplitude in the frontocentral region) is the typical EEG abnormality, but during sleep these complexes frequently becomes fragmented and may appear more focal.

Localization-Related Epilepsy (Partial Epilepsy) and Electroencephalography

Partial seizures can arise from any area of the brain, but those arising from the frontal and temporal lobes are the most likely to have a diurnal pattern.

Frontal Lobe Seizures

See Fig. 18.20.

- Clinically typified by an abrupt arousal with abnormal posturing of the body, the limbs flail violently and chaotically in a ballistic manner, the legs may make bicycling motions, and there is often vocalization.

- Involvement of specific regions of the frontal lobe may result in characteristic seizure "semiology" (clinical description), such as the supplementary motor area leading to tonic asymmetrical posturing of the limbs.
- Self-injury can occur; patients often opt to sleep close to the floor.
- An abrupt onset of extremely fast β activity with an apparent attenuation is classically associated with these seizures, although the EEG may not show a definite focus of onset, with muscle and movement artifact possibly obscuring the entire EEG tracing during the event.
- Generalization to tonic-clonic activity may occur but is not common.
- Patients have a very short postictal confusional stage, up to 1–2 min, and often rapidly return to sleep, amnestic to the event.
- Frontal lobe partial seizures commonly occur during sleep and are sometimes absent during wakefulness[13]; in this case they may be clinically unrecognized or be confused with night terrors, nocturnal parasomnias, or a conversion disorder.
- Etiology may be a migrational abnormality, acquired or genetic in nature (see later).

Autosomal Dominant Nocturnal Frontal Lobe Epilepsy

- A genetic syndrome in which nocturnal motor seizures occur.
- The seizures may be similar to the frontal lobe seizures described earlier, although there may be an associated aura of sensorimotor or experiential phenomena.

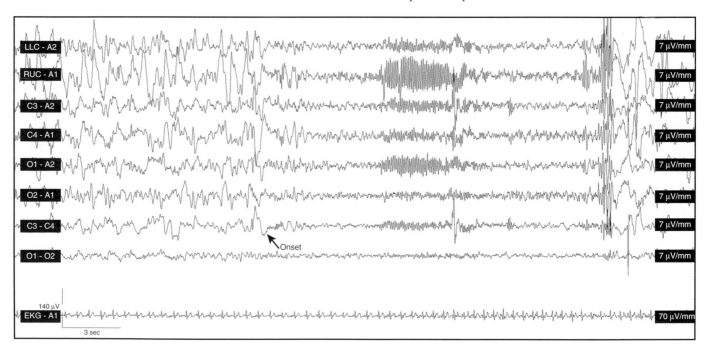

A

• **Figure 18.20** Frontal Lobe Seizure. The polysomnographic (at 10 mm/sec, **A**) and electroencephalographic (EEG) tracings (at 30 mm/sec, **B**) show a sudden change in background activity with a burst followed by diffuse attenuation *(arrows)* and then by a complex evolution of ictal activity: gradually increasing amplitude of fast activity, followed by another attenuation with fast β activity, before a final abrupt diffuse attenuation and slowing. In the latter stages of the seizure, there may be some lateralization to the right frontal region *(arrows)*, which is not definitive for localization of the onset. This patient had a tendency for the seizures to cluster, with another seizure before and another ensuing directly after. During the seizures, the patient exhibited mild bicycling of the legs, thrashing of the limbs, and irritability. She was amnestic to the details of the events. She is developmentally normal otherwise. The EEG electrode labels are from the modified 10-20 system (see Fig. 18.1).

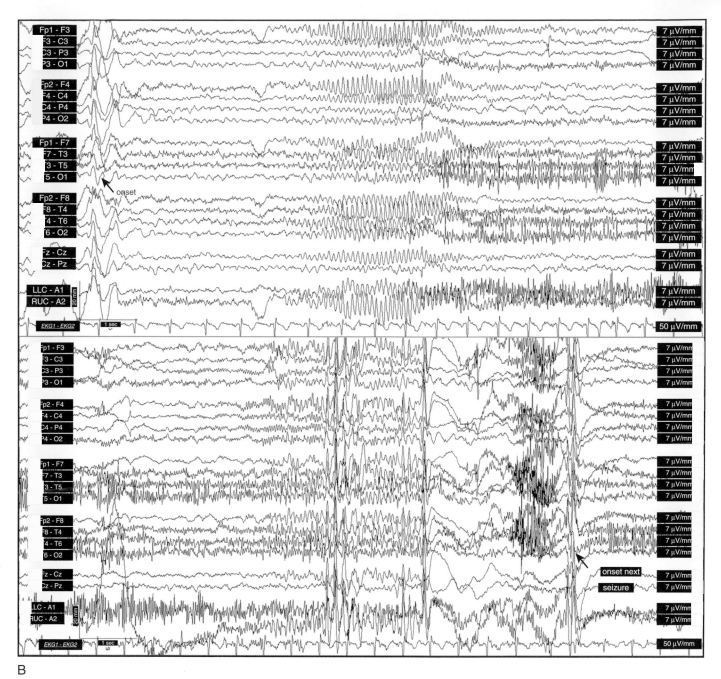

B

• **Figure 18.20, cont'd** B, EEG tracing in a long bipolar montage recorded at 30 mm/sec. Refer to Fig. 18.1 for electrode nomenclature. *EKG,* Electrocardiogram; *LLC,* left lower canthus; *RUC,* right upper canthus.

- Tendency to cluster and may occur several times nightly, frequently during NREM sleep.
- Seizures most commonly seen shortly after falling asleep or in the early morning, but they can also occur during daytime naps.
- EEG may not show interictal abnormalities, and similar to many frontal lobe seizures, an ictal pattern can be hard to appreciate because of movement artifact.
- There are many family lineages of autosomal dominant nocturnal frontal lobe epilepsy (ADNFLE), with the mutations affecting the coding for subunits of the nicotinic acetylcholine receptor.

- Most cases of ADNFLE have responded to treatment with anticonvulsants—in particular, carbamazepine.

Temporal Lobe Seizures

See Fig. 18.21.
- Can occur during sleep or wakefulness, with or without secondary generalization to tonic-clonic activity.[13]
- Patients are often unaware of their partial seizures without generalization.
- Nocturnally, they may cause only an arousal.
- Seizures involving the mesial temporal structures (hippocampus and amygdala) classically have a characteristic high-amplitude

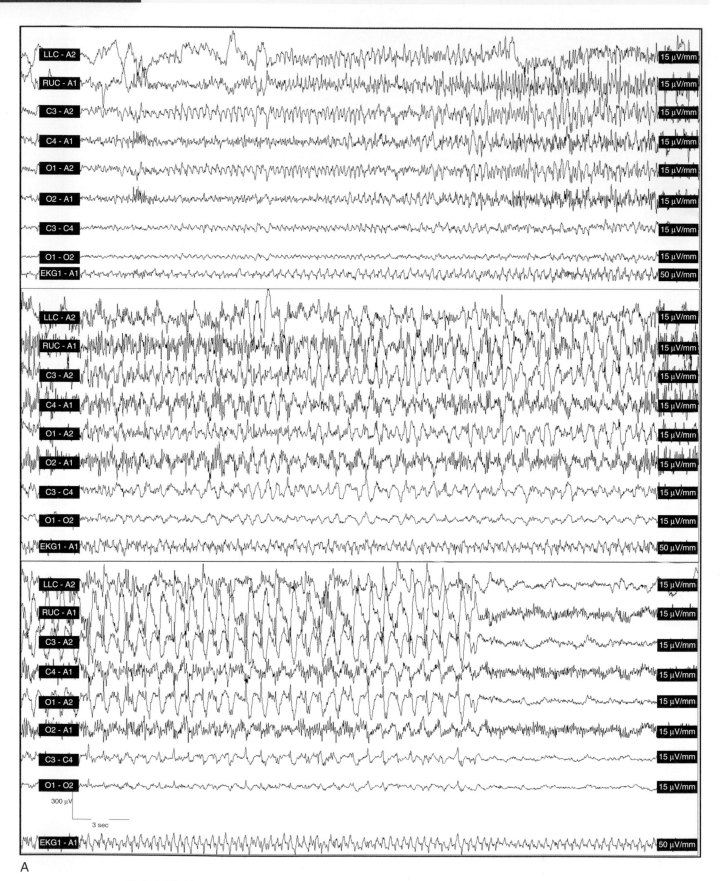

A

• **Figure 18.21 A,** Right temporal seizure on a typical polysomnogram at 10-mm/sec recording speed and limited scalp electrode coverage. Despite lacking dedicated temporal electrodes, the auricular references (A1-A2) pick up temporal activity. Here the rhythmic discharge contaminates the A2 reference: all channels referred to A2 (LLC-A2, C3-A2, O1-A2) demonstrate the seizure activity, which potentially appears to be left hemispheric. The same seizure is shown in B and is localizing to the right inferior temporal region. Note the evolution and abrupt offset of the rhythmic activity. Refer to Fig. 18.1 for electrode nomenclature.

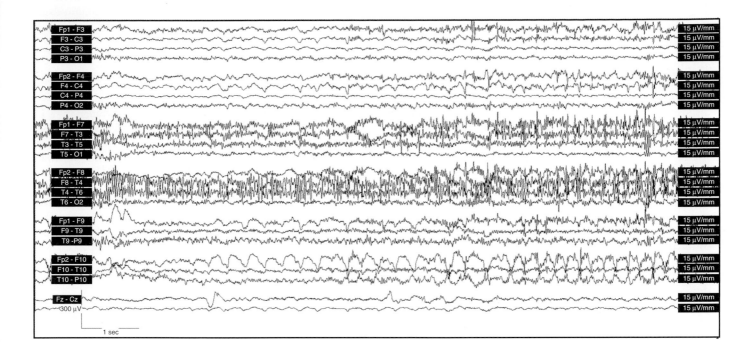

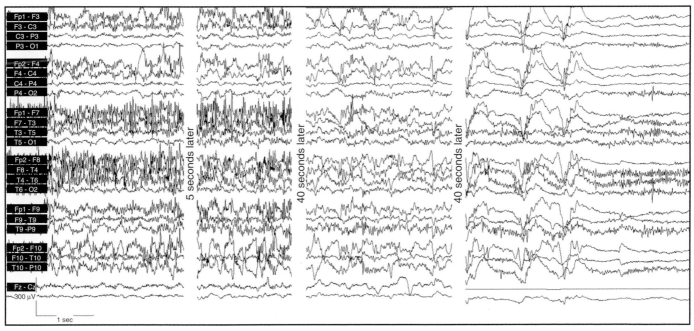

B

• **Figure 18.21, cont'd** B, Right temporal seizure in a long bipolar montage, including the inferior temporal chains. Note the electrographic evolution, initially rhythmic δ activity isolated to the right inferior temporal channels (Fp2-F10, F10-T10, T10-P10), with an increase in rhythmic frequency up to 7 Hz and spread in field to adjacent regions with an increase in amplitude. The end of the seizure is shown; large-amplitude, rhythmic slow sharp–slow wave complexes are followed by postictal diffuse attenuation and slowing. This patient had nocturnal awakenings without tonic-clonic activity, in addition to daytime staring spells with oromotor automatisms (lip smacking). Refer to Fig. 18.1 for electrode nomenclature. *EKG,* Electrocardiogram; *LLC,* left lower canthus; *RUC,* right upper canthus.

rhythmic discharge in the 7–8-Hz range, termed "rhythmic theta-alpha" (RTA).

Other Notable Epilepsy Syndromes and Electroencephalography

Rolandic Epilepsy

See Fig. 18.22.

- An "idiopathic" partial epilepsy associated with a genetic predisposition, but it has an excellent prognosis. Age at onset is 2–12 years; seizures usually spontaneously remit at 15–18 years of age.
- About 75% of seizures occur during sleep, and they may be focal or generalized.[14]
- Seizures can consist of hemifacial twitching or hemiconvulsions, with characteristic seizures involving hypersalivation, gurgling, and speech arrest.
- Interictal EEG shows frequent central or temporal spikes with distinctive morphology that are unilateral in 70% of recordings, but they can vary in location from recording to recording.
- The spikes are often highly "activated" (more frequent) during drowsiness and sleep, and are typified by a dipole, with negativity focused centrotemporally and positivity maximally in the bifrontal region. Sleep architecture is normal in these otherwise neurologically normal patients.
- Also known as "benign childhood epilepsy with centrotemporal spikes" (BECTS)

Continuous Spike-Wave Activity During Sleep

See Fig. 18.23.

- A rare childhood syndrome with predominantly nocturnal seizures, either focal or generalized[14]
- Consists of diffuse slow spike-wave complexes accounting for at least 85% of NREM sleep
- The EEG during wakefulness may show a combination of focal and generalized spikes.
- Onset typically between the ages of 1 and 12 years. Although seizures tend to remit by the age of 20, intellectual deterioration and neuropsychologic impairment are frequent.
- Previously known as electrical status epilepticus during sleep (ESES) or epilepsy with continuous spikes and waves in SWS (electrical status epilepticus during SWS [ESESS]).

Landau-Kleffner Syndrome

- A rare form of childhood epilepsy characterized by progressive and severe language dysfunction in addition to behavioral difficulties.[14]
- Abnormal electrical activity is recorded in one or both temporal lobes, often with multifocal EEG spikes, and characteristically can occur nearly continuously for hours at a time during sleep, as in the continuous spike-wave activity during sleep (CSWS) just described.
- Sleep is very disturbed.
- Seizures are frequent initially and have a tendency to lessen with time.

Benign Variants and Artifact on Electroencephalography

The skill in EEG is differentiating benign variants and artifact from an actual abnormality.

- Many benign variants can appear epileptiform, and many noncerebral events can create an artifact that can appear rhythmic, epileptiform, or focal, thereby leading to overcalling findings and potentially subjecting the individual to unnecessary long-term treatments.

Benign Variants

Rhythmic Midtemporal Theta of Drowsiness

See Fig. 18.24.

- Rhythmic, sharply contoured, short runs of θ-range (5–7 Hz) activity are maximal at T7 (T3) or T8 (T4), bilateral synchronous or unilateral.
- Most common in adolescents and young adults, in awake, drowsy, or light sleep states, and should disappear with deeper sleep.
- Also known as "rhythmic temporal θ bursts of drowsiness," "rhythmic midtemporal discharges," and "psychomotor variant."
- Asymmetrical, prolonged runs (duration can be seconds to beyond a minute) can be mistaken for a seizure, especially when notched by faster frequencies
- Fragments that are of higher amplitude than the background can be mistaken for a spike or sharp wave.

Wicket Spikes or Wicket Rhythm

See Fig. 18.25.

- Monophasic *negative* discharges or trains of waves, anterior or midtemporal.
- Typically 8–11 Hz and 60–200 µV; often arch-shaped (arciform).
- Seen in adults and elderly in a drowsy state.
- Longer runs can occur, which is referred to as a wicket rhythm.
- Can be mistaken for an epileptiform discharge when one is of higher amplitude to stand out from the background. If the morphology of the larger discharge is similar to more obvious wickets, it should be considered benign. Wickets should not disrupt the background.

Benign Epileptiform Transients of Sleep/Small Sharp Spikes

See Fig. 18.26.

- Low-amplitude (<50 µV) spikes of very short duration (~50 msec) and usually simply configured monophasic or diphasic. May or may not have a small after-going slow wave, but does not alter the background.
- Usually broad field, typically unilateral, can be bilateral independent, and rarely bisynchronous
- Seen in drowsiness and early sleep; disappears with deepening stages (as opposed to epileptiform activity)
- They can be numerous in one overnight recording.
- Patient may or may not have epilepsy. There is no clinical significance.

Subclinical Rhythmic Electrographic Discharges in Adults

See Fig. 18.27.

- A rhythmic and sometimes evolving rhythmic electrographic discharge
- Typically up to the θ range and without postictal slowing or attenuation
- Very rare; seen only in adults more common in the elderly
- The abrupt onset and offset mimic electrographic seizures, but they generally occur during wakefulness and without any clinical correlate.

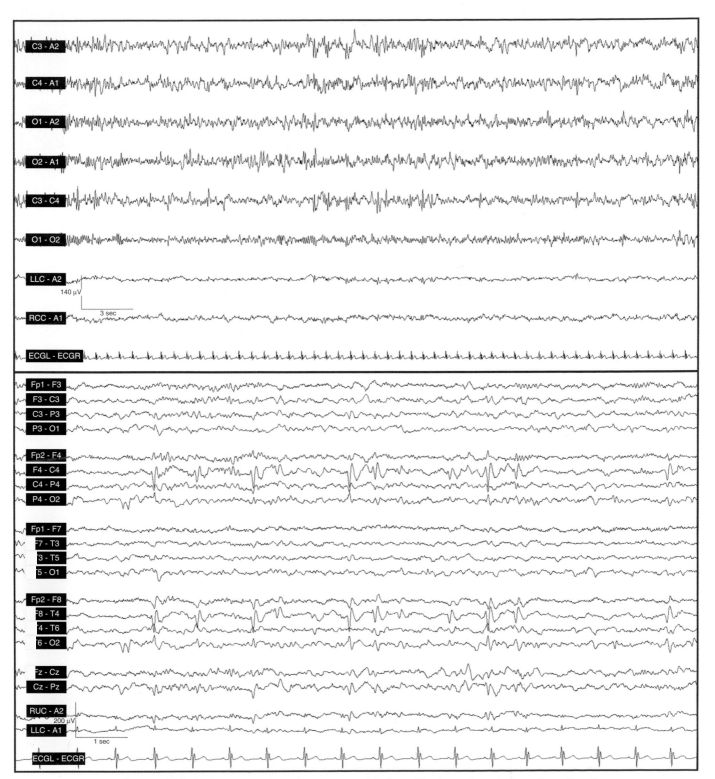

• **Figure 18.22** Benign Epileptiform Centrotemporal Spikes. Simply configured, triangular spike discharges in a 10-year-old boy are classic findings in the self-limited "rolandic" epilepsy syndrome. The example is shown at typical polysomnographic reading speed of 10 mm/sec (above) and a typical electroencephalographic reading speed of 30 mm/sec (below). Refer to Fig. 18.1 for electrode nomenclature.

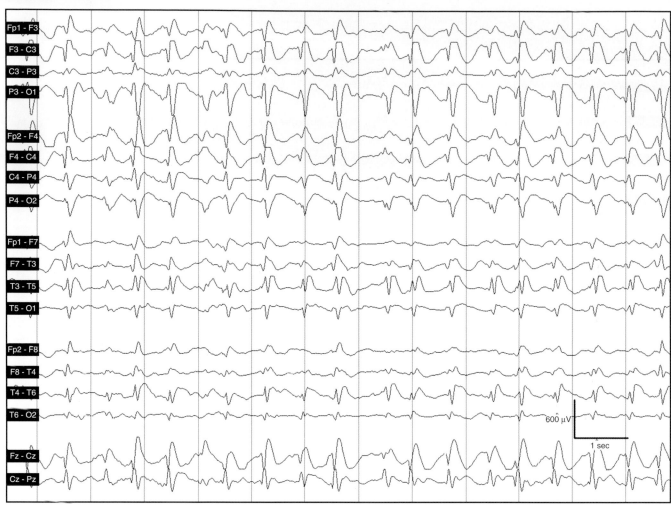

• **Figure 18.23** Continuous spike-wave activity during sleep (CSWS), previously known as electrical status epilepticus during sleep (ESES), seen on an electroencephalographic long bipolar montage recorded at 30 mm/sec. The patient was clinically asleep during these prolonged runs of epileptiform activity. Periodic spike-wave discharges are seen occurring at 1–2 Hz and occurred for greater than 85% of the nonrapid eye movement sleep recorded, which was thus classified as CSWS. Refer to Fig. 18.1 for electrode nomenclature.

- Long-term follow-up has shown no clinical significance of the pattern.

Artifacts

Please also refer to Chapter 32.

Physiologic Artifacts

The most common artifacts are physiologic but not of cerebral origin.

- Breach artifact (see Fig. 18.15): Defects in the skull from either fractures, unfused cranial sutures (from infancy), or previous cranial surgery will allow higher voltages to be recorded at the scalp. Typically the effect involves higher frequencies, and thus δ slowing in the same region, for instance, is usually due to underlying dysfunction and not the breach effect. Breach effect can also make normal activity appear sharper due to higher amplitude of normal β frequencies.

- Eye movement artifact: Movements of the eyes are recorded on eye channels during polysomnography, but these movements also cause changes on EEG. The cornea is electropositive in comparison to the negatively charged retina. Whatever direction the eye looks, a large positivity is seen on EEG. On a longitudinal bipolar montage, vertical eye movements are best demonstrated in the frontopolar leads (Fp1, Fp2), whereas horizontal movements are seen best at F7 and F8 (see Fig. 18.8).
- Glossokinetic artifact (Fig. 18.28): The tongue is also charged, with the tip being negative with respect to the base. Movements of the tongue, seen during speech, for instance, can create the appearance of focal slowing in the temporal regions, which can be quite difficult to distinguish from cerebral dysfunction.
- Muscle artifact: Muscle within the scalp also causes electrical activity (EMG), but it is usually easy to distinguish because of the typically sharper and higher frequency waveforms that are impossible for the brain to transmit to the scalp.

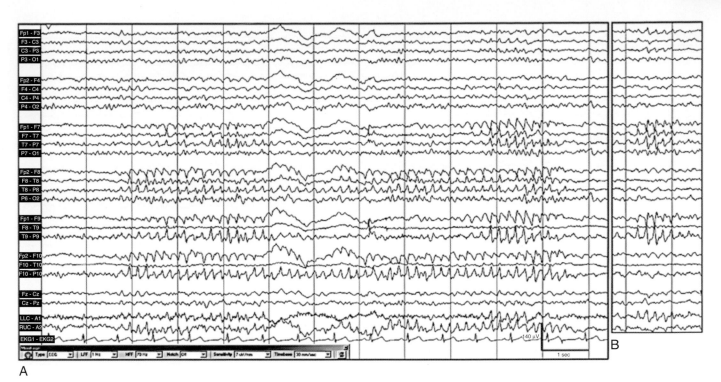

• **Figure 18.24** Rhythmic midtemporal θ of drowsiness (RMTD) is a benign variant that can be confused with epileptiform activity. RMTD can occur as a single waveform, similar to a spike, or in longer runs, which may mimic seizure activity. A longer run with bilateral involvement **(A)** and a short burst **(B)** was recorded at 30 mm/sec, with the left inferior temporal channels (Fp1-F9, F9-T9, T9-P9) better demonstrating the notched morphology. Refer to Fig. 18.1 for electrode nomenclature. *EKG,* Electrocardiogram; *LLC,* left lower canthus; *RUC,* right upper canthus.

• Chewing and bruxism (Fig. 18.29): Because the temporal chain resides over the temporalis muscles, activation of the muscle generates large-amplitude, very fast activity. During chewing it is very rhythmic, with bruxism classically producing a "checkerboard" pattern consisting of muscle artifact alternating side to side.

• Electrocardiographic (ECG) artifact (Fig. 18.30): The EEG leads are often contaminated by electrical impulses from the heart. The degree of contamination can vary during a recording, depending on the position of the patient, presumably as the position of the heart shifts in comparison to the leads. The left ear or mastoid lead, A1/M1, has a tendency to record the greatest amount of artifact. If it becomes problematic, a bipolar montage or a different reference electrode should be used. It is also possible to "link the ears" to remove the artifact by combining the signals from A1 and A2 to "average out" the ECG signal. This can be accomplished either mechanically (using a wire bridge) or electronically (computerized).

• Pulse artifact (Fig. 18.31): Arteries and veins within the scalp can cause physical movement of a lead, which can appear as a periodic discharge, often as a δ wave. The field will typically be restricted to a single lead and should be temporally linked to the ECG recording.

• Cardioballistic artifact: Similar to a pulse artifact, movement of blood rushing to the head with each cardiac compression can cause minute movements of the head or body, which will create the appearance of a periodic discharge, frequently in the leads that the patient is resting on.

• Respiratory artifact: Not typically seen in healthy individuals, a respiratory artifact can appear as large slow waves, particularly when electrodes are loosened by sweat. This effect is more common while viewing the recording in a PSG montage.

• Positive pressure apparatuses: The machine itself may create an artifact because of high-frequency oscillations of the breathing apparatus. Water trapped within the tubing can also vibrate with airflow and cause a periodic high-frequency artifact that is timed with respirations. This effect is seen more often in patients who are intubated than in patients managed with noninvasive ventilation or continuous positive airway pressure.

Nonphysiologic Artifacts

• Movement artifact: Any movement of the wires can cause an artifact; thus, when the patient moves, there will frequently be a correlate on EEG that is not of cerebral origin.

• Lead impedance/60-Hz artifact (Fig. 18.32): The electrodes will record the signal with least resistance. With failing conductance between the scalp and electrode, signals from the surroundings are instead transmitted and then amplified. Power supplies in North America run on a 60-Hz cycle, and a 60-Hz sinusoidal wave can be seen in the channels affected by poor electrical impedance or in extreme situations (e.g., intensive care units). This artifact can overrun the entire recording. In the latter case, a notch filter can help eliminate this artifact.

• Electrode pop artifact (Fig. 18.33): When an electrode intermittently loses proper contact with the scalp, relatively

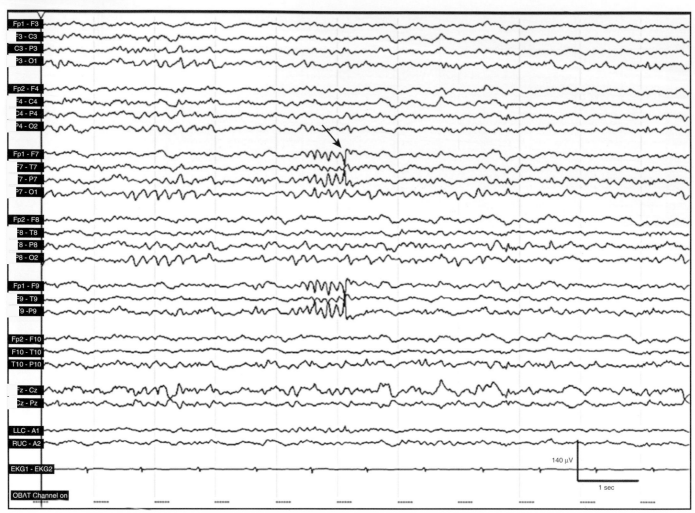

• **Figure 18.25** Wicket rhythm/spikes are sharply contoured, negative discharges or trains of waves, typically 8–11 Hz and 60–200 μV. The morphology is often arch shaped and typically a simply configured diphasic waveform with a symmetrical upstroke and downstroke. When found, they are usually anterior or midtemporal, and seen in adults and the elderly in a drowsy state. They are benign findings but can be mistaken for an epileptiform discharge. The *arrow* shows a higher-amplitude, sharply contoured discharge that stands out from the background, but the morphology remains arciform and clearly arises from a train of wickets. Longer runs can occur, which is referred to as a wicket rhythm. The montage was long bipolar, with a paper speed of 30 mm/sec and sensitivity of 7 μV. The electroencephalographic nomenclature is as per Fig. 18.1 with additional inferior electrodes on the left (T9, P9) and right (T10, P10). *EKG*, Electrocardiogram; *LLC*, left lower canthus; *RUC*, right upper canthus.

high-amplitude deflections will be recorded, but only from that electrode.

Limitations to Scalp Electroencephalogram

1. Information is lost when translating the three-dimensional structure of the brain into a two-dimensional array.
   a. Sulci and other cortical surfaces irregularities (including the insula, the mesial surfaces of the temporal lobes and the hemispheres, and the entire inferior surface of the brain) are electrically obscured due to tangential direction of electrical field, inability to place electrodes directly above these areas, physical distance, or excess intervening tissue.
   b. Electrical signal that is properly oriented for electrode recording and close to the skull is attenuated by the surrounding cerebrospinal fluid, meninges, skull, and scalp leading to a small signal that is prone to artifact. The signal that is recorded at the scalp is thus a relatively crude aggregate of regional cortical activity, with an estimated 10 neurons contributing to the electrical field at a given electrode.[1,2] Despite these limitations, technologic advances have helped the EEG improve, and currently the EEG supplies crucial and unique information about brain function over time that is helpful to epileptologists and sleep medicine experts and is not available by other tests.

Reporting the Electroencephalogram

• The age and clinical state are clinically relevant. The EEG changes dramatically from the newborn period to early childhood through

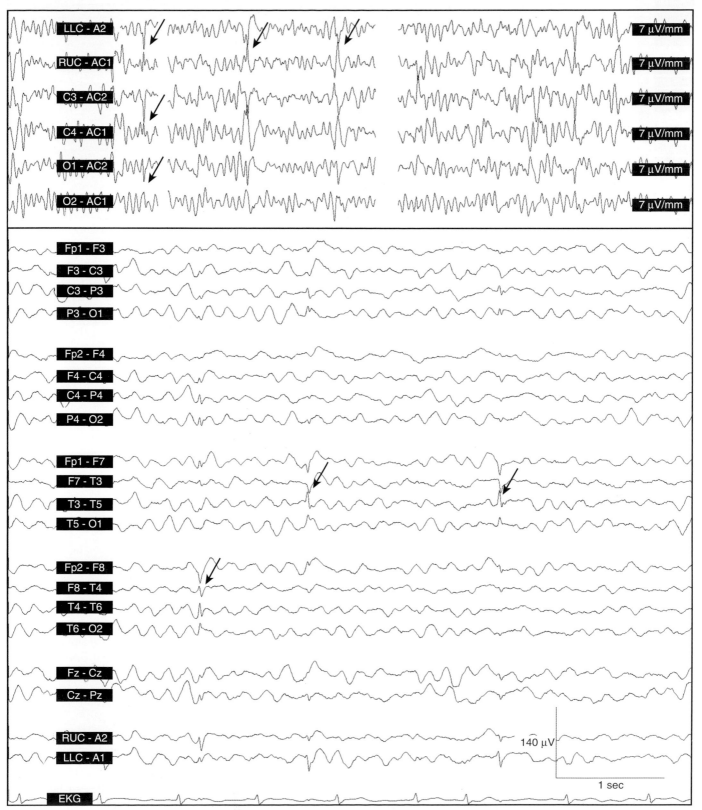

• **Figure 18.26** Benign Epileptiform Transients of Sleep/Small Sharp Spikes (arrows). Simply configured, low-amplitude (typically <50 μV) waveforms with rapid upstrokes and downstrokes may meet the formal duration criteria for spikes (20–70 msec) but are a benign finding, not associated with epilepsy. They are often broadly distributed on either or both hemispheres and should be seen only during sleep. This long bipolar montage was recorded at 30 mm/sec. Refer to Fig. 18.1 for electrode nomenclature. *EKG,* Electrocardiogram; *LLC,* left lower canthus; *RUC,* right upper canthus.

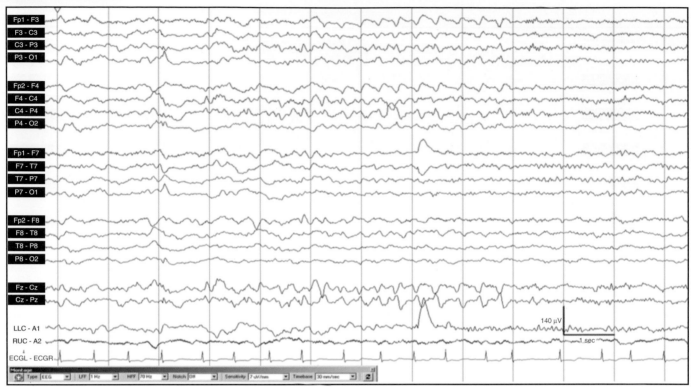

• **Figure 18.27** Subclinical rhythmic electrographic discharges in adults (SREDA) are seen rarely. It consists of a rhythmic and sometimes evolving pattern that typically reaches the θ range without postictal slowing or attenuation. The abrupt onset and offset have the appearance of a seizure, but they usually take place during wakefulness and without clinical correlate. SREDA are typically more common in the elderly and are considered benign. This long bipolar montage was recorded at 30 mm/sec. Refer to Fig. 18.1 for electrode nomenclature. *LLC,* Left lower canthus; *RUC,* right upper canthus.

adolescence. The basics of awake and sleep EEG through the ages are discussed briefly in this section and summarized in Fig. 18.6.

- A description of the awake background activity, in terms of frequency, amplitude, localization, quantity, organization, and variability, with abnormalities described in similar terms
- Indication of whether N2 sleep was seen, and the symmetry and synchrony of the sleep transients
- Highlight any focal abnormalities or asymmetries in the awake or sleep background.
- Description and abundance of epileptiform activity, if any, or significant benign variants
- Note any clinical events or electrographic events concerning seizure activity.
- An interpretation of the findings. Was there evidence of cerebral dysfunction that was global or focal? Epileptiform discharges indicate an elevated risk for seizures.

Sleep-Related Epilepsy

According to the *International Classification of Sleep Disorders*, 2nd edition (ICSD-3),[15] a diagnosis of sleep-related epilepsy requires that at least 70% of the episodes occur during sleep. Polysomnographic monitoring must demonstrate either an epileptiform discharge associated with the symptom or interictal epileptiform EEG activity during sleep. In addition, at least two of the following must be present and related to a seizure:

1. Abrupt awakenings from sleep
2. GTC movements of the limbs
3. Focal limb movement
4. Facial twitching
5. Automatisms such as lip smacking, orofacial movements, or picking movements
6. Incontinence
7. Tongue biting
8. Postictal confusion/lethargy

Cases of suspected sleep-related epilepsy must also not be better explained by another sleep disorder, medical disorder, mental disorder, medication use, or substance use disorder.

Epilepsy Syndromes and Sleep

- There are several epilepsy syndromes in which seizures are largely or completely restricted to sleep. Perhaps the most important from a diagnostic standpoint is nocturnal frontal lobe epilepsy (FLE), which consists of brief episodes of rocking or violent movements during sleep, sometimes followed by postictal confusion. Accordingly, this can be confused with arousal disorders (particularly if the seizure itself is unwitnessed). In this particular syndrome, findings on EEG may be normal even during the actual seizure, thus adding to the diagnostic confusion.
- Other important syndromes include juvenile myoclonic epilepsy, benign rolandic epilepsy of childhood, and Landau-Kleffner

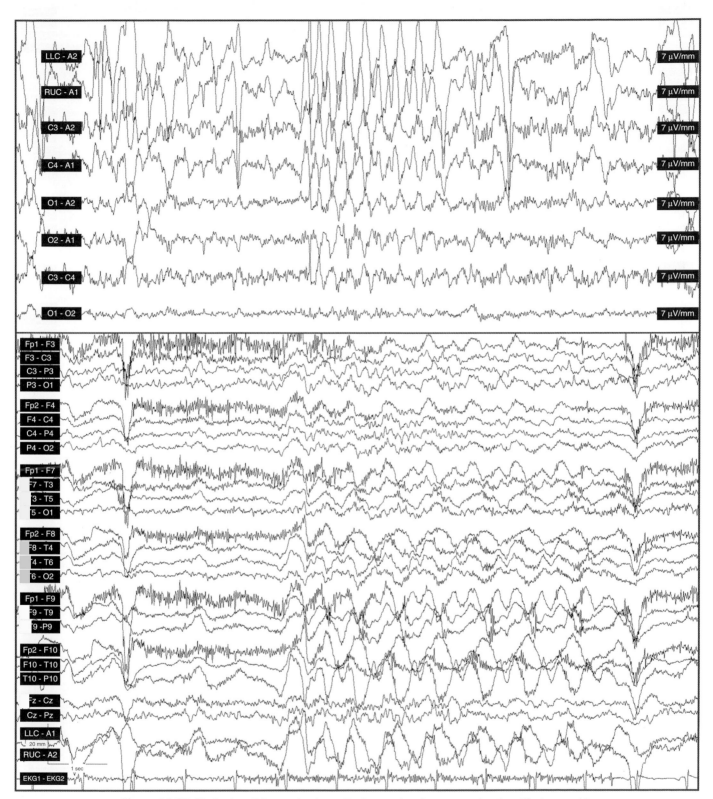

• **Figure 18.28** Rhythmic activity, maximal over the temporal regions, secondary to artifact caused by drinking water. The tongue and oropharynx can cause rhythmic artifacts during talking, drinking, and snoring that can be mistaken for epileptiform activity. In this case the rhythmic activity starts and stops abruptly, without evolution of the frequency of discharges, spread of the electrical field, or increase in voltage, thus making this easier to identify as artifact. This long bipolar montage was recorded at 30 mm/ sec. Refer to Fig. 18.1 for electrode nomenclature. *EKG,* Electrocardiogram; *LLC,* left lower canthus; *RUC,* right upper canthus.

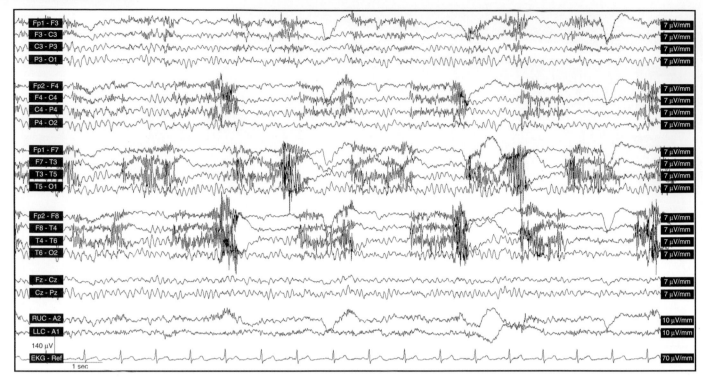

• **Figure 18.29** Bruxism. This child exhibits the typical checkerboard pattern of muscle artifact alternating between the left and right sides, as seen in a long bipolar montage recorded at 30 mm/sec. The pattern could not be identified on a typical polysomnographic montage. Bruxism is typically seen during sleep; however, this child is awake (note the eye blinks) but developmentally delayed. Refer to Fig. 18.1 for electrode nomenclature. *EKG*, Electrocardiogram; *LLC*, left lower canthus; *RUC*, right upper canthus.

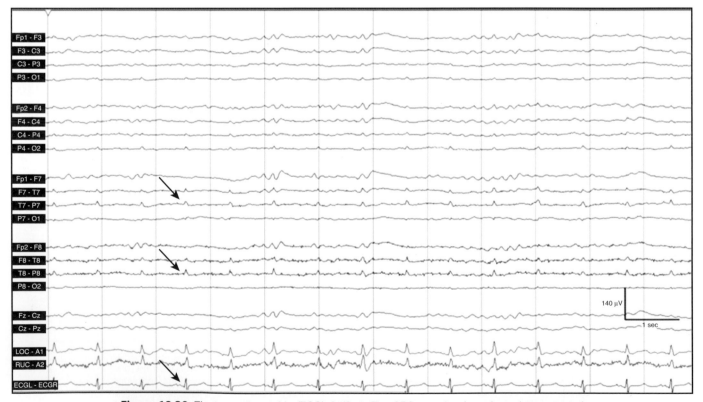

• **Figure 18.30** Electrocardiographic (ECG) Artifact. The QRS complex *(arrow)* can be seen on the electrocardiographic (ECG) tracing, but this electrical activity of the heart can also contaminate the electroencephalogram (EEG) tracing *(barbed arrows)*. When assessing periodic discharges on the EEG, ECG artifact should always be ruled out as a potential cause. This long bipolar montage was recorded at 30 mm/sec. Refer to Fig. 18.1 for electrode nomenclature. *RUC*, Right upper canthus.

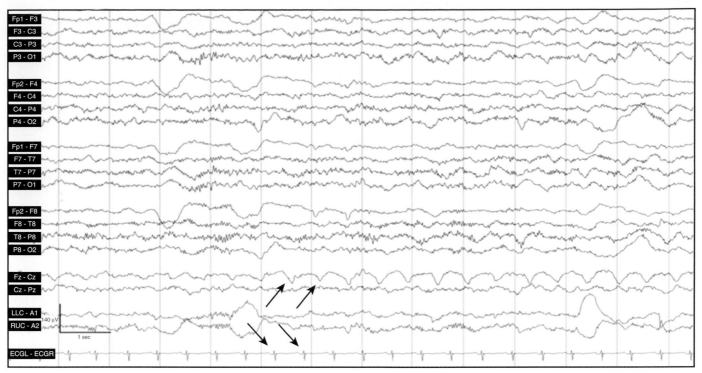

• **Figure 18.31** Pulse Artifact. An electrode may be in close proximity to an artery or vein within the scalp and be physically moved with every pulse. Movement of the electrode will cause an artifact, which can appear as a periodic discharge, often as a δ wave. The field will typically be restricted to a single lead and should be temporally linked to the electrocardiographic recording, although there may be a slight delay, as seen here between the QRS complex *(arrows)* and the δ wave *(barbed arrows)* at Cz. This long bipolar montage was recorded at 30 mm/sec. Refer to Fig. 18.1 for electrode nomenclature. *LLC,* Left lower canthus; *RUC,* right upper canthus.

syndrome/CSWS, all discussed earlier. Other epilepsy syndromes can also be manifested as sleep-related epilepsy.

• The interictal epileptiform discharges and the seizures themselves of focal and generalized seizure disorders have tendencies to occur at specific times in the circadian rhythm and sleep stage (Fig. 18.34).

Evaluation of Sleep-Related Epilepsy

• Sleep-related epilepsy can result in severe disruption of sleep structure and is commonly associated with daytime fatigue and somnolence. Injury and cognitive dysfunction can occur. Diagnosis of the condition may be difficult, particularly when diurnal episodes are completely absent.

• Patterns of occurrence can be helpful in distinguishing seizures from NREM parasomnias.[16] NREM parasomnias tend to occur predominantly during SWS (N3), in the first third of the night; are clinically variable; and usually decrease or stop in adolescence. A good description of the events, when available, will often reliably differentiate NREM parasomnias, sleep talking, bruxism, and rhythmic movement disorder from seizures.

• REM behavior disorder is typically easily distinguished from seizures by the variability and the association with dream images; however, diagnosis can be misleading when the patient does not recall the dream sequence and only a description of confused nocturnal behavior, possibly ictal or postictal, is obtained.

• When sleep-related epilepsy is suspected, EEG with at least 16 channels should be performed either during polysomnography or independently to look for interictal epileptiform activity suggestive of seizures. The EEG characteristics of particular syndromes were discussed earlier; it should be stressed, however, that normal findings on interictal EEG do not rule out the presence of epilepsy. If the diagnosis remains in doubt, video-EEG recording of the actual nocturnal episodes is the "gold standard." Most seizures will show a rhythmic EEG discharge during the event, whereas sleep starts, periodic limb movements during sleep, dyskinesia, or jerking with anoxia as a result of prolonged events in patients with obstructive sleep apnea (OSA) do not.

Obstructive Sleep Apnea and Epilepsy

• OSA is common in the general population, and evidence from subjective scales suggests that this disorder may be disproportionately responsible for the excessive sleepiness seen in patients with epilepsy.[17] In selected epilepsy patients referred for polysomnography, up to 70% are found to have OSA.[18,19] Sleep apnea may be particularly associated with late onset and refractory epilepsy.[20]

• Small series of epilepsy patients have also shown that diagnosis and treatment of OSA can improve seizures in patients with epilepsy,[18] but the overall prevalence of the disorder and impact on quality of life are less clear.

• In one prospective PSG study of 39 unselected patients with highly refractory epilepsy undergoing evaluation for epilepsy surgery, none of whom had a previous diagnosis of a sleep disorder,[21] one-third were found to have OSA as defined by a respiratory disturbance index (RDI) greater than 5, and 13%

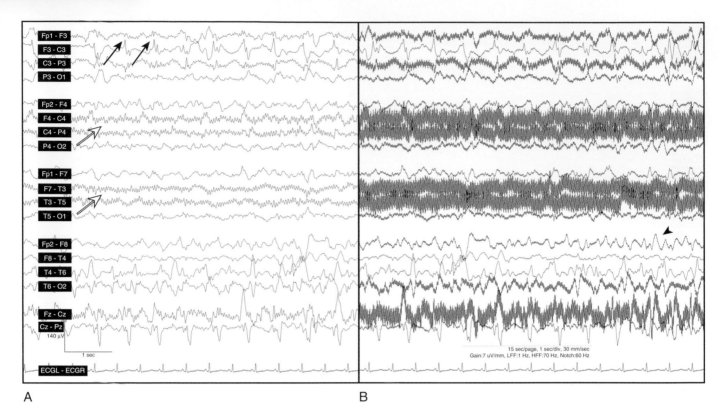

Figure 18.32 Overzealous use of filters can be misleading. Technicians may record with a 60-Hz notch filter to improve the aesthetic appearance of the electroencephalogram (EEG), but this can hide important information about poorly functioning electrodes. **A,** The notch filter alters artifactual signal from electrodes with high impedance (poor scalp connectivity) and results in a fictitious well-regulated appearing α frequency, which is particularly well seen from derivations including the C4 and T3 electrodes *(open arrows)*. This is a filtered artifact. Conversely, true spikes may be deemed to be artifact. In the left frontal region, the spike-like waveforms *(barbed arrows)* may be ignored, because there is no clear phase reversal. Positivity should be seen at Fp1-F3 with each spike, but it is not seen on the EEG because of electrode failure. **B,** Removal of the 60-Hz notch filter reveals not only the abundant artifact from failing C4 and T3 electrode contact but also artifact at the Fp1 and P3 electrode, thus indicating that they are also flooded with noncerebral signal, which explains the lack of clear phase reversals. In this example, these left frontal repetitive spikes have evolved to a rhythmic ictal pattern in the frontal regions *(arrowhead)*, accompanied by a clinical seizure. The signal from derivations including Fp1, P3, C4, T3, O1, and O2 are all contaminated by artifact and should be interpreted cautiously or even ignored. The electrode derivations are from a standard 10-20 long bipolar montage (see Fig. 18.3A) at a standard EEG speed of 30 mm/sec.

had moderate to severe OSA. This study, though small, suggests that OSA may be more common in patients with refractory epilepsy than in the general population. Although these authors also did not evaluate the relationship between apneas and seizures, oxygen desaturation could result in cerebral irritation, or chronic sleep deprivation could worsen the seizures. OSA is known to increase the risk for stroke and death[22]; however, it is not known whether this condition contributes to death in epilepsy or to sudden unexplained death in epilepsy.

Effects of Antiepileptic Drugs on Sleep

Many anticonvulsant drugs have been shown to affect sleep structure (in both positive and negative ways), usually through testing in normal subjects:

- Benzodiazepines and barbiturates are used less commonly for the chronic treatment of seizure disorders, but they reduce sleep latency and also decrease the amount of REM sleep, and benzodiazepines additionally reduce SWS.[23]

- Phenytoin increases light sleep and decreases sleep efficiency, and most studies show decreased REM sleep.[23,24]
- Findings for carbamazepine are more variable, but there also seems to be a reduction in REM sleep, particularly with acute treatment.[25]
- Valproate may increase stage 1 sleep[24] and (at least theoretically) could worsen OSA through weight gain.
- Lamotrigine was shown to have no effect on sleep in one study.[26]
- Gabapentin, pregabalin, and tiagabine enhance SWS and sleep continuity.[24,25,27]
- A study of levetiracetam showed an increase in sleep continuity and SWS.[28]

Antiepileptic Drugs Effects on Sleep Disorders

- Gabapentin and pregabalin are effective in the treatment of one common sleep disorder, restless legs syndrome,[29,30] although carbamazepine and lamotrigine have also been used.

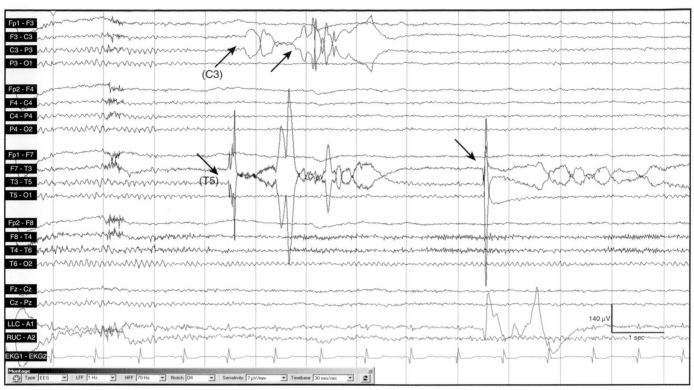

• Figure 18.33 A pop artifact can be seen at the left central (C3, *barbed arrows*) and left midtemporal (T5, *arrows*), electrodes with typical characteristics such as high-amplitude activity without a surrounding field in adjacent electrodes, and the activity seen within the artifact is a mirrored in the two adjacent channels containing these electrodes. Electrodes that demonstrate a pop artifact are at high risk for other artifacts, such as from movement and impedance, and can provide misleading information, even when the pop artifact is not obvious. They require proper reattachment to the scalp. This long bipolar montage was recorded at 30 mm/sec. Refer to Fig. 18.1 for electrode nomenclature. *EKG,* Electrocardiogram; *LLC,* left lower canthus; *RUC,* right upper canthus.

- Patients taking anticonvulsants known to disrupt sleep (phenobarbital, phenytoin, carbamazepine, or valproic acid) have increased daytime drowsiness in comparison to epilepsy patients who are not taking anticonvulsants.[31]
- Sedatives, including barbiturates and benzodiazepines, are known to worsen OSA.
- Agents that tend to cause weight gain (valproate, pregabalin) could also potentially worsen OSA in this way, whereas those that cause weight loss (felbamate, topiramate, zonisamide) could improve OSA.

The effects of anticonvulsants on sleep and sleep disorders are summarized in Table 18.2.

Effects of Hypnotics on Seizures

- Barbiturates and benzodiazepines are used to treat seizures, but abrupt withdrawal can result in exacerbation.
- Nonbenzodiazepine hypnotics (eszopiclone, zaleplon, zolpidem) at standard doses have no known effects on seizure threshold or risks for withdrawal seizures.
- Antidepressant drugs, including selective serotonin reuptake inhibitors and tricyclic antidepressants, can carry a slight risk for seizure exacerbation, but are generally outweighed by benefits. This risk is slightly greater with bupropion, particularly immediate release. Withdrawal should be supervised by a competent practitioner. The effects of hypnotics and antidepressants on seizures are summarized in Table 18.3.

TABLE 18.3	Effects of Hypnotics and Antidepressants on Seizures	
	EFFECTS ON SEIZURES	
Hypnotic	**Positive**	**Negative**
Benzodiazepines	Treats seizures, especially acutely	Risk for withdrawal seizure
Nonbenzodiazepine hypnotics (zolpidem, zaleplon, eszopiclone)	None	None
Antidepressants (tricyclic antidepressants, selective serotonin reuptake inhibitors, atypical)	None	May be minimal risk for exacerbation
Bupropion	None	Mild risk for exacerbation

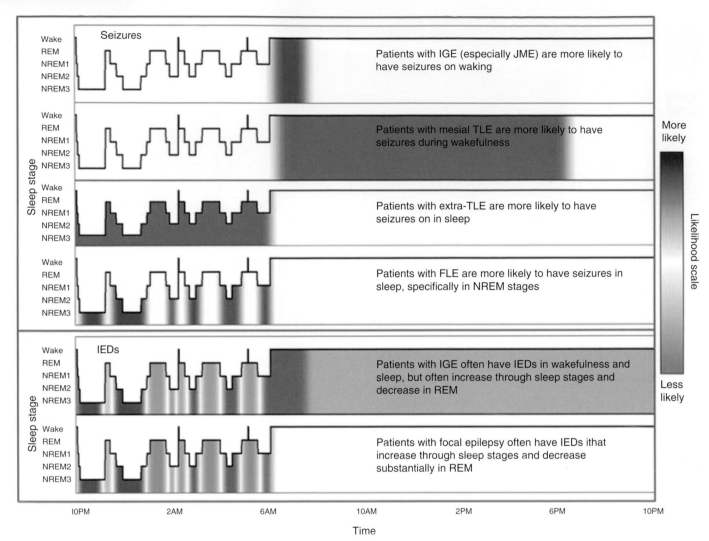

• **Figure 18.34** A diagram summarizing the tendency of seizures and interictal epileptiform discharges (IEDs) through a 24-hour sleep-wake cycle and a typified hypnogram. *FLE,* Frontal lobe epilepsy; *IGE,* idiopathic generalized epilepsy; *JME,* juvenile myoclonic epilepsy; *TLE,* temporal lobe epilepsy. (From Badawy RA, Freestone DR, Lai A, Cook MJ. Epilepsy: ever-changing states of cortical excitability. *Neuroscience.* 2012;222:89–99.)

Suggested Reading

Herman ST, Walczak TS, Bazil CW. Distribution of partial seizures during the sleep-wake cycle: differences by seizure onset site. *Neurology.* 2001;56(11):1453-1459.

Malow BA, Fromes GA, Aldrich MS. Usefulness of polysomnography in epilepsy patients. *Neurology.* 1997;48(5):1389-1394.

Malow BA, Levy K, Maturen K, Bowes R. Obstructive sleep apnea is common in medically refractory epilepsy patients. *Neurology.* 2000;55(7):1002-1007.

Placidi F, Diomedi M, Scalise A, et al. Effect of anticonvulsants on nocturnal sleep in epilepsy. *Neurology.* 2000;54(5 suppl 1):S25-S32.

Sammaritano M, Gigli GL, Gotman J. Interictal spiking during wakefulness and sleep and the localization of foci in temporal lobe epilepsy. *Neurology.* 1991;41(2 Pt 1):290-297.

19

Sleep and Neurological Disorders

MADELEINE M. GRIGG-DAMBERGER

Introduction

We sleep for the brain. Sleep is a function of and generated by the brain. The suprachiasmatic nucleus (SCN) in the lateral hypothalamus is our endogenous circadian pacemaker.[1] The preoptic area of hypothalamus drives nonrapid eye movement (NREM) sleep. The posterolateral perifornical region controls wakefulness through the hypocretin/orexin neuronal pathway. The subcoeruleus region of the pons is the major focus for rapid eye movement (REM) sleep generation. Fig. 19.1 summarizes the basic circuitry including key nodes in brain that underlie the regulation of sleep and wakefulness.

Of the many neurological disorders, almost all have complex bidirectional relationships with sleep. A wide range of derangements of sleep and/or wakefulness, sleep architecture, sleep-related breathing, or movements accompany many neurological disorders, phenotypic of the disorder in some. Worse yet, poor sleep can worsen many neurological disorders. Understanding these complex relationships is critical when evaluating and treating these patients.

Sleep/Wake Disorders in Stroke

Each year, more than 795,000 people in the United States have a stroke, and 610,000 of these are first or new strokes.[2,3] Stroke kills almost 130,000 Americans each year (1 of 20 deaths). The majority (87%) of strokes are ischemic. More than half of all stroke survivors have some type of sleep problem. Obstructive sleep apnea (OSA) is an independent risk factor for stroke, but often goes undiagnosed and untreated.[4]

Obstructive Sleep Apnea in Patients with Stroke or Transient Ischemic Attack

More than 50%–70% of patients with acute ischemic stroke or transient ischemic attack (TIA) have OSA. A 2010 meta-analysis of 29 case-control studies found 72% of 2343 patients with stroke or TIA had an apnea-hypopnea index (AHI) of ≥5 per hour in 72%, 38% greater than 20 per hour, 29% greater than 30 per hour, and 14% greater than 40 per hour.[5]

- OSA is associated with poorer outcomes after ischemic strokes. Several large well-designed prospective studies have shown that OSA independently increases risks of incident ischemic stroke, composite risk of stroke, TIA, and death.[6–9] OSA is an independent risk factor for ischemic stroke.[10–13]
- OSA is the predominant form of sleep-disordered breathing (SDB) in stroke, TIA, and intracerebral hemorrhage (Fig. 19.2).[14]

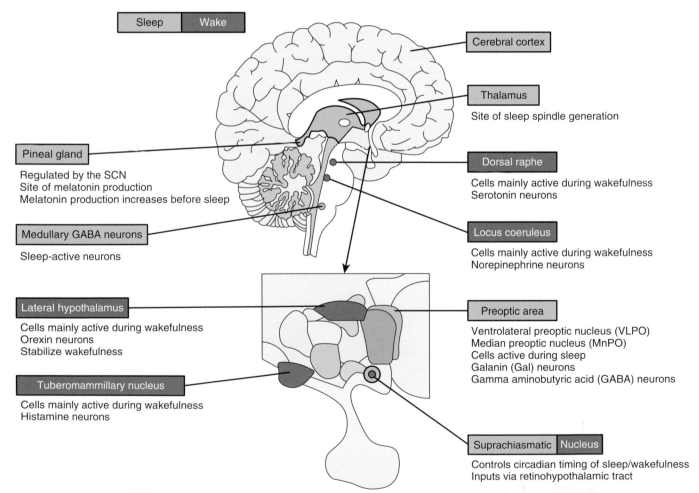

• **Figure 19.1** The basic circuitry, including key "nodes" in brain that underlie regulation of sleep and wakefulness and the transitions between these states in humans. *SCN*, Suprachiasmatic nucleus. (From Fuller PM, Zee PC, Buxton OM. Biology of sleep: sleep mechanisms. In: Kryger MH, Avidan AY, Berry RB, eds. *Atlas of Clinical Sleep Medicine*. 2nd ed. Philadelphia, PA: Elsevier Saunders; 2014.)

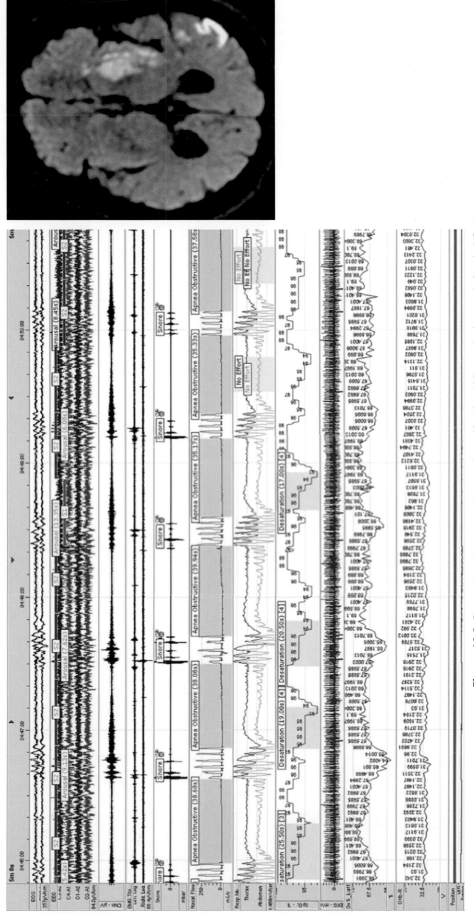

• **Figure 19.2** Obstructive sleep apnea in a patient with left middle cerebral artery ischemic infarct. (Magnetic resonance imaging pictures courtesy of Prof. G. Schroth, Institute of Neuroradiology, University Hospital, Bern, Switzerland. From Kryger MH, Roth T, Dement, WC, eds. *Principles and Practice of Sleep Medicine*. 5th ed. St. Louis: Elsevier Saunders; 2011.)

- OSA severity is typically unchanged 3 months poststroke (except those with dysphagia).[5,15]
  - Central sleep apnea (CSA) including Cheyne-Stokes respiration seen in 7%–26% of stroke patients acutely but typically disappears (Fig. 19.3).[16] The incidence of CSA increases in larger strokes and those associated with mass effect.[17]
  - Rare patterns of altered respiration can be seen with acute strokes (Table 19.1).[16,18]
- Stroke patients with OSA have worse outcomes than stroke patients without OSA (Fig. 19.4).[19–21]
- OSA in patients with atrial fibrillation is an independent predictor of stroke.[12] Prevalence of atrial fibrillation is 2–4 times higher in patients with OSA.[22] Patients with stroke and OSA were 5.3 times more likely to have atrial fibrillation, even after controlling for other variables.[23]
- The American Heart Association/American Stroke Association (AHA/ASA) published guidelines in 2014 that recommend a sleep study be considered (and continuous positive airway pressure [CPAP] if needed) for patients with ischemic stroke or TIA on the basis of the very high prevalence of sleep apnea in this population, and the strength of the evidence that the treatment of sleep apnea improves outcomes in the general population.[24]

- Most ischemic strokes (myocardial infarcts and sudden cardiac death) occur when awake between 6 AM and noon, and the lowest risk is between midnight and 6 AM.[25]
  - One study found OSA (AHI ≥15) was an independent predictor of nocturnal stroke in 152 patients with acute ischemic stroke.[26]
  - Severe OSA (AHI ≥ 40 per hour) increased the risk for sudden cardiac death during sleep 2.6 times compared with those with AHI 5–39 per hour, and far more than would be predicted in the general population or even by chance.[27]
  - Recent studies suggest that OSA may be the only independent variable predisposing to so-called wake-up strokes.[28–30]
  - A recent meta-analysis showed that patients with stroke have significantly poorer sleep than controls with lower sleep efficiency (mean 75% vs. 84%), shorter total-sleep time (309 vs. 340 min), more wake-after-sleep onset (WASO, 97 vs. 54 min), more time in NREM 1 (13% vs. 10%), and less time in NREM 2 (36% vs. 45%) and NREM 3 sleep (10% vs. 12%).[31]
  - Transient reductions in REM sleep occur in the first days after supratentorial stroke.[32–34] Sawtooth waves can be decreased bilaterally in large hemispheric strokes (especially those which involve the right hemisphere).[34] Low sleep

TABLE 19.1 Abnormal Patterns of Respiration Occasionally Seen with Strokes

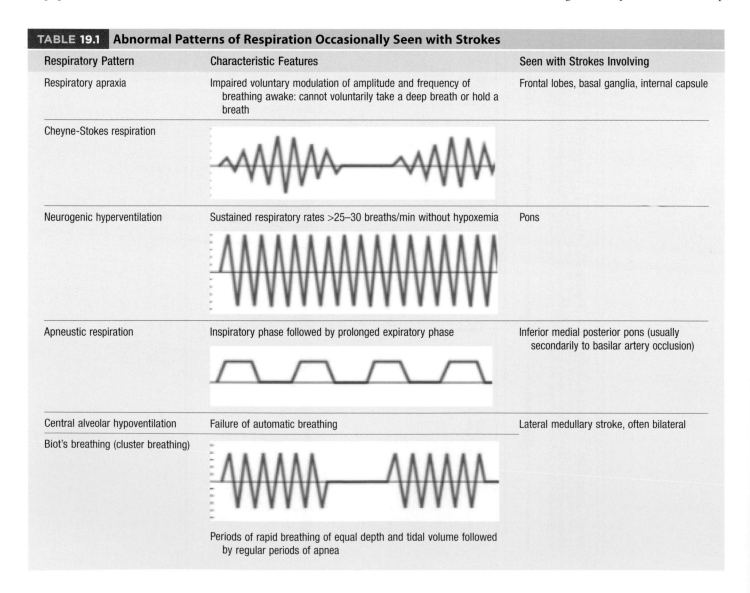

Respiratory Pattern	Characteristic Features	Seen with Strokes Involving
Respiratory apraxia	Impaired voluntary modulation of amplitude and frequency of breathing awake: cannot voluntarily take a deep breath or hold a breath	Frontal lobes, basal ganglia, internal capsule
Cheyne-Stokes respiration		
Neurogenic hyperventilation	Sustained respiratory rates >25–30 breaths/min without hypoxemia	Pons
Apneustic respiration	Inspiratory phase followed by prolonged expiratory phase	Inferior medial posterior pons (usually secondarily to basilar artery occlusion)
Central alveolar hypoventilation	Failure of automatic breathing	Lateral medullary stroke, often bilateral
Biot's breathing (cluster breathing)	Periods of rapid breathing of equal depth and tidal volume followed by regular periods of apnea	

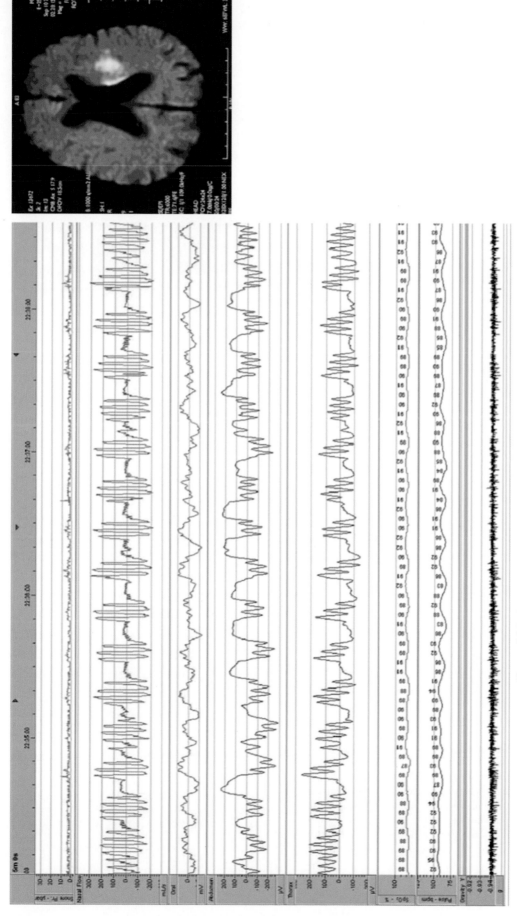

• **Figure 19.3** Central sleep apnea in acute ischemic stroke. (Magnetic resonance imaging pictures courtesy of Prof. G. Schroth, Institute of Neuroradiology, University Hospital, Bern, Switzerland. From Kryger MH, Roth T, Dement WC, eds. *Principles and Practice of Sleep Medicine.* 5th ed. St. Louis: Elsevier Saunders; 2011.)

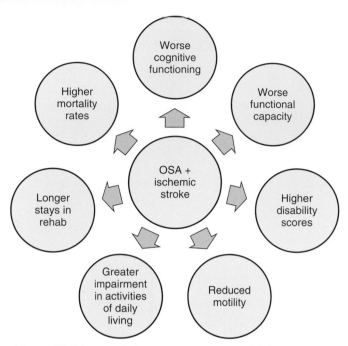

• **Figure 19.4** Impact of obstructive sleep apnea (OSA) on stroke outcomes compared with those without OSA.

efficiency, decreased sleep spindles, K-complexes, and REM sleep predict poor outcome after hemispheric strokes.[35]
- Treating OSA in acute ischemic stroke remains a challenge.[36] Recruitment of stroke patients willing to use CPAP has been limited,[37] further complicated by ethical issues.[38]
  - Stroke patients with OSA as a group do not report lower levels of sleep quality or higher levels of sleepiness, fatigue, and depressed mood than stroke patients without OSA.[21,39] They have poor tolerance of CPAP interfaces, and difficulty putting masks back on during the night.[40,41]
  - Different treatment strategies are needed including patient education and behavioral therapies, positional therapy, nasotracheal suction mechanical ventilation, oral appliances, high-flow humidity, oxygen, hypoglossal nerve stimulation, and weight loss.[41]

Other Primary Sleep Disorders in Patients with Stroke

Other primary sleep disorders besides SDB occur in 20%–50% of patients with stroke.[42] These include insomnia, hypersomnia, excessive daytime sleepiness (EDS), and fatigue.
- De novo hypersomnia after stroke[43–45]
  - In a study of 285 consecutive patients a mean of 21 months after stroke found 27% slept ≥10 hours per day (hypersomnia) and 28% had an Epworth Sleepiness Scale (ESS) score ≥10.[46] Thirty to seventy percent of patients report poststroke fatigue.
  - Hypersomnia is more likely to occur after bilateral thalamic, subthalamic, and hypothalamic, tegmental midbrain, or pons lesions affecting the ascending reticular activating system.
  - Paramedian thalamic infarcts can result in severe hypersomnia with sudden onset of stupor but responsive to stimulation (Fig. 19.5).
  - Hypersomnia in some stroke patients evolves to extreme apathy, slowness, and poverty of movement presleep behaviors

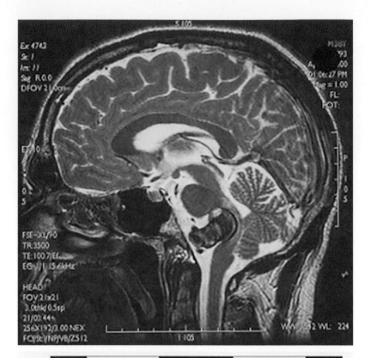

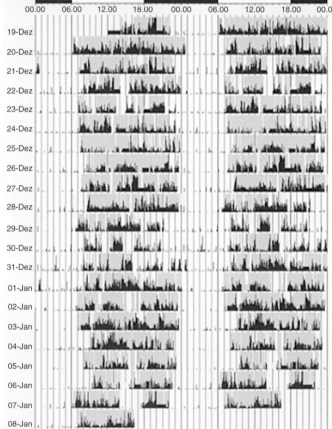

• **Figure 19.5** Hypersomnia after a paramedian thalamic stroke. (Magnetic resonance imaging pictures courtesy of Prof. A. Valavanis, Institute of Neuroradiology, University Hospital, Zürich, Switzerland. From Kryger MH, Roth T, Dement WC, eds. *Principles and Practice of Sleep Medicine.* 5th ed. St. Louis: Elsevier Saunders; 2011.)

can be seen in patients with hypersomnia and thalamic or deep subcortical strokes, characterized by repetitive yawning, stretching, curling up in sleep position, and constantly complaining of the urge to sleep.

- A study showed stroke patients with hypersomnia were 10 times more likely to be discharged from rehab to a nursing home and had significantly worse functional outcomes.[45]
- Treatment of hypersomnia in stroke patients is more often ineffective. A multicenter trial is planned, studying whether modafinil improves hypersomnia and/or fatigue after stroke, and improves rehabilitation outcomes.[47–49]

- De novo insomnia after stroke[50,51]
  - A study of 277 consecutive patients evaluated 3 months after stroke found 57% reported insomnia.[50] Insomnia appeared after the stroke in 18%. Insomnia after stroke is more common in women than in men.
  - On occasion, strokes involving the midbrain and pons can cause almost complete insomnia. Insomnia in stroke is often associated with agitation, reversal of sleep/wake cycles, and EDS.
  - Inversion of sleep/wake cycles can occur with strokes involving the thalamus, midbrain, and pontine tegmentum.
  - Insomnia increases the likelihood of stroke and other cardiovascular events compared with individuals who deny insomnia.
  - Insomnia after stroke increases risk of subsequent stroke, worsens psychological health, physical disability, and anxiety, and is associated with an increased risk of suicide.
  - Treatment of poststroke insomnia should include placing individuals in private quiet rooms at night, protecting them from nocturnal noise and light, increased mobilization during the day, and exposure to light in the day. If insomnia remains, only then consider the least sedating of hypnotics (e.g., zolpidem, zopiclone). Benzodiazepines may inhibit neuroplasticity and stroke recovery.

- De novo restless legs syndrome (RLS) and periodic limb movements during sleep (PLMS) following stroke
  - A recent in-hospital case-control cross-sectional study found RLS was much more common in patients with acute stroke/TIA than controls (15% of 149 acute stroke/TIA patients vs. 3% of 298 controls).[52] Using multivariate regression analyses, the researchers showed RLS increased the risk for acute stroke/TIA by six- to sevenfold after adjusting for cardiovascular and/or RLS risk factors.
  - The presence of RLS affects stroke outcome. RLS was found in 12.5% of 96 patients with acute ischemic stroke.[53] All had symptoms of RLS before stroke. Stroke outcome was significantly worse at 3 and 12 months in those with RLS, even after adjusting for diabetes mellitus and body mass index (BMI).
  - PLMS presented in 38% of 40 patients with a history of stroke compared with 13% of 40 controls.[54] The average PLMS index was higher in those with a history of stroke versus controls (12 ± 3 vs. 2 ± 0.7 per hour of sleep).
  - RLS developing following stroke is more likely to occur, and was diagnosed in 12% of 137 patients 1 month after acute ischemic strokes. Anatomic location of lesions associated with stroke-related RLS were most often located in the basal ganglia/corona radiata, occasionally in the pons, and rarely in the internal capsule or thalamus.[55]

- Further research is needed to explore the relationships among RLS, PLMS, and cardiovascular and cerebrovascular disease.[56–59] Symptomatic RLS associated with the Sleep Heart Health Study reported higher incidence of cardiovascular and coronary artery disease, and poorer health-related quality of life in patients with symptomatic RLS.[60,61]
- Increased sympathetic activity accompanying the PLMS-related arousal may explain the association among RLS, cardiovascular, and cerebrovascular disorders.
- Serum ferritin levels are warranted in patients with RLS following stroke.
- Treatments for RLS in patients with stroke include dopamine agonists, gabapentin enacarbil, and pregabalin (although only the first two agents are currently US Food and Drug Administration approved for RLS). Ropirinole (0.125–1 mg/d) and pramipexole (0.125–0.5 mg/d) have been shown to improve RLS in stroke patients.[62,63]

- De novo parasomnias following stroke
  - On rare occasion, a bilateral pontine tegmental stroke can trigger REM sleep behavior disorder (RBD).[64,65]
  - Visual hallucinations at sleep onset have been reported with infarcts in the paramedial thalamus, midbrain, or pontine tegmentum.[66]
  - Nightmares or increased dreaming have also been reported with strokes involving the occipital, temporal, parietal, or thalamus.[67]
  - Pharmacological treatment for RBD are clonazepam and/or exogenous melatonin.[68–70] Clonazepam increases the risk of falls.[71] Benzodiazepines in general may impair stroke recovery and neuroplasticity.[72] Safety interventions, such as removing sharp objects and barricading nightstands, should be reviewed with patients and family members.

Sleep in Neurodegenerative Disorders

Sleep disorders are common in patients with neurodegenerative disorders and are typically complex, multifactorial, and interactive. Common neurodegenerative disorders include Alzheimer's disease (AD), diffuse Lewy body disease (DLB), Parkinson's disease (PD), multiple system atrophy (MSA), spinocerebellar ataxias (SCA), progressive supranuclear palsy (PSP), and Huntington's disease (HD).

Some sleep disorders are red flags for specific neurodegenerative diseases:[73]

- Inspiratory stridor (IS) warrants consideration of MSA.
- Chronic RBD is common in DLB, MSA, PD, and SCA.
- The absence of RBD in a patient with parkinsonism suggests PD rather than MSA, because RBD presents early in the course of MSA.

Despite common misperception, inappropriate motor activity in diurnal movement disorders recurs during sleep:[73]

- Studies have shown that abnormal diurnal movements recur "occasionally" during sleep in the majority of patients with PD, HD, primary/secondary dystonia, or Tourette syndrome.

A classic study recorded video-electroencephalographic (EEG) in groups of 52 patients with PD, HD, primary or secondary dystonia, or Tourette syndrome, and compared them with 10 normal controls.[74]

- Abnormal diurnal movements recurred "occasionally" during sleep in 50 of 52 patients.
- Movements recurred in sleep after awakenings, in NREM 1, or in shifts to lighter stages of sleep.

TABLE 19.2	**Diagnostic Criteria for Dementia Syndrome and Probable Alzheimer's Disease**
Diagnostic Criteria for Dementia Syndrome	**Diagnostic Criteria for Probable Alzheimer's Disease**
• Objective cognitive or behavioral impairment in ≥2 of the following: • Memory • Reasoning and handling complex tasks • Visuospatial abilities • Language functions • Personality, behavior, or comportment • Decline from previous level of functioning • Functional impairment	• Criteria for dementia met; insidious onset with gradual progression • Initial symptoms: amnestic; nonamnestic (language, executive) • No other neurologic, psychiatric, or general medical disorders of severity can interfere with cognition. • Positive biomarkers (e.g., low CSF amyloid-β [Aβ] levels, positive amyloid PET scan, hippocampal atrophy on brain MRI)

CSF, Cerebrospinal fluid; *MRI,* magnetic resonance imaging; *PET,* positron emission tomography.

TABLE 19.3	**Biomarkers Which Predict Minimal Cognitive Impairment Likely to Progress to Alzheimer's Disease**
• Atrophy of medial temporal lobe on brain MRI • Posterior predominant hypometabolism with involvement of posterior cingulate gyrus on FDG-PET scan • Positive amyloid PET scan • Tau has spread outside medial temporal to lateral temporal structures on tau PET scan • Low CSF levels of Aβ42 and ↑ CSF levels of total tau and phosphorylated tau • APOE4 ε4 genotype useful in research, less so clinical practice	

CSF, Cerebrospinal fluid; *FDG,* fludeoxyglucose; *MRI,* magnetic resonance imaging; *PET,* positron emission tomography.

• Abnormal movements in sleep either occurred after an awakening or were preceded by a brief EEG arousal, sleep spindles, or slow waves.
• Abnormal movements were rarely seen in NREM 3 sleep.
• Video-polysomnographic (PSG) studies on 16 individuals with hemifacial spasm found the amplitude and duration of hemifacial muscle activity compared with wakefulness decreased 74% in NREM stage N1, 53% NREM stage N2, 51%–56% NREM stage N3, and 42% REM sleep.[75]
• Palatal myoclonus (PM) is a diurnal movement disorder that persists unchanged in sleep.[76]
   • PM is involuntary rhythmic movements of soft palate and pharynx at rate of 1.5–3 Hz.
   • Patients with PM often complain of hearing clicking noises in ear because of rhythmic contraction of tensor veli palatini muscle.
   • PM arises from lesions in the Guillain-Mollaret triangle. Lesions are usually found in dentate nucleus or its outflow tract, and in the central tegmental tract. Pathological finding is olivary hypertrophy.

Alzheimer's Disease

Basic Information[77–80]

• AD is the most common dementia and is characterized by neuronal loss and deposition of amyloid beta, neurofibrillary tangles, and tau in the hippocampus and cerebral cortex.[77,78] AD is the fifth most common cause of death in US adults age ≥65 years.[79] Eleven percent of adults ≥65 years (1 in 9) have AD. Among adults 85 years or older, 32% (1:3) have AD. Diagnostic criteria for dementia syndrome and probable AD are summarized in Table 19.2.[80] Neuropathology leading to AD begins 40 years prior. If poor sleep contributes to minimal cognitive impairment (MCI) and AD, it needs to be identified long before AD.

Minimal Cognitive Impairment[81]

• MCI was first defined as memory concern beyond that expected for age and slight memory impairment but patient does not meet criteria for dementia;
   • A diagnosis of MCI begins subjective cognitive complaint(s). Objective neuropsychological testing demonstrates the patient's cognitive function is not normal for age, and has declined from a higher baseline, but the individual does not meet criteria for dementia and functions normally in activities of daily living.
   • Epidemiology of MCI: 12%–18% of persons greater than 60 years. The Mayo Clinic Study of Aging reported MCI observed in 16% of adults ≥70 years; these patients were followed for a median of 5 years; 5%–6% with MCI progressed per year to AD. Rates for progression to AD are lower in younger subjects and rise considerably with age. Biomarkers that predict when MCI is likely to progress to AD are summarized in Table 19.3.
   • MCI often presents with memory impairment (amnestic MCI) but may not (nonamnestic MCI). MCI may affect only single cognitive domains (e.g., memory) or multiple cognitive domains (and still fulfill criteria for MCI). Logopenic aphasia, frontal lobe dysexecutive, and posterior cortical atrophy/visual variant are other presentations for MCI.
   • Amnestic MCI is a typical prodromal stage of dementia for AD but other phenotypes.
   • Not all MCI is early AD, especially when presents with multiple cognitive domains are affected.
   • When multiple cognitive domains are affected, consider vascular cognitive impairment (VCI), depression, DLB, or frontotemporal dementia (FTD).

The clinical evaluation for MCI, AD, and dementia is summarized in Table 19.4. The differential etiology of MCI in Table 19.5.

Changes in Sleep Architecture and Circadian Rhythms That Occur in Asymptomatic Healthy Older Adults

• Changes in sleep architecture observed in healthy asymptomatic older adults that occur with normal aging[82–84]
   • Decreased NREM 3 sleep (more so in older men than older women)
   • Increased sleep latency, nocturnal awakenings, and WASO (twofold higher than among young adults)

TABLE 19.4	Clinical Evaluation for Minimal Cognitive Impairment, Alzheimer's Disease, and Dementia

- Obtain history from patient and confirm with someone who knows the patient
- Change in cognitive performance, not lifelong low cognitive function
- Forgetfulness relatively new (e.g., 6–12 mon)
- Other cognitive domains (e.g., attention, language problems, functional performance)
- Screen with Montreal Cognitive Assessment (MoCA) or Short Test of Mental Status
- Formal neuropsychological testing to differentiate cognitive dysfunction seen in normal aging from minimal cognitive impairment, Alzheimer's disease, or dementia

TABLE 19.5	Differential Etiology of Minimal Cognitive Impairment

- Vascular risk factors; consider vascular cognitive impairment (VCI)
- OSA and intermittent nocturnal hypoxemia important considerations here
- Uncompensated CHF, COPD, and poorly controlled DM2 contribute to cognitive impairment
- Depression may have dyscognitive features, but also prodrome of MCI and dementias
- Attention, concentration, visuospatial difficulties; consider diffuse Lewy body disease (DLB)
- Behavior changes, inappropriate behavior, apathy, lack of insight, impaired attention/concentration; consider frontotemporal dementia

CHF, Congestive heart failure; *COPD*, chronic obstructive pulmonary disease; *MCI*, minimal cognitive impairment; *OSA*, obstructive sleep apnea.

- Daytime napping more common (>50% take ≥1 nap a day)
- Changes in circadian rhythms with age in healthy asymptomatic older adults[85]
  - Decreased amplitude and reduced period length of circadian rhythms
  - Increased intradaily and decreased interdaily stability of circadian rhythms
  - Increased internal desynchronization of circadian rhythms
  - Decreased amplitude of melatonin rhythms
  - Phase advance core body temperature and melatonin rhythms
  - Increased plasma cortisol levels at night lead to increased 24-hour mean cortisol level and reduced cortisol rhythm amplitude.

An older adult who complains of poor sleep is a red flag:
- Older women more likely to complain of poor sleep quality than older men; they also go to bed earlier and wake earlier.
- Insomnia is more common in women across the lifespan.
- A red flag is an elder who voices "sleep concerns" and warrants evaluation, but do not advise normal aging.
- Risk factors for insomnia in older adults include chronic illness, mood disturbance, less physical activity, physical disability.

Sleep/Wake Problems in People with Alzheimer's Disease

- Reported up to 25% with mild to moderate AD and about 50% with moderate to severe AD. Sleep/wake complaints include excessive nocturnal awakenings, napping greater than 1 hour per day, early morning awakening, and EDS.
- EDS is associated with greater impairments in AD patients, independent of the level of cognitive impairment.[86] Sleep disturbances are a common cause of early nursing home placement.
- SDB is more common in people with AD than age-matched general population (Fig. 19.6).[87] A recent quantitative meta-analysis found the aggregate odds ratio for OSA in patients with AD was five times in AD, compared with healthy controls.

Polysomnographic Findings in Alzheimer's Disease[84,88–90]

- Certain changes in sleep architecture in AD at first glance seem an exaggeration of those seen with aging (decreased sleep efficiency, increased number and duration of nocturnal awakenings, increased percent of NREM N1 sleep time, greater decrease in percent NREM N3 sleep).
- However, decreased percent REM sleep time is *not* a feature of healthy aging. REM sleep time decreases in AD, due to shortened REM sleep duration.
- REM sleep atonia and REM density are preserved in AD. The reduced percent of REM sleep time in AD is attributed to selective atrophy of the cholinergic nucleus basalis of Meynert.
- With increasing duration of AD, the number, amplitude, morphology, and duration of sleep spindle and K-complexes decrease such that in moderate to severe AD it becomes difficult to distinguish NREM N1 from NREM N2 sleep.
- Indeterminate NREM sleep (absence of sleep spindles, K-complexes, and slow wave activity) is common in severe AD.
- AD accounts for a greater percentage of sleep during day, greater wakefulness at night, and worsens with increasing dementia severity.
- Studies of EEG in early AD report that waking dominant posterior rhythm is typically normal till AD is moderate or severe. Increased percentage and slower frequencies of theta in waking EEG have been reported. There can be excessive intermixed slow activity during tonic REM sleep (>90% specificity and sensitivity for early AD).[91]

Emerging Concepts of Relationships Between Alzheimer's Disease and Poor Sleep[84,85,88,92,93]

See Fig. 19.7.
- Sleep and circadian rhythm disturbances increase risk for MCI, AD, and cognitive decline in older adults.
- Sleep problems are early biomarkers for AD dementia.
- Poor sleep is associated with AD neuropathologies, and *directly* contributes to neurodegenerative processes. The brain needs time to clean itself of amyloid beta. Insufficient sleep leads to accumulation of AD neuropathology.
- Sleep fragmentation in community-dwelling older adults predicts incident depression and fall risk, and correlates with poor quality of life and poorer cognition.
- Altered rest-activity patterns predict incident (later) MCI and/or AD. There is a twofold increased risk for early and more severe cognitive decline in AD who have sleep disturbances. EDS, nighttime sleep duration less than 6.5 hours and frequent awakenings predict cognitive decline in older adults.
- A longitudinal study of 346 adults followed for 8 years found insomnia increased the odds ratio 2.4 times for later AD.[94] After excluding the confounder of depression, insomnia

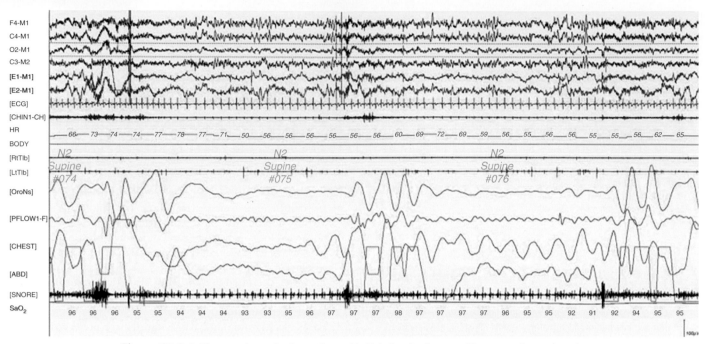

• **Figure 19.6** A 90-second epoch of a patient with Alzheimer's disease with severe obstructive sleep apnea. (From Chokroverty S, Bhat S, Provini F. Sleep dysfunction and sleep-disordered breathing in miscellaneous neurological disorders. In: Chokroverty S, Thomas RJ, eds. *Atlas of Sleep Medicine.* 2nd ed. Philadelphia, PA: Elsevier/Saunders; 2014.)

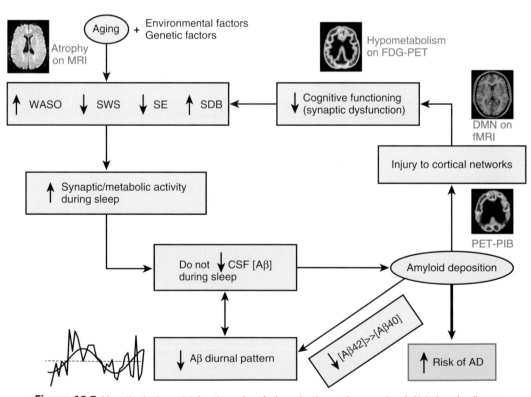

• **Figure 19.7** Hypothetical model for the role of sleep in the pathogenesis of Alzheimer's disease. *AD*, Alzheimer's disease; *CSF*, cerebrospinal fluid; *DMN*, dorsal motor nucleus; *FDG*, fludeoxyglucose; *MRI*, magnetic resonance imaging; *PET*, positron emission tomography; *SDB*, sleep-disordered breathing; *SE*, sleep efficiency; *SWS*, slow wave (NREM 3) sleep; *WASO*, wake-after-sleep onset. (From Lucey BP, Bateman RJ. Amyloid-β diurnal pattern: possible role of sleep in Alzheimer disease pathogenesis. *Neurobiol Aging.* 2014;35:S29–S34.)

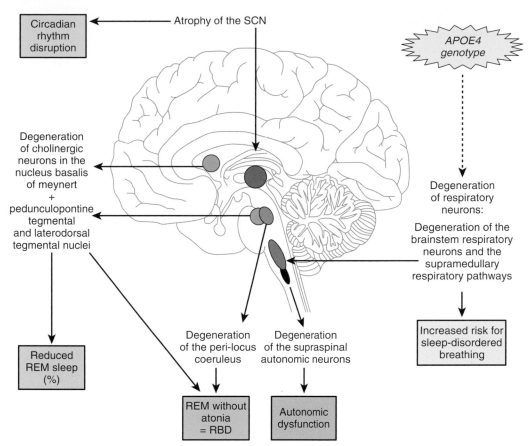

• **Figure 19.8** Pathophysiology of sleep disruption in patients with Alzheimer's dementia: potential environmental and intrinsic factors. *RBD,* REM sleep behavior disorder; *REM,* rapid eye movement; *SCN,* suprachiasmatic nucleus. (Copyright Alon Y. Avidan, MD, MPH.)

increased the risk for AD 3.3 times. Dementia progressed more rapidly in AD patients with insomnia than AD without insomnia.

- Longitudinal study ($n = 1574$ men age 50, follow-up 1029 age 90): Self-reported sleep disturbances at age 50 increased the risk for later AD 51% and for dementia 33%.[95] The greatest risk presented in those who first reported sleep disturbances ≥70 years (192% increased risk).
- OSA and/or intermittent hypoxia activates AD pathology in brain. In the PREADVISE study (Prevention of Alzheimer Disease by Vitamin E and Selenium) of 7547 older adults, self-reported sleep apnea in the absence of APOE ε4 was associated with a 66% higher risk for developing dementia.[96] Conversely, self-reported apnea did not confer additional risk for participants with an ε4 allele.
- Elevated orexin/hypocretin levels in patients with AD may predispose them to insomnia. Fig. 19.8 summarizes the relationships between sleep and AD neuropathology.

Circadian Rhythm Disorders Far Greater in Patients with Alzheimer's Disease Than Healthy Aged[85,97]

- Decreased amplitude of rest-activity cycle
- Nocturnal sleep duration reduced and fragmented
- Increased daytime napping
- Reversal of normal rest-activity documented by actigraphy
- Positive correlation between circadian rhythm disorder (CRD) and degree of dementia in AD
- CRD is a major cause for nursing home placement in AD.

Why Circadian Rhythm Pathology so Prevalent and Severe in Alzheimer's Disease?[85]

- AD pathology targets SCN, pineal gland, and melanopsin-containing retinal ganglion cells with neuronal cell loss and atrophy beginning early.
- Decreased cerebrospinal fluid (CSF) melatonin levels in preclinical AD are comparable with age-matched controls (and continue to fall with disease progression).
- Autopsy studies of patients with AD find neuronal loss in SCN, reduced numbers of melatonin receptors, vasoactive intestinal polypeptide (VIP), and neurotensin. Amyloid-beta and neurofibrillary tangles are also found near the areas of degeneration. VIP neurons may be important in circadian entrainment and maintaining circadian rhythms of activity.

Clinical Evaluation of Older Adults with Sleep/Wake Complaints and Cognitive Concerns

- Questions to ask when evaluating sleep/wake complaints in older adults:
  - Sleep/wake complaint(s)?
    - EDS; early bedtimes; late bedtimes; early morning awakenings; too little sleep per 24 hours; sleeping at wrong times
  - Stressors or environmental effects that contribute?
    - Too much light, noisy dog, hot bedroom, snoring, nocturia, or RBD bed partner

- Poor sleep habits that predispose?
  - Excessive time in bed awake, daytime naps
- Symptoms suggest which primary sleep disorders?
  - OSA, CSA, RLS, RBD
- Medications affecting sleep/wakefulness?
- Underlying medical and/or neurological conditions predisposing to sleep/wake disorders?

Diagnostic Tools When Evaluating Sleep/Wake Complaints in Older Adults[98]

- Sleep log (± actigraphy) is helpful.
- Supplement with information from bed partner and/or validated sleep questionnaire
- Focused physical exam guided by history
- Mental status testing (Montreal Cognitive Assessment)
- Home sleep apnea test (HSAT) if high pretest probability for OSA without other significant comorbid sleep or medical disorders; PSG for suspected RBD, PLMS, sleep-related violence, atypical parasomnia(s), CSA, sleep-related hypoventilation, following stroke, significant cardiopulmonary disease, and/or other comorbidities.

Treating Sleep Disorders in Patients with Alzheimer's Disease or Minimal Cognitive Impairment[99–101]

- Identify and treat risk and lifestyle factors that contribute to AD:
  - Insulin resistance, obesity, DM2, cerebrovascular and/or cardiovascular disease
  - Insufficient or fragmented sleep; sleep apnea; intermittent nocturnal hypoxia
  - Sedentary activity
- Nonpharmacological treatment of sleep problems in patients with AD:
  - Regular daily exercise ≥30 min and walking outdoors
  - Do not rest in bed; bedroom reserved for sleep (and sex).
  - Nocturnal light and noise exposure should be minimized.
  - Discourage daytime naps greater than 1 hour.
  - Avoid caffeinated beverages after 2 PM.
  - Identify and treat SDB.
- Value of daily exercise in aged, MCI, and AD:
  - Physical exercise has emerged as a potent enhancer of adult hippocampal neurogenesis and preservation of cognition in older adults.[102]
  - Exercise promotes cognitive function and neuroplasticity; leads to better sleep quality and lessens EDS (best 4–8 hours before bed). Evening exercise phase advances, whereas exercise during the habitual sleep time phase delays.
  - A study of physically active late-middle age adults in Wisconsin Registry for AD found exercise lessened the key biomarkers of AD pathophysiology.[103]
  - A pilot randomized controlled study showed improved cognition when subjects with AD used a treadmill for 30 min twice a week for 16 weeks.[104]
  - A randomized controlled trial showed increased walking and bright light exposure improved sleep in community-dwelling persons with AD.[105]
- Pharmacological treatment of sleep problems in AD:
  - A paucity of evidence for medications to treat sleep/wake problems in patients with AD was found in a 2014 Cochrane Review.[106] A 2016 review of the efficacy and safety of sleep medicines in older adults may suffice in lieu of other evidence.[107]

- Cholinesterase inhibitors: Improvements in REM sleep (increased percent REM sleep, REM density and decreased REM latency and EEG slowing in REM sleep) in patients with moderate AD. Dose in AM to reduce nightmares and respect physiological decrease of acetylcholine that normally occurs in NREM 3 sleep.
- Melatonin: Efficacy to improve sleep in AD is equivocal, but with no significant side effects.
- Antipsychotics: Best avoided in older adults, especially those with cognitive impairment, associated with increased risk of falls secondary to sedation. Risk of serious cardiac effects, especially with second-generation antipsychotics.
- Antihistamines: Wide range of side effects include sedation, cognitive impairment, increased daytime sleepiness, and other anticholinergic effects.
- Hypnotics: Non-BZP hypnotics less often associated with residual morning sedation or fall risk. Suvorexant (an orexin receptor antagonist) promising hypnotic in AD?

Parkinson's Disease

Basic Information

PD is a progressive neurodegenerative disease in which parkinsonism is asymmetric in onset and severity and response to levodopa robust.[108,109] The motor features of PD are easiest to recognize: resting tremor, bradykinesia, postural instability, and rigidity (Fig. 19.9). Other classic features of PD are monotonic hypophonic speech, masking of facial features, decreased automatic movements, and gait difficulties. However, PD is associated with many nonmotor symptoms, some of which can precede motor symptoms by years. Nonmotor symptoms of PD are also prominent, contribute to its pathology, and often first appear before the motor signs. Sleep disorders are one of the nonmotor (dopamine-nonresponsive) symptoms of PD (Table 19.6).[110–112]

Recent data suggest PD may begin in genetically susceptible patients as a cascade of α-synuclein aggregation, which reaches the brain via the olfactory or enteric system and then spreading.[113]

However, nonmotor symptoms of PD are also prominent, contribute to its pathology, and often first appear before the motor signs. Sleep disorders are one of the nonmotor (dopamine-nonresponsive) symptoms of PD (see Table 19.6).[110–112]

TABLE 19.6	Non-motor Symptoms of Parkinson's Disease

- Sleep disturbances and fatigue
- Rapid eye movement sleep behavior disorder
- Cognitive impairment (mild memory difficulties to dementia)
- Apathy, hallucinations
- Bradyphrenia (slowed thinking)
- Depression and anxiety
- Loss of smell, impaired color discrimination
- Constipation, gastroparesis, bladder urgency, and erectile dysfunction
- Hypophonic monotonic speech, drooling and swallowing problems
- Unexplained pain
- Orthostatic hypotension, hyperhidrosis

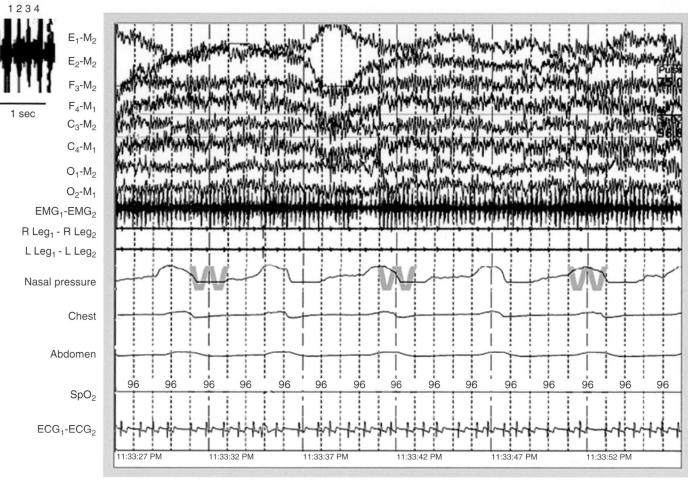

• **Figure 19.9** Polysomnographic recording during wakefulness, which shows a 4-Hz rest tremor in a patient with Parkinson's disease. (From Berry RB, ed. *Fundamentals of Sleep Medicine*. Philadelphia, PA: Elsevier Saunders; 2012.)

Sleep Disorders Common in Patients with Parkinson's Disease[114]

- Sleep disorders affect 60%–90% of patients with PD, correlate with disease severity, and have a negative impact on quality of life measures for patients with PD and their caregivers.
- Poor quality sleep and locomotor disability are their two major sources of dissatisfaction with quality of life in people with PD.
- One study of 689 patients with PD found 81% reported disrupted sleep, 40% early morning awakenings, 38% unrefreshing sleep, 31% nocturnal awakenings, and 18% difficulty falling asleep.[115]
- Sleep complaints in PD are thought to be multifactorial. Some are due to damage and functional dysregulation of brainstem structures that regulate sleep, wakefulness, and movement during sleep. Medication effects, depression (which often precedes the clinical onset of PD), anxiety, and dementia contribute. Fig. 19.10 summarizes factors contributing to sleep disorders in patients with PD.
- Reduced quantity and quality of nocturnal sleep in PD is associated with daytime fatigue but not EDS.[116]

Video-Polysomnographic Findings in Parkinson's Disease

- Nocturnal PSG findings in PD include increased sleep latency, reduced total sleep time and sleep efficiency, decreased NREM 3 and REM sleep time, reduced or loss of sleep spindles and K-complexes, RBD, PLMS, and RBD.
- PSG in early PD may show increased muscle tone, abnormal movements in sleep including increased blinking, blepharospasm, tremor, PLMS, and RBD. An amazing range of movements during sleep and sleep disorders are seen in patients with PD (Table 19.7).

Insomnia in Parkinson's Disease

- Insomnia is the most common sleep complaint in idiopathic PD. One study involving 689 patients with PD found 81% reported disrupted sleep, 40% early morning awakenings, 38% nonrestorative sleep, 31% nocturnal awakenings, and 18% trouble falling asleep.[115] Fig. 19.11 illustrates a characteristic hypnogram from a patient with PD highlighting respiratory disturbances, fragmentation of sleep architecture, frequent awakenings, and lack of slow wave sleep. The prevalence of insomnia increased with the severity and duration of the PD.
- Depression, anxiety, severe parkinsonism, dyskinesia, and RLS contribute to sleep onset insomnia in patients with PD.[117] Depression and early morning dystonia of the foot or trunk can cause early awakening in PD.[117]
- Poor quality and reduced duration of nighttime sleep were associated with daytime fatigue, not EDS.[116]

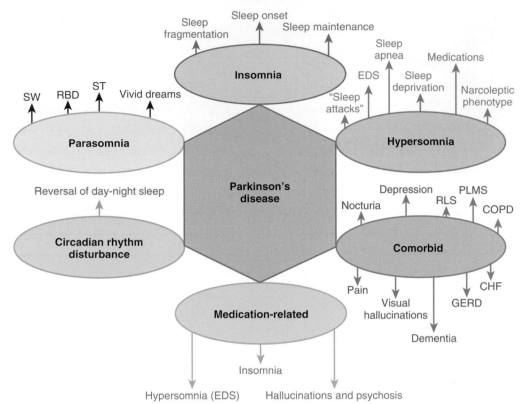

• **Figure 19.10** Spectrum of sleep dysfunction in Parkinson's disease. *CHF*, Congestive heart failure; *COPD*, chronic obstructive pulmonary disease; *EDS*, excessive daytime sleepiness; *GERD*, gastroesophageal reflux disease; *PLMS*, periodic limb movements during sleep; *RLS*, restless legs syndrome; *RBD*, REM sleep behavior disorder; *ST*, sleep terror; *SW*, sleepwalking. (From Chokroverty S, Bhat S, Provini F. Sleep dysfunction and sleep-disordered breathing in miscellaneous neurological disorders. In: Chokroverty S, Thomas RJ, eds. *Atlas of Sleep Medicine.* 2nd ed. Philadelphia, PA: Elsevier/Saunders; 2014.)

TABLE 19.7	Range of Sleep-Related Movements and Sleep/Wake Complaints in Patients with Parkinson's Disease

- Fragmented sleep, insomnia, nocturia, akathisia, stiffness, difficulty turning over in bed, confusional arousals, visual hallucinations, dream enactment behaviors, nightmares, snoring, respiratory pauses, or respiratory dyskinesias
- Excessive periodic and isolated leg jerks and twitches compared with age-matched controls; sleep-related leg cramps; repeated eye blinking at sleep onset; rapid eye movements (REMs) during nonrapid eye movement (NREM) sleep; blepharospasm at REM sleep onset; increased tonic muscle activity, episodic rigidity and dystonia in NREM and REM sleep
- Painful early morning dystonia prior to waking; episodic prolonged sustained extension or flexion of one or more limbs during NREM sleep; myoclonus; loss of REM sleep muscle atonia; and REM sleep behavior disorder (RBD)

- Reduced and fragmented sleep in PD is most often caused by parkinsonian symptoms during sleep (see Table 19.7). For example, rest tremor tends to disappear with sleep onset; this is rarely seen in deeper NREM sleep. Tremor amplitude is usually less than half that experienced during wakefulness, but bursts of tremor lasting less than 15 sec recur, most often after awakenings, transitions to and from REM sleep, stage NREM

N1 sleep, or during bursts of REMs. Tremor is often less or even absent the first 1–2 hours after awakening from sleep (so-called sleep benefit). Fig. 19.12A shows right leg tremor during NREM 1 sleep in a patient with PD. The tremor is of lower amplitude than when awake. Fig. 19.13 shows how the amplitude of the tremor lessens even more during REM sleep (see Fig. 19.12B).

- Patients with PD may complain of tremor, dystonia, difficulty rolling over, stiffness, restlessness, and nocturnal hallucinations fragmenting their sleep. Nocturia can make nocturnal mobility even more distressing. Depression and early morning dystonia may contribute to early morning awakenings.

Sleep Benefit in Parkinson's Disease[118–121]

- Sleep benefit is a subjective (less often objective) improvement in mobility upon awakening in patients with PD.
- Sleep benefit has been observed in 10%–55% of patients, lasting 30 min to greater than 3 hours and postponing morning levodopa/carbidopa.[121]
- Sleep benefit in PD tends to be observed in patients with PD who are younger at disease onset; exhibit less cognitive and physical disability; have longer disease duration; take less levodopa; have paradoxically shorter total nocturnal sleep times; and longer sleep latencies.[121]
- Prospective studies have found improvement in motor function after sleep in PD is mostly subjective, not borne out by objective testing.[119]

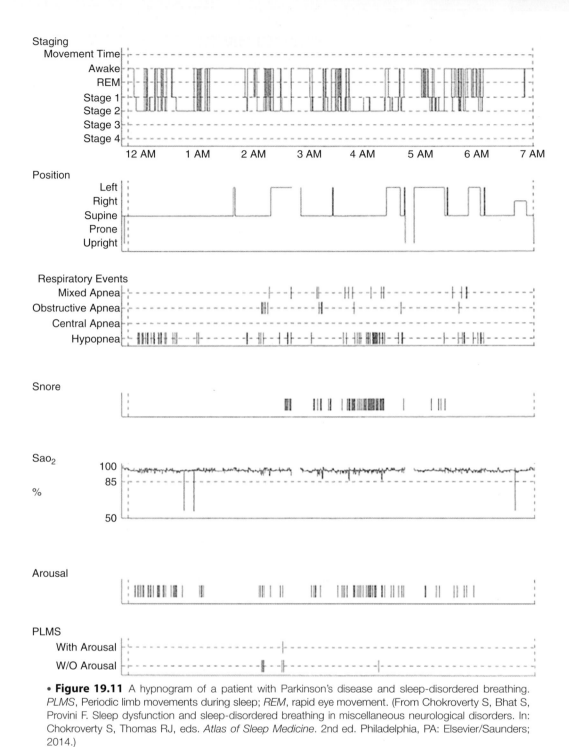

• **Figure 19.11** A hypnogram of a patient with Parkinson's disease and sleep-disordered breathing. *PLMS*, Periodic limb movements during sleep; *REM*, rapid eye movement. (From Chokroverty S, Bhat S, Provini F. Sleep dysfunction and sleep-disordered breathing in miscellaneous neurological disorders. In: Chokroverty S, Thomas RJ, eds. *Atlas of Sleep Medicine*. 2nd ed. Philadelphia, PA: Elsevier/Saunders; 2014.)

Excessive Daytime Sleepiness in Parkinson's Disease

- EDS is highly prevalent in patients with PD, and prevalence increases with disease duration. A large longitudinal cohort of greater than 400 PD patients examined annually for 5 years found 43% at baseline had EDS; another 46% developed it later.[122]
- EDS in PD can manifest as either continuous hypersomnia or episodes of sudden sleep onset (sleep attacks).
- One study of 134 subjects with PD found 46% reported subjective EDS, but only 15% had objective EDS evidenced by short mean sleep latencies on multiple sleep latency test (MSLT).[123]

- Risk factors for EDS in PD include PD severity, dementia, lower scores on cognitive tests, greater PD-related disability, anxiety, impulsive behavior, psychosis, hyposmia, worse subjective sleep, hallucinations, longer duration of dopaminergic therapy, and autonomic dysfunction.[124]
- People with PD occasionally report sudden, unexpected, and irresistible sleep attacks.
  - Sudden, unexpected, and irresistible sleep attacks reported in 177 (1%) of 2952 patients with PD (and in 91 without appropriate warning signs).[125] A high ESS score, dopamine agonists, and duration of PD were the main influencing

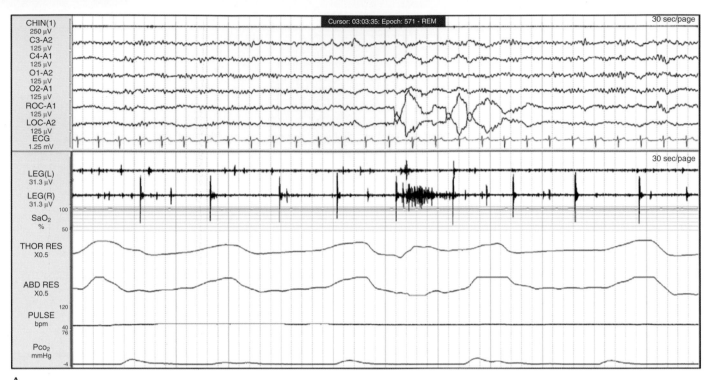

A

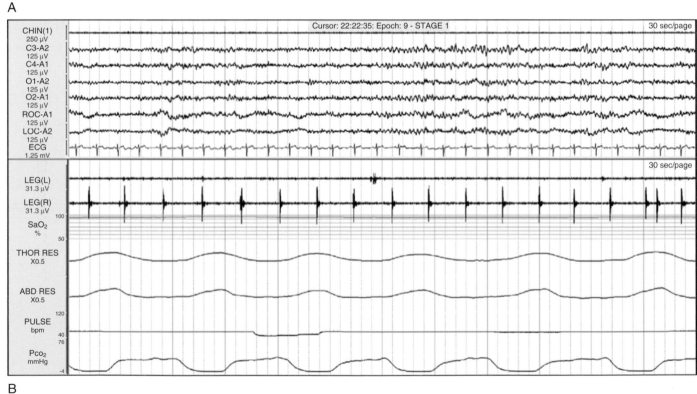

B

• **Figure 19.12** A and B, Effect of sleep on rest tremor in a patient with Parkinson's disease. (From Kryger MH, Avidan AY, Berry RB, eds. *Atlas of Clinical Sleep Medicine.* 2nd ed. Philadelphia, PA: Elsevier Saunders; 2014.)

factors for the occurrence of sleep attacks. The odds ratio for dopamine agonist therapy was 2.9 compared with 1.9 in L-dopa therapy and 1.05 for a 1-year-longer disease duration.

• A case-control study of 176 patients with PD and 174 controls found the same proportion of PD patients (27%) and controls

(32%) reported sleep attacks, but these were much more frequent in PD patients and occurred more frequently in situations requiring attention (11% vs. 2%).[126] Duration of levodopa therapy best predicted sleep attacks in PD.

• Sleep attacks often reported to occur several days/weeks after starting a particular dopaminergic drug, and improve/remit

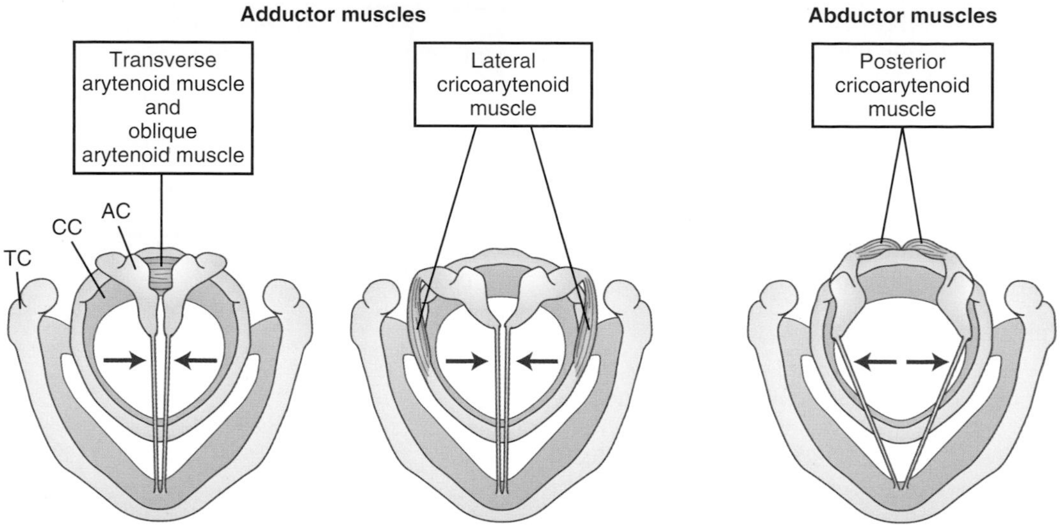

Adductor muscles | Abductor muscles

Transverse arytenoid muscle and oblique arytenoid muscle

Lateral cricoarytenoid muscle

Posterior cricoarytenoid muscle

• **Figure 19.13** Fundamental functional anatomy of the intrinsic laryngeal muscles, which may play a role in the mechanisms causing laryngeal stridor. (From Ozawa T, Sekiya K, Aizawa N, Terajima K, Nishizawa M. Laryngeal stridor in multiple system atrophy: clinicopathological features and causal hypotheses. *J Neurol Sci.* 2016;361:243–249.)

after reduction, withdrawal, or substitution for the drug.[127] Sleep attacks can lead to motor vehicle accidents.

- What predisposes patients with PD to EDS?[108]
  - Sleepiness in PD is thought to be an integral part of the disease, reflecting the extent of neurodegeneration.
  - Progressive cell loss of mesolimbic dopaminergic and nondopaminergic networks that modulate sleep mechanisms
  - Dopaminergic medications have sedative effects: EDS is associated with low doses of levodopa and higher doses of dopamine agonists.
  - A subset of patients with PD have findings on MSLT that resemble those seen with narcolepsy. Cataplexy is not seen in patients with PD and EDS. CSF levels of hypocretin are normal in PD with EDS.
- EDS in patients with PD warrant consideration of video-PSG, especially those with symptoms suggestive of SDB and/or RBD.

Rapid Eye Movement Sleep Behavior Disorder in Parkinson's Disease

- RBD occurs in approximately 40%–50% of patients with PD; 20% of cases of RBD occur before the onset of parkinsonism; and 65% of patients with PD are unaware of RBD behaviors and 20% do not recall unpleasant dreams.[117]
- Patients with PD and RBD compared with those without RBD are more likely to have:[124]
  - Longer disease duration, more axial (as opposed to limb) involvement, greater propensity to fall, more dyskinesia, worse outcomes after deep brain stimulation, more symmetry of motor manifestations, greater motor fluctuations, and increased cognitive impairment, of psychosis, depression, fatigue, reduced heart rate variability, orthostatic hypotention, and erectile dysfunction.
  - Sleep-related injury, EDS, nightmares, sleep talking, abnormalities of circadian rhythm, and sudden sleep attacks, leading to motor vehicle accidents

TABLE 19.8	Clinical or Subclinical Abnormalities Often Found in Patients with Chronic Idiopathic Rapid Eye Movement Sleep Behavior Disorder

- Impaired olfactory function and/or color vision
- Subtle cognitive deficits in executive function, visuospatial, and memory
- Excessive amounts of intermixed slowing in wake EEGs
- Reduced arm swing or masked facies
- Autonomic dysfunction (orthostatic hypotension, erective dysfunction, systolic blood pressure drop, decreased heart rate variability)
- Decreased dopamine transporter function in striatum (especially the left putamen)
- Reduced sympathetic function on ^{123}I-MBIG cardiac scintigraphy
- Hyperechogenicity of substantia nigra
- Hypoechogenicity of brainstem raphe
- Decreased cortical and increased pontine perfusion
- Reduce postprandial ghrelin response
- Episodes of acute psychosis or delirium after even minor surgery

- Longitudinal studies show most patients with chronic idiopathic RBD (iRBD) will eventually develop synucleinopathies (more often DLB dementia, PD, or MSA).[128–130]
  - Patients with iRBD at increased risk for PD often have clinical and subclinical abnormalities which suggest they are at greater risk to develop PD (Table 19.8).[131]
  - Voice changes (monotonic hypophonic speech) and masking of facial features are often the first signs of PD to develop in patients with iRBD, later followed by rigidity, gait abnormalities, and bradykinesia.
- RBD in PD is associated with male gender, impulse control disorders, cognitive impairment, freezing, falls, long duration of parkinsonism, and older age.

- A 2014 study found the frequency and severity of RBD in PD was not greater in patients with nontremor-dominant (akinetic-rigid) PD and tremor-predominant PD.[132]
- Video-PSG studies have demonstrated that PD patients with RBD move better in REM sleep than they do when awake. Purposeful movements in REM sleep in PD patients during RBD were surprisingly fast, ample, coordinated and symmetrical, and without obvious sign of parkinsonism. RBD movements in PD were jerky, violent, often repetitive, and six times more likely to involve the upper than lower limbs.

Circadian Rhythm Disorders in Parkinson's Disease[133–135]

- Patients with PD have a tendency toward phase advance, which predisposes them to EDS in the early evening and early morning awakenings.
- May be due to reduced amplitude of melatonin secretion, reduced nocturnal melatonin levels, hypercortisolemia, altered peripheral clock gene expression, depression, and/or dementia.
  Sleep apnea occurs in ~25% of patients with PD, more often obstructive in type.
- The incidence of OSA in PD is less prevalent than initially thought. One study found only 21% of 92 patients with PD had OSA on overnight PSG, using AHI cutoffs of greater than 5 or greater than 15.[136]
- Spending more time sleeping supine and less body position shifts can predispose patients with PD to more severe OSA.[137] Levodopa can improve upper airway obstruction; awake and sustained release levodopa-carbidopa before bed was shown to reduce OSA severity in patients with PD who had OSA.[138]
- A recent study found OSA on overnight PSG in 86 patients with PD, and also found OSA was associated with poor cognition in 38 patients.[139]
- The number of apneas and hypopneas per hour of sleep in PD is not related to BMI.
- PD patients do not move chest as well as they should (restrictive pulmonary defect) due to chest wall rigidity and faulty automatic reflex controls of lungs.
- Can observe diaphragmatic dyskinesias or upper airway obstruction with tremor-like oscillations in PD

Restless Legs Syndrome and Periodic Limb Movements During Sleep in Parkinson's Disease[117,140–145]

- Debates continue as to whether RLS is more common in patients with PD than age-matched controls.[140]
- PLMS in PD are present but not more frequent than seen in age-matched controls.[146] Patients with idiopathic RLS do not progress to PD. Postmortem brain studies do not find PD pathology in patients with idiopathic RLS.[143]
- In patients with PD who have comorbid RLS, parkinsonism most often precedes the onset of RLS, family history of RLS is uncommon, RLS age of onset is older, and RLS severity is mild.[117]
- Akathisia, dystonia, and leg cramps common in PD may be misdiagnosed as RLS.[141,142]
- PLMS in PD usually do not cause arousal, and not considered a major cause for sleep fragmentation or arousal in PD.[144] PLMS occur in patients with PD but are not more frequent than controls.[145]

Sleep Disorders in Hereditary Forms of Parkinson's Disease

- Patients with PD due to Parkin gene mutations can have RBD or RLS.[147]

TABLE 19.9	Adverse Effects of Medications Used to Treat Parkinson's Disease
Medication	**Adverse Effect on Sleep**
Levodopa	Reduces rapid eye movement (REM) sleep time Increases REM latency Hallucinations
COMT inhibitors	Enhance levodopa-induced adverse effects
Dopamine agonists	Low dose: insomnia High dose: daytime sleepiness
Anticholinergics	Alerting effects when taken at night Sedative effect when used in day
Selegiline	Metabolized to amphetamine

- Sleep/wake complaints are common in patients with PD, due to mutations of the leucine-rich repeat kinase 2 (LRRK2-PD) gene. One study of 18 PD subjects with LRRK2-PD found 78% reported poor quality sleep, 56% sleep fragmentation, 39% early morning awakening, and 33% sleep onset insomnia.[148] Short sleep latencies were noted on MSLT among those who complained of EDS. Sleep attacks without cataplexy were reported in three. RBD and EDS began after the onset of parkinsonism. Compared with idiopathic PD, sleep onset insomnia was more frequently reported, EDS similar, but RBD was less frequent and less severe in patients with PD and LRRK2-PD.

Treating Sleep Disorders in Patients with Parkinson's Disease[108,124,149]

- First assess whether the medications the patient is prescribed are contributing to the sleep/wake complaints. Table 19.9 lists adverse effects of PD medications on sleep.
- For patients with PD who complain their PD symptoms fragment their nighttime sleep, consider small doses of levodopa-carbidopa at bedtime or during the night, or extended release formulas of levodopa at bedtime can reduce nighttime rigidity and tremor.
- Nocturnal continuous subcutaneous apomorphine infusion was shown to improve insomnia, sleep quality, neurological function, and reduce daytime sleepiness in patients with severe PD.[150]
- A recent prospective study found adding rasagiline 1 mg/day (a selective irreversible monoamine oxidase B inhibitor) to 200–300 mg/d of levodopa increased total sleep time and shortened sleep latency compared with controls with PD taking levodopa alone.[151] Monoamine oxidase B inhibitors may increase melatonin levels in the pineal gland.
- Alternatively, consider drug delivery systems that provide more constant plasma concentrations of dopamine such as rotigotine transdermal patch, ropinirole prolonged release, levodopa/carbidopa intestinal gel infusion,[152] or subthalamic nucleus deep brain stimulation.[152,153] Rotigotine transdermal patch may improve mood and early morning motor function in patients with severe PD.[153]
- Deep brain stimulation therapy has been shown to improve the symptoms of PD, less motor fluctuations; improve sleep quality; and reduce sleep fragmentation in PD.[154]
- Insomnia in PD may respond to cognitive behavioral insomnia therapy, bright light treatment, and sleep-facilitating medications

dosed at bedtime (e.g., melatonin, trazodone, doxepin, eszopiclone, and quetiapine).

- RBD can be treated with melatonin (3–12 mg qhs) or clonazepam (1–4 mg qhs).
- Melatonin (3 mg) before bed can be tried to treat circadian rhythm disturbances in PD. A small double blind placebo controlled trial of melatonin in PD showed subjective improvement of sleep quality but no improvement in objective PSG measures compared with placebo.
- Treating EDS in PD should include good sleep hygiene, established bed- and wake-times, and exposure to sufficient light in the day and darkness at night. Physical exercise appropriate for level of disability can be beneficial.
- If the patient with PD has too early bedtime and early morning awakenings, bright light therapy at night could be tried. A small double-blind placebo controlled trial of bright light (7500 lux) to placebo (950 lux) showed improvements in nonmotor symptoms and depression, but no improvement in EDS compared with placebo.[155] Bright light therapy in PD might slow the degenerative process.[156]
- CPAP can lessen EDS in patients with PD and OSA, and improve sleep architecture, but compliance in patients with severe PD remains a challenge.
- Increased doses of dopaminergic agents can increase EDS. Reducing or discontinuing daytime doses of dopamine agonists (if tolerated) can lessen EDS (e.g., holding or delaying taking a dopamine agonist on an afternoon when the patient needs to drive a motor vehicle).
- Modafinil has been tried with modest success in some patients with PD and EDS, typically after reducing, changing, or substituting one dopaminergic agonist for another. A placebo controlled study of modafinil in PD failed to show improvement in ESS scores or based upon objective MSLT measures.[157]
- If serum ferritin levels are low (<50), a 2–3-month course of oral iron (with vitamin C to improve absorption) is warranted, and shown to be efficacious in patients with RLS who do not have PD. RLS in PD can be treated with a higher evening dose of dopaminergic agonist, and use of extended release formulas of dopaminergic agonists. If RLS augmentation is suspected, avoid levodopa, and consider gabapentin enacarbil, pregabalin, or oxycodone.
- A retrospective review of 203 consecutive iRBD seen at one sleep center over 24 years found 80% were men with a median age at iRBD diagnosis of 68 years (range 50–85 years).[158] When first diagnosed, 44% were unaware of their dream behaviors and 70% reported good quality sleep. Video-PSG had to be repeated to confirm REM sleep without atonia in 16% because of artifact from sleep apnea or insufficient REM sleep. Some patients with comorbid OSA reported a partial improvement in their RBD with CPAP therapy.

Diffuse Lewy Body Dementia

A neurodegenerative synucleinopathy characterized by pronounced variations in attention, alertness, and vigilance; recurrent detailed and well-formed visual hallucinations; visuospatial impairments; parkinsonism; and progression to dementia.[159–161] Autonomic dysfunction is common and often an early symptom. Lewy bodies extend beyond the brainstem and olfactory regions (of PD) into the limbic and/or cortical regions. DLB is the third most common dementia (after AD and vascular dementia).

It is difficult to distinguish DLB dementia from PD with dementia. Forty percent of patients with PD develop cognitive problems.

- Diagnosis of PD with dementia is made when the onset of cognitive problems is greater than 1 year after the onset of parkinsonism.
- PD with dementia is typically less severe than DLB.

Clinical Symptoms That Suggest Diffuse Lewy Body Dementia[160,161]

- Visual hallucinations are seen in two-thirds of patients with DLB, usually early. These are typically vivid, usually involve people or animals, and can be extracampine ("somebody looking over my shoulder").
- Fluctuating cognitive function with varying levels of alertness and attention (daytime drowsiness lasting greater than 2 hours, prolonged staring into space for long periods, episodes of disorganized speech, lucid periods when seem normal and alert).
- Parkinsonian signs of bradykinesia, rigidity, or gait disorders are seen in 70%–90% of patients with DLB.
- RBD, extreme sensitivity to the side effects of neuroleptics, early loss of smell, and low dopamine transporter uptake in basal ganglia by single photon emission computed tomography (SPECT) and positron emission tomography (PET) imaging are common features.
- Dysautonomia, orthostatic hypotension, urinary incontinence/retention, constipation, and impotence are often early symptoms of DLB.
- Eighty to ninety percent of patients with DLB have severe sensitivity to neuroleptics, causing parkinsonism (sometimes irreversible), impaired consciousness, sometimes combined with symptoms of neuroleptic malignant syndrome.
- Cognitive deficits in DLB: Deficits in frontal lobe executive functions and visuospatial impairments are more prominent. Patients with DLB do relatively well with confrontation naming tests but poorly on tests of visuospatial skills (e.g., drawing a clock, copying figures). Memory retrieval worse than memory storage.
- Resting tremor is common in PD and less common in DLB. May exhibit myoclonus before severe dementia.
  Sleep disorders affect ~80% of patients with DLB.[161,162]
- Compared with patients with AD and controls, patients with DLB had more severe daytime sleepiness or dysfunction due to sleepiness, longer nighttime sleep, more daytime naps, and more daytime fluctuations of attention.[163]
- Fifty percent of patients with DLB had EDS based on elevated ESS scores.[164]
- Sleep disorders in patients with DLB include insomnia, early morning awakenings, RBD, nocturnal hallucinations, confusional arousals with nocturnal wandering, and frequent daytime napping. RBD occurs in 70%–80% of patients with DLB, and precedes dementia in 70% of cases.[161,162]
- A study of sleep problems in patients with DLB using PSG found 77% had a sleep efficiency, 88% AHI greater than 5 per hour, and 74% PLM arousal indexes greater than 15 per hour.[165]
- RBD is common in patients with DLB; presence of RBD suggests DLB. RBD in men with dementia suggests DLB, because RBD is rare in tauopathies such as AD, PSP, and FTD.
- Quantitative EEG studies report slowing of the dominant posterior EEG rhythm and increased theta activity in the waking EEG of patients with DLB correlates with the degree of dementia.[166,167]

- Patients with DLB with daytime sleepiness had normal CSF orexin-1 levels.[168]
- Patients with DLB have a good response to cholinesterase inhibitors, reducing their delusions and improving nocturnal sleep.[169]

Multiple System Atrophy

Basic Information

MSA is a neurodegenerative disease characterized by parkinsonism, early and severe autonomic dysfunction, and/or cerebellar dysfunction. A distinctive feature of MSA is nocturnal IS causing life-threatening OSA.[170]

- Parkinsonism in MSA is typically an axial rigid syndrome, and less often a jerky postural tremor.
- Symptomatic orthostatic hypotension or urinary incontinence is less than 1 year after onset of parkinsonism.
- Early erectile dysfunction is almost universal in MSA.
- Early postural instability and falls less than 3 years after onset
- Rapid progression to wheelchair less than 5 years, despite dopaminergic (wheelchair sign)
- Mean survival less than 10 years; causes of death are bronchopneumonia (48%) and sudden death during wake or sleep (21%).
- A recent review of the literature regarding sudden death in MSA cited bronchopneumonia; disordered central respiration; suffocation by sputum/food; upper airway obstruction from nocturnal positive airway pressure (PAP) acting on floppy epiglottis, and cardiac autonomic factors.[171] Sudden death in MSA usually occurred during sleep, often then attributed to suffocation from vocal cord abductor paralysis. However, neither positive airway ventilation nor tracheostomy has prevented sudden death.

Seventy percent of patients with MSA report sleep problems.[117]

- Sleep disorders are common: reduced nocturnal sleep time and quality, EDS, RBD, and SDB are highly prevalent.
- Sleep onset insomnia and fragmented sleep occur in ~50% and EDS in 28%.
  - Almost all patients with MSA have RBD; often it is an initial symptom.[172] RBD is a red flag symptom for MSA, especially in older women who present with RBD. The absence of RBD should make you question the diagnosis of MSA.
  - A case-control study comparing 19 patients with MSA to 10 patients with OSA found among the patients with MSA, 42% had nocturnal stridor; 53% diurnal/nocturnal irregular breathing (snoring, gasping); and 63% RBD.[173] Sleep architecture in patients with MSA showed markedly decreased sleep efficiency (52%), decreased NREM 3 (12%) but relative preservation of REM sleep (25%). All MSA patients snored; only 37% had a respiratory disturbance index greater than 10 per hour. OSA was mild (mean RDI 11 per hour, 12 per hour NREM vs. 6 per hour REM sleep). Mean sleep SpO_2 was 93%, nadir SpO_2 82% but not especially worse in REM sleep. Expiratory noise with expiratory intercostal activation was observed in 74%. Decreased heart rate variability, increased heart rates, and respiratory rates during sleep were noted in those with MSA.
- Many different forms of SDB besides IS are common in patients with MSA: intermittent involuntary gasping and irregular breathing awake, impaired hypoxic and hypercapnic ventilatory responses, CSA, OSA, and Cheyne-Stokes respiration.

- Impaired control of laryngeal function in MSA awake and asleep predisposes them to IS, OSA, dyspnea awake, respiratory failure, and death.
- IS is a distinctive and life-threatening feature of MSA, seen in about 20% (13%–42%) of patients with MSA on video-PSG.[174–176]
- IS is characterized by high-pitched sound and thought either a dystonia of thryoarytenoid muscles, which adduct vocal cords or paralysis of posterior cricoarytenoid muscles and abduct the vocal cords.[174–176] Vocal cords normally abduct fully during inspiration, and adduct with expiration or phonation.
- IS in MSA is produced by vocal cord abduction restriction during inspiration, which is more often bilateral (partial or complete) and less often unilateral (partial or complete). The presence of IS in MSA is confirmed by laryngoscopy while awake.
- IS initially presents in sleep, and may antedate all other symptoms; there is no relation with MSA subtype, disease severity, or duration. Diurnal stridor may develop later, with increasing reduction in the glottis aperture.
- IS is associated with OSA, vocal cord paresis, subacute respiratory failure, sudden death in sleep, and a marker of short survival if untreated.
- Treatment of IS in MSA is obligatory; options include nasal CPAP (5–10 cm water pressure),[177] botulinum toxin injection into adductors, or tracheostomy. Botox increases risk for aspiration and dysphonia, and requires electromyogram (EMG) guidance and repeated injections (q 3 months). Tracheostomy for IS in MSA can be life-saving but is frequently refused.
- In a recent retrospective study of 136 patients with MSA, 42 had IS (early onset in 22). Twelve with early onset stridor were treated with tracheostomy, 19 with CPAP. Overall survival did not differ between patients with or without stridor, nor how stridor was treated. Early onset stridor was an unfavorable survival predictor.[178]
- In MSA, upper airway resistance increases because of activation of the adductors in the presence of abductor paralysis and laryngeal narrowing. This explains the increased muscle activity in the thyroarytenoid muscles seen on EMG in patients with MSA and IS. It also explains why moderate CPAP pressures (5–10 cm water pressure) may abolish IS, and botulinum toxin into these adductors increases laryngeal diameter. Fig. 19.13 shows the fundamental functional anatomy of the intrinsic laryngeal muscles, which may play a role in the mechanisms causing laryngeal stridor.

Progressive Supranuclear Palsy[179]

PSP is another neurodegenerative disease that typically presents between ages 50 and 70 years with cognitive problems, frequent propulsive falls, and difficulty with voluntary vertical eye movements (initially cannot look down, and then cannot look up).[179] It is later followed by axial rigidity, gait disorders, personality change, executive dysfunction, bradyphrenia, and dementia. It is typically sporadic, but some families have a mutation in the MAPT gene on chromosome 1q31.

Sleep Problems Are Common in Patients with Progressive Supranuclear Palsy[117]

- Difficulty falling and staying asleep are the most common sleep complaints.[180]

- PSG studies in patients with PSP show they have reduced total sleep time, decreased percentage of REM sleep time, and reduced numbers of sleep spindles and K-complexes.[181,182] In severe cases, the dominant alpha rhythm may be absent, and wake/sleep states are difficult to differentiate.
- REM sleep without atonia is observed in as many as 20% of patients with PSP.[183] RBD occurs in at most 10%–20%. RBD in PSP is usually mild in severity and develops after the onset of the dementia.
- Confusional arousals and nocturnal wandering are common when patients are still ambulatory.

Hereditary Spinocerebellar Ataxias[117]

Hereditary SCAs present with progressive ataxia and combinations of parkinsonism and polyneuropathy, and due to different gene mutations. Machado-Joseph disease (MJD), also known as spinocerebellar ataxia type 3 (SCA3), is the most common SCA worldwide.

Sleep disorders are common in SCAs, including RBD, RLS, insomnia, excessive fragmentary myoclonus, nocturnal cramps, snoring, nocturnal apnea, and fatigue.[184,185] OSA and EDS are not common in SCAs.

- RLS has been reported with SCA 1, 2, 3, and 6.
- Nocturnal stridor caused by vocal cord abnormalities has been reported in SCA3 and SCA1.
- RBD occurs in up to 50% of patients with SCA3. REM sleep without atonia is observed in patients with SCA2 without overt dream enactment behaviors.[186]
- A recent case-control PSG study of 47 patients with SCA3/MJD and 47 controls found the MJD/SCA3 patients had more frequent arousals from NREM 3, NREM arousal parasomnia complaints, nightmares, REM sleep without atonia, and higher PLM indexes.[187]
- A case-control study compared sleep/wake complaints and video-PSG in 32 patients with SCA type 2 and age- and gender-matched controls.[188] They found REM sleep without atonia, reduced percent of REM sleep time, and reduced REM density. The percentage of REM sleep without atonia correlated with the number of CAG repeats. RBD was not observed. PLMS were observed in 38%, and associated with ataxia scores and disease duration but not CAG repeats.

Huntington's Disease

HD is an autosomal dominant neurodegenerative disease characterized by progressive chorea, dystonia, incoordination, cognitive, behavioral, and psychiatric disturbances and dementia linked to expanded CAG repeats in the Huntington gene on the short arm of chromosome 4.[189] It is associated with severe atrophy of the putamen and caudate, and to a lesser extent, the cerebral cortex. Symptoms usually begin between ages 25 and 45 years (but can occur in childhood or old age).

- Slowness of thinking and frontal lobe executive dysfunction are typically the first cognitive symptoms.
- Depression and suicidal ideation are common in more advanced stages of HD.
- Paternal inheritance is associated with higher penetrance, younger onset, and more severe deficits.

The majority of patients with HD have sleep complaints (up to 87%), especially in later stages of the disease.[117]

- Patients with even mild to moderate HD have more movements when sleeping. Choreic or dystonic movements of HD were typically suppressed at sleep onset, but often recurred during NREM 1, NREM 2, or with arousals. Sleep complaints increased with progression of disease and atrophy of caudate nuclei.
- Insomnia, frequent nocturnal awakenings, EDS, delayed or advanced sleep phase type CRD with early morning awakenings are common in patients with HD and worsen with progression of the disease. RBD, OSA, and RLS are uncommon in PD.
- Patients with HD have disrupted night/day patterns. Transgenic mice carrying the HD also showed disruption of night/day activity and circadian timing, which worsened as the disease progressed and was associated with a marked reduction in expression of *mPer2* and disrupted expression of *Bmal1* in the SCN.[190]
- A case-control study comparing overnight PSG in 16 in-patients with HD with healthy controls found patients with HD had increased sleep onset latency, reduced sleep efficiency, frequent nocturnal awakenings, more WASO, less NREM 3 sleep, and increased density of sleep spindles.[191] Sleep disturbances correlated with caudate atrophy and severity of HD symptoms.
- A case-control study of 25 patients with HD comparing their sleep/wake complaints and PSG and MSLT results with patients with narcolepsy type 1 and healthy controls.[192] The patients with HD had sleep onset, lower sleep efficiency, increased NREM 1 sleep, delayed and shortened REM sleep, and increased PLMS. RBD was present in three (12%) HD patients. Four HD patients had abnormally low (<8 min) daytime sleep latencies but none had multiple sleep-onset REM periods. SDB is not common in patients with HD. Fig. 19.14 shows prolonged obstructive apnea during REM sleep in a woman with HD.
- Disintegration of sleep may occur early in HD. Asymptomatic HD gene carriers have more fragmented sleep than age-matched controls. Reduced REM sleep duration (but not RBD) was found in premanifest carriers and patients with very mild HD, and worsened with disease severity.[192]
- A recent cross-sectional cohort study performed structural interviews, validated questionnaires, and recorded overnight video-PSG in 30 patients with HD, and compared them with 30 matched healthy controls.[193] Compared with controls, subjects with HD had shorter sleep, reduced sleep efficiency, and increased arousals and awakenings. They found PLMS were observed during wake and sleep in all HD patients. No OSA, RBD, or REM sleep without atonia on PSG was noted in those with HD.
- Another recent study recorded video-PSG on 29 subjects with HD, and compared them with gender-matched healthy controls.[194] They found no correlation between CAG repeat length and sleep measures (as have others).[192] Total sleep time and sleep efficiency were more reduced in those with moderate compared with milder HD. Giant sleep spindles (>65 mV) were observed in 24% with HD and one control. Arousals from sleep in HD were often violent and harmful opisthotonus-like movements from either NREM or REM sleep. Only 2 of 29 subjects had REM sleep without atonia, and none had RBD.
- No treatment yet identified for HD.

Fatal Familial Insomnia[195–197]

Fatal familial insomnia (FFI) is a rare autosomal dominant prion disease due to missense mutation of codon 178 of prion protein

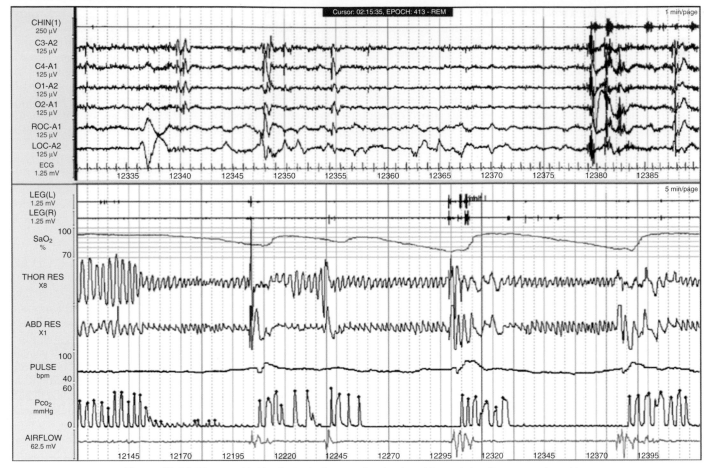

• **Figure 19.14** Woman with Huntington's disease who developed long obstructive apneas in rapid eye movement sleep. (From Kryger MH, Avidan AY, Berry RB, eds. *Atlas of Clinical Sleep Medicine*. 2nd ed. Philadelphia, PA: Elsevier Saunders; 2014.)

gene (PRNP) on chromosome 20 with the methionine at codon 129 of the mutated allele. Sporadic cases of FFI have been reported but very rare.

• FFI often starts around age 50, leads to death after 8–72 months, courses more rapidly (<11 months) in patients who express methionine at codon 129 of both mutated, and have a two- to threefold longer disease duration.

• At onset of FFI, patients become increasingly taciturn and apathetic. Neuropsychological testing shows an early progressive impairment in attention and vigilance, sparing intellectual function till the late stages of the disease.

• Trouble sleeping is one of the earliest features of FFI, which includes difficulty falling asleep, frequent nocturnal awakenings, and inability to nap in the day.

• Hallucinatory behavior, which represents dream enactment, is seen early in the disease. Patients mimic daily life activities (oneiric stupor).

• Sympathetic overactivity evident with elevated heart and respiratory rates, core body temperature, and arterial blood pressure are seen 24/7.

• Ataxia-abasia (unsteady gait), dysarthria, and dysphagia are seen as the disease develops.

• Mild fever and transient diplopia (and impotence in males) are seen when the disease is fully established.

• Patients lose weight and die from either infections or sudden cardiorespiratory failure.

• PSG documents early loss of sleep spindles and K-complexes 24/7. Later in the disease, the dominant EEG pattern is NREM 1, interspersed with short periods of REM sleep. No normal patterns of sleep architecture are seen. Motor activity is markedly increased 24/7 without any circadian pattern.

• Fig. 19.15 demonstrates PSG and hypnogram finding from a patient with FFI.

• Persistently elevated concentrations of cortisol and norepinephrine and lack of a nocturnal rise of melatonin secretion

• Magnetic resonance imaging (MRI) brain shows only mild cerebral and cerebellar atrophy in late clinical stages.

• However, an fludeoxyglucose (FDG)-PET scan shows profound reduction in metabolism in thalamus bilaterally (and to a lesser extent in the cingulate gyri). Later in the disease course, hypometabolism is seen in the entire cerebral cortex and basal ganglia.

• FFI is regarded as a predominantly thalamo-limbic hypometabolic state. Impaired thalamic metabolism on FDG-PET scans identifies preclinical FFI mutation carriers.

• Neuropathological findings of FFI: selective loss (up to 80%) of mesial mediodorsal and anteroventral thalamic nuclei.

• No known treatments for FFI. A prospective trial of doxycycline (100 mg/day) on 10 carriers of the FFI gene is underway.[198]

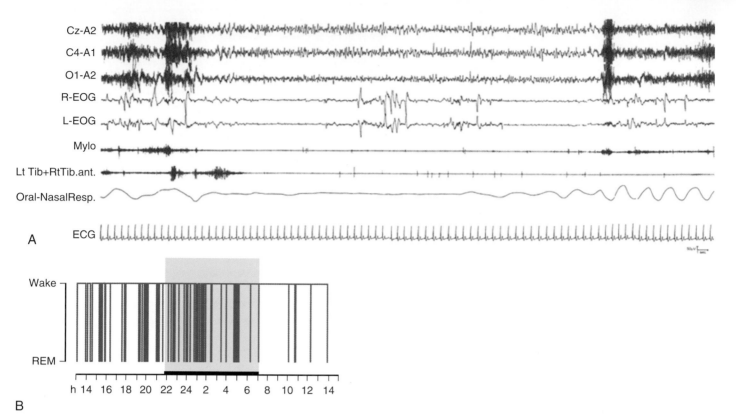

• **Figure 19.15** **A** and **B,** Polysomnographic sample and hypnogram from a patient with fatal familial insomnia. *REM,* Rapid eye movement. (From Chokroverty S, Bhat S, Provini F. Sleep dysfunction and sleep-disordered breathing in miscellaneous neurological disorders. In: Chokroverty S, Thomas RJ, eds. *Atlas of Sleep Medicine.* 2nd ed. Philadelphia, PA: Elsevier/Saunders; 2014.)

Niemann-Pick Type C Disease[199]

Niemann-Pick type C disease (NPC) is a rare progressive autosomal recessive disease characterized by accumulation of unesterified cholesterol in many tissues, and storage of sphingolipids in brain and liver.

- Laughter-induced cataplexy is one of the characteristic symptoms of NPC, particularly in the late infantile and juvenile forms.[199,200] The combination of cataplexy, splenomegaly, and vertical gaze supranuclear palsy should prompt consideration of NPC.[199]
- Adults with NPC exhibit ataxia, dystonia, dementia, vertical gaze palsy, and hepatosplenomegaly. In adolescent and adult patients, when intellectual deterioration progresses and emotional reactions become flat, cataplexy usually disappears.[199]
- Reduced CSF orexin/hypocretin levels are seen in patients with NPC and cataplexy.[201]
- Cataplexy in NPC responds to imipramine[202] and miglustat.[203]
- Pathological findings in the brainstem in the NPC mouse model are compatible with the patients' symptoms, including cataplexy.[199]

Limbic Encephalitis and Morvan Syndrome

Cases of autoimmune or paraneoplastic limbic encephalitis are increasingly recognized and diagnosed.[204,205] These typically present with a subacute encephalopathy, often with psychiatric features, seizure, and amnesia. Antibodies to *N*-methyl-D-aspartate receptor

(NMDA-R), AMPA receptor, voltage-gated potassium channels (VGKC), or antibodies to Ma or Hu are found.

- Sleep-wake disturbances (SWDs) are a prominent feature seen early in the acute phase of the illness.
- Hypersomnia with fragmented nocturnal sleep has been reported in patients with anti-MA encephalitis.
- Patients with NMDA-R encephalitis can present with reduced levels of consciousness and hypoventilation requiring mechanical ventilation.
- RBD has been observed in patients with VGKC limbic encephalitis, which disappeared with successful IV-IG therapy.
- Limbic encephalitis is treated first with a course of high-dose corticosteroids, and if ineffective, then a course of IV-IG.
- Insomnia may persist in some long-term survivors of limbic encephalitis.

Morvan syndrome is an even rarer disorder (100 cases in literature as of 2013) than FFI, and thought to be an autoimmune disorder associated with antibodies to VGKC.[206–208]

- Like FFI, it is characterized by acute severe insomnia associated with myokymias and muscle cramps, skin miliari, and autonomic hyperactivity (profuse sweating, tachycardia, hypertension, and increased body temperature).
- Like limbic encephalitis, Morvan syndrome often resolves in a few weeks or months, but progresses to death in some.
- Like FFI, Morvan syndrome is associated with episodes of oneiric stupor (similar to those seen in FFI), which herald other disease signs in Morvan syndrome. During these,

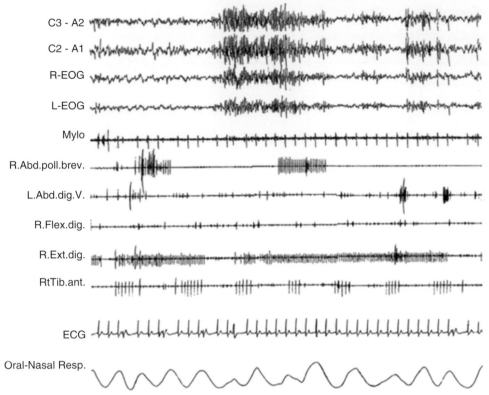

• **Figure 19.16** Polysomnogram of a patient with Morvan syndrome. (From Chokroverty S, Bhat S, Provini F. Sleep dysfunction and sleep-disordered breathing in miscellaneous neurological disorders. In: Chokroverty S, Thomas RJ, eds. *Atlas of Sleep Medicine*. 2nd ed. Philadelphia, PA: Elsevier/Saunders; 2014.)

patients make simple automatic gestures mimicking activities of daily life (e.g., eating, drinking, or manipulating nonexistent objects).

- Like FFI, the PSG in Morvan syndrome demonstrates a mixed state of theta activity and slow eye movements (NREM 1) and REM sleep. Sleep spindles and K-complexes are absent.
- Autopsy findings in one case suggest the VGKC antibodies attack the thalamic neurons involved in sleep/wake regulation.
- Fig. 19.16 shows an illustrative example of a polysomnogram in a patient with Morvan syndrome.
- Agrypia excitata (AE) is a syndrome characterized by loss of sleep, accompanied by persistent motor and autonomic sympathetic activation with marked persistent elevation of norepinephrine levels and loss of the normal nocturnal peak of melatonin secretion.[197,209–211]
  - The features of this syndrome have been described previously and are seen in patients with FFI, autosomal dominant prion diseases, autoimmune encephalitis, and alcohol withdrawal.
  - NREM N3 and sleep spindles disappear in AE; REM sleep persists but appears as brief isolated fragments or within NREM N1 sleep.
  - AE lumps together FFI, VGKC limbic encephalitis, and delirium tremens based on the presence of insomnia, PSG findings of a mixed state of NREM N1 with REM sleep intrusions, oneiric stupor, and sympathetic hyperactivity.

Creutzfeldt-Jakob Disease

Creutzfeldt-Jakob disease (CJD) is a devastating spongiform encephalopathy associated with an abnormal isoform of the prion protein that misfolds into insoluble fibrils, causing neuronal damage. CJD causes a rapidly progressive dementia with extrapyramidal signs and startled myoclonus. CJD usually begins between the fifth and seventh decades of life, with a mean survival of 4–8 months (although 5%–10% have a clinical course of 2 or more years, especially those with familial forms). Younger age of onset is associated with increased likelihood of sleep disturbances.[212] The majority of cases of SJD are sporadic; 5%–15% are familial.

- CJD typically presents as rapidly progressive cognitive decline over months with abnormalities in attention, behavior, judgment, and perception. Apathy and depression are common, but anxiety, euphoria, or emotional lability may also occur. Myoclonus (often provoked by startle) is present in 90% (although appearance of it may be delayed till later). Bradykinesia, nystagmus, or ataxia is seen in two-thirds of patients, and pyramidal signs in 40%–80%.
- Prognosis poor; with no treatment, death typically within a year

Sleep disorders in CJD:
- Two case series found half of CJD patients have sleep disturbances, most often severe insomnia.[213,214]
- PSG studies show disorganized sleep patterns in patients with CJD with abrupt transitions between sleep stages, reduced numbers of sleep spindles and K-complexes, decreased slow

wave activity, reduced REM density, and REM sleep time.[215,216] Indeterminate sleep states have been observed in some patients.

- Episodes of nocturnal oneiric, sometimes aggressive behavior with dream-reality confusion, have been reported in some patients.[213]
- Periodic sharp wave complexes while awake are the most distinctive EEG feature of classic CJD. These are usually present within 1–3 months after the onset of symptoms.[217]

Sleep problems occur in at least half of patients with CJD:

- Two large case series of patients with CJD found sleep disturbances (primarily insomnia) were reported in half of patients with CJD. Sleep disturbances were a prodromal or presenting symptom in 15%.
- The EEG pattern of classic CJD are periodic sharp wave complexes on a background of low-voltage generalized slow activity. These are seen in about two-thirds of patients, usually within 1–3 months after onset of symptoms, and have a high specificity (seen in only 9% of patients with another neurodegenerative disorder, often then an autoimmune encephalitis or lithium toxicity).

Traumatic Brain Injury[218]

Traumatic brain injury (TBI) affects 1.7 million people every year in the United States. SWDs are among the most prevalent and persistent sequelae of TBI.[219–221]

- The core neurological deficit in acute TBI is a quantitative and qualitative impairment in vigilance, ranging from coma in severe TBI to drowsiness and inattention in mild TBI.[218]
- A recent meta-analysis indicated about half of TBI patients have SWDs after TBI, most often insomnia, EDS, fragmented sleep, and increased sleep need.[222] Insomnia is reported by 50%, difficulty maintaining sleep by 50%, poor sleep efficiency on PSG by 49%, early morning awakening by 38%, and nightmares by 27%.
- A recent questionnaire-based study of 98 TBI patients (mild TBI 70%; moderate 15%, severe in 15%) found SWDs in 38%, insomnia in 29%, and posttraumatic hypersomnia in 9%.[223]
  - Of those with insomnia: 18% have difficulty falling asleep, 29% difficulty staying asleep, and 53% both.
  - Risk factors for insomnia include headache (HA) and/or dizziness, symptoms of anxiety, and depression.
  - Insomnia was the more common SWD after mild TBI. Hypersomnia was uncommon after mild TBI.
- Potential contributing factors for insomnia after TBI include pain, depression, anxiety, medicolegal issues, medication effects, posttraumatic epilepsy, and brain damage.[218]
- A recent prospective study of 205 patients with severe TBI admitted to acute rehab hospital found 84% had SWDs upon admission, with 66% at 1 month postinjury.[224]
  - The presence of moderate/severe SWDs 1 month postinjury predicted duration of posttraumatic amnesia and rehabilitation hospital length of stay.
- SWDs are often persistent following mild TBI.
  - A recent study assessed SWDs in 374 mild TBI patients. They found 72% reported SWDs ≤3 months postinjury, and 54% at 1 year.[225] Persistent sleep disturbance and higher symptom burden 6 months postinjury were independent predictors of outcome.
  - Six months after TBI, de novo SWDs were seen in 72% of 65 consecutive patients with TBI. Arousal disorders were the most common type: EDS or fatigue in 55%, and

pleiosomnia (needing ≥2 hour of sleep per 24 hours compared with before TBI).[226]

- Insomnia occurs in a third with mild TBI due to unrecognized CRDs, most often with delayed sleep phase or irregular sleep/wake types.[227]
  - Diagnosis: Structured interviews, questionnaires, actigraphy with sleep log, dim light melatonin onset, and/or core body temperature measurements
  - Treatment: Consider bright light therapy in morning and oral melatonin in evening.[228]
- SWDs after TBI predict cognitive recovery, anxiety, depression, and pain, suggesting a causal role of SWD in subsequent recovery. SWDs increase long-term sequelae, intensify comorbid conditions, limit recovery potential, reduce rehabilitation participation, heighten irritability, slow cognitive processing, exacerbate pain, and further impair attention.[219–221]
  - Identifying and treating SWD in TBI is important, and can promote maximal functional recovery.[229]
  - One needs to identify and treat comorbid conditions such as pain and depression to lessen insomnia after TBI.
- Posttraumatic EDS:
  - EDS is reported in 25%–60% of TBI patients, irrespective of trauma severity.
  - Factors contributing to EDS in TBI include PLMS, sleep fragmentation, insufficient sleep, irregular sleep/wake schedules, medication effects, mood disorders, and damage to wake-promoting brain centers.[218]
  - A recent prospective study found 57% of first-ever TBI patients 6 months postinjury and 19% of healthy controls had objective daytime sleepiness.[230] The average sleep need per 24 hours as assessed by actigraphy was greater in TBI patients versus controls (8.3 ± 1.1 hour vs. 7.1 ± 0.8 hour), and the average sleep latency is shorter (9 ± 5 min vs. 12 ± 5 min).[230] Patients with TBI tend to subjectively underestimate their EDS and increased sleep needs.
  - Intracranial hemorrhage is associated with posttraumatic hypersomnia.[230]
  - There are no convincing reports of posttraumatic narcolepsy with cataplexy in the medical literature.
- Diagnosis of SWD in TBI is based on structured interview, sleep questionnaire, supplemented by sleep log and actigraphy, and followed by overnight PSG and MSLT.[231]
- Treatment for SWD after TBI:
  - Cognitive behavioral therapy[232]
  - A few studies have reported improvement with modafinil (100–200 mg) or armodfinil (250 mg).[233]
  - A randomized placebo controlled trial of blue light therapy lessened EDS in subjects with posttraumatic EDS.[231]
  - Medications for insomnia after TBI[231]: Use medications that will not produce dependency and have minimal adverse effects for TBI patients. Short term is preferred, and it is best to avoid benzodiazepines, which impair brain plasticity.

Sleep/Wake Disorders in Patients with Down Syndrome (Trisomy 21)

Basic Information[234]

- Down syndrome (DS) is the most common genetic cause of intellectual disability (ID) and accounts for ~30% of all cases of moderate to severe ID. Most often caused by a partial duplication of distinct regions of chromosome 21 (21q22.3).

- Phenotypic expression of the Trisomy 21 genotype shows great interindividual variability, modified by allelic variation, genomic imbalances, epigenetic, but also early intervention programs and parental nurturing.

Sleep/Wake Problems in Down Syndrome

- Children with DS have significantly more sleep problems compared with the general pediatric population: greater bedtime resistance, sleep anxiety, night waking, parasomnias, SDB, and EDS compared with the general pediatric population.[235]
- OSA is highly prevalent in children, with DS ranges from 30% to 60% compared with 2%–3% of the general pediatric population.[236] A prospective cohort study reported that 57% of DS children ages 2–4 years had OSA.[237] Prevalence of OSA among 122 children with DS referred for PSG was 66%; half had AHI greater than 10 per hour. Sex and BMI did not correlate with AHI. Younger age was associated with more severe OSA.

Physical Findings That Predispose Children and Adults with Down Syndrome to Sleep Apnea[238–240]

- Smaller airway volumes, smaller mid- and lower face skeletons, shorter hard palates, and smaller mandible volumes compared with age-matched controls predispose DS children to OSA.
- The volume of their tonsils/adenoids is not larger in DS children than controls, but the upper airway space is smaller in them than controls.
- OSA in infants with DS is most often due to laryngomalacia (often with gastroesophageal reflux).[241]
- Adenotonsillar hypertrophy (complicated by gastroesophageal reflux disease [GERD] in nearly two-thirds) is more likely the cause of upper airway obstruction in DS children older than 2 years.
- Many young children with DS have pharyngeal hypotonia, oral aversion, dysphagia, laryngomalacia, tracheomalacia, and/or tracheal abnormalities.
- Because of impaired cellular immunity, children with DS have a 12-fold greater risk for infections, especially pneumonia.
- Obesity, pulmonary arterial hypertension, and hypothyroidism may further predispose to SDB.[239]
- Children with DS are thought to be at increased risk for pulmonary arterial hypertension because of reduced number of alveoli, thinner media of pulmonary arterioles, and impaired endothelial function.[242,243]
- Reduced hypoxic drive in some may lead to sleep-related hypoventilation, central apneas, and rarely respiratory failure.[244]

Diagnosis of Sleep-Disordered Breathing in Down Syndrome

- Overnight comprehensive PSG with end-tidal and transcutaneous CO_2 monitoring is the best way to identify OSA in children with DS.[245] Sometimes, other patterns of SDB are also seen, including sleep-related hypoxemia, sleep-related central and/or obstructive hypoventilation, and/or CSA.
- A pattern of long runs of central apneas in NREM sleep and/or bradypnea on a PSG in a child with DS warrants ordering a brain MRI with attention to the posterior fossa for Chiari malformation. Chiari malformation occurs with a higher frequency in children with DS than the general population.

Treatment of Sleep-Disordered Breathing in Down Syndrome

- Adenotonsillectomy is the initial treatment of choice for DS children with OSA and relatively enlarged tonsils and/or adenoids.[246] Before surgery, however, cervical x-rays in extension and lateral flexion are recommended to screen for atlantoaxial subluxation or cervical ligament instability (present in 10%–20% of infants and children with DS).[247]
- Children with DS in general, and particularly those with OSA, are at increased risk for postoperative respiratory complications and require overnight hospitalization after upper airway surgery.[248]
- A repeat PSG should be considered 2–3 months after AT in children with DS, because significant residual OSA may be found despite parental report of subjective cure.[249,250]
- One study found OSA resolved sufficiently to require no further treatment in 27% of the children with DS, while 73% required further treatment (CPAP, bilevel PAP [BPAP], or oxygen) for significant residual obstruction.[251]
- Many children with DS have difficulty tolerating PAP or even supplemental oxygen via nasal cannula, disliking anything covering their face. PAP desensitization with help by Child Life specialists is worth trying, especially if the residual OSA is severe and symptomatic.
- Residual (or recurrence) of OSA following AT in a child with DS warrants evaluation for the presence of lingual tonsils, regrowth of adenoidal tissue, and/or macroglossia.[252] Lingual tonsillectomy can be beneficial, further reducing the AHI.[253]
- Oral appliances should be considered for older children with DS who will not tolerate or use PAP, but often there are similar issues of compliance.[254]
- Weight management, good dental care, and medical treatment of rhinitis and allergies may also help when indicated clinically.[255–257]
- For infants and young children with DS who have severe persistent OSA and have severe retrognathia, mid-face hypoplasia, and/or macroglossia, but do not tolerate PAP, upper airway surgeries such as mandibular distraction osteogenesis, tongue base reduction, maxillary/midface advancement, or tracheostomy may be considered.[239,258–260]

Autistic Spectrum Disorders

Basic Information

- Autistic spectrum disorders (ASDs) are a group of clinically heterogeneous NDD that share common features of impaired socialization/communication and restricted, repetitive stereotyped behaviors. Etiology of ASD is undetermined, multifactorial, and most likely involves a complex interplay of polygenetic, epigenetic, and/or environmental factors. ASD is inheritable but probably polygenetic.[261]
- Abnormally low levels of melatonin and/or its urinary metabolic derivatives have been found in ASD and correlate with the severity of sleep problems and autistic behaviors.[262]
- Mutations in circadian clock genes are more frequent in patients with ASD than in controls, and contribute to sleep problems in them.[263]

Sleep/Wake Problems in Autistic Spectrum Disorder

- Sleep problems are common in children with ASD, and present in greater than 50%. ASD children often take more than an hour to fall asleep, and many have nocturnal awakenings as long as 2–3 hours.[264–266]
- The most common sleep problems are sleep-onset delay, frequent nighttime awakenings, and reduced sleep duration.[267]
- As opposed to typically developing children, sleep problems in ASD tend to persist past midpuberty, and even adulthood.[268]

Physical Findings and Problems in Children with Autistic Spectrum Disorder

- Children with ASD often have multiple physical, behavioral, and health problems. One prospective study of 54 children with ASD (mean age 6.8 ± 3.0 years) found 96% had eating disorders, 92% obsessive-compulsive behaviors, 89% behavioral problems, 85% sensory processing issues, 74% anxiety/fear 67% hyperactivity, 57% incontinence and sleep problems, 48% gastrointestinal disturbances, and 26% lethargy.[269]

Diagnosis/Evaluation of Sleep/Wake Disorders in Children with Autistic Spectrum Disorder[270]

- An in-laboratory PSG is not the best initial test in ASD unless symptoms suggestive of SDB, frequent paroxysmal nocturnal behaviors, PLMD, and/or RBD are suspected.[270] Actigraphy with sleep logs are useful, providing objective data for evaluating and treating their insomnia.
- Overnight PSG in 60 consecutive children with ASD (ages 2–13) who were selected without regard to sleep/wake problems showed children with ASD compared with normal controls had significantly shorter sleep times, greater percentage of NREM 3 sleep, and markedly decreased percentage of REM sleep time (15% vs. 23%).[271]
- It is crucial to identify and treat concomitant epilepsy, gastroesophageal reflux, iron deficiency, or other primary sleep disorders (e.g., OSA, PLMS, CRD) in ASD.[270]
- Complaints of excessive motor restlessness, frequent limb jerks, restless legs, and/or recording PLMS on PSG in children with ASD should prompt ordering serum ferritin levels.[270]

Treatment of Sleep/Wake Disorders in Children with Autistic Spectrum Disorder[270]

- Decreased iron and ferritin levels are common in children with ASD and should be treated with supplemental iron (taken with orange juice/vitamin C to improve absorption).
- Cognitive behavioral therapy for insomnia (CBTi) and oral melatonin extended release (doses ranging from 1–6 mg) given 1 hour before bed have been helpful in treating insomnia in children with ASD.
- Hyperactivity, stereotyped body movements, self-stimulation, hypervigilance, and impulsivity in ASD may respond to treatment with alpha-2-adrenergic receptor agonists (clonidine or guanfacine), or selective norepinephrine reuptake inhibitors (atomoxetine).

- Oral clonidine (0.1–0.2 mg) 30 min before bed reduced sleep latency and lessened nocturnal awakenings, especially in ASD children who are overly aroused or mildly anxious at bedtime.
- Guanfacine (3 mg by mouth) significantly improved aberrant behaviors and lessened hyperactivity in 5 of 11 children with ASD, but caused some drowsiness and irritability.
- Anxiety, obsessive-compulsive, repetitive behaviors, irritability, or behavioral rigidity may respond to treatment with liquid fluoxetine (mean final dose: 10 ± 4 mg/day) or other selective serotonin reuptake inhibitors (SSRIs).
- SSRIs may cause insomnia or sleepiness, and timing of dosing may need adjustment, depending on whether there is, for example, morning sleepiness or evening insomnia.
- SSRIs may also trigger sleepwalking, and worsen PLMS or RLS symptoms. Insomnia caused by SSRIs may respond to clonazepam (0.25–1 mg 30 min before bed), but may cause disinhibition in some.
- Repetitive behaviors may respond to valproate or fluoxetine with weight gain—a significant side effect especially with valproate.
- Trazodone for insomnia can cause priapism, best avoided in ASD pubertal males unable to report it.
- Aggression, irritability, self-injury, and explosive outbursts often respond to neuroleptics such as aripiprazole or risperidone, but weight gain leading to obesity and OSA are major adverse effects for them. Sedation with risperidone may be used to advantage by dosing it all at night.

Prader-Willi Syndrome

Basic Information[272,273]

- Prader-Willi syndrome (PWS) is a genetic disorder caused by absent or deficient expression of paternally derived imprinted genes on chromosome 15q 11-q13; in 70% there is a sporadic microdeletion on the long arm of the paternal chromosome 15 at q11q13, and 20% inherit both copies of chromosome 15 from their mother (maternal uniparental disomy).[273–275] Molecular genetic testing confirms the genetic mutation in n greater than 99%.
- PWS is the most frequent cause of *secondary* obesity in children, occurring in about 1 of 15,000 births.[274,275]
- During infancy, PWS is characterized initially by severe central hypotonia and feeding difficulties with poor suck, weak cry, decreased movement, and lethargy.[272,273]
- Between ages 1 and 6 years, symptoms of hyperphagia and insatiable appetite develop and lead to morbid central obesity.[272] Motor milestones and language development are delayed.
- Some degree of cognitive impairment is usually present. A distinctive behavioral phenotype (with temper tantrums, skin-picking, food-foraging, stubbornness, manipulative behavior, and obsessive-compulsive characteristics) is common.[273]
- Short stature is usually present (50% are ≤ 3rd percentile for age) if not treated with growth hormone (GH).[273] Hypogonadism is present in both males and females, and manifests as genital hypoplasia, incomplete pubertal development, and in most, infertility.[273] Characteristic facial features, strabismus, and scoliosis are often present.

Sleep/Wake Complaints in Prader-Willi Syndrome

- Patients with PWS are referred to sleep specialists most often to evaluate hypersomnia and/or SDB.
- EDS has been reported in the majority of people with PWS, often persists after successful treatment of SDB, and is thought to be due to central hypothalamic dysfunction (but not an orexin/hypocretin deficiency) and manifest as persistent generalized hypoarousal.[276]
- EDS in PWS is closely associated with problematic behaviors (food foraging and hoarding, skin picking, repetitive ritualistic behaviors).[277–280] Treating SDB in PWS can lessen these behavioral problems.
- SDB is common in PWS, even in those without sleep/wake complaints.[281]
- Hypoventilation in PWS is thought to reflect a primary disorder of ventilatory control.[282]
  - Absent or depressed peripheral chemoreceptor function responses to acute hypoxic and hypercapnic challenges have been found in children with PWS, whether obese or not.[283]
  - PWS subjects compared with controls rarely aroused from NREM sleep in response to hypoxia and failed to demonstrate the appropriate tachycardia response to it.[284]
  - The level of pCO_2 needed to provoke an arousal from sleep has been shown to be much higher in subjects with PWS compared with controls.[285]

Diagnosis/Evaluation

- Sleep-related alveolar hypercapnic central hypoventilation (either primarily or exclusively in REM sleep) is the most common pattern of SDB in patients with PWS (the risk for it increased by hypotonia and obesity).[281]
- One study of 19 adolescents and adults with PWS found 47% had obesity hypoventilation, 95% had an AHI greater than 5, but only 21% had an AHI greater than 30 per hour.[286] Patients with PWS, as compared with a control group, had significantly greater amounts of nocturnal hypoxemia, lower nadir SpO_2, and higher percentages of sleep time with oxyhemoglobin saturation less than 80%.
- Sleep-related hypoventilation with hypercapnea is often present, and will go undetected without reliable carbon dioxide (CO_2) monitoring (simultaneously recording end-tidal and transcutaneous CO_2 recommended).
- Respiratory events observed in overnight PSG of PWS patients are more often central apneas in type, but obstructive hypopneas are seen with considerable frequency.[287]
- OSA is found in only 10%–20% of patients with PWS, and often only mild (AHI <5–10 per hour)[288–290]
- Higher BMI correlated with higher AHI and lower arterial oxygen desaturations on the PSG of 43 children and adults with PWS.[291]
- CSA is common in infants with PWS who are not overweight but have hypotonia (see Fig. 19.3).[292,293] One study found 43% of infants with PWS had CSA, and supplemental oxygen reduced their central apnea index from a mean of 14 per hour to 1 per hour.[293]
- Hypotonia in PWS improves with age, but PWS adults remain mildly hypotonic, and are often prone to develop scoliosis.[294,295] Scoliosis in an adult with PWS may add a pulmonary restrictive component to the person's SDB.

- Children with PWS on PSG compared with controls had shorter REM latency, decreased duration of N3 sleep, and increased NREM instability.
- MSLT studies done in PWS patients with hypersomnia are often abnormal (mean sleep latencies of less than 5 min in 50% and sleep onset REM periods in some).[296]

Treatment Strategies for Sleep/Wake Disorders in Prader-Willi Syndrome

- Reducing the likelihood and severity of sleep-related hypoventilation in PWS begins with avoiding or reducing obesity.
  - Stringent caloric intake and restricting access to food is needed for a child or adolescent with PWS to avoid or lose excessive weight gain.[297,298] This often makes them unhappy.[299]
  - Early recognition of the diagnosis by genetic testing in a floppy infant, early introduction of exogenous GH therapy, and strict caloric restriction has reduced, but not eliminated, obesity or excessive weight among children with PWS.
- OSA without sleep-related central hypoventilation in patients with PWS may respond to CPAP.[288,300]
- Sleep-related central hypoventilation in PWS (with or without a component of OSA) is usually best treated by BPAP, sometimes requiring a timed or backup rate.
- Treating SDB in children with PWS improved their cognitive function, and improved daytime performance and sleep quality.[301]
- If significant adenotonsillar hypertrophy and OSA on the PSG are present, AT can be considered. Recent studies show AT improves quality of life in children with PWS and OSA.[302] However, PWS patients are at increased risk for postoperative complications,[303,304] and residual SDB is likely to remain following surgery, requiring PAP.[304]
- Central hypersomnia that occurs without concomitant SDB or that persists after successful treatment of SDB warrants consideration of trials of modafinil, armodafinil, or other CNS stimulants.
- Treatment of their behavior problems and depression often helped by SSRIs

Exogenous Growth Hormone Therapy in Prader-Willi Syndrome Can Affect Sleep Disordered Breathing in Prader-Willi Syndrome

- Many individuals with PWS have a deficiency of GH. A randomized placebo-controlled trial of exogenous GH therapy in PWS children has found significantly increased height velocity, decreased mean body fat, increased mean lean body mass, improved physical strength, respiratory muscle function, and lipid profiles.[305,306] GH therapy is recommended for children with PWS, preferably starting it before age 3.[307]
- The dosage of GH actually recommended in children with PWS is 1 mg/m^2/daily, to be reached within the first weeks and months, after a first period of treatment at a lower dose. The goal of GH treatment is to obtain a significant increase of serum IGF-I concentrations within the upper limits of the normal range (maximum + 2 SDS), in order to avoid potential side effects due to exaggerated GH therapy.[308,309]
- Individuals with PWS have an annual death rate of 3% and are at increased risk for sudden death. A large case series found respiratory failure or infections were the most common cause of death in PWS, present in 61% of 64 PWS children.[287] Impaired central (hypothalamic) body temperature regulation may contribute to sudden death in infants and children with

PWS, respiratory failure, pulmonary embolism, and cellulitis or other complications of morbid obesity in adults with PWS.[310]

- Sleep specialists are often asked to evaluate infants and children with PWS for OSA before starting, and again after starting exogenous GH therapy. The presence of OSA may require holding the GH therapy, treating the OSA, and then retesting to ensure that OSA has remitted or needs treatment before resuming GH therapy.[308,309,311,312] GH therapy can cause tonsillar hypertrophy and precipitate OSA.[311,312]
- Other endocrine abnormalities are common in PWS, including central adrenal insufficiency, hypothyroidism, glucose intolerance, and diabetes mellitus.[273] Identification and treatment is important. Central adrenal insufficiency is rare in PWS.[313]

Other Neurodevelopmental Disorders in Which Sleep Problems Are so Common as to Be Phenotypic

Severe persistent difficult-to-treat insomnia is so common in particular neurodevelopmental disorders as to be included in diagnostic criteria for the syndrome.

Rett Syndrome

Basic Information[314,315]

- Rett syndrome (RS) is an X-linked dominant neurogenetic disorder primarily affecting girls and characterized by loss of spoken language and hand use, replaced by repetitive stereotypic hand movements. After seemingly normal development in the first 6–18 months of life, skill stagnation and then rapid severe regression follows.
- RS is the second most common cause of genetic ID in females (after DS), with a prevalence of 1 in 10,000 live female births and 1 in 8500 females by age 15.
- More than 95% of RS is due to sporadic mutations in the MECP2 (methyl-CpG binding protein gene on the X-chromosome; Xq28).

Sleep/Wake Problems in Rett Syndrome

- The clinical hallmark of RS is severe arrhythmic breathing awake.[316] Multiple types of irregular breathing are typically seen. The most striking are episodes of hyperventilation interspersed with breath-holding.[317] Breath-holding often lasts greater than 20 sec, causes desaturations less than 50%, and severe hypocapnea, often accompanied by Valsalva maneuvers.
- Sleep disturbances reported in greater than 80% of females with RS and include: irregular sleep/wake patterns, excessive daytime naps, and especially problematic nighttime behaviors (nocturnal laughter, bruxism, long spells of screaming, and/or inconsolable crying, nocturnal seizures, sleep terrors, and sleep talking.[318] Sleep problems tend to persist: daytime napping in 85%, frequent nocturnal awakenings in 40%, and nocturnal screaming in 30% at age 18.
- SDB (central and/or obstructive events, irregular breathing, and runs of tachypnea/bradypnea, tachycardia/bradycardia) have been observed in overnight PSG of patients with RS. Other PSG abnormalities include significantly more awakenings and stage shifts per hour of sleep, more WASO, greater percentage of NREM 3, less REM sleep, and higher PLM-I.

- A 2013 case-control study found significantly reduced NREM 3, increased WASO and stage shifts, and much higher central and obstructive apnea indexes on overnight PSG in 13 patients with RS compared with 40 healthy controls.[319]
- A recent parent-reported sleep questionnaire study found night waking was the most prevalent sleep problem, affecting more than 80%, with 48% waking often at night.[320] Difficulty falling and staying asleep was most disturbed in younger children and those with a p.Arg294* mutation. Severe seizure activity was associated with poor sleep after adjusting for age, mutation type, and mobility.
- Epilepsy occurs in 50%–90% of patients with RS, and seizures are more often nocturnal and refractory.[321,322] Video-PSG with expanded EEG montages is useful to distinguish focal or generalized seizures from episodes of apnea and hyperventilation, laughing, screaming, and vacant staring spells awake and asleep.
- Sudden unexpected death occurs with greater frequency in RS; may be due to respiratory abnormalities, prolonged QTc, and aberrant cardiorespiratory autonomic function.[323–325]

Treatment of Sleep Disorders in Rett Syndrome

- A 2015 longitudinal study found sleep problems in RS were present in more than 80%, often persisted into adulthood, and were not improved by treatment.[326] Those with a large deletion had a higher prevalence of night laughing.
- Behavioral insomnia and problematic nighttime behaviors in RS may respond to be graduated extinction and other behavioral treatments, and oral melatonin.[270]
- Sleep-related hypoxemia can be treated with supplemental oxygen. On occasion, PAP therapy can be tried for significant SDB, if the patient will tolerate it.

Angelman Syndrome

Basic Information

- Angelman syndrome (AS) is characterized by severe ID, a unique behavior of frequent inappropriate laughter, smiling easy excitability, and hand-flapping coupled with a peculiar ataxic gait, prompting them to be called *happy puppets*.[327–329]
- AS occurs in 1 in 12,000–20,000 people and accounts for 6% of all children with severe cognitive disability and epilepsy.[329] It is caused by a lack of expression of the UBE3A gene on chromosome 15q.
- Other clinical features in AS are widely spaced teeth, an open mouth, tongue protrusion, microcephaly, fair skin and hair, little/no speech, hyperactivity, medically refractory epilepsies, and problems sleeping.

Sleep/Wake Problems

- Sleep problems are so common they are regarded as phenotypic of the syndrome.[330,331] These include difficulty falling and staying asleep, frequent nighttime awakenings, irregular sleep/wake cycles, CRDs, and reduced sleep duration with increased WASO. They also have heightened sensitivity to their sleep environment, are easily aroused by noise, and exhibit problematic nocturnal behaviors including nocturnal laughing, sleepwalking/sleep terrors, bruxism, seizures, and PLMs.

  Sleep problems in AS tend to persist well past mid-puberty but improve in adulthood.[331,332]
- Low nocturnal melatonin levels may predispose AS children to chronic insomnia and CRDs (irregular sleep/wake, delayed sleep onset or free-running).[333]

Treatment of Sleep/Wake Problems

- CBTi has been used to treat the insomnia and oral melatonin dosed between 6 and 7 PM to improve nocturnal sleep in children with AS.[334,335]

Smith-Magenis Syndrome

Basic Information

- Smith-Magenis syndrome (SMS) occurs in 1 of 25,000 births, characterized by a developmental delay with later IQs in the 40s–60s, short stature, scoliosis, a hoarse deep voice, obesity, scoliosis, a distinctive face (deep close-set eyes, midfacial hypoplasia, a cupid bow-shaped mouth, and a broad, square-shaped face), and peripheral neuropathy.[336,337]
- Striking behaviors in SMS are (1) self-injury with a low sensitivity to pain; (2) peculiar motor stereotypies including upper body self-hugging, compulsive finger licking, and book or magazine page flipping; (3) temper tantrums, oppositional defiant behaviors, and ADHD; and (4) disrupted circadian rhythm patterns and maladaptive sleep behaviors.[336,337]
- SMS is caused by a mutation or small interstitial deletion in a crucial transcriptional regulator gene of the mammalian circadian clock, RAI1 (retinoic acid induced), on chromosome 17p11.2.[336,337]

Sleep/Wake Problems

- CRDs in SMS are thought to be related to disturbance regulation of downstream circadian clock genes.[336,337]
- Children and adults with SMS more often have inverted endogenous secretion of melatonin, peaking the day rather than at night.[338–340]

Treatment Strategies for Insomnia and Circadian Rhythm Disorders in Angelman Syndrome

- Oral acebutolol (a beta1-adrenergic antagonist, 10 mg/kg) given in the early morning (to suppress the daytime melatonin secretion) coupled with an evening dose of melatonin (to replace the normal nighttime peak) improved sleep/wake complaints in a small group of SMS patients.[341]
- CBTi often also needed to improve insomnia.[270,342]
- Patients with SMS should be screened for symptoms of OSA, given their midfacial hypoplasia and obesity.[343]

Williams Syndrome

Basic Information

- Williams syndrome (WS) is a multisystem genetic disorder characterized by distinctive facial features (full cheeks and lips, broad nasal tip, widely spaced teeth), cognitive profile (visual spatial deficits, relatively preserved expressive language, and IQs in the 60s and 70s), personality profile (social, friendly, gregarious, empathetic, loquacious, difficulty interpreting social cues, and prone to worries and fears), and various cardiovascular, skeletal, connective tissue, growth, and endocrine abnormalities (elastin arteriopathy, peripheral pulmonic stenosis, supravalvular aortic stenosis, hypertension, hypercalcemia, hypothyroidism, early puberty, hyperextensible joints).
- WS occurs in 1 in 7500 births and is caused by a contiguous gene deletion of the Williams-Beuren syndrome critical region, which includes the elastin gene (ELN) on chromosome 7q11.23.

Sleep/Wake Complaints

- Children with WS have (1) greater bedtime resistance, sleep anxiety, night waking, and daytime sleepiness; (2) sleep onset insomnia, enuresis, and body pain; and (3) decreased sleep efficiency, increased respiratory-related arousals and increased slow wave sleep, more difficulty falling asleep, with greater restlessness and more arousals from sleep.[344]

Treatment of Sleep/Wake Disorders in Williams Syndrome

- Clonazepam and cognitive behavioral insomnia therapy can be used to improve their sleep quality.[270]

Fragile X Syndrome

Basic Information[345]

- Fragile X syndrome (FXS) is the most common cause of genetically acquired ID and is due to a mutation in the fragile X mental retardation 1 gene (FMR1) on the X chromosome at Xq23.7. Severity of the phenotype is influenced by the length of the CGG triplet repeats in the gene; the full mutation typically greater than 200 CGG repeats.
- Individuals with FXS often have social anxiety, agitation, and outbursts of physical or verbal aggression, inattention, mood swings, and 30% have ASD. ID in FXS is often more severe in males. Males with FXS have mild to severe ID with IQs greater than 70 in only 15%. Whereas 40% of women with FXS are cognitively normal, 35% have borderline intelligence and only 25% have an IQ less than 70.

Sleep/Wake Problems in Fragile X Syndrome

- Sleep problems are common in children with FXS (reported in 32%–47%)—most often difficulty falling asleep or frequent nocturnal awakenings.
- Case-control study of adolescents with FXS (mean age 13.1 years) found those with FXS had reduced time in bed, a higher percentage of NREM 1 sleep, a lower percentage of REM sleep, and more disrupted sleep compared with age-matched controls and children with DS.[346]

Treatment of Insomnia in Fragile X Syndrome[347]

- Oral melatonin 4 mg before bed lessened insomnia in a randomized controlled trial of its use in children with FXS. CBTi helped behavioral insomnia in boys with FXS and ASD.[348,349]

Intellectual Disability

Sleep problems are very common in children with ID.

- One study found 16% of children with mild to profound ID had at least one type of sleep problem: 4% had severe settling problems, 11% night waking, and 4% early morning awakening.[350]
  - They found that the children with severe sleep problems tended to have more severe ID, cerebral palsy (CP) and/or epilepsy, daytime sleepiness, and problem behaviors (aggression, hyperactivity, and opposition) compared with those children without a severe sleep problem.[350]
- Particularly debilitating for caregivers, sleep problems in children with severe ID tend to be persistent.[351]
- Teaching CBI therapy to caregivers of sleepless ID children improved sleep, increased sense of control, and reduced stress of the sleep-deprived caregivers.[352]

- One study found 16% of children with mild to profound ID had insomnia.
- Severe sleep problems were seen more often in children who were younger, needed medication more often, or had CP, epilepsy, more severe ID, daytime sleepiness with napping, and daytime problem behaviors (aggression, hyperactivity, and opposition).
- Sleep problems in children with severe ID tend to be persistent.
- CBTi and oral melatonin has been used with success to treat insomnia in children with ID.

Cerebral Palsy

Sleep/Wake Disorders in Children with Cerebral Palsy

- Forty-four percent of children with CP (mean age 8.8 years) had at least one sleep problem compared with 5% of the general pediatric population.[353] Dyskinetic CP increases the risk for a sleep disorder in a child with CP by 21-fold, active epilepsy by 17-fold, visual impairment, or spastic quadriplegia 13-fold.[353]
- PSG studies in children with CP have shown they are more likely to have altered sleep architecture, increased arousals, delayed REM sleep latency, decreased numbers of gross body movements, fewer body position shifts, and decreased duration of REM sleep compared with healthy controls.[354,355]
- SDB in children with severe CP often consists of varying combinations of obstructive and central events, central and obstructive hypoventilation, and hypoxemia during REM sleep.
- Children with CP are more likely to have poor quality sleep, altered sleep architecture, increased arousals, delayed REM sleep latency, decreased numbers of gross body movements, fewer body position shifts, and decreased duration of REM sleep compared with age-matched healthy controls.
- Recurrent aspiration, airway colonization with pathogenic bacteria, bronchiectasis, and SDB are major contributors to mortality and morbidity in individuals with CP.

Treatment of Sleep Disordered Breathing in Cerebral Palsy

- Adenotonsillectomy is usually the first treatment option for children with CP, OSA, and adenotonsillar hypertrophy.[356] Such children are at higher risk for postoperative complications and need to be hospitalized overnight after surgery.[357–359]
- OSA is less likely to remit with adenotonsillectomy in CP. Repeat PSG 2–3 months following upper airway surgery for OSA as needed in CP.[357–359] Since residual postoperative OSA is likely to remain, a PSG should be performed 2–3 months following surgery.[358]
- If significant SDB persists, consider (1) a repeat sleep study titrating CPAP for OSA, or BPAP if needed for tolerance or concomitant hypoventilation, best preceded by a PAP desensitization trial; (2) for pediatric ENT re-evaluation consider, whether other upper airway surgeries (including mandibular distraction, tongue base reduction, and/or skeletal advancement or expansion) would be useful (especially if PAP is not well-tolerated);[356,360–362] and (3) aggressive treatment of comorbidities, including excessive oral secretions, swallowing problems, epilepsy, and reflux to possibly improve overall sleep quality.[363]
- Other treatment strategies for SDB in children with CP, with or without ID or spastic quadriparesis, are (1) nocturnal postural devices, as long as they do not worsen the SDB[364]; (2) oral appliances[365]; and (3) botulinum toxin injections of submandibular salivary glands to reduce hypersalivation.[366]

Sleep in Neuromuscular Disorders

Sleep-related alveolar hypercapnic hypoventilation is the most common form of chronic SDB in patients with neuromuscular disorders (NMD), and typically first develops during REM sleep.[367,368]

- The diaphragm is a primary muscle of inspiration, awake and asleep.
- NMD patients with significant diaphragmatic weakness depend on their intercostal and accessory muscles to breathe; hypoventilation occurs during REM sleep when accessory respiratory muscles are atonic.
- Sleep hypoventilation is likely to occur in patients with NMD when the forced vital capacity (FVC) is less than 50% predicted; can occur at FVC of 60%–70% when patients are obese, have concomitant pulmonary disease, and/or kyphoscoliosis.[369]
- A prospective study of 48 children and adolescents with progressive NMD noted the presence of scoliosis and an FVC less than 70% or a forced expiratory volume in 1 sec (FEV_1) less than 65% predicted that sleep hypoventilation would be found on their overnight PSG.[370]
- Weak pharyngeal muscles, weak cough reflexes, obesity, pulmonary restrictive disease, kyphoscoliosis, obesity, malnutrition, opiates, respiratory fatigue, and impaired central respiratory control can predispose NMD to sleep-related hypoventilation at FVC of 60%–70%.

Clinical Presentation[367,368,371]

- Studies have shown sleep/wake symptoms poorly predict which NMD patients will have SDB, even when using a structured sleep questionnaire. Too often patients with NMD deny sleep/wake complaints (often when confined to wheelchairs, they little to tax them).
- The symptom that suggests sleep-related hypoventilation is difficulty breathing when supine, immersed in water, bending over, and/or sleeping. In the absence of congestive heart failure (CHF), this suggests significant diaphragmatic weakness/dysfunction.
- Weak cough, difficulty speaking or swallowing, coughing when eating or drinking suggests bulbar weakness. Bulbar weakness in NMD predisposes to difficulty clearing secretion, recurrent aspiration, frequent lower respiratory infections, and secondary lung disease. Other red flag symptoms for sleep-related hypoventilation in NMD are summarized in Table 19.10.
- The most important findings on physical examination that predict sleep-related hypoventilation are likely paradoxical breathing supine awake; SpO_2 ≤91% awake, seated, at rest, breathing room air; and/or ≥25% fall in FVC sitting versus supine. Paradoxical breathing supine (abdomen flattens/moves inward during inspiration) is not obvious until diaphragmatic strength less than 25% of normal strength.
- The FVC normally falls ~10% supine versus sitting in healthy subjects. Paradoxical breathing occurs because accessory muscles of inspiration to create negative intrathoracic pressure that pulls the weakened diaphragm superiorly.

TABLE 19.10	Red Flag Symptoms for Sleep-Related Hypoventilation in Neuromuscular Disorders

- Orthopnea (breathlessness), bending over or immersed in water, lying supine, or sleeping
- New onset of sleep complaints: frequent nocturnal awakenings (>3 per night), restlessness or unrefreshing sleep, vivid dreams, daytime sleepiness, lethargy, poor concentration, mood disturbance, sweating, or difficulty awakening
- Headache upon awakening
- Daytime tiredness or generalized fatigue; decreased stamina or endurance without increased weakness
- Shallow/noisy breathing; apnea, gasps, snorts, tachypnea, or cyanosis when sleeping
- Coughing during/after eating/drinking; problems with speech, swallowing, recurrent aspiration, frequent lower respiratory infections, weak cough, and reduced clearance of secretions

TABLE 19.11	Abnormalities in Pulmonary Function Tests May Help Predict Which Patients with Neuromuscular Disorders Most Likely to Have Sleep-Related Hypoventilation

- Forced vital capacity (FVC) < 50% predicted (<60% if obese, have concomitant pulmonary disease, and/or kyphoscoliosis)
- Paradoxical breathing supine
- ≥25% decrease in FVC changing from sitting to supine
- SpO_2 awake < 91% breathing room air
- $PaCO_2$ > 45 mmHg (>6 kPA) awake
- SpO_2 < 88% more than 5 consecutive minutes on nocturnal pulse oximetry
- Maximal inspiratory pressure (MIP) < 40 cm H_2O
- SNIP < –60 cm H_2O

- Other findings on exam that suggest sleep hypoventilation is more likely are use of accessory muscles to breathe, ineffective cough, soft voice, cannot finish sentence because of dyspnea, tachypnea supine and/or with exertion, bell-shaped chest deformity, and chest paradox.
- NMD patients with only mild limb weakness can have severe sleep hypoventilation, particularly those who have mitochondrial or other metabolic myopathies that can predispose to respiratory muscle fatigue or individuals with myotonic dystrophy in whom myotonia of the tongue and diaphragm delays muscle relaxation, thereby impairing ventilation.[372]

Diagnosis and Evaluation of Sleep-Related Hypoventilation in Neuromuscular Disorders[371,373]

- PSG with CO_2 monitoring is indicated in patients with NMD who have symptoms suggestive of sleep-related hypoventilation (especially morning HA, fatigue, orthopnea, or dyspnea) or in asymptomatic patients with daytime hypercapnia or significant defects on pulmonary function tests (PFTs; Table 19.11).

- PSG findings in patients with NMD are often missed if only looking for discrete events or low SpO_2:[369,371,373–375]
  - Abrupt sleep-related fall in baseline SaO_2 with sleep onset (e.g., 96%–92%)
  - Elevated mean end-tidal CO_2 (etCO_2) and low mean SpO_2 initially present only during REM sleep and later seen in all stages of sleep; periods of nonapneic oxygen desaturation and intermittent periodic or shallow breathing;
  - Hypoventilation, especially or only during REM sleep
  - May only see a few apneas or hypopneas (most often central) and often then only in REM sleep; obstructive events are uncommon, if seen often myotonic dystrophy 1, marked bulbar weakness, and/or obesity.
  - Tachycardia and tachypnea as they work to breathe, particularly in NREM 3 sleep
  - Fig. 19.17 shows recurrent periods of central apneas, many of which are prolonged, followed by irregular ventilatory cycles that resemble ataxic breathing accompanied by severe oxygen desaturation and sleep hypoxemia during REM sleep.
  - A hypnogram characteristic of patients with myotonic dystrophy showing hypoventilation with hypoxemia occurring primarily during REM sleep in shown in Fig. 19.18.
- Bilevel positive airway pressure with spontaneous or timed mode (BPAP-ST) is most often used as initial therapy for sleep-related hypoventilation in NMD.[371]
- When to start BPAP-S/T in patients with NMD: Consider BPAP-S/T in patients with NMD after they become symptomatic (otherwise compliance is often poor, and many often deny symptoms) and in asymptomatic patients who have an FVC less than 50% of predicted, an MIP or sniff pressure that fails to generate less than –40 cm H_2O, and/or a waking $PaCO_2$ more than 45 mmHg (>6.0 kPa).[371]
- Backup rate needed in NMD with sleep-related hypoventilation who have episodically low respiratory efforts and tidal volume caused by muscle weakness or increased work of breathing; frequent central apneas at baseline or during noninvasive positive pressure ventilation (NPPV) titration/treatment; inappropriately low respiratory rates; respiratory muscle rest not achieved with maximum pressure support (PS) or maximum tolerated PS; and/or adequate ventilation not achieved with maximum PS or maximum tolerated PS.[371]
- Setting backup rates for patients with NMD and sleep-related hypoventilation:[371]
  - Initial backup or timed rate should be equal or slightly less (e.g., 10%) than the spontaneous respiratory rate during sleep (minimum 10 breaths per minute).
  - Patients with NMD often like high respiratory rates.
  - Inspiratory time should be set based on respiratory rate to provide IPAP time between 30% and 40% of cycle time (60 per respiratory rate in breaths per minute).
  - Some patients require modest increases in their backup or timed rates to achieve optimal respiration during sleep. We do this in 1–2 breath per minute increments.
  - Beneficial for patients with NMD and sleep-related hypoventilation to use BPAP-S/T with pure timed rates. Using pure timed rate is associated with threefold longer survival rates, significantly reduced $PaCO_2$, increased daytime PaO_2, and improved maximum respiratory muscle strength.[371]
- In-laboratory PSG monitoring facilitates determination of the best ventilator settings, but subsequent home sleep studies may also help optimize NPPV treatment.

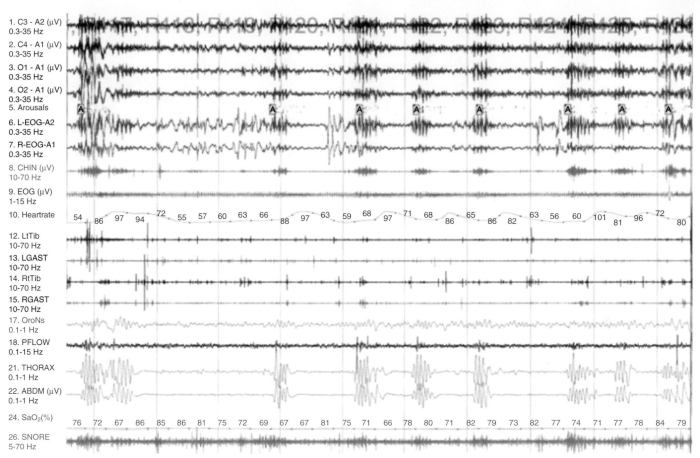

• Figure 19.17 Overnight polysomnographic recording from a patient with amyotrophic lateral sclerosis. (From In: Chokroverty S, Thomas RJ, eds. *Atlas of Sleep Medicine*. 2nd ed. Philadelphia, PA: Elsevier/ Saunders; 2014.)

- Accumulating studies demonstrate that assisted nocturnal ventilation contributes to longer survival in NMD patients once they develop hypoventilation.[376–381]
- Benefits of BPAP-S/T for NMD with sleep-related hypoventilation:
  - Lessened daytime sleepiness and morning HA
  - Improved daytime and nighttime arterial blood gases
  - Improved sleep architecture
  - Decreased hospitalization rates
  - Enhanced exercise capacity
  - Improved survival and quality of life
- The mean age of survival in males with DMD who used NPPV increased from 19 to 25 years in one study,[382] and in a more recent study, 39.6 years;[377] in patients with type 1 spinal muscular atrophy, age of survival increased from 10 ± 4 months to 65 ± 46 months.[383]
- BPAP-S/T prolonged survival in patients with amyotrophic lateral sclerosis (ALS) who did not have severe bulbar dysfunction.[384] BPAP-S/T does not prolong survival in ALS with severe bulbar dysfunction (and who have difficulty tolerating BPAP).
- A prospective randomized control trial in 48 patients with DMD with FVC less than 50% predicted and nocturnal hypercapnia (PtcCO$_2$ >45 mmHg) randomized 26 subjects to BPAP-S/T compared with 22 control patients who received no nocturnal ventilatory support.[385]

- The percentage of the night during which PtcCO$_2$ was greater than 45 mmHg decreased an average of 58%, and the mean SpO$_2$ increased 3% in the BPAP group but not in the controls.
- Ninety percent of the (initially untreated) controls developed diurnal hypercapnia or respiratory complications and subsequently met criteria for starting NPPV after a mean of 8 ± 7 months.
- Studies in patients with DMD and ALS show no benefit of prophylactic use of BPAP-S/T as a strategy aiming to prevent respiratory decline or at improving long-term survival.
- Increased survival in DMD due to proactive management:
  - Long-term oral corticosteroids (prednisone, deflazacort)
  - More common use of BPAP-S/T
  - Aggressive treatment of respiratory infections
  - Transition to 24/7 assisted ventilation typically FVC ≤15%–20% of predicted
  - Avoid malnutrition and obesity.
  - Identify and pretreat DMD cardiomyopathy.
- Absolute contraindications to using BPAP-S/T in patients with NMD and sleep-related hypoventilation:
  - Anatomical features prevent appropriate mask placement; uncontrollable secretion retention; unable to achieve adequate peak cough flow, even with assistance; unable to fit or tolerate mask

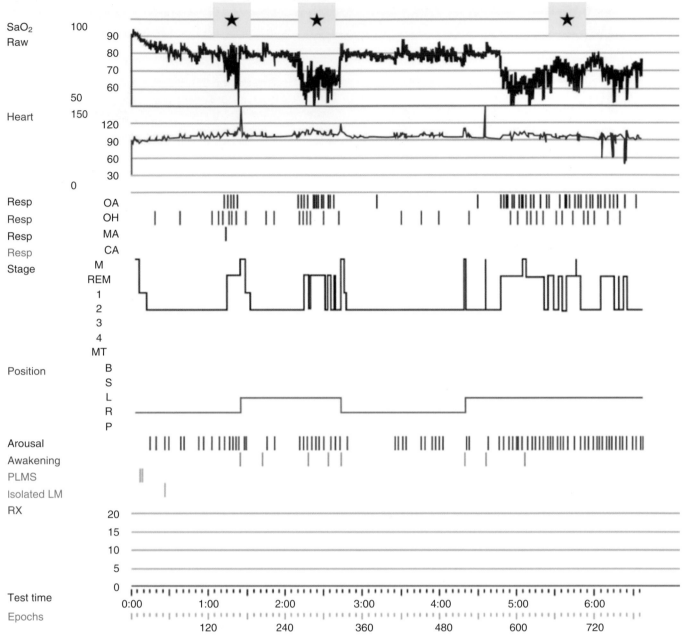

• **Figure 19.18** A hypnogram characteristic of patients with myotonic dystrophy showing hypoventilation with hypoxemia occurring primarily during rapid eye movement sleep. (From Kryger MH, Avidan AY, Berry RB, eds. *Atlas of Clinical Sleep Medicine.* 2nd ed. Philadelphia, PA: Elsevier Saunders; 2014.)

- Challenges for patients with NMD and sleep-related hypoventilation for using BPAP-S/T:
  - Inability to protect airway including inefficient cough, severe dysphagia with chronic aspiration, excessive bronchial secretions, and/or need for continuous or near continuous ventilation
  - Lack of patient and/or family/caregiver support or motivation and/or inability of patient to cooperate, understand, accept, or tolerate noninvasive ventilation.
- Cardiomyopathy in Duchenne muscular dystrophy[386–388]
  - Sinus tachycardia and abnormal electrocardiogram (EKG) majority at an early age

- 95% develop cardiomyopathy by age 20; limits survival in 20%
- Cardiac echo shows progressive LV wall fibrosis, loss of contractility, dilated cardiomyopathy, and heart failure, which can lead to sudden death.
- Early referral to cardiologist, cardiac medications, and tailored exercise program is critical.
- Patient-ventilator asynchrony (PVA) in NMD:
  - PVA, especially during sleep, is a common problem in patients with NMD, especially those prescribed BPAP-ST without in-laboratory titration during sleep.[368,389,390]

- Type of PVA in NMD:
  - Ineffective breath: presence of inspiratory effort without an assisted ventilator cycle
  - Prolonged cycle: ventilator cycle that spanned two inspiratory efforts
  - Double triggering: two consecutive ventilator cycles during a single inspiratory effort
  - Autotriggering: occurrence of one to several consecutive and rapid ventilator-derived breaths without a concomitant respiratory effort
- Too often patients with ALS are prescribed BPAP-ST without in-laboratory determination during sleep of optimal settings.
- One study found ALS patients empirically prescribed BPAP-S/T without in-laboratory PSG titration were likely to have PVA: mean asynchrony index 69 ± 46 per hour, mean asynchrony time as a percentage of the nocturnal recording time 17% ± 19%, mean nadir SpO$_2$ 85% ± 7%.[390]
- Another study found PVA events averaged 4.3 per hour in 18 NMD patients who had in-laboratory titration.[389] PVA was significantly more likely to occur (and go untreated) during subsequent home sleep studies. PVA at home was most often due to air leaks.
- Auto-triggering was the most common cause of asynchrony, followed by ineffective inspiratory efforts and failure to trigger the transition from IPAP to EPAP.[389]
- All types of PVA occurred more often in NREM than in REM sleep.[389]
- Auto-triggering and ineffective inspiratory efforts were more often associated with arousals than failure to transition to EPAP.[389]
- Only 13% of arousals and awakenings were due to PVA, but PVA events of all types are often associated with arousals.[389] Ineffective effort was the most frequent problem.
- Strategies for managing PVA in NMD:[371]
  - DMD patients whose PS ventilators were set when awake often had asynchrony when sleeping
  - Incorrect titration of inspiratory support or PEEPe may impede trigger of mechanical breath.
  - NMD patients sent home with ventilator should have PSG to optimally titrate ventilator settings when sleeping.
- Fig. 19.19 summarizes neuromuscular control of upper airway patency that predisposes neuromuscular patients to SDB.

Sleep in Primary Headache Disorders[391–395]

Complex bidirectional relationships between sleep and primary HA disorders. The most common sleep disorders associated with primary HA disorders are insomnia, SDB, and CRDs. HA disorders worsened or caused by sleep disorders are migraine, cluster, chronic tension-type, and paroxysmal hemicranias. Sleep disorders associated with HA include insomnia, SDB, sleep bruxism, sleepwalking, RLS, and CRDs. Sleep often terminates HA, but too much or too little sleep can trigger a migraine. Disrupted sleep regulation can contribute migraine, tension-type headache (TTH), cluster, and chronic daily HA.

Epidemiology

- Seventeen percent of patients seen in HA clinic report either nocturnal or early morning before awakening HAs.[396] A specific

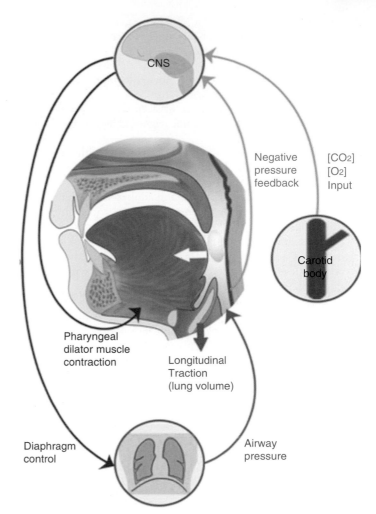

• **Figure 19.19** Neuromuscular control of upper airway patency. (From Jen R, Grander MA, Malhotra A. Future of sleep-disordered breathing therapy using a mechanistic approach. *Can J Cardiol.* 2015;31[7]: 880–888.)

sleep disorder was identified by PSG in 54% of migraineurs who reported sleep-related migraines.
- Insomnia is common in patients with chronic HAs.[397] Patients with chronic HA are 1.4–1.7 times more likely to complain of insomnia, and 2–2.6 times more likely if their HAs are chronic or severe.[397] Sleep disorders are two- to eightfold more common in patients with primary HA disorders than the general population.
- Chronic daily or morning HA patterns suggest concomitant primary sleep disorders.[394]
- Habitual snoring reported in 24% with chronic daily HAs compared with 14% controls.[398]
- Twelve to 20% of people with OSA complain of HA upon awakening versus 5%–8% of the general population.[399]
- Adults with sleep bruxism are 3–4 times more likely to complain of migraine or TTH.[400]

Migraine

- Insomnia is most prevalent sleep disorder in migraine. More than one-third of migraineurs sleep less than 6 hours/night, and nearly half have difficulty falling or staying asleep.[401] Patients with chronic migraine had a 17-fold greater risk for insomnia. Severity and prevalence of insomnia increases proportionally to HA frequency. Insomnia in people with migraine is not merely a function of comorbid psychiatric disorders.

- Sleep is often effective treatment for acute migraine, especially in children younger than age 8.[402]
- A 30%–55% higher incidence of sleep terrors, sleepwalking, enuresis in children with migraine (eightfold higher than general population)[403]
- Higher incidence of chronic HAs in patients with narcolepsy type 1.[395] One study found 54% of patients with narcolepsy type 1 report migraine (64% women, 35% men).[404]
- Good sleep hygiene in children and adolescents with migraine can significantly reduce the mean duration and frequency of their HAs.[405]
- Delayed nocturnal melatonin peak, lower melatonin levels, decreased nocturnal prolactin peak, and increased nocturnal cortisol levels have been observed in patients with chronic migraine.[406]
- Migraine may occur during nocturnal or daytime sleep, and can be precipitated by sleep deprivation (<6 hours), sleep fragmentation, or prolonged sleep (>8.5 hours).
- Migraines that awaken the patient from sleep are associated with abnormal REM sleep duration during the previous night.
- Patients with migraine attacks are more likely to awaken with them between 4 and 9 AM.
- A recent randomized double-blind placebo controlled trial of eszopiclone 3 mg nightly for 6 weeks only reduced sleep latency in patients with chronic migraine, but did improve sleep quality, total sleep time, and HA frequency, intensity, or duration.[407]
- CBTi can improve sleep in patients with migraine and insomnia. Those treated with CBTi at 6 weeks had fewer HAs than sham controls, although the difference did not reach statistical significance.[408]
- Recent studies find simvastatin 20 mg daily plus vitamin D 1000 international units twice daily effective for episodic migraine.

Sleep Apnea Headache

- Sleep apnea headache (SAH) is diffuse pressing mild to moderate intensity head pain that typically resolves within 30 min–4 hours after awakening. SAH is most often associated with OSA, but can be seen in patients with any type of SDB.
- Twenty percent of OSA patients complain of morning HA (most often chronic TTH); it resolves within 60% in less than 30 min, and 81% by 4 hours.[409]
- OSA patients with SAH compared with those without SAH had more time in overnight PSG with SpO_2 less than 90%, greater desaturations, and lower nadir SpO_2.[410] These differences were statistically significant but numerically modest. No particular PSG characteristics identify which patients with OSA will complain of SAHs.
- Some OSA with SAH report improvement in HA with PAP use (more so if PAP-adherent).[411]

Cluster Headache

- Cluster headache (CH) is the primary HA disorder with the strongest chronobiological traits.[412] A majority of CH occur from sleep.

- OSA is 8–24 times more common in patients with CH. A case-control study recorded overnight PSG in 42 patients with CH and 28 controls.[413] They found 29% with CH had OSA versus 7% of controls. Central apneas were seen in CH, but only during CH periods.
- A recent study compared 275 patients with CH and 145 controls: sleep was the most common trigger for CH (80%).[414] CH recurred at a particular time of day in 82% and annually in 56%. Sleep quality was worse and sleepiness greater during a cluster cycle. Sleep quality improved when a cluster remitted, but sleep was still pathological in patients with CH compared with controls even when their last CH happened one year earlier.
- Insomnia can worsen CHs.[415] Complaints of insomnia may herald the onset of a CH bout. Repeated nocturnal awakenings can be a warning sign of impending cluster period. Poor quality sleep in-between cluster cycles but much worse during active bouts.
- Another recent study found patients during active cluster periods had decreased percent REM sleep time, increased REM sleep latency, decreased arousal index, modest but significant increase in AHI, and PLMs during a cluster HA bout.[416] Very limited evidence of the effect of CPAP on CH reports it helps some; others complained it made their CH worse.

Tension-Type Headache Disorders

- Chronic TTH in 2%–3% of the general population.[393] A majority also complain of insomnia. Chronic TTH is the most common HA type in patients with sleep apnea.
- Insomnia is a risk factor for new-onset TTH and progression of new-onset TTH to chronic TTH.[393]
- Overnight PSG study in chronic TTH patients showed they need more sleep than healthy controls.[417]
- Inadequate sleep may contribute to increased pain sensitivity and HA frequency in TTH.[418]

Idiopathic Hypnic Headache[419]

- HA of idiopathic hypnic headache (IHH) occurs exclusively during sleep (often even the same time of night) but can occur also during naps.[419] IHH typically last 10–180 min, often need to stand for relief, are diffuse in two-thirds, most often mild to moderate intensity (severe in one-third) and usually occur only once in a 24-hour period. IHH can begin from NREM or REM sleep. Patients with IHH are usually over age 50.
- Need to exclude SDB or nocturnal HTN as cause and distinguish from cluster HA by lack of cranial autonomic symptoms.
- Brain MRI warranted to rule out pituitary, intracranial, or parasellar lesion.
- Treatments tried for IHH include caffeine, lithium, indomethacin, melatonin, flunarizine.

Sleep-Related Exploding Head Syndrome Is Not Headache[420]

- Exploding head syndrome are attacks of sudden noise or explosive feeling in head that occur in transition from wake to sleep, or sleep to wake.[420,421] Other symptoms are reported: fear and flashing lights inside head. Mean age of onset 54 years, modestly more common in women.

- Regarded as a benign condition. PSG does not show particular patterns with it.
- First treated by reassurance; some find tricyclic antidepressants helpful.

Effects of Drugs Used to Treat Headache on Sleep[422]

- Indomethacin at high doses can worsen SDB.
- Oral sumatriptan causes sleepiness in 5% of patients with migraine, typically only then at high doses; not seen for intranasal or subcutaneous formulations.
- $5-HT_{2A}$ antagonists (mirtazapine and trazodone) can increase NREM 3 sleep.
- Lipophilic beta-blockers (propranolol) more adverse sleep effects than hydrophilic (atenolol). Propranolol given to normal individuals associated with increased remembered awakenings and dreams while recording PSG (not observed with atenolol or placebo). Beta-blockers associated with nightmares but reported by less than 10% of patients. Beta-blockers may lower amplitude of endogenous melatonin secretion.
- Tricyclic (TCA) and SSRI antidepressants increase REM sleep onset latency, decrease REM, and increase total sleep time. Reduced dream recall with SSRI and TCAs. Nightmares are more likely to be reported with TCA than SSRIs. Excessive dreaming and REM sleep rebound after TCA withdrawal thought, due to anticholinergic effect.
- Imipramine and clomipramine have stronger REM sleep suppressing effects than amitriptyline.
- With exception of bupropion, all antidepressants' propensity is to worsen or precipitate symptoms of RLS and PLMS.
- Fluoxetine may worse bruxism and exacerbate TMJ-related HA.
- REM sleep without atonia may manifest or worsen RBD, especially with venlafaxine, fluoxetine, and mirtazapine.
- Topiramate successfully used to treat cluster HA and sleep-related eating disorder. Eight percent of patients taking topiramate reported somnolence versus 2% treated with placebo.
- Valproate can delay or advance circadian rhythms of clock gene expression in vitro (whereas lithium lengthens the circadian period).
- Lamotrigine occasionally causes insomnia (perhaps in those predisposed), can increase REM sleep, and/or reduced NREM 3 sleep.
- Gabapentin or pregabalin tend to increase NREM 3 sleep and reduce REM latency, which reduces nocturnal awakenings. Both have been used to treat RLS and reduce PLMs. Gabapentin can be helpful in treating perimenopausal insomnia.

Multiple Sclerosis

Basic Information

- Multiple sclerosis (MS) is a chronic neurodegenerative, demyelinating autoimmune disease of the central nervous system, which is characterized by relapsing and/or progressive multifocal neurological deficits. It is the leading cause of nontraumatic disability in young adults.

- Different clinical courses are observed in individuals with MS: relapsing-remitting, primary progressive, secondary progressive, and progressive-relapsing.
- Common symptoms in MS include impaired vision, sensory disturbances, paresis, gait difficulties, bladder dysfunction, cognitive decline, and fatigue.

Sleep Disorders in Multiple Sclerosis

- Sleep disorders are common in MS.[423] Nocturnal sleep in patients with MS can be disturbed by spasticity, nocturia, RLS, PLMS, depression, deconditioning, pain, and medication effects.
- Fatigue is a common and distressing symptom in patients with MS, present in about 50% of patients, leading to significant disability and reduced quality of life.
- A recent cross-sectional study of 102 patients with MS found patients reporting poor sleep quality were more frequently fatigued, and had a higher prevalence of EDS, sleep/wake, and RLS symptoms.[424]
- RLS is significantly associated with MS, especially in patients with severe pyramidal and sensory disability. A case-control study of 861 patients with MS found the prevalence of RLS was 19% in MS, compared with 4.2% in control subjects.[425] RLS in MS may be associated with infratentorial lesions on brain MRI.
  - MS patients with RLS often have more neurological disability than those without it. RLS and PLMS in MS are frequently associated with spinal cord lesions, spasticity, pain, and muscle spasms.
  - Iron/ferritin deficiency may contribute to RLS in MS. When present, this should be treated with iron supplement coupled with vitamin C to improve iron absorption.
  - Medications typically prescribed for treating RLS can be used with good response in patients with MS and RLS.
- Far fewer patients with MS complain about EDS. When they do, comorbid potentially treatable primary sleep disorders are often undiagnosed, and need to be identified and treated (such as OSA, CSA, RLS, PLMS, and/or insomnia). Fig. 19.20 shows a hypnogram of a patient with MS and SDB.
- Patients with MS describe their sensory symptoms as burning, itching, electric/formicatory pain involving their legs, feet, trunk, arms, or face, and can be challenging to distinguish from RLS, which most often affects the lower extremities.

Diagnosis/Treatment of Sleep Disorders in Multiple Sclerosis

- An overnight PSG case-control study in 25 patients with definite MS showed they had significantly reduced sleep efficiency and more awakenings during sleep.[426] PLMs were found in 36% with MS and 8% of controls.
- If SDB is suspected, overnight PSG with CO_2 monitoring indicated. If hypersomnia and/or fatigue present, after excluding treatable primary sleep disorders on PSG, multiple sleep latency testing may be warranted. If RBD is suspected, overnight video-PSG with wrist extensor EMG is warranted.
- Wake-promoting medications such as modafinil, amantadine, and methylphenidate can be tried to treat sleepiness or fatigue in MS, but often are no more effective than placebo.[427]

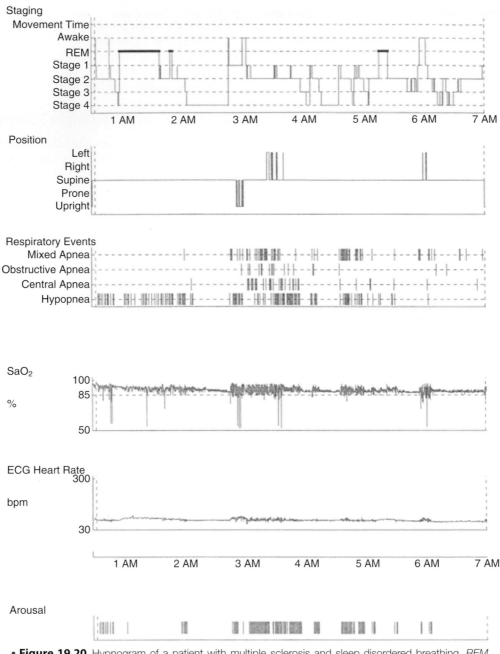

• **Figure 19.20** Hypnogram of a patient with multiple sclerosis and sleep disordered breathing. *REM*, Rapid eye movement. (From Chokroverty S, Bhat S, Provini F. Sleep dysfunction and sleep-disordered breathing in miscellaneous neurological disorders. In: Chokroverty S, Thomas RJ, eds. *Atlas of Sleep Medicine*. 2nd ed. Philadelphia, PA: Elsevier/Saunders; 2014.)

Sleep Disorders in Chiari Malformations and Other Craniocervical Junction Disorders

- The craniocervical junction (CCJ) is an intricate pathway of interlocking muscles, ligaments, and skeletal components that act in concert to preserve neurological function.
- Infants and children with CCJ disorders are at increased risk for sleep apnea, prolonged breath holding, and sudden death.
- Children or adolescents at risk for CCJ dysfunction include those with Chiari 1 malformations (CM1) but also craniofacial syndromes such as Conradi, Goldenhar, Klippel-Feil, Larsen, Morquio, Weaver, and Pierre-Robin[428]
- Early diagnosis and prevention of neurological compromise is critical.
- IS, CSA with/without OSA in varying combinations are often present in patients with CCJ disorders, and may be the *sole* manifestation of potentially life-threatening cervicomedullary junction compression. Early diagnosis and prevention of neurological compromise are crucial.
- Individuals with Chiari malformations (CM) often have varying combinations of spina bifida, meningomyelocele, syringomyelia, bilateral abductor vocal cord paralysis, SDB, prolonged

breath-holding spells, and sudden death due to compression at the cervico-medullary junction.
- Chiari 1 (CM1) is defined as a caudal herniation of the cerebellar tonsils 5 mm below the foramen magnum.
- Chiari 2 (CM2) is a caudal herniation of the brain stem, caudal cerebellar vermis, and fourth ventricle thorough the foramen magnum into the cervical spinal canal.
- Patients with CM2 are more likely than those with CM1 to have spina bifida, meningomyelocele, and spastic paraparesis with neurogenic bladder.
- Syringomyelia is a central cavitation or tubular fluid-filled cavity in several spinal cord segments present in 40%–75% of cases of CM1 (occurring as early as 12 months), and 90% of patients with syringomyelia have Chiari malformations.

Clinical Presentation of Cervical-Medullary Compression

- Symptoms of cervico-medullary compression include suboccipital HA (which may increase with coughing, sneezing, or bowel movement), neck pain (continuous burning, deep-seated discomfort in the shoulders, nape, chest, and/or arms, which often worsens with Valsalva maneuvers), vertigo (especially positional or triggered by head movements, often with tinnitus, aural fullness, and sometimes mild sensorineural hearing loss), and basilar migraine.
- SDB in patients with CCJ disorders can be obstructive and/or CSA, bradypnea, sleep-related alveolar hypercapnic hypoventilation, or sleep-exacerbated restrictive lung disease, causing sleep-related hypoxemia with apnea or hypercapnia.[429–432]
- Other clinical signs of CCJ compression include myelopathy (mono-, hemi-, para-, or quadriparesis), which may develop acutely following a seemingly mild head or neck injury, abnormal sensation in hands or feet (possibly presenting, in an infant or young child, as constant rubbing of the affected limbs), transient visual field deficits, vertigo, altered consciousness or confusional states (sometimes provoked by neck extension or rotation), uni- or bilateral paralysis or dysfunction of soft palate or pharynx, basilar migraine, downbeat nystagmus, hearing loss and SDB, apneic episodes, breath holding, or sudden death in sleep.

Diagnosis of Cervico-Medullary Compression in Chiari Malformations

- Begins with a thorough neurological and sleep history and examination followed by neuro-imaging, beginning with cervical x-rays in flexion and extension.
- Symptoms suggestive of SDB and/or cervicomedullary junction compression in individuals with CM warrants comprehensive overnight PSG with CO_2 monitoring evaluates for OSA, CSA, stridor, central, or obstructive sleep-related hypoventilation, and/or pulmonary restrictive disease.
- Unexpectedly observing long runs of central apnea and/or marked bradypnea during NREM sleep in a PSG warrants ordering a brain MRI to exclude posterior fossa compression. Fig. 19.21 shows a case of SDB in a patient with Chiari 1 malformation.
- Brain MRI is initially the best choice for neuroimaging (evaluates soft tissue structures, ligaments, and brain); computed tomography scan of the CCJ is useful for evaluating bony structures. Static or dynamic MRI of CCJ evaluates soft tissue structures, ligaments, and the brain.

Treating Sleep-Disordered Breathing in Chiari Malformations

- PSG is recommended to evaluate the SDB. Treatment with CPAP, BPAP, BPAP-ST, and/or supplemental oxygen is often needed and tried, depending upon the SDB found. When evaluating the need for decompression, posterior fossa/cervicomedullary junction neuroimaging identifies and quantifies brain stem compression.
- Posterior fossa decompression in patients with symptomatic CM1 often improves or stabilizes symptoms, including the SDB and HA. Syrinxes would usually stabilize (and sometimes decrease) in size.
- Acute hydrocephalus sometimes develops in the immediate postoperative period, heralded by worsening of the SDB. PAP therapy is often then needed or resumed.
- Better outcomes follow if decompression is performed while symptoms are present less than 2 years.
- Posterior fossa decompression in symptomatic CM2 may reverse obstructive hydrocephalus, vocal cord paralysis, and CSA.
- Sometimes SDB does not fully remit after posterior fossa decompression in CM. Persistent SDB in CM may be secondary to developmentally immature brainstem networks and respiratory centers, lower brainstem cranial nerve nuclei aplasia or hypoplasia, ischemic or hemorrhagic changes in the brainstem, and chronic chemical meningitis and arachnoiditis.
- Some patients with posterior fossa decompression have recurrence years later. Recurrence of SDB may herald this.
- Neuroimaging is indicated to rule out "unexpected" posterior fossa compression in children with CM and adenotonsillar hypertrophy before proceeding to adenotonsillectomy.

Achondroplasia

Basic Information[433,434]

- Achondroplasia (AC) is the most common cause of short-limbed dwarfism, affects greater than 250,000 individuals worldwide, and occurs in 1 of 10,000–40,000 live births.
- AC is due to a heterozygous mutation in the FGFR3 gene on chromosome 4p16.3 that codes for production of the FGFR3 (fibroblast growth receptor-3) protein.
- FGFR3 protein is a negative regulator of linear bone growth inhibiting chondrocyte proliferation. The FGFR3 mutant gene causes a gain of function by increasing FGFR3 protein activity that severely inhibits bone and cartilage growth.
- Phenotypic expression of the mutant gene in AC is 100%.
- Patients with AC have short stature (average adult height 4 feet), large heads with frontal bossing set on a short cranial base, short squat long bones, and short proximal limbs. Intelligence is usually normal.
- AC infants usually have thoracolumbar kyphosis (gibbus) attributed to a combination of a large head, cervical ligamentous laxity, and delayed motor milestones.
- AC infants exhibit poor head control, which improves by 3–4 months of age. Lumbar kyphosis is usually replaced by an exaggerated lumbar lordosis, once the children begin to walk (typically by 24–36 months).
- Infants, children, and young adults with AC have higher mortality rates compared with the age-matched general population. Sudden death occurs in 2%–7.5% of young AC children.

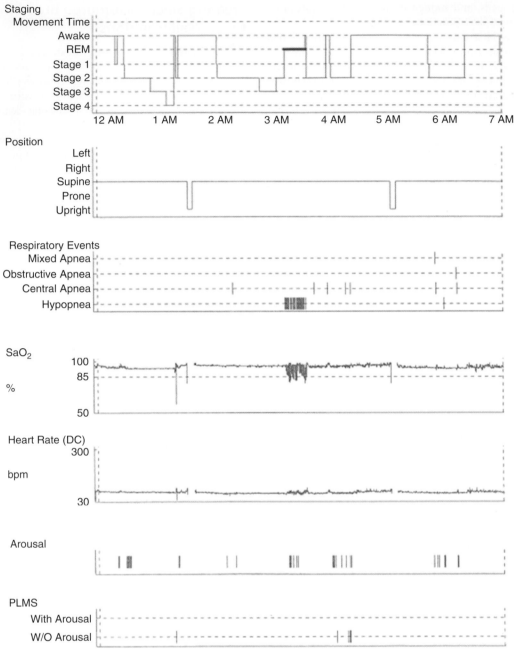

• **Figure 19.21** A case of Chiari 1 malformation with sleep disordered breathing. *PLMS*, Periodic limb movements during sleep; *REM*, rapid eye movement. (From Chokroverty S, Bhat S, Provini F. Sleep dysfunction and sleep-disordered breathing in miscellaneous neurological disorders. *Atlas of Sleep Medicine*. 2nd ed. 2014.)

- Sudden death is responsible for most of the mortality seen in those younger than 4 years, and brainstem compression has been identified as the cause in half.
- Foramen magnum stenosis in AC infants can cause brainstem compression with apnea and sudden death. Other possible causes of sudden death include compression of the pontomedullary junction, obstruction of the Sylvian aqueduct, ischemic injury to vital brainstem nuclei, and cranio-cervical dislocations from minor trauma with poor neck support.
- Young adults with AC continue to have a higher incidence of accidental, neurological, or cardiac-related deaths, and a life

expectancy 10 years less than the general population, despite advances in their medical care.

Sleep-Disordered Breathing in Achondroplasia

- SDB is present in a third to nearly half of children or adults with AC and is characterized by varying combinations of pulmonary restrictive disease, OSA, CSA, and abnormal activity of accessory muscles[435–437]
- One study of 88 AC children (1 month–12.6 years) found 44% had nocturnal hypoxemia (attributed to pulmonary

restrictive disease); only 4% had OSA, but it was severe enough to require treatment with CPAP in two, and tracheotomy in three patients.[438] The authors argued that SDB in AC was most often nocturnal hypoxemia due to pulmonary restrictive disease. Sisk et al. (1999) found OSA in 38% of 95 AC children (mean age 3.7 years).[439] Symptoms that best predicted OSA on their PSG were snoring, observed apnea, glottal stops, and apneic episodes during wakefulness. Severe (4+) tonsillar hypertrophy, a small oropharyngeal size, or redundant oropharyngeal tissue did not predict OSA.

- Evaluation for foramen magnum stenosis is recommended before adenotonsillectomy in AC children with OSA—even those without CSA on PSG.[437,440–443]
- Another study found CSA on PSG was a common and distinctive pattern of SDB in AC infants and children with symptomatic cervicomedullary compression (which presented before age 2 in 14 of their 18 cases).[444] CSA was present in preoperative PSG in 12 of 18 children who had pre- and postoperative PSGs. CSA improved or resolved following surgery in all but one child. Persistence of CSA following surgery prompted at least in part early reoperation. With further decompression, the CSA resolved. Eleven percent of the AC children needed their decompressive surgeries repeated years later (mean age 5.5 years). The need for repeat decompressive surgery in older children with AC was often heralded by the return of the central apnea.
- Untreated SDB in AC increase the risk for sudden infant death and neuropsychological deficits.[442] Sudden death in AC is most common in infants and children. Cardiovascular events are the main cause of mortality in adults.

Summary

As mentioned at the beginning of this review, and evident by this point, sleep disorders are more prevalent in almost every neurological disorder. Untreated SDB greatly affects the morbidity and mortality of many neurological disorders (particularly stroke and neuromuscular diseases). Complex behavioral insomnia is prevalent among many neurodevelopmental disorders as to be phenotypic of the particular neurodevelopmental disorder. Chronic idiopathic RBD heralds the likely development of a synucleionpathy. IS appearing first asleep warrants consideration of MSA. Studying the wide range of sleep disorders in neurological diseases provides a good review of all sleep disorders, since they span the breadth of them.

Suggested Reading

Kotagal S. Sleep in neurodevelopmental and neurodegenerative disorders. *Semin Pediatr Neurol.* 2015;22(2):126-129.

Leu RM. Sleep-related breathing disorders and the Chiari 1 malformation. *Chest.* 2015;148(5):1346-1352.

Lyashenko EA, Poluektov MG, Levin OS, Pchelina PV. Age-related sleep changes and its implication in neurodegenerative diseases. *Curr Aging Sci.* 2016;9(1):26-33.

Videnovic A, Willis GL. Circadian system—a novel diagnostic and therapeutic target in Parkinson's disease? *Mov Disord.* 2016;31(3):260-269.

Wickwire EM, Williams SG, Roth T, et al. Sleep, sleep disorders, and mild traumatic brain injury. What we know and what we need to know: findings from a National Working Group. *Neurother.* 2016;13(2):403-417.

20

Sleep and Psychiatric Disorders

MAX HIRSHKOWITZ, JOHN HERMAN

Introduction

Scope-Psychiatric Disorders and Sleep Disturbance

This review will focus on the relationship between psychiatric disorders and sleep disturbances. Psychiatric disorders cover a wide spectrum of illnesses, ranging from neurodevelopmental disorders to iatrogenic problems induced by medication. In this chapter we will focus specifically on those disorders marked by sleep complaints and polysomnographic sleep aberrations.

- Early on, clinicians recognized the co-occurrence of sleep and psychiatric disorders.[1]
- Insomnia runs rampant in patients with mood disorders. Some estimates indicate as many as 90% of patients with major depressive disorders (MDDs) report having insomnia.[2]
- Many clinicians considered early morning awakening with inability to return to sleep to be pathognomonic for depression.[4]

Patients with anxiety disorders commonly report difficulty falling asleep, maintaining sleep, and falling back to sleep after multiple awakenings at night.[5] These problems were often attributed to anxiety, worry, and ruminations. Similarly, schizophrenia and sleep problems correlated highly.[6] A wide variety of fanciful theories attempted to explain this relationship. Section II enumerates the intersection between psychiatric disorders and symptoms of sleep disturbance.

When polysomnographic techniques became reliable and somewhat standardized, research-minded psychiatrists and psychologists began describing sleep physiology in several major patient groupings. These researchers paid particular attention to:

- Mood disorders
- Anxiety disorders
- Thought disorders

In part, this focus belies the belief that such disorders have a biologic basis and therefore should be reflected by neurophysiologic alterations of sleep architecture (Fig. 20.1). This research avenue was productive, results were encouraging, and connections between other psychiatric diagnoses and disrupted sleep were demonstrated polysomnographically. Section III provides a tabulation of major findings.

Vulnerability Hypothesis for Psychiatric Disorders

Psychiatrists and mental health professionals are keenly aware of the high prevalence of sleep disorders in their patient population.[1,7]

- Sleep problems occur more often in patients with psychiatric disorders than in the general population.
- Sleep disruption often exacerbates psychiatric pathology.
- Correlations between mental and sleep disorders, however, do not prove causality.

Theoretical models concerning sleep's role in regulating mood and maintaining coping mechanisms abound. One such hypothesis, the Stress-Vulnerability Coping Model, postulates that in those who are more vulnerable to mental illness, disrupted sleep might pose a risk factor.[7]

Some individuals are biologically at risk for certain psychiatric conditions, including: major depression, schizophrenia, anxiety disorders, and bipolar disorder. This vulnerability may stem from:

- Genetic predisposition
- Prenatal or perinatal problems
- Developmental experiences, especially trauma

The vernacular aphorism is that the particular problem "runs in the family." However, not all family members necessarily develop an illness. In this model, stressful events are thought to catalyze the process. Problems with sleep insufficiency and/or quality (and the subsequent adverse daytime effects) act as potent neurophysiologic, neuroendocrine, and behavioral risk factors for the development of mental disorders.

In a study of more than 116,000 military veterans with sleep apnea[8]:

- 21.8% had comorbid depression
- 16.7% had anxiety disorders
- 11.9% had posttraumatic stress disorder (PTSD)

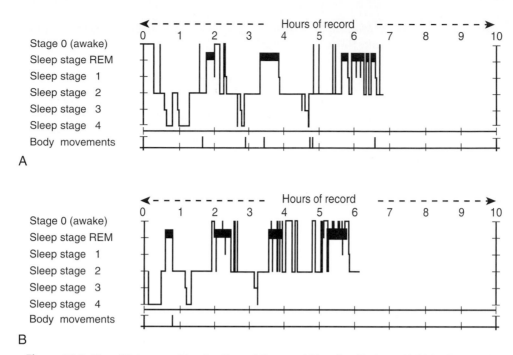

• **Figure 20.1** Sleep Histograms Showing Normal Sleep and Sleep in a Patient with Major Depressive Disorder. Sleep stage histograms comparing normal sleep **(A)** with that found in a patient with major depressive disorders **(B)**. Difficulty maintaining sleep and early morning awakenings are common complaints in patients with depression. **B** illustrates the electrophysiologic correlates of these complaints beginning, in this case, after approximately two hours of sleep. Sleep continuity becomes disrupted as morning approaches. Also present is a markedly reduced latency to rapid eye movement (REM) sleep. This sleep feature is characteristic of this patient population and is thought by some to reflect cholinergic-aminergic imbalance. (From Hirshkowitz M, Seplowitz-Hafkin RG and Sharafkhaneh A, Sleep Disorders In: Sadock BJ, Sadock VA, Ruiz P (Eds.) Kaplan and Sadock's Comprehensive Textbook of Psychiatry, 9th edition. Philadelphia, PA: Lippincott Williams and Wilkins; 2009, page 2153.)

- 5.1% had psychosis
- 3.3% had bipolar disorders

Compared with patients from the same population not diagnosed with sleep apnea, mood disorders, anxiety, PTSD, psychosis, and dementia were significantly more common ($P < .0001$).[8]

Causality, Comorbidity, and/or Synergy

- In most cases, a worsening sleep disorder and/or increased sleep disruption exacerbates the ongoing psychiatric problem.
- Increasing sleep duration and/or improving sleep quality is usually therapeutically beneficial.
- However, in some psychiatric disorders (e.g., MDD), the underlying sleep architecture does not necessarily normalize when psychiatric status improves.
- Furthermore, the sleep complaint may still be present.

For many years, insomnia was considered a "symptom" of the psychiatric condition and therefore was thought to be "secondary" insomnia. Even after this notion was judged incorrect, the term "primary insomnia" remains. For this reason, the term "comorbid insomnia" is now encouraged. Perhaps more interestingly, longitudinal studies find that[1,9]:

- Insomnia predates the development of mood disorders, but
- Anxiety disorders usually predate the onset of insomnia.

Thus there appears to be a disorder-specific synergy between psychiatric and sleep disorders.

Psychiatric Disorders Associated with Sleep Disturbance

Overview

As previously mentioned, many psychiatric disorders frequently are associated sleep problems, excessive daytime sleepiness, or both. Table 20.1 provides an overview of various psychiatric disorders and their related sleep problems.[1] The table also notes when a comorbid sleep disorders is prevalent within a particular patient group.

Clinical and research interest concerning the intersection of sleep and psychiatric disorders has long focused on insomnia. This is especially true for mood and anxiety disorders.[4,5,10] Insomnia in different mood disorders can present differently. The same holds for anxiety disorders. These differences are highlighted in the following section, with a comparison of insomnia and sleep complaints in MDDs compared with insomnia in bipolar disorders. This is followed by an appraisal of insomnia in generalized anxiety disorders (GADs), contrasted with sleep disturbance in PTSD.

Insomnia in Specific Mood Disorders

Major Depressive Disorder

MDD is diagnosed when an individual exhibits a depressed mood or loss of interest or pleasure for at least 2 weeks' duration compared with the patient's normal mood.[1,7] The depressed mood is present most of the day, nearly every day. Depressed mood may be described

TABLE 20.1	*Diagnostic and Statistical Manual for Mental Disorders* (Fifth Edition) Diagnostic Categories and Recognized Sleep and Wakefulness Problems	
Overall Diagnostic Category	**Specific Diagnostic Entities**[a]	**Sleep and Wakefulness Problems**
Neurodevelopmental disorders	Intellectual disabilities, communication disorders, ASD, ADHD, specific learning disorder, and motor disorders	The two disorders in this group receiving attention from sleep researchers are ASD and ADHD. Sleep problems occur in an estimated 80% of children with ASD. Children with ASD also often resist going to bed at bedtime. Insufficient sleep can exacerbate aggressive behavior. Children with ADHD suffer from many sleep problems, including: difficulty initiating sleep and maintaining sleep, sleepwalking, snoring, sleep-disordered breathing, delayed sleep phase, insufficient sleep, and daytime sleepiness. Some of the above findings are more prevalent in sleep diary studies and not as frequently observed with PSG.
Schizophrenia spectrum and other psychotic disorders	Schizotypal (personality) disorder, delusional disorder, brief psychotic disorder, schizophreniform disorder, schizophrenia, schizoaffective disorder, and catatonia disorders	Schizophrenia is associated with reduced need for sleep, insomnia, and daytime sleepiness. The insomnia can be severe during the acute phase of the illness and the patient may remain awake for extended time periods. There can be a reversal of the normal nighttime-sleeping, daytime-awake pattern. Nightmares and frightening dreams are often reported. Sometimes, the patient may report being unable to determine if he or she is awake or asleep.
Bipolar and related disorders	Bipolar I disorder, bipolar II, and cyclothymic disorder	During the manic phase, total sleep time is reduced as is apparent sleep requirement. During the depressive phase, time in bed and sleep time is prolonged. Patients also complain of nightmares.
Depressive disorders	Disruptive mood dysregulation disorder, MDD, persistent depressive disorder (dysthymia), and premenstrual dysphoric disorder	The vast majority of patients with MDD report sleep onset insomnia, sleep maintenance insomnia, early morning awakenings, and decreased appetite. Patients with atypical depression may also complain of daytime sleepiness and fatigue (characterized by increased appetite and weight gain).
Anxiety disorders	Separation anxiety disorder, selective mutism, specific phobias, social anxiety disorder, panic disorder, agoraphobia, GAD	Common sleep symptoms include sleep onset insomnia, frequent nocturnal awakenings, and anxiety-provoking dreams. GAD is the most studied of the anxiety disorders.
Obsessive-compulsive and related disorders	Obsessive-compulsive disorder, body dysmorphic disorder, hording disorder, trichotillomania (hair pulling), and excoriation (skin picking) disorder	Insomnia is common as obsessive rumination interferes with sleep.
Trauma- and stressor-related disorders	Reactive attachment disorder, disinhibited social engagement disorder, PTSD, acute stress disorder, and adjustment disorders	Nightmares, sleep terrors, and/or dream anxiety attacks are part of the diagnostic criteria. Insomnia may develop in response to a fear of sleeping and having nightmares and/or the patient's general hypervigilant/hyperarousal state.
Dissociative disorders	Dissociative identity disorder, dissociative, amnesia, and depersonalization/derealization disorder	Little sleep research has been done but sleep deprivation is known to exacerbate the condition.
Somatic symptom and related disorders	Somatic symptom disorder, illness anxiety disorder, conversion disorder, and factitious disorder	Little sleep research has been done on these disorders.
Feeding and eating disorders	Pica, rumination disorder, avoidant/restrictive food intake disorder, anorexia nervosa, bulimia nervosa, and binge-eating disorder	Insomnia and nocturnal awakenings are reported. In rare cases, sleep-related eating disorder occurs which can be part of REM sleep behavior disorder.
Elimination disorders	Enuresis and encopresis	Enuresis is a well-established sleep disorder that can sometimes be treated behaviorally and/or with medication.
Sleep-wake disorders	Insomnia disorder, hypersomnolence disorder, narcolepsy, breathing-related sleep disorders, circadian rhythm disorders, and parasomnias	The sleep disorders nosology listed in DSM, 5th Edition, is somewhat comparable to the ICSD, 3rd Edition. The notable difference is that ICSD lists additional specific diagnostic entities and includes a distinct category for sleep-related movement disorders.

TABLE 20.1	*Diagnostic and Statistical Manual for Mental Disorders* (Fifth Edition) Diagnostic Categories and Recognized Sleep and Wakefulness Problems—cont'd	
Overall Diagnostic Category	**Specific Diagnostic Entities[a]**	**Sleep and Wakefulness Problems**
Sexual dysfunctions	Delayed ejaculation, erectile dysfunction, female orgasmic disorder, female sexual interest/arousal disorder, genito-pelvic pain/penetration disorder, male hypoactive sexual desire disorder, and premature ejaculation	These disorders mostly have not been studied with respect to sleep disturbance, with the exception of erectile dysfunction and nocturnal painful penile erections. Polysomnographic findings are listed in Table 20.3.
Gender dysphoria	Gender dysphoria	Little or no sleep research has been done on these disorders.
Disruptive, impulse-control, and conduct disorders	Oppositional defiant disorder, intermittent explosive disorder, conduct disorder, antisocial personality disorder, pyromania, and kleptomania	Little sleep research has been done on these disorders; however, in general, it is thought that sleep deprivation exacerbates the symptoms and characteristics. A common expression, "The bad sleep well," the title of a Japanese film, has no empirical support for this claim.
Substance-related and addictive disorders	Alcohol-related, caffeine-related, cannabis-related, hallucinogen-related, inhalant-related, opioid-related, sedative- hypnotic- or anxiolytic-related, stimulant-related, and tobacco-related disorders	The sleep effects depend upon the particular substance, the dose, and the phase of use (acute or chronic use, intoxication, or withdrawal). Stimulants (e.g., amphetamines, cocaine, and caffeine) produce alertness and reduce sleep time while depressants (e.g., sedatives and hypnotics) produce sedation and sleepiness. Opioids and tobacco depending on usage chronicity. Different types of cannabis produce different outcomes ranging from increased alertness to significant sedation.
NCD	Delirium, NCD due to Alzheimer's disease, frontotemporal neurocognitive disorder, NCD with Lewy bodies, Vascular neurocognitive disorder, NCD due to traumatic brain injury, NCD due to HIV infection, NCD due to Parkinson's disease, NCD due to Huntington's disease	Sleep disorders and daytime sleepiness are associated with the various neurocognitive disorders. As with most neurodegenerative diseases, the phase of illness determines the severity of sleep symptoms. Some NCDs, especially Parkinson's disease, are associated with REM behavior disorder in which a patient literally acts out their dreams (often becoming injured or injuring their bed partner in the process).
PD	Paranoid PD, Schizoid PD, Schizotypal PD, Antisocial PD, Borderline PD, Histrionic PD, Narcissistic PD, and Cluster C PD	Short REM latency, nightmares, and poor sleep have been reported in patients with borderline PD but not other PDs. Little sleep research has been done on most of these disorders.
Paraphilic disorders	Voyeuristic disorder, exhibitionistic disorder, frotteuristic disorder, sexual masochism disorder, sexual sadism disorder, pedophilic disorder, fetishistic disorder, and transvestic disorder	Little sleep research has been done on these disorders.

[a]In addition to the specific diagnostic entities listed, each grouping also contains (a) disorder(s) due to another medical condition and other or unspecified types.

ADHD, Attention-deficit/hyperactivity disorder; *ASD,* autism spectrum disorder; *DSM,* Diagnostic and Statistical Manual; *GAD,* generalized anxiety disorder; *ICSD,* International Classification of Sleep Disorders; *MDD,* major depressive disorder; *NCD,* neurocognitive disorders; *PD,* personality disorders; *PSG,* polysomnography; *PTSD,* posttraumatic stress disorder; *REM,* rapid eye movement.

by the patient (feels sad or empty) or may be reported by others (appears tearful). Marked loss of interest or pleasure in nearly all activities is present most of the day nearly every day during the 2 weeks. At least four of the following must be present in addition during this same 2-week period:

- Significant weight loss or gain (5% change in body weight)
- Insomnia or hypersomnia almost every day
- Psychomotor agitation or retardation (observable by others)
- Fatigue or loss of energy nearly every day
- Feelings of worthlessness or excessive guilt (which may be delusional) nearly every day
- Diminished ability to think or concentrate or indecisiveness nearly daily
- Recurrent thoughts of death, suicidal ideation, a suicide plan or a suicide attempt

To meet diagnostic criteria, the symptoms listed cause clinically significant distress or impairment in social, occupational, or other important areas of functioning. MDD is diagnosed as seasonal (affective) pattern if there is:

- A recurrent association between the onset of MDD, bipolar I, or bipolar II disorder at a particular time of year, typically autumn or winter.

- Full remission must also occur at a specific time of year, typically spring.
- The above pattern must occur at least twice or be the majority of all episodes the patient experiences in his or her lifetime.

Problems with sleep are among the most common and earliest symptoms of depression. Frequent sleep complaints include sleep onset and sleep maintenance insomnia, early morning awakenings, and nonrestorative sleep.[2,4,10] Increased sleep (hypersomnia) is also reported. Disturbing dreams frequently accompany MDD.

- Approximately 15%–20% of individuals with insomnia and 10% of individuals with hypersomnia have comorbid MDD.
- In individuals with no sleep complaints, the incidence of MDD is less than 1%.
- The more severe an individual's insomnia or hypersomnia, the more severe the MDD is likely to be.

Insomnia often precedes the onset of a first episode of MDD which goes against the concept that the depression causes insomnia. Especially in the elderly, the onset of insomnia is likely to precede an episode of MDD. If a patient has had a prior episode of MDD, bipolar I, or II disorder, the onset of insomnia is likely to be a harbinger of recurrence of the disorder. Episodes of depression recur throughout the lifespan. It is estimated that:

- One-third of patients with MDD recover fully (with treatment).
- One-third only obtain partial remission (despite treatment).
- One-third do not respond to treatment.
- In the one-third of patients who recover fully, sleep is not significantly different from nondepressed individuals, whereas about half of the patients with partial remission continue to experience sleep difficulties.

Polysomnographic findings in depression include[2]:

- Reduced rapid eye movement (REM) sleep latency
- Reduced stage N3 sleep
- Increased frequency of awakenings and arousals
- Early morning awakenings

Bipolar Disorder

Bipolar disorder has a lifetime prevalence of approximately 5%, making it a widely prevalent as well as a devastating psychiatric disorder. Recurrent episodes of mania, hypomania, and depression extract an enormous toll. Once an individual is hospitalized for an episode of bipolar disorder, he or she is likely to spend 20% of his or her life in recurrent episodes, and 50% of his or her life with dysthymic symptoms.

Bipolar I disorder is diagnosed when a patient suffers from[1,7]:

- Mania lasting at least 1 week that is characterized by a distinct and abnormal elevated or irritable mood
- Mania severe enough to disrupt occupational and interpersonal activities and clearly observable by others

Bipolar II disorder is diagnosed when a patient has experienced at least one episode of hypomania in addition to one episode meeting criteria for MDD. Despite good patient adherence to medication and therapy, bipolar patients remain symptomatic between episodes and the likelihood of recurrence is high.

The diagnostic criteria for bipolar disorder, including manic, hypomanic, and depressive episodes, encompass multiple symptoms of sleep and circadian rhythm disruption. A worsening of sleep disturbances may be a harbinger of a first bipolar episode, as disrupted sleep frequently precedes the onset of the disorder by at least 1 year. Approximately three quarters of patients with

bipolar disorder continue to suffer sleep disturbances between episodes.

A classic presentation of a manic episode is characterized by a reduced need for sleep in which the patient sleeps little and remains manic while awake. This reduced need for sleep has been verified by polysomnography (PSG) studies.[10]

Other sleep symptoms of bipolar disorder include:

- Insomnia
- Hypersomnia
- Delayed sleep phase (Fig. 20.2)
- An irregular sleeping pattern
- Insomnia is nearly universal during depressive episodes, and over half of patients experience insomnia when in remission from depressive episodes.

Conversely, episodes of depression may be accompanied by:

- Vegetative hypersomnia rendering the patient virtually immobile for periods of time as the patient remains in bed for much of the 24 hour period.
- In some cases, the hypersomnia (sleeping throughout the day) may be mixed with periods of insomnia (inability to sleep at night).
- Delayed sleep phase may be present concurrently as the patient has great difficulty getting out of bed.

A worsening of insomnia, hypersomnia, or circadian rhythm delay frequently precedes a recurrence of a bipolar episode. The appearance of these symptoms makes it extremely difficult to manage bipolar patients.

Differences in Sleep Between Major Depressive Disorder and Bipolar Disorder

In general, sleep is more disturbed in bipolar disorder than in MDD both during episodes and between episodes, although there is much overlap. The distinctive hallmark of bipolar disorder not seen in MDD is the loss of a need for sleep observed in bipolar I patients during manic episodes. Greater variability in the quality of sleep and the timing of sleep is present during bipolar episodes and between bipolar episodes compared with MDD or normal controls.

Insomnia in Specific Anxiety Disorders

Generalized Anxiety Disorder

GAD is characterized by excessive anxiety and worry that are difficult to control and cause clinically significant distress or impairment in social, occupational, or other important areas of functioning. Diagnosis requires that the symptoms have been present for 6 or more months. This disorder is twice as frequent in females as in males. Three of the following six symptoms must be present[1,7]:

- Restlessness
- Being easily fatigued
- Difficulty concentrating or mind going blank
- Irritability
- Muscle tension
- Disturbed sleep, including sleep onset insomnia, sleep maintenance insomnia, or nonrestorative sleep

Insomnia and GAD are frequently comorbid conditions, which is to be expected, as disturbed sleep is one of the six core symptoms for diagnosing GAD. Individuals with GAD frequently describe their worrying increasing as bedtime approaches.[5]

In contrast, in primary insomnia, the patient worries about getting a good night's sleep, whereas in GAD the worry focuses on areas that have been concerns during the day. Individuals with

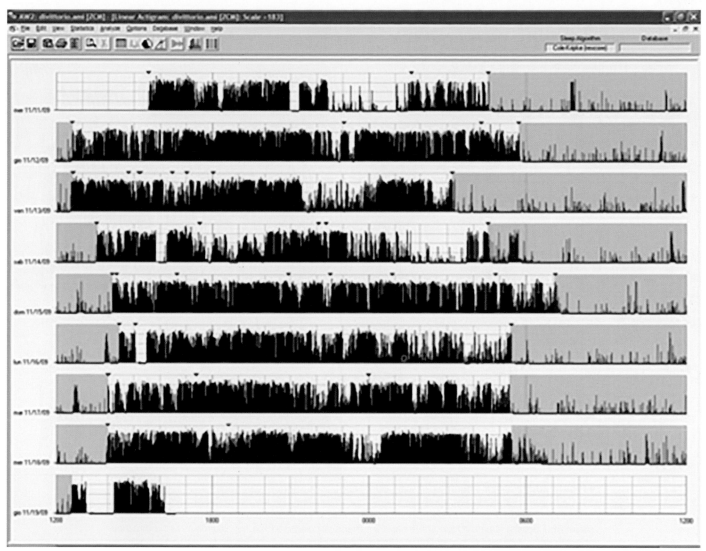

• **Figure 20.2** Delayed Sleep Phase Disorder. A 55-year-old woman with a tendency to have difficulty falling asleep at night and a tendency to fall asleep during the day since childhood. She experienced progression of the disorder with age and chose a work schedule from 11 AM to 7 PM. There is a family history for evening type (brother). The sleep diary showed sleep from 4:30 AM to 5 AM until noon to 1 PM if free running. Actigraphy for 8 day-night periods confirmed a delayed sleep (range 4:30 AM to 6 AM to 12:30 PM to 2 PM), with an estimated sleep efficiency above 90% in all of the nights except the last night (79.8%). Note an attempt to sleep in the evening/night on two occasions (first and fourth nights), with short duration and increased activity, indicating poor sleep quality. Treatment with melatonin in the evening and bright light in the morning was started. Comparison of mean periodic leg movement index during sleep by group. Values indicate Mean ± SE. *SE,* Standard error; *SSRIs,* selective serotonin reuptake inhibitors. *$P < .001$, control, bupropion versus venlafaxine, SSRIs; **$P < .0001$, control versus venlafaxine, SSRIs. (From Chokroverty S, Zucconi M. Specialized techniques. In *Atlas of Sleep Medicine.* Philadelphia, PA: Elsevier; 2;2014:255–299.)

GAD have increased sleep latency, increased wake after sleep onset, lower sleep efficiency, and decreased total sleep time.

Posttraumatic Stress Disorder

PTSD occurs after an individual is exposed to a traumatic event during which the person witnessed or was confronted with the threat of death, serious injury, or a threat to the physical integrity of self or others. The person's response included intense fear, helplessness, or horror. The diagnosis of PTSD involves the traumatic event being persistently experienced as[1,7]:

- Recurrent and intrusive images, thoughts or perceptions of the event
- Recurrent distressing dreams of the event
- Acting or feeling as if the traumatic event were recurring, including flashbacks and hallucinations
- Intense psychologic and/or physiologic distress following exposure to cues that symbolize or resemble an aspect of the traumatic event

Individuals with PTSD persistently avoid stimuli associated with the trauma as evidenced by:

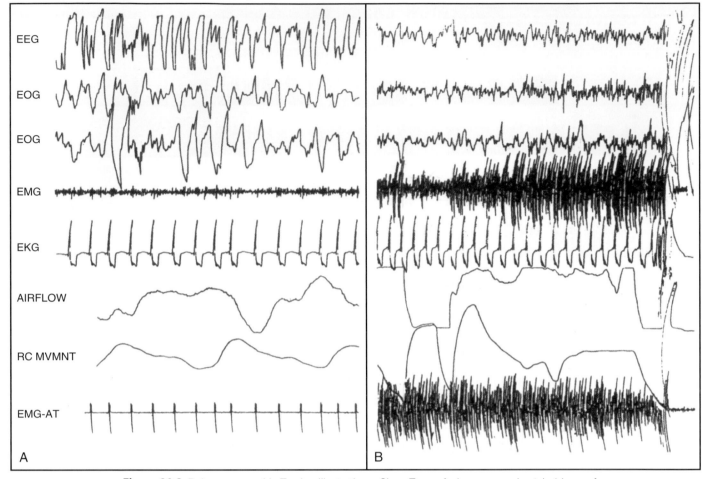

EEG

EOG

EOG

EMG

EKG

AIRFLOW

RC MVMNT

EMG-AT

A

B

• **Figure 20.3** Polysomnographic Tracing Illustrating a Sleep Terror. **A** shows approximately 14 sec of tracing occurring immediately before the sleep terror. Prominent EEG slow wave activity and other characteristics of stage 4 sleep are seen. **B** shows the awakening, accompanied by tachycardia and movement. EEG activity is ambiguous and the patient eventually disconnected his electrodes as he thrashed about in bed (visible at far right of figure). Although the patient was screaming and greatly agitated, there was no report of dreaming. In the morning, there was little recollection of anything having occurred during the night. *EEG,* Electroencephalogram; *EOG,* electrooculogram; *EMG,* submentalis electromyogram; *EKG,* electrocardiogram; *RC MVMNT,* rib cage movement; *EMG-AT,* anterior tibialis electromyogram. (From Hirshkowitz M, Seplowitz-Hafkin RG and Sharafkhaneh A, Sleep Disorders In: Sadock BJ, Sadock VA, Ruiz P (Eds.) Kaplan and Sadock's Comprehensive Textbook of Psychiatry, 9th edition. Philadelphia, PA: Lippincott Williams and Wilkins; 2009, page 2166.)

- Efforts to avoid thoughts, feelings, or conversations associated with the trauma
- Efforts to avoid activities, places, or people that arouse recollections of the trauma
- Inability to recall an important aspect of the trauma
- Diminished interest or participation in significant activities
- Feelings of detachment from others
- Loss of the ability to experience significant feelings, such as love
- Loss of anticipation of a significant future, including career, marriage, or children

Other symptoms include sleep onset or maintenance insomnia, irritability, outbursts of anger, difficulty concentrating, hypervigilance, or an exaggerated startle response. These symptoms are present for greater than 1 month. PTSD is twice as frequent in females.

In addition to the insomnia that is a diagnostic criterion for PTSD, sleep disturbances include nightmares, often frequent and associated with frightening awakenings.[5]

The sleep of patients with PTSD is also associated with:
- Nightmares
- Sleep terrors
- Violent or injurious activities during sleep
- Sleep talking
- Hypnogogic or hypnopompic hallucinations
- Heightened arousal during sleep including excessive movements and arousals (Figs. 20.3 and 20.4)

PTSD patients experience awakenings with somatic anxiety symptoms. Episodes of sleep paralysis are reported with PTSD.

Distinctions Between Insomnia with Generalized Anxiety Disorder and Insomnia with Posttraumatic Stress Disorder

Insomnia comorbid with GAD is remarkably different from insomnia comorbid with PTSD. Insomnia with GAD is typically sleep onset insomnia, sleep maintenance insomnia, and early morning awakenings. There is evidence that insomnia comorbid with GAD is associated with increased cortisol levels present both

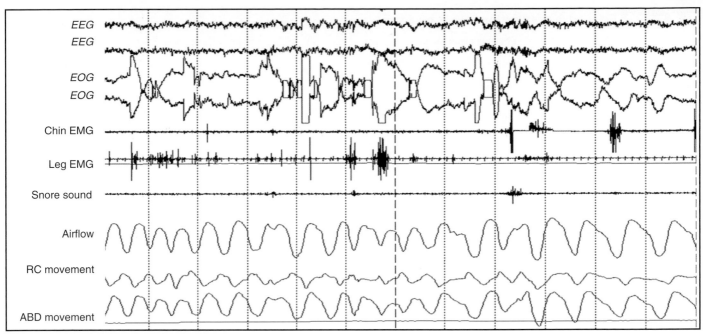

• **Figure 20.4** One-Minute Polysomnographic Tracing Illustrating High Rapid Eye Movement (REM) Density and Phasic Electromyogram Activity. This pattern of activity is often associated with REM sleep behavior disorder. It has been found in combat veterans with posttraumatic stress disorder. *EEG,* Electroencephalogram; *EOG,* electrooculogram; *Chin EMG,* submentalis electromyogram; *Leg EMG,* anterior tibialis electromyogram; *RC,* rib cage; *ABD,* abdominal.

awake and asleep, making it difficult for these patients to nap. In fact, the inability to nap after sleeping for 2–3 hours during the night is almost pathognomonic of insomnia with GAD.

Insomnia associated with PTSD has been shown to be related to increased sympathetic activity and increased release of noradrenalin. Nightmares often associated with frequent arousals are distinctive to PTSD as are the violent or injurious activities during sleep. Sleep talking and awakenings with somatic anxiety symptoms are associated with PTSD and not with GAD.

Polysomnographic Characteristics in Patients with Psychiatric Disorders

Beginning in the 1960s there was a flurry of research activity aimed at describing sleep electrophysiologically. The technique "polysomnography" was applied to determine objective sleep changes associated with age, sex, sleep deprivation, and clinical conditions.

Early psychiatric sleep research enthusiasm was bolstered by:
• The hope that neurophysiologic activity underlying sleep alterations could shed light on mental disorders
• Anticipation that sleep pattern changes produced by medications might be applied to normalize any detected sleep abnormalities
• The idea that sleep normalization might be used to objectively gauge therapeutic success

An early theory posited schizophrenia being REM sleep intrusion into wakefulness. The dream-like hallucinatory activity associated with REM sleep led researchers to investigate whether REM sleep abnormalities existed in patients with thought disorders.[6] Although it became clear that REM intrusion into wakefulness is associated with narcolepsy rather than schizophrenia, the paradigm was established for examining sleep to investigate mental illnesses.

MDD always struck researchers as likely organically based. Sleep electrophysiology seemed fertile ground for study. And indeed sleep structural differences were discovered. PSG studies show that the majority of patients with MDD have objective sleep disturbances and alterations (see Fig. 20.1). There is a greater than 50 year history of considering sleep abnormalities as a biologic marker of MDD. In PSG studies, patients with MDD show[9]:
• Increased latency to sleep onset
• Decreased latency from sleep onset to the first occurrence of REM sleep
• Increased wake after sleep onset
• Decreased sleep efficiency
• Increased sleep fragmentation
• Early morning awakenings
• Decreased slow wave sleep duration and percentage (of total sleep time)
• Decreased electroencephalogram (EEG) delta-bandwidth power (most notable in the first non-REM sleep [NREM] cycle but persisting throughout the night)

This second feature (short REM latency) is perhaps the most notable characteristic of sleep in depression. This finding has been the focus of much speculation on the relationship between REM sleep and MDD.

Additional REM sleep abnormalities include:
• An abnormally long first REM period
• Increased eye movement density (the number of eye movements per unit time) in early REM episodes
• REM sleep duration that is greater in MDD as a percentage of total sleep time

These results supported the "cholinergic overdrive" hypothesis,[2] in which it is suggested that:
• REM sleep is a time when brain cholinergic activity becomes activated and monoaminergic activity is suppressed.

TABLE 20.2 **Psychiatric Medication Effects on Sleep**

Rx Class	Subclass	Pharmacologic Agent	N3	REM	Wake	Other Sleep Effects
Antidepressants	SSRIs	Fluoxetine, Citalopram, Escitalopram, Fluvoxamine, Dapoxetine	↓	↓	↑	Can be associated with REMs intruding into NREM sleep (nicknamed Prozac Eyes) and increased EMG activity during REM sleep
		Paroxetine	↓	↓↓	↑↑	
		Sertraline	↔	↓↓	↔	
	TCAs	Amitryptiline, Nortryptiline, Clomipramine	↑	↓↓↓	↓↓↓↓	Increases PLMs and sleep-related movements, may cause RLS-like symptoms
		Doxepin	↑↑	↓↓	↓↓↓↓	
		Clomipramine	↑	↓↓↓↓	↔	
	MAOIs	Phenelzine	↓	↓↓↓↓	↑↑	Prominent REM sleep rebound on withdrawal
		Tranylcypromine	↓	↓↓↓	↑↑↑	
Sedative-hypnotics and anxiolytics	BZDs	Diazepam, Lorazepam, Midazolam	↓↓	↓	↓↓↓	Tolerance and rebound on discontinuation
	BZRAs	Zopiclone, Zolpidem, Eszopoclone, Zaleplon	↔	↔	↓↓↓	Low overdose liability, minor AE on withdrawal
Antipsychotics	Traditional	Haloperidol, Thioridazine Chlorpromazine	↑	↑	↓↓↓	Increase PLMs and RLS-like symptoms
	Atypical	Clozapine, Risperdal, Olanzapine	↓	↔	↓	Increase PLMs and RLS-like symptoms
		Quetiapine	↔	↓a	↓↓	Increase PLMs and RLS-like symptoms
Stimulants		Cocaine, Amphetamine, Amphetamine Salts	↓↓	↓↓	↑↑↑	Hypersomnolence and prominent REM sleep rebound on withdrawal, bruxism may occur
Other Rx used in psychiatry	SNRIs	Duloxetine	↑	↓	↑	May exacerbate PLMs
		Venlafaxine, Desvenlafaxine, Milnacipran	↑	↓↓	↑	May exacerbate
	5-HT$_{1A}$ partial agonist	Buspirone	↔	↓	↔	Reportedly a treatment for SSRI-induced bruxism
	AChE inhibitors	Physostigmine, Rivastigmine, Galantamine, Donepezil	↔	↑	↓	Shortens REM sleep latency
	Adrenergic α$_1$ antagonist	Prazosin	↔	↑a	↓	Decreases nightmare distress in patients with PTSD
	Adrenergic β antagonist	Propranolol	↓	↓	↑	Sometimes used to treat performance anxiety; can provoke nightmares

aChange found in some studies on clinical populations but no difference or mixed results in normal.

ACh, Acetyl choline; AChE, acetyl cholinesterase; BZD, benzodiazepines; BZRAs, Benzodiazepine receptor agonists; EMG, electromyogram; 5-HT, 5-hydroxytriptamine (serotonin); MAOIs, monoamine oxidase inhibitors; N3, Slow wave sleep; PLMs, periodic leg movements; PTSD, posttraumatic stress disorder; REM, rapid eye movement; RLS, restless legs syndrome; SNRIs, selective norepinepherine reuptake inhibitors; SSRI, selective serotonin reuptake inhibitor; TCA, tricyclic antidepressant; ↓, decreases; ↑, increases; ↔, no differences or mixed results.

- Catacholinergic activity is not properly balanced with cholinergic activity in the brain.

Evidence supporting the "cholinergic overdrive" hypothesis include[11]:

- Cholinergic agonists infusion (e.g., arecoline) during sleep will provoke REM sleep in patients predisposed to or who have mood disorders. Control subjects do not respond in this manner.
- Most antidepressant medications suppress REM sleep through anticholinergic or proaminergic actions (Table 20.2).
- Studies also revealed that instrumentally depriving a patient of REM sleep by awakening them during a major depressive episode reduced depressed mood.

Some researchers hypothesized that REM sleep was depressionogenic in patients with mood disorders. Nevertheless, a few of the second and third generation NREM suppressing antidepressants (e.g., bupropion and nefazodone) indicate it is not necessary to suppress REM sleep to elevate mood. However, it apparently remains sufficient to suppress REM sleep to achieve an antidepressant effect.

PSG findings in bipolar disorder are similar to those in MDD, including:

- A reduced latency from sleep onset to the first REM period and increased REM density.
- These alterations in REM architecture reportedly accompany manic, hypomanic, and depressive episodes.
- Reduced EEG delta bandwidth power and slow wave sleep appear to accompany manic episodes.

However, PSG studies of bipolar disorder need replication. Study limitations include heterogeneity of diagnoses (bipolar I and II), differing episode types (manic, hypomanic, and depressive), the episodic nature of the disease, and small sample sizes.

- The similarities between bipolar disorder and MDD in REM architecture suggest a commonality in the neurobiology between these two psychiatric illnesses.
- The continued presence of sleep and circadian rhythm disturbances in-between bipolar I and II episodes suggests that a subsyndromal manifestation of the disorder is present continuously.

In contrast to the normalization of sleep that occurs with the one-third of fully remitted patients who have suffered an episode of MDD, the vast majority of patients with bipolar disorder will continue to experience sleep difficulties throughout their lifespan.

While mood, anxiety, and thought disorders held center stage for polysomnographic research in psychiatry, other mental disorders have been explored. Table 20.3 summarizes results of available research.

In some cases, sleep alterations follow patterns similar to those found in mood disorders. In other cases, different profiles appear.

By contrast, sleep appears normal (at least according to measures applied) in some psychiatric conditions, such as the personality disorders. We also note in the next section when PSG uncovers comorbid sleep disorders within a particular patient group. Finally, some diagnostic groups remain polysomnographically unexplored or manifest inconsistent findings.

TABLE 20.3　Polysomnographic Findings in Patients with Psychiatric and Mental Disorders

Overall Diagnostic Category	Subcategory	Polysomnographic Findings
Neurodevelopmental disorders	ASD	Shorter REM latency; decreased TST versus controls Lower CAP rate during N3 sleep
	ADHD	SRBD, PLMD, and RLS found in many patients. If the underlying cause of the ADHD is treated, such as tonsillectomy for children with hypertrophic tonsils, ADHD symptoms frequently resolve.[3]
Schizophrenia spectrum and other psychotic disorders	Schizophrenia	Decrease N3 sleep. Short REM sleep latency and decreased eye movement intensity in REM sleep (may normalize with therapy) Decreased REM sleep rebound after REM sleep deprivation Decreased TST and REM sleep during active phases (may normalize during remission)
Bipolar and related disorders	Bipolar disorder	Short REM sleep latency during depressive phase Increased TST during depressive phase notwithstanding reported daytime sleepiness and fatigue Decreased TST during manic phase
	Manic disorder	Decreased N3 Sleep Short REM sleep latency Increase eye movement density during REM sleep
Depressive disorders	MDD	Difficulty initiating sleep and disrupted sleep Short REM sleep latency (may persist after episode remits) Increase eye movement density during REM sleep Decrease N3 sleep, especially during first NREM/REM sleep cycle (may persist after depressive episode remits) "Reverse REM Sleep Architecture," i.e., longer REM episodes early in the night and shorter episodes toward end of the night
	Atypical depression	Short REM sleep latency Increased time in bed and TST notwithstanding reported daytime sleepiness and fatigue
	Seasonal affective disorder, in DSM V called MDD, seasonal pattern	Circadian rhythm variation between fall-winter and spring-summer phases
Anxiety disorders	Various	Difficulty initiating sleep Decreased N3 sleep and REM sleep
	Panic disorder	Prolonged sleep latency and reduced SEI in some patients
Obsessive-compulsive and related disorders	Obsessive-compulsive disorder	Some possible subtle sleep disturbances No differences in sleep architecture
Trauma- and stressor-related disorders	PTSD	Decreased N3 and REM sleep Increased phasic activity during REM sleep, transitions from REM sleep to wakefulness REM fragmentation, and N1 sleep RBD-like activity in combat veterans
Dissociative disorders	Sleep related	Rare cases of sleep-related dissociative disorders have been reported in the literature
Somatic symptom and related disorders	Various	No systematic data
Feeding and eating disorders	Anorexia	Possibly decreased REM and N3 sleep but findings are inconsistent
Elimination disorders	Enuresis	Sometimes provoked by SRBD
Sleep-wake disorders	Sleep disorders[a]	Different PSG findings for different disorders. PSG is useful to diagnose SRBD, narcolepsy, nocturnal seizure disorder, and some parasomnias

Continued

TABLE 20.3	Polysomnographic Findings in Patients with Psychiatric and Mental Disorders—cont'd	
Overall Diagnostic Category	Subcategory	Polysomnographic Findings
Sexual Dysfunctions	ED	Before pharmacotherapy for ED, surgical penile prosthetic implantation was a popular treatment. Evaluating REM sleep-related penile erections served as an objective diagnostic technique to differentiate psychogenic from organic ED.
Gender dysphoria	Various	No systematic data
Disruptive, impulse-control, and conduct disorders	Various	No reliable systematic data
Substance-related and addictive disorders	Various substances	The stimulants amphetamine and cocaine decrease TST, REM sleep and NREM sleep. Provokes REM rebound (sometimes massive) during withdrawal. Many sedatives, hypnotics, and anxiolytic medications reduce N3 sleep and increase sleep spindle activity. In general, they shorten latency to sleep onset and increase sleep efficiency, some in the first half of the sleep episode. Sleep disturbances commonly return upon discontinuation. Alcohol can transiently increase N3 sleep early in the night and reduce REM sleep early in the sleep period; however, REM increases as alcohol blood level declines. Alcohol initially reduces wakefulness but during withdrawal it is associated with increased arousals Caffeine decreases TST and increases wakefulness awakenings, especially in the later part of the night. Small amounts of morning caffeine have no effect on sleep or sleep stages, but increase waking brainwaves (beta and gamma) during sleep. Tobacco increases sleep latency initially and during withdrawal Opioids can produce sedation but disturb sleep architecture, especially during withdrawal which is associated with REM and N3 rebound.
NCD	Alzheimer's disease	Decreased REM sleep Decreased eye movement density in REM sleep
	Parkinson's disease	Increased sleep latency Decreased TST and SEI Decreased N3 sleep, REM sleep, and REM latency Circadian rhythm disturbance and higher prevalence of sleep apnea noted
	NCD with Lewy bodies	Sleep-related movement disorders
	Traumatic brain injury	Mixed findings
	HIV infection	Decreased TST and SEI; longer sleep latency Increased N1 sleep. Increased N3 sleep in later part of night
	Huntington's disease	Decreased SEI, increased N1 sleep, decreased REM sleep and longer REM sleep latency PLMs and RBD also noted
PD	General	Decreased REM sleep latency
Paraphilic disorders	Various	No systematic data

[a]Sleep disorders are not necessarily psychiatric disorders; however, they are included because DSM is a widely used sleep disorders nosology.

ADHD, Attention-deficit/hyperactivity disorder; *ASD,* autism spectrum disorder; *CAP,* cyclic alternating pattern; *DSM,* Diagnostic and Statistical Manual; *ED,* erectile dysfunction; *MDD,* major depressive disorder; *NREM,* non-REM sleep; *NCD,* neurocognitive disorders; *PD,* personality disorders; *PSG,* polysomnography; *PLMs,* periodic leg movements; *PTSD,* posttraumatic stress disorder; *RBD,* REM behavior disorder; *RLS,* restless legs syndrome; *REM,* rapid eye movement; *SEI,* sleep efficiency index; *SRBD,* sleep-related breathing disorders; *TST,* total sleep time.

Polysomnographic Features Associated with Psychiatric Medications

- Many psychoactive substances used pharmacotherapeutically in psychiatry alter sleep continuity, integrity, and architecture.
- Many medications produce sedation as a main effect or as an unwanted side effect.
- Sedative hypnotic medications can alter sleep microarchitecture (e.g., benzodiazepines can greatly increase sleep spindle activity [Fig. 20.5]).
- Many medications reduce particular sleep stages (e.g., N3 and/or REM sleep).

- A small number of medications increase N3 sleep (sometimes indirectly by raising core body temperature).
- A small number of medications increase REM sleep (via pro-cholinergic mechanisms).
- Some antidepressants may worsen periodic leg movements in sleep (PLMS) (i.e., selective serotonin reuptake inhibitors), some may have particular propensity to worsen PLMS (venlafaxine), while others may be PLMS sparing (bupropion; Fig. 20.6).

Table 20.2 summarizes sleep alterations associated with commonly used psychiatric medications. It is also noted when a medication appears to provoke or exacerbate a sleep disorder or enhance the underlying pathophysiologies associated with a sleep disorder.[11,12]

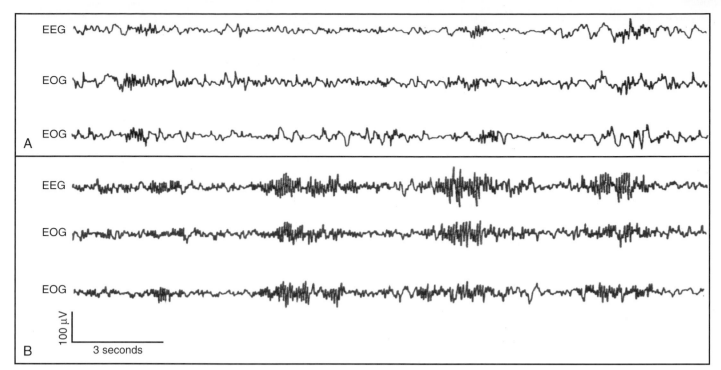

• **Figure 20.5** Polysomnographic Tracings Illustrating Normal and Excessive Spindle Activity. Polysomnographic tracings comparing normal sleep spindle electroencephalogram (EEG) activity during stage 2 sleep **(A)** with that of a patient chronically using a benzodiazepine **(B)**. This patient, who had been treated with benzodiazepines for more than a decade (and currently taking an extremely high dose), before being seen at the sleep disorders center. Sleep was grossly abnormal. The most obvious aberration was the tremendous increase in the frequency, magnitude, and duration of EEG spindle activity (see **B**). In addition, slow wave sleep was absent, stage 2 was grossly elevated, and spindles even intruded into rapid eye movement sleep. *EEG,* Electroencephalogram; *EOG,* electrooculogram. (From Hirshkowitz M, Seplowitz-Hafkin RG and Sharafkhaneh A, Sleep Disorders In: Sadock BJ, Sadock VA, Ruiz P (Eds.) Kaplan and Sadock's Comprehensive Textbook of Psychiatry, 9th edition. Philadelphia, PA: Lippincott Williams and Wilkins; 2009, page 2175.)

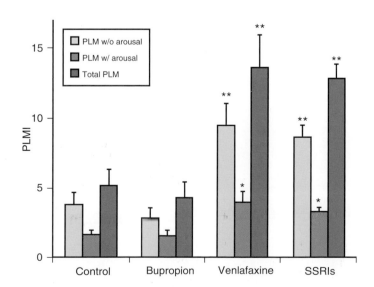

• **Figure 20.6** Comparison of Mean Periodic Leg Movement Index During Sleep by Group. Values indicate Mean ± SE. *PLMI,* Periodic leg movement index; *SE,* Standard error; *SSRIs,* selective serotonin reuptake inhibitors. *$P < .001$, control, bupropion versus venlafaxine, SSRIs; **$P < .0001$, control versus venlafaxine, SSRIs. (Reprinted by permission of Elsevier from Antidepressants and Periodic Leg Movements of Sleep, by Changkook Yang, David P. White, John W. Windelman, Biological Psychiatry, 58[6], 510–514, 2005 by the Society of Biological Psychiatry.)

Summary

In this chapter we reviewed the relationship between psychiatric disorders and sleep disturbances. The psychiatric and mental disorders span a wide range of illnesses. Using the *Diagnostic and Statistical Manual, 5th Edition*, nosology we summarized sleep symptoms and polysomnographic findings (where available) for each major classification from neurodevelopmental disorders to iatrogenic problems induced by medication. We also included a review of sleep alterations provoked by medications commonly used in psychiatry.

Suggested Reading

Hirshkowitz M, Rose MW, Sharafkhaneh A. Neurotransmitters, neurochemistry, and clinical pharmacology of sleep. In: Chokroverty S, ed. *Sleep Disorders Medicine: Basic Science Technical Considerations, and Clinical Aspects.* 3rd ed. Philadelphia, PA: Saunders Elsevier; 2009:67-79.

Krystal AD, Stein MB, Szabo ST. Anxiety disorders and posttraumatic stress disorder. In: Kryger MH, Roth T, Dement WC, eds. *Principles and Practice of Sleep Medicine.* 6th ed. Philadelphia, PA: Elsevier; 2017:1341-1351.

Lee-Chiong T. *Somnology 2.* CreateSpace Independent Publishing Platform; 1st ed. (August 28, 2011).

Reynolds CF, Kupfer DJ. Sleep research in affective illness: state of the art circa 1987. *Sleep.* 1987;10:199-215.

Sharafkhaneh A, Giray N, Richardson P, et al. Association of psychiatric disorders and sleep apnea in a large cohort. *Sleep.* 2005;28:1405-1411.

21

Sleep in Medical Disorders and Special Populations

QANTA A. AHMED, MICHAEL WEINSTEIN

O sleep, O gentle sleep, Nature's soft nurse, how have I frightened thee. That thou no more will weigh my eyelids down, And steep my senses in forgetfulness?

—WILLIAM SHAKESPEARE, *HENRY IV*, PART 2

Sleep Medicine: A New Clinical Frontier

Until 1973, when Stanford University declared the study of clinical sleep medicine a new field, our understanding of illness and health had been confined to the waking patient over centuries of medical study and practice. A mere 20 years after rapid eye movement (REM) sleep was first identified, clinical sleep medicine opened enquiry of both clinical physiology and pathology of the sleeping patient, creating new frontiers in the understanding of disease. In many respects, sleep medicine can be considered a new frontier.

While collective focus has been primarily on the physiology, circadian biology, and mechanisms of both normal sleep and primary sleep disorders themselves, insights into the impact of systemic disease on sleep and vice versa are only beginning to come into view.

- Sleep disorder specialists will encounter diverse patient populations in both adult and pediatric practice.
- Sleep disorder specialists must be familiar with sleep disorders in systemic disease and sleep disorders found in special populations.

- Knowledge of specific sleep disorders alone is not sufficient; their interaction and impact in the setting of systemic disease is critical to understanding both the sleep disorder and the systemic disease.
- Above all, sleep disorder specialists in their best capacities become experts informing the broad medical community; recognizing common sleep disorders in systemic medical disorders provides a vital education to other specialists who can then educate their own patient populations and other practitioners, raising awareness both of the nature of sleep disorders and their impacts on populations with specific medical conditions.

Sleep Is a Biological Necessity, Not an Expendable Luxury

Sleep deprivation is only recently recognized as a physiologic stressor. In the contemporary culture of "sleep machismo" defining postindustrial societies such as the United States, Japan, and Western Europe, society continues to see sleep as an expendable luxury rather than a biological necessity.[1]

- The pathophysiology of sleep deprivation was most emphatically shown in the landmark sleep deprivation studies performed by Rechtschaffen et al. using a rat model.
- Rats were placed on rotating platforms suspended in water tanks. When sleepy, the rat would fall into the water, requiring it to wake and return to the platform.
- Sustained sleep was thus impossible. The findings have become sentinel indicators of the pathology of sleep deprivation.
- Within several weeks total sleep deprivation resulted in the death of all rat subjects.
- Prior to death, rats demonstrated weight loss despite hyperphagia.
- Skin lesions on both the fur of the body and the tail suggested breakdown of host immunity; lesions in the gastrointestinal tract were also noted.
- Prior to death, rats lost thermoregulatory control developing hypothermia. Further enquiry suggested the rats died of complications of sepsis underlining the fatal impact on host immunity.

Rechtschaffen's investigations were among the first and most emphatic confirming that sleep is a biological necessity and that sleep deprivation, whether total or chronic partial deprivation, posed a serious risk for basic metabolic function. Bacterial invasion and gastrointestinal erosions seen in the rats prior to death mimic the findings of many critically ill patients in intensive care units—environments notorious for sleep deprivation—who go on to die of sepsis and multiorgan failure.

Sleep Deprivation Has Increased Over the 20th Century

- With the advent of electricity, the average major sleep period has diminished by approximately 20% in the last century because of the inexorable advance of a 24/7 culture. Consequences can be physiologically catastrophic for the individual and societally for the community.
- Notorious public health disasters have been caused by sleep deprivation. The Exxon Valdez oil spill (often wrongly attributed to the inebriation of the captain) was due to the sleep-deprived shipmate who assumed control of the doomed vessel because of the captain's inebriation.
- On March 28, 1979, at the Three Mile Island Plant Unit 2 Reactor in Pennsylvania, shift workers on duty between the 4 AM and 6 AM hour failed to recognize and react to the lack of core coolant, which had been obstructed by a defective valve. While the mechanical problem of a dysfunctional valve was to blame for the near meltdown, Mitler and colleagues determined it was worker fatigue and sleep loss that resulted in the human error of omission and risked a catastrophic accident with untold public health effects.
- Much more common than meltdowns in nuclear reactors are motor vehicle accidents. We examine the impact of sleep disorders and sleep deprivation in the commercial driver—and by extension all drivers—later in this chapter. With the high prevalence of driving in the United States, sleepy driving poses a tremendous public health burden: the National Transportation Safety Board estimates more than 100,000 motor vehicle accidents each year can be attributed to drowsiness at the wheel or "fatigue."

Sleep Disorders Are Highly Prevalent

While sleep deprivation is widely experienced in both adult and pediatric populations, *primary sleep disorders themselves* are extremely common.

- The recently revised International Classification of Sleep Disorders (ICSD-3) includes 74 sleep-related disorders, including "sleep-related medical and neurologic disorders."[2]
- While most people will experience insomnia occasionally, more than one in three adults regard their insomnia as significant and problematic and, of these, more than half report it to be serious in nature.
- Similarly, snoring is so prevalent that many sufferers consider it a normal variant and fail to seek medical attention, even when it frequently impacts the bed partner's sleep.
- Obstructive sleep apnea (OSA) syndrome by some studies may affect as many as 1 in 4 Americans, largely consequent to the obesity pandemic.
- Restless legs syndrome, with an estimated prevalence of 5%–10%, likewise, is highly prevalent but underdiagnosed.

Sleep Disorders in Systemic Disease Are Common and Numerous

The ICSD-3 includes six conditions under the heading of "sleep-related medical and neurological disorders":

- Fatal familial insomnia
- Sleep-related epilepsy
- Sleep-related headaches
- Sleep-related laryngospasm
- Sleep-related gastroesophageal reflux
- Sleep-related myocardial ischemia
- These disorders are distinct from primary sleep disorders, which can coexist with medical disorders.
- Common sleep disorders can have systemic manifestations that may contribute to the pathophysiology of underlying medical conditions.[3]
- The impact of medical treatments for systemic disorders on sleep quality and physiology must be considered in evaluating the patient's complaints.

TABLE 21.1	General Medical Causes of Hypersomnolence

Hepatic, renal or respiratory failure
Electrolyte disturbances
Congestive cardiac failure
Severe anemia
Endocrinological disease: acromegaly, hypothyroidism, Addison's disease
Diabetes mellitus—both hypoglycemia and hyperglycemia

Presentation of the Medical Patient with Sleep Disturbances and Sleep Disorders

- Most patients with medical disorders will present to the sleep medicine physician with reports of insomnia and/or hypersomnolence.
- Insomnia is defined as difficulty initiating or maintaining sleep, early morning awakening, or nonrestorative sleep.
- More than one manifestation of insomnia may be present in a patient.
- Hypersomnolence may be consequent to the insomnia due to sleep deprivation or a medication effect, or may be related to an underlying sleep disorder. Medical causes of hypersomnolence are listed in Table 21.1.

Considering Sleep in Specific Systemic Diseases

Sleep and Pain

- There is a complex interrelationship between pain and sleep that is frequently neglected by clinicians.
- Imaging studies for pain and sleep reveal considerable overlap in the neuromatrix of pain (Figs. 21.1 and 21.2).
- Many Americans experience sleep disruption related to chronic pain disorders.
- A 1996 National Sleep Foundation survey found 56 million Americans reporting chronic pain interfering with sleep onset or sleep maintenance.
- Next day pain was associated with either less than 6 hours of sleep the night before or more than 9 hours of sleep.
- Sleep deprivation has been found to be predictive of hyperalgesia in carefully designed experiments on normal subjects—that is, subjects without chronic pain disorders—suggesting that consolidated sleep and adequate sleep may be analgesic.[4]
- Chronic partial sleep deprivation caused by painful syndromes may result in hyperalgesia, exacerbating those painful syndromes.
- The interaction between pain and sleep is bidirectional and reinforcing.
- Pain interferes with and fragments sleep; fragmented sleep escalates painful disorders due to the hyperalgesic impact of fragmented sleep.
- Assessing patients with painful disorders for primary sleep disorders is therefore important to search for reversible causes of sleep fragmentation, which can increase sleep consolidation and not only improve insomnia but have a positive impact on the primary pain disorder.

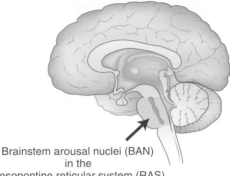

Two key sleep-wake centers

Brainstem arousal nuclei (BAN) in the Mesopontine reticular system (RAS)
1. Locus ceruleus (LC)
2. Dorsal raphe nuclei (DRN)
3. Pedunculopontine tegmentum (PPT)

• **Figure 21.1** The Brainstem Arousal Nuclei in the Mesopontine Reticular Activating System (RAS). The area of the brainstem arousal nuclei and the neurotransmitters associated with the brainstem arousal nuclei subnuclei that are also active in pain modulation. (From Merrill RL. Orofacial pain and sleep. *Sleep Med Clin*. 2010;5[1]:131–144.)

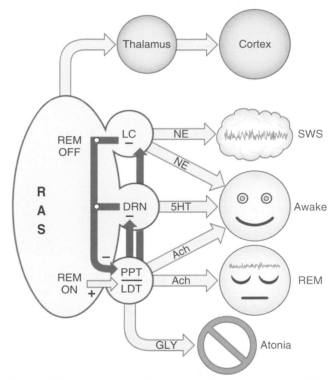

• **Figure 21.2** Reticular Activating System Neurotransmitters of Sleep and Pain. The reticular activating system (RAS) oversees the wakefulness state through activity of four subnuclei: (1) the locus ceruleus (LC), which releases norepinephrine; (2) the dorsal raphe nuclei (DRN), which release serotonin (5HT); (3) the pedunculopontine (PPT); and (4) the laterodorsal tegmentum (LDT), which are associated with acetylcholine (Ach). The PPT-LDT neurons are active not only in wakefulness but also in REM sleep, and are thought to be the REM on-switch. Lesions in the PPT-LDT area do not affect wakefulness but lead to loss of REM sleep. SWS is modulated through LC and DRN by decreasing the release of NE. Wakefulness is achieved through the combined activity of the PPT, LC, and DRN nuclei releasing Ach, norepinephrine, and serotonin, respectively. The primary neurotransmitter of REM is Ach. SWS is achieved through suppression of the wakefulness neurotransmitters NE and 5HT and release of Ach. (From Merrill RL. Orofacial pain and sleep. *Sleep Med Clin*. 2010;5[1]:131–144.)

- A sizeable proportion of patients with chronic pain are found to have disrupted sleep, with estimates ranging from 50%–80%, suggesting that all patients with chronic pain disorders should have a careful sleep history and, based on the findings, referral for formal sleep evaluation.
- Furthermore, many of these patients will have primary sleep disorders, including restless legs syndrome, periodic limb movement disorder, and obstructive sleep apnea syndrome.

Sleep and Orofacial Pain

Orofacial pain syndromes comprise head, neck, and temporomandibular pain syndromes, all of which are commonly encountered in a sleep medicine practice.[5,6]
- Patients with orofacial pain syndromes are likely to have sleep disruption. Often these patients present after long and complex evaluations with other specialists before referral for sleep consultation.
- Patients frequently experience more than one orofacial pain syndrome at once.
- Proximity to the brain, and the intense innervation of the face and head, may lead these syndromes to cause severe pain and severe sleep disruption, resulting in marked morbidity.

Sleep and Headache Disorders

- Obstructive sleep apnea syndrome is associated with both early morning headaches noted on awakening and sleep-related headaches that can interrupt the major sleep period.
- These headaches resolve on treatment of underlying sleep-disordered breathing. Headaches occurring during the night are frequently associated with a primary sleep disorder and should be quickly referred for sleep medicine evaluation.

Sleep and Temporomandibular Joint Disorders Disorders

- An expert sleep history always entails taking a detailed dental history.
- Extraction of wisdom teeth, orthodontic work including braces, and other clues that malocclusion was corrected suggest an anatomically crowded airway.
- In our practice, we customarily enquire about all of the previously listed items as well as bruxism, a history of which can be elicited by a prior dental diagnosis (including treatment with an oral bruxism guard), morning jaw pain or dental pain, or overt sounds of bruxism observed by a family member or bed partner.
 Temporomandibular joint (TMJ) disorders can be considered in three distinct categories:
- Mechanical disruption of the TMJ
- Problems related to the muscles around the TMJ
- Arthritides impacting the TMJ
 Masticatory muscles can become painful due to the preferred sleeping position.
- Patients with untreated sleep-disordered breathing often prefer sleeping in the decubitus position or even prone position.
- A nonsupine position can aggravate masticatory pain and TMJ pain due to pressure on the dependent TMJ and jaw.

- Patients may note morning "locked" jaw on mouth opening, which resolves shortly after awakening.
- TMJ arthritis is also common and can be exacerbated by decubitus sleeping.
- Some patients are predisposed to TMJ *disc dislocation.*
- Supine sleeping precipitates disc dislocation, since jaw muscles relax with onset of sleep, allowing the jaw to slide posteriorly due to gravity.
- On awakening, jaw locking on mouth opening follows, which is in general a temporary condition, but one that may eventually need the intervention of a TMJ specialist.
 Bruxism is a parafunctional jaw behavior related to TMJ and is defined as a sleep-related non-REM sleep parasomnia.
- Bruxism is so common it is considered a "parafunction," affecting approximately 1 in 10 in the general population, but its impacts are considerable.
- Patients are most often identified by dentists who recognize abnormal tooth wear, abfractures (dental enamel fractures), dental hypersensitivity, and (on interview) masticatory muscle discomfort, pain, and temporomandibular disorders.
- Despite its extensive prevalence and morbidity, etiology and mechanisms of bruxism remain unknown.
- Polysomnographic findings are characterized by repetitive jaw muscle contractions, termed rhythmic masticatory muscle activity (RMMA).
- RMMA consists either of a series of repetitive contractions (phasic muscle contractions) or sustained jaw clenching (tonic contractions).
- Contractions are typically associated with tooth-grinding sounds, the history of which can often be elicited from a bed partner as well as being recorded on video PSG.
- Some patients will present with bruxism and obstructive sleep apnea. Treatment of the obstructive sleep apnea syndrome often improves bruxism symptoms.
- Bruxism can be seen in the setting of sleep-related GERD, and treatment of GERD has been reported to improve symptoms of sleep bruxism[7] (Fig. 21.3).

Sleep and the Eye

The eye is well known to exhibit signs and impacts of systemic disease, but few recognize the specific association of disorders of the eye with disorders of sleep.
- OSA has been associated with the following conditions:
  - Floppy eyelid syndrome
  - Preglaucoma
  - Glaucoma
  - Nonarteritic anterior ischemic optic neuropathy
- Sleep specialists should seek out expert ophthalmologic and oculoplastic consultation to facilitate diagnosis and management of these disorders.
- Conversely, ophthalmologists must be aware of the association of specific eye disorders with OSA.
- The most commonly encountered eye disorder in a sleep medicine practice is floppy eyelid syndrome.

Sleep and Floppy Eyelid Syndrome

See Fig. 21.4.
- Floppy eyelid syndrome refers to an abnormal laxity of the eyelid leading to pseudoptosis, reduced peripheral vision, and

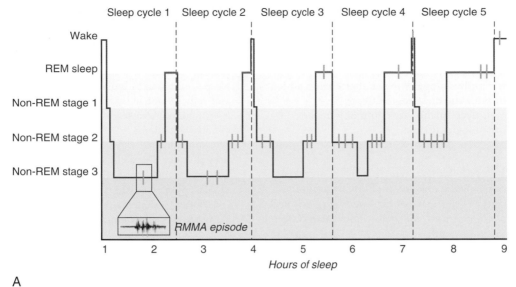

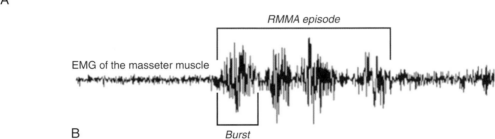

• **Figure 21.3** Hypnogram Representing the Schematic Distribution Over the Sleep Cycles of Rhythmic Masticatory Muscle Activity (RMMA) Episodes. **A,** A full-night hypnogram showing the sleep stage distribution over five non–rapid eye movement (REM)/REM sleep cycles. Green vertical lines represent episodes of RMMA. As schematically displayed, RMMA episodes are observed more frequently during non-REM sleep stages 1 and 2, sleep stage shift, and pre-REM sleep periods. **B,** Example of an RMMA episode, defined on the masseter and/or temporalis electromyographic channels as an activity of at least three consecutive electromyographic bursts (frequency 1 Hz) lasting ≥0.25 sec. (From Carra MC, Huynh, N, Fleury B, Lavigne G. Overview on Sleep Bruxism for Sleep Medicine Clinicians. *Sleep Med Clin.* 2015;10[3]:375–384.)

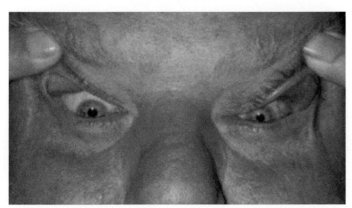

• **Figure 21.4** Rubbery, floppy, and easily everted upper eyelids in a patient with floppy eyelid syndrome. (From Leibovitch I, Selva D. Floppy eyelid syndrome: clinical features and the association with obstructive sleep apnea. *Sleep Med.* 2006;7[2]:117–122.)

propensity for eye irritation, episcleritis, foreign body sensation, and eye trauma, due to an inefficient eyelid that can no longer effectively protect the globe during wake or sleep.[8]
• Patients may be unaware of their symptoms until these findings are noted for them during careful interviews.

• On later questioning, patients recall they may raise their eyebrows for photographs and they may notice a familial preference for cosmetic blepharoplasty—with the suggestion that floppy eyelid syndrome may cluster in family members.

The pathophysiology of floppy eyelid syndrome is incompletely understood, but there is a remarkable association with OSA, with an estimated 21%–100% of patients with floppy eyelids having OSA.
• An increase in matrix metalloproteinases has been noted, possibly precipitated by recurrent hypoxemia, and may account for the loss of elastic tissue.[9] Histopathologic studies of floppy eyelid syndrome patients reveal depleted levels of elastin within the tarsal plate of the eyelid, in the skin of the eyelid and adjacent to the lash roots.
• Recognition of floppy eyelid syndrome should prompt screening and referral for the evaluation of sleep-disordered breathing.
• Treatment consists of therapeutic blepharoplasty to restore peripheral vision and treatment of underlying obstructive sleep apnea syndrome.
• Referral to an ophthalmologist for floppy eyelid syndrome in our practice has also resulted in early diagnosis of silent retinal detachment in evolution, saving one patient's vision.

Sleep and Autoimmune Rheumatic Disease

Autoimmune rheumatologic diseases are characterized by multisystem involvement and defined immunologic abnormalities, often with overlapping clinical and immunological features.

- Sleep deprivation is a physiologic stressor that creates added impact on the host with rheumatologic disease.
- Fatigue and impaired sleep quality are commonly reported by patients with rheumatologic disease.
- An assessment of sleep is helpful to identify treatment opportunities.
- Patients frequently report fatigue, which is often mistakenly ascribed to the primary rheumatologic condition or medications used in its treatment before searches for underlying primary sleep disorders are commenced and before preventable sleep deprivation has been addressed.

Commonly encountered rheumatologic conditions include:

- Rheumatoid arthritis
- Sjogren's syndrome
- Systemic lupus erythematosus
- Fibromyalgia

Activation of the immune system may exert impacts on sleep.[10]

- Various peptides have been found to exercise immune-modulatory impact on sleep, including alpha interferon (IFNalpha), tumor necrosis factor (TNF), interleukins IL-1 and IL2, vasoactive peptides, and prostaglandins.
- Cellular, humoral, and natural killer cell immunity are altered during sleep.
- Sleep-deprived animal models have increased circulatory levels of corticosteroids and sleep-deprived adults demonstrate exaggerated morning cortisol levels without afternoon dip, mimicking aging, both suggesting that sleep loss directly impacts the hypothalamic pituitary axis.

See Table 21.2.

Sleep and Systemic Lupus Erythematosus

Sleep and systemic lupus erythematosus (SLE) patients frequently report nonrefreshing sleep and sleep disturbance, in addition to frequent reports of fatigue.

- Sleep disorders and sleep-related complaints are more common in the SLE patient than in the general population.

Fatigue correlates strongly with disability and poor quality of life in the SLE patient, emphasizing the importance of identifying sleep disorders and sleep-related problems in this population, as treatment may diminish disabilities and morbidities.

- Sleep complaints are common in the SLE population.
- Cross-sectional data of a series of 129 SLE patients showed 72% to report poor sleep quality and more than 37% reporting fatigue.
- Valencia-Flores et al. studied patients with validated questionnaires and polysomnography, finding that SLE patients experienced more sleep interruptions and sleep stage shifting, and

were objectively sleepier in the daytime than normative controls.

- Disease activity correlated with declining sleep measures—reduced sleep efficiency, reduced N3 sleep, and increased sleep fragmentation, all correlating with increased disease activity.
- Sleep disorders in SLE may also correlate with increasing dyspnea and reflux esophagitis severity.

It is important to assess the SLE patient's symptoms both during sleep and wakefulness.

- Screening for obstructive sleep apnea syndrome and other primary sleep disorders should be aggressively pursued in the SLE patient.
- Untreated obstructive sleep apnea syndrome can dramatically increase sleep-related GERD, increase acid contact time, and contribute to sleep fragmentation.
- Eliminating factors contributing to sleep-related GERD in the SLE patient can improve quality of life and mitigate risks of Barrett's esophagus and bronchospasm caused by chronic GERD.

Sleep and Osteoarthritis

Osteoarthritis is a common condition that increases in prevalence with age.

- Patients frequently experience nighttime awakenings attributed to joint pain but often do not self-report, assuming this to be part of the normal disease process.
- Osteoarthritis patients have more frequent sleep stage shifts on polysomnography, more arousals, and more nocturnal awakenings during sleep. Treatment of the underlying arthropathy improves sleep.
- Patients frequently report sleep quality improving after joint replacement.
- Patients with osteoarthritis should be screened for commonly occurring sleep disorders, which can contribute to nocturnal sleep disruption; this may improve quality of sleep and daytime function. Improvement of sleep may also favorably impact the perception of pain, extensive investigations showing consolidated sleep to exert an analgesic effect, and sleep deprivation to lower pain threshold.

Sleep and Rheumatoid Arthritis

While many sleep disorders can coexist with rheumatoid arthritis (RA), including insomnia, obstructive sleep apnea, sleep-related GERD, periodic limb movement disorder, and others, more than one in three patients meets diagnostic criteria for restless legs syndrome (RLS).

Physicians frequently overlook this diagnosis. RA patients can distinguish typical RA symptoms from RLS symptoms. Symptoms of RLS in the RA patient are as reported in all RLS patients.

Four features should be confirmed on careful interview, and serial interview may be necessary (Table 21.3).

Sleep and Fibromyalgia

Fibromyalgia syndrome (FMS) is characterized by diffuse myalgias and pains unrelated to specific diseases of the joints bones or connective tissue.

- Pathognomonic of FMS are bilateral tender points elicited on examination. Common sites include the neck and shoulder joints, and sacrospinal and gluteal regions.
- Patients often report daytime fatigue and insomnia including nonrefreshing sleep and sleep maintenance insomnia.

TABLE 21.2	Sleep and Autoimmune Disease

Sleep deprivation is common in autoimmune rheumatologic disease
Sleep deprivation can trigger cytokine and antibody production
Sleep deprivation correlates with disease activity in autoimmune diseases

TABLE 21.3	Pathognomonic Features of Restless Legs Syndrome

Urge to move the legs—usually associated with a difficult to articulate sensation of discomfort in lower extremities

Circadian distribution of symptoms with worsening in the early to late evening

Onset or worsening of symptoms at rest or inactivity

Relief of discomfort with movement

TABLE 21.4	Conditions Associated with Alpha Delta Sleep

Fibromyalgia

Other rheumatologic conditions

Chronic fatigue syndrome

Chronic pain syndrome

Postviral syndromes, febrile individuals

Temporal lobe epilepsy

Psychiatric disorders

Major depressive disorder, schizophrenia, schizoaffective disorder, narcotic addiction

Normal variant in patients without medical comorbidities

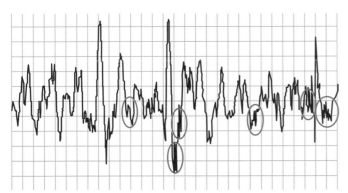

Alpha intrusions in SWS

• **Figure 21.5** Alpha Intrusions Into Slow Wave Sleep (SWS). This figure shows alpha wave intrusions circled in the pattern of slow wave sleep. The alpha intrusions represent cortical arousal activity in response to sleep-disturbing signals. (From Merrill RL. Orofacial pain and sleep. *Sleep Med Clin.* 2010;5[1]:131–144.)

- Polysomnography shows reduced sleep efficiency increased sleep fragmentation and increased wake after sleep onset.

Intriguingly, FMS is one of the few medical conditions with a characteristic, *though nonspecific*, finding on polysomnography: "alpha-sleep" (originally described as "alpha-delta sleep").[11,12]

- Alpha wave activity, measured at 8–12 Hz frequency, is characteristic of relaxed wakefulness.
- Alpha activity is enhanced when individuals close their eyes and the occipital region loses visual stimulus.
- Alpha-delta sleep is the intrusion of an alpha wave electroencephalogram (EEG) pattern on an established slow wave sleep pattern.
- While not pathognomonic for FMS (alpha sleep is found in other disorders as well as in familial clusters), alpha delta sleep is seen more often in fibromyalgia than any other condition (Table 21.4 and Figs. 21.3 and 21.5).

Other conditions in which alpha-delta sleep has been reported include:
- Neuro-psychiatric conditions
  - Schizophrenia
  - Depression
  - Schizoaffective disorder
  Alpha-delta sleep can also be seen in:
- Narcotic addiction
- Seizure disorders in the form of temporal epilepsy
- Chronic fatigue syndrome
- Chronic pain syndromes

Alpha wave intrusion correlates with pain severity, suggesting a potential role as a surrogate in determining response to therapy (Fig. 21.6).

Sleep and the Endocrine System

The endocrine system is composed of specialized organs or glands that secrete hormones directly into the circulation. These hormones are critical in maintaining growth essential hormonal function and metabolic homeostasis.

- Sleep is a key influence on human homeostasis and impacts hormone secretion by imposing a circadian rhythmicity on hormone release determined by the body's internal clock, the suprachiasmatic nucleus.
- Sleep and the endocrine system are closely interlinked.
- Disorders of the endocrine system frequently present with sleep and/or daytime fatigue symptoms, rendering it important to consider primary sleep disorders and sleep deprivation as possible contributors to these symptoms.
- These patients may present initially to the sleep disorders specialist before diagnosis of an endocrine disorder is considered.

Sleep and Thyroid Disease

Hyper- or hypothyroidism may cause systemic metabolic dysfunction.

- Patients with thyroid disease report fatigue, diminished mental acuity, and somnolence, among other systemic manifestations.
- Severe hypothyroidism can cause myxedema coma, which presents with profound coma and obtundation, typically preceded by progressive and severe hypersomnolence.
- The hyperthyroid patient may present with agitation, anxiety, and sleep initiation and sleep maintenance insomnia.
- Patients may report nocturnal palpitations contributing to the complaint of "insomnia."
  Thyroid disease can also impact the airway mechanically.
- Less commonly, sleep can be disturbed by the mechanical effects of an enlarged thyroid (goiter), with patients reporting symptoms of positional apnea, which is typically worse in the supine position and relieved by assuming the decubitus position.
- Complications from thyroid surgery can also alter upper airway anatomy and sometimes contribute to the development of symptoms of obstructive sleep apnea syndrome.
  Thyroxine supplementation can cause sleep disruption.
- Patients can present with insomnia in relation to initiation of supplemental thyroxine akin to findings associated with hyperthyroidism.
- Sleep onset insomnia is more common than sleep maintenance insomnia.

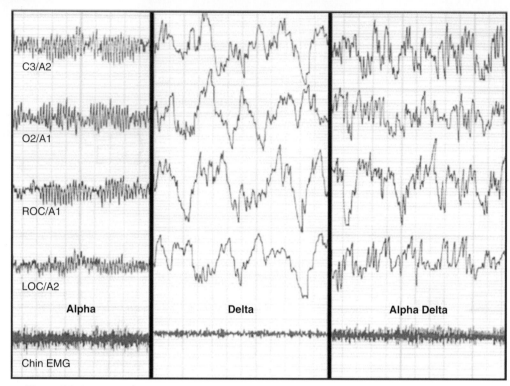

• **Figure 21.6** Three consecutive representative polygraph samples displaying awake, δ sleep and α-EEG sleep (i.e., α intrusion in δ sleep). (From Rains JC, Penzien DB. Sleep and chronic pain: challenges to the α-EEG sleep pattern as a pain specific sleep anomaly. *J Psychosom Res*. 2003;54[1]:77–83.)

- Excess thyroid hormone can trigger symptoms of restless leg syndrome in association with increased agitation and restlessness.
- Symptoms resolve with adjustment of thyroxine dose, although occasionally insomnia can become chronic and require additional behavioral and pharmacological therapies.

Sleep and the Pituitary Gonadal and Adrenal Axis

Adrenal insufficiency, whether primary or secondary (from pituitary failure), causes fatigue, lethargy, and hypersomnolence. Once replacement therapy is commenced, symptoms resolve and carefully adjusted steroid replacement therapy is required chronically. Pituitary insufficiency causes numerous hormonal disorders, including secondary adrenal failure, secondary hypothyroidism, growth hormone deficiency, secondary hypogonadism, and diabetes inspidus.

- Most of these disorders are associated with fatigue and sleep disruption.
- In diabetes inspidus, polyuria causes nocturnal awakenings and sleep deprivation, mandating appropriate intervention with desmopressin to consolidate nighttime sleep.

Hypogonadism may be either primary or secondary and may impact men or women.

- Hypogonadism is associated with reduced lethargy and fatigue.
- With the availability of FDA-approved testosterone replacement therapy, clinician and patient awareness of the possibility of low testosterone levels has grown.

- Patients diagnosed with low testosterone should be screened for obstructive sleep apnea syndrome, which is a well-documented cause of reversible central hypogonadism.
- Treatment of obstructive sleep apnea syndrome improves endogenous testosterone levels; however, replacement therapy should not be commenced until underlying obstructive sleep apnea syndrome has been treated, since untreated sleep-disordered breathing may be worsened by testosterone administration.

Sleep and Acromegaly

Acromegaly is the clinical syndrome resulting from excessive endogenous growth hormone secretion. Acromegaly is associated with distinctive physical findings, including elongated digits, coarsening of the facial features associated with frontal bossing, and other features.

- Acromegaly predisposes to obstructive sleep apnea syndrome as a result of associated macroglossia, elongation, redundancy, and thickening of the soft palate, swelling and thickening of the pharyngeal walls, and thickening of both the true and false vocal cords.
- Craniofacial abnormalities that continue throughout life result in an increased longitudinal axis of the face with excessive vertical growth, resulting in more posterior tongue position, further narrowing the upper airway. Increased inferiority of the hyoid bone adds to the destabilization of the upper airway.
- High prevalence of obstructive sleep apnea is noted in the acromegaly population, with clinical features of snoring and daytime sleepiness noted as early as the late 1800s—almost a century before obstructive sleep apnea was recognized as a clinical syndrome.

- Australian data suggest that more than 60% of acromegalic patients have obstructive sleep apnea syndrome; in the same population, 33% were found to have central sleep apnea syndrome, likely related to increased hypercapnic ventilatory response.[13]
- Even after treatment, whether surgical with transphenoidal hypophysectomy with or without radiation or with octreotide, prevalence of obstructive sleep apnea syndrome remains high at 20% (and central sleep apnea seems to persist), likely related to irreversible anatomic, ventilatory, and craniofacial changes.

Sleep and Diabetes Mellitus

Diabetes mellitus is not directly linked to sleep disorders, but symptoms of uncontrolled diabetes can disrupt sleep due to both polyuria and polydipsia. Nocturnal awakenings associated with hypoglycemia can manifest with diaphoresis, nausea, pallor, and weakness. Patients with brittle diabetes may seek to preempt these episodes of hypoglycemia and set their alarm for deliberate awakenings to check their glucose level, and perhaps to eat, in addition to disrupting sleep. Judicious management of medications and nutrition can greatly impact sleep in patients with diabetes.

Sleep, insulin, and glucose control are tightly linked and easily disrupted by stressors.

- Sleep deprivation promotes insulin resistance and elevated circulating glucose levels. This is the likely mechanism for insulin resistance seen in the untreated obstructive sleep apnea patient.
- Decreased glucose tolerance is noted during sleep—a protective mechanism perhaps to avert nocturnal hypoglycemia.
- Reduced glucose tolerance during sleep is due to decreased cerebral glucose utilization, reduced utilization of glucose by muscle tissue, and the antiinsulin effects of the release of growth hormone that is tightly coupled to slow wave sleep.
- Insulin sensitivity improves close to the end of the major sleep period, due to increased metabolism during wakefulness and REM sleep, which increases in percentage toward the end of the major sleep period.

Sleep in Pulmonary Overlap Syndromes

The term "pulmonary overlap syndrome" (OVS) was first used in reference to patients with comorbid COPD and obstructive sleep apnea syndrome, though now the definition is extended to patients with comorbid obstructive sleep apnea syndrome and other chronic lung diseases, including interstitial lung disease.[14]

- A distinct definition remains lacking, and the patient population with OVS remains diverse, encompassing both chronic lung disease and obstructive sleep apnea syndrome of any severity, both of which span a broad spectrum.
- The current definitions of obstructive sleep apnea syndrome may be insufficiently rigorous for assessing obstructive sleep apnea in the setting of chronic hypoxemic lung disease, particularly as obstructive sleep apnea syndrome is defined by specific desaturation criteria and distinguishing hypoxemia due to chronic lung disease from concurrent sleep-disordered breathing event may be difficult.
- Basic interactions between chronic obstructive pulmonary disease (COPD) and OSA syndrome are not completely understood, including, for example, the full spectrum of effects of COPD on upper airway collapsibility.
  Therapeutic goals for these patients are undefined.
- Most practitioners seek to eliminate sleep-disordered breathing both by objective criteria as well as by patient-defined outcomes

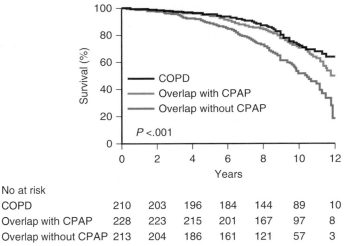

No at risk							
COPD	210	203	196	184	144	89	10
Overlap with CPAP	228	223	215	201	167	97	8
Overlap without CPAP	213	204	186	161	121	57	3

• **Figure 21.7** Kaplan-Meier Survival Curves for Patients with COPD. Patients with OVS on CPAP, and patients with OVS not on CPAP. Treatment with CPAP seems to prevent against the excess mortality in patients with OVS. Note these data are observational. (From Dudley KA, Owens RL, Malhotra A. Pulmonary overlap syndromes, with a focus on COPD and ILD. *Sleep Med Clin.* 2014;9[3]:365–379.)

of sleep satisfaction and improved quality of life, much the same as we seek in other patient populations. While patients with severe COPD may benefit from treatment with bilevel positive airway pressure due to improvement in nocturnal ventilation, for other patients conventional treatment with CPAP may be adequate.

- Nonetheless, despite these unknowns, it is important to recognize patterns of sleep and sleep disorders in this patient population, which will be readily encountered in any sleep disorders' medicine practice due to the widespread prevalence of both obstructive sleep apnea and COPD (Fig. 21.7).

Sleep and COPD

A majority of patients with COPD report sleep difficulties, in part due to nocturnal symptoms of their respiratory disease—nocturnal cough, dyspnea and wheezing—and also because of coexisting sleep disorders in the form of insomnia, sleep-disordered breathing, movement disorders, and other abnormalities.

- Clinical insomnia is very common in the COPD patient population, and sleep symptoms are typically chronic and longstanding.
- As COPD disease severity increases, insomnia complaints worsen.
- Sleep architecture is objectively seen to change in severe COPD patients with reduced sleep efficiency, delayed sleep latency at sleep onset, increased wakefulness after sleep onset (WASO), increased arousals, nocturnal awakenings, diminished REM sleep, increased N1 and N2 sleep, reduced N3 sleep, and more frequent sleep stage transitions and EEG arousals.
- COPD patients have been found to have a high prevalence of RLS; more than one-third of patients with COPD report RLS symptoms, and frequent periodic limb movements have also been found in these patients. Treatment with dopaminergic agents is effective as in other patient populations. Sedative hypnotics can provide relief and may improve sleep initiation and maintenance difficulties, but may worsen nocturnal hypoventilation and oxygenation and should be used with caution.

Sleep and Interstitial Lung Disease

Interstitial lung disease (ILD) includes a diverse array of lung disorders characterized by restrictive lung physiology.
ILDs include:
- Idiopathic pulmonary fibrosis
- Sarcoidosis
- Autoimmune-related pulmonary disorders such as systemic sclerosis and hypersensitivity pneumonitis or restrictive lung disease following drug exposure such as amiodarone
- Sleep has been most widely examined among these conditions in the setting of idiopathic pulmonary fibrosis (IPF).

Sleep and Idiopathic Pulmonary Fibrosis

IPF is, by definition, without known cause, characterized by a chronic and unremitting course with episodes of relapses—acute exacerbations and associated acute decline in lung function interspersed with periods of stability. Prognosis tends to be very poor. Histologically these patients are defined by findings of usual interstitial pneumonitis. Unlike COPD, IPF is relatively uncommon, rendering investigation of sleep and sleep disorders more difficult.
- Patients with IPF report impaired sleep quality, excessive daytime sleepiness, increased sleep maintenance insomnia, reduced sleep efficiency, reduced total sleep time, and reduced REM sleep percentages.
- Nocturnal cough maybe a prime contributor to sleep disruption, as well as the impact of medications, including corticosteroids, which are well known to cause insomnia. Comorbid depression and other affective disorders are commonly seen in the IPF patient, which further impacts sleep and increases likelihood of insomnia.
- Medications used to treat these comorbid affective disorders may further impact daytime function and increase daytime sleepiness.
- Sleep-disordered breathing is found to be extremely prevalent in the IPF patient population; reports range from more than two-thirds of all patients to more than 90% of patients studied.[15]
- Patients are noted to have nocturnal tachypnea in IPF compared with normal controls. Nocturnal desaturations during sleep can be more severe than the desaturations seen during exercise, suggesting that sleep is a major stressor to the IPF patient.
- If challenged with obstructive sleep apnea syndrome, in addition, sleep in the IPF patient can become severely disrupted.
- Treatment goals remain the same as treatment of other patients with obstructive sleep apnea, and improving sleep quality in these patients offers a chance to reduce morbidity for patients with a poor long-term prognosis and escalating short term morbidities.

Sleep and Chronic Kidney Disease

Patients with chronic kidney disease commonly report fatigue and exhibit specific sleep disorders, particularly when dialysis dependent.
- Insomnia is the most common finding, but daytime sleepiness, typically multifactorial, can also be present.
- Daytime sleepiness is multifactorial.
  - Often daytime sleepiness is due to untreated primary sleep disorders, including obstructive sleep apnea syndrome, periodic limb movement disorder, and restless leg syndrome
  - Daytime sleepiness can also be behavioral due to early morning dialysis sessions and the long journeys required to reach the dialysis center, resulting in sleep deprivation.
- Adequate sleep hygiene is critical, and effort should be made to arrange for the patient's travel to the dialysis center to be as unobtrusive as possible to the major sleep period.
- Careful sleep evaluation can elucidate primary sleep disorders, though secondary RLS is best treated by treating the underlying renal disease, anemia, and iron deficiency.
- Treatment of RLS with dopaminergic medications is effective and may also help ameliorate symptoms of periodic limb movement disorder, but requires adjustment of dosing.
- Hypersomnolence in these patients should always raise the suspicion for uremia and also evolving sepsis, both of which could be life threatening if unrecognized, though common causes including medications and sleep-disordered breathing are more often the culprits.

Fatigue in the chronic kidney disease patient is often multifactorial and needs to be distinguished from hypersomnolence clinically and sometimes even objectively.

Table 21.5 lists the common causes of fatigue in the CKD patient.

Sleep and Gastrointestinal Disease

GERD is a common disorder impacting up to 20% of Americans.
- The vast majority of these patients—more than 74%—will experience nocturnal symptoms reporting impaired sleep with subsequent daytime impact.
- Reflux during sleep is not as well recognized by patients, as waking symptoms of GERD and sleep pose *increased risk* for GERD, with reduced acid clearance times, reduced swallowing frequency, and reduced frequency of peristalsis, mechanical disadvantages of the recumbent position, and suppression of salivation.
- Longer durations of reflux are associated with worsening sleep quality.
- In some cases, underlying obstructive sleep apnea may precipitate or worsen GERD.

Sleep and Peptic Ulcer Disease

Peptic ulcer disease is commonly seen in the sleep apnea patient.
- A large study of nearly 35,000 Taiwanese obstructive sleep apnea patients documented a 2.4-fold higher risk for peptic ulcer bleeding.
- Investigators suggested the repeated hypoxemia associated with sleep-disordered breathing as a factor in greater severity of gastric erosion and propensity for peptic ulcer formation.
- The intense sympathomimetic activation triggered by obstructive sleep apnea is an additional risk factor for peptic ulcer disease formation through damage caused to the gastric mucosa, likely due to sympathomimetic vasoconstriction.

Sleep in Inflammatory Bowel Disease

Patients with inflammatory bowel disease have been found to have impaired sleep quality defined by self reported validated scores.[16]

TABLE 21.5	Common Causes of Fatigue in the CKD Patient	
Underlying Etiology	**Mechanism of Effect**	**Treatment**
Anemia	Reduced erythropoietin Blood loss from HD Iron deficiency Disturbed iron metabolism Shortened RBC lifespan	Stimulate erythropoietin Supplement iron
Mineral and bone disorders	Phosphate retention due to reduced GFR Secondary hypothyroidism Vitamin D deficiency	Supplement vitamin D Restrict phosphates Phosphate binding
Depression	Disrupted social life Poor quality of life Comorbidities	Cautious medical treatments with antidepressants
Protein energy wasting	Diminished oral intake Increased metabolic rate Insulin resistance Deranged appetite hormones Inability to use free amino acids	Nutritional correction Manage metabolic acidosis
Uremia uremic milieu	Systemic inflammation Altered cytokine state Increased oxidative stress	Treat underlying renal disease. Renal replacement therapy as needed.

- Using the Pittsburgh Sleep Quality Index—a nineteen-point, five-domain validated self-report survey—investigators have found patients to report subjective complaints of insomnia, indicating prolonged sleep latency, reduced daytime energy, and increased use of sleep aids.
- Crohn's disease patients experiencing sleep loss may be at increased risk of relapse, with such patients carrying twice the usual risk of active disease in a 6 month period compared with those patients reporting no sleep loss.
- Animal models have confirmed these findings using sleep deprivation models in mice with colitis—both acute and chronic sleep loss in these mice models worsened colitis.

Sleep and Irritable Bowel Syndrome

Irritable bowel syndrome (IBS) is a common disorder impacting 10%–15% of North Americans.
- Sleep disruption is often seen in association to IBS symptoms, which is perhaps unsurprising since IBS is known to be associated with anxiety and perceived stress.
- Lower sleep quality was associated with altered sphincter function and lower thresholds for rectal sensitivity.
- Mechanistically it is conceivable that sleep disruption in the IBS patient could result in the hyperalgesic effect shown in normal subjects experiencing sleep loss and thereby exacerbating IBS symptoms.

Sleep and Colon Cancer

Colon cancer is extraordinarily common. Worldwide it is the most commonly diagnosed cancer in women and the third most common diagnosed in men.
- Among patients with colon cancer, fatigue is a prime symptom prior to diagnosis, as well as during and after treatment.

- Tumor formation has been associated with circadian rhythm disorders in animal studies, and concerns grow that shift work that denies patients of usual melatonin release and thereby decreases melatonin levels could be an independent risk factor for tumor genesis.
- Investigators examining patients with colon cancer noted that a shorter sleep duration increased risk of colorectal adenomas by 50%, and these adenomas can frequently be precursors to colon cancers.[17]

In our 24/7 world, shift work is inevitable for many in the workforce. This together with abnormal expression of the *clock* gene and other causes of circadian rhythm disorders are also emerging as risk factors for malignancy.
- Among women working nightshifts, investigators have found a greater risk of colon cancer.[18]
- Melatonin's antiproliferative effects may well be serious risk factors, suppressed by light. Melatonin suppression through night shift work may be a preventable risk factor for cancer formation.

Sleep and Liver Disease

Disrupted sleep is common in the patient with cirrhosis of the liver.
- Over 47% of patients with cirrhosis report sleep dissatisfaction.
- Sleep wake cycle reversal is also commonly seen in this patient population with daytime sleepiness and nighttime insomnia.
- Women with primary biliary cirrhosis sleep twice as much during the daytime than normal controls.
- Patients with hepatitis C have been noted to frequently report sleep disruption in as many as 65% of affected patients.
- Interferon-alpha, used to treat hepatitis C, can also cause sleep disruption escalating risk for insomnia and daytime sleepiness.

- Hepatic encephalopathy associated with cirrhosis of the liver may present as hypersomnolence to the sleep specialist. In our practice we have seen at least one patient diagnosed with cirrhosis of the liver following routine level I attended polysomnography performed for hypersomnolence in an older woman with hepatic encephalopathy. The excessive delta waves disproportionate to age were seen on polysomnography, triggering clinical suspicion and intervention.

In addition, accumulating evidence, including noninvasive serum markers of liver injury and liver biopsies, strongly suggest that OSA, via the mechanism of chronic intermittent hypoxemia, may contribute to the development and progression of nonalcoholic fatty liver disease (NAFLD). Conversely, the absence of OSA may be protective against developing NAFLD in morbidly obese patients.[19]

Occupational Sleep Medicine: Managing Sleep and Sleep Disorders in Special Populations

A novel field, occupational sleep medicine encompasses (1) the science of sleep, (2) sleep and performance measurement in the operational environment, and (3) the clinical practice of sleep medicine to mitigate impact of sleep and sleep disorders on impaired performance, reduced productivity, workplace errors and incidents, and propensity to workplace accident.

- Occupational sleep medicine is critical in managing fatigue in the workplace and ensuring longer term worker well-being and health.
- In common practice, sleep disorder specialists will frequently encounter commercial drivers, commercial and recreational pilots, air-traffic controllers, first responders (including enforcement, firefighters, and military personnel), and other individuals working in high risk jobs that also pose a societal risk if the worker is performing under sleep duress.
- Many of these roles mandate the worker perform on rotating shifts, in a setting with chronic understaffing, switching shifts with short turnaround time, working back-to-back shifts, operating heavy machinery and heavy goods vehicles, and sometimes operating firearms and other lethal instruments.

Some industries have legislated worker hours rigidly, including for the commercial driver and the aviation pilot. Even recreational pilots are subject to the same rigors of testing as commercial pilots by the FAA licensing authorities. Yet the social and occupational deterrents to seek treatment are so great that patients may present late through significant fear of losing employment. The sleep disorders specialist must always emphasize that he or she is foremost an advocate for the patient's safety and well-being, and secondarily as a public duty to society; rarely does the latter supersede the former, but occasionally duty to society may supersede duty to the patient in our practices. This has not yet transpired, as we have found patients enormously responsible and ready to comply with treatment recommendations once they have access to proper sleep education. Many of them become excellent ambassadors for good sleep practice and safety, encouraging colleagues to seek evaluation and promoting an overall healthier workplace. In managing the occupational sleep patient, the physician may need to act as an advocate for the patient to ensure employment is not inappropriately terminated.

Sleep and the Commercial Driver

A major risk due to sleep deprivation is drowsy driving.

- Commercial drivers are subject to shift work that compels the driver to drive outside of his preferred circadian periods of alertness, to drive when involuntarily sleep deprived, and to drive when drowsy.
- Globally 25% of fatal motor vehicle accidents are related to drowsy driving.
- Professional drivers are often found to be driving drowsy, with studies showing they report a mean sleep duration of 4.78 hours a day, dangerously below the median norms of sleep for healthy adults, which approaches 7.4 hours.

Sleepiness while driving has been documented by the National Sleep Foundation.

- Among transportation drivers, an NSF poll showed 15% of truck drivers, 28% of train drivers, and 10% of bus, taxi, and limousine drivers are driving when sleepy, reporting their work affected at least once weekly due to sleepiness.
- EEG monitoring of truck drivers when driving showed that more than half demonstrated physiologically objective measures of sleepiness at the wheel. Two drivers in this study were recorded in stage 1 sleep while operating their vehicles.
- Other than sleepiness, drowsy drivers confront other risks that escalate motor vehicle collision risks:
  - Delayed reaction time
  - Attention lapses
  - Impaired decision making
- Driving simulator studies show driving after 21 hours of wakefulness mimics driving when intoxicated with alcohol as legally defined (>BAC 0.08%).
- Driving simulator studies show there is increased variability in speed, decreased ability to maintain central lane position, and increased lane drifting.

This is consistent with known impacts of sleepiness: decreased vigilance, increased errors due to impaired cognitive performance, reduced brain processing speed causing slower response times on diverse tasks, and diminished logical reasoning.

Sleep disorder specialists must take every opportunity to educate all patient drivers on driving safety, but with special emphasis for this education on the commercial driver who has greater driving exposure—more miles and hours of driving—and may often be driving large vehicles carrying dangerous payloads at times of increased circadian propensity of sleepiness when other sleepy drivers will also be on the road.

- This education must be repeated at every visit, and patients should be interviewed for their understanding of driving safety.
- Patients should be educated to pull off the road when tired, take planned naps as needed, consume caffeine after these naps, and avoid reinitiating driving until sleep inertia has worn off.
- If necessary, drivers may be well advised to continue driving on local roads, not express roads, to allow for frequent stops, lower operating speeds, and avoidance of driving monotony, which can itself promote sleep (what drivers in our practice often refer to colloquially as "Road Hypnosis").
- If the driver recognizes he is too fatigued to drive, he must not present for work, and sleep physicians should be ready to provide documentation that the patient is under the care of a sleep specialist.

Obstructive Sleep Apnea and Drowsy Driving

Critically important is the recognition, treatment, and compliance with treatment of sleep apnea in the commercial driver.

- Patients with even mild obstructive sleep apnea syndrome with an apnea-hypopnea index (AHI) of 10/hour or more carry a two to six times greater risk of motor vehicle collision, independent of any added risks patients may have due to sleep deprivation or working out of alignment with their intrinsic circadian rhythm.
- Treating a commercial driver not only improves his own morbidity and mortality but also offsets an enormous public health burden.

Conclusion

Sleep impacts all aspects of systemic disease, and a sleep specialist is likely to encounter patients from diverse disease populations in diverse stages of life and work.

- Treatment of systemic disorders must always address impact on sleep and evidence of organic sleep disorders comorbid to the primary systemic disease.

- Primary care physicians will encounter numerous sleep disorders as part of their practice and will benefit from an informed sleep specialist.
- Sleep specialists must be familiar with the many manifestations of sleep disorders in diverse populations with comorbid systemic disease.
- Sleep specialists must be familiar with the risks posed by sleep disorders in specific populations.

Suggested Reading

Abad VC, Sarinas P, Guilleminault C. Sleep and rheumatologic disorders. *Sleep Med Rev.* 2008;12(3):211-228.

Majid H, Shabbir-Moosajee M, Nadeem S. Fatigue in other medical disorders. *Sleep Med Clin.* 2013;8(2):241-253.

Waller EA, Bendel RE, Kaplan J. Sleep disorders and the eye. *Mayo Clin Proc.* 2008;83(11):1251-1261.

Winkelman JW, Plante DT. Polysomnographic features of medical and psychiatric disorders and their treatments. *Sleep Med Clin.* 2009;4(3):407-419.

Young T, Palta M, Dempsey J, et al. The occurrence of sleep-disordered breathing among middle-aged adults. *N Engl J Med.* 1993;328:1230-1235.

22

Pediatric Sleep–Wake Disorders

SURESH KOTAGAL, ROBIN LLOYD

History

- Electroencephalogram (EEG) Monitoring: In 1929 Berger recorded electrical activity from the exposed surface of the cerebral cortex in a patient who had a piece of skull removed.[1] In 1937 Loomis et al. reported their findings on all-night sleep studies in humans.[2] They observed that sleep consisted of alternating stages that could be differentiated by their EEG pattern.
- Rapid eye movement (REM) sleep: In 1953 Aserinsky and Kleitman identified a novel EEG pattern consisting of low-voltage, fast activity that occurred in conjunction with bursts of REMs.[3] Dement and Kleitman then recognized that this state was associated with dreaming.[4] They coined the term REM sleep.
- Maturation of human sleep: In 1966 Roffwarg et al. reported on the maturation of human sleep from a developmental perspective.[5] In 1970 Dreyfus-Brisac observed that active (REM) sleep could be identified on polygraphic tracings by 32 weeks' gestation, because of the presence of frequent body movements, irregular respiration, and REMs while the eyes were closed.[6] In 1972 Parmelee and Stern recognized quiet or nonrapid eye movement (NREM) sleep after 36 weeks' gestation, and characterized it by the presence of closed eyes with no eye

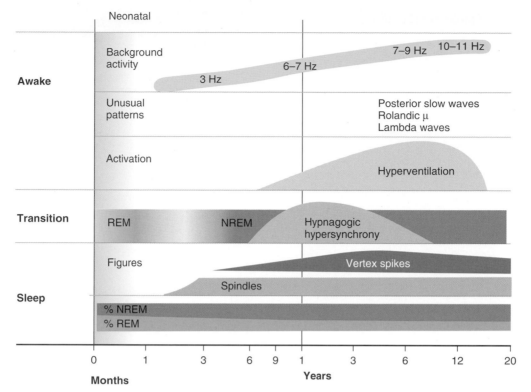

• **Figure 22.1** Electroencephalogram maturational stages. *NREM,* Nonrapid eye movement; *REM,* Rapid eye movement. (From Eisermann M, Kaminska A, Moutard ML, Soufflet C, Plouin P. *Neurophysiologi Clinique/Clinical Neurophysiology,* 43[1]:35–65.)

movements, no body movements, and very regular respiration.[7] The relationship of NREM sleep to release of growth hormone was reported in by Shaywitz et al. in 1971.[8] The EEG undergoes maturational changes across childhood (Fig. 22.1).

• Clinical sleep disorders in childhood remained largely obscure until the pioneering studies of Guilleminault in the late 1970s and early 1980s, when he documented obstructive sleep apnea (OSA) in children.[9] In 1981 Weitzman et al. described the first case of delayed sleep phase syndrome in a medical student at Montefiore Hospital in New York, thereby ushering in the era of understanding circadian rhythm sleep disorders.[10] In 1992 the American Academy of Pediatrics (AAP) initiated the "Back to Sleep" campaign, which recommended supine sleep in all infants when they are placed in bed in an effort to prevent sudden infant death syndrome (SIDS).[11] The relationship between prone sleeping, rebreathing of exhaled air, and SIDS was also elucidated by Kemp et al.[12] The use of home apnea monitors, which had flourished dramatically in the 1980s when these devices were prescribed routinely for siblings of SIDS babies and for infants with recurrent apnea, fell dramatically in the late 1990s after the "Back to Sleep" recommendations of the AAP.

The Anders manual for the scoring of sleep in newborns was first developed by Anders et al. in 1971.[13] The American Academy of Sleep Medicine published new infant scoring rules in July of 2015.[14] The past decade and a half has ushered in technological advances in the laboratory assessment of childhood sleep–wake disorders, with nasal thermocouples and thermistors giving way to nasal pressure transducers as the "gold standard" for monitoring nasal respiration. Respiratory inductance plethysmography has replaced mercury-filled strain gauges for the measurement of thoracic and abdominal respiratory effort. Analog polygraphs have largely been replaced by digital systems.

The molecular biological and genetic era of sleep medicine was ushered in by observations such as those of de Lecea et al., who in 1998 recognized the hypocretin system in the central nervous system and its alerting effects.[15] Subsequently, Lin et al. demonstrated that canine narcolepsy was associated with mutations in the hypocretin-2 receptor gene.[16] Nishino et al. demonstrated a deficiency of hypocretin-1 in the cerebrospinal fluid (CSF) of humans with narcolepsy.[17] Thannickal et al. demonstrated in postmortem studies a reduced number of hypocretin neurons in the hypothalamus of humans with narcolepsy.[18] Increasing recognition of the neurobehavioral aspects of sleep disturbances by Beebe and Gozal[19] has further broadened the field of pediatric sleep medicine. This chapter addresses some key sleep–wake issues in infancy, childhood, and adolescence.

The Pediatric Sleep Consultation

• Consultation requests must be triaged in advance of the sleep clinic visit in order to gauge the nature and urgency of the sleep complaint, as well as to facilitate scheduling of diagnostic procedures in advance. A questionnaire concerning the patient's sleep–wake function should be completed by family members before the visit. The items that should be addressed in the sleep history are shown in Table 22.1. Components of the pediatric sleep-related examination are listed in Table 22.2.

• A provisional sleep diagnosis should be established on completion of the history and examination. A plan for investigations is drawn up and the studies completed, subsequent to which the patient returns for discussion of the test results and for formulation of a management plan, which includes patient and family education.

TABLE 22.1 Pediatric Sleep History Items

Nature and duration of the sleep complaint
Activities carried out in the 2–3 h before bedtime
Rituals around bedtime (e.g., rocking, patting, reading in bed)
Bed-onset time (weekdays and weekends)
Any sensation of restlessness in the legs before sleep onset?
Estimated sleep-onset time
Sleeping position (e.g., prone/supine)
Habitual snoring, mouth breathing, observed apnea, excessive sweating
Dysphagia, salivary drooling
Restless sleep
Estimated number and length of night time awakenings and behavior during awakenings
Nocturnal enuresis
Any behavior that is suggestive of parasomnias or seizures
Final morning awakening time (weekdays and weekends)
Does the child feel refreshed or tired on awakening?
School start time
Days of school missed because of sleepiness during the current academic year
Daytime sleepiness, voluntary and involuntary naps; their duration
Dream-like feelings during these daytime naps
Impaired concentration, mood swings, and declining grades
Episodes suggestive of cataplexy or sleep paralysis
Afternoon and evening activities, including after-school employment
A review of other systems
Medications used (past and present)
Allergies
Quantify exposure to caffeinated beverages, exposure to passive smoke, electronic media use close to bedtime
Previous diagnostic procedures and their results
Life stresses, history of anxiety, depression, substance use

TABLE 22.2 Sleep-Related Examination

Pulse, blood pressure, body mass index, head circumference
Craniofacial abnormalities, tonsil size, mouth breathing, inflammation and narrowing of the anterior nasal passages, deviated nasal septum, enlargement of the tongue base, soft palate mobility
Neck and submandibular lymph node enlargement
Thyromegaly
Lungs and heart auscultation
Abdominal palpation for mass or tenderness
Higher cortical functions: digit span (for attention span), recall of recent information, mood, memory, speech comprehension and expressive ability, involuntary movements, gait

Normal Sleep and Breathing During Infancy

Newborns and Infants: EEG activity can clearly be recorded from the fetus by 24 weeks' gestation. Wakefulness can be differentiated from sleep by 27–28 weeks' postconceptional age. By 30–32 weeks' postconceptional age, the low-voltage and irregular EEG pattern of active (REM) sleep can clearly be distinguished from the high-voltage and slow wave EEG pattern of quiet (NREM) sleep (Figs. 22.2 and 22.3). At this age, close to 80% of total sleep time is spent in active sleep. By full term or 40 weeks' postconceptional age, the proportion of time spent in active sleep decreases to approximately 55%–65% of the total sleep time, with a corresponding increase in quiet sleep.[20] The transition from wakefulness in healthy term infants is typically directly into REM sleep until 2–3 months of age. Sleep spindles are

TABLE 22.3 Typical Sleep Architecture Values for Normal Children Aged 1–18 Years

Parameter	Usual Value	References
Sleep efficiency (1%)	89%, large variability	26;41;42
Sleep latency (min)	23, large variability	26;41;42
REM latency (min)	87–155 (<10 years of age) 136–156 (>10 years of age)	41;42
Arousal index (N/hour)	9–16	26;41;42
Stage N1 (%TST)	4–5	26;33;42
Stage N2 (%TST)	44–56	26;33;42
Stage N3 (%TST)	29–32 (<10 years of age) 20 (>10 years of age)	26;33;42
Stage R (%TST)	17–21 (can be higher in young children)	26;33;42

Data are approximated from mean and median values provided in references from large studies of normal children. Sleep stage distributions from reference[41] are not provided as data in that study are quoted as percent of total sleep period and not %TST. *TST*, Total sleep time.
From *Sleep Med Clin.* 2009;4(3):393–406.

present by 4–6 weeks postterm and K complexes 3–6 months postterm, such that NREM sleep can be scored as stage N1, N2, or N3 in most infants by 5–6 months (Table 22.3).

Cerebral blood flow and the metabolic rate are higher during active sleep than during quiet sleep. Respiration during active sleep is irregular, with intermittent inhibition of the striated muscle of the upper airway and rib cage. Diaphragmatic activity remains relatively unaltered, however. The incoordination between the intercostal muscles and the diaphragm during active sleep predisposes to paradoxical chest and abdominal wall motion, inefficient breathing, and oxygen desaturation. The paradoxical chest and abdominal wall movement pattern is most prominent during the active sleep of premature infants, gradually subsides over the first 5–6 months of life, and disappears by the age of 3 years. By contrast, respiration during quiet (NREM) sleep is deep and regular. The responsiveness of the brainstem chemoreceptors to hypercapnia is blunted during active sleep as compared with quiet sleep.[21]

Respiratory control: The carotid body contains receptors that have oxygen-sensitive K^+ channels,[22] as well as carbon dioxide–sensing properties. The carotid sinus nerve carries hypoxia- and hypercapnia-mediated afferent impulses from the carotid body to the petrosal sinus, and hence via the glossopharyngeal nerve to the nucleus of the tractus solitarius in the medulla.[23] Exposure to high levels of nicotine prenatally or to perinatal hyperoxia reduces the size of the carotid body, with possible blunting of the compensatory responses to hypoxia,[24] thus underscoring the critical role of the peripheral chemoreceptors of the carotid body in terminating apnea and initiating normal breathing. The role of an exaggerated laryngeal chemoreflex in the pathogenesis of apnea in preterm infants should also be emphasized.[25] This reflex is characterized by central apnea, glottic closure, and bradycardia in response to the instillation of water, saline, or milk into the pharynx. This vagally mediated laryngeal reflex may become

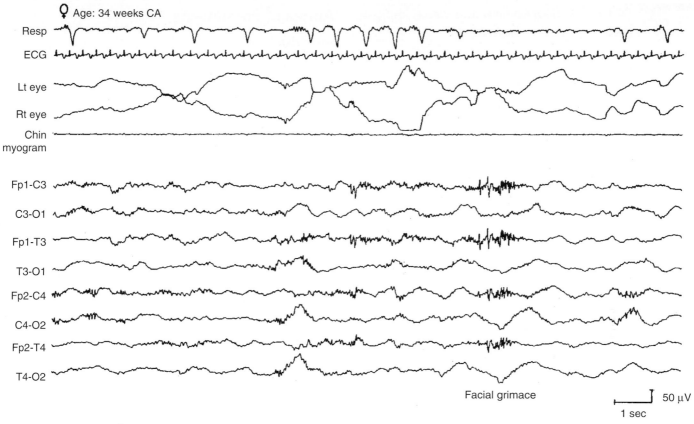

• **Figure 22.2** REM (or active) sleep in a normal 34 week premature infant with low-voltage, mixed-frequency pattern. *CA,* Conceptual age; *ECG,* electrocardiogram.

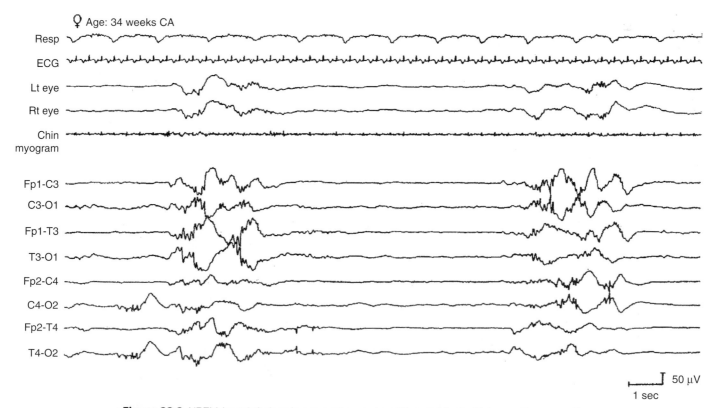

• **Figure 22.3** NREM (or quiet) sleep in a normal premature 34 week infant with trace alternans pattern-periods of high-voltage cortical activity that alternate with low-amplitude periods. *CA,* Conceptual age; *ECG,* electrocardiogram.

TABLE 22.4	Typical Sleep Architecture Values and Recommended Normative Polysomnographic Values for Normal Children Aged 1–18 Years
Parameter	**Usual Value**
Sleep efficiency (%)	89%, large variablility
Sleep latency (min)	23, large variablility
REM latency (min)	87–155 (<10 years of age) 136–156 (>10 years of age)
Arousal index (N/hr)	9–16
Stage N1 (%TST)	4–5
Stage N2 (%TST)	44–56
Stage N3 (%TST)	29–32 (<10 years of age) 20 (>10 years of age)
Stage R (%TST)	17–21 (can be higher in young children)
Obstructive AHI (N/hr)	≤1.4
Central apnea index (N/hr)	≤0.4
Time with SpO$_2$ <90% (%TST)	0
SpO$_2$ nadir (%)	≥91
Time with peak PCO$_2$ ≥ 50 mm Hg (%TST)	<25%
Periodic limb movement index (N/hr)	≤4.3

TST, Total Sleep Time; *AHI*, Apnea Hypopnea Index; *N*, Number; *hr*, hour; *mm Hg*, millimeter of Mercury; *PCO$_2$*, partial pressure of carbon dioxide (CO$_2$).
Adapted from Beck SE, Marcus CL. Pediatric Polysomnography *Sleep Med Clin.* 2009; 4(3): 393–406.

more prominent during upper respiratory infections. It is most prominent during the neonatal period and gradually subsides during infancy.

Adults prefer to breathe through the nose. Infants do have the ability to switch to mouth breathing if necessary, although this ability is not fully developed in preterm infants. Periodic breathing is a normal variant that is defined as three or more apnea episodes lasting 3 sec or longer with an intervening period of 20 sec or less. It is most prevalent during active sleep in preterm infants and gradually resolves during infancy. Prolonged periodic breathing may be associated with oxygen desaturation.

Patterns of apnea vary with the age of the infant; premature infants are more likely to exhibit mixed or obstructive apnea, whereas term infants are more likely to have central apnea. Central apneas are considered significant only if they last 20 sec or longer, or if they last at least two missed breaths but are associated with arousal or oxygen desaturation of 3% or greater. In preterm infants, the frequency of apneic pauses decreases by more than 80% between 40 and 52 weeks' postconceptional age, and ultimately matches that of infants who have been born at full term.

Reference values for pediatric polysomnography (PSG) are listed in Table 22.4.

Apnea of Prematurity

Introduction

This disorder of respiratory control affects 70%–90% of premature infants less than 1500 g birth weight or less than 28 weeks' gestation. It is characterized by prolonged apneas of 20 or more sec, or shorter respiratory pauses that are accompanied by decreases in oxyhemoglobin saturation and/or bradycardia (heart rate less than 100/min).[26] There is lingering concern that recurrent events may have an impact on the brainstem neural structures that regulate respiration. Also of concern is the possible occurrence of long-term cognitive and behavioral disturbances.

Patients may exhibit central, obstructive, or mixed apneas, or a combination thereof. There may be recurrent episodes of periodic breathing, oxygen desaturation, and bradycardia.[27] In periodic breathing, between 5- and 10-sec periods of apnea alternate with regular breathing. It is most often observed during active sleep and may predispose to oxygen desaturation and longer episodes of apnea.

Pathophysiology

Apnea of prematurity is complex and multifactorial, and reflects immaturity of respiratory control. Passive collapse of the hypotonic upper airway of premature infants predisposes them to obstructive apnea. Furthermore, preterm infants of 30–32 weeks' postconceptional age spend close to 80% of their total sleep time in active (REM) sleep, and thus have an increased likelihood of hypotonic collapse of the upper airway when asleep. Their central control of ventilation is immature, being characterized by a blunted central ventilatory response to the accumulation of carbon dioxide.[27] There is also immaturity of the excitatory *N*-methyl-D-aspartate (NMDA) receptors located in the nucleus of the tractus solitarius in the medulla. These receptors increase ventilation in response to recurrent hypoxia.[28] In addition, exposure to hypoxia usually increases ventilation via enhanced expression in the brainstem of neuronal nitric oxide synthase activity. This compensatory mechanism may be insufficiently developed in preterm infants and can predispose to recurrent central apneic spells. Another important causative factor is that preterm infants respond by decreasing ventilation when challenged with hypoxia. This is most likely a consequence of suppression of the central ventilatory drive by hypoxia. Adenosine probably plays a role in mediating this inhibition.[29] Caffeine (used frequently to treat apnea of prematurity) is an inhibitor of adenosine metabolism. Paradoxical chest and abdominal wall motion is common during the active sleep of premature infants, and this may further exacerbate inefficient breathing. Yet another contributing factor might be immaturity of the Hering-Breuer reflex—small increases in lung volume may thus trigger apnea.[30] Gastroesophageal reflux disease (GERD) is a factor in some patients. Although "cardiorespiratory events" and GERD are common in preterm infants, they are not causally related.[31] Perhaps they are dual manifestations of central autonomic nervous system immaturity. The influence of inherited factors in the pathogenesis of apnea of prematurity has also been recognized recently. Bloch-Salisbury et al. retrospectively evaluated 317 premature twin pairs between 2000 and 2008.[32] They found greater concordance for apnea of prematurity in monozygotic twin pairs (87%) than in same-gender dizygotic twins (62%), which suggests a genetic predisposition. The mechanisms that might be impacted by this genetic predisposition are at this point unclear.

Clinical approach: Apnea of prematurity is considered a diagnosis of exclusion. It is important to evaluate for other potential causes of apnea especially in an infant who has been apnea-free then resumes having apnea after having an apnea-free period.

The *diagnostic workup* usually includes:
- A detailed antepartum and neonatal history evaluating for exposure to opiates or anesthesia, risk factors for infection, or trauma/perinatal asphyxia.
- Physical exam should assess for signs and symptoms of infection, hypoglycemia, congenital anomalies of the upper airway, and neurologic deficit. Laboratory evaluation for sepsis, hypoglycemia, anemia, and metabolic disorder should be considered.
- EEG to exclude the possibility of a seizure disorder
- Esophageal pH study to evaluate for GERD
- Otolaryngology consultation to exclude structural airway lesions such as partial choanal atresia, and a chest radiograph may be appropriate. Laryngoscopy might reveal a "cobblestone" appearance of the mucosa secondary to GERD. Neuroimaging should be considered if concern for hemorrhage.

Management

The mainstay of treatment for apnea of prematurity is:
- Supportive care—Focused on eliminating factors that increase the risk of apnea, including maintenance of a stable thermal environment, transfusion for significant anemia, tactile stimulation as needed, maintaining nasal patency, avoidance of extreme neck flexion, and extension.
- Caffeine therapy—Caffeine citrate is the preferred agent because of its longer half-life and wider safety margin. The recommended dose is a 20-mg/kg intravenous or oral loading dose, followed by 5 mg/kg per day by mouth or the intravenous route, and may be increased to 10 mg/kg per day for persistent apnea.[33] Improved long-term outcomes from the standpoint of cognitive and motor function have also been reported with the use of caffeine in the newborn period.[34]
- Nasal continuous positive airway pressure (CPAP), in general provided via prongs
- Although the respiratory stimulant doxapram appears to have some immediate and short-lived efficacy, long-term benefit has not been established.[35]
- If medical therapy fails, consideration can be given to the use of CPAP. High-flow nasal cannula or nasal intermittent positive pressure ventilation may be acceptable options for CPAP but further study is needed.
- Levocarnitine has also been tried, but without proven benefit.[36]

Clinical Course

Apneic events subside spontaneously and resolve after 46–48 weeks' postconceptional age. The benefits of home apnea monitoring are uncertain, but monitoring can be provided to cover the risk period.

Sudden Infant Death Syndrome

Introduction

SIDS is defined as the sudden death of an infant younger than 1 year that remains unexplained after a complete clinical review, autopsy, and death scene investigation.[37] SIDS is the leading cause of infant mortality from 1 month to 1 year of age in the United States, and about 1500 infants died of SIDS in 2014.[38] Since

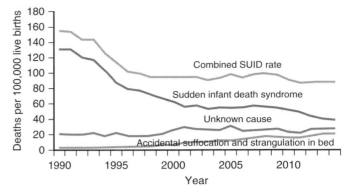

• **Figure 22.4** Trends in Sudden Unexpected Infant Death by Cause, 1990–2014. *SUID,* Sudden unexpected infant death. (Source: CDC/NCHS, National Vital Statistics System, Compressed Mortality File.)

introduction of the "Back to Sleep" campaign in the early 1990s, there has been a significant decline in the incidence of SIDS in the United States. It is currently estimated at 0.8 per 1000 live births. This decline has leveled off, despite widespread adoption of the supine sleeping position for babies, thus suggesting that SIDS is multifactorial in etiology, with persistence of congenital or additional, undetermined environmental risk factors (Fig. 22.4).[38]

Epidemiology

Ninety percent of SIDS occurs between birth and 4 months of age, which suggests that this is the most vulnerable period.
- Major epidemiological risk factors for SIDS are related to maternal factors and infant/environmental factors: young maternal age, late or no prenatal care, maternal anemia, maternal illicit drug use during pregnancy, maternal smoking, prematurity and or low birth weight prone sleeping, soft sleep surface and/or bedding, bed-sharing, and blunting of central arousal mechanisms by an overheated environment.[39–42] Many of these risk factors are modifiable. The prone sleeping position is a major contributor, with infants younger than 2–2.5 months being unable to change body position sufficiently to overcome suffocation from being placed prone on a soft mattress. This predisposes to rebreathing, hypercapnia, and consequent depression of the central ventilatory drive. Systemic infections may also alter the arousal threshold.[43]

Pathophysiology

- Filiano and Kinney proposed a triple-risk model that considers epidemiological, physiological, and autopsy data.[44] This model proposes that SIDS is likely to occur only when exogenous stressors affect homeostatic control in a vulnerable infant (Fig. 22.5). They established that the critical region for ventilatory control is the arcuate nucleus, which is derived from the caudal raphe system and located over the ventromedial aspect of the medulla. Using tissue autoradiography, they also demonstrated decreased binding of ^{3}H-lysergide (H-LSD) to the serotonergic receptors 5-hydroxytryptophan 1A–1D (5-HT$_{1A-D}$) and 5-HT$_{2A}$ in the arcuate nuclei of patients with SIDS, in comparison with that of age-matched controls.[45] Furthermore, application of a 5-HT$_{1A}$ serotonin agonist called *8-hydroxy-2-(di-n-propylamino) tetralin (8-OH-DPAT)* to the ventral surface of the cat medulla increases the respiratory rate,[45] which confirms the role of the medullary

TRIPLE RISK MODEL FOR SIDS

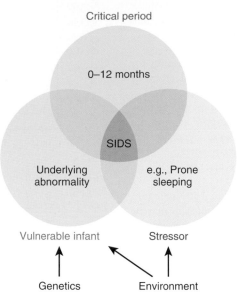

• **Figure 22.5** Triple Risk Model for SIDS Demonstrating Genetic-Environmental Interactions. The Triple Risk Model for SIDS proposes that death occurs when three factors simultaneously impinge upon the infant: 1) an underlying vulnerability in the infant; 2) a critical developmental period, i.e., the first year of life; and 3) an exogenous stressor, e.g., prone sleep. According to this model, normal infants do not die of SIDS, but rather, only infants with an underlying disease process. Gene variants are thought to contribute to SIDS risk either by directly causing or contributing to the failure of homeostatic mechanisms or by rendering the infant less resilient to environmental stressors. (From Paterson DS. Serotonin gene variants are unlikely to play a significant role in the pathogenesis of the sudden infant death syndrome. *Respir Physiol & Neurobiol* 2013;189[2]:301–314.)

serotonergic network in the control of breathing. These findings might ultimately lead to an understanding of molecular factors that regulate the proliferation, migration, and maturation of cells from the caudal raphe system to the medullary arcuate nucleus.

- A small percentage of SIDS cases are of cardiac etiology. At the Mayo Clinic, Ackerman et al. studied postmortem cardiac tissue from 93 patients with SIDS, as well as from 400 controls, and found two distinct mutant alleles in 2 of 93 subjects in the voltage-gated sodium channel, type V, α subunit (SCN5A), which predisposed to prolongation of the QT interval.[46] Furthermore, when the mutant alleles were introduced in vitro into wild-type human heart sodium channels, voltage clamp studies showed that rates of voltage conductance were significantly slowed.

Prevention

The management strategy for prevention of SIDS will continue to be one of risk reduction, with emphasis on:
- Preventing prenatal exposure to nicotine
- Educating underserved and low-socioeconomic populations about the dangers of the prone sleeping position in infants
- Avoidance of excessive swaddling and overheating that tend to blunt the central arousal response

Congenital Central Hypoventilation Syndrome

Congenital central hypoventilation syndrome (CCHS) is characterized by defective automatic control of breathing during sleep. In general, patients become symptomatic at birth or shortly thereafter, but a late-onset childhood form has also been reported.[47]

Etiology

The primary form of CCHS is linked to mutations in the homeobox gene *PHOX2B*, which maps to chromosome 4p12 and is transmitted in an autosomal dominant manner.[48] The gene encodes a highly conserved transcription factor. Approximately 92% of primary CCHS patients carry this mutation.[49] About 20% of CCHS patients have coexisting Hirschsprung's disease, a disorder of bowel motility resulting from a defect in development of the autonomic ganglia of the wall of a segment of the large bowel. This combination of CCHS and Hirschsprung's disease is called Haddad syndrome. There is also an association between CCHS and neural crest tumors such as ganglioglioma and neuroblastoma, which are seen in 5%–10% of CCHS cases. Frameshift and missense *PHOX2B* mutations predispose to neuroblastoma.[49] It is been postulated that CCHS is a neural crest disorder in which there is defective fetal development because brainstem neurons that regulate chemosensitivity are derived from the neural crest.

Secondary forms of central hypoventilation, though infrequent, may be related to subtle or overt developmental malformations of the brainstem, head injury, bulbar poliomyelitis, syringobulbia, Arnold-Chiari type II malformation, Zellweger syndrome, and mitochondrial disorders such as Leigh syndrome. In some instances, no specific cause is identifiable. The report of mother-to-daughter transmission of the disorder suggests an autosomal dominant transmission in some families.[50]

Pathology

Common sites of hypoplasia or neurodegeneration include the arcuate nucleus of the medulla (regulates chemosensitivity), the ventrolateral nucleus of the tractus solitarius, the nucleus ambiguus or nucleus retroambiguus, and the nucleus parabrachialis in the dorsolateral pons.

Clinical Features

The respiratory rate and depth are initially normal during wakefulness, but shallow and infrequent breathing, hypercapnia, and oxygen desaturation initially appear during NREM sleep and subsequently during REM sleep. $PaCO_2$ is higher than 60 mm Hg during sleep, despite the absence of pulmonary, neuromuscular, or cardiac disease. Ventilatory challenge with inhalation of a mixture of 5% CO_2 and 95% O_2 during NREM sleep fails to evoke the physiological, three- to fivefold increase in minute volume.

Management

The American Thoracic Society has developed a comprehensive evaluation and management strategy for CCHS.[51] Prompt recognition, evaluation, and initiation of treatment are recommended; otherwise patients may die in infancy or early childhood.

- Ventilatory support is of utmost importance, and in most cases tracheostomy with positive pressure ventilation is the safest way to manage afflicted infants. In more severely affected patients, assisted ventilation may be needed during both sleep and wakefulness.
- Diaphragmatic pacing may be considered in these patients during wakefulness to improve quality of life. In milder cases where gas exchange during wakefulness is adequate, noninvasive positive pressure ventilation with a mask during sleep may be an option.
- Patients with CCHS require vigilant home care and monitoring. Typical breath-holding spells in young children may require resuscitation in CCHS patients, as can underwater swimming. Any CNS depressants such as alcohol or anesthesia may cause problematic respiratory depression.
- Careful long-term surveillance for adequate ventilation during sleep with biannual PSG during the first 3 years of life followed by annual PSG is recommended.[51] Similarly, echocardiogram looking for cor pulmonale should be conducted. Additionally, hematologic monitoring for polycythemia and respiratory acidosis, Holter evaluations for arrhythmias, surveillance for neural crest tumors, and neurocognitive testing should be part of the longitudinal care of these medically complex children.

Brief Resolved Unexplained Events (Brue; Formerly Apparent Life-Threatening Events)

Experts at the AAP have recently published a clinical guideline, which recommends dropping the previously used term ALTE. This term was subjective, nonspecific, and predisposed to unnecessary hospitalizations, diagnostic tests, and burdensome and low-yield home apnea monitoring.[52–54] This new guideline was developed to help clinicians identify low risk patients. It also provides evidence-based guidelines for evaluation and management, with the intent of reducing unnecessary and costly medical interventions and improving patient outcomes. Instead, the events are to be

TABLE 22.5	Potential Etiologies for Brief Resolved Unexplained Events (BRUE; Previously Termed Apparent Life-Threatening Episodes)
Category	**Disorder**
Respiratory	Upper airway infections—e.g., respiratory syncytial virus
	Upper airway obstruction—retrognathia, adenoidal hypertrophy
	Lower airway closure or obstruction—tracheomalacia
	Intrapulmonary shunting—cyanotic breath-holding spells
Neurological	Partial seizures with orbitofrontal onset
	Intracranial hemorrhage—shaken infant syndrome
	Central hypoventilation—congenital, drug mediated
	Neuromuscular disease—botulism
Infective	Sepsis
	Meningoencephalitis
Autonomic	Vasovagal
	Gastroesophageal reflux disease
Cardiac	Wolff-Parkinson-White syndrome
	Long QT syndrome
	Congenital heart disease
Inborn errors of metabolism	Medium- and long-chain acyl coenzyme A dehydrogenase deficiency

characterized henceforth as BRUE, which is an evidence-based term.[55] BRUE is defined as:

- An event occurring in an infant <12 months of age
- Brief, <1 minute episode of apnea or cyanosis that resolves spontaneously
- Association with a reassuring history and normal physical examination
- The patient is afebrile, and there is no history of choking or gagging to suggest GERD

Potential etiologies for BRUE are listed in Table 22.5. It is appropriate to obtain a 12-lead ECG on the patient with straightforward BRUE, but outside of that, additional measures may not be warranted. Nocturnal PSG, EEG, and neuroimaging tests are not required in patients with uncomplicated, simple BRUE.

Higher risk patients in whom more detailed evaluation may be necessary include those with:

- Possible child abuse[56]
- Family history of sudden death, with need to exclude a cardiac arrhythmia
- Fever and concerns about an underlying infection
- Choking and spitting up suggesting GERD

Restless Legs Syndrome

Introduction

In 1994 Walters and colleagues described restless legs syndrome (RLS) in a mother and her three children aged 1, 4, and 6 years, as well as in a 16-year-old from an unrelated family.[57] The disorder exhibited autosomal transmission. The patients experienced leg

TABLE 22.6	International Restless Legs Syndrome Study Group Consensus Diagnostic Criteria for Restless Legs Syndrome

1. An urge to move the legs, usually but not always accompanied by or felt to be caused by uncomfortable or unpleasant sensations in the legs
2. The urge to move the legs and any accompanying unpleasant sensations begin to worsen during periods of rest or inactivity such as lying down or sitting[a]
3. The urge to move the legs and any accompanying unpleasant sensations are partially or totally relieved by movement, such as walking or stretching at least as long as the activity continues
4. The urge to move the legs and any accompanying unpleasant sensations during rest or inactivity only occur or are worse during the evening or night than during the day
5. The occurrence of the above features is not solely accounted for as symptoms primary to another medical or behavioral condition (e.g., myalgia, venous stasis, leg edema, arthritis, leg cramps, positional leg discomfort, habitual foot tapping)

Specifiers for Clinical Significance of RLS

The symptoms of RLS cause significant distress or impairment in social, occupational, educational, or other important areas of functioning by the impact on sleep, energy/vitality, daily activities, behavior, cognition or mood

Specifiers for clinical course of RLS[b]
A. Chronic-persistent RLS: symptoms when not treated would occur on average at least twice weekly for the past year
B. Intermittent RLS: symptoms when not treated would occur on average <2/week for the past year, with least five lifetime events

[a]For children, the description should be in the child's own words.
[b]The clinical course criteria do not apply for pediatric cases or for some special cases of provoked RLS such as pregnancy or drug-induced RLS, in which the frequency may be high or limited due to the duration of the provocative condition.
RLS, Restless legs syndrome.
From Picchietti DL, Bruni O, de Weerd A, et al., on behalf of the International Restless Legs Study Group (IRLSSG). Pediatric restless legs syndrome diagnostic criteria: an update by the International Restless Legs Syndrome Study Group. *Sleep Med.* 2013;14:1253–1259.

TABLE 22.7	A Comparison Between Pediatric and Adult-Onset RLS	
Feature	Pediatric RLS	Adult RLS
Common description by patients	"Owwies", "oucchies", feel like kicking, feel like I have to move	Feel like moving, discomfort made worse by keeping limbs still, relieved somewhat by movement
Polysomnography	Frequently indicated for documenting periodic limb movements	Less frequently indicated
Iron deficiency	+++	++
Family history of RLS	Present in ~75% of patients	Variable
Daytime symptoms	Hyperactivity, inattentiveness	Insomnia, nonrestorative sleep
Pharmacotherapy	Iron supplements, gabapentin	Iron supplements, gabapentin, ropinirole, pramipexole

RLS, Restless legs syndrome.

discomfort and nocturnal motor restlessness, with temporary relief afforded by voluntary movement. They also observed that on nocturnal PSG, children with RLS tended to have periodic limb movements in sleep (PLMS), which are defined as a series of four or more limb electromyographic discharges 0.5–10 sec in duration that are separated by intervals of 5–90 sec. The presence of PLMS is not essential for the diagnosis of RLS, although close to 80% of RLS patients are found to have PLMS on nocturnal PSG. Because of the subjective nature of RLS, it may be difficult to accurately diagnose RLS in young or nonverbal children. The current diagnostic criteria for RLS are shown in in Table 22.6.[58]

Clinical Features

- Children may describe a "creepy" or "crawling" feeling in their limbs that appears late in the evening or at night. Terms commonly used by children to describe their limb discomfort include "owwies," "ouchhies," and "tickles." It is important to inquire of RLS symptoms using child-appropriate terms.
- There is an irresistible urge to move the legs.
- This sensorimotor disturbance shows a circadian variation, being most prominent in the evenings and at night.[59]

- It is relieved by movement of the limbs and stretching and exacerbated by rest.[59]
- The increased sleep fragmentation from RLS may provoke disorders of partial arousal such as confusional arousals or sleepwalking. The child may be tired and unrefreshed on awakening in the morning. Attention-deficit/hyperactivity disorder (ADHD), a condition characterized by inattentiveness, hyperactivity, and impulsivity, and RLS are comorbid conditions—between 25% and 30% of patients with ADHD exhibit coexisting RLS.[60]
- Differences between pediatric and adult RLS are shown in Table 22.7.

Pathogenesis

- A positive family history for RLS is present in approximately 75% of children with RLS.[59] RLS most likely develops in children when genetic predisposition interacts with environmental factors that have yet to be fully established. Applying complex segregation analysis to predominantly adult RLS patients and their relatives, Winkelmann and associates found that patients with an age at the onset of symptoms of younger than 30 years showed single-gene, autosomal dominant transmission with a multifactorial component.[61]
- Periodic limb movement disorder (PLMD), a core component of RLS, appears to be linked to systemic iron deficiency.[62] In a prospective study of 39 children with a mean age of 7.5 years (standard deviation [SD] of 3.1 years), Simakajornboon et al. found that patients with serum ferritin levels less than 50 μg/dL had a significantly higher periodic limb movement index (PLMI) than those with serum iron levels higher than 50 μg/dL (42.8 ± 18.3 vs. 23.1 ± 10.1; $P = .02$).[62] Furthermore, the PLMI was reduced following oral iron replacement therapy. Iron is a co-factor for tyrosine hydroxylase synthesis, which is the rate-limiting step in the synthesis of dopamine. The end

result of iron deficiency appears to be a relative lowering of central nervous system levels of dopamine.

- Using whole genome analysis in a cohort drawn from Iceland and the United States, Stefansson and associates found periodic limb movements (PLM) to be associated with an intronic variant on the *BTBD9* gene, which has been localized to chromosome 6p21.2.[63]
- The term "growing pains" is applied to a conglomeration of symptoms of discomfort in the limbs that are seen in children, usually at night, and may be secondary to arthritic or nonarthritic conditions. Rajaram et al. pointed out the heterogeneous nature of "growing pains," and that a subset of children with "growing pains" might actually have RLS.[64] The differential diagnosis of growing pains includes positional discomfort, myalgia, tendinitis, dermatitis, fibromyalgia, and drug-induced akathisia.[58] Of note, myalgia and tendinitis are usually made worse by movement, whereas the discomfort of RLS improves with movement.

Diagnosis

As in adults, childhood RLS is a clinical diagnosis that is based on the sleep history and family history.

- Nocturnal PSG is utilized more often than in adults, simply because children are at times unable to provide a reliable history, and because a PLMI value higher than 5 is one of the supportive diagnostic criteria under the present classification.
- An inexpensive and useful diagnostic aid is a videotape of the child's sleep in the home environment, which may show (PLM). Drawings of the discomfort experienced by children with RLS are often very helpful in establishing the diagnosis, particularly since younger children may not be able to clearly describe the sensorimotor disturbance.[65]
- Serum ferritin levels should be checked to ensure that it is above 50 µg/dL.
- ADHD may be an important comorbidity necessitating neuropsychological assessment.

Treatment

Large, prospective studies on the treatment of childhood RLS are lacking. Drugs commonly used to treat adults with RLS have been prescribed for children as well on an off-label basis, in general with a favorable response.

- Iron replacement therapy is in general the first step in pediatric RLS management.[66] Infants and young children may be prescribed liquid preparations of ferrous sulfate, whereas tablets of ferrous sulfate, 325 mg daily, are recommended for older children. The iron supplement should be administered on an empty stomach, with vitamin C or orange juice to enhance absorption. The side effects of oral iron include constipation and abdominal discomfort. In patients with significant iron deficiency and intolerance to oral iron, intravenous iron sucrose, 6 mg/kg as a single dose, can be provided over a 2-hour period, with careful monitoring for anaphylaxis.[67] The fact that the improvement in RLS following oral iron therapy is gradual (over a period of months) should be emphasized to the patient and the family, lest they develop unrealistic expectations about a prompt response.
- Gabapentin, 50–100 mg at bedtime, may also help in symptomatic relief of the discomfort associated with RLS. Somnolence and weight gain are potential side effects of gabapentin.[68]
- Dopamine agonists like ropinirole (0.25–0.5 mg at bedtime) or pramipexole (0.125–0.25 mg at bedtime) are third line

TABLE 22.8	**Medical Conditions Associated with Childhood Obstructive Sleep Apnea**
Craniofacial syndromes	Crouzon syndrome Apert syndrome Treacher-Collins syndrome Goldenhar syndrome Pierre Robin syndrome
Neurologic diseases	Arnold-Chiari malformation Meningomyelocele Cerebral palsy Duchenne muscular dystrophy
Conditions with abnormal muscle tone	Down syndrome Prader-Willi syndrome Hypothyroidism
Conditions with reduced upper airway patency	Adenotonisllar hypertrophy Obesity Allergic rhinitis Macroglossia Laryngomalacia Subglottic stenosis Mucopolysaccharidoses/metabolic storage diseases

drugs for pediatric RLS. Potential side effects are tremor, confusion, and augmentation (reappearance of RLS symptoms earlier in the evening). Walters and co-authors described the response of six children with ADHD and RLS to treatment with levodopa/carbidopa or pergolide.[69] All six subjects showed subjective improvement in their sleep, as well as a significantly reduced PLMI and arousals from sleep. The daytime behavior also improved to the point that three of the six no longer met the diagnostic criteria for ADHD. In addition, a welcome development was the resolution of associated oppositional defiant disorder, as verified with the Connors subscale and the Oppositional Defiant Disorder Scale.[69] The long-term outcome of childhood RLS is unknown, especially in terms of characteristics that predict its resolution/persistence over time.

Sleep-Related Breathing Disturbances

Introduction

OSA is characterized by recurrent episodes of oxygen desaturation and limitation of nasal airflow with preserved thoracic and abdominal respiratory effort.[70] OSA has a prevalence rate of 2%–4%[71] and is more common in those born prematurely, and in those of African American or Hispanic ethnicity.[72] It is equally prevalent in boys and girls.

- The most common etiological factors are adenotonsillar hypertrophy, neuromuscular disorders, nasal allergies, exposure to passive smoke, and craniofacial syndromes that are associated anomalies such as midface hypoplasia, retrognathia, and macroglossia (Table 22.8). Complex upper airway problems such as unilateral choanal atresia, macroglossia, laryngomalacia, vocal cord paresis, laryngeal clefts, and tracheoesophageal fistula are considerations in infants.[73] Obesity accompanies childhood OSA less often than in adults, although it is now starting to become a significant risk factor in adolescents, given the significant increase in obesity in this age group (Fig. 22.6).

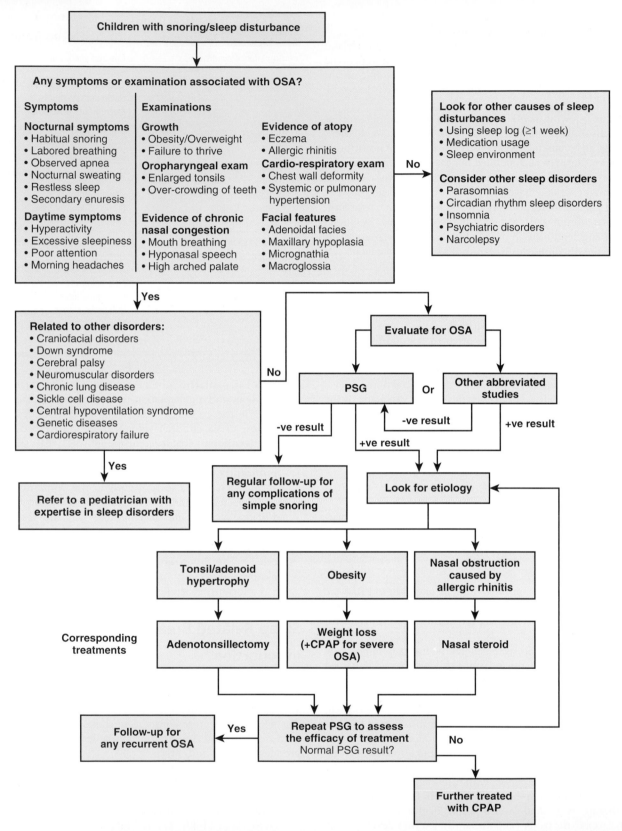

• **Figure 22.6** Diagnosis and Treatment of Childhood Obstructive Sleep Apnea (OSA). This figure illustrates the timing of sleep from preadolescence through adolescent development, highlighting the factors that affect sleep as described in the text. Thus sleep is relatively long and timed at an early hour for preadolescents, but maturational changes to intrinsic bioregulatory factors—the circadian phase delay arising from the circadian timing system and a slowed rise of sleep pressure stemming from sleep–wake homeostasis—push for a delay of the timing of sleep. Such psychosocial factors as self-selected bedtimes, response to academic pressure, and the availability and use of technology and social networking in the evening also push for a delay in the timing of sleep. Note that the length of sleep is not affected by these processes. Societal pressures that push for an early rise time—most notably an early start to the school day—are the forces that limit amount of time available for sleep. As a consequence, adolescents sleep too little and are asked to be awake at an inappropriate circadian phase. *CPAP*, continuous positive airway pressure; *PSG*, Polysomnography. (From Au CT, Li AM. Obstructive Sleep Breathing Disorders. *Pediatr Clin North Am.* 2009;56[1]:243–259.)

TABLE 22.9	Comparison of Obstructive Sleep Apnea in Children and Adults	
	Children	Adults
Estimated prevalence	1%–4%	2%–4%
Peak age	2–8 years	30–60 years
Gender (male/female)	1:1	3:1
Weight	Normal, decreased, increased	Overweight
Major cause	Adenotonsillar hypertrophy	Obesity
Gas exchange abnormalities	Always	Always
Duration of obstructive apneas	Any	>10 sec
Abnormal AI (per hour)	>1	>5
Abnormal AHI (per hour)	>1	>10
Sleep architecture	Preserved	Always altered
Arousals	Occasional	Always
Daytime sleepiness	30%	>90%
Neurocognitive problems	Common	Less common
Common treatment	Adenotonsillectomy	CPAP

AHI, Apnea-hypopnea index; *AI*, apnea index; *CPAP*, continuous positive airway pressure.

- Childhood OSA also differs from adult OSA, in that there is a greater likelihood of partial airway obstruction than frank apneas. Additionally, the duration of obstructive events is in general 5–10 sec rather than 10 sec or longer, as encountered in adults (Table 22.9).
- Primary snoring is characterized by habitual snoring that is not accompanied by sleep–wake complaints. It occurs in about 10%–12% of children. Though initially thought to be benign and of no pathological significance, it has been linked to neurobehavioral disturbances.[74] Childhood sleep-related breathing disturbances (SRBDs) constitute a spectrum ranging from primary snoring to OSA. An intermediate form of SRBD between primary snoring and OSA is the upper airway resistance syndrome (UARS), which is characterized by habitual snoring, increased negative intrathoracic pressure on esophageal manometry, and an increased frequency of respiratory event-related arousals (RERAs; Fig. 22.7). The mean critical pressure at which the upper airway collapses (Pcrit) is higher (1 cm H_2O, SD 3) in children with OSA syndrome than in those with primary snoring (Pcrit of –20 cm H_2O, SD 9).[75]

Clinical Features

- The *nocturnal features of OSA* include habitual snoring, mouth breathing, periods of observed apnea, restless sleep, and urinary incontinence. There is no correlation between how loudly a child snores and the presence or severity of sleep-disordered breathing. Infants with OSA may not snore, but may present with excessive sweating in sleep. Also, infants with OSA may

have significant GERD, which predisposes to chronic upper airway inflammation. Hypoventilation may accompany OSA in obesity, neuromuscular disorders, Prader-Willi syndrome (PWS), and Down syndrome. It is most reliably documented by measuring end-tidal CO_2 levels during PSG. Sleep-related hypoventilation, defined as end-tidal CO_2 greater than 50 mm for 25% or greater of the total sleep time. Early morning headaches may accompany OSA; they may develop either from sleep fragmentation and fluctuating cerebral blood flow velocities or due to hypercapnia secondary to hypoventilation.
- The *daytime features* of childhood OSA include waking up feeling nonrefreshed, mood swings, hyperactivity, inattentiveness, and hypersomnolence. In some children, an attention deficit disorder may be mistakenly diagnosed. It is thus important to take a detailed sleep–wake history in every patient undergoing evaluation for inattentiveness. The neurobehavioral abnormalities in children with OSA are a consequence of frontal lobe dysfunction and may include hyperactivity, inattentiveness, and impaired executive function.[76] An increased inflammatory response in the upper airway (as evidenced by elevated levels of C-reactive protein) and neurocognitive dysfunction may also develop as a consequence of OSA.[77]
- At examination, the height, weight, and blood pressure should be recorded, and the body mass index calculated. Failure to thrive and poor weight gain are now observed less often than in the past, perhaps because of increased awareness of OSA and its more timely diagnosis (Fig. 22.8). Evaluation for craniofacial abnormalities such as retrognathia or dental malocclusion, enlarged tongue size, swelling of the uvula, crowded oropharynx, mouth breathing, inflamed nasal mucous membranes, polyps, deviated nasal septum, and thyroid gland enlargement is also recommended. Tonsillar size (hypertrophy) should be graded on a 0–IV grade scale developed by Brodsky[78] (grade 0 = tonsils within the tonsillar fossa, grade 1 = tonsils just outside the tonsillar fossa and occupying 25% of the oropharyngeal width, grade 2 = tonsils occupying 26%–50% of the oropharyngeal width, grade 3 = tonsils occupying 51%–75% of the oropharyngeal width, and grade 4 = tonsils occupying >75% of the oropharyngeal width).

Laboratory Investigations

Oximetry: In a patient with severe tonsil hypertrophy and a history that is classic for OSA, documentation of recurrent episodes of oxygen desaturation of 4% or higher on an overnight oximetry study is sufficient to establish the diagnosis. A "normal" overnight oximetry study does not, however, rule out mild or moderate OSA, and based on the history, one might still need to resort to a nocturnal polysomnogram. In the context of a sleep laboratory, a high pretest probability of OSA in children with a positive oximetry trend (defined as three or more clusters of oxygen desaturation and at least three desaturations below 90%) had a positive predictive value of 97% for OSA and could pave the way for adenotonsillectomy. In contrast, a patient with a negative or inconclusive oximetry study had a posttest probability of 47%, thus necessitating the need for PSG in this set of patients.[79,80]

Nocturnal PSG: This is the gold standard for diagnosing SRBD, because it can detect and quantify respiratory events accurately. Ideally, respiration is investigated by using a combination of a nasal pressure transducer, oronasal thermocouple, thoracic and abdominal respiratory inductance plethysmography, pulse oximetry, and end-tidal CO_2. Infants and toddlers may not tolerate nasal

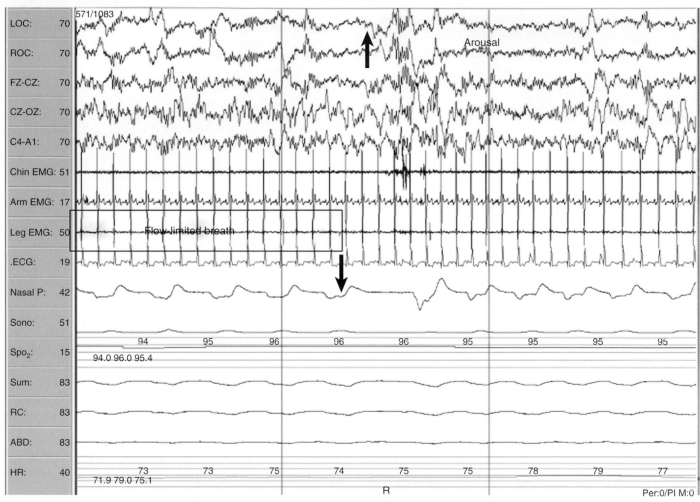

• **Figure 22.7** Nocturnal Polysomnogram Showing Upper Airway Resistance Syndrome. Notice the change in configuration of the nasal pressure transducer tracing, which shows a flow-limited breath *(down arrow)* that is followed by an electroencephalographic arousal *(up arrow)* and acceleration of the heart rate. *ABD,* Abdomen; *ECG,* electrocardiogram; *EMG,* electromyogram; *HR,* heart rate; *LOC,* left outer canthus; *Nasal P,* nasal pressure; *RC,* rib cage; *ROC,* right outer canthus; *Sono,* snore channel.

TABLE 22.10	A Comparison Between Pediatric and Adult Obstructive Sleep Apnea	
Feature	**Pediatric OSA**	**Adult OSA**
Prevalence	2% of the general population	10%–20% of the general population
Etiology (in order of frequency)	Adenotonsillar hypertrophy Craniofacial anomalies Neuromuscular disorders Obesity	Obesity Craniofacial anomalies Neuromuscular disorders
Polysomnogram findings	Partial obstructions with arousals more common than classic obstructive apnea events; duration of obstructive apneas is ≥5 or seconds; hypoventilation, with end-tidal CO_2 > 50 mm for at least 25% of recording time is more common than in adults	Classic OSA events more common; duration of obstructive apneas is ≥10 seconds; obstructive hypoventilation is less common
Management (in order of approach)	Adenotonsillectomy (A-T) For mild OSA persisting after A-T: topical nasal corticosteroids + monteleukast; For moderate to severe OSA persisting after A-T: consider CPAP	CPAP Weight reduction measures Dental devices (for mild residual OSA with craniofacial anomalies)

CPAP, Continuous positive airway pressure; *OSA,* obstructive sleep apnea.

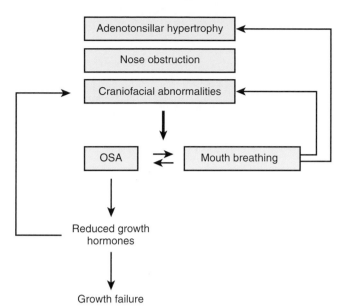

• **Figure 22.8** Mechanisms of Growth Failure in Childhood Sleep Apnea. (From Spicuzza L, Leonardi S, La Rosa M. Pediatric sleep apnea: early onset of the "syndrome"? *Sleep Med Rev.* 2009;13[2]:111–122.)

pressure cannulae, so one may have to rely only on the nasal signal from the thermocouple. According to the scoring manual of the American Academy of Sleep Medicine, apnea is defined as an event that lasts at least two missed breaths (or the duration of two missed breaths).[81] Furthermore, the event must be associated with greater than a 90% reduction in amplitude for more than 90% of the entire respiratory event, as compared with the pre-event baseline breath amplitude. Central apneas last 20 sec or longer or the duration of two or more missed breaths, along with an oxygen desaturation of 3% or higher (Fig. 22.9).[81] Hypopneas are events with greater than a 50% fall in nasal pressure amplitude or an alternative signal in comparison with the pre-event baseline excursion.[81] The event lasts at least two missed breaths or the duration of two breaths. Furthermore, the event is associated with oxygen desaturation of 3% or more (Fig. 22.10). RERAs are scored if there is a discernible fall in the amplitude of the signal on the nasal pressure sensor, but it is less than 50% in comparison with the baseline; there is flattening of the nasal pressure waveform; the event is accompanied by a snore, noisy breathing, elevation in end-tidal CO_2, or visual evidence of increased work of breathing; and the duration is that of two breath cycles or greater.[81] Nasal thermistors and thermocouples are not sensitive enough to detect RERAs. It is thus critical to use nasal pressure transducers, which

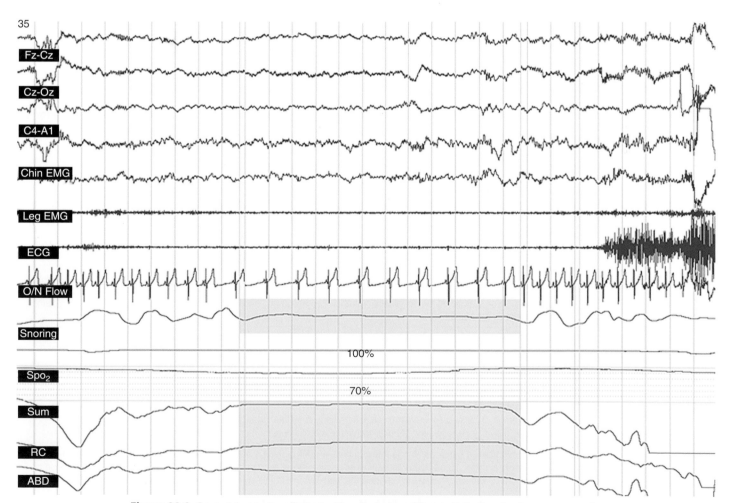

• **Figure 22.9** Central Apnea in a Patient with a Brainstem Glioma. Note the simultaneous cessation of signal from the thermocouple and the thoracic and abdominal *(ABD)* effort channels. The duration is 12 sec, and the event is followed by an arousal. *ECG,* Electrocardiogram; *EMG,* electromyogram; *O/N,* oral/nasal; *RC,* rib cage.

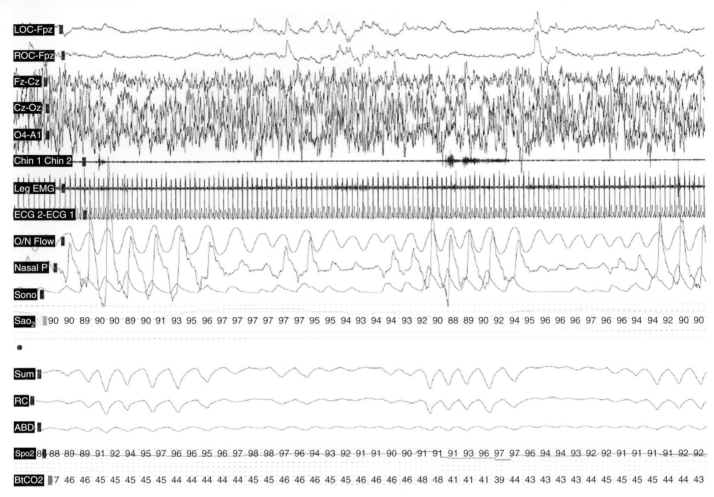

- **Figure 22.10** Hypopnea in a 12-Year-Old Child with Medically Complicated Obesity. Note the approximately 50% fall in amplitude of the nasal pressure (nasal P) signal, duration of at least two missed breaths, and oxygen desaturation of 3% or greater. *ABD*, Abdomen; *ECG*, electrocardiogram; *EMG*, electromyogram; *LOC*, left outer canthus; *RC*, rib cage; *ROC*, right outer canthus; *Sono*, snore channel.

TABLE 22.11	Some Common Comorbid Conditions in Childhood Obstructive Sleep Apnea
Condition	**Additional Comments**
Down syndrome	Trisomy 21; maxillary hypoplasia, macroglossia, hypotonic collapse of the upper airway, weak chest wall, altered central control of respiration
Prader-Willi syndrome	Absence of expression of the paternally inherited gene on 15q11-13. Patients exhibit hypotonic collapse of the upper airway, leading to OSA or obstructive hypoventilation. Central sleep apnea and hypersomnia on the basis of central nervous system dysfunction may also occur.
Pierre Robin (Robin) sequence	Multifactorial; micrognathia, posterior displacement of the tongue; pulmonary hypertension secondary to severe OSA
Crouzon syndrome	Mutations in the fibroblast growth factor receptor gene 2 gene; maxillary hypoplasia, decreased antero-posterior diameter of the oropharynx
MPS	At least six subtypes (1–6), each with absence of a distinct lysosomal enzyme that degrades a certain mucopolysaccharide. There is storage of heparin sulfate/dermatan sulfate/keratan sulfate in the soft tissue of the tongue, nasopharynx and oropharynx; this may be reversible in Hurler syndrome after early bone marrow transplantation (MPS-type 1)
Spinal muscular atrophy types 1 and 2	Deletions or mutations in the survival motor neuron gene 1 (SMN1). Type 1 presents in the newborn period or early infancy; type 2 in early childhood; both types show marked oropharyngeal and chest wall weakness leading to hypotonic collapse of the upper airway and sleep-related hypoventilation; non-invasive ventilation at home is recommended.
Duchenne muscular dystrophy	Deletion/mutation on Xp21 involving the dystrophin gene; marked oropharyngeal and chest wall weakness leading to hypotonic collapse of the upper airway and sleep-related hypoventilation; noninvasive ventilation at home is recommended.
Achondroplasia	Mutations in the fibroblast growth factor receptor 3 gene; misshapen foramen magnum, brainstem compression, midface hypoplasia, thoracic cage restriction

MPS, Mucopolysaccharidoses; *OSA*, obstructive sleep apnea.

will show the pattern of flow limitation immediately preceding the EEG arousal (see Fig. 22.7). Differences between adult and pediatric OSA are shown in Table 22.10.[82] Based on the obstructive apnea-hypopnea index (OAHI), the severity of pediatric OSA can be graded as mild (OAHI of 2–5), moderate (OAHI of 5–10), and severe (OAHI >10).[83]

The EEG manifestations of OSA consist of decreased sleep efficiency, suppression of the proportion of time spent in REM or N3 sleep, and an increase in the number of RERAs to more than 10%–12% of the total arousal index.

Important syndromes associated with OSA are shown in Table 22.11.

- *Cardiopulmonary assessment:* Sinus arrhythmia and a tachycardia-bradycardia pattern may accompany OSA. If uncorrected, the recurrent episodes of oxygen desaturation may lead to significant pulmonary vasoconstriction, right ventricular hypertrophy, and cor pulmonale. Patients with severe OSA (OAHI >10, oxygen saturation nadir below 80%) may therefore need a chest radiograph, electrocardiogram, and echocardiogram to evaluate for right heart failure consequent to pulmonary hypertension.

- *Evaluation of autonomic disturbance:* Apneic events provoke oxygen desaturation, as well as shifts in the frequency of the EEG waveforms, and these are denoted as RERAs. The traditional polysomnographic method of visual analysis and scoring of respiratory events is, however, not sensitive enough. Using spectral array EEG analysis, Bandla and Gozal detected changes during apneas suggestive of arousal that could not be picked up on the routine scalp EEG study.[84]

- *Neuropsychological assessment:* Though not routinely indicated, neuropsychological assessment should be considered on a case-by-case basis. The neuropsychological sequelae of classic childhood OSA are presumed to be secondary to sleep fragmentation. O'Brien and coauthors reported on 35 children with OSA (mean age, 6.7 years) and an equal number of closely matched controls.[85] Those with OSA had significant deficits in attention span, executive function, phonological processing, visual attention, and general conceptual ability in comparison with controls. Also worrisome is the fact that phonological processing is a basic building block in learning to read.

- *Endoscopy:* Direct visualization of the upper airway with flexible endoscopy under topical anesthesia allows detection of areas of narrowing from the nasal passages down to the glottis. It has the advantage of being a dynamic assessment that is especially useful in evaluating children with stridor and hoarseness.[73] In children with suspected subglottic stenosis secondary to lesions such as hemangioma (often accompanied by stridor in early infancy), rigid bronchoscopy may be necessary.

Management

- In general, adenotonsillectomy is the first step in management. Monopolar or bipolar electrocautery, the harmonic scalpel, and co-ablation have now taken technical precedence over traditional snare and cold knife techniques. Complications include bleeding, hemodynamic compromise, postoperative pain with decreased oral intake, nasopharyngeal stenosis, and hyponasality.[86] Although adenotonsillectomy is widely applied as initial therapy, its benefit has not been firmly established through evidence-based research. In about a fifth of patients younger than 36 months, dangerous postoperative airway edema develops following this procedure. All children younger than 36 months or those with severe OSA, craniofacial anomalies, and neuromuscular disorders should undergo close postoperative observation for at least 24 hours in the intensive care unit setting for airway compromise from edema.

About 21%–73% of patients fail to show complete resolution of SRBDs after adenotonsillectomy.[87]

- Three clinical parameters confer an independent risk for recurrence of OSA after adenotonsillectomy: the velocity of gain in body mass index, African American ethnicity, and obesity.[87] The group in which SRBDs do not resolve following adenotonsillectomy also includes patients with Down syndrome, neuromuscular problems, and craniofacial anomalies. In this group of subjects, repeat nocturnal PSG is helpful in establishing the degree of resolution.

- Positive airway pressure (PAP) is recommended if there is persistence of significant SRBD after adenotonsillectomy. PAP works by splinting the upper airway and thus keeping it patent. CPAP or bilevel positive airway pressure (BPAP) breathing can be titrated during the nocturnal polysomnogram to assess optimum pressure settings and mask type and size. The AAP recommends CPAP for children with OSA in whom surgery is not an option and for those with postoperative residual sleep apnea.[88] It is less invasive than surgery and has been approved by the US Food and Drug Administration for children older than 7 years; however, efficacy has also been documented in younger children (class II efficacy; i.e., evidence provided by a well-designed, matched-group cohort study, or by a randomized controlled clinical trial lacking in one design).[89]

  - Anxiety can limit adaptation to CPAP. A desensitization program aimed at reducing anxiety about using CPAP that is directed by a sleep technologist or nursing staff can be very helpful. In such a program, the child is initially exposed to the mask interface alone, followed by the addition of airway pressure during wakefulness and finally during sleep. The entire process may take a few days to weeks. The child may require considerable reassurance and positive reinforcement during this period. Diligent parental support is a key to success of CPAP use in the home environment. Patients with hypoventilation related to obesity and neuromuscular disorders may benefit from BPAP rather than CPAP. Decreased pressure during expiration is available in several CPAP devices and can facilitate tolerance by easing subjective exhalation against pressure. Side effects of positive pressure breathing include dryness of the nose and mouth. There are anecdotal reports of flattening of the midface because of long-term use of the mask.

- Weight reduction has been helpful in adults with obesity and OSA. Clear evidence of improvement in children following correction of obesity is not available. There is class III evidence (i.e., provided by other controlled trials such as those with natural history controls or patients serving as their own controls, with independent outcome assessments) in children, suggesting that weight reduction improves OSA.[90–92] It is, however, inconclusive from the standpoint of a strong direct association.[92] The relationship is further compounded by factors such as age and ethnicity.

- *Pharmacological measures:* A combination of nasal steroids and leukotriene antagonist therapy has been documented to benefit mild residual sleep apnea (apnea-hypopnea index of 2–5 per hour) following adenotonsillectomy in children.[93] A commonly recommended steroid is budesonide, 32 μg in each nostril at bedtime. The safety and efficacy of budesonide in children younger than 6 years has not been established. The leukotriene antagonist montelukast may be provided in a dose of 4 mg for children 2–6 years of age and 5 mg for children 6–11 years of age. Treatment with this agent can reduce the size of the adenoids and the apnea-hypopnea index.[94]

- *Dental appliances and procedures:* There is insufficient evidence to draw conclusions regarding the efficacy of oral appliances for the treatment of OSA in children.[95] Rapid maxillary distraction can be attempted in patients with high arched palates that predispose to narrowing of the nasal passages. A distractor bar anchored to the molars on either side of the upper jaw is used to apply constant pressure on the maxillary halves to induce bone growth from the borders of the midline cartilage. This procedure enlarges the nasal passages and lowers the height of the soft palate via maxillary widening.[96] Mandibular distraction osteogenesis has been used successfully for syndromic craniofacial deformities associated with mandibular hypoplasia, and secondary upper airway obstruction.[97]

Sleep in Patients with Central Nervous System Disorders

Alterations in sleep–wake function vary, depending on the anatomic location of the neurological lesion. For example, patients with Chiari malformations are likely to exhibit central apnea, obstructive apnea, hypoventilation, or bradypnea as a result of the altered development of the medulla and medullary compression, whereas those with mental retardation may exhibit cortical dysfunction in the form of excessive awakening and daytime or nighttime seizures. The severity of alterations in sleep–wake function also depends on the extent of the lesion, and whether it is static or progressive. Medications used to treat neurological disorders can influence sleep architecture; for example, benzodiazepines and barbiturates used for the treatment of seizures may suppress REM sleep. Fragmentation of sleep is in general quite common in children with neurological disorders. Treatment of the sleep–wake disorder may enhance the quality of life of these children.

Cerebral Palsy

Cerebral palsy is defined as a static insult to the developing central nervous system that may have been acquired prenatally, perinatally, or during early infancy. The incidence of cerebral palsy is approximately 1.2 per 1000 live births. Risk factors for its development include birth weight less than 2500 g, maternal mental retardation, breech presentation, and multiple congenital anomalies. The disorder leads to abnormalities in muscle tone, resting posture, muscle coordination, and joints. Cerebral palsy may be of the spastic, dyskinetic, or hypotonic types. Spastic cerebral palsy can be further subcategorized into the hemiplegic, diplegic, or quadriplegic types. Although their exact incidence has not been established, SRBDs are commonly encountered in patients with cerebral palsy.

- The upper airway may collapse as a consequence of neuromuscular incoordination, associated craniofacial abnormalities, or adenotonsillar hypertrophy. Children with spastic cerebral palsy may exhibit daytime irritability, fragmented sleep with frequent nighttime awakenings, and nocturnal oxygen desaturation.[98]

The inability to compensate for the disordered breathing by changes in body position makes OSA an especially dangerous condition in this group of patients. Patients may also be at risk for GERD and aspiration pneumonia. Periodic change in body position at night by the caretaker might be indicated. Coexisting seizures can also increase sleep fragmentation. Treating epilepsy with phenytoin should perhaps be avoided in children with cerebral palsy, because of its tendency to cause adenotonsillar hypertrophy as a result of lymphoid hyperplasia. Circadian rhythm abnormalities and sleep-related epilepsy (see later) might also complicate sleep–wake function in children with cerebral palsy.

Mental Retardation

Patients with severe mental retardation may have prolonged initial REM sleep latency and suppression of the proportion of time spent in REM sleep. Decreased REMs and spindle density, as well as the presence of "undifferentiated" sleep, correlate with low levels of intelligence. There may be difficulty falling asleep and staying asleep. Depression may coexist with mild mental retardation, in which case it may lead to early morning awakenings. Physical problems such as OSA and seizures may also coexist. Group-delivered interventions involving the parents may be helpful in improving sleep in this population[99] It is important to exclude physical problems such as sleep apnea before attempting cognitive and behavioral treatments such as ignoring the child, use of reward systems,[100] or short-term hypnotic therapy.

Down Syndrome

- OSA may develop as a consequence of macroglossia, midface hypoplasia, hypothyroidism, and hypotonic upper airway musculature.[101] Obesity may also coexist. Superimposed on this might be an element of chronic hypoventilation as a result of retention of CO_2, because of the hypotonic intercostal and diaphragmatic musculature. Sleep architecture is frequently abnormal, with decreased sleep efficiency, increased arousals, and suppression of slow wave and REM sleep. Behavioral problems in children with Down syndrome may in part be linked to these abnormalities in respiratory function. Central sleep apnea has also been observed in those with Down syndrome.

- Once nocturnal PSG has confirmed OSA or obstructive hypoventilation, a stepwise management approach is recommended—adenotonsillectomy is usually the first step, followed a few weeks later by repeat clinical and polysomnographic assessment and a trial of CPAP or BPAP for any residual OSA. Behavioral conditioning techniques may be needed for facilitating patient compliance with the mask and positive pressure ventilation.

Autism Spectrum Disorders

About two-thirds of children with an autism spectrum disorder (ASD) have sleep–wake problems.[102]

- In a sleep diary study, Richdale and Prior found that those with a higher intelligence quotient (IQ) had more severe sleep problems.[103] Anxiety from communication difficulties and obsessive-compulsive behavior occur frequently in children with ASDs, and may underlie at least some of the sleep initiation and maintenance problems in this population.

- Polygraphic studies have shown prolonged initial sleep latency, decreased sleep efficiency, and low early morning awakening spontaneous arousal thresholds. Melatonin deficiency and circadian rhythm disturbance might also contribute to the sleep disturbance.[104]
- Management usually involves identifying the key factors (organic or behavioral), supplementation with melatonin at bedtime, counseling the parents, and providing respite care, if necessary.

Rett Syndrome

This X-linked dominant neurodegenerative disorder occurs exclusively in girls. It is characterized by progressive speech and cognitive regression during early childhood, in association with stereotypic hand-wringing movements and gait apraxia that seem to develop during the first 6–18 months of life. About 80% of patients with Rett syndrome have a mutation in the methyl-CpG-binding protein 2 (*MECP2*) gene, which regulates transcriptional silencing. It is located on Xq28. The Rett trait is lethal in males. Sekul and Percy reported that sleep problems develop in more than 80% of children with Rett syndrome, with irregular sleep–wake rhythms being the most common.[105] Nighttime screaming, crying, and episodes of laughter have also been reported.[106] As a group, patients with Rett syndrome may have less sleep at night and increased sleep fragmentation, combined with carry-over sleepiness into the daytime. There have been isolated case reports of the success of melatonin in ameliorating this sleep disruption. Patients with Rett syndrome also display episodic hyperventilation during wakefulness, but the respiratory rate and rhythm remain unaffected during sleep. About 50% of patients have partial or generalized seizures, some of which may include apnea as an ictal manifestation.

Prader-Willi Syndrome

- This syndrome of congenital hypotonia, hypogonadism, and cognitive dysfunction is linked to microdeletion of the paternally contributed region of chromosome 15q11.2-q13. During the neonatal period and infancy, patients manifest severe hypotonia, anorexia, and feeding difficulties to the point of requiring nasogastric tube feedings. Around early childhood, however, there is an increase in appetite, to the extent that it becomes almost voracious and may become associated with morbid obesity. Patients with PWS may have elevated ghrelin levels, which might contribute to their hyperphagia.[107] Although it has not been systematically evaluated, mild to moderate daytime sleepiness is common in PWS and affects perhaps half the subjects. It may be associated with sleep-onset REM periods (SOREMPs) on the multiple sleep latency test (MSLT).[108]
- Results of nocturnal PSG are highly variable. Sleep apnea seems to be relatively infrequent, however, and does not contribute to the daytime sleepiness, which appears to be a consequence of hypothalamic dysfunction. In support of this is the finding of low CSF levels of hypocretin-1 in a patient with combined PWS and Kleine-Levin syndrome who was tested at the time of increased sleepiness.[109]
- Lately, it has been recognized that treatment of PWS with growth hormone promotes an increase in muscle mass and motor development. The long-term impact of growth hormone therapy on PWS has not been clearly established. These patients need to be monitored closely in a multidisciplinary setting for the development of obstructive apnea secondary to growth hormone therapy, because deaths have occurred in patients receiving growth hormone, although the exact underlying mechanism has not been established.[110]

Blindness

- Blindness associated with loss of light perception as a result of lesions of the eye or the optic nerves and chiasm can disrupt circadian rhythms and neuroendocrine functions. The resultant "free running" sleep–wake cycles are longer than 24.2 hours and tend to shift toward progressively later and later times around the clock.[111] The basis for the free-running cycles seems to be dysregulation of the secretion of melatonin, which is a light-sensitive hormone secreted by the pineal gland and dependent on an intact retinohypothalamic pathway. In sighted individuals, secretion of melatonin is low during the daytime, but its plasma levels rise immediately before bedtime and during the night. It has important sleep induction and maintenance properties. Children with severe retinopathy of prematurity, congenital bilateral glaucoma, septo-optic dysplasia, or severe bilateral optic neuritis may have "free-running" or non-24-hour sleep–wake cycles because of the lack of light perception. In a questionnaire survey of 77 blind children ranging in age from 3 to 18 years and sighted controls, Leger and co-workers found that 17% of blind children reported sleeping less than 7 hours at night, as compared with 2.6% of controls, with blind children awakening much earlier in the morning; they also exhibited increased daytime sleepiness.[112] In turn, daytime sleepiness may have an impact on attention, concentration, and the behavior of blind children. The presence of multiple associated physical and neurological handicaps can further complicate management.
- Administration of 0.5–5 mg of melatonin 1 hour before bedtime seems to facilitate sleep onset, increase total sleep time, and reduce awake time at night.[111] Manipulation of nonphotic "zeitgebers" such as food, music, physical activity, and exercise might also be of some value in establishing sleep–wake schedules when circadian rhythms are disrupted in blind children.

Arnold-Chiari Malformations

Myelomeningocele is invariably associated with Arnold-Chiari malformation type II, a condition in which a segment of the medulla and the fourth ventricle are congenitally displaced below the foramen magnum (in general at the C1–2 level), along with hydrocephalus. About two-thirds of children with Chiari type II malformation have a history of breathing disturbance.

- Mechanisms underlying the SRBD include developmental malformations of the brainstem respiratory areas, mechanical compression of the brainstem as a result of a small posterior fossa, combined with downward compression from the supratentorial compartment due to hydrocephalus. There may also be unilateral vocal cord paralysis, obstructive apnea from adenotonsillar hypertrophy/hypotonic collapse of the upper airway, and hypoventilation due to obesity and intercostal muscle paralysis. Patients with thoracic or thoracolumbar myelomeningocele and those with abnormalities in pulmonary function secondary to kyphoscoliosis can have persistent sleep-related breathing abnormalities such as OSA, obstructive hypoventilation, and central sleep apnea. The respiratory abnormalities in Chiari malformations are in general more severe during REM sleep than during NREM sleep.

- Adenotonsillectomy is the initial step in managing OSA, but patients may ultimately need CPAP or BPAP breathing devices. Counseling of preteens about the importance of avoiding excessive weight obesity around adolescence is also recommended. Collaboration of care with the neurosurgeon is required to ensure that the brainstem is not being compressed due to raised intracranial pressure from obstructive hydrocephalus.
- Type I Chiari malformation is characterized by descent only of the cerebellar tonsils below the plane of the foramen magnum, with a normally positioned fourth ventricle. There is no accompanying hydrocephalus or myelomeningocele. The abnormally positioned cerebellar tonsils may compress the medulla and lead to brainstem related respiratory compromise. Some patients may exhibit swallowing difficulties and vocal cord paresis. Severe cases of Chiari type I malformation may show a cervical syrinx (fluid-filled cavity within the spinal cord). The diagnosis of Chiari type I malformation is made on the basis of head and cervical spinal cord MRI scan. Nocturnal polysomnogram findings in Chiari type I malformation include obstructive apnea, obstructive hypoventilation, central apnea, or bradypnea. Significant respiratory dysfunction may necessitate posterior fossa decompression.[113]

The Relationship Between Sleep and Epilepsy

Seizures are events characterized by paroxysmal, repetitive, and excessive neuronal discharges from the cerebral cortex. The onset of sleep may be associated with build-up of spikes, which are the basic building block or precedent for seizures.[114] A tendency to experience repetitive, unprovoked seizures over time is termed epilepsy. Frontal and temporal lobe seizures are especially likely to occur in sleep and to spread bilaterally (exhibit secondary generalization). Nocturnal seizures are in general more likely to occur during stage N2, followed by stage N1 and stage N3 of NREM sleep, in that order, and least likely to occur during REM sleep.

- The syndrome of *electrical status epilepticus in slow wave sleep (ESES)* is characterized by continuous spike and wave discharges during 85% or more of nocturnal NREM sleep, in association with cognitive and behavioral regression.
- *Landau-Kleffner syndrome* is typified by regression in language function (auditory verbal agnosia) in association with focal or generalized epileptiform (slow spike and wave) activity during wakefulness and sleep.
- Patients with *Lennox-Gastaut syndrome* may exhibit tonic seizures in sleep in association with generalized, 0.5–2 Hz spike and wave discharges (slow spike and waves).
- *Benign Rolandic epilepsy of childhood* develops typically around age 5–6 years in children who manifest predominantly sleep-activated focal seizures that are characterized by unilateral facial twitching with preserved consciousness. Seizures with onset in the hemisphere that is dominant for language may also exhibit aphasia during the seizure (ictal aphasia). Neurodevelopment and examination are normal. The EEG shows repetitive spikes and sharp waves localized over the central or midtemporal regions. Owing to the benign nature of the epilepsy that tends to resolve spontaneously over time, antiepileptic drug therapy is prescribed only if there are a significant number of seizures (more than 3–4 over a lifetime).
- Seizures tend to suppress REM sleep, with a corresponding increase in slow wave sleep. This effect may persist for as long

TABLE 22.12 Common Causes of Daytime Sleepiness in Childhood

Insufficient sleep at night (e.g., from abnormal sleep hygiene)
Delayed sleep phase syndrome
Drugs (over the counter/prescription; hypnotics and sedatives/psychostimulants)
Depression
Obstructive hypoventilation
Upper airway resistance syndrome
Narcolepsy
Idiopathic hypersomnia
Kleine-Levin syndrome
Restless legs syndrome
Posttraumatic hypersomnia

as 24 hours after the seizure event. Frequent nocturnal seizures tend to disrupt sleep, with an increased number of arousals.
- Sleep disorders can also have an adverse impact on seizure control. Deprivation of sleep may trigger seizures. Patients with OSA may manifest poor seizure control, which is improved following correction of OSA.[115] In some instances, daytime somnolence is mistaken for a side effect of antiepileptic therapy, when in fact it may be the consequence of an underlying sleep disorder.
- Antiepileptic drugs in general lead to stabilization of sleep, with a decrease in the amount of sleep fragmentation. There may be no change or decreased N3 sleep and increased spindle density with phenobarbital, and there is decreased REM sleep with phenytoin/carbamazepine and decreased N2 and N3 sleep with benzodiazepines. Lamotrigine causes either no change or a decrease in REM sleep. Felbamate is associated with insomnia in about 9% of cases.

Daytime Sleepiness—General Comments

Excessive daytime sleepiness is a common, disabling, and frequently underrecognized symptom of diverse etiology.[116] Many of the underlying disorders are treatable. Questionnaire surveys indicate a prevalence of 4%–20%. Most teenagers are chronically sleep deprived and report sleep lengths of 6.5–7.5 hours, in contrast to the optimum amount of sleep necessary to maintain adequate daytime alertness of around 8.5–9.5 hours.

Consequences

Sleepiness interferes with the consolidation of short-term memory into long-term memory. It also leads to loss of "affect control" because of disinhibition of the prefrontal cortex, with resultant mood swings, inattentiveness, and impulsivity. Motor speed and judgment also become impaired and result in an increased propensity for accidents. Common causes of daytime sleepiness are listed in Table 22.12. Multiple factors contributing to daytime sleepiness may coexist (e.g., inadequate sleep hygiene in a teen with apnea hypopnea syndrome).

Assessment

The sleep history may elicit unrefreshed night sleep, tendency to fall asleep easily at school or while being driven in a car, mood swings, increasing forgetfulness, and tendency for automatic daytime behaviors that the patient may not recall. Survey instruments that can be used for evaluating sleepiness include the Pediatric Daytime Sleepiness Scale, the Sleep Disturbance Scale for Children, and the modified Epworth Sleepiness Scale. Ambulatory procedures like maintenance of sleep logs and simultaneous wrist actigraphy for 2–3 weeks are helpful in evaluating for causes of daytime sleepiness like inadequate sleep hygiene and circadian rhythm sleep disorders. Nocturnal PSG, which may or may not be followed by the MSLT, are other tests required for the objective assessment of sleepiness. The laboratory tests are tailored to the specific underlying problem. Urine drug screens are recommended when there a suspicion of drug-seeking behavior. Psychological assessment and child psychiatric consultation are also helpful when emotional and behavioral issues are present. Human leukocyte antigen (HLA) typing and CSF hypocretin analysis may be indicated in selected patients with suspected narcolepsy-cataplexy. Narcolepsy is characterized by a relatively early appearance of REM sleep on the nocturnal polysomnogram, sleep fragmentation, periodic leg movements, marked shortening of the daytime mean sleep latency on the MSLT (<5 minutes in contrast to a normal value of 16–18 minutes), and two or more associated SOREMPs.

Periodic Hypersomnia

Also termed the *Kleine-Levin syndrome*, in general this disorder is seen in adolescents, with male preponderance.

- There are periods of hypersomnolence lasting 1–2 weeks, during which patients may sleep 18–20 hours a day and manifest cognitive and mood disturbances, compulsive hyperphagia and hypersexual behavior, with an intervening 2–4 months of normal alertness and behavior.[117] The hyperphagia may be in the form of binge eating and can actually be associated with a 2–5-kg increase in body weight.
- Variants of the syndrome have also been recognized, with anorexia, feelings of depersonalization, and absence of hypersexual behavior. Nocturnal PSG during the symptomatic periods shows decreased sleep efficiency, shortened REM sleep latency, and a decreased percentage of time spent in stage N3 sleep. The MSLT may show moderately shortened mean sleep latency in the 5–10-minute range, but without the two or more SOREMPs that are typical of patients with narcolepsy. The periodic hypersomnia gradually subsides over a period of several years, or may evolve into classic depression. A disturbance in hypothalamic-thalamic function has been postulated, but not established. The association of Kleine-Levin syndrome with HLA-DQB1*0201, the occasional precipitation after systemic infections, and the relapsing and remitting nature suggest the possibility of an underlying autoimmune disturbance.[118]
- There is no satisfactory treatment, although lithium has been reported to be effective than other agents like lamotrigine and sodium valproate.[119]

Narcolepsy

- Overwhelming and chronic daytime sleepiness, fragmented night sleep, superimposition of REM sleep onto wakefulness in the form of hypnagogic hallucinations (vivid dreams at sleep onset), sleep paralysis, and cataplexy (sudden loss of skeletal muscle tone in response to emotional triggers such as laughter, fright, or surprise) are the characteristic clinical features of narcolepsy. Type 1 narcolepsy is with cataplexy, and type 2 is narcolepsy without cataplexy. Children are more likely to manifest type 1

narcolepsy. The overall incidence of narcolepsy in the United States is about 1.37 per 100,000 persons per year (1.72 for men and 1.05 for women).[120] The incidence is highest in the second and third decades, followed by a gradual decline thereafter. About a third of narcolepsy has onset of symptoms in childhood. The prevalence is approximately 56 per 100,000 persons.[120] Although the age at onset in children is in the latter half of the first decade or the second decade, rare cases with an onset in infancy or early childhood have also been reported.[121] The daytime sleepiness may initially be overlooked by parents, school teachers, and physicians alike. Sleepy children can be mistaken for being "lazy," and may exhibit mood swings and inattentiveness.

- Cataplexy is present in about two-thirds of all patients with narcolepsy. In general, cataplexy attacks last 1–5 minutes, and are characterized by skeletal muscle atonia and absence of muscle tendon reflexes during emotional events such as laughter, excitement, or the anticipation of reward. Facial weakness with the jaw dropping open or a slight rolling movement of the head and neck are most common. Episodes of more severe muscle weakness leading to falls may also occur, but are less common. Children younger than 7 or 8 years may be unable to provide a reliable history of hypnagogic hallucinations or sleep paralysis.
- The night sleep is fragmented, with frequent arousals. REM sleep without atonia and REM sleep behavior disorder (RBD) may occur in type 1 narcolepsy. PLMS are also common.[122] Patients exhibit less circadian drive–dependent alertness during the daytime and also less sleepiness at night.[123] In rare instances, secondary narcolepsy may develop in patients following closed head injury, primary brain tumors, lymphomas, and encephalitis (secondary or symptomatic narcolepsy).[124]
- The presence of HLA-DQB1*0602 in close to 100% of persons with type 1 narcolepsy, as compared with 12%–32% prevalence in the general population, indicates a genetic susceptibility, which per se is insufficient to precipitate the clinical syndrome. For instance, monozygotic twins may remain discordant for narcolepsy, which suggests a role for epigenetic factors in precipitating narcolepsy.[125] In genetically susceptible individuals, however, acquired life stresses such as minor head injury, systemic illnesses such as infectious mononucleosis, and bereavement may trigger narcolepsy, perhaps by altering cell-mediated immunity.[126] They have been reported to occur in about two-thirds of subjects—the "two-hit hypothesis."
- The key pathophysiological event in narcolepsy type 1 is hypocretin deficiency.[127] Hypocretin (orexin) is a peptide that is produced by neurons of the dorsolateral hypothalamus. Hypocretin-1 and hypocretin-2 (synonymous with orexin-A and orexin-B) are peptides synthesized from preprohypocretin. Hypocretin neurons have widespread projections to the forebrain and brainstem. Hypocretin promotes alertness and increases motor activity and the basal metabolic rate. Of significance is the observation made in human postmortem brains of narcolepsy patients by Thannickal et al. of a 85%–95% reduction in the number of hypocretin neurons in the hypothalamus, as compared with controls,[18] with the intermingled melanin-concentrating neurons remaining unaffected. This suggests selective vulnerability for a targeted neurodegenerative process. It is hypothesized that degeneration of the hypocretin-producing cells of the hypothalamus (possibly disrupted cell mediated immunity, perhaps predisposed to by HLA-DQB1*0602 due to mechanisms not yet fully defined) provokes a decrease in forebrain noradrenergic activation, which decreases alertness. A corresponding decrease in noradrenergic activity in the brainstem leads to disinhibition

of the brainstem cholinergic systems, thus triggering cataplexy and other phenomena of REM sleep such as hypnagogic hallucinations and sleep paralysis.

The decrease in hypocretin-1 levels that is characteristic of type 1 narcolepsy is also reflected in the CSF. Using a radioimmunoassay, Nishino et al. found that the mean CSF level of hypocretin-1 in healthy controls was 280.3 ± 33.0 pg/mL; in neurological controls it was 260.5 ± 37.1 pg/mL, and in those with narcolepsy type 1 (narcolepsy with cataplexy) the hypocretin-1 was either undetectable or below 100 pg/mL.[126] Low to absent CSF hypocretin levels were found in 32 of 38 narcolepsy type 1 patients, who were all also HLA-DQB10*0602 positive. Narcolepsy patients who were HLA-DQB1*0602 antigen negative tended to have normal to high CSF hypocretin-1 levels. In another study of narcolepsy type 1, narcolepsy type 2 (narcolepsy without cataplexy), and idiopathic hypersomnia, Kanbayashi and co-workers found that their nine CSF hypocretin-deficient narcolepsy-cataplexy patients were all HLA-DQB1*0602 positive, including three preadolescents.[128] In contrast, patients with narcolepsy without cataplexy and idiopathic hypersomnia had normal CSF hypocretin levels (Fig. 22.11). The CSF hypocretin

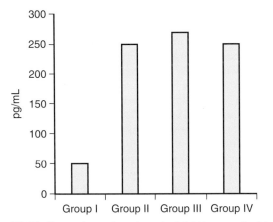

• **Figure 22.11** Comparison of cerebrospinal fluid hypocretin-1 levels in HLA-DQB1*0602–positive narcolepsy-cataplexy (group I), narcolepsy-cataplexy that is HLA-DQB1*0602 negative (group II), narcolepsy without cataplexy (group III), and idiopathic hypersomnia (group IV). (Data adapted from Kanbayashi T, Inoue Y, Chiba S, et al. CSF hypocretin-1 (orexin A) concentrations in narcolepsy with and without cataplexy and idiopathic hypersomnia. *J Sleep Res.* 2002;11:91–93.)

assay is most useful in an HLA-DQB1*0602–positive patient with suspected narcolepsy-cataplexy who is younger than 5 years (because the MSLT is invalid at this age) or is receiving central nervous stimulants/selective serotonin reuptake inhibitors, the discontinuation of which for the purpose of obtaining PSG and an MSLT may be unsafe or impractical.

• Since it is most readily available, the combined battery of a nocturnal polysomnogram and MSLT is still the recommended method for the diagnosis of narcolepsy, however. The nocturnal polysomnogram shows a short sleep onset latency, possible SOREMP (onset within 15 minutes of falling asleep), possible decreased initial REM sleep latency of less than 70 minutes (time from sleep onset to onset of the first REM sleep epoch; the normal value in teenagers is around 140 minutes), increased tendency for spontaneous arousals, and increased PLMS. Type 1 narcolepsy may also be accompanied by REM sleep without atonia or RBD. Other sleep pathologies like obstructive hypoventilation are absent. The MSLT is initiated on the morning after the nocturnal polysomnogram. In narcolepsy, the MSLT, in general, shows a mean sleep-onset latency on four nap opportunities of less than 8 minutes after "lights out,"[129] whereas the reference value for children is approximately 14–16 minutes.[130] MSLT SOREMPs are also seen during at least two of the four nap opportunities. Since narcolepsy is a lifelong condition, the diagnostic test results need to be absolutely certain. A urine drug screen may be obtained in between the nap opportunities if one suspects that the sleepiness might be related to drug-seeking behavior.

The management requires a combination of lifestyle changes and pharmacotherapy.[131,132]

• A planned daytime nap of 20–30 minutes at school and another one in the afternoon on return home may enhance alertness. The patient should observe regular sleep-onset and morning wake-up times, avoid alcohol, and exercise regularly. To minimize the risk for accidents, the patient should stay away from sharp, moving objects such as conveyor belts or working at heights. Driving should be avoided until daytime alertness has been brought into the normal or nearly normal range.

• Drugs commonly used for the management of daytime sleepiness and cataplexy are listed in Table 22.13. The emotional and behavioral problems that commonly accompany childhood narcolepsy may require supportive psychotherapy and the

TABLE 22.13	Pharmacotherapy for Childhood Narcolepsy	
Target Symptom	**Drug**	**Dose Range**
Sleepiness	Methylphenidate, regular or extended release	20–60 mg/day in two divided doses
	Dextroamphetamine, regular or extended release	10–30 mg/day in two divided doses
	Modafinil	100–400 mg in two divided doses
Cataplexy	Protriptyline	5–10 mg in two divided doses
	Clomipramine	25–50 mg once a day
	Sodium oxybate	3–6 g at night in two divided doses given 2–3 hours apart
Emotional/behavioral problems	Fluoxetine	10–30 mg/day
	Sertraline	25–50 mg/day
Periodic limb movement disorder/restless legs	Clonazepam	0.5–1.0 mg at bedtime
	Pramipexole	0.125–0.25 mg at bedtime
	Ropinirole	0.25–0.5 mg at bedtime

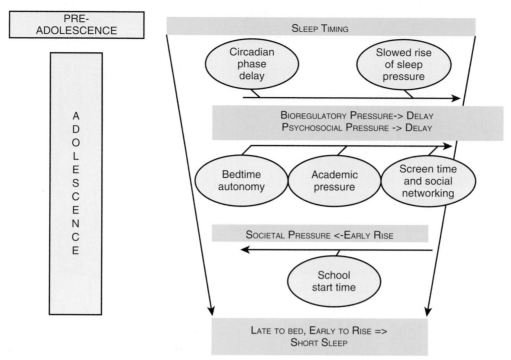

• **Figure 22.12** Adolescent Development and Sleep: the Perfect Storm. This figure illustrates the timing of sleep from preadolescence through adolescent development, highlighting the factors that affect sleep as described in the text. Thus sleep is relatively long and timed at an early hour for preadolescents, but maturational changes to intrinsic bioregulatory factors—the circadian phase delay arising from the circadian timing system and a slowed rise of sleep pressure stemming from sleep–wake homeostasis—push for a delay of the timing of sleep. Such psychosocial factors as self-selected bedtimes, response to academic pressure, and the availability and use of technology and social networking in the evening also push for a delay in the timing of sleep. Note that the length of sleep is not affected by these processes. Societal pressures that push for an early rise time—most notably an early start to the school day—are the forces that limit amount of time available for sleep. As a consequence, adolescents sleep too little and are asked to be awake at an inappropriate circadian phase. (From Clarskadon MA. Sleep in adolescents: the perfect storm. *Pediatr Clin North Am.* 2011;58[3]:637–647.)

prescription of selective serotonin reuptake inhibitors. Support groups like the Narcolepsy Network and Wake-Up Narcolepsy may be able to provide emotional support to patients and families.

Circadian Rhythm Sleep Disorders

Delayed Sleep Phase Disorder

Delayed sleep phase disorder (DSPD) is a circadian rhythm disorder related to dysfunction of the suprachiasmatic nucleus, which serves as our circadian timekeeper.[133,134] It typically has onset in adolescence, with a male preponderance (Fig. 22.12). Patients have a constitutional difficulty in phase-advancing sleep, and can fall asleep only at progressively later and later times at night (Fig. 22.13). DSPD is frequently misdiagnosed as severe insomnia. The patient may be unable to fall asleep till midnight or the early morning hours. Once asleep, and if allowed to sleep uninterrupted, patients show normal sleep quantity and quality. In general, most patients are obligated to wake up by 6:30 or 7:00 AM to attend school, which results in chronic sleep deprivation, sleep "drunkenness" on awakening, and variable degrees of depression and changes in personality. Polymorphisms in the *hPer*, arylalkamine *N*-acetyltransferase, HLA-DR1, and *Clock* genes have been associated with an increased predisposition to DSPD.[134] There is increased clustering of DSPD within some families. DSPD must

be differentiated from the school avoidance behavior seen in truant adolescents, as the latter individuals may be able to fall asleep at an earlier hour at night in a controlled environment.

- Sleep logs for 2–3 weeks combined with wrist actigraphy are helpful in making a diagnosis of DSPD.
- "Bright light" therapy is helpful in advancing the sleep-onset time.[135] It consists of the provision of 6000–8000 lux of bright light via a "light box" for 20–30 minutes immediately on awakening in the morning. The light box is kept at a distance of 18–24 inches from the face. It leads to a gradual advancement (shifting back) of the sleep-onset time at night. Bright light therapy may be combined with melatonin, 0.5 mg, given 5.5–6 hours before the required bedtime in a dose of 0.5–1 mg. Decreasing the intensity of light in the evening may facilitate earlier sleep onset at night. Another therapeutic approach is to progressively delay bedtime by 3–4 hours/day, until it becomes synchronized with socially acceptable sleep–wake times, and then adhering to this schedule (chronotherapy). This may take 1–2 weeks to achieve. Over time, however, all patients with DSPD are at risk for drifting to progressively later and later bedtimes. Daytime stimulants such as modafinil (100–400 mg/day in two divided doses) may also improve the level of daytime alertness. The physician may need to communicate with the school to explain that absences from school before the diagnosis may have been on medical grounds, and request a slightly later (midmorning) school start time.

Time of day

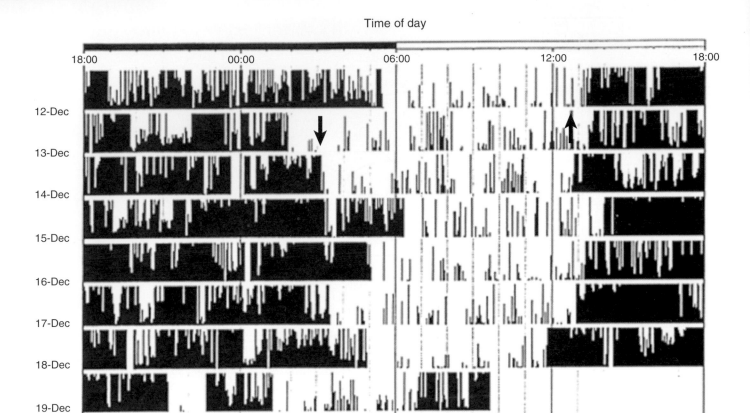

• **Figure 22.13** Actigram in an Adolescent Boy with Delayed Sleep Phase Syndrome. Note the persistence of muscle activity until late at night, which correlates with remaining awake. Sleep-onset time is indicated by the *down arrow*. The early afternoon wake-up time is indicated by the *up arrow*. (From Kotagal S. Sleep disorders in childhood. *Neurol Clin*. 2003;21:1–21.)

Irregular Sleep–Wake Rhythms

This disorder tends to occur in patients with chronic neurological disorders like cerebral palsy, autism, or sequelae of head injury or encephalitis.[135] Patients may have a hard time trying to fall asleep at a scheduled time of the night and may manifest three or more major periods of sleep over a 24-hour period. The total sleep time over the 24-hour period is, however, essentially within normal limits. Lack of exposure to orienting light (sunlight) during the daytime may play a causative role. The diagnosis can be established on the basis of sleep logs and actigraphy, with the latter demonstrating multiple irregular periods of sleep onset. Treatment consists of providing a consistent bed-onset and morning wake-up time, and exposure to bright light immediately on awakening. Melatonin or melatonin receptor agonists like ramelteon or tasimelteon may also be helpful in facilitating sleep.

Non-24-Hour Sleep Cycles

Also termed free-running disorder, this circadian rhythm disorder is characterized by conformity of the sleep–wake schedule to the endogenous, 24.3-hour period average (rather than the extraneous 24-hour clock). This leads to a progressive stair-stepwise delay in the sleep onset time from one night to the next. If allowed to ad lib, patients may fall asleep at progressively later and later times on the 24-hour clock.[135] This disorder is seen most often in blind patients with absent light perception, though rare cases have also been reported after closed head

injury. The diagnosis can be made by using a combination of sleep logs and actigraphy. The management can be difficult and frustrating, but in general, the adherence to a fixed morning wake-up schedule; provision of time cues such as breakfast, lunch, exercise, and bedtime; and provision of melatonin 2 hours prior to desired bed onset or the use of melatonin receptor agonists is recommended.

Parasomnias

Events that occur at the sleep–wake interface or during sleep are termed parasomnias.

- Common sleep–wake transition disorders include hypnic starts and rhythmic movement disorder (head banging, head rolling, or body rocking).
- Parasomnias of NREM sleep include confusional arousals, sleep terrors, and sleepwalking.[136,137] NREM parasomnias are consequent to partial arousal from stage N3. They are most likely to occur in the first third of the night's sleep. Sleep deprivation, fever, underlying OSA, PLM, RLS, and GERD might predispose to NREM parasomnias by activating arousals. There can be a familial predisposition to NREM parasomnias.[138] In contrast to sleepwalking and sleep terrors, patients with confusional arousals exhibit less motor and autonomic activity. Sweating, flushing of the face, and agitation are prominent, however, in patients with sleep terrors and sleepwalking. The duration of NREM parasomnias may be 5–30 minutes. Even though the sleep of the parents may be disrupted by severe NREM

parasomnias, the child is typically amnestic for these events upon awakening the following morning.

- *Nightmares* and *RBD*[139–141] are common parasomnias of REM sleep. By virtue of occurrence during REM sleep phenomena, they are more likely to occur in the early morning hours. Recurrent nightmares may be a marker for underlying anxiety or posttraumatic stress disorder. Psychological counseling, including cognitive behavioral therapy, is helpful in the management of nightmares. RBD of childhood is associated with narcolepsy, the use of selective serotonin reuptake inhibitors, and neurodevelopmental disorders like autism. Unlike in adults with RBD, there is no association with synuclein-related degenerative disorders like Lewy Body disease. The patients may yell out in sleep or flail the extremities. The history is of key importance in diagnosing most NREM and REM parasomnias. A home videotape that has captured the event may be helpful. Nocturnal PSG with synchronized video monitoring and a 16-channel EEG montage is required if the diagnosis cannot be established on the basis of the history, and when an additional sleep disorder such as OSA or PLMD that may be triggering partial arousals is suspected. Nocturnal frontal lobe seizures are sometimes mistaken for parasomnias, but tend to occur out of sleep stages N1 and N2, and hence develop randomly throughout the night's sleep. They are also much shorter in duration than parasomnias, typically 30–60 sec long. They may occur on multiple occasions during the same night. In contrast to parasomnias, patients with seizures are often tired on awakening in the morning.
- *Management:* Infrequently occurring parasomnias do not warrant specific therapy because they are benign events. On the other hand, recurrent parasomnias may increase the risk of injury to the patient, and also disrupt the sleep of other family members. Recurrent parasomnias need investigation with nocturnal PSG, also because they may serve as a marker for underlying sleep pathology (such as OSA and RLS) or psychiatric disease (such as anxiety or posttraumatic stress disorder [PTSD]).
- Environmental safety issues such as placing dead bolts on the doors and removal of sharp objects from the customary path should be considered in individuals with sleep walking.
- Underlying OSA and RLS should be treated when they are triggering NREM parasomnias.
- The technique of "anticipatory awakening" has been tried in patients with NREM parasomnias with mixed results—the parent awakens the child about 15–20 minutes before the usual time of occurrence of the NREM parasomnia, in general, by wiping the child's face with a wet washcloth in an effort to shift the patient from deep sleep into a lighter stage, and thus aborting the event. Some parents like this technique because it is non-pharmacological. Its effectiveness is, however, not established as it has not been evaluated systematically.
- Clonazepam in a dose of 0.125–0.5 mg at bedtime is effective in preventing most parasomnias, probably by virtue of its tendency to consolidate sleep and decrease arousals.

Sleep Enuresis

From a developmental perspective, complete control of the bladder is usually achieved by the age of 4–5 years; thus bed-wetting in children below this age is probably physiological.[141] Enuresis as a parasomnia in those over 5–6 years of age may occur from all sleep stages.

- It is categorized as *primary* when the patient has not achieved bladder control during sleep for 6 or more months and *secondary* when the patient has relapse of bed-wetting after initially having achieved bladder control for 6 or more months. Primary enuresis is present in about 10% of 6-year-olds, 5% of 10-year-olds, and 1%–2% of 18-year-olds.[142] Primary enuresis may be associated with ADHD, living in disorganized families, insufficient rise in nocturnal vasopressin secretion, elevated arousal threshold, relatively uninhibited detrusor muscle contractility, or a decreased bladder capacity.
- Secondary enuresis may accompany significant psychosocial stress, chronic constipation, severe OSA, and urinary tract infections. For both forms of enuresis, deficits in central arousal and in control of the micturition reflex because of brainstem dysfunction have also been causally implicated.[142] Negative emotional feedback about the enuresis, whether overt or self-perceived, may undermine the child's self-image.
- Sleep enuresis is in general more common in boys than girls by a 3:2 ratio. There is a higher incidence of other family members with a similar disturbance in primary enuresis. On the basis of segregation analyses, multiple modes of inheritance such as autosomal dominant with high penetrance, autosomal dominant with low penetrance, and autosomal recessive modes of inheritance have been postulated.[143] Linkage analysis has shown association with chromosome 4 (in autosomal dominant families), as well as with chromosomes 8q, 12q, 13q, and 22q. Individual genes and mutations have not yet been identified.[143]
- The spontaneous remission rate for bed-wetting in childhood is 14%–19% per year[140]—this natural history should be kept in mind when counseling parents about the prognosis and assessing the effectiveness of various treatment modalities.
- The first step in management is to exclude a chronic urinary tract infection.
- One can then prescribe an alarm system with a moisture-sensing buzzer that is applied to the perineal area at bedtime. It works by operant conditioning. It arouses the patient when moisture is sensed, at which point the patient is trained to get out of bed and void in the toilet. Alarms for enuresis are helpful in children who are motivated and cooperative. The resolution rate for enuresis with conditioning devices varies from 65% to 80%.[140]
- Limiting the fluid intake after dinnertime is also recommended.
- Medications such as imipramine, 10–25 mg at bedtime, may lessen enuresis by decreasing detrusor muscle contractility (anticholinergic effect), but there may be relapse after an initial favorable response. The vasopressin analogue, desmopressin, given in a dose of 0.1–0.2 mg at bedtime as a nasal spray or tablet is also effective, and works by promoting fluid retention. Combining operant conditioning with medication may also help in the short term.[144]

Behavioral Insomnia of Childhood

These syndromes are characterized by difficulty falling asleep and staying asleep owing to due to maladaptive behaviors, to which that the infant or toddler has become habitually accustomed. In the *sleep-onset association* type, the infant or child starts to link falling asleep to extraneous stimuli, for example, being held, rocked patted to sleep. Upon awakening in the middle of the night, the child will once again require the extraneous stimuli to fall back to sleep. This leads to considerable stress in the child and parent alike.

The *limit-setting type* of behavioral insomnia is exemplified by refusal to go to sleep, with protests, and making unreasonable demands (e.g., another glass of milk, another drink of water, another bedtime story).

Behavioral insomnia affects 20%–30% of all preschool age children. The etiology is complex, and related to a combination of:

- Biological factors
- Circadian factors
- Neurodevelopmental factors

As in adult psychophysiologic insomnia, there may be a variety of predisposing, precipitating, and perpetuating factors.[145]

Management techniques recommended by the American Academy of Sleep Medicine[146] include:

- *Unmodified extinction*—Putting the child to sleep and leaving the child alone till the morning wake-up time (four level I controlled trials and two level II studies in support of this recommendation).
- *Graduated extinction*—Involves ignoring bedtime crying and protests for predetermined periods before intervening. For night awakenings, ignoring for progressively longer before intervening is recommended. The objective to train the child to "self-soothe" independently and fall back to sleep on his/her own (two level I studies and one level II study in support of this recommendation).

- *Positive routines and faded bedtime*—Involves the parent creating a set of enjoyable and quiet activities to facilitate behavioral calm; also the bedtime is temporarily delayed to coincide with the child's intrinsic sleep onset time (based on one level I study).
- *Delaying bedtime to allow the child becoming more sleepy* and removal from the bed in case the child is not falling asleep (one level I study in favor).

Suggested Reading

American Academy of Pediatrics. Clinical practice guideline: diagnosis and management of childhood obstructive sleep apnea syndrome. *Pediatrics*. 2012;130:576-584.

Kotagal S, Paruthi S. Narcolepsy in childhood. In: Goswami M, Pandi-Perumal SR, Thorpy MJ, eds. *Narcolepsy: A Clinical Guide*. 2nd ed. New York: Springer; 2016:51-67.

Kotagal S. Parasomnias in children. *Sleep Med Rev*. 2009;13(2):157-168.

Picchietti DL, Bruni O, de Weerd A, et al. Pediatric restless legs syndrome diagnostic criteria: an update by the International Restless Legs Syndrome Study Group. *Sleep Med*. 2013;14:1253-1259.

Task Force on Sudden Infant Death Syndrome, Moon RY. SIDS and other sleep-related infant deaths: expansion of recommendations for a safe infant sleeping environment. *Pediatrics*. 2011;128(5):1030.

23

Synopsis of Geriatric Sleep Disorders

JOSEPH M. DZIERZEWSKI, JUAN CARLOS RODRIGUEZ TAPIA, CATHY A. ALESSI

Introduction

Late life sleep disorders are common, yet they are often unrecognized and may carry serious adverse physical, mental, and social consequences.[1-3] At least 50% of older adults suffer from one of several different sleep disorders. The most common sleep disorders in older adults are insomnia and sleep apnea, but age-related changes in sleep, comorbidity, and other causes of sleep disturbance must also be considered in the older patient.

Age-Related Changes in Sleep

- Predictable changes in sleep timing, sleep architecture, and sleep quantity that occur throughout the lifespan, including changes with advanced age (Fig. 23.1 and Table 23.1)[4-7]
- Older adults often display an advanced circadian tendency, exhibiting an earlier sleep initiation and an earlier wake-up time (Fig. 23.2).

- Advanced age is associated with increased morningness based on the Horne ± Ostberg Morningness ± Eveningness Questionnaire (MEQ), which classifies people as morning-type (M-type), neither-type (N-type), or evening-type (E-type).
- Tendency toward M-type, which is characterized by an earlier sleep schedule and an earlier circadian temperature phase, as may be an important mediator of this and other age-associated changes in sleep[8]
- With advanced age, sleep architecture changes, which results in lighter and less restorative sleep (Fig. 23.3). These changes include:
  - Increased proportion of time in Stage N1 sleep
  - Increased proportion of time in Stage N2 sleep
  - Decreased proportion of time in Stage N3 sleep, a finding that is more pronounced in older men than older women.[9] Delta amplitude is even more impacted by aging than delta incidence.[10]
  - Decreased proportion of time in rapid eye movement (REM) sleep
- Compared with younger adults, older adults spend less total time asleep and experience more time awake during the night (Fig. 23.4).[7]

Insomnia in Aging

- In older adults, insomnia is most often comorbid with other physical/medical (Fig. 23.5)[11] and mental health conditions, including other sleep disorders. The co-occurrence of insomnia with comorbid medical or psychiatric disorders does not preclude diagnosis or treatment of insomnia in older adults.
- In community-living older adults, the prevalence of insomnia symptoms is 60%. This figure is higher in nursing homes and other institutional settings, among women, and in older adults with multiple comorbid conditions.[4,12]
- Evidence suggests that the higher prevalence rates of insomnia in older compared with younger adults is largely conferred through and related to the increased medical and psychiatric comorbidities (Fig. 23.6).[13]
- Insomnia is typically chronic in late life, with an average duration of several years.[14]
- Negative consequences of insomnia in late life include:[15-20]
  - Decreased quality of life
  - Increased risk for falls
  - Cognitive impairment and increased risk of dementia
  - Greater physical difficulties and more functional status impairment
  - Increased health services utilization and costs

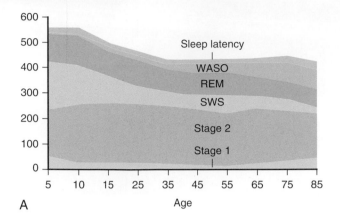

A

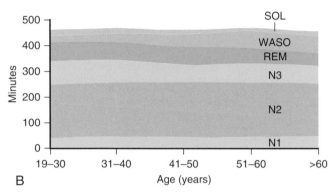

B

• **Figure 23.1** Changes in Sleep with Age. **A,** Time (in minutes) for sleep latency and wake after sleep onset (WASO) and for rapid eye movement (REM) sleep and nonrapid eye movement (NREM) sleep stages 1, 2, and slow wave sleep (SWS). Summary values are given for ages 5–85 years. **B,** Changes in sleep in adults using the current AASM scoping standards. Time (in minutes) for sleep latency and WASO, and for REM sleep and NREM sleep stages N1, N2, and N3. Values are medians. (**A,** From Ohayon M, Carskadon MA, Guilleminault C, Vitiello MV. Meta-analysis of quantitative sleep parameters from childhood to old age in healthy individuals: developing normative sleep values across the human lifespan. *Sleep*. 2004;27:1255–1273; **B,** Data from Mitterling T, Högl B, Schönwald SV, et al. Sleep and respiration in 100 healthy Caucasian sleepers—a polysomnographic study according to American Academy of Sleep Medicine standards. *Sleep*. 2015;38:867–875).

TABLE 23.1	Change in Sleep Parameters from Young Adulthood to Old Age[6]
Sleep Parameter	Change in Sleep Parameter
Total sleep time	Decrease
Sleep latency	Slight increase
Wake time during night	Decrease
Sleep efficiency	Decrease
Stage N1 sleep	Increase
Stage N2 sleep	Increase
Stage N3 sleep	Decrease
REM sleep	Decrease

REM, Rapid eye movement.

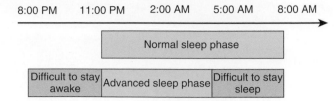

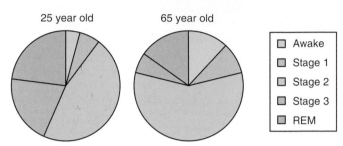

• **Figure 23.2** Illustration of an advanced sleep phase. This phase shift is common among older adults.

• **Figure 23.3** Typical changes in sleep architecture found with advanced age. (From Ohayon MM, Carskadon MA, Guilleminaulty C, Vitiello MV. Meta-analysis of qualitative sleep parameters from childhood to old age in healthy individuals: developing normative sleep values across the human lifespan. *Sleep*. 2004;27:1255–1273.)

- Increased risk for nursing home placement
- Increased mortality
- As in younger adults, in older adults insomnia can be conceptualized using the 3P model.[21] When considering the 3P model of insomnia, factors of unique or particular importance in older adults include:
  - *Predisposing factors*: Related to genetics, hyperarousal phenotype, poor physical and mental health, low socioeconomic status
  - *Precipitating factors*: Consist of recent lifetime events that induce insomnia over the threshold (e.g., depressive episode, hospitalization, bereavement, loss of a loved one, moving residence).
  - *Perpetuating factors*: Include functional status impairment, limited mobility with difficulty moving in and out of bed, decreased physical activity, frailty, social isolation, decreased bright light exposure, noise, and nighttime nursing activities in institutional settings that keep insomnia above threshold.

Diagnosis

- Due to the high prevalence and negative consequences of insomnia in older adults, screening for insomnia and other sleep disorders should be included in the routine examination. Particular attention should be paid to the following items:
  - Nature of associated daytime consequences, which may present as suspicion for cognitive impairment or other common conditions of aging
  - Physical and mental health conditions and symptoms associated with the sleep complaint
- As in younger adults, use of a sleep diary and/or structured sleep questionnaires (e.g., Insomnia Severity Index,[22] Pittsburg Sleep Quality Index[23]) is appropriate in older adults, but those with significant vision or hearing impairment, problems with

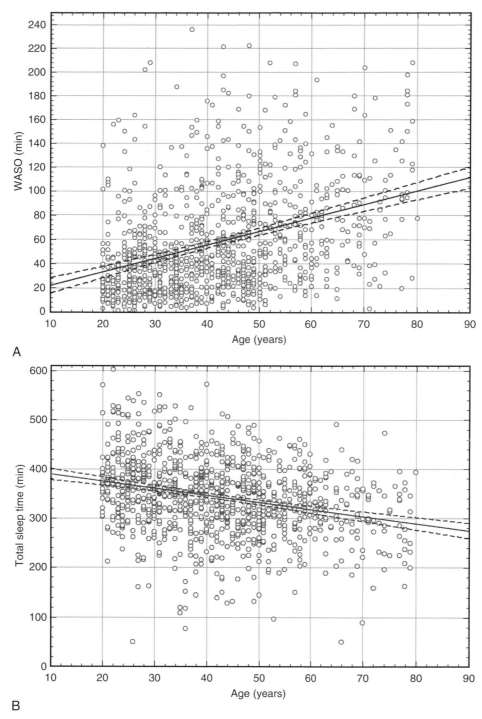

• **Figure 23.4** Correlation between age and (**A**) wake after sleep onset (WASO) and (**B**) total sleep time (TST). (From Moraes W, Piovezan R, Poyares D, Bittencourt LR, Santos-Silva R, Tufic S. Effects of aging on sleep structure throughout adulthood: a population-based study. *Sleep Med.* 2014;15:401–409.)

manual dexterity, or other symptoms may have difficulty with these diagnostic methods.

- Objectively verifiable indicators of sleep (e.g., wrist actigraphy, polysomnography) are appropriate for use in older adults with snoring, apneic spells, dream enactment behaviors, disruptive nocturnal movements, and persistently abnormal circadian schedule, which results in insomnia or hypersomnia.

Treatment

Treatment of sleep problems in older adults includes the range of options available for younger people. For insomnia, several recommending bodies suggest behavioral/psychological treatments should be first-line treatment for insomnia in older adults.[24,25]

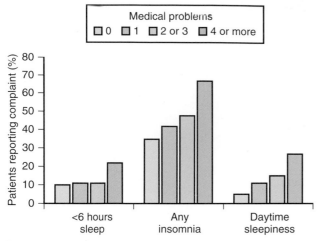

• **Figure 23.5** The association between sleep problems and medical conditions. (From Ancoli-Isreal S. Sleep and its disorders in aging populations. *Sleep Med*. 2009;10:S7–S11.)

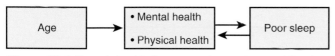

• **Figure 23.6** The relationship between aging and sleep difficulties is likely mediated by mental and physical health changes.

Psychological Treatment

- Treatment techniques with a strong foundation in behavioral theory and practice have proven very effective in the treatment of insomnia in older adults, including those with comorbidity (Table 23.2).
- Psychological treatment techniques for insomnia that have empirical evidence supporting their use as standalone treatment in older adults include:
  - *Stimulus control* is based on classical conditioning principles; the individual is instructed to limit use of the bed for sleep and sex, and this treatment has a strong evidence base.[26,27]
  - *Sleep restriction* is aimed at matching the amount of time in bed with the actual amount of time asleep; uses a consistent sleep schedule and limits time in bed. This treatment modality has a moderate evidence base; results have been mixed in older adults.[26,27]
- Psychological treatment techniques for insomnia that have little empirical evidence supporting their use as standalone treatment options in older adults include:
  - *Sleep education* provides information about normal sleep changes with age to patients.
  - *Cognitive therapy* includes in its approach modification of challenging maladaptive thoughts, beliefs, and attitudes that can negatively impact sleep as a way to reduce thoughts and emotions that disrupt sleep.
  - *Sleep hygiene* provides instruction to avoid substances and behaviors that interfere with sleep, such as caffeine and

TABLE 23.2	**Psychological Treatment for Insomnia in Older Adults**
Technique	**Level of Support**
Sleep education Information regarding normal sleep changes with age. Aimed at normalizing current sleep, improving expectations, and reducing anxiety	Low*; not an evidence-based practice†; not a recommendation‡
Cognitive therapy Maladaptive thoughts, beliefs, and attitudes can negatively impact sleep. Challenging these thoughts can help promote sleep through a reduction in sleep disruptive thoughts and emotions	Low*; not an evidence-based practice†; not a recommendation‡
Sleep hygiene Instruction to avoid or limit sleep disruptive substances and behaviors, including caffeine, alcohol, nicotine, exercising, and heavy meals at night	Low*; not an evidence-based practice†; not a recommendation‡
Relaxation strategies Active or passive relaxation techniques all aimed at reducing physiological or mental arousal that may be interfering with sleep	Moderate*; not an evidence-based practice†; standard recommendation‡
Stimulus control Behavioral technique based on classical conditioning principles. Instructs an individual to limit use of the bed to sleep and sex, and to limit the amount of time spent awake in bed.	Strong*; not an evidence-based practice†; standard recommendation‡
Sleep restriction Behavioral strategy aimed at matching the amount of time one spends in bed with the actual amount of time asleep. A consistent sleep schedule and time in bed is collaboratively prescribed and adjusted as needed.	Strong*; evidence-based practice†; guideline recommendation‡
Multicomponent treatment packages (CBTI) Combine several individual components into a treatment package. Usually consist of stimulus control, sleep restriction, sleep education. Sometimes include cognitive therapy, relaxation techniques, or sleep hygiene recommendations.	Strong*; evidence-based practice†; standard recommendation‡

*Based on authors' critical review of empirical evidence and clinical practice with older adults.
†Criteria for an intervention to be considered evidence-based include: 50% of the outcome measures must demonstrate significant treatment effects with between-group effect sizes of at least 0.20.[26]
‡American Academy of Sleep Medicine (AASM) Practice Parameters.[27]

alcohol consumption, nicotine, nighttime exercising, and heavy meals.
- Relaxation strategies might have some benefit for improving the sleep of older adults, but appear to be most useful in combination with other psychological treatments.
- Multicomponent treatment packages (e.g., cognitive behavioral therapy for insomnia, CBTI) have the strongest evidence for insomnia in older adults.[26,27] Typically, CBTI includes (at least):
  - Stimulus control
  - Sleep restriction
  - Sleep education
- In qualitative research, older adults report preference of behavioral treatment to use of sedative hypnotic medications.

Pharmacotherapy

- Older adults are twice as likely to be prescribed pharmacotherapy for insomnia as younger adults.[28]
- Most guidelines recommend avoiding the use of sedative hypnotic medications in older adults.
- Evidence suggests that sedative hypnotic medications in older adults carry increased risk of:
  - Drug side effects. The evidence is based on meta-analyses. Older adults have increased risk of falls; cognitive adverse events such as memory loss, confusion, disorientation, and residual morning sedation; and morning impairment as measured by performance tasks such as reaction time or hand-eye coordination tasks.
  - Drug-drug interactions, particularly since older adults are more likely to have polypharmacy and exposure to more medications
  - Increased risk for tolerance and misuse, which may in part be due to greater likelihood of prolonged use in older compared with younger adults
  - There is limited empirical evidence to support the use of pharmacotherapy in older adults with insomnia, particularly in patients who are frail, of very advanced age, or those with medical comorbidities.
- Commonly cited recommendations to minimize risks when using sedative hypnotics in older adults is to prescribe the smallest effective dose of the agent, with the lowest risk of adverse effects, for the shortest period of time appropriate.
- Issues to consider in prescribing sedative hypnotics in older adults:
  - Longer-acting direct benzodiazepines should be avoided due to risks of daytime sedation, falls, and confusion.[29]
  - Due to a shorter duration of action, most nonbenzodiazepines are believed to carry a lower risk of side effects in older adults, but there is limited evidence in older patients of very advanced age, and in those with underlying cognitive impairment and/or significant comorbidities.
  - Sedating antidepressants (e.g., trazodone and mirtazapine) are commonly prescribed for sleep in older adults, but there is limited empirical evidence to support this practice.
  - Agents with anticholinergic side effects (e.g., amitryptiline) should be avoided in older adults, due to risks of central and/or peripheral anticholinergic toxicity.
  - The American Geriatrics Society's Beer's criteria for potentially inappropriate medication use in older adults recommends the following:

- Avoid benzodiazepines (e.g., estazolam, temazepam, and numerous others, with a strong recommendation against use) and nonbenzodiazepine benzodiazepine receptor agonist hypnotics (e.g., eszopiclone, zolpidem, zaleplon), with a strong recommendation against use in older adults.[30]
- Many other medications that are used off-label for insomnia in older adults are also not recommended (e.g., first-generation antihistamines, antidepressants with anticholinergic side effects, antipsychotic medications).
- Doxepin ≤6 mg per day is described as having a safety profile comparable with that of placebo.
- In a subsequent publication providing alternatives to medications that are potentially inappropriate in older adults, the American Geriatrics Society provides no medication(s) as alternatives, and instead recommends nonpharmacological options (i.e., behavioral treatment) to treat insomnia in older adults (initially).[31]
- Table 23.3 provides a list of hypnotic agents commonly used for insomnia in older adults (≥65 years of age).

Sleep Apnea in Older Adults

- The prevalence of sleep apnea increases with age. Reported prevalence rates in older adults vary, but one community-based sample reported 24.2% of men and 15.9% of women aged 60–70 years had an AHI of ≥15.[32]
- Sleep apnea is more common in older patients with multiple comorbidities, especially in patients with dementia.
- In older adults, sleep apnea is associated with the following conditions: hypertension, coronary artery disease, depression, falls, nocturia, cognitive impairment, stroke, and increased mortality.[33,34]
- Sleep apnea in older adults is partly attributed to increased propensity for airway collapse.
- Aging is associated with a decrease in the negative pressure reflex, particularly in men; increased deposition of parapharyngeal fat in both men and women; elongation of the soft palate, particularly in women; and remodeling in the bony shape surrounding the pharynx.[35]
- Both older men and women experience an increased in the parapharyngeal fat pad size independent of body mass index (BMI).[35] This is summarized in Fig. 23.7A and B.
- Although obesity is a significant risk factor for obstructive apnea at any age, data in older adults illustrate that deposition of adipose tissue around the airway occurs independently of age-related changes in body adipose.[35]
- Fig. 23.7C illustrates an observation of decrease in negative pressure reflex with increasing age. With increasing age, there was a significant decrease in the genioglossal response to negative intrapharyngeal pressure pulses. Fig. 23.7D depicts a significant increase in the size of the fat pads with increasing age, independent of BMI.
- Unique aspects of sleep apnea in older adults include:
  - Daytime symptoms may be mistaken for cognitive impairment.
  - Increased BMI is less tightly linked with sleep apnea in older compared with younger adults, and many older adults with sleep apnea are not obese.
  - The clinical consequences of mild, asymptomatic sleep apnea in older adults are unclear.
  - Sleep-disordered breathing with excessive daytime sleepiness is a risk factor for increased mortality in older adults,[36] even

TABLE 23.3 | **Examples of Medications Commonly Used for Insomnia in Older Adults**

Generic Name	Drug Class	Initial Dosage (mg)	Usual Dosage	Half-Life (in Hours)	Comments
Eszopiclone	Nonbenzodiazepine, immediate release	1	1–2	6 (~9 in elderly)	Approved for long-term use (not specific to older patients); may cause unpleasant taste (gustatory side effect), somnolence, and headaches.
Zolpidem	Nonbenzodiazepine, immediate release	2.5	5	~2.5	Drowsiness, lightheadedness; risk of complex nocturnal behaviors
Zaleplon	Short-acting nonbenzodiazepine	5	5–10	1	Drowsiness, lightheadedness, dizziness
Temazepam	Benzodiazepine, intermediate-acting	7.5	7.5–15	3.5–18.4	Psychomotor impairment; risk of falls
Ramelteon	Melatonin receptor agonist	8	8	1–2.6	Not scheduled; little rebound insomnia or withdrawal; dizziness, myalgia, and headaches; approved for sleep initiation
Doxepin	Selective H_1 receptor antagonist (sedating antidepressant)	3	3–6	15.3	Not scheduled, treatment of insomnia characterized by difficulties with sleep maintenance. Should not be taken within 3 hours of eating.
Suvorexant	Dual orexin/hypocretin receptor antagonist	5	10–15, 15–20	12	Not scheduled, treatment of insomnia characterized by difficulties with sleep initiation of maintenance. Somnolence, depression.
Trazodone*	Sedating antidepressant	25	25–150	2–4	Off-label use; insomnia + depression; low anticholinergic effects; orthostatic hypotension
Mirtazapine*	Sedating antidepressant	7.5	7.5–45	31–39	Off-label use; insomnia + depression; increased appetite, weight gain, headache; akathisia

*Off-label use; no FDA indication for insomnia, although frequently used in the management of insomnia in older adults.

when adjusted for other risk factors such as prolonged sleep duration.
- Cognitively impaired older adults with sleep apnea may be relatively asymptomatic, or symptoms may be attributed to another cause.
- Sleep apnea is also a risk factor for cognitive impairment. For example, in one study women with sleep apnea were 1.85 times more likely to develop mild cognitive impairment or dementia within 5 years of follow-up, whereas measures of sleep fragmentation and sleep duration were not associated with increased risk of cognitive impairment.[37]
- For a listing of potential age-dependent risk factors and outcomes of sleep apnea in late life, please review Fig. 23.8.[38]

Diagnosis

- Issues of particular importance in the diagnosis of sleep apnea in older adults include:
  - Sleep apnea is often unrecognized in older adults.
  - Sleep apnea is common among older adults presenting with symptoms of insomnia.
  - Ambulatory monitoring can be successfully completed in older adults, but factors such as sensory deficits, arthritis, or other functional limitations may need to be addressed to help ensure successful completion of the monitoring.

- Sleep apnea screening questionnaires can be useful in older adults, but there is less evidence for their use in older adults with significant comorbidities.

Treatment

- Positive airway pressure (PAP) therapy can be effectively used in older adults, and is associated with a decreased risk of stroke, cardiovascular disease, and mortality in older patients.[39,40]
- Regardless of the age of the patient, sleep apnea should be treated when it is associated with negative consequences (e.g., excessive daytime sleepiness, decreased quality of life, cognitive impairment, nocturia, hypertension, cardiovascular disease).[41]
- Measures to improve PAP adherence in younger patients (e.g., bilevel PAP, proper fitting of the correct interface, concomitant behavioral therapy) can also be effective in older adults, and should be considered.
- Special issues regarding use of alternative (non-PAP) treatments for older adults who refuse or do not tolerate PAP include:
  - Oral appliances can be effective, but may not be appropriate in older patients who are edentulous.
  - There is very little evidence to support surgical procedures (including uvulopalatopharyngoplasty, bimaxillary advancement) for sleep apnea in older adults, particularly for patients with advanced age or with significant underlying comorbidities.

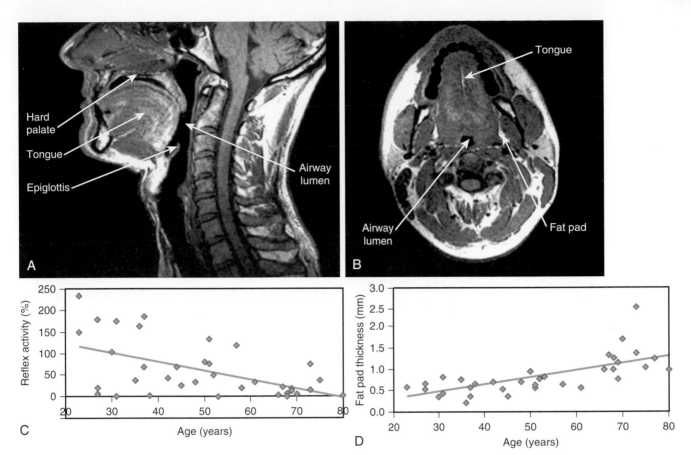

• **Figure 23.7** **A,** Midsagittal magnetic resonance image (MRI) illustrating anatomical structures of interest. **B,** Axial MRI illustrating structures relevant to pharyngeal collapse. **C,** The decrease in negative pressure reflex with increasing age for the sample. With increasing age, there was a significant decrease in the genioglossal response to negative intrapharyngeal pressure pulses ($R = -0.55$; $P = .001$). **D,** The graph shows a significant increase in the size of the fat pads with increasing age, independent of body mass index ($R = 0.59$; $P = .005$). (From Atul M, Yaqi H, Robert F, et al. Aging influences on pharyngeal anatomy and physiology: the predisposition to pharyngeal collapse. *Am J Med.* 2006;119[1]:72.e9–72.e14.)

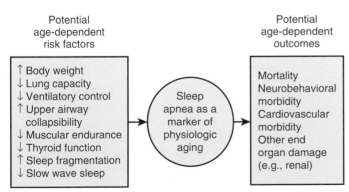

• **Figure 23.8** Potential age-dependent risk factors and outcomes of sleep apnea in older adults. (From Bliwise D. Epidemiology of age-dependence in sleep-disordered breathing in old age: they bay area sleep cohort. *Sleep Med Clin.* 2009;4:57–64.)

• Evidence for the effectiveness of these treatments in older adults is limited, since most empirical studies have excluded older adults.[42]
• Examples of specific outcomes of treatment of sleep apnea in older adults that have been reported include:[43]

• Reduces or eliminates apneas and hypopneas
• Improves sleep architecture
• Improves daytime sleepiness
• Improves self-reported symptoms (snoring and gasping)
• Improves motor speed and nonverbal learning and memory
• Improves vascular resistance, platelet coagulability, and other factors affecting cardiac function
• Has a positive effect on nocturia, reducing the number of voids per night
• Evidence supports the treatment of sleep apnea among older adults with dementia. For example, in one study of patients with mild to moderate Alzheimer's disease who had sleep apnea, those treated with continuous positive airway pressure (CPAP) had decreases in wake after sleep onset (WASO), percent stage N1 sleep, arousals, and an increase in stage N3 sleep.[44]

Circadian Rhythm Disorder in Older Adults

• Circadian rhythm sleep disorders, especially advanced sleep phase disorder, are more common in older adults compared with younger adults.[45]

- Circadian rhythm sleep disorders may be due to endogenous factors in late life:
  - Degeneration of the suprachiasmatic nucleus[46]
  - Reductions in melatonin production by the pineal glad[47]
  - Cataracts may hinder normal sleep-wake regulation because of the selective blue light photosensitivity of the retinal ganglion cells governing circadian photoentrainment.[48]
- Circadian rhythm sleep disorders may also be due to exogenous factors in late life:
  - Reduced exposure to bright light[49]
  - Increased sedentary behavior[50]
  - Reduced social activity levels
- Treatment for advanced sleep-wake phase disorder (ASPD) in older adults may include:
  - Timed exposure to bright light[51]
  - Behavioral strategies (e.g., deliberate timing of bedtime, sleep restriction, planned daytime social activities)
  - Although melatonin supplementation therapy may be used in other circadian disorders such as delayed sleep-wake phase disorder (DSWPD), non-24 circadian disorder, and jet lag disorder, no systematic reports of melatonin administration for ASPD currently exist.[52]
  - There may be theoretical utility for administering melatonin in the morning for delaying circadian rhythms in patients with ASPD, but one must consider the safety of taking a potentially sleep-promoting supplement in the morning; this may be associated with adverse effects, particularly in the older adults who are more likely to suffer from ASPD and daytime sleepiness.[52]

Sleep-Related Movement Disorders in Older Adults

Restless Legs Syndrome

- Epidemiologic studies suggest restless legs syndrome (RLS) prevalence and symptoms typically increase with advanced age, but is routinely underdiagnosed or misdiagnosed. It is important to consider RLS in the differential diagnosis of any older patient with nocturnal leg cramps, peripheral neuropathy, and paraesthesias of the limbs who fail to respond to treatment.
- Unlike REM sleep behavior disorder (RBD), RLS does not appear to be a precursor to Parkinson's disease (PD), and in fact, there is some evidence that RLS might delay the onset of PD.[53]
- The following single item has been validated for the diagnosis of RLS in a sample with a high representation of older adults (about 50% older than 60; mean age 60.7 years).[54]
  - *When you try to relax in the evening or sleep at night, do you ever have unpleasant, restless feelings in your legs that can be relieved by walking or movement?*
- Given that RLS diagnosis involves a clinical interview, it can be difficult to diagnose RLS in older adults with dementia. For example, nighttime agitation (sometimes referred to as "sundowning") may be a presentation of RLS in dementia. Therefore family/caregiver history is particularly important. Some indirect signs of RLS in dementia patients may include wandering behavior and leg discomfort that is alleviated with leg massage.
- Older adults should avoid the following agents that may induce or worsen RLS symptoms:

- Antipsychotic and other neuroleptic agents
- Antidepressants, particularly tricyclic, tetracyclic, or selective serotonin reuptake inhibiting antidepressants
- Antiemetic drugs
- Lithium
- Iron deficiency in older adults may be related to the following factors:
- Causes of iron-deficiency anemia in the elderly
  - Nutritional issues: Malnutrition
  - Impaired efficiency of iron absorption
  - Occult blood loss: Gastrointestinal malignancy, peptic ulcer disease, hiatus hernia, colonic vascular ecstasy, Crohn's disease
  - Chronic inflammatory disease
  - Gastrointestinal disease not associated with bleeding: Atrophic gastritis, celiac disease, and *Helicobacter pylori* infection
  - Institutionalization[55]
- Medications: Aspirin, nonsteroidal antiinflammatory drugs

Treatment of Restless Legs Syndrome in Older Adults

Management of RLS is depicted in the algorithm in Fig. 23.9.
- As in younger adults, iron repletion (if ferritin is low) and nonpharmacological treatments such as mental activity (e.g., lecture, crosswords, and Sudoku), physical activity, and avoidance of precipitating factors should always be considered in older patients with RLS.
- Nonergotamine dopamine-receptor agonists including pramipexole, ropinirole, and rotigotine, and the alpha-2-delta ligand, gabapentin enacarbil, are FDA approved for the management of primary moderate to severe RLS in adults and older adults above age 65.[55]
- Pharmacological therapy considerations in treating RLS in older adults include:
  - When alpha-2-delta ligands (e.g., gabapentin enacarbil) are chosen, side effects, such as oversedation and problems with balance, should be carefully monitored. Dose should be adjusted in patients with impaired creatinine clearance, which is common in older adults with renal disease.[55]
  - Given adverse side effects and lack of clinical trials, benzodiazepines should be avoided for treatment of RLS in older adults. Drugs such as clonazepam can induce confusional state, agitation, disorientation, impairment of memory, and cognition.
  - The dopamine precursor levodopa and dopamine-receptor agonists are associated with augmentation.
  - RLS associated with painful symptoms may respond more favorably to alpha-2-delta ligand, but sedation is a limitation.
- Alpha-2-ligand related adverse effects include:[55]
  - Weight gain
  - Neurologic: Sleepiness, dizziness; common: ataxia, tremors, dysarthria, cognitive impairment (memory and attention), sedation, paresthesia, and balance impairment
  - Psychiatric: Euphoria, confusion, irritability, disorientation, insomnia
  - Cardiovascular: Tachycardia, first-degree atrioventricular block, peripheral edema (gabapentin)
- Dopaminergic agents are associated with the following side effects:[55]
  - Primarily visual hallucinations
  - Excessive sleepiness, fatigue, and sleep attack

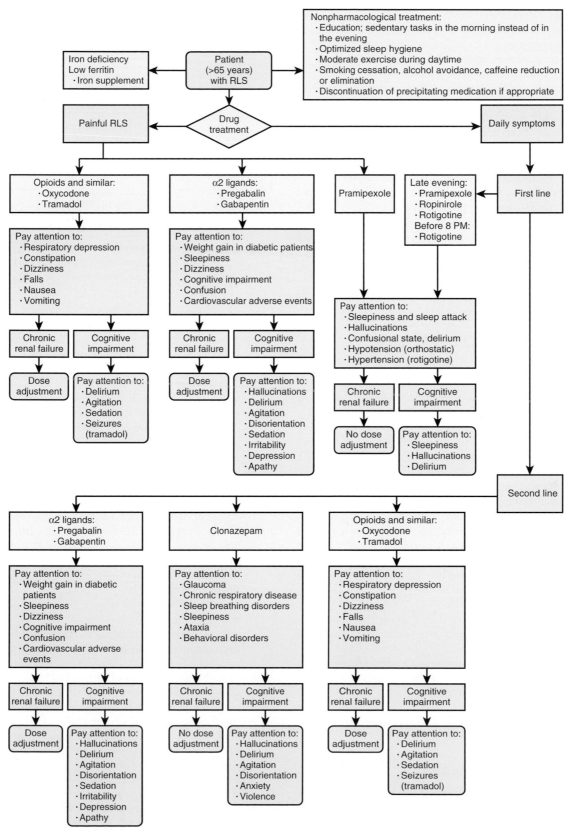

• **Figure 23.9** Treatment algorithm of (restless legs syndrome) RLS, in older patients. (From Figorilli M, Puligheddu M, Ferri R. Restless legs syndrome/Willis–Ekbom disease and periodic limb movements in sleep in the elderly with and without dementia. *Sleep Med Clin.* 2015;10[3]:331–342.)

- Impulsive control behaviors (i.e., compulsive shopping)
- Delirium and confusional state
- Dizziness
- Cardiovascular: Orthostatic hypotension or hypertension (related to rotigotine)
- Nausea, constipation, and vomiting
- Peripheral edema
- Skin irritation reaction (in relationship to the patch delivery system in rotigotine)
- Opioids and hypnosedatives are sometimes helpful, but cardiovascular side effects are limited in the elderly.
  Opioids-related side effects include:
  - Neurologic: Excessive sleepiness, dizziness, sedation, cognitive impairment, seizure (particularly with tramadol)
  - Psychiatric: Mood disorders, confusion, amnesia; uncommon: hallucinations, tolerance, and addiction
  - Cardiovascular: Hypotension
  - Respiratory: Depressed respiratory drive, dyspnea, worsening of sleep apnea
  - Gastrointestinal: Constipation, nausea, vomiting, xerostomia, abdominal pain, dyspepsia
  - Skin: Rash, pruritus, hyperhidrosis
  - Urinary retention

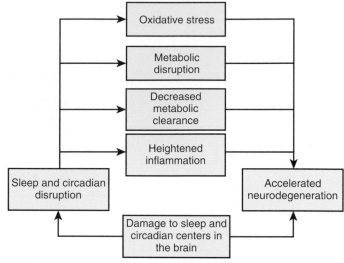

• **Figure 23.10** Conceptual model linking sleep and circadian disruption and neurodegeneration. (Adapted from Mattis J. Circadian rhythms, sleep, and disorders of aging. *Trends Endocrinol Metab.* 2016;27:192–203.)

Napping Behavior in Older Adults

- About 25% of older adults take naps; however, there is significant variation in the reported prevalence of napping.
- It is important to consider that older adults tend to underestimate the number and duration of their naps.[56]
- Insomnia and sleep apnea are common causes of daytime sleepiness and compensatory naps in older adults, and should be considered in the older patient who presents with napping.
- At the time of writing this review, there is controversy in the literature about the clinical impact of napping on sleep quality, health status, cognition, and quality of life in older adults.
- Short naps have been demonstrated to improve cognitive performance, but there is concern that napping, when prolonged (>20–30 min) and occurring outside the hours of 1 to 3 PM (which can decrease the homeostatic drive for sleep that occurs with prolonged wakefulness), may interfere with nighttime sleep.
- Given the lack of consistent evidence about the benefits or harms of napping, individuals' preferences should be considered in a patient-centered approach.
- Some older adults resist napping because they associate naps with unproductive and unhealthy aging. Others see napping as beneficial to keeping an active life.[57]

Sleep in Common Clinical Disorders of Late Life

Sleep Disorders and Dementia

- Various models have been conceptualized to explain the link between sleep and circadian disruption, and cognitive dysfunction and dementia (Fig. 23.10).[58]
- Sleep disorders are common in older adults with dementia, and may be associated with loss of function, accelerated cognitive impairment, caregiver burden, and predisposition for institutionalization.[59]

- Sundowning has been described as an altered behavioral state (e.g., anxiety, agitation, wandering) that is more prevalent during the late evening hours.
- Sundowning in older adults with dementia is hypothesized to be related to biological factors, environmental factors, and/or caregivers' perceptions at the end of the day.[56]
- As described previously, sundowning may be a presentation of RLS.
- Treatment of sleep/wake disturbance in dementia should focus on both the identified cause(s) of the sleep disturbance in conjunction with interventions to address the sleep symptom(s).
- Examples of nonpharmacological techniques recommended to improve sleep/wake disturbance in older adults with dementia:
  - Bright light exposure (although the most appropriate timing and duration of bright light exposure is controversial)
  - Physical exercise
  - Social activities (which may be important zeitgebers in the setting of dementia)
- Pharmacotherapy is generally not recommended for the treatment of sleep disturbances in older adults with dementia. If pharmacotherapy is necessary, consider the following:
  - Trazodone in low doses (50 mg) has been demonstrated to improve total nocturnal sleep time and sleep efficiency in older adults with Alzheimer's disease.[60] However, given that this finding was based on one study, and trazodone is associated with alpha 2-adrenergic blocking activity and potential orthostatic hypotension, its use in older patient cohorts should be supervised with care.
  - Evidence for use of either melatonin or ramelteon in dementia is conflicting.
  - At present, there is no evidence supporting the use of most sedative hypnotic drugs (e.g., benzodiazepines, nonbenzodiazepines hypnotics, other antidepressants, and antipsychotics agents) in patients with Alzheimer's disease.[61]
- In the absence of a dementing disorder, poor sleep can still have a negative impact on late-life cognitive functioning.[62]

Psychiatric Disorders

- Sleep disorders are more common among older adults with comorbid psychiatric conditions (particularly depression or anxiety) than in older adults without such comorbidities. In fact, over 30% of older adults with insomnia also have a psychiatric disorder.[63]
- The prevalence of sleep complaints in late life drops to approximately 2% when excluding all older adults with a comorbid psychological or physical condition.[13]
- The presence of a sleep condition in the context of one or more psychiatric conditions can alter clinical presentation, interfere with appropriate diagnosis, and impact treatment.
- Sleep disturbances in older adults are commonly comorbid with other conditions, such as pain, depression, and other common problems.[64]
  - Sleep disturbances are not merely the symptom of a psychiatric disorder, even when they co-occur. In addition to management of the psychiatric disorder, the sleep disturbance should also be addressed.
  - Unless treated, sleep problems often persist following successful treatment of the psychiatric condition.
- Depression is a common psychiatric disorder in late life and is associated with sleep disruption.
  - Sleep changes commonly observed with aging are more pronounced in older adults with depression.[65]
  - Early morning awakenings are the most frequent sleep disturbance in older adults with depression.[66]
  - When insomnia and depression co-occur, the prognosis is worse than either disorder in isolation.[67]
  - Growing evidence suggests that CBTI is the treatment of choice for insomnia in older adults with comorbid depression.
- Anxiety disorders are also common in older adults, and approximately 50% of older adults with an anxiety disorder also suffer from poor sleep.[62]
  - Severity of anxiety symptoms and severity of sleep disturbances are directly related.[6]
  - Difficulty initiating sleep is the most common sleep disturbance in older adults with anxiety disorders.
  - Growing evidence suggests that CBTI is the treatment of choice for insomnia in older adults with comorbid anxiety disorders.
- There is a lack of research directly investigating bipolar disorders and sleep in older adults.[59]
- Older adults with schizophrenia have high rates of disturbed sleep,[68] including changes in the following sleep parameters:
  - Increased time spent in bed
  - Greater nighttime awakening
  - More awake time during the night
  - Increased napping behavior[64]
  - More research is needed on treatment of sleep problems in this challenging clinical population.

Contextual Factors Impacting Sleep in Older Adults

Hospitalization and institutionalization are common in late life and are associated with increased rates of sleep disorders when compared with that seen in community-dwelling older adults.

Sleep Disorders in Hospitalized Older Adults

- Sleep disorders are frequent and generally under-recognized in hospitalized older adults.
- There are many patient-level factors associated with the increased prevalence of insomnia in hospitalized older adults, including:
  - Dyspnea and cough due to acute pulmonary and cardiac diseases, pain, delirium, and anxiety
- There are also environmental-level factors (i.e., those related to the hospital environment) that can have a negative impact on the sleep of hospitalized older adults, including:
  - Nighttime nursing care activities, such as administration of medications and the measurement of vital signs
  - Excessive noise and light exposure at night, such as related to nursing care activities (as described previously) and/or roommates
  - Unfamiliar bed and lack of usual bedtime routines
- Stimulating medications (e.g., bronchodilators) given in the evening can also be problematic.
- Addressing environmental-level factors (as mentioned previously) should be preferred over pharmacological treatments in patients with sleep complaints during the hospital stay.
- The overall prevalence of sleep apnea in the hospital setting is unknown; however, in specific populations such as stroke patients, it is as high as 60%.[69]
- Adverse outcomes are more frequent in hospitalized patients with sleep apnea, and include: intra- and postoperative complications, prolonged length of stay, and possibly increased mortality.[70,71]
- Screening questionnaires can be used to assess the risk of undiagnosed sleep apnea in hospitalized patients.
- As in younger patients, older hospitalized patients who have been previously diagnosed with sleep apnea and were prescribed PAP therapy should use it during hospitalization.

Sleep Disorders in the Nursing Home

- Sleep disorders are more frequent in nursing home residents than in community-dwelling older adults.
- A common sleep presentation in a nursing home resident is an irregular sleep pattern with:
  - Several episodes of napping during the day
  - Fragmented sleep at night
- Factors associated with the altered sleep patterns in nursing home residents include:
  - Patient-level factors:
    - Older age
    - Medical comorbidities
    - Psychiatric comorbidities
  - Environmental-level factors:
    - Lack of daytime exposure to sunlight and physical activity
    - Increased amount of time spent in bed during the day
    - Use of medications with effects on the central nervous system
- Sleep disorders in nursing home patients are associated with many negative consequences, including:
  - Poor quality of life
  - Reduced involvement in social activities
  - Increased mortality[72,73]

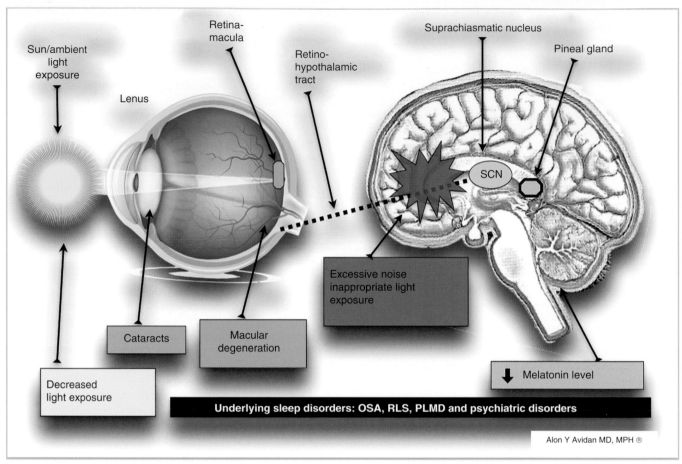

• **Figure 23.11** Pathophysiology of sleep and circadian in aging based on underlying external factors (environmental-related such as inappropriate or insufficient light exposure) and internal (patient-related factors, such at contacts). *SCN,* Suprachiasmatic nucleus. (Copyright Alon Y. Avidan, MD, MPH.)

• When poor sleep is identified in nursing home residents, a multidimensional treatment approach should be considered. Treatment strategies with some evidence of efficacy in improving the sleep of nursing home residents include:
  • Increased daytime light exposure (e.g., outdoor light exposure, bright light boxes), but the most appropriate timing and intensity of light has varied
  • Participation in physical activity, such as activity programs provided in the facility or increasing physical activity around the time of nursing care activities
  • Nighttime reductions in noise and light
  • Multicomponent treatment packages combining light exposure, time out of bed, and increased physical activity[74]
• Sedative hypnotic medications may have limited benefit in improving sleep of nursing home residents,[69] and should be avoided given potential side effects, risks, and the complex metabolism of these drugs in frail older adults.
• Treatment of sleep problems in nursing home patients requires buy-in and adherence from nursing home staff.

Fig. 23.11 summarizes the pathophysiology of sleep and circadian in aging based on underlying external factors (environmental-related such as inappropriate or insufficient light exposure) and internal (patient-related factors, such as contacts).

Conclusions

• Older adults experience sleep disorders at very high rates, which are associated with serious adverse physical, mental, and social consequences, and generally occur in the setting of significant medical/physical and mental comorbidity.
• Insomnia and sleep apnea are the two most common sleep disorders in older adults.
• Poor sleep can be very deleterious to general health and quality of life in older patients.
• Recognition and appropriate management of sleep problems in older adults is essential to optimal health and function in later life.

Acknowledgment

This work was supported by UCLA Claude D. Pepper Older Americans Independence Center (NIA 5P30 AG028748), NIH/NCATS UCLA CTSI (UL1TR000124), NIH/NIA (K23AG049955, PI: Dzierzewski), and the Geriatric Research, Education, and Clinical Center (GRECC), VA Greater Los Angeles Healthcare System.

Suggested Reading

Figorilli M, Puligheddu M, Ferri R. Restless legs syndrome /Willis-Ekbom Disease and periodic limb movements in sleep in the elderly with and without dementia. *Sleep Med Clin*. 2015;10:331-342, xiv-xv.

Kay DB, Dzierzewski JM. Sleep in the context of healthy aging and psychiatric syndromes. *Sleep Med Clin*. 2015;10:11-15.

Lopez-Pousa S, Garre-Olmo J, Vilalta-Franch J, et al. Trazodone for Alzheimer's disease: a naturalistic follow-up study. *Arch Gerontol Geriatr*. 2008;47:207-215.

Malhotra A, Huang Y, Fogel R, et al. Aging influences on pharyngeal anatomy and physiology: the predisposition to pharyngeal collapse. *Am J Med*. 2006;119(72):e9-e14.

McCurry SM, Logsdon RG, Teri L, Vitiello MV. Evidence-based psychological treatments for insomnia in older adults. *Psychol Aging*. 2007;22:18-27.

Morgan K. Sleep and aging. In: Lichstein K, Morin C, eds. *Treatment of Late-Life Insomnia*. Thousand Oaks, CA: Sage Publications; 2000.

Rodriguez JC, Dzierzewski JM, Alessi CA. Sleep problems in the elderly. *Med Clin North Am*. 2015;99:431-439.

Scullin MK, Bliwise DL. Sleep, cognition, and normal aging: integrating a half century of multidisciplinary research. *Perspect Psychol Sci*. 2015;10:97-137.

Zee PC. Melantonin for the treatment of advanced sleep phase disorder. *Sleep*. 2008;31:923. author reply 925.

24

Cardiac Monitoring and Scoring in Polysomnography

SEAN M. CAPLES, VIREND K. SOMERS

With an increasing interest in and recognition of the association between cardiovascular (CV) disease and sleep disorders, particularly sleep-disordered breathing, abnormal cardiac rhythms are likely to be regularly encountered in clinical practice. This review will discuss physiologic underpinnings of normal and aberrant cardiac recordings and recommended methods of cardiac scoring during polysomnography (PSG).

Cardiovascular Homeostasis During Normal Sleep—Nonrapid Eye Movement

- Compared with wakefulness, nonrapid eye movement (NREM) sleep is characterized by CV stability marked by a reduction in blood pressure (BP) and heart rate (HR); the lowest BP and HR in a 24-hour period is most likely to occur during NREM. Slowing of the HR is primarily under the influence of heightened vagal tone.
- Sinus arrhythmia is common during NREM, as cardiac output couples with the respiratory rhythm. With inspiration, as venous return to the heart increases, there is an acceleration of HR followed by a deceleration with exhalation.
- Further reduction in sympathetic neural traffic is seen during slow wave (N3) sleep; the output may be half that encountered in wakefulness.[1] Stage N2 sleep is punctuated by characteristic "K-complexes," high-amplitude electroencephalogram (EEG) discharges associated with transient increases in peripheral sympathetic neural activity, and an attendant rise in BP.[2] Bursts of vagal activity sometimes accompany the transition out of NREM, resulting in HR pauses.[3]
- Heightened parasympathetic tone during NREM in healthy individuals can result in HR slowing, sinus arrhythmia, sinus pauses, and slowed conduction through the atrioventricular (AV) node. Low-grade AV block (first degree and type I second degree) can result. These are seen across gender and age groups,[4,5] and have been demonstrated in young and older athletes.[6,7]
- Normative data from the literature led the American Academy of Sleep Medicine (AASM) to recommend lowering the threshold HR for the diagnosis of bradycardia during sleep from the traditional 60 to 40 beats per minute (bpm) (see later).[8]

Cardiovascular Homeostasis During Normal Sleep—Rapid Eye Movement

- Rapid eye movement (REM) sleep is considered a state of autonomic instability, marked by surges in both sympathetic and vagal activity with attendant variations in HR, BP, and peripheral vascular resistance.[9,10] Changes may be more prominent in association with transient muscle activity (TMA), previously referred to as phasic REM, where darting eye movements and muscle twitches, predominantly seen in the extremities and face, break through skeletal muscle atonia.
- Animal and human studies have demonstrated more concentrated autonomic changes associated with TMA, during which intense electrical discharges have been recorded from the brain stem.[11]
- Animal experiments have demonstrated marked HR instability during REM. Increments in HR of more than 30% are seen in association with TMA, and are often accompanied by an elevation in BP,[12,13] particularly concentrated during sleep epochs where a muscle twitch was recorded.[14]
- In humans, the average HR is higher during REM than NREM sleep,[15] as is sympathetic neural output, although there is some evidence that sympathetic activation is not a global phenomenon during REM. Case reports and series suggest that healthy young adults, sometimes athletes,[16] have periods of exaggerated vagal tone during REM sleep, manifesting as first- or second-degree AV block[17] or sinus pauses that may exceed 9 seconds in duration.[18,19] REM therefore appears to be marked by fluctuations in autonomic activity, both to the cardiac conduction system as well as to peripheral blood vessels.[20]

Mechanisms of Arrhythmias During Sleep, Including Sleep Apnea

- Those with established cardiac conduction disease may have distinct pathophysiologic mechanisms during sleep. A study of a small group of subjects with preexisting AV block demonstrated shortening of AV delay during periods of REM.[21]
- Ambulatory cardiac monitoring (nonpolysomnographic) data in an elderly populations report less common occurrences of sinus pauses and AV blocks during sleep episodes, with relatively common supraventricular and ventricular ectopic beats.[5,22]
- The circadian variation in paroxysmal atrial fibrillation (AF) noted by some, with clustering of events in the early morning hours, suggests a potential influence of the autonomic nervous system.[23,24] Analysis of HR variability in patients with AF demonstrated abrupt shifts in sympathovagal balance preceding the onset of the arrhythmia.[25–27]
- Gender-selective effects of REM on cardiac electrical activity have been demonstrated, with measured prolongation of the QT interval exclusive to women.[28]
- In animals with coronary-artery stenosis, REM sleep causes further decrements in coronary-artery blood flow.[29] These findings were prevented with sympathectomy, suggesting an effect attributable to sympathetic overdrive rather than parasympathetic withdrawal.
- Obesity, diabetes, dyslipidemia, hypertension, ischemic heart disease, and systolic and diastolic heart failure all cluster with obstructive sleep apnea (OSA). Therefore, simply by association

with these conditions, the risk of arrhythmias is increased in patients with sleep-disordered breathing. The physiologic stressors associated with repetitive upper airway collapse (hypoxemia, swings in intrathoracic pressure) and central nervous system arousals in OSA further heighten acute CV risk that may predispose to arrhythmias.

- In individuals with OSA, apnea and hypoxemia activate the physiologic "diving reflex," so named from observations of marine mammals that must conserve oxygen during prolonged water submersion.[30] The reflex results in peripheral vasoconstriction and bradycardia during hypoxemia. With resumption of breathing as the apnea terminates, the vagolytic effects of lung inflation coupled with the arousal from sleep cause a transient increase in HR.[31] This common finding has been described as the "brady-tachy" phenomenon of OSA (not to be confused with the so-called tachy-brady syndrome associated with pathologic sinus node dysfunction; Fig. 24.1). Not infrequently, patients who are found to have bradycardias associated with sleep apnea have gone on to have normal cardiac electrophysiologic studies, reflecting the powerful influence of autonomic changes that occur in OSA.[32]

The Scoring of Cardiac Events During Polysomnography

- The AASM sleep scoring manual includes an entry outlining recommendations for the scoring of cardiac events during sleep.[8]
- With no prior published standards to guide acquisition, interpretation, or reporting of cardiac events during sleep, the

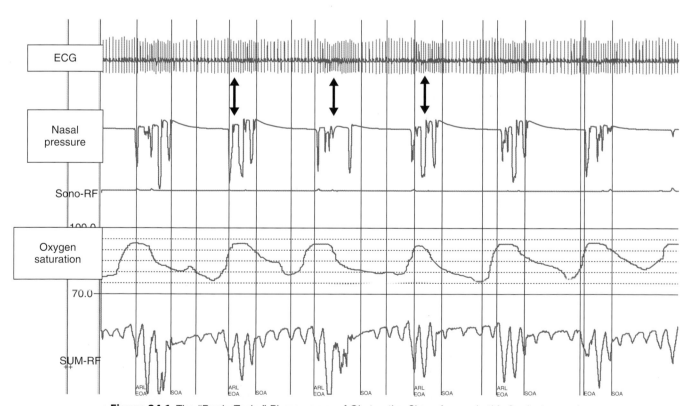

- **Figure 24.1** The "Brady-Tachy" Phenomenon of Obstructive Sleep Apnea. In this 3-minute epoch, repetitive apneas (as defined by flat nasal pressure tracings and oxyhemoglobin desaturations to near 70%) are associated with the slowing of the heart rate on the electrocardiogram (ECG) tracing. Immediate increases in heart rate are coupled with resumption of ventilation (arrows).

AASM task force considered and incorporated recommendations for ambulatory cardiac recordings from existing guidelines from the American Heart Association (AHA) and American College of Cardiology (ACC),[33,34] as appropriate. For example, guidelines related to electrocardiogram (ECG) lead placement during stress testing were informative.

Electrocardiogram Lead Choice

- In formulating the cardiac scoring manual, it was assumed (though not systematically verified) that the vast majority of sleep laboratories utilize a single ECG lead during PSG. In recommending a specific single lead, the committee placed primacy on determination of HR, basic rhythm recognition (sinus or otherwise), and detection of ectopy.
- Based upon existing AHA recommendations in ambulatory patients to utilize proximally placed limb electrodes (such as during exercise testing), and because the vector of limb lead II probably best captures atrial (and therefore sinus node) activity (Fig. 24.2), lead II with torso electrode placement is the recommended single lead of choice during PSG (Figs. 24.2 and 24.3).
- At the discretion of the clinician, adjustments to this lead positioning or additional lead placement may occasionally be warranted. For example, the left-sided lead may be placed almost anywhere on the lateral left thorax in parallel to the left hip. Fig. 24.4 demonstrates the morphologic changes evident in p wave tracing output when utilizing lead I compared with lead II in a sleeping 70-year-old woman.
- There are two important caveats to the use of a single limb ECG lead in PSG monitoring. First, a single limb lead is poorly sensitive and an unreliable indicator of cardiac ischemia by ST segment recording. Furthermore, fluctuations in the ST segment are known to occur in association with position changes that are often part and parcel of sleep testing, and are therefore not specific for cardiac ischemia. Therefore the single lead alone should not be used as a sole indicator of myocardial ischemia,

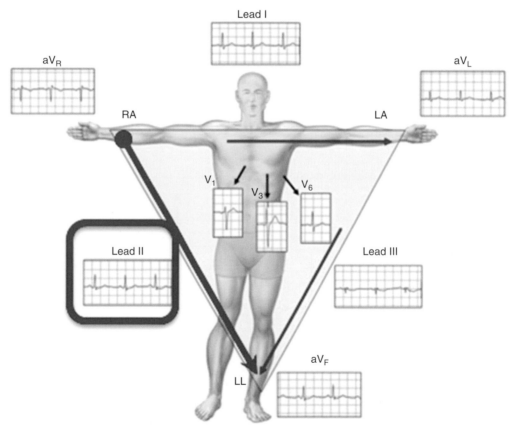

• **Figure 24.2** Einthoven's triangle is formed by three skin electrodes on the right arm (RA), left arm (LA), and left leg (LL). It is an inverted equilateral triangle with the heart lying in the center. **Lead I** is created between the negative potential RA electrode and the positive potential LA electrode and in the normal subject is upright with current flowing from right to left *(red arrow)*. **Lead II** is created between a negative RA electrode and a positive LL electrode, whereas **Lead III** is between LA and LL electrodes and in both cases the LL electrode is positive with current flowing downward *(red arrows)*. The typical ECG appearance of the bipolar limb leads and the unipolar augmented leads; aVR, aVL, and aVF are shown as are three of the unipolar chest leads, V1, V3, and V6. Lead II with torso electrode placement is the recommended single lead of choice during polysomnography. (From Mond HG, Garcia J, Visagathilagar T. Twisted leads: the footprints of malpositioned electrocardiographic leads. *Heart Lung Circ*. 2016;25[1]: 61–67.)

but could be used as an adjunct to the clinical assessment in a patient suspected of having ischemia.

- Second, the single limb lead should not be considered a reliable indicator of the origin of a wide QRS complex (i.e., supraventricular versus ventricular).

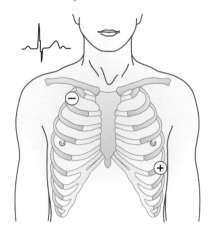

A single modified elctrocardiograph lead II using torso electrode placement is recommended

Notes:
1. Additional leads may be placed if clinically-indicated at the discretion of the practitioner.
2. Increasing image size on display may improve detection of arrhythmias.
3. While classically lead II is derived from electrodes placed on the right arm and left leg, the electrodes may be placed on the torso aligned in parallel to the right shoulder and left hip.
4. Standard ECG electrode applications are superior to EEG electrodes in minimizing artifact.

• **Figure 24.3** Electrode placement for the recommended electrocardiogram (ECG) lead II. While classically placed on the right arm and left leg, the electrodes may be placed on the torso aligned in parallel to the right shoulder and left hip. (Adapted from Wagner GS. *Marriott's Practical Electrocardiography*. 9th ed. Baltimore, MD: Williams and Wilkins; 1994.)

Scoring of Bradycardia in Adults

- Traditionally, bradycardia during wakefulness has been defined as a HR < 60 bpm. However, because the lowest HR encountered over a 24-hour period in normal individuals is most likely to occur during NREM sleep, this daytime standard may not be appropriate for the sleep period.
- Unpublished normative data from the Sleep Heart Health Study (SHHS) reveals HR from 43–48 bpm captured within two standard deviations from the mean (Redline, S., personal communication, 2005), with women consistently showing a slightly higher HR than men.
- Based upon these data and expert consensus, the recommended operational definition of bradycardia in adults is a HR less than 40 bpm.[8]
- Cardiac rhythms associated with a low HR that the clinician may encounter during sleep testing include sinus bradycardia and AV blocks (Figs. 24.5–24.7). Bradycardias are not uncommon in the setting of untreated OSA, though it should be noted that AHA/ACC designates AV block associated with apneic events during sleep as a Class III indication ("not useful/ effective or may be harmful") for a pacemaker.[35]
- Asystole (systolic pauses) of less than or equal to 2 seconds are felt to occur in normal adults. In trained athletes, pauses may be longer. The AHA defines asystolic pauses greater than 3 seconds as pathologic in those with attributable symptoms.

Scoring of Sinus Tachycardia

- By tradition, the definition of tachycardia has been an HR greater than 100 bpm, although it has been argued that this threshold is too high, advocating a revision to 90 bpm (during wakefulness, without regard to sleep).[36] However, as in scoring bradycardia, because of the autonomic changes that occur during sleep, applying similar HR thresholds to wakefulness and sleep is not appropriate.
- Unpublished data from the SHHS shows upper limits of the 95% confidence interval HR in women of 84.7 and 80.8 bpm in men.

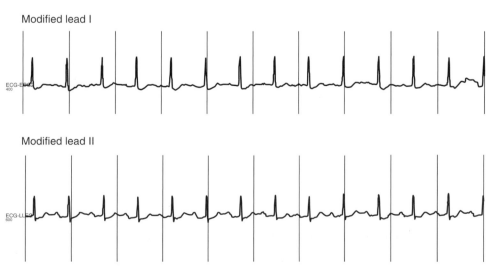

Modified lead I

Modified lead II

• **Figure 24.4** Identical electrocardiogram (ECG) tracing in a 70-year-old woman. The upper panel is output from modified lead I (left clavicle +, right clavicle −), the lower panel modified lead II (right clavicle −, left leg +). Note the sharper p waves in lead II. The lack of obvious p waves in the upper panel might be mistaken for atrial fibrillation.

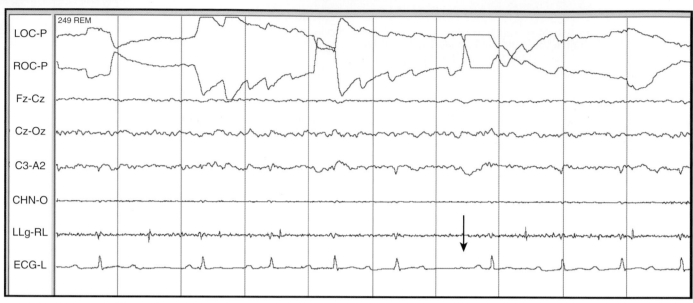

• **Figure 24.5** An example of Mobitz type I (Wenckebach) second-degree atrioventricular block. Note the progressively increasing PR interval and decreasing R-R interval until a P wave is not conducted (arrow).

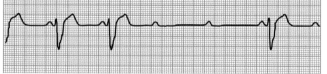

• **Figure 24.6** Second-degree atrioventricular (AV) block type II (Mobitz II). The site of block is below the AV node (infranodal). Conduction through AV node is normal, so QRS is dropped without prolongation of the PR interval. QRS is often widened.

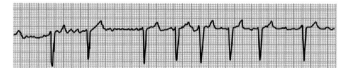

• **Figure 24.8** Atrial fibrillation. P waves are replaced by rapid oscillations or waves that vary in size, shape, and timing, with a resultant irregular ventricular rhythm. (From Bontemp LJ, Goralnic E. Atrial Fibrillation. *Emerg Med Clin of North Am* 2011;29[4]:747–748.)

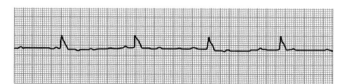

• **Figure 24.7** Third-degree atrioventricular (AV) block. No relationship exists between P waves and ventricular escape beats ("AV dissociation"). The QRS is usually widened but can be narrow if the AV block is above the AV node.

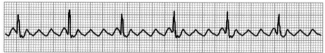

• **Figure 24.9** Atrial flutter, a somewhat more organized rhythm than atrial fibrillation, where the atrioventricular block may be more constant (4 : 1 or 3 : 1), resulting in the characteristic "sawtooth" atrial waves. (From Goralnick E, Bontempo LJ. Atrial Fibrillation. *Emerg Med Clin of North Am* 2015;33[3]:597–612.)

• The AASM has recommended that the threshold for sinus tachycardia during sleep be defined as greater than 90 bpm.

Scoring of Tachyarrhythmias Other Than Sinus

• Consensus guidelines from the AHA typically classify tachyarrhythmias as wide or narrow complex, utilizing a cutoff of 120 mssec to differentiate the two. While this is an appropriate operational definition, it should be noted that the distinction can be difficult when utilizing a single lead ECG during PSG.

• The most common narrow complex tachycardia (and most common arrhythmia overall) is AF. As the atrial rate approaches 600 bpm, p waves are replaced by rapid oscillations or waves that vary in size, shape, and timing, with a resultant irregular ventricular rhythm (Fig. 24.8).

• Atrial flutter represents a somewhat more organized atrial rhythm, where atrial activity may manifest as flutter or sawtooth waves (Fig. 24.9).

• Supraventricular tachycardia (SVT), which usually represents a re-entry phenomenon in the proximal conducting system,

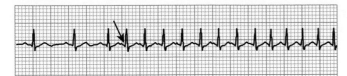

• Figure 24.10 Reentry supraventricular tachycardia. The arrow shows arrhythmia initiation. Reentry refers to repeated recycling of the electrical impulse through the atrioventricular node. Heart rate usually greater than 150 bpm, with a narrow QRS. Usually undetectable p waves, which may be buried in preceding T waves.

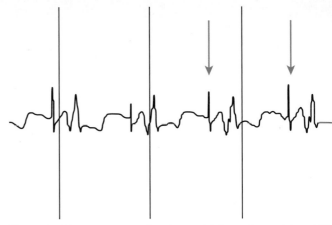

• Figure 24.11 Pacemaker spikes *(arrows)* followed by a widened QRS complex. The vertical black lines represent 1-second intervals during polysomnography, so this pacemaker is set at 60 bpm.

will manifest as a narrow complex tachycardia that tends to be regular in ventricular rhythm (in distinction to AF; Fig. 24.10).

- Wide QRS complexes may represent a ventricular origin of the cardiac impulse or may originate from the atria or sinus node in the setting of disease of the conducting system.
- A wide complex QRS is typically seen with ventricular pacemakers (Fig. 24.11).
- Considering the limitations of utilizing the single ECG lead in deciphering the impulse origin as outlined previously, labeling wide complex tachycardias with a specific diagnosis (such as "ventricular tachycardia" or "supraventricular tachycardia with aberrancy") during PSG is dubious. The clinical context might provide clues, however. In those over 40 years of age who have structural heart disease, a wide complex tachycardia is more likely to be ventricular in origin.
- The AASM guidelines utilize conventional definitions for scoring tachyarrhythmias. A wide complex tachycardia is a sustained rhythm (lasting more than 3 cardiac cycles) with a QRS duration ≥120 msec and a rate greater than 100 bpm. A narrow complex tachycardia is a sustained rhythm lasting more than 3 cardiac cycles, with a QRS duration less than 120 msec and a rate greater than 100 bpm. AF is an irregularly irregular ventricular rhythm associated with the replacement of P waves, with rapid oscillations or waves that vary in size, shape, and timing.

Cardiac Scoring in Children

- Very little normative HR data during sleep exist in pediatric populations, though there is a well-recognized reduction in the HR as age advances to young adulthood, as drawn from data of resting children during wakefulness.[8]
- Because vagal tone is often higher in children and adolescents, HRs during sleep are expected to be significantly lower compared with resting wakefulness, when compared with adults.

- Normative HRs were measured during sleep testing of ethnically diverse 6–11-year-old populations studied in Tucson and Cleveland. Faster sleeping HRs were noted in younger children, African Americans, females, and those who were obese.[37] A subsequent study of Hispanic and Caucasian children into adolescence (up to 17 years of age) showed a continued trend of decreasing HR as age increased. Females, on average, had HR 5 bpm faster than males. HR during REM was higher than in NREM. The level of fitness was found to explain some of the difference between genders.[38]

Suggested Reading

Archbold KH, Johnson NL, Goodwin JL, et al. Normative heart rate parameters during sleep for children aged 6 to 11 years. *J Clin Sleep Med*. 2010;6(1):47-50.

Caples SM, Somers V, Rosen C, et al. The scoring of cardiac events during sleep. *J Clin Sleep Med*. 2007;3(2):147-154.

Kadish AH, Buxton AE, Kennedy HL, et al. ACC/AHA clinical competence statement on electrocardiography and ambulatory electrocardiography: a report of the ACC/AHA/ACP-ASIM task force on clinical competence (ACC/AHA Committee to develop a clinical competence statement on electrocardiography and ambulatory electrocardiography) endorsed by the International Society for Holter and noninvasive electrocardiology. *Circulation*. 2001;104(25):3169-3178.

Spodick DH. Normal sinus heart rate: appropriate rate thresholds for sinus tachycardia and bradycardia. *South Med J*. 1996;89(7):666-667.

25

Pharmacotherapy of Sleep Promoting Agents

THOMAS ROTH, TIMOTHY V. ROEHRS

Defining Hypnotic Efficacy

Therapeutic Endpoints

- In defining the efficacy of hypnotics, it is important to distinguish between disturbed sleep and insomnia.
- Disturbed sleep refers to objective signs of sleep disruption, including excessive wakefulness before, during, and after the sleep period, as well as the intrusion of arousals and awakenings from sleep per se.
- Insomnia is defined as a report of difficulty falling asleep, staying asleep, or nonrefreshing sleep, associated with some daytime consequence.
- Evaluations of hypnotic efficacy must assess both endpoints.
- Clinical trials have in general neglected the areas of daytime function and patient estimates of the adequacy of sleep.

There are three dimensions along which hypnotic efficacy can be defined:
1. Objective measures versus patient reports
2. Nocturnal sleep versus diurnal functioning
3. Nature of the patient population (primary vs. comorbid insomnia)

Objectives Assays of Sleep

- Laboratory based polysomnography (PSG) is recognized as the gold standard for the objective measurement of sleep. This is considered the standard, as it provides quantitative data on all important aspects of sleep physiology in a controlled environment.[1] Increasingly, studies on insomnia are using home PSGs.
- The advantage of home recordings is that they are a closer approximation of the actual clinical situation.
- In attempts to assay sleep outside of the laboratory, a variety of other methods have been attempted.
- The most widely used non-PSG surrogate of sleep is the measurement of movement or actigraphy. Actigraphy has been used in a variety of sleep research contexts.
- Utility of actigraphy seems to be greater in measuring sleep duration, as opposed to sleep initiation.

Subjective Reports

- In the laboratory setting, postsleep questionnaires are most often used.

- In home studies, diaries are used to assay sleep over weeks and even months.
- Caregiver observations (nurses, caregivers of the cognitively impaired) are commonly used in mild cognitive impairment (MCI) trials, as these are not typically recommended in efficacy trials.
- Global measures such as patient and clinician global impressions of improvement are widely used in clinical trials in many areas and need to be used more frequently in insomnia.
- Insomnia scales such as the Insomnia Severity Index are critical to our determining of response and remission rates.[2]

Daytime Efficacy Measures

- The daytime benefits associated with improvements in sleep and insomnia are the most neglected area in hypnotic efficacy trials.
- This is due to the fact that insomnia morbidity research has, to date, failed to identify potential outcomes that might be improved with the successful treatment of insomnia.
- Studies evaluating quality of life have met with some mixed success. In contrast, objective measure of daytime function such as memory, psychomotor, and vigilance performance, and physiological measures of alertness (i.e., Multiple Sleep Latency Test [MSLT]), have not met with much success.
- The exceptions to this are isolated studies in transient insomnia and insomnia associated with pain.[3]
- This lack of consistent results suggests that insomnia morbidity is different than that of sleep loss.

Efficacy Populations

- The vast majority of insomnia trials have been performed in patients with primary insomnia. However, in both population and clinic-based studies, it is estimated that primary insomnia accounts for about 10%–25% of the chronic insomnia population.
- Populations that have been studied and show promise include insomnia associated with psychiatric disorders, pain conditions, and circadian rhythm disorders.[4–6]
- In these populations it is important to study how improvements in sleep modify the course of the comorbid conditions.

Pharmacology

See Table 25.1 for therapeutic targets and Table 25.2 for therapeutic categories.

Herbals

- According to the 2002 National Health Interview Survey of the general population, 17% of respondents reported past-year insomnia and approximately 5% of those reported using various alternative treatments for their insomnia, with the majority being the use of herbals.
- There is a paucity of rigorous scientific investigation of the efficacy and safety of the use of herbals to treat insomnia.[7]

Valerian

- Valerian is a root occurring in several species (i.e., *Valeriana officinalis*, *Valeriana wallichii*, *Valeriana edulis*) that is extracted and prepared in different methods, producing differing chemical constituents in the final product.[8]

TABLE 25.1	Therapeutic Targets of Sleep Medications
SLEEP/WAKE NEUROTRANSMITTERS AND MODULATORS: TARGETS FOR PHARMACOLOGIC INTERVENTIONS	
Wake (Antagonists)	**Sleep (Agonists)**
Norepinephrine	Adenosine
Serotonin	GABA
Acetylcholine	Galanin
Histamine	Melatonin
Orexin/hypocretin	

GABA, γ-Aminobutyric acid.

TABLE 25.2	Therapeutic Categories of Sleep Medications

- FDA-approved drugs
  - Benzodiazepine receptor agonists
  - Melatonin receptor agonists
  - Orexin antagonists
- Drugs used off-label (not FDA approved for insomnia)
  - Sedating antidepressants
  - Antipsychotics
- Self-medication
  - Alcohol
  - H1 antihistamines (over-the-counter sleep aids)
  - Herbal remedies

- The mechanism of action for valerian's hypnotic effect is not certain, although one study suggests that valerian has agonistic activity at the adenosine A_1 receptor.
- Twenty-nine controlled trials of the efficacy of valerian in insomniacs have been done and concluded that relative to placebo, regardless of preparation, valerian did not improve self-rated or PSG sleep.

St. John's Wort

- An herbal taken for a variety of conditions, including depression, anxiety, and sleep disturbances is St. John's Wort.[8]
- St. John's Wort is a flowering herb that is also available in a number of different preparations, although the active ingredient is thought to be hyperforin. Hyperforin inhibits reuptake of serotonin, norepinephrine, dopamine, L-glutamate, and γ-aminobutyric acid (GABA).
- Trials of its efficacy in depression have been conducted, but there are no trials in primary insomnia. The two studies of its hypnotic activity in healthy normals are equivocal.

Melatonin

- Melatonin (*N*-acetyl-5-methoxytryptamine) is produced by the pineal gland.
- Synthesis and secretion occurs nocturnally in darkness and is inhibited by light, a specific time that suggests its involvement in modulating circadian rhythms. Normal melatonin secretion starts in the evening and falls during the morning hours.[9]

- Some people who have trouble sleeping may have low endogenous levels of melatonin or a delayed secretion, and it is thought that supplementing melatonin might assist with sleep.
- Exogenous melatonin (dietary supplements) is used for a variety of reasons: circadian rhythm sleep disorder, to combat jet lag and shift work disorder, and for disrupted sleep, with inconsistent evidence of its effectiveness.[10]
- Made synthetically, melatonin supplements are available in liquid, sublingual lozenge, and immediate and time-release tablets.
- The half-life of melatonin ranges from 0.54–2 hours, with doses ranging from 0.3–5 mg; it is less likely to cause residual daytime drowsiness. Side effects include headache, odd taste in mouth, dizziness, and poor sleep quality.
- Decreases in nighttime melatonin concentrations and a delay in melatonin secretion have been reported in insomniacs.
- Double blind placebo controlled studies have failed to show the effectiveness of supplemental melatonin in treating insomnia. Melatonin is more effective in reducing sleep initiation in patients with delayed sleep phase syndrome than in those with primary insomnia.[10]

Alcohol

- Alcohol is a sedative that disturbs sleep and has a myriad of effects on the central nervous system (CNS).[11]

Mechanism

- As a depressant, alcohol enhances the inhibitory neurotransmitter GABA, resulting in an overall decrease in brain excitability.[12]

Effects on Sleep

- The initial sedative effects following alcohol consumption contributes to the self-mediated use of alcohol consumption as a sleep aid. The use of alcohol as a sleep aid is common.
- Alcohol causes does-dependent decreases in sleep latency, increases in stage 3–4 sleep (slow wave), with the first half relative to the second half of the sleep period and initial REM suppression.[12]
- The metabolism of alcohol during the second portion of the night leads to rebound increases in sleep fragmentation or nighttime wakefulness, REM rebound, and increases in dreams and nightmares.[12]
- Tolerance to the sedative effects of alcohol can lead to dependence and/or abuse.[13]
- Alcohol consumption can worsen sleep-disordered breathing and various parasomnias.

Over-the-Counter Agents

- An immune response to a normally innocuous substance (e.g., pollen, dust) can cause the release of histamines, which generates the classic allergic response.
- Antihistamines are indicated for effective control of seasonal and environmental allergies.
- In terms of sleep-wake function, these drugs block histamine receptors, a major alerting CNS neurotransmitter.

- First-generation H_1 antihistamines are lipophilic and cross the blood-brain barrier to antagonize cholinergic muscarinic, alpha-adrenergic, and serotoninergic receptors. Second-generation antihistamines do not enter the brain well, and hence do not cause sedation. Diphenhydramine and doxylamine are H_1 receptor antagonists, thereby producing sedation. This, in part, mediates the activity of many over-the-counter (OTC) sleep aids.[14]

Diphenhydramine

- A limited number of subject reports or PSG are limited trials.
- Diphenhydramine is to be taken 30 minutes prior to bed, and peak plasma concentration occurs 2–3 hours after administration.
- Overall, improvements in sleep when reported are seen with 50 mg.
- Does have a long half-life with potential for daytime impairment.
- Tolerance has been shown to develop following 3 days of administration.[15]

Doxylamine

- Doxylamine is indicated as a short-term insomnia treatment.[16]
- Doxylamine is to be taken 30 minutes before retiring to bed.
- Sleep is usually achieved within 45–60 minutes after oral administration, with peak plasma concentration occurring after 90 minutes.
- There is little evidence supporting efficacy.
- Given the long half-life, it is associated with daytime impairment.
- Commonly reported side effects are next-day drowsiness, grogginess, dry mouth, and tiredness.

Over-the-Counter Combination Products

- Diphenhydramine and doxylamine are combined with other medications to provide multiple symptom relief.[16]
- Diphenhydramine combination preparations include analgesics, such as acetaminophen, ibuprofen, and aspirin.
- Doxylamine is combined with various cold preparations to provide relief of cold symptoms and sleeplessness.
- Patients with concomitant hypertension, cardiovascular, and/or respiratory disease should take precautions in taking diphenhydramine or doxylamine.
- Additive CNS effects occur when H_1 antihistamines are taken concurrently with alcohol, other sedative-hypnotics, anxiolytics, narcotic analgesics, and neuroleptic drugs.
- Significant interactions may occur if these drugs are taken concomitantly with anticholinergic agents or tricyclic antidepressants.
- Geriatric patients and those sensitive to sedative and anticholinergic properties of H_1 antihistamines are particularly vulnerable populations and should use caution when using diphenhydramine or doxylamine.

Prescription Medications

See Tables 25.3 and 25.4 for the most commonly prescribed medications for insomnia, as well as their pattern of use. As can be concluded, most patients (up to two-thirds) are more likely to use hypnotic agents for less than 2 weeks.

TABLE 25.3 Most Frequently Prescribed Hypnotics

DRUGS MOST COMMONLY USED FOR INSOMNIA IN 2002

Drug	Occurrences (Millions)
Trazodone	2.730
Zolpidem	2.074
Amitriptyline	0.774
Mirtazepine	0.662
Temezepam	0.558
Quetiapine	0.459
Zaleplon	0.405
Clonazepam	0.394
Hydroxyzine	0.293
Alprazolam	0.287
Lorazepam	0.277
Olazepine	0.216
Flurazepam	0.205
Doxepin	0.199
Cyclobenzaprine	0.195
Diphenhydramine	0.192

Verispan PDDA; desired action of "hypnotic," "promote sleep," or "sedate night."
From Walsh JK. Drugs used to treat insomnia in 2002: regulatory-based rather than evidence-based medicine. *Sleep.* 2004;27:1441–1442.

TABLE 25.4 Patterns of Prescribed Hypnotic Use

Longest Period of Continuous Use	% Of Total Hypnotic Users
1–2 days	54
3–13 days	20
2–3 weeks	4
1–3 months	6
4–11 months	6
≥12 months	11

From Balter MB, Manheimer DI, Mellinger GD, Uhlenhuth EH. A cross-national comparison of anti-anxiety/sedative drug use. *Curr Med Res Opin.* 1984;8(suppl 4):5–20.

TABLE 25.5 γ-Aminobutyric Acid: the Principal Inhibitory Neuronal Transmitter

- GABA
- 30% of all brain synapses use GABA as transmitter
- Binds to and activates $GABA_A$ receptors
- Controls flow of chloride ions across neuronal membrane through receptor channels
- Resulting ion flux causes membrane hyperpolarization and neuronal inhibition

GABA, γ-Aminobutyric acid; *GABA$_A$*, gaminobutyric acid type A.

TABLE 25.6 Pharmacological Properties of US FDA-Approved Hypnotics Benzodiazepine Receptor Agonists

FDA-APPROVED HYPNOTICS BENZODIAZEPINE RECEPTOR AGONISTS

Drug	Dose (mg)	$T_{1/2}$ (h)	Metabolism
Triazolam	0.25	2–4	Oxidation
Temazepam	15–30	8–20	Conjugation
Estazolam	1–2	10–24	Oxidation
Quazepam	15	25–41	Oxidation
Flurazepam	15–30	24–100	Oxidation
Zaleplon	10	1	Oxidation
Zolpidem	5–10	1.5–2.5	Oxidation
Eszopiclone	1–3	5–7	Oxidation

which is a widely distributed, inhibitory neurotransmitter in the CNS.

- BzRAs act allosterically, meaning that GABA must also be present on the receptor complex for BzRAs to have their inhibitory effects, which in part explains their wide therapeutic index (e.g., efficacy to safety ratio).[17]
- The BzRAs include drugs that have the benzodiazepine chemical structure (i.e., flurazepam, triazolam, temazepam, estazolam, and quazepam) and those that do not, but yet act at the benzodiazepine receptor (i.e., zolpidem, zaleplon, eszopiclone, zolpidem CR, and zolpidem sublingual; see Fig. 25.1 and Table 25.6).

Pharmacology

- The BzRAs differ on two pharmacologic dimensions: their pharmacokinetics and their alpha receptor subtype (see Table 25.7).
- Fig. 25.2 illustrates the gaminobutyric acid type A receptors ($GABA_A$R), with BDZ-specific pharmacology, as it relates to clinically relevant effects and side effects.
- All the BzRAs are rapidly absorbed, having a T_{max} of 0.5–2 hours, which accounts for their capacity to hasten sleep onset.
- They differ widely in their half-lives, and half-life is predictive of the likelihood of producing residual effects.

Benzodiazepine Receptor Agonists

Mechanism

- Benzodiazepine receptor agonists (BzRAs) have been the drugs of choice for the treatment of insomnia since their introduction approximately 50 years ago.
- These drugs occupy benzodiazepine alpha receptors of the $GABA_A$ receptor complex, hence their name BzRAs (see Table 25.5).
- Occupation of the receptor results in opening the chloride ion channel and facilitation of the inhibitory action of GABA,

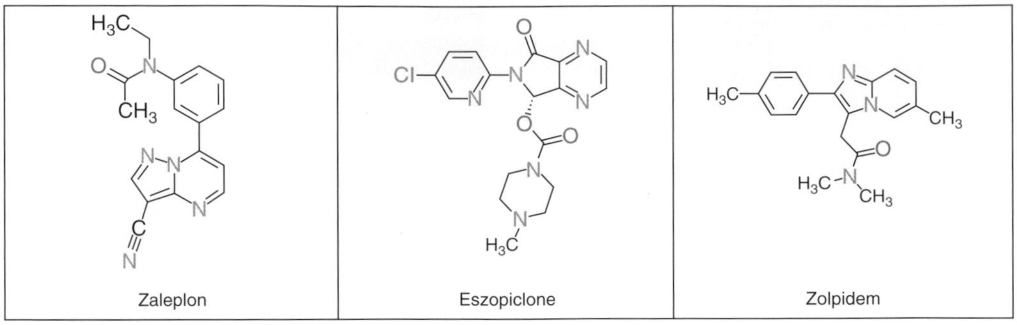

• **Figure 25.1** Chemical Structure of Z Drugs. (From Ciraulo DA, Oldham M. Sedative hypnotics. In: Madras B, Kuhar M, eds. *The Effects of Drug Abuse on the Human Nervous System*. Boston, MA: Elsevier; 2014:499–532.)

TABLE 25.7	Gaminobutyric Acid Type A Receptor Subtypes	
α Subtype	% Of Central Nervous System Gaminobutyric Acid Receptors	Action Mediated
α_1	60	Sedation, amnesia, partial anticonvulsant
α_2	15–20	Anxiolytic, myorelaxation
α_3	10–15	Myorelaxation (only at high doses)
α_4	<5	Insensitive to BzRAs
α_5	<5	Partial myorelaxation
α_6	<5	Insensitive to BzRAs

BzRAs, Benzodiazepine receptor agonists.

TABLE 25.8	Effects of the Benzodiazepines
• Sleep induction • Sleep maintenance • Sleep consolidation • Sleep stage changes • EEG changes • Motor activity • Ataxia	• Amnesia • Rebound • Withdrawal • Anticonvulsant • Myo-relaxant • Anxiolytic (subtypes)

• Among the benzodiazepines, only triazolam has a short half-life. Temazepam and estazolam have intermediate half-lives, while flurazepam and quazepam have long half-lives. All of these intermediate and long-acting benzodiazepines have been shown to have residual effects.

Nonbenzodiazepines

(See Fig. 25.1.)
• Among the "nonbenzodiazepines," zaleplon has an ultra-short half-life (1 hour), zolpidem and its different formulations have short half-lives (1.5–2.5 hours), while eszopiclone has an intermediate half-life (5–7 hours).

Benzodiazepine Receptor Agonist Receptor Subtypes

• A major pharmacologic difference among the BzRAs is in their alpha receptor subtype binding (see Table 25.7). For the alpha receptor of the GABA$_A$ complex, six subtypes have been identified.[18]
• All of the benzodiazepines demonstrate similar affinity to the alpha 1, 2, 3, and 5 receptor subtypes.

• Zolpidem and zaleplon have higher affinity for alpha 1 than the other subtypes.
• Eszopiclone shows a decreased preference for the alpha 1 subtype, having a greater affinity to alpha 2 and 3.
• Based on the animal studies, it is hypothesized that alpha 1 mediates sleep and amnesic effects, while alpha 2 and 3 are involved in anxiolytic, muscle relaxation, and possibly antidepressant effects (see Fig. 25.2).
• In human studies, eszopiclone (alpha 2 and 3), but not zolpidem, has been shown to augment an antidepressant response in patients with insomnia comorbid with depression, as well as anxiolytic response in patients with insomnia comorbid with generalized anxiety disorder (GAD).

Efficacy of Benzodiazepine Receptor Agonists

• The hypnotic efficacy of the FDA-approved BzRAs have been well documented using objective PSG and subjective measures of sleep induction and duration in clinical trials, and in meta-analyses of trials using various benzodiazepines and zolpidem (see Table 25.8). It can be concluded they are effective.
• Note the hypnotic effects have been shown to be dose-related and the studies have been conducted in both young and elderly adults. Depending on their different pharmacokinetics (i.e., T_{max} and $T_{1/2}$) and dose, the BzRAs induce and maintain sleep.[19,20]

FDA Indications for Use

• The FDA indications given to the BzRAs are mostly general and nonspecific as to insomnia subtype (i.e., "for treatment of insomnia," or "for treatment of insomnia including sleep onset, sleep, and maintenance").

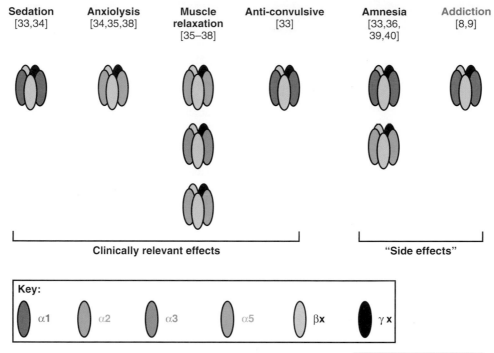

| Sedation [33,34] | Anxiolysis [34,35,38] | Muscle relaxation [35–38] | Anti-convulsive [33] | Amnesia [33,36, 39,40] | Addiction [8,9] |

Clinically relevant effects   **"Side effects"**

Key:

α1   α2   α3   α5   βx   γ x

TRENDS in neurosciences

• **Figure 25.2** Gaminobutyric Acid Type A Receptors BDZ-Specific Pharmacology. The past decade has seen an emerging understanding of the specific gaminobutyric acid type A receptors (GABAAR) subtypes responsible for mediating the diverse spectrum of BDZ pharmacological effects. For example, the sedative actions are known to be mediated by α1-containing GABAARs, whereas the anxiolytic actions are mediated by α2-containing GABAARs. (From Tan KR, Rudolph U, Lüscher C. Hooked on benzodiazepines: GABA$_A$ receptor subtypes and addiction. *Trends Neurosci.* 2011;34:188–197.)

- Among the nonbenzodiazepines, based on FDA labeling, zaleplon, zolpidem, and zolpidem sublingual are specifically indicated for sleep induction, while eszopiclone and zolpidem CR are indicated for both sleep induction and sleep maintenance.
- A recently introduced low-dose (1.75 and 3.5) buffered zolpidem formulation bypassing first pass metabolism has recently been approved for treating insomnia characterized by difficulty falling asleep after a middle of the night awakening, provided that 4 additional hours in bed are available.

Tolerance

- Tolerance is defined as the loss of effects with repeated use of a stable dose, or the need to increase dose to maintain effects over repeated use.
- Efficacy studies have been short and intermediate term in duration (i.e., ≤6 weeks) and given a paucity of controlled long-term data and many uncontrolled clinical observations, tolerance development has remained an area of controversy.
- Recent double-blind, placebo controlled studies using self-reports have shown eszopiclone is effective for 6–12 months of nightly use and in a PSG study zolpidem remained effective for 8 months of nightly use.[21,22]
- Studies reporting tolerance development reveals that the sleep of the drug treated group remained stable over time, while the sleep of the placebo group improves, the result being statistically significant group differences were lost, suggesting tolerance had developed.

- The placebo group improvement may reflect a placebo response or a sleep hygiene effect (i.e., adherence to a regular sleep schedule, avoidance of alcohol, etc.) required by the study restrictions of the clinical trial.

Efficacy in Daytime Functioning

- Patient reports of quality of life, work impairment, absenteeism, daytime fatigue, and daytime sleepiness have all found impairment among insomniacs relative to age-matched healthy controls.
- Studies have now shown that the improvement in nocturnal sleep is associated with improvement in some aspects of daytime function.
- With eszopiclone, self-reports of daytime alertness, ability to function during the daytime, and physical well-being all improved in the eszopiclone-treated versus the placebo-treated group.
- Studies have shown positive effects of BzRAs on comorbid conditions, including major depression disorder (MDD), GAD, pain disorders, and menopause.[4,5]

Safety

Adverse Events

(See Table 25.9.)

- In general, adverse reactions to BzRAs in clinical practice and clinical trials are mild, of short duration, and occur in a minority of patients.

TABLE 25.9	Benzodiazepine Receptor Agonist Adverse Events and Safety Consideration

- Determinants
  - C_{max} $T_{1/2}$
- Adverse events:
  - Somnolence
  - Ataxia
  - Amnesia
  - Dizziness
  - Taste
  - Nausea
- Discontinuation effects
  - Rebound insomnia, withdrawal syndrome
- Dependence liability
  - Dose escalation, self-administration outside therapeutic context

Aes, Adverse events.

- Many of the adverse effects of BzRAs are mediated by their desired pharmacological activity and sedation.

Residual Effects

- Residual effects refer to the experience of impaired functions in the morning after using a hypnotic. It is important to recognize that all BzRAs can impair many aspects of human performance while there are significant blood levels.
- Assessments have included psychomotor tests like digit symbol substitution, simple and complex reaction time tests, measures of daytime sleepiness such as the MSLT, and on-the-road automobile driving (Fig. 25.3).[23]
- At peak plasma concentration, the degree of impairment relates to dose and time since ingestion.
- The duration of the impairment relates to the half-life and dose of the hypnotic. Intermediate and long half-life drugs are more likely to exhibit residual effects. But even short half-life drugs,

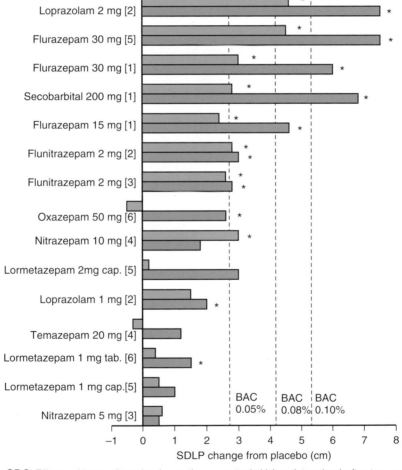

- **Figure 25.3** Effects of benzodiazepine hypnotics on actual driving determined after two successive treatment nights. Standard deviation of lateral position (SDLP) corresponds to the amount of weaving of the car. SDLP changes from placebo (cm) are shown for the morning test sessions (10–11 hours after bedtime administration; black bars) and the afternoon test sessions (16–17 hours after bedtime administration; open bars). Significant differences from placebo are indicated by an asterisk (*). *BAC*, Blood alcohol concentration; *cap.*, capsules; *tab.*, tablets; for study numbers, the most important references are denoted by an asterisk (*). 1, 2, 3, 4, 5, and 6 are shown between brackets. (From Verster JC, Veldhuijzen DS, Volkerts ER. Residual effects of sleep medication on driving ability. *Sleep Med Rev.* 2004;8[4]:309–325.)

taken at high doses beyond the therapeutic dose, can produce residual effects. Such effects have been reported with 20 mg of zolpidem and 0.5 mg of triazolam, with both doses being above the clinically recommended dose.[24]

Falls

- Falls in the elderly are considered as a special case of psychomotor impairment associated with BzRAs, either due to elevated peak plasma concentrations or residual effects.
- Data suggest falls in the elderly are not a significant BzRA risk among insomniacs.
- Studies have shown that in the elderly insomniacs, the risk for falls is due to insomnia and not BzRAs.[25]
- Given an awakening during peak plasma, there is a clear increase in ataxia associated with BzRAs.
- This risk is not unique to BzRAs and can be seen with many sedating and anticholinergic drugs.

Amnesia

- Anterograde amnesia is an inability to remember information presented after drug administration, as is a characteristic of all BzRAs.
- It can be mediated by attention and consolidation failures in the memory process.
- The severity of the amnesia is related to plasma concentration at the time of stimulus presentation, which is determined by dose and time since drug ingestion.[26]
- Animal knock-in studies have shown that the benzodiazepine alpha 1 receptor of the GABA$_A$ complex mediates both sleep and amnesia.
- As there currently are no BzRAs that do not bind to the alpha 1 receptor, all available BzRAs are associated with amnesia.
- Beyond BzRA receptor pharmacology, many sedating drugs with other pharmacological mechanisms also produce amnesia. Amnesia is reported with sedating antidepressants, sedating antipsychotics, antihistamines, and alcohol.
- While there have been reports of "global" amnesia, a total loss of memory for events over a long period of time the day after taking a BzRA hypnotic, these have now been systematically verified or studied.

Benzodiazepine—Discontinuation Effects

(See Table 25.10.)
- The most frequently reported discontinuation effect associated with BzRAs is rebound insomnia.
- Rebound insomnia is defined as worsened sleep for 1 or 2 nights after discontinuation relative to baseline.
- The most important determinant of rebound insomnia is dose. Clinical doses are rarely associated with rebound, while doses above the clinical dose are more likely to produce rebound.[27]
- Duration of use of clinical doses is not associated with an enhanced likelihood of rebound. Several long-term studies have now shown that 6 months of eszopiclone 3 mg or 12 months of zolpidem 10 mg were not associated with rebound.
- Rebound was seen after 1–2 nights of a supraclinical dose of triazolam (0.5 mg), as well as with zolpidem (15 mg), which do not produce withdrawal signs and symptoms.

TABLE 25.10	Signs and Symptoms of Benzodiazepine Discontinuation Syndrome

Benzodiazepine—Discontinuation Effects

- Rebound insomnia
  - Single symptom
  - Exacerbation relative to baseline
  - One–two night duration
- Withdrawal syndrome
- Recrudescence
  - Return of original symptom(s)
  - At basal level of severity
  - Complex of symptoms
  - Longer duration

- Half-life is also a determinant of rebound with the short- and intermediate-acting drugs more likely to produce rebound. Rebound is unlikely to occur with long-acting drugs, due to the gradual decline in plasma concentrations inherent to their pharmacokinetics.
- Clinically rebound after short- and intermediate-acting drugs can be avoided by tapering the dose.
- Rebound insomnia does not alter the subsequent likelihood of self-administration and hence is not associated with abuse.

Abuse

- There has long been concern that behavioral and/or physical dependence develops with chronic use of BzRAs, which leads to their abuse.[28]
- There is little question that individuals with a drug abuse history will abuse BzRAs.
- 6–12 months of nightly BzRA short half-life hypnotic use did not lead to a withdrawal syndrome.[29]
- BzRA withdrawal involves supraclinical doses and longer durations of use (18–90 months).
- Epidemiological studies indicate the majority of hypnotic users report using hypnotics for 2 weeks or less, and they rarely escalate the dose beyond what was initially prescribed.

FDA Scheduling

- The FDA has designated BzRA hypnotics as controlled substances, giving them a schedule IV designation, which indicates these drugs have an abuse liability in at risk individuals.

Abnormal Behaviors During Sleep

- Reports of parasomnia-like episodes with associated amnesia have appeared in the literature, which has led the FDA to issue a "black-box" warning. The behaviors reported have included sleep eating, sleep walking, sleep driving, and even violent behaviors.[30]
- They have been reported with zolpidem, zaleplon, zopiclone (a drug not available in the United States), and triazolam.
- Their occurrence is associated with high doses (i.e., doses much greater than the clinical dose), sleep deprivation, and

co-ingestion of alcohol and other CNS depressant drugs, including alcohol.

Melatonin Agonist

Mechanism

- Ramelteon is the first FDA-approved selective melatonin receptor agonist that has high affinity for melatonin MT_1 and MT_2 receptors of the suprachiasmatic nucleus (SCN).
- Activation of the MT_1 receptor is believed to regulate sleepiness and sleep initiation. In contrast, the MT_2 receptor mediates phase shifting effects of melatonin on circadian rhythms.[31]

Efficacy

- Ramelteon is indicated for sleep onset insomnia, due in part to its short elimination half-life.
- In clinical trials, ramelteon has evidence of inducing sleep with minimal next-day residual effects, rebound insomnia, and withdrawal effects, with discontinuation.[32] Thus this hypnotic is not a controlled substance by the FDA.

In clinical trials in chronic insomniacs, PSG-defined measures of sleep efficiency show that ramelteon reduced sleep initiation and increased sleep duration.

Safety

- Ramelteon does not bind to the GABA receptor; thus its side effect profile differs from that of BzRAs.
- The incidence of adverse effects is low and moderate in severity. Reported adverse effects included somnolence, fatigue, dizziness, headache, and exacerbated insomnia, with incidence of these effects being similar in both ramelteon and placebo treatment groups.

H1 Receptor Agonists (Low Dose Doxepin)

Mechanism

- Doxepin is a tricyclic antidepressant that is frequently used off-label as a hypnotic in antidepressant doses (25–150 mg). Over this dose range, doxepin has antihistaminic, anticholinergic, antiserotonergic, and antiadrenergic effects.[33]
- In the CNS histamine is a major alerting neurotransmitter, and doxepin has its greatest affinity for the H_1 histaminic receptor, which when antagonized produces its sedating effects.
- At the "ultra-low" doses approved for insomnia (3 and 6 mg), doxepin is thought to be a relatively pure H_1 antagonist, without anticholinergic, antiserotonergic, and antiadrenergic activity.
- The T_{max} for doxepin is relatively long, and its metabolite's half-life is similarly long.

Efficacy

- The FDA indication given to low-dose doxepin is for sleep maintenance insomnia. This is consistent with its pharmacokinetics and the efficacy data available. It has been shown in both adults and the elderly to maintain sleep, particularly in the last 2 hours of the night, unlike the BzRAs.[34]
- Clinical trials of the short and intermediate term (≤3 months) show sustained efficacy.

Safety

- Doxepin at 3 and 6 mg does not produce residual effects, which given its half-life, seems counterintuitive.

- It is hypothesized that the normal circadian raise in histamine in the morning (recall histamine is a major alerting neurotransmitter) overrides the sedative effects of low doses of doxepin in the morning.
- Adverse events associated with low-dose doxepin are similar to those seen with placebo. And the anticholinergic side effects typically seen with antidepressant doses were not seen with 3 and 6 mg.
- Doxepin is not a scheduled drug and is considered to not have an abuse liability. However, these considerations are based on antidepressant doses, which have the additional and considerably aversive anticholinergic side effects.

Orexin Antagonists

Mechanism

- Orexin/hypocretin peptides are produced by a cluster of hypothalamic neurons. This small cluster of cells have projections to many brain regions, especially those associated with arousal and motivation, including the histaminergic neurons of the tuberomammilary nucleus, noradrenergic neurons of the locus coeruleus, serotonergic neurons of the raphe nucleus, and dopaminergic neurons of the ventral tegmental area (as illustrated in Fig. 25.4A and B).
- Orexin neurons are responsive to a variety of inputs including the amygdala, nucleus accumbens, as well as the dorsomedial nucleus of hypothalamus (see Fig. 25.4A and B). Thus orexin neurons are responsive to stress, autonomic activity, hunger, satiety, reward system, sleep-wake homeostasis, and circadian timing.
- Effects on sleep-wake are well documented, with antagonist improving sleep onset and maintenance effects, while agonists producing sustained wakefulness and reversal of sleep deprivation effects.
- The improvement in sleep is seen an advance in insomnia therapy, given the nature of insomnia and the mode of action of orexin. With the use of orexin antagonists, there is the potential to avoid the side effects of broad CNS depressant drugs, which are the mainstay of current insomnia therapies.
- The presence of elevated levels of orexin in the morning allows for using longer half-life drugs, thereby having greater impact on sleep maintenance without a morning "hangover."[35]

Efficacy

In a double-blinded placebo, controlled trials for up to 1 year of nightly administration in primary insomniacs suvorexant produced a significant dose-response in PSG-defined measures of sleep onset and maintenance.[36]

- Suvorexant produces more robust seep maintenance effects than sleep initiation, demonstrating efficacy through the last hour of the night.
- Objective assays of sleep show a more robust seep effect than patient reports. This is the opposite of what is seen with BzRAs.

Safety

- Despite its 12-hour half-life, it was free of residual effects. This is felt to be due to the rise of circulating orexin levels in the morning.
- Suvorexant like other sleep agents is a schedule IV drug.
- It is contraindicated in patients with narcolepsy.

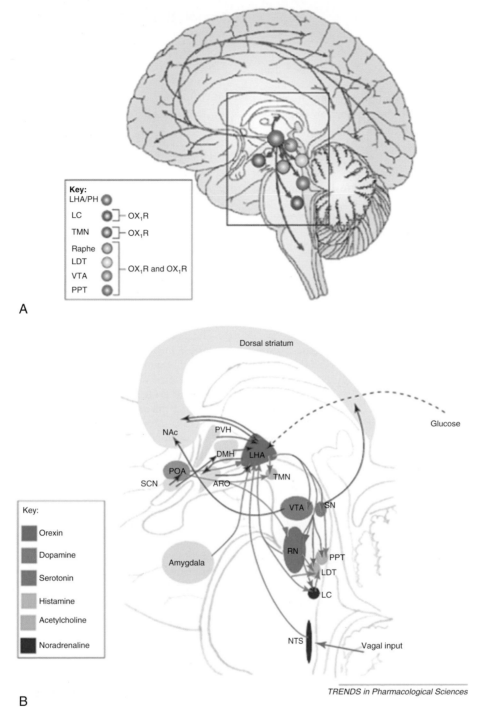

TRENDS in Pharmacological Sciences

• **Figure 25.4** Connections of Orexin Neurons with Other Regions. Orexin Neurons in the Lateral Hypothalamic Area Provide a Link Between the Limbic System, Energy Homeostasis, and the Brain Stem Nuclei. **A,** Major projections of orexin neurons. Modified from Sakurai.[4] Circles show major target sites for orexins. Included in these are the LC (containing noradrenaline, NA), TMN (containing histamine, HA), raphe nuclei (Raphe, containing 5HT), VTA (containing dopamine, DA), and PPT/LDT (containing Ach). Orexin neurons promote wakefulness through the monoaminergic/cholinergic nuclei that are wake-active. **B,** Schematic presentations of output and input of orexin neurons shown in regions of the rectangle in (**A**). Connection between dopaminergic centers and orexin neurons modulates the reward systems. Input from the limbic system might be important to regulate the activity of orexin neurons upon emotional stimuli to evoke emotional arousal or fear-related responses. Sleep-active neurons in the POA send inhibitory influences to monoaminergic/cholinergic neurons and orexin neurons. Orexin neurons send both direct excitatory input to cholinergic neurons in the LDT/PPT and indirect inhibitory input to these cells through GABAergic local interneurons and GABAergic neurons in the substantia nigra pars reticulata.[41] Noradrenergic neurons in the LC and serotonergic neurons in the RN also send inhibitory influences to these cholinergic neurons. Blood glucose levels also affect the activity of orexin neurons through fluctuations of glucose levels in the CSF and vagal afferent. *ARC,* Arcuate nucleus; *DMH,* dorsomedial hypothalamus; *LC,* locus coeruleus; *LDT,* laterodorsal tegmental nucleus; *LHA,* lateral hypothalamic area; *NAc,* nucleus accumbens; *PPT,* pedunculopontine tegmental nucleus; *PVH,* paraventricular hypothalamic nucleus; *RN,* raphe nucleus; *SCN,* suprachiasmatic nucleus; *SN,* substantia nigra; *TMN,* tuberomammillary nucleus; *VTA,* ventral tegmental area.

Off Label Drug Use

Antidepressants

Mechanism

- Tricyclic antidepressants are the most commonly used drugs off-label for the treatment of insomnia.[37]
- Trazodone is the most widely used antidepressant, prescribed at "lower doses" for insomnia than its standard antidepressant dose.
- Amitriptyline and mirtazapine are similarly used at increased doses for sleep.
- These drugs have complex and different neural receptor binding profiles; their commonality in having antihistaminic and antiserotonergic activity is thought to be responsible for their sedating effects.[38]

Efficacy

- The safe and effective hypnotic dose of these drugs has not been established. There are no studies in primary insomnia with amitriptyline or mirtazapine, and only two studies with trazodone.
- Trazodone 150 mg failed to reduce sleep latency or increase total sleep time, although it did decrease wake after sleep onset over the 3-week study.[39]
- In another study, trazodone at a threefold lower dose, 50 mg, reduced sleep latency and increased total sleep time, but the effect on total sleep time was present for only 1 week.
- The inconsistency in dose effects on total sleep time and the apparent tolerance development raise concerns regarding the dose related effects trazodone as a hypnotic.
- The issue of proper hypnotic dose is also illustrated with doxepin. Before doxepin was developed as a hypnotic, the doses recommended for use as a hypnotic were "low," 25–50 mg. As described previously, the approved hypnotic doses (3 and 6 mg) ended up being four to eight times lower.

Safety

- The information regarding the safety of antidepressants comes from their use at antidepressant doses. At such doses, a variety of serious side effects ranging from suicidality, residual effects, anticholinergic effects (i.e., dry mouth, urinary retention, and hallucinations), orthostatic hypotension, priapism, and cardiac arrhythmias and conduction abnormalities have been reported.[40]
- Whether "low doses" would carry the same risk profile is unknown.

Antipsychotics

- The atypical antipsychotics quetiapine and olanzapine are also frequently used for the treatment of insomnia in nonpsychiatric patients.
- As with the antidepressants, these drugs affect multiple transmitter systems, but their sleep promoting effects are thought to be mediated by their antihistaminic activity.

Efficacy

- There is limited information regarding efficacious and safe doses. There have been three open label studies in primary or comorbid insomnia, suggesting improvement in self-reported sleep.[41]
- Their safety is unknown. While the risks of dopamine-associated movement disorders characteristic of typical antipsychotics are reduced with these atypical antipsychotics, a metabolic disorder is a known risk.[42]

Anxiolytics

Anxiolytic BzRAs are also often used as hypnotics with clonazepam, alprazolam, and lorazepam, the most commonly used off-label BzRAs.

Mechanism

- They share the same mechanism of action with the hypnotic BzRAs,
- Their hypnotic doses are not known, and given the pharmacokinetics of those that are long-acting (i.e., clonazepam and lorazepam), they are likely to produce residual effects.
- There is no advantage to using BzRAs anxiolytics off-label as hypnotics.

Treatment Considerations

Comorbid Insomnia

- There has always been a clear agreement that the FDA-approved hypnotics are the appropriate pharmacological treatment for transient and short-term insomnia.
- The 2005 NIH consensus conference has led to a paradigm shift in understanding chronic insomnia and its treatment. With this conference, the use of hypnotics in comorbid insomnia has become clinically more important.
- There is evidence that improved sleep is associated with a more rapid antidepressant response and a reduced suicide risk.[43]
- There is some evidence that treating insomnia comorbid with various medical disorders improves the status of the medical, especially pain, condition.

Chronic Use

- Thus there is no medical or scientific reason to withhold or to withdraw effective long-term pharmacotherapy for chronic primary or comorbid insomnia. But this requires that physicians carefully discuss with their patients the chronic nature of their insomnia and the benefits and risks associated with chronic treatment.
- The treatment plan should also include instructions about the timing of drug administration, nightly versus PRN use, and the various precautions.

Insomnia Phenotype

- Insomnia complaints include initiating sleep, maintaining sleep, early morning awakening, or nonrestorative sleep.
- Patients may present with single or multiple sleep complaints, and the nature of the complaints may vary with various patient characteristics.
- Sleep onset problems are often seen in younger insomniacs, while sleep maintenance problems are more characteristic of insomnia in middle age or elderly patients.
- Sleep maintenance difficulty is often associated with sleep-related breathing disturbances or periodic leg movements, or it can be comorbid with chronic pain disorders.
- Early morning awakening is a complaint often associated with depression as well as phase advance syndromes in the elderly.
- The specificity or nonspecificity of the patient's sleep complaint can guide the physician in the choice of hypnotics. Some of the hypnotics have indications for sleep onset, some for sleep

maintenance, some for both, and more recently for falling back to sleep after an awakening.

Dose Management

- The lowest clinically indicated dose is chosen in light of the patient's age, comorbid medical conditions, and medications.
- Recently it has been shown that females metabolize zolpidem more slowly, and hence the maximum recommend dose for women is 5 mg.
- The physician in consultation with the patient should make dose adjustments in the first week of treatment. In general, the patient should not be allowed to self-initiate dose adjustments.

Pattern of Use

- Typically hypnotics have been used nightly before sleep.
- Nonnightly zolpidem was effective on nights it was taken, and on the off-nights rebound insomnia was not experienced.
- Nonnightly treatment regimens have been suggested due to concerns regarding tolerance development and development of physical/behavioral dependence.[44]
- There is no clear advantage to nonnightly treatment regimens, at least regarding the risk of tolerance or abuse.

Middle of the Night Use

- The principal complaint of some insomniacs is difficulty returning to sleep after a major middle of the night awakening.
- Recently a low-dose sublingual buffered zolpidem has been approved by the FDA for middle-of-the-night use.[45]
- Studies show that this drug with short duration of action and a novel formulation will hasten return to sleep after a middle-of-the night awakening.
- To avoid residual effects, caution is made that the patient is able to remain in bed for an additional 4–5 hours after taking the medication.

Abuse Liability Signs

- There is an abuse liability associated with the BzRA hypnotics.
- The two FDA-approved hypnotics that are not scheduled have limitations regarding their indications, ramelteon being only for sleep onset and low dose doxepin only for sleep maintenance insomnia.

- Two important signs have been identified for potential abuse identified. In the first week of treatment, the dose is escalated much beyond the indicated clinical hypnotic dose.
- The second sign was that the drug was used during the daytime again, suggesting nonhypnotic drug effects were being sought.

Cautions and Contraindications

- Important contraindications for hypnotic pharmacotherapy include advanced hepatic disease and pregnancy.
- Precautions include concomitant illnesses such as sleep apnea syndrome and concomitant sedating medications.
- Special consideration is needed in patients with alcohol or drug abuse histories, as difficulty with sleep, particularly sleep maintenance, is a chief complaint among abstinent alcohol and drug abuse patients, which can continue to a year and more.
- The non-BzRA, low-dose doxepin may be an option.
- If the physician considers use of a BzRA hypnotic in an outpatient setting, the patient must be monitored closely.

Suggested Reading

Buysse DJ, Tyagi S. Clinical pharmacology of other drugs used as hypnotics. In: Kryger MH, Roth T, Dement WC, eds. *Principles and Practice of Sleep Medicine*. 6th ed. Part II. Philadelphia, PA: Elsevier Saunders; 2016.

Greenblatt D, Roth T. Zolpidem for insomnia. *Expert Opin Pharmacother*. 2012;13(6):879-893.

Herring WJ, Connor KM, Ivgy-May N, et al. Suvorexant in patients with insomnia: results from two 3-month randomized controlled clinical trials. *Biol Psychiatry*. 2016;79:136-148.

Meolie AL, Rosen C, Kristo D, et al. Oral nonprescription treatment for insomnia: an evaluation of products with limited evidence. *J Clin Sleep Med*. 2005;1(2):173-187.

Mohler H, Crestani F, Rudolph U. GABA-A receptor subtypes: a new pharmacology. *Curr Opin Pharmacol*. 2001;1:22-25.

National Institutes of Health (NIH). National Institutes of Health State of the Science conference statement on manifestations and management of chronic insomnia in adults, June 13–15, 2005. *Sleep*. 2005;28:1049-1057.

Roehrs T, Roth T. Medication and substance abuse. In: Kryger MH, Roth T, Dement WC, eds. *Principles and Practice of Sleep Medicine*. 6th ed. Part II, Section 17. Philadelphia, PA: Elsevier Saunders; 2016:1380-1389.

Verster JC, van de Loo AJ, Roth T. Effects of hypnotic drugs on driving performance. In: Kryger MH, Roth T, Dement WC, eds. *Principles and Practice of Sleep Medicine*. 6th ed. Part I, Section 6. Philadelphia, PA: Elsevier Saunders; 2016:499-505.

Walsh JK, Roth T. Pharmacologic treatment of insomnia: benzodiazepine receptor agonists. In: Kryger MH, Roth T, Dement WC, eds. *Principles and Practice of Sleep Medicine*. 6th ed. Part II, Section 11. Philadelphia, PA: Elsevier Saunders; 2016:832-841.

26
Medication Effects on Sleep

PAULA K. SCHWEITZER, KARA S. GRIFFIN

Introduction

Medications or substances that act on brain mechanisms involved in sleep-wake regulation may have therapeutic or impairing effects on sleep-wake behavior. These effects may include changes in:

- Alertness
- The duration, timing, or architecture of sleep
- The propensity for abnormalities during sleep, such as restless legs symptoms, periodic limb movements (PLMs), nightmares, disordered breathing, or abnormal behaviors

This chapter reviews the effects of drugs on sleep-wake behavior, with a principal focus on side effects pertinent to sleep and wakefulness.

Receptor and Pharmacological Mechanisms

- Dose, time to peak concentration, and half-life determine the rapidity of onset and the duration of a drug's clinical effect, while the receptor binding profile determines both mechanism of action and adverse events. These properties as well as timing of drug administration determine whether a drug's action is a desired clinical effect or a side effect. For example, sedation may be desirable to promote sleep at night, but undesirable if it occurs during waking hours.
- Receptor mechanisms relevant to sleep-wake behavior are listed in Table 26.1.[1-5] Drugs that enhance γ–aminobutyric acid (GABA) or inhibit arousal systems containing histamine, orexin, norepinephrine, serotonin (5HT), acetylcholine, or dopamine promote sleep but may adversely affect wake behavior. Conversely, drugs that activate arousal systems promote wake but may disrupt sleep. Activation of these arousal systems typically occurs via reuptake inhibition of dopamine, serotonin, or norepinephrine. A number of drugs affect both sleep-promoting and wake-promoting mechanisms to varying degrees (e.g., antidepressants, antipsychotics), with the net effect determining the likelihood of sedation or arousal.
- Effects on neurotransmitters and neuronal systems involved in the generation of slow wave sleep (SWS) and rapid eye movement (REM) sleep can affect sleep architecture. REM suppression may occur with blockade of cholinergic receptors and increased 5HT binding to 5HT$_{1A}$ receptors. NREM and SWS may increase via blockade of 5HT$_2$ receptors.
- Medications and sleep architectural effects: Table 26.2 summarizes effects of drugs on sleep architecture. It is important to note that a number of other factors may affect sleep architecture, such as comorbid disease or sleep disorder, circadian time, duration of prior sleep, age, and sex. In addition, improvement in sleep latency or sleep continuity may be the result of improved symptom control rather than a direct consequence of the drug on sleep (e.g., improved sleep with dopamine agonist treatment of restless legs symptoms). Polysomnographic data is limited or unavailable for many drugs that have effects on sleep-wake behavior.

Drugs Used to Treat Insomnia

- Most hypnotics with an FDA indication for insomnia (Table 26.3) facilitate sleep by enhancement of GABA,[6] but there are three drugs with other mechanisms. Low-dose doxepin selectively antagonizes histamine$_1$ (H$_1$) receptors,[7] suvorexant antagonizes orexin (hypocretin)$_{1,2}$ receptors,[8] and ramelteon has agonistic

TABLE 26.1	Pharmacologic Mechanisms of Drug Effects on Sleep and Wake Behavior			
Mechanism	**Promotes Sleep**	**Promotes Wake**	**Suppresses REM**	**Increases SWS**
Adenosine agonism	X	—	—	—
GABA$_A$ agonism	X	—	—	—
Galanin agonism	X	—	—	—
Glycine agonism	X	—	—	—
Melatonin$_{1,2}$ agonism	X	—	—	—
Acetylcholine antagonism	X	—	X	—
Alpha$_2$ (α_2)-adrenergic agonism	X	—	—	—
Alpha$_1$ (α_1)-adrenergic antagonism	X	—	—	—
Dopamine$_{1,2}$ antagonism	X	—	—	—
Histamine$_1$ (H$_1$) antagonism	X	—	—	—
Orexin$_{1,2}$ antagonism	X	—	—	—
Serotonin$_2$ (5HT$_2$) antagonism	X	—	—	X
Dopamine agonism	—	X	—	—
Orexin$_{1,2}$ agonism	—	X	—	—
Serotonin$_{1A}$ (5HT$_{1A}$) agonism	—	X	X	—
Adenosine antagonism	—	X	—	—
Alpha$_2$ (α_2)-adrenergic antagonism	—	X	—	—
Beta$_2$ (β_2)-adrenergic antagonism	—	X	X	—
Dopamine reuptake inhibition	—	X	—	—
Histamine$_3$ (H$_3$) antagonism	—	X	—	—
Monoamine oxidase inhibition	—	X	X	—
Norepinephrine reuptake inhibition	—	X	—	—
Serotonin (5HT) reuptake inhibition	—	X	X	—

GABA$_A$, γ-aminobutyric acid type A; *REM*, rapid eye movement; *SWS*, slow wave sleep.

activity at melatonin type 1 (MT-1) and type 2 (MT-2) receptors.[9]

- Most prescription drugs used "off-label" for the treatment of insomnia (Table 26.4) promote sleep by antagonism of H$_1$, alpha$_1$ (α_1)-adrenergic, or 5HT$_{2A}$ receptors.[10] However, most of these drugs affect multiple receptors, resulting in variable effects on sleep-wake behavior, as well as side effects not associated with sleep-wake mechanisms.
- Mechanisms for sedation of the over-the-counter agents diphenhydramine and melatonin are H$_1$ antagonism and melatonin agonism, respectively. The mechanisms for the herbal remedies valerian, kava, and chamomile are unclear, but may involve effects on GABA.[11] Valerian extracts have been reported to increase release, decrease reuptake, and decrease degradation of GABA. Kava pyrones have been reported to inhibit sodium channels, increase GABA$_A$ receptor density, block norepinephrine reuptake, and suppress glutamate release. Components of chamomile abstract have also been reported to bind to GABA receptors. Herbal remedies are commonly used for insomnia, but evidence for efficacy is lacking.[12]
- Kava kava may be associated with hepatic toxicity.[13]
- Drugs with short half-lives may be ineffective in maintaining sleep throughout the night, while drugs with intermediate to long half-lives are more likely to promote sleep toward the end of the night. However, long half-life drugs are likely to produce residual sedation during waking hours.

Drugs Used to Promote Wakefulness

- Amphetamine and amphetamine-like compounds (dextroamphetamine, methamphetamine, methylphenidate) promote wakefulness primarily by blocking dopamine and norepinephrine reuptake and inducing dopamine and norepinephrine release via the dopamine and norepinephrine transporters (DAT, NET).[14] The mechanism of action for modafinil and armodafinil is likely via DAT inhibition.[14] The antidepressant bupropion, which blocks dopamine uptake and is a weak inhibitor of

TABLE 26.2 Effects of Drugs on Sleep Architecture

Drug Class/Drug	Sleep Latency	Sleep Continuity*	SWS	REM†
Hypnotics with FDA-indication for Insomnia				
Estazolam, flurazepam, quazepam, temazepam, triazolam	↓	↑	↓	↓
Eszopiclone	↓	↑	↔	↔
Zaleplon	↓	↔	↔	↔
Zolpidem	↓	↑	↔	↓
Doxepin	↓	↑	↔	↔
Ramelteon	↓	↔	↔	↔
Suvorexant	↓	↑	↔	↑
Psychotherapeutic Drugs				
Antidepressant Drugs				
Tricyclics				
Amitriptyline, clomipramine, doxepin, imipramine, trimipramine	↓	↑	↔	↓
Desipramine, nortriptyline	↔	↔		↓
SSRIs				
Citalopram, escitalopram, fluoxetine, fluvoxamine, paroxetine, sertraline	↑	↓	↔↓	↓
SNRIs				
Duloxetine, venlafaxine	—	↓	↓	↓
MAOIs				
Phenelzine, tranylcypromine	↔↑	↓	—	↓↓
Moclobemide	—	↓	—	↔
Isocarboxazid, selegiline	—	↓	—	↔
Other Antidepressants				
Mirtazapine	↓	↑	↔	↔
Nefazodone		↑	↔	↔
Trazodone	↓	↔↑	↑	↔↓
Lithium	—	↑	↔↑	↔↓
Antipsychotic Drugs				
Chlorpromazine, clozapine, haloperidol, risperidone, thioridazine, thiothixene, ziprasidone	↔↓	↑	↑	↓
Quetiapine	↓	↑	↑	↓
Olanzapine	↓	↑	↑↑	↑
Antianxiety Drugs: Benzodiazepines				
Alprazolam, clorazepate, chlordiazepoxide, clonazepam, diazepam, lorazepam, oxazepam	↓	↑	↓	↓
Antiepileptic Drugs				
Benzodiazepines				
Clonazepam, clorazepate, diazepam, lorazepam, midazolam	↓	↑	↓	↓
Other				
Phenobarbital	↓	↑	↓	↓
Carbamazepine	?↓	↑	↑	?↓
Ethosuximide		↓	↓	↔↑
Gabapentin	↔	↑	↑	↔↑
Lamotrigine	—	—	↔↓	↔↑
Levetiracetam	↔	↑	↑	↓
Phenytoin	↓		↓	↓

TABLE 26.2 Effects of Drugs on Sleep Architecture—cont'd

Drug Class/Drug	Sleep Latency	Sleep Continuity*	SWS	REM[†]
Pregabalin	↓	↑	↑	↓
Tiagabine	↔↓	↑	↑	↔
Valproate, valproic acid	—	?↑	↔	↔
Antihypertensive Drugs				
α₁-adrenergic Antagonist				
Prazosin	—	↑	—	↑
α₂-adrenergic Agonists				
Clonidine	—	↔↑	↑	↓
Methyldopa	—	↑	↓	↑↓
Angiotensin Converting Enzyme Inhibitors				
Enalapril, captopril, lisinopril	↔	↔	↔	↔
β-Antagonists				
Atenolol, metoprolol, propranolol	—	↓		↓
Dopamine Agonists				
Benzotropine, hyoscyamine	—	↔↓	↔↑	↓
Levodopa	—	↓	↔↑	↔↓
Pergolide	↓	↑	—	—
Pramipexole	—	—	?↑	↓
Ropinirole	↓	↑	↔	↔
Other Drugs				
Alcohol				
Acute ingestion	↓	↑	↑	↓
Withdrawal	↑	↓	↓	↑
Antihistamines				
Chlorpheniramine, diphenhydramine, doxylamine, hydroxyzine	↔↓	↑↔	↔	↔↓
Pain Medications				
Aspirin, ibuprofen	—	↓	↓	↔
Opioids	—	↓	↓	↓
Stimulants				
Amphetamine, methamphetamine, methylphenidate	↑	↓	↔↓	↓
Modafinil	↔↓	?	↔	—
Caffeine	↑	↓	↓	—
Nicotine	↑	↓	—	↓
Other				
Corticosteroids	—	↓	↔↓	↓
Melatonin	↓	↔↑	↔	↔↓
Pseudoephedrine	?↑	↓	—	—
Sodium oxybate	↓	↑	↑	↔↓
Tasimelteon[‡]	↓	↑	↔	↔
Theophylline	—	↓	↓	—
Valerian	↔↓	↔↑	↑	↔↑

*Sleep continuity refers to the proportion of sleep relative to wakefulness, as reflected by sleep efficiency. Thus ↑ indicates improvement in sleep continuity, as would be reflected by increased sleep efficiency or decreased wakefulness.

[†]Decreased REM is typically accompanied by increased REM latency and vice versa.

[‡]Improvement in sleep with tasimelteon (indicated for treatment of non-24-hour sleep-wake disorder) may be the result of circadian entrainment rather than a direct action of the drug on sleep.

ACE, Angiotensin-converting enzyme; *MAOI*, monoamine oxidase inhibitor; *NSAID*, non-steroidal anti-inflammatory drug; *REM*, rapid eye movement; *SNRI*, serotonin-norepinephrine reuptake inhibitor; *SSRI*, selective serotonin reuptake inhibitor; *SWS*, slow wave sleep; ↑, increase; ↓, decrease; ↔, no change; ?, mixed results.

TABLE 26.3 Pharmacology of Drugs with Food and Drug Administration (FDA) Indication for Insomnia

| Generic Name | Trade Name | RECEPTOR BINDING PROFILE | | | | | $T_{1/2}$ (hours) |
		$GABA_A$ Specificity	MT_1-MT_2	Anti-OX_1-OX_2	Anti-H_1	Anti-M_1	
Benzodiazepine Receptor Agonists							
Estazolam	Prosom	Nonspecific	—	—	—	—	10–24
Flurazepam	Dalmane	Nonspecific	—	—	—	—	48–120[†]
Quazepam	Doral	Nonspecific	—	—	—	—	39–73[†]
Temazepam	Restoril	Nonspecific	—	—	—	—	8–20
Triazolam	Halcion	Nonspecific	—	—	—	—	2–6
Eszopiclone	Lunesta	$\alpha_1 > \alpha_2 > \alpha_3$	—	—	—	—	6–7
Zaleplon	Sonata	$\alpha_1 > \alpha_{2,3,5}$	—	—	—	—	1
Zolpidem	Ambien	$\alpha_1 \gg \alpha_{2,3,5}$	—	—	—	—	1.5–2.4
Zolpidem modified release	Ambien CR	$\alpha_1 \gg \alpha_{2,3}$	—	—	—	—	1.6–4.5
Zolpidem sublingual	Intermezzo	$\alpha_1 \gg \alpha_{2,3}$	—	—	—	—	1.5–2.4
Zolpidem sublingual	Edluar	$\alpha_1 \gg \alpha_{2,3}$	—	—	—	—	2.6–2.8
Zolpidem oral spray	Zolpimist	$\alpha_1 \gg \alpha_{2,3}$	—	—	—	—	2.7–2.8
Melatonin Receptor Agonist							
Ramelteon	Rozerem	—	+++	—	—	—	0.8–2
Orexin Receptor Antagonist							
Suvorexant	Belsomra	—	—	+++	—	—	12
Histamine Receptor Antagonists							
Doxepin*	Silenor*	—	—	—	+++	—	15.3–31[†]
Diphenhydramine	Benadryl	—	—	—	+++	+++	5–11
Doxylamine	Unisom	—	—	—	+++	+++	10–12

*At the low doses used in Silenor (≤6 mg), doxepin binds with high specificity and affinity to the H_1 receptor, with negligible binding to $5HT_{2A}$, α_1, NET, and 5HTT, unlike the higher doses of doxepin used for treatment of depression and off-label use for insomnia (See Tables 26.4 and 26.6.)

[†]Includes active metabolites.

Anti-H_1, Histamine 1 receptor antagonism; Anti-M_1, muscarinic anticholinergic receptor antagonism; Anti-OX_1-OX_2, orexin 1 and 2 receptor antagonism; $GABA_A$, γ-aminobutyric acid type A receptor agonist; MT_1-MT_2, melatonin 1 and 2 receptor agonism; $T_{1/2}$, elimination half-life.

Adapted from Schweitzer PK, Feren SD. Pharmacological treatment of insomnia. In: Attarian HP, ed. *Clinical Handbook of Insomnia*. 3rd ed. Switzerland: Springer; 2017:97–132.

norepinephrine reuptake,[14] is sometimes used off-label to treat sleepiness.

- Atomoxetine, an antidepressant used primarily for treatment of attention-deficit hyperactivity disorder (ADHD), is wake promoting in adults but may have sedative side effects in children. Atomoxetine is a selective norepinephrine reuptake inhibitor (SNRI).[14]
- The mechanism by which sodium oxybate improves alertness is unknown, but may be related to changes in nocturnal sleep architecture, including increased SWS and decreased arousal frequency.[15]
- Selegeline, a monoamine oxidase B inhibitor, is metabolized into L-amphetamine and L-methamphetamine.[14]
- The alerting effects of caffeine are mediated primarily through antagonism of adenosine receptors, which indirectly affects the release of norepinephrine, dopamine, acetylcholine, serotonin, glutamate, and GABA. While the mean half-life of caffeine is 5 hours, it can range from 1.5–9.5 hours because of physiologic and environmental influences such as obesity, pregnancy, altitude, and other medications.[14]

- Novel wake-promoting drugs include histamine₃ receptor inverse agonist/antagonist selective for the H3 subtype (e.g., pitolisant, not yet approved by the US Food and Drug Administration) and negative allosteric modulators of $GABA_A$ receptors such as flumazenil and clarithromycin.[14,15]
- Wake-promoting drugs may cause sleep-onset or maintenance difficulties if taken too close to bedtime. Withdrawal may produce rebound sleepiness.

Drugs Used in the Treatment of Circadian Rhythm Disorders

- Drugs that shift the phase of the endogenous circadian clock include endogenous melatonin,[16] prolonged-release melatonin,[17] and the melatonin agonists ramelteon[18] and tasimelteon.[19] FDA indication for ramelteon and tasimelteon, respectively, are insomnia and non-24-hour sleep-wake disorder.
- Hypnotics and wake-promoting drugs (discussed elsewhere) may be used to treat insomnia and sleepiness that occur as a

TABLE 26.4 Pharmacology of Drugs Used Off-Label for Insomnia

Generic Name	Trade Name	FDA Indication	RECEPTOR BINDING PROFILE							$T_{1/2}$ (hours)	Dose Range for Insomnia (mg)	Likelihood of Residual Sedation
			GABA$_A$	MT$_1$-MT$_2$	Anti-H$_1$	Anti-5HT$_2$	Anti-α$_1$	Anti-D	Anti-M			
Benzodiazepines												
Alprazolam	Xanax	Anxiety	+++	—	—	—	—	—	—	12–14	0.25–1.0	+
Alprazolam extended release	Xanax XR	Anxiety	+++	—	—	—	—	—	—	6.3–27	0.5–3	++
Chlordiazepoxide	Librium	Anxiety, alcohol withdrawal	+++	—	—	—	—	—	—	5–100	5–10	+++
Clonazepam	Klonopin	Anxiety, seizures	+++	—	—	—	—	—	—	35–40	0.25–2.0	+++
Ddiazepam	Valium	Anxiety, spasm, seizures	+++	—	—	—	—	—	—	20–50	2–10	+++
Lorazepam	Ativan	Anxiety	+++	—	—	—	—	—	—	12–15	0.25–2	++
Antidepressants												
Amitriptyline*	Elavil	Depression	—	—	++++	++	++	—	++	5–45	25–150	++
Doxepin*	Sinequan	Depression, anxiety	—	—	++++	—	—	—	—	10–30	10–150	+++
Trimipramine†	Surmontil	Depression	—	—	+++	—	—	—	—	15–40	25–150	+++
Mirtazapine	Remeron	Depression	—	—	+++	++	+	—	—	20–40	7.5–30	+++
Trazodone†,‡	Desyrel	Depression	—	—	+	++	++	—	—	7–15	25–150	++
Antipsychotics												
Olanzapine	Zyprexa	Schizophrenia, bipolar disorder	—	—	+++	+++	+	++	++	30	2.5–20	+++
Quetiapine	Seroquel	Schizophrenia	—	—	+++	+	++	+	+	7	25–250	++
Anticonvulsants												
Gabapentin	Neurontin	Seizures, neuropathic pain	—	—	—	—	—	—	—	5–7	300	+
Pregabalin	Lyrica	Seizures, neuropathic pain	—	—	—	—	—	—	—	6.3	100	+
Tiagabine	Gabitril	Seizures	—	——	—	—	—	—	—	2–9	2–12	+
Other												
Melatonin	—	None	—	+++	—	—	—	—	—	1–3	0.1–75	—
Prazosin	Minipress	Hypertension	—	—	—	—	+++	—	—	2–3	2–20	—
Valerian	—	NA (herbal)	?	—	—	—	—	—	—	1.1?	400–600	—

*Also has potent serotonin and norepinephrine transporter reuptake inhibition (Table 26.6).
†Also has weak 5HTT reuptake inhibition (Table 26.6).
‡At low doses trazodone exhibits H$_1$, α$_1$, and 5HT$_{2A}$ antagonism. At moderate to high doses there is also 5HT$_{2C}$ and 5HTT inhibition.
Anti-5HT$_2$, Serotonin type 2 receptor antagonist; *Anti-α$_1$*, alpha adrenergic type 1 receptor antagonist; *Anti-D*, dopamine receptor antagonist; *Anti-H$_1$*, histamine 1 receptor antagonist; *Anti-M*, muscarinic anticholinergic receptor antagonist; *GABA$_A$*, γ[gamma]-aminobutyric acid type A receptor agonist; *MT$_1$-MT$_2$*, melatonin 1 and 2 receptor agonist; *T$_{1/2}$*, elimination half-life.
Adapted from Schweitzer PK, Feren SD. Pharmacological treatment of insomnia. In: Attarian HP, ed. *Clinical Handbook of Insomnia*. 3rd ed. Switzerland: Springer; 2017:97–132.

TABLE 26.5 **Drugs with Sedating Side Effects**

Antidepressants*	Antipsychotics†	Antiepileptics‡	Opioids
Tricyclics	**Typical**	**Conventional**	Codeine
Amitriptyline	Chlorpromazine	*Benzodiazepines*	Methadone
Amoxapine	Fluphenazine	Clonazepam	Morphine
Clomipramine	Haloperidol	Diazepam	Oxycodone
Desipramine	Loxapine	Lorazepam	Propoxyphene
Doxepin	Perphenazine		
Imipramine	Pimozide	*Other*	**Triptans**
Nortriptyline	Thioridazine	Carbamazepine	Andrizatriptan
Trimipramine	Thiothixene	Ethosuximide	Eletriptan
	Trifluoperazine	Phenobarbital	Zolmitriptan
Tetracyclic		Phenytoin	
Maprotiline	**Atypical**	Primidone	**Muscle Relaxants**
	Aripiprazole	Valproate	Baclofen
NaSSA	Asenapine	Valproic acid	Carisoprodol
Mirtazapine	Clozapine		Cyclobenzaprine
	Iloperidone	**New Generation**	Dicyclomine
SARI	Lurasidone	Eslicarbazepine	Orphenadrine
Trazodone	Olanzapine	Ezogabine	
	Paliperidone	Felbamate	**Antihistamines**
SNRI	Quetiapine	Fosphenytoin	Cetirizine
Duloxetine	Risperidone	Gabapentin	Chlorpheniramine
	Ziprasidone	Lacosamide	Clemastine
SSRI		Lamotrigine	Cyproheptadine
Citalopram	**Antiemetics**	Levetiracetam	Diphenhydramine
Fluvoxamine	Droperidol	Oxcarbazepine	Doxylamine
	Metoclopramide	Perampanel	Hydroxyzine
Dopamine Agonists	Ondansetron	Pregabalin	
Apomorphine	Prochlorperazine	Rufinamide	**Antihypertensives**
Bromocriptine		Tiagabine	Clonidine
Cabergoline			Methyldopa
Lisuride			
Pergolide			
Pramipexole			
Ropinirole			

*See Table 26.6.
†See Table 26.7.
‡See Table 26.8.
NaSSA, Noradrenergic and specific serotonergic antidepressant; *SARI*, serotonin antagonist and reuptake inhibitor; *SNRI*, serotonin-norepinephrine reuptake inhibitor; *SSRI*, selective serotonin reuptake inhibitor.

result of circadian misalignment in shift work sleep disorder or in jet lag.

Drugs with Sedating Side Effects

Sedation is a side effect of numerous drugs that have antagonistic effects at H_1, $5HT_2$, α_1-adrenergic, or muscarinic cholinergic (M) receptors. Other mechanisms of sedation include GABA enhancement and activation of opioid μ and κ receptors (Table 26.5).

Antidepressant Drugs

- Antidepressants vary considerably in the relative affinity for receptors associated with sleep-wake regulation (Table 26.6). Sedating antidepressants vary in their antagonism of H_1, $5HT_2$, α_1, and M receptors. Most antidepressants also exhibit reuptake inhibition of serotonin and norepinephrine transporters (5HTT, NET), which is the likely

mechanism for their therapeutic effect, but may promote wakefulness. Drugs that more selectively inhibit reuptake of 5HTT (selective serotonin reuptake inhibitors [SSRI]) or NET (SNRI) are unlikely to be sedating and may produce insomnia.
- The most sedating antidepressants include the tricyclic antidepressants amitriptyline, trimipramine, and doxepin, which have potent antihistaminergic and anticholinergic activity.[10] Drugs with less affinity for H_1 receptors (e.g., desipramine, nortriptyline, protriptyline) are less sedating. Half-lives generally range from 15–30 hours, with active metabolites having slightly longer half-lives.
- Mirtazapine also has effects on a number of receptors, but sedation likely results from potent antagonism of H_1 and $5HT_2$ receptors.[10] Half-life is 7.5–15 hours.
- Trazodone has complex effects on the 5HT system, but moderate H_1 and α_1 antagonism are the mechanisms for sedation.[10] At low doses, trazodone exhibits H_1, α_1, and $5HT_{2A}$ antagonism. At moderate to high doses, there is also

TABLE 26.6 Antidepressant Drugs: Receptor Binding Affinity Profiles and Likelihood of Sedation or Insomnia

Drug	Class	Sedation	Insomnia	H$_1$	5HT$_{2A}$	5HT$_{2C}$	α$_1$	M	D$_1$	D$_2$	5HTT	NET	DAT
				\multicolumn{10}{c}{RECEPTOR/TRANSPORTER}									
Amitriptyline	Tricyclic	+++	+	—	—	—	—	—	—	—	—	—	—
Amoxapine	Tricyclic	+++	+	—	—	—	—	—	—	—	—	—	—
Doxepin	Tricyclic	+++	—	—	—	—	—	—	—	—	—	—	—
Imipramine	Tricyclic	+++	+	—	—	—	—	—	—	—	—	—	—
Trimipramine	Tricyclic	+++	+	—	—	—	—	—	—	—	—	—	—
Clomipramine	Tricyclic	++		—	—	—	—	—	—	—	—	—	—
Desipramine	Tricyclic	+	+	—	—	—	—	—	—	—	—	—	—
Nortriptyline	Tricyclic	+	+	—	—	—	—	—	—	—	—	—	—
Protriptyline	Tricyclic	—	+	—	—	—	—	—	—	—	—	—	—
Maprotiline	Tetracyclic	++	—	—	—	—	—	—	—	—	—	—	—
Mirtazapine	NaSSA	+++	—	—	—	—	—	—	—	—	—	—	—
Trazodone	SARI	++	—	—	—	—	—	—	—	—	—	—	—
Citalopram	SSRI	+	+	—	—	—	—	—	—	—	—	—	—
Fluvoxamine	SSRI	++	++	—	—	—	—	—	—	—	—	—	—
Escitalopram	SSRI	—	+	—	—	—	—	—	—	—	—	—	—
Paroxetine	SSRI	—	++	—	—	—	—	—	—	—	—	—	—
Sertraline	SSRI	—	++	—	—	—	—	—	—	—	—	—	—
Fluoxetine	SSRI	+	+++	—	—	—	—	—	—	—	—	—	—
Levomilnacipran	SNRI	—	—	—	—	—	—	—	—	—	—	—	—
Milnacipran	SNRI	—	+	—	—	—	—	—	—	—	—	—	—
Desvenlafaxine	SNRI	—	+++	—	—	—	—	—	—	—	—	—	—
Duloxetine	SNRI	—	++	—	—	—	—	—	—	—	—	—	—
Venlafaxine	SNRI	++	++	—	—	—	—	—	—	—	—	—	—
Atomoxetine*	NRI	+	+	—	—	—	—	—	—	—	—	—	—
Bupropion	NDRI	—	++	—	—	—	—	—	—	—	—	—	—
Vortioxetine	MMAD	—	—	—	—	—	—	—	—	—	—	—	—
Vilazodone	MMAD	—	++	—	—	—	—	—	—	—	—	—	—
Affinity		\multicolumn{2}{c}{Very high}		\multicolumn{2}{c}{High}		\multicolumn{2}{c}{Moderate}		\multicolumn{2}{c}{Low}		\multicolumn{2}{c}{Negligible}	

Binding affinities (pK_i values) range from 5 (negligible, white) to 9.8 (very high, dark blue).
*Sedation in children, insomnia in adults.

5HT$_{2A}$, Serotonin 2A receptor; *5HT$_{2C}$*, serotonin 2C receptor; *5HTT*, serotonin transporter; α$_1$, alpha adrenergic type 1 receptor; *D$_1$* dopamine 1 receptor; *D$_2$* dopamine 2 receptor; *H$_1$* histamine 1 receptor; *M* acetylcholine muscarinic receptor; *MMAD*, multimodal antidepressant; *NaSSA*, noradrenergic and specific serotonergic antidepressant; *NET*, norepinephrine transporter; *NDRI*, norepinephrine-dopamine reuptake inhibitor; *NRI*, norepinephrine reuptake inhibitor; *SARI*, serotonin antagonist and reuptake inhibitor; *SNRI*, serotonin-norepinephrine reuptake inhibitor; *SSRI*, selective serotonin reuptake inhibitor.

Affinity profiles were extracted from the Psychoactive Drugs Screening Program (PDSP) K_i database (pdspdb.unc.edu; Roth BL Lopez E, Patel S, Kroeze WK. The multiplicity of serotonin receptors: uselessly diverse molecules or an embarrassment of riches? *Neuroscientist.* 2000;6:252–262.)

TABLE 26.7 | **Antipsychotic Drugs: Receptor Binding Affinity Profiles and Likelihood of Sedation**

Drug	Class	Sedation	H$_1$	5HT$_{2A}$	5HT$_{2C}$	α$_1$	M	D$_1$	D$_2$	5HTT	NET
Chlorpromazine	Typical	++++	—	—	—	—	—	—	—	—	—
Clozapine	Atypical	++++	—	—	—	—	—	—	—	—	—
Loxapine	Typical	++++	—	—	—	—	—	—	—	—	—
Asenapine	Atypical	+++	—	—	—	—	—	—	—	—	—
Olanzapine	Atypical	+++	—	—	—	—	—	—	—	—	—
Perphenazine	Typical	+++	—	—	—	—	—	—	—	—	—
Quetiapine	Atypical	+++	—	—	—	—	—	—	—	—	—
Risperidone	Atypical	+++	—	—	—	—	—	—	—	—	—
Thioridazine	Typical	+++	—	—	—	—	—	—	—	—	—
Haloperidol	Typical	++	—	—	—	—	—	—	—	—	—
Pimozide	Typical	++	—	—	—	—	—	—	—	—	—
Iloperidone	Atypical	++	—	—	—	—	—	—	—	—	—
Thiothixene	Typical	++	—	—	—	—	—	—	—	—	—
Ziprasidone	Atypical	++	—	—	—	—	—	—	—	—	—
Aripiprazole	Atypical	+	—	—	—	—	—	—	—	—	—
Fluphenazine	Typical	+	—	—	—	—	—	—	—	—	—
Lurasidone	Atypical	+	—	—	—	—	—	—	—	—	—
Paliperidone	Atypical	+	—	—	—	—	—	—	—	—	—
Trifluoperazine	Typical	+	—	—	—	—	—	—	—	—	—
Affinity		Very high	High		Moderate		Low		Negligible		

Binding affinities (pK_i values) range from 5 (negligible, white) to 9.8 (very high, dark blue).

5HT$_{2A}$, Serotonin 2A receptor; 5HT$_{2C}$, serotonin 2C receptor; 5HTT, serotonin transporter; α$_1$, alpha adrenergic type 1 receptor, D$_1$, dopamine 1 receptor; D$_2$, dopamine 2 receptor; H$_1$, histamine 1 receptor; M, acetylcholine muscarinic receptor; NET, norepinephrine transporter.

Affinity profiles were extracted from the Psychoactive Drugs Screening Program (PDSP) K_i database (pdspdb.unc.edu; Roth BL, Lopez E, Patel S, Kroeze WK. The multiplicity of serotonin receptors: uselessly diverse molecules or an embarrassment of riches? *Neuroscientist.* 2000;6:252–262.)

5HT$_{2C}$ and 5HTT inhibition. Half-life is 5–9 hours, but half-life of its active metabolite is 4–14 hours.

- Sedation is not common with most SSRIs. However, in placebo-controlled studies, the incidence of sedation was as high with fluvoxamine, possibly because of inhibition of melatonin degradation. Much lower incidences of sedation have been reported with the SSRI citalopram and the SNRI duloxetine. The sedating effects may be explained by citalopram's mild H$_1$ and 5HT$_{2C}$ antagonism, and by duloxetine's slight 5HT$_{2A,2C}$ antagonism.
- Sedation is sometimes reported with monoamine oxidase inhibitors (MAOI), but the mechanism for sedation is unclear.

Anxiolytic Drugs

- Drugs with sedating side effects used in the treatment of anxiety include benzodiazepines, antidepressants, antiepileptics, and

antipsychotics. GABA agonism is the mechanism for sedation of benzodiazepines. Mechanisms of sedation for other drug classes are discussed elsewhere. Most of these drugs have intermediate to long half-lives.

Antipsychotic Drugs

- Antipsychotic drugs, particularly the newer generation (atypical) drugs, have complex pharmacological profiles (Table 26.7).[20] The antipsychotic effects of these drugs are thought to be mediated primarily by antagonism of dopamine D$_2$ receptors. Sedation is more likely in drugs with relatively more potent antagonism of H$_1$, α$_1$-adrenergic, or 5HT$_2$ receptors compared with antagonism of D$_2$ receptors.
- Clozapine, a strong antagonist of H$_1$, α$_1$, and 5HT$_{2A}$, is the most sedating among these compounds. Haloperidol and pimozide, which have much lower affinity for these receptors,

are much less sedating. However, dose is also relevant in determining the degree of sedation. While the older compounds chlorpromazine and thioridazine have lower affinity for H_1, higher doses are required for therapeutic efficacy, increasing the sedating side effect.

- The atypical drugs quetiapine and, to a lesser extent, olanzapine are used off-label in the treatment of insomnia. Quetiapine and aripiprazole are sometimes used off-label to treat anxiety.

Antiepileptic Drugs

- Sedation is common with antiepileptic drugs (Table 26.8),[21,22] particularly for drugs that affect GABAergic neurotransmission (e.g., benzodiazepines, barbiturates, gabapentin, vigabatrin), although tiagabine, which blocks GABA uptake, appears to be an exception. The incidence of sedation is less frequent with drugs acting primarily via sodium channel blockade (e.g., carbamazapine, phenytoin, pregabalin). Sedation is moderately high to high for drugs that act on calcium channels or drugs that have multiple mechanisms of action (e.g., felbamate, lacosamide, levetiracetam, zonisamide).

Antihistamines (H_1 Antagonists)

- Sedation is a common side effect of the first-generation antihistamines (e.g., diphenhydramine, hydroxyzine), which are lipophilic molecules that easily penetrate the central nervous system (CNS).[23] There is some data that tolerance to daytime sedation may develop.[24] Diphenhydramine may cause residual sedation when used as a sleep aid.
- Second-generation antihistamines (e.g., cetirizine, fexofenadine) are less lipophilic and more selective in their binding than the classic antihistamines, and thus unlikely to be sedating. The exception is cetirizine, which has moderate affinity for the H_1 receptor.[25]

Dopamine Agonists

- Dopamine agonists differ in their selectivity for dopamine receptor subtypes.[26] The ergot agonists (e.g., pergolide, apomorphine) activate both D_1 and D_2 receptors, while the non-ergot agonists (e.g., pramipexole, ropinirole, rotigotine) are more selective for D_2 and have higher specificity for the D_3 subtype. Ergot-derived drugs also demonstrate $5HT_{2A}$ and $5HT_{2B}$ agonism, and have been associated with valvular heart disease.
- The cause of sleepiness and sudden "sleep attacks" with these drugs is not well understood. Studies in rats and humans have detected selective loss of orexin-immunoreactive neurons with the use of non-ergot dopamine D_2 agonists, possibly caused by suppression of glutamatergic input to orexin neurons.[27]
- There are some data suggesting that low doses of dopaminergic medications tend to improve sleep, while higher doses are likely to disrupt sleep.[27] PSG studies have shown mixed results, including both increased and decreased REM sleep and SWS. Decreases in sleep latency may be the result of improved symptom control rather than a direct consequence of the drug on sleep.

Antihypertensive Drugs

- Sedation is the most common side effect of clonidine and methyldopa, centrally acting α_2-adrenergic agonists. Sleepiness usually occurs at treatment initiation and may diminish with time in some individuals.[28]

Pain Medications

- Medications used to treat pain include opioids, skeletal muscle relaxants, nonsteroidal anti-inflammatory drugs (NSAIDs), antidepressants, and antiepileptics.
- The mechanism of action for analgesia of opioid-type medications involves the μ, κ, and δ opioid receptors, while the mechanism for sedation involves the μ and κ receptors.[29] Sedation is a common side effect of this type of drug although objective data are limited. Magnitude of sedation is affected by dose, duration of use, patient age, and severity of condition. Opioids may also disrupt sleep.
- Skeletal muscle relaxants vary in their mechanism of action, but most have CNS activity.[30] Baclofen is a GABA derivative, and tizanidine is an α_2 agonist. Cyclobenzaprine is similar in structure to amitriptyline, while orphenadrine is a muscarinic antagonist that binds to the H_1 receptor. The antispasmodic dicyclomine is a muscarinic antagonist.
- Triptans, used in the treatment of migraine headaches, activate $5HT_{1B}$ and $5HT_{1D}$ receptors and are sometimes sedating. Somnolence is highest with eletriptan, zolmitriptan, and rizatriptan, all of which are highly lipophilic and have active metabolites.[31]
- NSAIDs may affect sleep because they decrease the synthesis of prostaglandin D_2, suppress the normal nocturnal surge in melatonin synthesis, and attenuate the normal nocturnal decrease in body temperature.[32]

Other Medications

- Sedation is a side effect of antiemetic drugs such as droperidol and metoclopramide, which antagonize central and peripheral dopamine receptors.
- Amantadine, used for flu prophylaxis and for control of drug-induced extrapyramidal reactions, is a weak N-Methyl-D-aspartate (NMDA) receptor antagonist, appears to have effects on dopamine receptors, and exhibits anticholinergic side effects such as dry mouth.

Drugs with Insomnia Side Effects

- Insomnia may be a side effect of drugs whose mechanisms include reuptake inhibition of dopamine, norepinephrine, or serotonin. Wake-promoting drugs, including caffeine (an adenosine antagonist; see Table 26.1), may cause insomnia if taken too close to bedtime. Drugs that promote or exacerbate restless legs symptoms may cause insomnia indirectly (Table 26.9).
- Among antidepressants, bupropion, which weakly inhibits DAT and, to a lesser extent, NET, is most likely to cause insomnia.[33] In fact, this drug is sometimes used to promote alertness. Other second-generation antidepressants likely to cause insomnia include the SNRIs, particularly desvenlafaxine and venlafaxine.[34] Insomnia has been reported with SSRIs, particularly fluoxetine, fluvoxamine, and sertraline, and MAOIs such as phenelzine and selegeline.[34] Vilazodone, a 5HTT

TABLE 26.8 Antiepileptic Drugs: Likelihood of Sedation and Mechanism of Action

Drug	Sedation	GABA Enhancement*	Ca²⁺ Channel Blockade	Na⁺ Channel Blockade	SV2A Release	Glutamate Blockade†	Carbonic Anhydrase Inhibition	K⁺ Channel Opening
Benzodiazepines‡	++++	Primary	—	—	—	—	—	—
Brivaracetam	++++	—	—	—	Primary	—	—	—
Levetiracetam	++++	Possible	—	—	Probable	—	—	—
Phenobarbital	++++	Primary	—	—	—	—	Probable	—
Primidone	++++	Primary	—	—	—	—	—	—
Vigabatrin	++++	Primary	—	—	—	—	—	—
Gabapentin§	+++	Possible	Probable	—	—	—	—	—
Perampanel	+++	—	—	—	—	Primary	—	—
Topiramate	+++	Probable	—	—	—	—	Possible	—
Ezogabine	++	—	—	—	—	—	—	Primary
Felbamate**	++	Probable	—	—	—	Probable	—	—
Fosphenytoin	++	—	—	Primary	—	—	—	—
Lacosamide	++	—	—	Primary	—	—	—	—
Pregabalin§	++	—	Probable	—	—	—	—	—
Phenytoin	++	—	—	Primary	—	—	—	—
Rufinamide	++	—	—	Probable	—	—	—	—
Tiagabine	++	Primary	—	—	—	—	—	—
Zonisamide	++	—	Probable	Primary	—	—	—	—
Carbamazepine	+	—	—	Primary	—	—	—	—
Eslicarbazepine	+	—	—	Primary	—	—	—	—
Ethosuximide	+	—	Primary	—	—	—	—	—
Lamotrigine	+	—	Probable	Primary	—	—	—	—
Oxcarbazepine	+	—	—	Primary	—	—	—	—
Valproate	+	Probable	—	Probable	—	—	—	—

Mechanism of Action

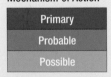

Primary
Probable
Possible

*GABA enhancement can occur by direct binding to GABA_A receptors (benzodiazepines, phenobarbital), blockade of presynaptic GABA uptake (tiagabine), inhibition of GABA metabolism by GABA transaminase (vigabatrin), increased synthesis of GABA (gabapentin, valproate).
†Glutamate blockade can occur via N-methyl-D-aspartate (NMDA) receptors and AMPA/kainite receptors.
‡Benzodiazepines include clonazepam, diazepam, lorazepam.
§Gabapentin and pregabalin bind to the alpha₂-delta subunit of voltage-activated calcium channels.
**Insomnia is also reported with felbamate.
Ca²⁺, Calcium; GABA, gamma-aminobutyric acid; K⁺, potassium; Na⁺ sodium; SV2A, synaptic vesicle protein 2A.

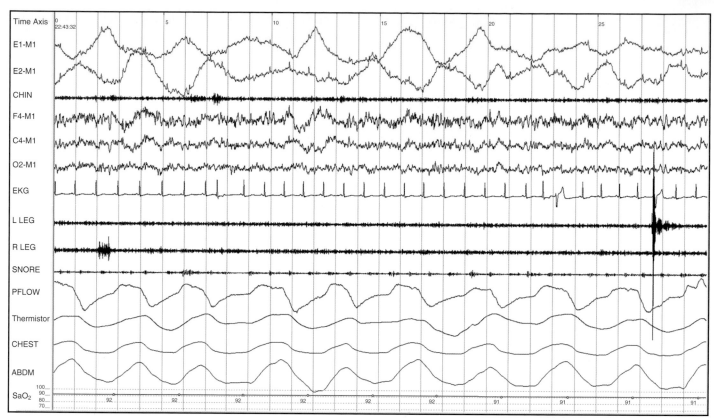

• **Figure 26.1** Slow eye movements during nonrapid eye movement sleep seen in a patient treated with the selective serotonin reuptake inhibitors sertraline.

inhibitor and $5HT_{1A}$ partial agonist, may also disrupt sleep.[34] Fluoxetine has been associated with the presence of prominent slow eye movements during sleep, the so-called Prozac or SSRI-eyes (Fig. 26.1).[35]

• While most antipsychotic drugs are more likely to be sedating, insomnia has occasionally been reported. It is more commonly reported with haloperidol, thioridazine, and aripiprazole, but the mechanism is unclear.

• Insomnia with β-blockers used in the treatment of hypertension is more likely with highly lipophilic compounds that are nonselective for β_1 and β_2 receptors.[36] Drugs selective for β_1 receptors have lower affinity for 5HT receptors. Among these drugs, propranolol, which has high lipid solubility and high 5HT affinity, is most commonly associated with disturbed sleep.

• Data mining studies suggest that hypolipidemic drugs, particularly the more lipophilic compounds, are associated with both insomnia and parasomnias.[37] However, meta-analyses of polysomnographic studies show no adverse effects on sleep.[38]

• Insomnia is frequently reported with oral corticosteroid use, but the results of objective studies are inconsistent.[39]

• Pseudoephedrine and phenylpropanolamine are α-adrenergic agonists. Both drugs disturb sleep.[39] Phenylpropanolamine has been reported to increase plasma caffeine levels.

• Theophylline, a respiratory stimulant and bronchodilator, is chemically related to caffeine and frequently associated with insomnia.[39] Among weight loss drugs, insomnia is common with diethylpropion and the combination drugs phentermine/topiramate and naltrexone/bupropion.[39] Phentermine and diethylpropion are sympathetic amines with pharmacologic

activity similar to amphetamine. Naltrexone is an opioid antagonist, and bupropion is a weak inhibitor of DAT and NET.

Drugs That May Cause Nightmares

• Nightmares or vivid dreams have been reported with numerous drugs (Table 26.10).[40,41] Data quality is variable, however, with much of the information coming from case reports. There are very few studies that include drug withdrawal and rechallenge to confirm the relationship.

• Nightmares appear to be more common with drugs which have effects on dopamine, serotonin, and norepinephrine and less common with drugs affecting GABA, acetylcholine, and histamine.[41] However, the pharmacological mechanisms of drug-induced nightmares are unknown. The brainstem and hypothalamus contain "REM-on" and "REM-off" cells, which are maximally and minimally active, respectively, during REM. Neurotransmitters used by subgroups of REM-on cells include GABA, acetylcholine, and glutamate; neurotransmitters used by subgroups of REM-off cells include norepinephrine, serotonin, histamine, and GABA. Thus drugs that affect these neurotransmitters can affect REM sleep in a variety of ways. The role of dopamine is unclear.

• Dream recall frequency is often decreased with antidepressants, probably because of the decrease in REM caused by these drugs. However, dream detail may be more vivid. Nightmares occur more commonly upon withdrawal of these drugs, likely because of REM rebound. Other REM-suppressant drugs with nightmares on withdrawal include alcohol, barbiturates, and benzodiazepines.

TABLE 26.9 Drugs with Insomnia Side Effects

Antidepressants*	Antihypertensive Drugs	Wake Promoting Drugs
SSRIs	**β-Antagonists†**	**Sympathetic Amines**
Citalopram	Carvedilol	Amphetamine
Escitalopram	Labetalol	Dextroamphetamine
Fluoxetine	Metoprolol	Lisdexamfetamine
Fluvoxamine	Nadolol	Methamphetamine
Paroxetine	Pindolol	Methylphenidate
Sertraline	Propranolol	**Other**
SNRIs	Sotalol	Armodafinil
Desvenlafaxine	Timolol	Modafinil
Duloxetine	**Antipsychotics**	Atmoxetine
Levomilnacipran	Aripiprazole	Bupropion
Milnacipran	Fluphenazine	Selegiline
Venlafaxine	Haloperidol	Caffeine
NDRI	Thioridazine	**Other Drugs**
Bupropion	Trifluoperazine	Corticosteroid
MAOIs	**Weight Loss Drugs**	Lovastatin
Phenelzine	Diethylpropion	Phenylpropanolamine
Selegeline	Naltrexone/bupropion	Pseudoephedrine
Tranylcypromine	Phentermine/topiramate	Theophylline
Other		
Vilazodone		

*See Table 26.6.
†Insomnia is more likely with propranolol, metoprolol, and labetol than with other β-antagonists.
MAOI, Monoamine oxidase inhibitor; *NDRI,* norepinephrine dopamine reuptake inhibitor; *SNRI,* serotonin-norepinephrine reuptake inhibitor; *SSRI,* selective serotonin reuptake inhibitor.

- Bupropion, which increases REM sleep, is the antidepressant most frequently associated with nightmares. Although dream recall frequency may be decreased with tricyclic antidepressants, nightmares are commonly reported, likely because of effects on cholinergic mechanisms. Other drugs associated with nightmares include centrally acting antihypertensive medications such as β-blockers and α₂ agonists.

Drugs Associated with Restless Legs Syndrome Symptoms or Periodic Limb Movements

- There are numerous reports of pharmacologically induced restless legs syndrome (RLS) and PLMs, but the quality of the available evidence is variable and much of the data come from case reports (Table 26.11). PLM data are limited by the need for polysomnography or actigraphy to document occurrence.
- There is good evidence to support that RLS may be induced or exacerbated by SSRIs, SNRIs, tricyclic antidepressants, and

mirtazapine, and that PLMs may be induced or exacerbated by SSRIs, the SNRI venlafaxine, and mirtazapine.[42,43] There is moderate evidence to support inducement/exacerbation of PLMs for other SNRIs and tricyclic antidepressants.[42,43] Bupropion is an exception among antidepressants; it does not exacerbate RLS or PLMs, and in fact, may improve RLS symptoms, likely because of DAT inhibition.[44] Among antipsychotic drugs, there is moderate evidence that RLS and PLMs may be induced or exacerbated by olanzapine.[42] There are a few case reports implicating risperidone and quetiapine in RLS symptoms. Caffeine and alcohol may exacerbate RLS symptoms.
- Augmentation of restless legs symptoms may occur following RLS treatment with levodopa and dopamine agonists. There are some case reports of augmentation with tramadol.
- Caffeine and alcohol are believed to exacerbate RLS and PLMs. There is some epidemiologic data that support that caffeine consumption is higher in individuals with PLMs and alcohol intake is higher in those with RLS, but there are also studies that report no relationship of caffeine and alcohol consumption with RLS/PLM incidence.

Drugs That May Cause Rapid Eye Movement Sleep Without Atonia or Rapid Eye Movement Behavior Disorder

- There is an increased prevalence of Rapid Eye Movement Sleep Without Atonia (RSWA) and Rapid Eye Movement Behavior Disorder (RBD) in patients taking antidepressant medication (Fig. 26.2).[42,45,46] This includes patients with narcolepsy who take antidepressants for treatment of cataplexy.[48] Drugs include tricyclic antidepressants, the SSRIs citalopram, fluoxetine, paroxetine, and sertraline, the SNRIs duloxetine and venlafaxine, the MAOI inhibitors phenelzine and selegeline, as well as trazodone and mirtazapine (Table 26.11).
- The likely mechanism is interference with the normal inhibition of motor neurons during REM via increases in serotonin or norepinephrine, or via a blockade of cholinergic activity.
- Patients in whom RBD symptoms developed after ingestion of antidepressants appear to be less likely to develop neurodegenerative disease than idiopathic RBD patients.[47,48] Longer-term follow-up is needed for more definitive conclusions. There is also data to suggest that antidepressant use may unmask RBD rather than cause it. RBD patients with or without antidepressants have higher RSWA than non-RBD patients on antidepressants, and show a different pattern of tonic and phasic muscle activity.[48]
- RSWA, but not RBD, has been reported with bupropion. Thus bupropion may be the drug of choice for treatment of depression in patients with RBD and comorbid depression. Melatonin and clonazepam reduce but rarely completely eliminate RBD symptoms.[49] There are case reports but no definitive studies that levodopa, dopamine agonists, and quetiapine may improve RBD symptoms.

Conclusion

Drugs with pharmacological effects on brain mechanisms involved in sleep-wake regulation may improve or impair sleep and waking function. Effects on sleep may include changes in sleep duration, timing, or sleep architecture, as well as abnormalities such as

TABLE 26.10	Drugs That May Cause Vivid Dreams or Nightmares During Use or Withdrawal		
Drug Class	**Drug**	**With Use**	**On Withdrawal***
Alcohol		X	X
Antibiotics	Ciprofloxacin, erythromycin, levofoxacin, moxifoxacin	X	—
Antivirals	Amantadine, ganciclovir, efavirenz	X	—
Antidepressants			
Tricyclics	Amitriptyline, clomipramine, desipramine, doxepin, imipramine, nortriptyline	X	X
SSRIs[†]	Citalopram, escitalopram, fluoxetine, fluvoxamine, paroxetine, sertraline	X	X
SNRI	Desvenlafaxine, duloxetine, venlafaxine	X	X
NaSSA	Mirtazapine	X	—
NDRI[‡]	Bupropion	X	—
MAOIs	Phenelzine, tranylcypromine	—	X
Other	Vilazodone, vortioxetine	X	—
Antihypertensives			
ACE inhibitors	Enalapril, losartan, quinapril	X	—
α_2-adrenergic Agonists	Clonidine, methyldopa	X	—
β-Antagonists	Metoprolol, pindolol, propranolol,	X	—
Antipsychotics	Clozapine, risperidone	X	—
Barbiturates	Phenobarbital	—	X
Benzodiazepines	Estazolam, flurazepam, quazepam, temazepam, triazolam, zolpidem	—	X
Other drugs	Chlorpheniramine, naproxen, sibutramine	X	—

*REM rebound occurs on withdrawal with these drugs.
[†]Vivid dreams but decreased dream recall. Nightmares more frequent with paroxetine than with other SSRIs.
[‡]Nightmares more frequent with bupropion than with other antidepressants, possibly because of increase in REM.
ACE, Angiotensin converting enzyme; *NaSSA*, norepinephrine and specific serotonin antagonist; *REM*, rapid eye movement; *SNRI*, serotonin-norepinephrine reuptake inhibitor; *SSRI*, selective serotonin reuptake inhibitor.

TABLE 26.11 Drugs That May Be Associated with Restless Legs Symptoms, Periodic Limb Movements, Rapid Eye Movement Sleep Without Atonia, or Rapid Eye Movement Behavior Disorder, Grouped by Quality of Evidence*

Drug Class/Drug	RLS	PLMs	RSWA	RBD
Antidepressants				
TCAs				
Amitriptyline	—	—	—	—
Clomipramine	—	—	—	—
Imipramine	—	—	—	—
Nortriptyline	—	—	—	—
Trimipramine	—	—	—	—
SSRIs				
Citalopram	—	—	—	—
Escitalopram	—	—	—	—
Fluoxetine	—	—	—	—
Paroxetine	—	—	—	—
Sertraline	—	—	—	—
SNRIs				
Duloxetine	—	—	—	—
Venlafaxine	—	—	—	—
MAOIs				
Phenelzine	—	—	—	—
Selegiline	—	—	—	—
Other Antidepressants				
Bupropion	Not associated	Not associated	—	—
Mirtazapine	—	—	—	—
Trazodone	—	—	—	—
Antipsychotics				
Aripiprazole	—	—	—	—
Chlorpromazine	—	—	—	—
Clozapine	—	—	—	—
Haloperidol	—	—	—	—
Olanzapine	—	—	—	—
Quetiapine	—	—	—	—
Risperidone	—	—	—	—
Thioridazine	—	—	—	—
Thiothixene	—	—	—	—
Ziprasidone	—	—	—	—
Zonisamide	—	—	—	—
Other Drugs				
Dopamine Agonists				
Levodopa	—	—	—	—
Ropinirole	—	—	—	—
Pramipexole	—	—	—	—
Other				
Alcohol	—	—	—	—
Caffeine	—	—	—	—

*Dark color indicates there is good evidence to suggest a relationship. Light color indicates there is some evidence to support a relationship, typically in the form of case reports.

MAOI, Monoamine oxidase inhibitor; *PLMs*, periodic limb movements; *RBD*, rapid eye movement behavior disorder; *REM*, rapid eye movement; *RLS*, restless leg symptoms; *RSWA*, rapid eye movement sleep without atonia; *SNRI*, serotonin-norepinephrine reuptake inhibitor; *SSRI*, selective serotonin reuptake inhibitor.

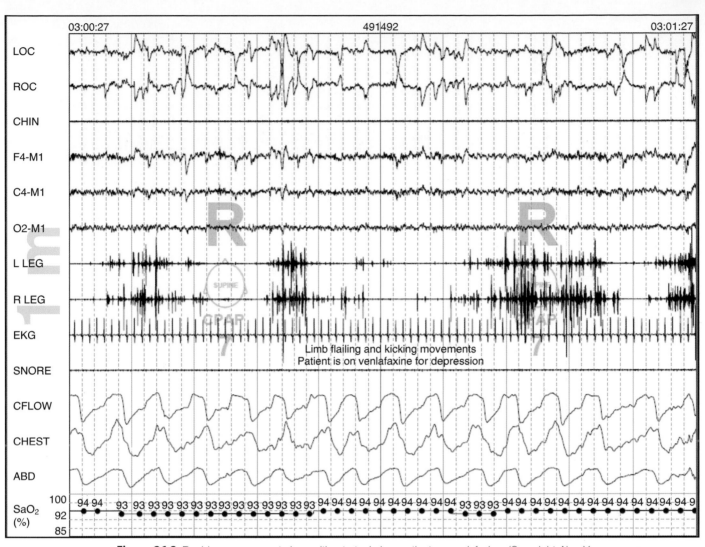

• **Figure 26.2** Rapid eye movement sleep without atonia in a patient on venlafaxine. (Copyright Alon Y. Avidan, MD, MPH.)

nightmares, restless legs, or abnormal behaviors. Effects on waking function may include changes in alertness and performance caused directly by drugs or indirectly by the effects of drugs on prior sleep.

Suggested Reading

Gulyani S, Salas RE, Gamaldo CE. Sleep medicine pharmacotherapeutics overview: today, tomorrow, and the future (Part 1: insomnia and circadian rhythm disorders). *Chest.* 2012;142(6):1659-1668.

Gulyani S, Salas RE, Gamaldo CE. Sleep medicine pharmacotherapeutics overview: today, tomorrow, and the future (Part 2: hypersomnia, parasomnia, and movement disorders). *Chest.* 2013;143(1):242-251.

Hoque R, Chesson AL. Pharmacologically induced/exacerbated Restless Legs Syndrome, periodic limb movements of sleep, and REM behavior disorder /REM sleep without atonia: literature review, qualitative scoring, and comparative analysis. *J Clin Sleep Med.* 2010;6(1):79-83.

Krystal AD. Antidepressant and antipsychotic drugs. *Sleep Med Clin.* 2010;5(4):571-589.

Pagel JF, Helfter P. Drug induced nightmares—an etiology based review. *Hum Psychopharmacol.* 2003;18:59-67.

Roux FJ, Kryger MH. Medication effects on sleep. *Clin Chest Med.* 2010;31(2):397-405.

Schweitzer PK, Randazzo AC. Drugs that disturb sleep and wakefulness. In: Kryger MH, Roth T, Dement WC, eds. *Principles and Practice of Sleep Medicine.* 6th ed. Philadelphia: Elsevier; 2017:480-498.

27

Overview of Sleep Practice Parameters

KIMBERLY NICOLE MIMS, DOUGLAS BENJAMIN KIRSCH

Highlights

The American Academy of Sleep Medicine (AASM) publishes practice parameters providing recommendations for evaluation, diagnosis, and treatment of sleep conditions. The practice parameters are intended to provide guidance and standardize care for clinicians involved in evaluating and managing sleep disorders. These practice parameters are updated as needed to reflect evolving diagnostics and therapy (at a minimum every 5 years). While the AASM tries to reflect current clinical standards by providing necessary addenda more often than every 5 years, it should be acknowledged that practice parameters approaching renewal may contain recommendations not representative of newly emerging clinical standards of care. The practice parameters are currently divided into eight sections, as follows: circadian rhythm sleep disorders (CRSD), diagnostics, hypersomnias, insomnia, parasomnias, pediatrics, sleep-related movement disorders, and sleep-related breathing disorders (SRBD). Within each section, there may be multiple publications detailing different aspects of diagnosis and therapy; for instance, the SRBDs section contains publications describing treatment for sleep apnea with oral appliances, positive airway pressure (PAP), and surgery in separate publications. The following lists a summary and highlights of each practice parameter and a table provided, with links to each practice parameter as of May 1, 2016 (Table 27.1):

- CRSD practice parameter provides recommendations for management of advanced sleep-wake phase disorder (ASWPD), delayed sleep-wake phase disorder (DSWPD), non-24-hour sleep-wake rhythm disorder (N24SWD), and irregular sleep-wake rhythm disorder (ISWRD). Highlighted recommendations include[1–4]:
  - Sleep diary and actigraphy are helpful for assessment and evaluation of treatment in patients with CRSD; polysomnography (PSG) is not indicated.
  - Evening light therapy is suggested for ASWPD.
  - Appropriately timed melatonin is appropriate in adults and children for DSWPD and for blind adults with N24SWD.
  - Light therapy for ISWRD is helpful in dementia patients; sleep-promoting medications and melatonin should be avoided.
  - Appropriately timed melatonin is useful for children with ISWRD.

- In shift work disorder, planned napping during night shift and wakefulness-promoting agents during night shift improve wakefulness. Timed light exposure (avoidance in morning, increased during night shift) and sleep-promoting agents improve daytime sleep.
- The diagnostics section of the practice parameters provides recommendations governing appropriate use of diagnostic tools like unattended portable monitors (PMs)—now referred to as home sleep apnea tests (HSATs), actigraphy, PSG, multiple sleep latency test (MSLT), and maintenance of wakefulness test (MWT). Recommendations include[5–11]:
  - HSATs are useful in patients with a high pretest probability of moderate to severe obstructive sleep apnea (OSA) and who have received an in-depth sleep evaluation. HSATs are not indicated in patients with comorbid medical conditions such as moderate to severe pulmonary disease, neuromuscular disease, or congestive heart failure. HSATs are not indicated for asymptomatic populations (Fig. 27.1).
  - An HSAT should record airflow, respiratory effort, and blood oxygenation at a minimum.
  - Actigraphy is useful to assess circadian rhythm disorders and insomnia and total sleep time in patients with obstructive sleep apnea.
  - PSG is indicated to evaluate patients suspected of having SRBD. PSG is not indicated for patients treated with continuous positive airway pressure (CPAP) with symptom resolution; however, if significant weight loss or weight gain occurs or clinical symptoms worsen despite continued PAP therapy, repeat polysomnogram should be considered. PSG requires recording at least electroencephalography (EEG), electrooculography (EOG), chin electromyography (EMG), airflow, arterial oxygen saturation, respiratory effort and electrocardiography (EKG), or heart rate.
  - PSG and a following day MSLT is indicated in patients with suspected narcolepsy. An MWT may be used to verify adequate treatment but is not a diagnostic test. HLA typing alone is not diagnostic for narcolepsy.
  - PSG is not indicated for patients with common, noninjurious parasomnias, but expanded EEG montage may be useful in patients suspected of having a sleep-related seizure disorder after a normal routine EEG. PSG is indicated in patients with sleep behaviors that are atypical because of the patient's age; time, duration, or frequency of behavior; or motor patterns are suspicious (i.e., stereotypical, repetitive or focal).

- PSG is not indicated to diagnose restless legs syndrome (RLS), but when observer complains of periodic limb movements or patient experiences unexplained arousals, PSG may be useful.
- Pharmacologic agents for depression often affect sleep, but removal of antidepressants and other mood-related medication is not typically recommended for PSG. Removal of antidepressants for an MSLT may be considered based on the patient's clinical condition, although it may not represent a patient's typical circumstances and symptoms.
- PSG is not generally indicated to assess patients with insomnia. Alpha-delta sleep is a nonspecific finding in PSG. PSG is indicated in patients with insomnia if behavioral or pharmacologic treatment is unsuccessful.
- In the practice parameters referring to hypersomnias, recommended treatments for narcolepsy and hypersomnia are provided. Recommendations include[12-13]:
  - For patients with narcolepsy, modafinil, amphetamine, methamphetamine, dextroamphetamine, and methylphenidate may effectively control sleepiness. Tricyclic antidepressants, selective serotonin reuptake inhibitors, and venlafaxine may effectively treat cataplexy, sleep paralysis, and hypnagogic hallucinations. Sodium oxybate is effective for cataplexy, daytime sleepiness, and disrupted sleep and may also improve hypnagogic hallucinations and sleep paralysis. Scheduled naps may improve daytime sleepiness in narcoleptics but rarely suffice as primary treatment.
  - Modafinil, amphetamine, methamphetamine, dextroamphetamine, and modafinil may be effective in hypersomnia that is idiopathic, recurrent, or due to a medical condition.
  - Modafinil may be used in patients with hypersomnia who also suffer from Parkinson's disease, multiple sclerosis, or myotonic dystrophy.
  - Lithium carbonate is effective for recurrent hypersomnia and behavioral symptoms of Kleine-Levin syndrome.
- The insomnia practice parameters detail treatment recommendations for different categories of insomnia. Briefly, these recommendations include[14-16]:
- Psychological and behavioral interventions are effective in the treatment of chronic and secondary insomnia.

TABLE 27.1	List of Practice Parameter Locations
Practice parameters	http://www.aasmnet.org/practiceguidelines.aspx
Circadian rhythm disorder	http://www.aasmnet.org/practiceparameters.aspx?cid=116
Diagnostics	http://www.aasmnet.org/practiceparameters.aspx?cid=120
Hypersomnias	http://www.aasmnet.org/practiceparameters.aspx?cid=118
Insomnia	http://www.aasmnet.org/practiceparameters.aspx?cid=109
Parasomnias	http://www.aasmnet.org/practiceparameters.aspx?cid=121
Pediatrics	http://www.aasmnet.org/practiceparameters.aspx?cid=100
Sleep-related movement disorders	http://www.aasmnet.org/practiceparameters.aspx?cid=119
Sleep-related breathing disorders	http://www.aasmnet.org/practiceparameters.aspx?cid=102

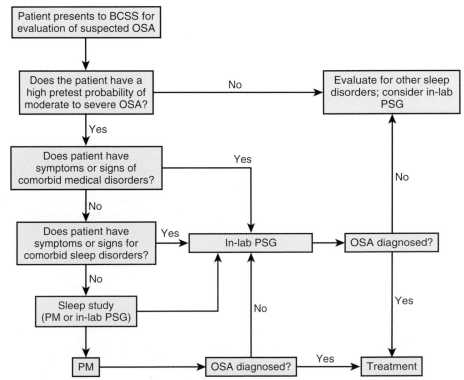

- **Figure 27.1** Portable Monitoring Decision Tree. *BCSS,* Board certified sleep specialist; *OSA,* obstructive sleep apnea; *PM,* portable monitors; *PSG,* polysomnography.

- Insufficient data are available to recommend sleep hygiene as a primary therapy for insomnia.
- Stimulus control therapy, relaxation training, and cognitive behavioral therapy are standard recommended treatments for chronic insomnia. Sleep restriction, multicomponent therapy (without cognitive therapy), bio-feedback, and paradoxical intention are efficacious for insomnia. Cognitive therapy as single therapy and imagery training lack sufficient data to meet recommendation criteria for insomnia.
- The parasomnia practice parameter reviews recommendations for specific types of parasomnias. For instance[17,18]:
  - Prazosin is recommended, and clonidine may be considered for posttraumatic stress disorder (PTSD)-associated nightmares. Other medications to be considered (but with less robust data supporting therapy) include trazodone, atypical antipsychotics, topiramate, low dose cortisol, fluvoxamine, triazolam and nitrazepam, phenelzine, gabapentin, cyproheptadine, and tricyclic antidepressants.
  - Nefazodone is not recommended for treatment of nightmares due to hepatotoxicity, and venlafaxine is not recommended for PTSD-associated nightmares.
  - Nonpharmacologic interventions for nightmare disorder include cognitive behavioral therapy, progressive deep muscle relaxation training, and eye movement desensitization and reprocessing. Hypnosis and testimony method may be considered.
  - For REM sleep behavior disorder (RBD), clonazepam is the most well studied and recommended, although caution is encouraged for patients with dementia, gait disorders, or sleep-disordered breathing. Monitoring for neurodegenerative disorders is suggested.
  - Melatonin may be considered for RBD. Pramipexole efficacy studies demonstrate contradictory results, and paroxetine and L-DOPA can induce or exacerbate RBD, so use cautiously. Acetylcholinesterase inhibitors can be considered in patients with concurrent synucleinopathy. Other medications with limited efficacy based on current evidence include zopiclone, benzodiazepines other than clonazepam, Yi-Gan San, desipramine, clozapine, carbamazepine, and sodium oxybate.
  - Modifying the sleep environment is suggested for patients with RBD who have or are likely to suffer sleep-related injuries.
- The pediatrics practice parameters identify recommended interventions for patients under age 18 suffering from different sleep disorders. These include[19–25]:
  - MSLT preceded by nocturnal polysomnogram is recommended for children with suspected narcolepsy and to evaluate excessive sleepiness.
  - Polysomnogram using expanded EEG montage is indicated to assess atypical or potentially injurious parasomnias and differentiate parasomnia from sleep-related epilepsy if the initial clinical history and routine EEG are inconclusive.
  - In children with recurrent enuresis or frequent parasomnias or epilepsy, a polysomnogram is recommended if suspicion for sleep-disordered breathing or periodic limb movement disorder (PLMD) exists.
  - PSG is indicated in infants who experience an apparent life-threatening event (ALTE) and clinical evidence of an SRBD exists.
  - In children considered for adenotonsillectomy (AT), a preceding polysomnogram is indicated. In children with mild OSA, if residual symptoms persist post-AT, a repeat polysomnogram is indicated. In children with moderate to severe OSA, obesity, craniofacial anomalies, or neurologic disorders, a repeat polysomnogram is indicated post-AT.
  - PSG is indicated in pediatric OSA treated with oral appliance, for initial titration of PAP therapy, for re-assessment of PAP therapy after child's growth or if symptoms recur, to adjust ventilator settings in children on mechanical ventilation, and in children with tracheostomies prior to decannulation.
  - PSG is unnecessary in children treated with supplemental oxygen unless sleep-related symptoms are notable. Unless clinical suspicion is present for an SRBD, PSG is not indicated in chronic asthma, cystic fibrosis, pulmonary hypertension, bronchopulmonary dysplasia, or chest wall abnormalities.
  - Behavioral interventions are effective and suggested to treat bedtime problems and nighttime awaking in young children. These interventions include unmodified extinction, modified extinction, parent education/prevention, graduated extinction, delayed bedtime, and scheduled awakenings.
- In the sleep-related movement disorders practice parameters, recommendations for treatment of RLS and PLMD are outlined. These include[26,27]:
  - Pramipexole and ropinirole should be used to treat patients with RLS. Levodopa with dopa decarboxylase inhibitor can be effective, usually in those with intermittent symptoms.
  - Pergolide and cabergoline should not be used due to potential for heart valve damage, unless all other agents tried and failed, and close clinical follow-up is available.
  - Opioids, gabapentin enacarbil, gabapentin, pregabalin, carbamazepine, rotigotine, and clonidine can be considered for patients with RLS.
  - Supplemental iron may be used in patients suffering from RLS with low iron levels.
- The sleep-related breathing practice parameter encapsulates different treatment paradigms for sleep-disordered breathing and provides recommendations for adequate PAP titrations, including[28–40]:
  - Oral appliances, rather than no therapy, should be used for primary snoring.
  - A custom, titrable oral device provided by a qualified dentist is recommended over noncustom oral appliances.
  - Periodic follow-up is recommended for the patient with both the dentist and sleep physician after initiation of oral appliance therapy.
  - All potential PAP titration candidates should receive PAP education, hands-on demonstration, mask fitting, and acclimatization prior to a titration.
  - During PAP titration, recording airflow signal via the PAP device or estimating airflow by measurement of pressure difference between mask and machine outlet using a pressure transducer are acceptable to detect respiratory events. Nasal airflow obtained from thermistor or thermocouple underneath PAP mask is unacceptable to confirm respiratory events (Table 27.2 and Fig. 27.2).
  - Increasing CPAP or inspiratory positive airway pressure (IPAP) should not exceed 5 cm of water above the pressure, which controls abnormalities, and if patient complains of pressure feeling too high, the pressure should be restarted at a lower CPAP or IPAP comfortable enough to allow patients to return to sleep. Down titration is not required.

TABLE 27.2	Positive Airway Pressure Titration Protocols (AASM Practice Parameter)	
	Patients <12 Years Old	Patients ≥12 Years Old
CPAP starting pressure	4	4
CPAP maximum pressure	15	20
CPAP increase intervals	1 cm H₂O every 5 min	1 cm H₂O every 5 min
Apnea increase criteria	Increase pressure if 1 obstructive apnea	Increase pressure if 2 obstructive apneas
Hypopnea increase criteria	1 hypopnea	3 hypopneas
RERA increase criteria	3 RERAs	5 RERAs
Snoring increase criteria	1 min of loud or unambiguous snoring	3 min of loud or unambiguous snoring
Starting IPAP/EPAP min	8/4	8/4
Maximum IPAP	20	30
Minimum IPAP-EPAP differential	4	4
Maximum IPAP-EPAP differential	10	10

CPAP, Continuous positive airway pressure; *EPAP*, expiratory positive airway pressure; *IPAP*, inspiratory positive airway pressure; *RERA*, respiratory-effort related arousal.

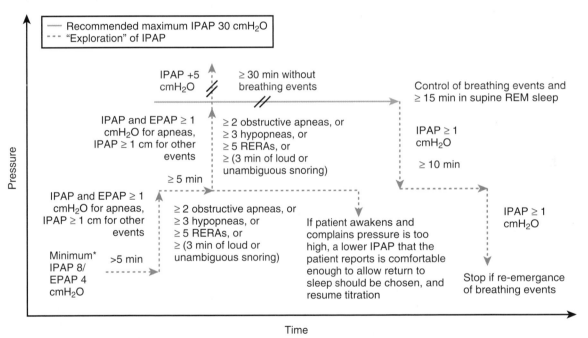

• **Figure 27.2** Positive Airway Pressure Titration Protocols for Adults (AASM Practice Parameter). *EPAP*, Expiratory positive airway pressure; *RERA*, respiratory-effort related arousal.

- Decrease in IPAP or setting BPAP in spontaneous-timed mode (ST) may help if treatment-emergent central apneas develop (Table 27.3).
- Supplemental oxygen should be added if during a PAP titration while the patient is awake, supine SpO₂ is less than 88% or is ≤88% for ≥5 min in the absence of respiratory events. Oxygen supplementation should be started at 1 L/min and increased until oxygen levels are between 88% and 94%.
- Adaptive servo-ventilation (ASV) should be considered if Cheyne-Stokes breathing is observed or if treatment-emergent central sleep apnea occurs. However, ASV is contraindicated in patients with symptomatic, chronic heart failure with left ventricular ejection fraction (LVEF) less than 45%, and moderate to severe predominantly central sleep apnea.

- Acetazolamide may be considered for treatment of primary central sleep apnea. Zolpidem and triazolam may be considered only if patient does not have underlying risk factors for respiratory depression.
- Nocturnal oxygen is indicated for treatment of central sleep apnea related to congestive heart failure.
- Acetazolamide and theophylline may be considered for central sleep apnea treatment in patients with congestive heart failure after optimization of medical therapy, and if PAP therapy is not tolerated.

TABLE 27.3	Grading of Positive Airway Pressure Titrations (American Academy of Sleep Medicine Practice Parameter)			
Titration Grading	RDI		Supine REM	Arousals
Optimal titration	RDI < 5 per hour for at least 15 min		Supine REM recorded	Decrease in spontaneous arousals or awakenings
Good titration	RDI ≤ 10 per hour or decreased by 50% if baseline RDI < 15 per hour		Supine REM recorded	Decrease in spontaneous arousals or awakenings
Adequate titration	RDI > 10 per hour but RDI reduced by 75% from baseline or RDI criteria meets optimal or good criteria		Supine REM not recorded	—

RDI, Respiratory disturbance index; *REM*, rapid eye movement.

TABLE 27.4	Surgical Interventions for OSA	
Surgical Procedures for OSA	Efficacy	Considerations
Tracheostomy	Effective single intervention for sleep apnea	Consider when other options failed, refused or clinical urgency
Maxillo-mandibular advancement	Severe OSA	Useful in patients failing PAP therapy or in patients with mild to moderate OSA who fail PAP + oral appliance
Uvulopalatopharyngoplasty	Ineffective	With or without tonsillectomy, does not reliably normalize AHI in moderate to severe OSA
Multi-level surgery	Effective in those with multiple sites of narrowing in upper airway	Considered in patients who initially failed UPPP as sole treatment
Laser-assisted uvuloplasty	Ineffective	Studies indicated no significant decrease and sometimes worsening in AHI after procedure
Radio-frequency ablation	Mild to Moderate OSA	Considered in patients failing PAP or oral appliance therapy
Palatal implants	Mild OSA	Considered in patients failing PAP or oral appliance therapy

PAP, Positive airway pressure; *UPPP*, uvulopalatopharyngoplasty.

- CPAP, supplemental oxygen, bicarbonate buffer use during dialysis, and nocturnal dialysis may be used to limit central sleep apnea related to end stage renal disease (Table 27.4).
- Postoperatively, after appropriate healing, patients should receive objective measure of presence and severity of sleep-disordered breathing and oxygen saturation.
- Auto-titrating PAP (APAP) therapy should not be used in patients with congestive heart failure, significant lung disease such as chronic obstructive pulmonary disease, patients having decreased oxygenation other than OSA, patients who do not snore, and patients with central sleep apnea.
- APAP may be used to determine an appropriate fixed pressure in patients with moderate to severe OSA without significant comorbidities.
- Weight reduction may improve the AHI in overweight patients with OSA. Dietary weight loss should be combined with a primary OSA treatment. Bariatric surgery may be adjunctive treatment in OSA.
- Selective serotonergic reuptake inhibitors, protriptyline, methylxanthine derivatives (aminophylline and theophylline), estrogen therapy, and oxygen supplementation are not recommended for treatment of OSA.
- Modafinil is recommended for treatment of residual daytime sleepiness in patients with OSA adequately treated with PAP therapy, and who lack other identifiable causes of sleepiness.
- Topical nasal corticosteroids may improve AHI in patients with OSA and concurrent rhinitis. Short-acting nasal decongestants should be avoided.
- Positional therapy may be effective in patients with a low AHI in the nonsupine versus the supine position, as a secondary therapy, or to supplement primary therapy for OSA.

Suggested Reading

Collop NA, Anderson WM, Boehlecke B, et al. Clinical guidelines for the use of unattended portable monitors in the diagnosis of obstructive sleep apnea in adult patients. *J Clin Sleep Med.* 2007;3(7):737-747.

Kushida CA, Littner MR, Morgenthaler T, et al. Practice parameters for the indications of polysomnography and related procedures: an update for 2005. *Sleep.* 2005;28(4):499-521.

Littner MR, Kushida C, Wise M, et al. Practice parameters for clinical use of the multiple sleep latency test and the maintenance of wakefulness test. *Sleep.* 2005;28(1):113-121.

Schutte-Rodin S. Clinical guideline for the evaluation and management of chronic insomnia in adults. *J Clin Sleep Med.* 2008;4(5):487-504.

Wise MS, Arand DL, Auger RR, et al. Treatment of narcolepsy and other hypersomnias of central origin. *Sleep.* 2007;30(12):1712-1727.

28

Mechanism and Disorders of Circadian Physiology

CHRISTOPHER S. COLWELL, ANDREW VOSKO

Questions

1. A 35-year-old woman arrives to the sleep disorders clinic complaining of "sleep problems." At night, she can fall asleep but has difficulties maintaining sleep. During the day, she feels constant fatigue and finds herself napping at inappropriate times. Actigraphy data indicate that there is no pronounced temporal pattern to the sleep-wake cycle, but when she is not forced to stay awake by any type of light-dark (LD) cycle regiment, she is asleep for about one-third of a 24-hour period. Also, during a constant routine protocol, you find there to be no consistent diurnal rhythm in core body temperature. What are the possible cellular deficits that could explain these symptoms?
   A. Loss of the melanopsin-containing retinal ganglion cells (RGCs)
   B. Disruption of communication between the RGCs and the suprachiasmatic nucleus of the hypothalamus (SCN)
   C. Loss of the ability to produce melatonin
   D. Disruption of communication between neurons in the SCN
   E. Abnormal rhythm in cortisol secretion

2. A young woman is referred to you after complaining of an abnormal sleep schedule. She wakes up extremely early every morning (3:00 AM) and cannot stay awake during the full day. She has tried forcing herself to go to bed later and wake up later to better coincide with the schedules of her friends, but she always finds herself eventually back at the same abnormal schedule (waking up at 3:00 AM). The patient reports that she had this sleeping problem all of her life. You suspect that:
   A. She has an unusually short free running period (FRP) or Tau.

B. She has an unusually long FRP.
   C. She cannot be treated with timed exposure to bright light.
   D. She can be treated with antidepressant drugs.
   E. She has a damaged SCN.

3. A 29-year-old man is referred to you after complaining of an abnormal sleep schedule. He wakes up late every day and has difficulty getting to work on time. He has tried forcing himself to go to bed earlier and wake up earlier to better coincide with his work schedule, but he always finds himself waking up late again after about a week. You suspect that:
   A. He has an unusually phase-delayed dim-light melatonin onset (DLMO).
   B. He has an unusually phase-advanced DLMO.
   C. He can be treated with psychomotor stimulants.
   D. He can be treated with biofeedback therapy.
   E. He has damage in his SCN.

4. A 23-year-old male patient arrives complaining of troubles sleeping. The symptoms are intermittent as the problems sleeping "come and go." Actigraphy data indicate that the patient is successively waking up 30–60 minutes later each day. Based on your understanding of the circadian system, which of the following brain regions are likely to be involved in the dysfunction?
   A. Melanopsin-containing RGCs
   B. SCN of the hypothalamus
   C. Paraventricular nucleus of the hypothalamus (PVN)
   D. Medial preoptic nucleus of the hypothalamus (MPN)
   E. Pineal gland

5. A 35-year-old blind patient arrives complaining that she sleeps normally some days but other days she cannot fall asleep until the early morning. To aid entrainment, you would:
   A. Suggest morning light exposure
   B. Suggest use of social cues like an alarm clock
   C. Suggest melatonin or melatonin agonist treatment
   D. Suggest use of a low fat diet to aid entrainment
   E. Suggest use of antidepressants to aid entrainment

6. A 14-year-old patient is brought in by her mother with the complaint of difficulty falling asleep. During the school week, the patient complained of difficulty staying awake during her early morning classes. In order to help relax before bedtime,

the patient reports spending the last hour or two of her day blogging online. Actigraphy and polysomnography measures taken from the sleep lab show a normal sleep-timing phenotype for an adolescent female. You would make the following suggestion:

A. "Don't worry" about the sleep difficulties because there is a normal phase delay in the sleep-wake cycle that accompanies puberty during adolescence.

B. Take 3 mg of melatonin upon awakening every morning to readjust the sleep-wake schedule.

C. Perform some type of active exercise following computer use to help induce fatigue.

D. Suggest minimizing late night computer use as it disrupts sleep-wake timing and is an arousing stimulus.

E. Raise the concern that the emitted light from the computer would depress the teenager.

7. Which of the following statements characterizes the human circadian system?

A. Humans have an endogenous clock with FRP around 23.5 hours.

B. Sleep-wake chronotypes cannot be predicted by studying an individual's cells.

C. The human pineal gland secretes melatonin rhythmically, even in constant light.

D. Rhythm desynchrony improves athletic and cognitive performance.

E. The human circadian system cannot adapt to all of the different artificial lighting schedules.

8. In an in-patient facility, you receive measurements of a 54-year-old man's cortisol levels in the morning and find that the values are high. You order another test later that day and find that the levels are much lower. Based on your understanding of the circadian system, you would:

A. Conclude that the morning measurements were abnormal

B. Order another measurement to be made the following morning

C. Be relieved that the patient's stress and anxiety were improving

D. Not worry as cortisol measurements are notoriously unreliable

E. Be concerned about a tumor in the adrenal glands

9. The melatonin concentration in human saliva shows a daily rhythm. Which of the following regulatory mechanisms is likely to be responsible for this pattern?

A. Direct photoreception by the pineal gland, which alters melatonin secretion

B. SCN-mediated regulation of pineal melatonin secretion

C. Direct SCN secretion of melatonin

D. The daily rhythm in the metabolism of melatonin to serotonin

E. Rhythmic production of melatonin from cells lining the oral cavity

10. Your pancreas shows robust daily rhythms in the secretion of insulin. Possible factors driving this rhythm include:

A. The daily rhythm in rapid eye movement (REM) sleep

B. Rhythms in daily locomotor activity

C. The total amount of fat in the diet

D. A photoreceptive pancreas that is directly masked by light cues

E. A peripheral circadian oscillator in the pancreas

11. Advanced age strongly contributes to which of the following phenotypes in the human circadian system?

A. Increased sleep efficiency at night

B. Ability to adjust to new time zones more quickly

C. Ability to generate more robust rhythms in behavior

D. Ability to generate more robust rhythms in electrical activity in the central clock

E. Ability to wake up earlier in the day

12. Your grandfather has decided to take up a new job as a security officer on the night shift of a local movie studio. Based on your understanding of circadian medicine, you would:

A. Suggest that he resume his diurnal schedule whenever he has the chance in order to offset the nocturnal zeitgebers he is exposed to from his job

B. Suggest that he consult a health care professional regarding an increased risk for cardiovascular diseases from the job

C. Assume that there is little to worry about with this new job because he spends many hours awake during the night normally

D. Suggest that he take sedative hypnotics during the day in order to help him get 8 hours of sleep during the daytime while engaged in the work week

E. Suggest he take "power naps" during his breaks in order to get enough sleep to function through the night

13. You are consulting for a local utility company. During which time of day should you be most concerned about operator errors?

A. 8:00 PM to 10:00 AM

B. 1:00–3:00 PM

C. 8:00–10:00 PM

D. 2:00–4:00 AM

E. None of the above, as time of day has negligible effects on human errors

14. You now work the night shift at the local hospital (7 days/week). Which of the following treatments may help you adjust to your new work hours?

A. Amphetamines in the late afternoon

B. Benzodiazepines at night

C. Bright light at night while at work

D. High dose of melatonin before work

E. Alcohol before bedtime

15. One of your patients suffers from asthma. You are concerned about respiratory failure. When should you monitor this patient most closely?

A. 2:00–4:00 AM

B. 8:00–10:00 AM

C. 1:00–3:00 PM

D. 8:00–10:00 PM

E. None of the above, as there is no rhythm in the reporting or severity of asthma attacks

16. A week after your sleep medicine board examination, you plan to travel to France (phase advance) for a 3-week-long vacation. Which of the following treatments may help your circadian system in order to preadjust to French time before your trip?

A. Drink coffee in the afternoon on your flight to help you stay awake later.

B. Expose yourself to bright light successively earlier during each morning for a few days before travel.

C. Expose yourself to bright light late at night (midnight) the day before you depart.

D. Expose yourself to bright light in the middle of the day (noon–4:00 PM) each day during the week before you leave.

E. Take a hypnotic to help you sleep on the plane.

17. Despite your best efforts to phase-shift your circadian system before your trip, upon arrival in France you are suffering from jet lag symptoms, including troubles with sleep and gastrointestinal disturbances. In order to get over the symptoms as soon as possible, you should do the following:

A. Have a glass of wine with dinner to help you fall asleep later.

B. Stay in your hotel room and sleep until you are rested.

C. Go outside as soon as it is morning in France.

D. Take melatonin as soon as it is morning in France.

E. Take long-acting sedative hypnotics to help you fall asleep during your duration in France.

18. Twice a year, most of the US population adjust their clocks by shifting them either an hour forward (daylight saving time) or an hour backward to correspond with changing daylight hours. Due to our own lighting schedules that we impose on top of such changes, these official clock shifts (adhered to in most states) tend to be abrupt to our systems. Which would best describe the characteristics of this shift?

A. It takes more time for the internal clock to adjust 1 hour ahead.

B. It takes more time for the internal clock to adjust 1 hour back.

C. Both types of time changes are internally resolved at the same rate.

D. Melatonin is not useful as a chronobiotic to aid in these time changes.

E. The core body temperature rhythm will be severely blunted in each case.

19. Delayed sleep-wake phase disorder (DSWPD) is characterized by patients having difficulty falling asleep before 3:00 AM and then sleeping late. Which of the following treatments might help?

A. Melatonin in the evening (8:00–10:00 PM)

B. Exercise at night (midnight–4:00 AM)

C. Bright light at night (midnight–4:00 AM)

D. Hot bath at night (midnight–4:00 AM)

E. Alcohol at night (midnight–4:00 AM)

20. You are advising students studying for their board exams. You find that your students plan to stay up all night cramming for an exam. Based on your understanding of circadian medicine, which of the following arguments would you make to these students?

A. Humans and other organisms show daily rhythms in cognitive performance. It will be much harder to learn new information during the "low point" in the daily cycle.

B. As long as REM sleep is preserved, learning will remain unaffected.

C. Sleep causes the loss of short-term memories. Performance will be better without sleep.

D. Studying in a well-lit area at night is recommended, as only light exposure at dawn, not at night, will shift daily rhythms.

E. Melatonin in the morning before the exam will help performance.

TABLE 28.1   Defining Features of the Circadian Timing System

- Endogenous
- Period close to but not equal to 24 hours
- Synchronized by light and other environmental cues
- Impact almost all biological processes
- Strong genetic control

21. When taking the personal histories of a patient with circadian rhythm disturbances, which of the following need to be considered?

A. Difficulty in falling asleep during night

B. Difficulty in staying awake during day

C. Difficulty in waking up in morning

D. Difficulty staying asleep at night

E. All of the above

Answers

1. **D. Disruption of communication between neurons in the SCN.**

Almost all organisms, including humans, exhibit daily rhythms in their behavior and physiology (Table 28.1). Endogenous, cellular networks composed of multiple circadian oscillators generate these rhythms, providing temporal information to an organism's physiological systems including the daily sleep-wake cycle. In mammals, the part of the nervous system responsible for most circadian behavior can be localized to a bilaterally paired structure in the hypothalamus known as the SCN (Fig. 28.1). Despite the existence of other circadian oscillators, the clock within the SCN exhibits a profound effect on temporal organization and represents the "master" oscillator coordinating daily rhythms throughout the mammalian body. Disruption of the SCN circuit or loss of these cells would produce an arrhythmic sleep/wake cycle. The symptoms described previously specifically point to a deficit in the timing and consolidation of sleep/wake, not in the initiation of either one, and the patient would be diagnosed as having an irregular sleep-wake rhythm timing disorder. Furthermore, since more than one major biological rhythm is affected, the deficit is likely at the point of the master oscillator; hence, D is the best answer.

The loss of melanopsin-containing RGCs or disruption of communication between the RGCs and the SCN would result in a patient who generated robust circadian rhythms, but these rhythms would be difficult to synchronize to the environment. This symptom set is sometimes referred to as non-24-hour sleep-wake disorder. In such a case, the patient would maintain consolidated periods of sleep and wake and also a robust core body temperature rhythm, but at times, these rhythms would not align with the ambient LD cycle. Therefore A and B would not be correct answers. The SCN regulates the rhythmic secretion of melatonin and cortisol. The loss of these hormonal rhythms would impact some of the outputs of the circadian system, but neither the loss of melatonin nor cortisol would by itself produce a behaviorally arrhythmic patient without a core body temperature rhythm. Therefore C and E are not the best answers.[1–3]

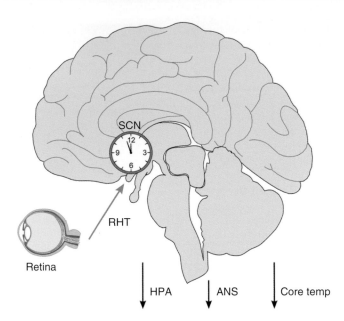

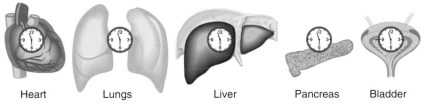

MAJOR ORGAN SYSTEMS ARE PERIPHERAL CLOCKS

Heart   Lungs   Liver   Pancreas   Bladder

• **Figure 28.1** Schematic Illustrating Key Components of the Circadian System. The circadian system is made up of a network of circadian oscillators. The central clock is located in the suprachiasmatic nucleus (SCN). The SCN is a small structure in the anterior hypothalamus and is enlarged in this schematic. SCN neurons receive light information from melanopsin expressing retinal ganglion cells found in our retina. They are most sensitive to blue wavelength light. The axons of these ganglion cells form the retino-hypothalamic tract that makes a direct synaptic connection onto cells in the SCN. These neurons integrate this photic information with other timing cues to generate robust circadian oscillations that are synchronized to the environment. Signals from the SCN travel out via the hypothalamic-pituitary adrenal axis, as well as through the autonomic nervous system, to coordinate regulate independent circadian oscillations found throughout the body.

2. **A. She has an unusually short FRP or Tau.**

The Tau (τ, FRP) is the time that it takes for the biological oscillator to complete one cycle (i.e., to go from start to finish; Fig. 28.2). In the case of circadian oscillators, Tau is close to, but not equal to, 24 hours. For diurnal organisms like humans, Tau is typically longer than 24 hours, while for nocturnal organisms, the period is typically less than 24 hours. Tau of circadian oscillations is largely determined by genetic factors, although there is also evidence for modest history-dependent regulation. While there a number of strategies for measurement of human sleep-wake cycle (Table 28.2), measurement of the FRP requires specialized research faculties and are not yet in common clinical practice.

For the circadian system, *entrainment* refers to the process by which a biological oscillator with a FRP that is close to 24 hours is adjusted to the exact 24-hour period (T) of the environment. When entrained, the FRP of the biological rhythm equals the period of the entraining stimuli, and the two oscillations exhibit a stable phase relationship. The daily cycle of light and dark is the dominant cue responsible for entrainment, though other environmental and social cues can

play a role. The entraining cue is referred to as a "zeitgeber" (translated from German "time giver").

If the FRP of the circadian system is shortened by a mutation, the entrainment process can still occur, but the phase relationship between the LD cycle and the rhythm will be altered. Therefore an individual with a short Tau will be phase advanced compared with the LD cycle with early bedtime and early awakenings, and so A is the best answer. In the case of having a long Tau, a patient would have a phase-delayed sleep-wake phase, waking up and going to sleep later than most others. Therefore B would not be the appropriate answer.

We should also point out that a shortened FRP is not the only reason that a patient may exhibit an advanced sleep-wake phase (Fig. 28.3). The phase relationship between one's endogenous rhythm and that of the LD cycle also can depend on the strength of light cues at specific times. Because light can be an effective tool to change the phase relationship between the clock and the LD cycle, C is not a good answer. While antidepressant drugs appear to be commonly used as a treatment for some sleep disorders (sometimes in spite of more effective and available insomnia- or other sleep disorder–specific

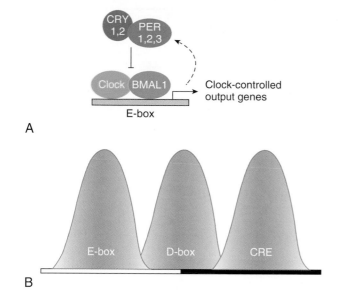

A

B

• **Figure 28.2** Schematic of Transcriptional-Translational Feedback Loop at the Core of the Molecular Clockwork Driving Rhythms in the Suprachiasmatic Nucleus and Throughout the Body. **A,** In the simplest formulation, CLOCK/BMAL1 activation of Per and Cry expression via their E-box regulatory sequences at the beginning of the circadian day. The accumulating mRNAs are translated into protein, which accumulate as dimers in the cytoplasm. By end of the circadian day, these proteins are translocated into the nucleus, and at that time, SCN neurons will have high levels of nuclear PER and CRY proteins. These proteins inhibit the binding of CLOCK and BMAL to the E-box and result in a decline in mRNA levels. This completes the negative feedback action of the accumulated PER/CRY complexes on their own transcriptional activation. By late circadian night, the existing PER/CRY complexes have been cleared from the nucleus. Thus the Clock/Bmal1 activity is de-repressed, and the new day begins. This molecular clockwork is found throughout the body. **B,** The molecular clockwork drives rhythms in E-box mediated transcription. So genes with an E-box in the promoter region will exhibit rhythms in transcription. In addition, other transcriptional regulators including the D-box and cAMP response element (CRE) will drive daily rhythms in transcription. At this point, it appears that most clock-controlled genes are regulated by combinations of these elements that fine-tune gene expression to a particular phase in the daily cycle.

TABLE 28.2	Possible Tools for the Measurement of Human Circadian Rhythms

- Actigraphy, including remote monitoring with smart phones and other electronic devices
- EEG recordings over several days
- Melatonin and other hormones
- Autonomic output including heart rate and blood pressure
- Clock gene expression from fiberblasts or other tissue samples

pharmacological options), they are not as effective for treating sleep-wake timing disorders, cannot be recommended for treatment of phase disorders of the circadian system, and so **D** is not a good answer either. Finally, as described previously, a damaged SCN would most likely produce an arrhythmic patient, whereas the patient in this case appears to be rhythmic, and so **E** is not the best answer.[4–8]

3. **A. He has a phase-delayed DLMO.**
   DLMO is used as a laboratory measure to determine relative phase of the circadian cycle (Fig. 28.4; see Table 28.2). The presence of melatonin in the saliva in the evening is a phase marker of an upcoming period of rest. When the DLMO appears during a relatively later time, it suggests a delayed phase relationship between light and activity in that individual. As this person goes to sleep and wakes up later than his schedule requires, it suggests that he is in a delayed phase relationship with daily light, and therefore A would be the best answer.

   Core body temperature minimum is also a laboratory measure to determine the relative phase of the circadian cycle. An earlier core body temperature minimum would suggest an advanced phase relationship between light and activity in that individual, which is not the case here, as this person goes to sleep and wakes up later than his schedule requires. Therefore B would not be the best answer. Also, as was described before, while antidepressant drugs are commonly used as a treatment for sleep disorders, they are not the appropriate treatment for phase disorders of the circadian system, and thus C is not the best answer. Similarly, biofeedback therapy can help a patient relax and may be beneficial for initiating sleep, but because the symptoms presented suggest a phase relationship disorder, the symptoms will persist and biofeedback is likely insufficient to treat in the long term. Therefore D is not the best answer. Finally, as described previously, a damaged SCN would most likely produce an arrhythmic patient, and therefore E is not an appropriate answer in this case either.[4–8]

4. **A. Melanopsin-containing RGCs.**
   Light reaches the SCN directly via a projection of intrinsically photosensitive RGC axons that contain the photopigment melanopsin (see Fig. 28.1). This pigment is most sensitive to light in the blue wavelength range (specifically at 480 nm) and is necessary for normal resetting of behavioral rhythms in animals following changes in their LD cycle. Animals missing these neurons have severe disruption when resynchronizing to light-based phase shifts. The human circadian system is most sensitive to resetting at light wavelengths around 460 nm, which coincides within the photoresponsive range of melanopsin. Interestingly, melanopsin-containing neurons not only project to the SCN, but also to the pretectum, where light acts independently of the circadian system to acutely induce sleep in nocturnal mammals during their active phase. A dysfunction in melanopsin-containing RGCs would result in a patient that exhibits a free-running rhythm when in an otherwise normal LD cycle, and the patient would be diagnosed as having a non-24-hour sleep-wake disorder. Since most people's FRP is longer than 24 hours, the patient would wake up 30–60 minutes later every cycle. Therefore A is the best answer.

   Specific lesions in the SCN would result in arrhythmic behaviors, as discussed in Question 1, but the current patient does not appear arrhythmic, just nonentrained, and so B is not an appropriate answer. While the PVN is an efferent target from the SCN, lesions in the PVN would impact specific circadian and noncircadian processes not described in the previous question, and therefore C is also inappropriate. These processes include stress responses and the ability of the posterior pituitary to regulate the secretion of oxytocin and vasopressin. Other PVN neurons control various anterior pituitary functions, while still others directly regulate appetite and autonomic functions in the brainstem and spinal cord. Similarly to the

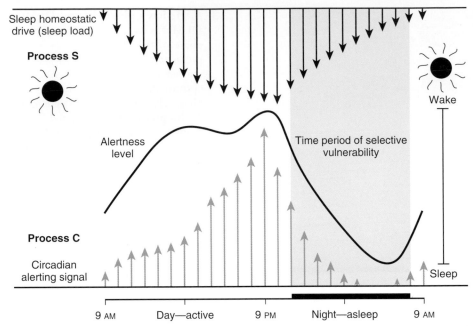

• **Figure 28.3** Schematic Illustrating How Sleep and Circadian Networks Work Together to Determine the Sleep-Wake Cycle in Humans. Process S (sleep load) represents a homeostatic sleep pressure that accumulates in a nonlinear progression from the time of last sleep episode. With a subsequent sleep episode, the signal strength representing Process S decays at an exponential rate. Juxtaposed against Process S is Process C, which in this case is represented by a circadian alerting signal. Process C follows a nearly sinusoidal pattern. While anatomically independent networks govern Process S and Process C, it is also clear that these centers are in communication and must work together to ensure a consolidated sleep/wake cycle. Performance will be at the lowest point near the middle of the sleep interval. (This figure is adapted from one originally presented by Kryger MH, Roth T, Dement WC. *Principles and Practice of Sleep Medicine*. 5th ed. Philadelphia, PA: Saunders/Elsevier; 2011.)

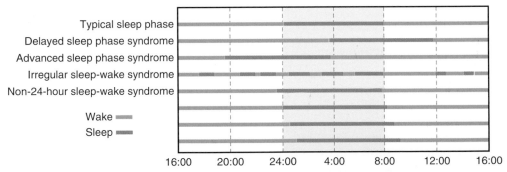

• **Figure 28.4** Types of Circadian Rhythms Disorders. The most obvious circadian rhythms disorders are delayed or advanced sleep-wake phase disorder, in which an individual's required or preferred sleep and wake times are significantly delayed or advanced with respect to conventional times. These individuals often present with symptoms of insomnia related to keeping to a work or school schedule. If patients are allowed to sleep during their preferred times, they exhibit normal sleep quality and duration for age. Irregular sleep-wake disorder is characterized by the absence of a clear consolidated sleep bout. The individual will instead have multiple separate sleep bouts during a 24-hour period. The total amount of sleep would be normal but the temporal patterning would be lost. Non-24-hour sleep-wake disorder is characterized by individuals who are unable to entrain to the 24-hour day and instead follow their endogenous circadian period (typically 24.5 hours). Their sleep-wake pattern moves progressively later each day, eventually alternating between sleeping during the night and sleeping during the day. These figures and the concepts behind them are adapted from the pioneering work of Dr. Zee. Finally, although not shown in this figure, we believe that low amplitude rhythms are quite common in the population. In animal models, low-amplitude rhythms are characteristic of aging and diseases of the nervous system. At present, in general there are no accepted diagnostic criteria for this condition. (From Abbott SM, Reid KJ, Zee PC. Circadian rhythm sleep-wake disorders. *Psychiatr Clin North Am*. 2015;38[4]:805–823.)

PVN, the preoptic area and nucleus also receive input from the SCN and regulate certain behaviors, but these are specific to thermoregulation and sleep initiation. The patient only presented sleep-wake timing abnormalities, not any other insomnia phenotypes. Thus D also is not the best answer to this question. Finally, the pineal gland secretes the hormone melatonin. The loss of melatonin may well impact the robustness of daily rhythms, but a dysfunctional pineal gland would not likely produce an individual who fails to entrain to the LD cycle. Although melatonin helps to synchronize rhythms to the ambient LD cycle, it is not necessary to do so, and so **E** is not the best answer.[9–11]

5. **C. Use of melatonin.**

As described previously (see answer to Question 4), conceptually it is useful to think of our retinas as containing both image-forming and nonimage-forming photoreceptors. A patient can be blind (i.e., unable to form images and still be able to perceive light), but these patients typically still have normal light regulation of the circadian system. There are also patients who have experienced retinal damage and the ability to perceive light, and these patients typically have great difficulty entraining or synchronizing to the LD cycle. Since we do not know the cause of blindness in this case, we cannot assume A as a correct answer.

Light is the primary zeitgeber entraining the human circadian system. There are other nonphotic means for entrainment, such as social cues, but these tend to be weaker and might not themselves be sufficient without light-based cues to entrain someone exposed to a day filled with variably timed activities. Therefore B is an inappropriate answer as well. Evidence from research suggests that retinally blind patients can be helped by nightly treatment with melatonin supplements (0.5–3 mg). Again, while melatonin is not necessary to entrain the master clock, it is sufficient to do so when other cues are removed. Therefore C is the best answer. Please note that melatonin is considered a dietary supplement in the United States.

A low-fat diet might be beneficial in the long term for a healthy lifestyle that includes more consolidated sleep, but the *timing* of meals would be more important for entraining the circadian system than the amount of fat in the meals. Therefore D is not the best answer. Also, for reasons described previously regarding antidepressant treatment as inappropriate for treating circadian phase disorders (in this case the inability to establish a consistent phase between activity and environment via normal entrainment mechanisms), E is an inappropriate answer as well.[12–14]

6. **D. Suggest minimizing late night computer use, as it disrupts sleep-wake timing and is an arousing stimulus.**

Based on our understanding of the circadian system, the light environment is the most important regulator of the human circadian system and is a critical component of sleep hygiene. Exposure to light (especially blue/green) during the night will stimulate the circadian system as well as other brain regions that receive nonvisual light information. This would result in a phase delay of behavioral rhythms (later sleep onset and wake times) as well as acutely contribute to general arousal. Therefore D would provide the best and easiest treatment.

While there is a natural phase delay in the sleep-wake cycle that accompanies puberty, actigraphy data from the lab suggested the patient had a normal "adult female" phase alignment.

This would suggest that the phase misalignment she experiences at home is likely due to something in her home environment. Therefore A is not the best answer.

If the patient's phase delay was endogenously controlled, low doses of melatonin would be a viable treatment option to try and help realign the sleep-wake cycle to better fit the patient's environment. However, the timing of melatonin administration is incorrect for the current scenario. Melatonin taken in the morning would phase delay the circadian clock, further exacerbating the patient's symptoms. Also, the higher dose (>3 mg) has been shown to have direct somnogenic (hypnotic) effects, so taking melatonin in the morning would promote inappropriately timed sleep in the day. Therefore B is not the correct answer.

The effects of exercise on the clock have been studied but results are inconsistent. Exercise at night would promote fatigue, but it could also be arousing, as well as further expose the individual to bright light at night (which phase delays the clock). Therefore C is not the best answer.

If the patient does need to be exposed to light during the night, there is an argument that red light would be less disruptive to the circadian system. There is some evidence that disruptions of the circadian system are associated with mood disorders including depression. Still the evidence linking light exposure at night to depression is not compelling, and E would not be the best answer.[15–18]

7. **E. The human circadian system cannot adapt to all of the different artificial lighting schedules.**

The first four statements are all false and represent central points in our understanding of the human circadian system. Studying human rhythms in constant conditions has revealed that both A and C are false. Recent evidence has also uncovered the existence of clocks persisting in individual cells in the human body. The periodicity of these clocks has been shown to correlate with behavioral chronotypes in humans. Therefore B is also false. Finally, studies have shown that sleep deprivation and phase shifting both lead to impaired cognitive and athletic performance, so D is false as well. The human circadian system, while somewhat adaptable, cannot completely adapt to many work schedules. The technological advances that allow artificial lighting do not allow us to escape our biology, and thus **E** is the best answer.[19–21]

8. **B. Order another measurement to be made the following morning.**

The entire hypothalamic-pituitary-adrenal axis (HPA) is under strong circadian control. One of the most robust circadian rhythms is the daily rise in circulating cortisol that occurs just prior to waking in mammalian species. It is postulated that this rise prepares an organism for the various stressors that are associated with activity onset, acting as a global timing cue for various processes like metabolism and the immune system. Glucocorticoid and mineralocorticoid receptors have a widespread distribution in the peripheral organs as well as throughout the central nervous system but are not found in the SCN, suggesting that the daily increase in cortisol concentration could act as a unidirectional output signal from the SCN. One of the important implications of this regulation is that time of day needs to be taken into account when interpreting results of measurements of cortisol as well as many other hormones in our body. Therefore B would be the best answer.

Knowing that there is a robust rhythm, it would not make sense to just discard an abnormal measurement without consideration for time of day. Therefore A and C are not good answers. Many measurements of hormones need to be interpreted with a clear understanding of impact of time of day as well as from ultradian rhythmic influences. Understanding these factors would make taking measurements of variable markers interpretable, so D is not a good option either. In general, pathology that alters secretion of a hormone would be expected to alter amplitude of rhythms. Therefore an adrenal tumor could result in high levels of cortisol in both the morning as well as later in the day, or at low levels during both times. Since there is no evidence of a damped rhythm, it would be premature to suspect a tumor, and so E is not the most appropriate answer.[22;23]

9. **B. SCN-mediated regulation of pineal melatonin secretion.**
Many SCN efferents are routed through the paraventricular hypothalamus, which signals to the autonomic intermediolateral cell column (IML) of the spinal cord, and eventually to the pineal gland to produce the "nocturnal" hormone melatonin. Melatonin is carried throughout the body with targets in both the brain and periphery, it exhibits a robust circadian rhythm, and it is synthesized in the pineal gland in the absence of light. The SCN has strong expression of melatonin receptors, and it is thought that melatonin is capable of phase shifting the circadian clock in the SCN. In other words, melatonin feeds back to the SCN and modulates the expression of its own rhythmic profile. Interestingly, the SCN has been shown to be important for both the circadian rhythm in melatonin synthesis as well as the light-induced suppression of melatonin. Therefore B is the best answer.

In humans and other mammals, the pineal is not directly photoreceptive (as it is in birds and reptiles), so A is incorrect. While the SCN is a neuroendocrine structure, melatonin is not directly secreted from SCN neurons, and so C is incorrect as well. Also, melatonin is not metabolized to produce serotonin (but, rather, serotonin is a precursor for melatonin), so D is incorrect. Finally, even though it is possible for individual clocks to produce a secreted factor in a rhythmic profile, melatonin is primarily produced in the pineal gland and in the retina, but not in cells lining the oral cavity, and so E is not the best answer.[24]

10. **E. A peripheral circadian oscillator in the pancreas.**
While the mechanisms are still unknown, the insulin-secreting beta cells in the pancreas exhibit the molecular clockwork necessary to drive circadian rhythms in transcription. Animal studies have shown that pancreas explants show both a rhythm in insulin secretion and intrinsic clock components that are necessary for the normal function of the pancreas and glucose tolerance. Therefore E is the correct answer.

While there are daily rhythms in REM sleep and activity, these rhythms are indirectly related to insulin secretion, and thus A and B are not the best answers. A high-fat diet does increase your risk for type II diabetes, and while mutations in some core clock genes are related to the onset of obesity and type II diabetes, a high-fat diet per se has not yet been shown to drive a rhythm in secretion of insulin, so C is not the best answer either. Note that there is data indicating that a high fat diet can disrupt the circadian rhythm in insulin in animal models. Finally, there is no evidence suggesting the pancreas as a photoreceptive organ so D is not a good answer.[25–27]

TABLE 28.3	Common Age-Related Changes in Circadian System

- Phase advance of sleep/wake cycle with earlier bedtimes and earlier awakenings
- Reduction of coherence of sleep/wake cycle with fragmentation of sleep particularly common
- Reduction in amplitude of rhythms in behavior and physiology

TABLE 28.4	Symptoms of the Dysfunction of the Circadian System

- Cognitive dysfunction including memory problems
- Affective disorders
- Metabolic dysfunctions including increased risk of type 2 diabetes
- Cardiovascular disease
- Gastrointestinal disturbances
- Inflammation
- Increased risk for certain cancers, specifically breast cancer

11. **E. Ability to wake up earlier in the day.**
In humans and other animals, aging is associated with disruptions in the coherence of the nocturnal sleep bout and, in many cases, a phase advance in the relationship between the LD cycle and sleep onset (Table 28.3). There is also consistent evidence for an age-related decline in the light-response of the circadian system, as measured by the speed of resynchronization of the activity cycle following a light-induced phase shift. The impact of aging on Tau (free running period) has been inconsistent, with some groups finding evidence for a shortened free-running period but not others. A weakening of the circadian system can account for certain aspects of these age-related sleep changes, and treating the circadian system in the elderly offers a potential target for ameliorating age-related changes in sleep and daytime alertness. An aged circadian system shows a reduction in its normal response to light, as well as a reduction in the output of the central clock. Attenuation of the circadian output signal could lead to both less consolidated sleep at night and alert wakefulness during the day. Therefore the best answer is E, as humans and other animals tend to awake earlier with age.

Sleep efficiency as well as the amplitude of behavior rhythms decline with age, so A and C are incorrect. It is not possible to measure electrical activity rhythms from the human SCN, so D is not a good answer either. Finally, evidence suggests that the ability to readjust to new LD cycles is compromised with aging, so B is incorrect as well.[28–31]

12. **B. Consult a health care professional regarding an increased risk for cardiovascular diseases from the job.**
This disruption of circadian output is likely to have profound consequences on an individual's health. It is becoming increasing clear that robust daily rhythms of sleep-wake are essential for well-being. A wide range of studies have demonstrated that disruption of the circadian system can lead to a cluster of symptoms, including cardiovascular problems (and also metabolic disease; see Table 28.4). This brings up the question as to the extent that circadian perturbations exacerbate the age-related alterations in the functions of other physiological systems. Therefore B is an appropriate answer.

One of the detriments of shift work is the desynchronization between one's own endogenous clock and the ambient LD cycle. While prolonged shift work can contribute to a host of cognitive and health impairments (see the following discussion for more detail), *rotating* shift work schedules, in which one only assumes a nocturnal schedule for part of the week, can be even more harmful. Answer choice A suggests trying to revert back to a diurnal schedule whenever possible during the nocturnal work week, which essentially forces the circadian clock to abruptly shift 180 degrees out of phase during multiple days in the week, like in rotating shift work. Clearly, this is not the best answer.

A misconception about sleeping patterns in the aged population is that the elderly need less sleep. There is no strong evidence that this is the case. While there are more difficulties in maintaining a consolidated period of sleep throughout the night, this might well be due to a circadian misalignment with the homeostatic pressures that normally initiate and help consolidate sleep at night. Even if an individual has trouble sleeping at night, they can still reasonably maintain circadian health by avoiding bright light and arousing stimuli that would reset their clocks. Therefore C would be an inappropriate answer.

Sedative hypnotics are often prescribed for elderly individuals with sleep difficulties, but this is not necessarily the most effective treatment for sleep disorders with a circadian etiology. The act of going to sleep itself contributes to entrainment, mostly by altering activity levels and avoiding light. There are data to suggest that sleep does have small phase shifting effects independent of light, but these are minor in comparison to those achieved by light alone. This is not to imply that treating sleep disturbance is ineffective, but in the case of shift work, sleep disturbance is just one target. Furthermore, only taking the hypnotics to aid in sleep during the work week leaves non-workdays open, where the circadian clock could be shifted to adjust to a LD cycle 180 degrees out phase with the work week. Therefore D is not the best answer.

Finally, the idea of "power naps" to help refresh a sleep-deprived individual without strongly disturbing his sleep homeostat is not a viable long-term solution for trying to accommodate shift work schedules. It is important to consider that appropriately timed sleep, not just total sleep amount, is important for normal, healthy function in an individual. Therefore E is not the best answer.[32–35]

13. **D. 2:00–4:00 AM.**
For most individuals, there is a robust daily rhythm in alertness with peaks in the morning and evening. In many people, there is a midday dip in alertness after lunch and lowest alertness found between 2:00 and 6:00 AM (see Fig. 28.2). These individual rhythms in alertness/fatigue are likely to lie at the heart of population data, suggesting that frequency of industrial accidents is also highest during this time. Therefore D is the best answer.

For most individuals, morning and evening would be times of relatively strong performance, so both A and C would not be correct answers. While there is in fact a post lunch dip in cognition, the magnitude of this would not be as high as in the middle of the night, and so B is not the best answer either. The last answer choice, E, is quite obviously incorrect. Most car accidents and hospital errors have been tracked to specific hours during the day, as well as major industrial accidents.[36,37]

| TABLE 28.5 | Types of Circadian Disorders |

- Delayed sleep-wake phase disorder
- Advanced sleep-wake phase disorder
- Irregular sleep-wake disorder
- Non-24-hour sleep-wake disorder
- Low amplitude sleep-wake disorder

14. **C. Bright light at night while at work.**
Bright light is directly stimulatory and will be the strongest cue to synchronize the circadian system (Table 28.5). When consistently working the night shift, the most effective way to adjust to this schedule is assuming a completely nocturnal schedule outside of work as well. This includes only exposing oneself to light during one's active phase and avoiding bright light during the resting phase. Therefore **C** is the best answer.

While amphetamines do promote arousal, in the absence of appropriately timed photic cues, their use is not going to offset the circadian disturbances caused from shift work. Similarly, benzodiazepines may promote sleep without addressing the circadian disturbances in shift work. Furthermore, both amphetamine and benzodiazepine use carry many side effects, and so A and B are not the best answers in this case.

In humans, increases in melatonin at the appropriate circadian phase are associated with inducing sleepiness and exogenous melatonin at higher also has a hypnotic effect. Therefore you would not want to take melatonin before a night shift and not at a high dose, and so D is not an appropriate answer either.

While alcohol can decrease sleep latency, it can also interfere with sleep maintenance and nocturnal breathing. It cannot be recommended as part of a strategy to adjust to a new night shift, and so E would be incorrect as well.[38,39]

15. **A. 2:00–4:00 AM.**
Like most physiological systems, there is a robust daily rhythm in respiratory functions. In animal studies, the airway tissues, including bronchus and lung, exhibit rhythmic expression of circadian genes and appear to contain a functional peripheral oscillator that is controlled by the SCN. Likely as a consequence of this endogenous rhythm as well as the strong rhythm in autonomic function, the bronchioles exhibit a daily rhythm in dilatation with highest risk for respiratory failure in the middle of the night. Therefore E is obviously incorrect, and A would be the best answer choice. While it is important to monitor the asthma patient at all times, the other times are not points of greatest risk so B, C, and D are not the best answers.[40–42]

16. **B. Expose yourself to bright light successively earlier during each morning for a few days before travel.**
There are a number of treatments for jet lag involving bright light exposure, melatonin, and the use of hypnotics, but their efficacy greatly depends on their time of use, the length of time in the new time zone, and the specific circadian disturbance involved. Because in this case the trip duration is longer, the best strategy would be to gradually readjust the internal clock so as to match the new LD cycle without abruptly desynchronizing from the current LD cycle. Light in the morning would help to advance the circadian system to the LD cycle in France and could be used pretrip to start this phase readjustment. Therefore B is the best answer.

Taking stimulants like caffeine to stay awake in the evening will not help in getting up early during the next cycle. Furthermore, the arousing effects of coffee often fragment sleep later on, so the symptoms of jet lag would possibly become more severe, and A would be inappropriate in this case. Light in the middle of the day is unlikely to alter the phase of the circadian system (because it is a "dead-zone" period in circadian responsiveness to light) while light late at night will produce delays of the circadian system. Therefore C and D are incorrect.

In the current scenario, it would in fact be important to avoid light during the relative night hours in France, as this would undo the phase advancing from the early morning light exposure. Finally, hypnotic use to help with sleep can be useful for short-term trips where complete phase shifts of the clock are not desirable. However, promoting sleep on the plane will mostly offset travel fatigue and not address the phase misalignment caused in jet lag. Jet lag involves desynchrony between clock systems within an individual, as well as desynchrony with the environment. While sleep disturbances are usually the most noticeable effects of jet lag, many physiological systems are affected, and therefore treating only the sleep disturbance does not sufficiently treat the cause, and answer choice E is therefore not the most appropriate.[43–45]

17. **C. Go outside as soon as it is morning in France.**
Again, there are a number of proposed treatments for jet lag involving bright light exposure, low-dose melatonin, and use of hypnotics, but their efficacy greatly depends on their time of use, the length of time in the new time zone, and the specific circadian disturbance involved. Going outside in the morning would expose you to light, social cues, exercise, and likely food. This combination of temporal cues would help advance the circadian system to the new time zone, and therefore C would be the best answer.

While alcohol is commonly used to help in initiating sleep, it interferes with sleep maintenance, and therefore choice A cannot be recommended. Staying in one's room and sleeping will prevent re-entrainment and prolong the duration of the symptoms, because it will avoid important temporal cues in the new environment, even though it will offset the fatigue from traveling and phase realignment. Because circadian phase-shifting is the only complete method to treat the symptoms of jet lag, B (similarly to A and E) would not be an appropriate answer. Likewise, because the short-term use of long-acting hypnotics has minimal effects on circadian realignment outside of treating insomnia, E may be useful, but it is not the best answer to this question and could worsen daytime function the next day. Melatonin in the morning actually phase delays the circadian clock. When traveling to France from the United States, the circadian system needs to align by advancing, not delaying, and so answer D would be incorrect. However, taking low-dose melatonin (0.5–3 mg) in the evening would further aid in the phase advancing process, especially if accompanied with bright light exposure in the early morning.[43–45]

18. **A. It takes more time for the internal clock to adjust 1-hour ahead.**
The changing of clocks twice a year is equivalent to experiencing jet lag over one time zone. During these particular shifts there are minor but rapid shifts in the LD cycle that transiently disrupt coordinated regulation of the body where (1) the clock network loses synchrony with the external environment, and

TABLE 28.6	Possible Tools for Strengthening the Circadian System

- Robust light/dark cycle with bright sunlight in day and darkness during sleep
- Schedule timing of meals
- Schedule timing of exercise
- Restrict intake of stimulants like caffeine
- Restrict intake of alcohol
- Short-term use of hypnotics
- Possible use of melatonin supplements

(2) the many oscillators within our bodies become desynchronized with each other.

As a general rule, it takes longer for the circadian system to adjust to a phase-advancing stimulus than it does a phase-delaying one. In the case of "jumping 1-hour ahead," the clock is advancing, and so A is the best choice. Therefore answers B and C can be immediately discounted. Taking low doses of melatonin at the appropriate times has been shown to aid in circadian re-entrainment and can certainly do so during 1-hour phase adjustments, so D would be incorrect. The rhythm in core body temperature is robust and is persistent as long as the central pacemaker outputs are intact. With a phase shift of only one hour, it is unlikely that this rhythm would be severely blunted, and so E is incorrect in this case.[38,39]

19. **A. Melatonin in the evening (8:00–10:00 PM).**
DSWPD is the one of the most common circadian sleep disorders and appears to be particularly prevalent among young adults (see Fig. 28.4; Table 28.5). Those individuals with DSWPD will have difficulty following a conventional sleep schedule and will experience sleep onset insomnia along with excessive sleepiness during the day. The underlying mechanisms responsible for DSWPD are unknown and are likely to due to a number of factors. Conceptually, a long FRP or alterations in the entrainment mechanisms by which light acts to entrain the circadian system are likely culprits. Based on first principles, several treatment approaches do exist (Table 28.6), including timed exposure to bright light in morning and treatment with melatonin or hypnotics at night. Melatonin taken in the evening, perhaps 2–3 hours before habitual sleep time, is likely to be most effective. Specifically, the actions of melatonin at night can be twofold: (1) At higher doses, melatonin has hypnotic effects and can help an individual get to sleep earlier, and (2) melatonin is a chronobiotic that phase advances the central clock when taken in the evening. Together, these two effects would promote a more advanced sleep phase. Therefore A is the best answer to this question.

Exercise at night would promote fatigue, but it could also be arousing, as well as further expose the individual to bright light at night (which phase delays the clock). Therefore exercising at night is not recommended, and B would not be the best answer. While light in the morning would be helpful, light at night would delay the circadian clock and would not be recommended, and so C is not the correct answer. Alcohol at night is commonly used to self-medicate for sleeping problems, but as mentioned previously, it interferes sleep maintenance. Finally, some patients provide anecdotal evidence that a hot bath at night helps them sleep. The bath may help individuals relax before bed, but the evidence for the use of a bath is not as compelling as the use of melatonin, so D would not be the best answer.[46,47]

20. **A. Humans and other organisms show daily rhythms in cognitive performance. It will be much harder to learn new information in the low point in the daily cycle.**

Circadian rhythms govern many aspects of physiology and behavior, including cognitive processes. Components of neural circuits involved in learning and memory (e.g., the amygdala and the hippocampus) exhibit circadian rhythms in gene expression and signaling pathways. The functional significance of these rhythms is still not understood. There are several lines of evidence that the circadian system can regulate cognitive functions—especially memory. Perhaps the most important is the observation that peak performance in the recall of a number of behavioral tasks varies with a diurnal rhythm. In addition, the disruption of the circadian cycle alters the ability to recall training (i.e., memory; see Table 28.4). Therefore A is the best answer to this question.

Staying up all night will most definitely result in a loss of both kinds of sleep, both NREM and REM, and the effects of sleep loss will surely affect one's ability to perform. The poor ability to learn during the night's low point, combined with the following day's fatigue, will together result in a negative outcome for the exam, and so B is incorrect. In a similar way, sleep deprivation has been shown to hurt performance on a number of memory tasks, and so C would also be incorrect. As was explained in the many examples listed here, light has direct and robust effects in altering the circadian system, and so D is clearly incorrect. Finally, melatonin in the morning will phase delay the circadian clock, which would not be helpful for performance on this exam. Furthermore, at higher doses, it would cause sleepiness, and so E would not be a reasonable answer either.[48–50]

21. **E. All of the above.**

The answers to all of these questions will help determine whether the patient has a sleep or circadian problem (see Table 28.5). Therefore E is the best answer.

Suggested Reading

Abbott SM, Reid KJ, Zee PC. Circadian rhythm sleep-wake disorders. *Psychiatr Clin North Am.* 2015;38(4):805-823.

Bass J. Circadian topology of metabolism. *Nature.* 2012;91(7424): 348-356.

Czeisler CA, Gooley JJ. Sleep and circadian rhythms in humans. *Cold Spring Harb Symp Quant Biol.* 2007;72:579-597.

Hastings MH, Brancaccio M, Maywood ES. Circadian pacemaking in cells and circuits of the suprachiasmatic nucleus. *J Neuroendocrinol.* 2014;26(1):2-10.

Martino TA, Young ME. Influence of the cardiomyocyte circadian clock on cardiac physiology and pathophysiology. *J Biol Rhythms.* 2015;30(3):183-205.

29

Tools in Clinical Sleep Medicine

KEVIN A. WALKER, ANITA V. SHELGIKAR

Questions, 436

Answers, 443

Suggested Reading, 452

Questions

1. Electrooculography (EOG) is an important tool in sleep staging. A sleep technician is training a new sleep medicine fellow on electrode placement for EOG. After placing the EOG electrodes on the patient according to the American Academy of Sleep Medicine (AASM) recommended position, the patient is asked to look horizontally and then vertically. What will the fellow see on the EOG tracing?
   A. Out-of-phase deflections regardless of what direction the patient looks
   B. In-phase deflections regardless of what direction the patient looks
   C. Out-of-phase deflections with horizontal eye movements and in-phase deflections with vertical eye movements
   D. In-phase deflections with horizontal eye movements and out-of-phase deflections with vertical eye movements

2. A sleep technician is training a new sleep medicine fellow on electrode placement for electroencephalography (EEG). He explains that electrodes are placed according to the International 10–20 System, which involves 21 electrodes, including the two reference electrodes. He further explains that for routine polysomnography (PSG), only 8 of the possible 21 electrodes are placed. Not including the reference electrodes, which of the following six electrodes is part of the recommended EEG derivation in PSG?
   A. Fp1, Fp2, C3, C4, Cz, Pz
   B. F7, F8, T3, T4, O1, O2
   C. F3, F4, C3, C4, O1, O2
   D. Fz, Cz, T3, T4, O1, O2
   E. F3, F4, C3, C4, P3, P4

3. During your first month of sleep medicine fellowship, one of your first tasks is to become very familiar with the AASM scoring manual in order to accurately identify sleep stages. As you review a 30-sec PSG epoch (Fig. 29.1), you correctly identify the stage of sleep. Which of the following statements is true regarding this stage of sleep?
   A. Sleep spindles are never seen during this stage of sleep.
   B. Greater than 50% of the epoch must consist of the characteristic waveform.
   C. The characteristic waveform of this sleep stage is best seen in the occipital leads.

   D. ≥20% of the epoch must consist of the characteristic waveform.
   E. The characteristic waveform is sharply contoured 2–6 Hz frequency.

4. You are scoring the sleep study of a 19-year-old male with excessive daytime sleepiness (EDS) who also describes a history of sleep paralysis and hypnagogic hallucinations. You recognize that it is important to correctly identify his rapid eye movement (REM) sleep latency. Fig. 29.2 shows a representation of five contiguous epochs of his PSG. Which epoch is the first epoch of REM sleep?
   A. 28
   B. 29
   C. 30
   D. 31
   E. 32

5. A 45-year-old obese male is undergoing a diagnostic PSG to evaluate for obstructive sleep apnea (OSA). During the night, the oronasal thermal airflow sensor signal becomes unreliable. In this situation, which of the following can be used to identify apneas?
   A. Esophageal manometry
   B. Nasal pressure transducer
   C. Transcutaneous carbon dioxide (CO_2)
   D. Apneas cannot be scored in this situation

6. You are performing PSG on a 32-year-old female who reports multiple sleep complaints including snoring, trouble falling asleep, frequent nighttime awakenings, occasional jerking leg movements observed by her husband, and feeling exhausted in the morning. She has a history of sleepwalking as a child. You observe the following pattern on her EEG during her PSG (Fig. 29.3). What is the appropriate next step in her evaluation and management?
   A. Check her medication list for benzodiazepines.
   B. Order brain magnetic resonance imaging (MRI) to look for Chiari malformation.
   C. Start her on levetiracetam and refer her to a neurologist for further seizure management.
   D. Check liver function tests.

7. As you spend a night working with a registered PSG technologist, you observe the following on a patient's EEG that is being done as part of the PSG (Fig. 29.4). You become concerned about the finding identified by the arrows. What is the appropriate next step?
   A. Stop the recording and reboot the computer.
   B. Have the patient move his left arm and monitor for suppression of this activity.

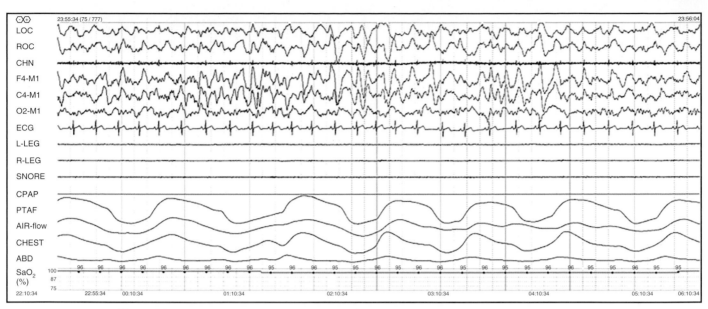

• **Figure 29.1** Thirty-second epoch of the patient's polysomnogram. *ABD*, Abdominal respiratory inductance plethysmography (RIP); *AIR-flow*, oronasal thermal airflow; *C4-M1*, right central electroencephalogram (EEG); *CHEST*, thoracic RIP; *CHN*, submental electromyogram (EMG); *CPAP*, continuous positive
airway pressure; *ECG*, electrocardiogram; *F4-M1*, right frontal EEG; *L-LEG*, left leg EMG; *LOC*, left outer
canthus; *M1*, left mastoid referential lead; *O2-M1*, right occipital EEG; *PTAF*, pressure transducer airflow;
R-LEG, right leg EMG; *ROC*, right outer canthus; *SaO₂*, oxygen saturation; *SNORE*, snore microphone.

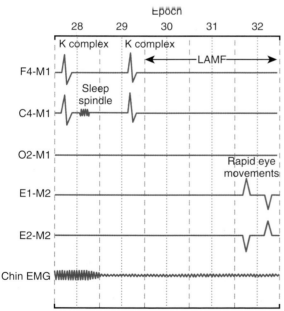

• **Figure 29.2** A representation of five contiguous epochs of the patient's
polysomnogram numbered 28 through 32. Dashed lines represent the
divisions between each 30-sec epoch, and dotted lines represent the
middle of each epoch. *C4-M1*, Right central electroencephalogram (EEG);
Chin EMG, submental electromyogram; *E1-M2/E2-M2*, left/right electrooculogram; *F4-M1*, right frontal EEG; *LAMF*, low-amplitude, mixed-
frequency EEG; *M1/M2*, mastoid referential leads; *O2-M1*, right
occipital EEG.

C. Do nothing and wait for the problem to resolve on its
own.

D. Reapply the affected electrodes to ensure secure contact
with the skin.

E. Apply a notch filter.

8. A 15-year-old healthy male is brought to clinic by his mother
who is concerned about his declining school performance. For
the past 6 months, he has had increasing difficulty falling asleep
at 10 PM, which had been his standard bedtime previously, and
he finds it almost impossible to wake up in the morning at 7 AM
for school despite setting three alarm clocks. In fact, he has missed
his first period class multiple times this year. Even when he gets
to school on time, he frequently sleeps through his first two classes
but does not have trouble staying awake in subsequent classes.
On weekends he typically goes to bed easily around midnight,
sleeps until 10 AM, and reports feeling better on awakening
those days. What is required to diagnose delayed sleep-wake
phase disorder (DSWPD) in this teenager?

A. A concurrent diagnosis of a mood disorder like
depression

B. Sleep logs for at least 7 days that include school days and
free days

C. Improvement in symptoms following initiation of melatonin
at bedtime

D. Scoring as an evening type on the Morningness-Eveningness
Questionnaire (MEQ)

E. Demonstration of a delay in the timing of dim-light melatonin onset (DLMO)

9. Actigraphy is a useful clinical tool in the diagnosis of circadian
rhythm disorders and is typically done in conjunction with
patient-recorded sleep logs. Fig. 29.5 is characteristic for a
specific circadian rhythm sleep-wake disorder. According to
current diagnostic criteria, actigraphy must be done for a

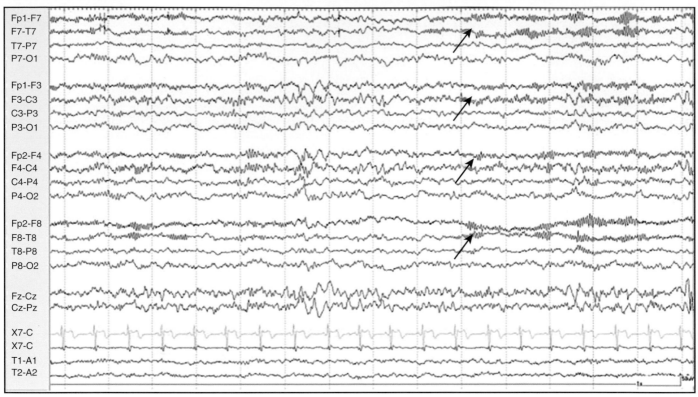

• **Figure 29.3** Fifteen-second epoch of the patient's electroencephalogram from her polysomnogram with each vertical dotted line representing 1 sec. *A*, Ear lobe; *C*, central; *Cz*, central midline; *F*, frontal; *Fp*, frontal polar; *Fz*, frontal midline; *P*, parietal; *Pz*, parietal midline; *O*, occipital; *T*, temporal; *X7-E and X1-E*, EKG. (From Vendrame M, Kothare SV. Recognizing normal, abnormal, and benign nonepileptiform electroencephalographic activity and patterns in polysomnographic recordings. *Sleep Med Clin.* 2012;7[1]:23–38.)

minimum of how many days to establish a diagnosis for this particular disorder?

A. 5
B. 7
C. 14
D. 21
E. 28

10. A 32-year-old otherwise healthy woman comes to your clinic complaining of severe insomnia for several years. She reports typically sleeping for only 2–3 hours per night. She is a light sleeper and wakes frequently during the night with a prolonged latency to return to sleep. Her sleep pattern is unchanged regardless of whether she sleeps home or elsewhere. Despite her sleep complaints, she works a full-time job and has performed well enough at work to recently earn a promotion. She snores lightly but denies feeling sleepy during the day. Her husband thinks she sleeps more than she realizes. What findings are most likely to be seen on PSG?

A. Significant underestimation of sleep onset latency reported by the patient compared with PSG recording of sleep onset latency
B. A prolonged first REM period and shorter subsequent REM periods
C. A REM latency of less than 15 min
D. Significant underestimation of total sleep time (TST) reported by the patient compared with PSG recording of TST

11. A 21-year-old college student presents with EDS. He is failing multiple classes, largely because he cannot stay awake in class or while studying, despite excessive caffeine consumption. In high school he also struggled to stay awake but attributed this to sleep deprivation. He reports multiple episodes of collapsing to the ground after hearing funny jokes but has never lost consciousness in these situations. He has a history of major depressive disorder that has worsened over the past few years and currently takes two antidepressant medications. You discuss diagnostic testing with him, and he is unwilling to discontinue antidepressant therapy even for a short time because of past suicidality. What testing should you pursue?

A. Human leukocyte antigen (HLA) DQB1*0601 subtype
B. Serum ferritin levels
C. No further testing because a diagnosis can be made on clinical history alone
D. PSG to look for REM sleep without atonia (RWA)
E. Cerebrospinal fluid (CSF) hypocretin-1 levels

12. A 25-year-old patient with EDS, sleep paralysis, episodic daytime sleep attacks, and possible cataplexy comes for sleep testing. During her multiple sleep latency test (MSLT), she has a mean sleep latency of 2.5 min but only one sleep onset REM period (SOREMP). According to the *International Classification of Sleep Disorders, Third Edition* (ICSD-3), what additional information from the preceding night's PSG supports a diagnosis of narcolepsy?

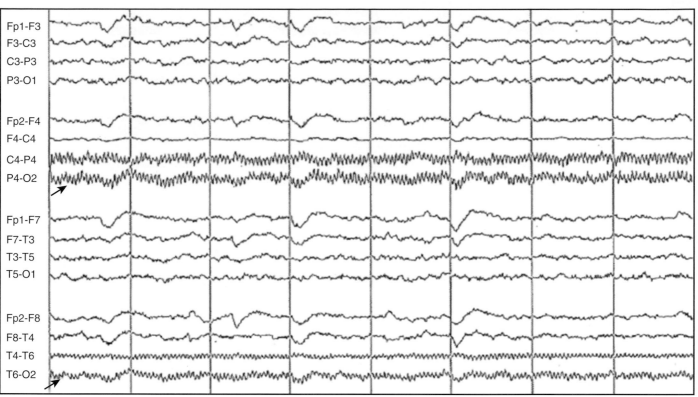

• **Figure 29.4** An 8-sec epoch of the patient's electroencephalogram with each vertical line representing 1 sec. *A*, Ear lobe; *C*, central; *Cz*, central midline; *F*, frontal; *Fp*, frontal polar; *Fz*, frontal midline; *P*, parietal; *Pz*, parietal midline; *O*, occipital; *T*, temporal. (From Vendrame M, Kothare SV. Recognizing normal, abnormal, and benign nonepileptiform electroencephalographic activity and patterns in polysomnographic recordings. *Sleep Med Clin.* 2012;7[1]:23–38.)

A. Minimum of 25% REM sleep
B. A REM latency of 10 min
C. RWA
D. A REM latency of 30 min
E. A sleep onset latency of 5 min with a REM latency of 45 min

13. Early in your sleep medicine fellowship, you became familiar with the diagnostic criteria for narcolepsy and learned of the role of the MSLT in diagnosis. You also learned of the many confounding factors that can influence the results of the MSLT. For correct interpretation of the MSLT, which of the following conditions is necessary?
    A. The patient must be free of drugs that influence sleep for at least 14 days prior to the MSLT.
    B. Nocturnal PSG should be performed within 1 week of the MSLT to rule out other sleep disorders.
    C. The sleep-wake schedule must have been standardized for 2 days before the MSLT.
    D. The patient must sleep for at least 9 hours the night prior to MSLT.

14. A 35-year-old otherwise healthy female presents to your clinic for evaluation of EDS that has been present since college. Sleep logs and actigraphy indicate a TST of 10 hours per night, despite which she struggles to stay awake at work during the day. She takes a 60- to 90-min nap almost daily, but naps are unrefreshing. She has no history of cataplexy. Her PSG shows normal sleep onset latency and REM latency, high sleep efficiency of 94%, normal sleep architecture, and absence of sleep-disordered breathing (SDB) and periodic limb movement

disorder (PLMD). The PSG is followed by a five-nap MSLT, during which no SOREMPs are observed. She does not fall asleep during nap 2, but her sleep onset latency during the other four naps is 3, 8, 3, and 6 min. What is her mean sleep latency?
    A. Indeterminate due to absence of sleep in nap 2
    B. 5 min
    C. 8 min
    D. 7 min
    E. 6 min

15. A 45-year-old healthy female CEO presents for EDS the past 6 months that is impacting her work performance; she dozes off during meetings and when working in her office. Due to the demands of her job, she often arrives at work at 6:30 AM and does not leave until 10 PM. She goes to bed between 11 and 11:30 PM, falls asleep almost immediately, and then gets up at 5 AM with an alarm to exercise for 30 min before getting ready for work. On the weekends she does not set her alarm and may sleep in until 10 AM. Despite this, she still feels tired on the weekends. Her weight is normal, she does not snore, and she does not report any symptoms of restless legs syndrome (RLS). Her mood is down, and she is increasingly relying on coffee to get her through the day. What testing would you recommend first?
    A. PSG
    B. MSLT
    C. CSF hypocretin-1 level
    D. Salivary DLMO measurements
    E. Two weeks of sleep logs and actigraphy

Time of day

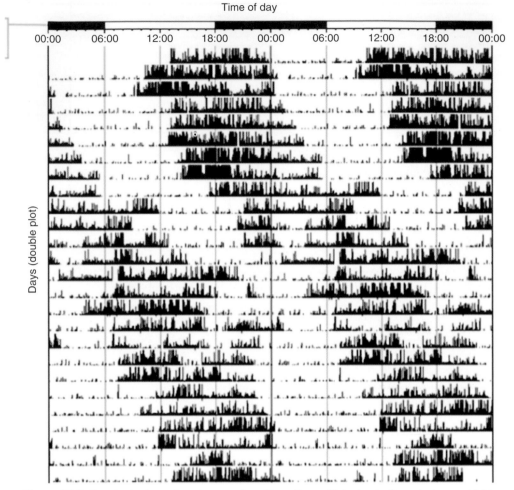

• **Figure 29.5** Twenty-six-day actigraphy recording. (From Dagan Y, Ayalon L. Case study: psychiatric misdiagnosis of non-24-hours sleep wake schedule disorder resolved by melatonin. *J Am Acad Child Adolesc Psychiatry*. 2005;44[12]:1271–1275.)

16. A 53-year-old airline pilot was diagnosed with OSA last year and has been on continuous positive airway pressure (CPAP) therapy for the past 13 months. He reports using CPAP nightly. Prior to his diagnosis and treatment, he reported significant daytime sleepiness reflected in an Epworth Sleepiness Scale (ESS) score of 18 out of 24. His ESS is now 5. However, you would like to obtain more objective data regarding his ability to stay awake. What test should you order?
    A. MSLT
    B. Actigraphy for 14 days
    C. PSG to measure his sleep onset latency
    D. Maintenance of wakefulness test (MWT)

17. For patients in occupations where OSA has significant safety implications, such as pilots and truck drivers, OSA treatment is of utmost importance. According to current Federal Aviation Administration guidelines, pilots with diagnosed OSA treated with positive airway pressure (PAP) therapy must use their device at least 75% of sleep periods for a minimum average of 6 hours per sleep period. Current Federal Motor Carrier Safety Administration guidelines recommend that commercial truck drivers with diagnosed moderate to severe OSA treated with PAP therapy must use their device at least 4 hours per night on at least 70% of the nights for a minimum of 1 week.

What is the most appropriate way to determine PAP compliance in these patients?
    A. Patient reported compliance during the clinic visit
    B. PAP device download showing usage over a specified time period
    C. Patient reported compliance during the clinic visit when verified by a reliable third party such as a spouse, other family member, or caregiver
    D. Sleep logs for a specified time period with patient documentation of PAP usage along with sleep duration

18. A 67-year-old male whose only medical history is hypertension presents to your clinic with a 3-year history of abnormal behaviors in his sleep. His wife says he starts to groan in his sleep and then seems to "grab at the air." On rare occasions he has unknowingly hit his wife in his sleep, and once even lunged out of bed while yelling, "Stop!" His wife is typically able to awaken him during these episodes, and he describes vivid dreams of being chased or threatened by people. These events typically happen toward the end of the night, with increased frequency over the past 6 months. What finding on PSG would confirm the diagnosis?
    A. Increased periodic limb movement index as measured by anterior tibialis electromyography (EMG)

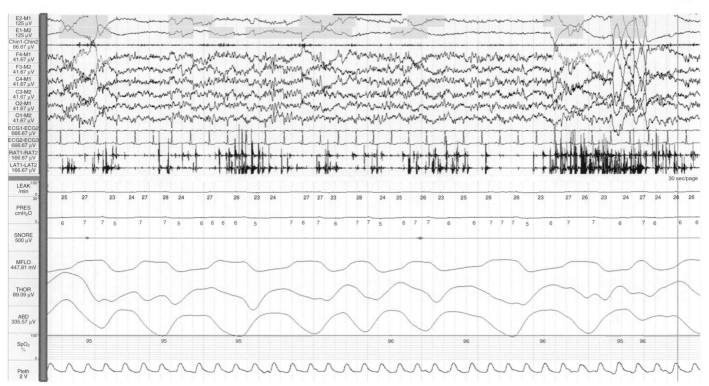

• **Figure 29.6** Thirty-second epoch of the patient's polysomnogram. *ABD*, Abdominal respiratory inductance plethysmography (RIP); *C4-M1/C3-M2*, right/left central electroencephalogram (EEG); *Chin1-Chin2*, submental electromyogram (EMG); *E2-M1/E1-M2*, right/left electro-oculogram; *ECG1-ECG2/ECG2-ECG3*, electrocardiogram; *F4-M1/F3-M2*, right/left frontal EEG; *LAT1-LAT2/RAT1-RAT2*, left/right anterior tibialis EMG; *LEAK*, mask leak; *M1/M2*, mastoid referential leads; *MFLO*, airflow derived from pressure signal; *O2-M1/O1/M2*, right/left occipital EEG; *Pleth*, plethysmography; *PRES*, CPAP pressure; *SpO₂*, oxygen saturation; *THOR*, thoracic RIP.

B. Spike-and-wave activity in the frontal EEG leads

C. Signs of autonomic arousal including mydriasis, tachycardia, and diaphoresis

D. Sustained muscle activity in REM sleep in the chin EMG

E. Shortened REM latency with increased REM duration and density

19. A 66-year-old woman with OSA presents to the sleep laboratory for her titration study. The following is observed during the study (Fig. 29.6), and the associated video shows the patient flailing and "punching" both arms while yelling incomprehensibly. What disorder is this patient most at risk to develop?
    A. Parkinson's disease
    B. Vascular dementia
    C. Multiple sclerosis
    D. Myasthenia gravis
    E. Amyotrophic lateral sclerosis

20. The parents of a 4-year-old girl bring her to the pediatric sleep medicine clinic because of disturbing nighttime events. A few nights per week, the girl starts screaming about 60 min after going to bed. When her parents enter the room, she is usually sitting up in bed with her eyes open. She is sweating, her heart is racing, and her breathing is very rapid. She becomes very agitated when they try to console her. Episodes typically last between 5 min and 10 min, after which the girl seems to calm down and falls back asleep. She does not remember these events in the morning. She is otherwise healthy with normal developmental milestones and no evidence of daytime sleepiness or impairment. She has no symptoms of or risk factors for SDB or sleep-related movement disorders. Which diagnostic procedure is indicated in this patient?
    A. EEG
    B. PSG
    C. Serum ferritin level
    D. HLA-DQB1*0602 genotyping
    E. No testing is indicated at this time

21. A 46-year-old woman reports a 10-year history of abnormal sensations in her legs that occur mostly in the evening when she is trying to fall asleep. She describes the sensations as "crawling" in her calves with a strong urge to move her legs. If she stands up and walks around, she gets immediate relief, but the symptoms recur when she lies down. The symptoms are progressively worsening and disrupting her sleep. Her neurologic exam is normal and she has no significant past medical history. Which laboratory test should you order?
    A. Serum magnesium
    B. Liver function tests
    C. Arterial blood gas (ABG)
    D. Serum iron studies

22. A 10-year-old female has overnight PSG due to EDS. She has a history of "growing pains" but does not report any other health issues. What is the primary PSG finding identified by the arrows in Fig. 29.7?
    A. Obstructive hypopneas
    B. Bruxism
    C. Periodic limb movements of sleep (PLMS)
    D. Non-specific arousals

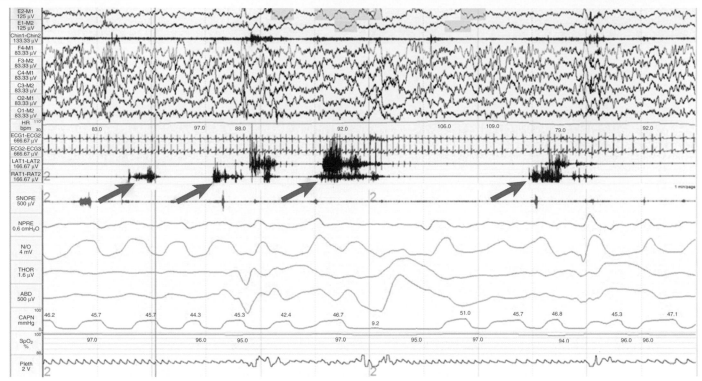

• **Figure 29.7** Thirty-second epoch from the patient's polysomnogram. *ABD*, Abdominal respiratory inductance plethysmography (RIP); *C4-M1/C3-M2*, right/left central electroencephalogram (EEG); *CAPN*, capnogram; *Chin1-Chin2*, submental electromyogram (EMG); *E2-M1/E1-M2*, right/left electro-oculogram; *ECG1-ECG2/ECG2-ECG3*, electrocardiogram; *F4-M1/F3-M2*, right/left frontal EEG; *HR*, heart rate; *LAT1-LAT2/RAT1-RAT2*, left/right anterior tibialis EMG; *M1/M2*, mastoid referential leads; *N/O*, oronasal thermistor; *NPRE*, nasal pressure transducer; *O2-M1/O1-M2*, right/left occipital EEG; *Pleth*, plethysmography; *SpO2*, oxygen saturation; *THOR*, thoracic RIP.

23. A 54-year-old obese hypertensive female has a long history of loud snoring, observed pauses in her breathing at night, and significant daytime sleepiness. During her home sleep apnea test (HSAT), the respiratory pattern in Fig. 29.8 is observed. What is required to score these respiratory events as obstructive apneas?
    A. An associated desaturation of ≥3%
    B. A drop in peak signal excursion by ≥90%
    C. A drop in peak signal excursion by ≥30%
    D. A duration of drop in sensor signal by ≥5 sec

24. A 45-year-old obese male presents with 5 years of loud snoring that progressively worsened with 50-pound weight gain. His wife has seen him stop breathing in his sleep, with several occasions during which he awakened gasping for air with associated palpitations and night sweats. His sleep is not refreshing, he feels sleepy throughout the day, and he frequently dozes while at his desk at work. He was involved in a minor motor vehicle accident when he fell asleep while driving and ran into a street sign. His physical exam is notable for a body mass index (BMI) of 39 kg/m^2, crowded oral airway with an inability to visualize the soft palate or uvula, neck circumference of 18.5 inches, and mild pitting edema in the bilateral lower extremities. He has a history of hypertension treated with four antihypertensive medications, diabetes, and hyperlipidemia. You order HSAT, which shows an apnea-hypopnea index (AHI) of 3 per hour with oxygen saturation mean of 90.5% and nadir of 88%. According to current clinical guidelines, what is the appropriate next step?

A. Pursue in-laboratory PSG.
B. No further testing is necessary as negative HSAT is adequate to confidently rule out sleep apnea in this patient.
C. Repeat HSAT.
D. Perform overnight oximetry for three consecutive nights to further screen for SDB.
E. Given the likelihood of a false negative test, start the patient on empiric CPAP given the high pretest probability of OSA.

25. Two methods for monitoring respiratory effort during PSG are currently recommended by the AASM. You are very familiar with one of these methods, dual thoracoabdominal respiratory inductance plethysmography (RIP), as this is routinely used in PSG. What is the other recommended method of measuring respiratory effort?
    A. Intercostal EMG
    B. Suprasternal pressure monitoring
    C. End-tidal CO$_2$ monitoring
    D. Esophageal pressure manometry
    E. Midsagittal jaw movement analysis

26. During your rotation in the pediatric sleep medicine clinic, you become familiar with the scoring rules for respiratory events in children and realize, to your chagrin, that there are some differences in the rules between adults and children. What is necessary to score a hypopnea in a child on PSG?
    A. A drop in peak signal excursion by ≥50% of the pre-event baseline
    B. A ≥4% oxygen desaturation associated with the event

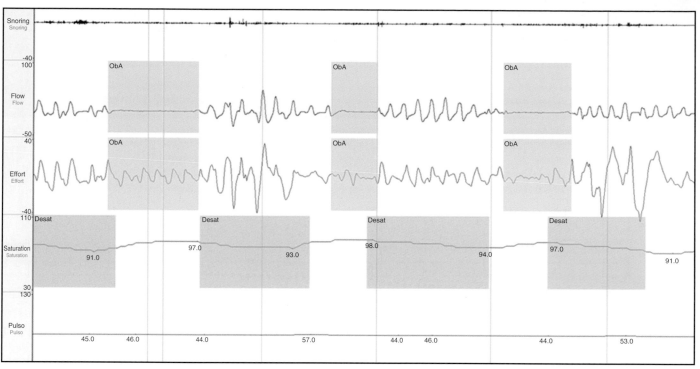

• **Figure 29.8** This home sleep apnea test segment shows six 30-sec epochs delineated by vertical gray lines. *Desat,* Desaturation; *ObA,* obstructive apnea.

C. A duration of ≥2 breaths

D. Snoring during the event

E. Thoracoabdominal paradox during the event

27. You are reviewing the PSG of a 65-year-old male. He has been experiencing significant daytime sleepiness and fatigue. He lives alone and no one routinely observes his sleep to determine if he snores. He complains of frequent nighttime awakenings and occasionally feels short of breath when he awakens. On physical exam his BMI is 23 kg/m², neck circumference is 14 inches, and he has a Mallampati Class II oral airway. Fig. 29.9 is an example from his PSG that is reflective of his breathing much of the night. What clinical condition is most likely in this patient?

A. High-dose opioid pain medication

B. Poorly controlled hypertension

C. Multiple system atrophy

D. Type 2 diabetes

E. Congestive heart failure

28. You are seeing a 48-year-old female who has a history of extremely loud snoring and progressively worsening hypersomnolence. She recently lost her job because she was frequently late to work. Even when she made it to work, she was found asleep at her desk multiple times over the course of the past few months. She has type 2 diabetes, hyperlipidemia, and hypertension. She takes medications for these conditions, is not on any other medications or supplements, and does not use any illicit substances or drink alcohol. She does not have any other pertinent medical history. She is 5 foot 8 inches tall and weighs 296 pounds, with a BMI of 45 kg/m². Recent pulmonary function tests revealed no abnormality. You are concerned that she may have obesity hypoventilation syndrome (OHS). What test is necessary to establish this diagnosis?

A. PSG to determine if her AHI is ≥5 per hour

B. ABG with a partial pressure of carbon dioxide ($PaCO_2$) greater than 45 mmHg

C. Overnight pulse oximetry that demonstrates a baseline oxygen saturation of 87%

D. Basic metabolic panel with a serum bicarbonate greater than 27 mEq/L

E. Complete blood count to determine if the hematocrit is greater than 55%

29. You are asked to consult on a newborn girl with cyanosis, breath-holding spells, and feeding difficulties. The baby was born full term at 40 weeks following an uncomplicated pregnancy and delivery. The baby has been hypoxemic since birth despite normal appearance, and the hypoxemia worsens during sleep. Her chest x-ray shows no clear cause for hypoxemia. ABG is notable for a $PaCO_2$ of 46 mmHg while the baby is awake. You request a repeat ABG while she is sleeping that demonstrates a $PaCO_2$ of 61 mmHg. What would you expect to find on further testing?

A. HLA-DQB1*0602 positivity

B. Serum ferritin level of 10 ng/mL

C. PHOX2B gene mutation

D. D178N PRNP gene mutation

Answers

1. **The correct answer is A.**

Out-of-phase deflections regardless of which direction the patient looks. The eye has a corneoretinal potential difference, with the retina being negative with respect to the cornea. Thus as the eye moves, the EOG tracing reflects this movement. The AASM recommended electrode position for E1 is 1 cm

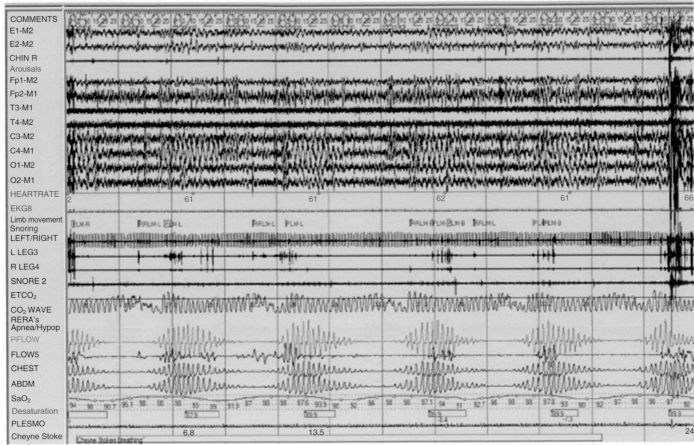

• **Figure 29.9** A 6-min segment from the patient's polysomnogram with vertical red lines delineating 30-sec epochs. *ABDM*, Abdominal respiratory inductance plethysmography (RIP); *C3-M2/C4-M1*, left/right central electroencephalogram (EEG); *CHEST*, thoracic RIP; *CHIN R*, submental electromyogram (EMG); *E1-M2/E2-M2*, left/right electro-oculogram; *EKG*, electrocardiogram; *ETCO₂*, end tidal carbon dioxide; *Fp1-M2/Fp2-M1*, left/right frontal polar EEG; *L LEG3/R LEG4*, left/right anterior tibialis EMG; *M1/M2*, mastoid referential leads; *O1-M2/O2-M1*, left/right occipital EEG; *PLESMO*, plethysmography; *RERA's*, respiratory effort-related arousals; *SaO₂*, oxygen saturation; *T3-M1/T4-M2*, left/right temporal EEG. (From Castriotta RJ, Majid R. Complex sleep apnea. *Sleep Med Clin.* 2013;8[4]:463–475.)

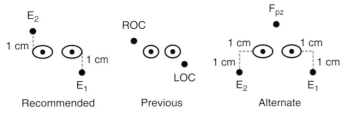

• **Figure 29.10** Recommended, previous, and alternate eye movement electrode positions. *LOC,* Left outer canthus; *ROC,* right outer canthus. (From Berry RB. Sleep stages and basic sleep monitoring. In: Goolsby J, Pritchard J, eds. *Fundamentals of Sleep Medicine.* Philadelphia, PA: Saunders Elsevier; 2012:1–11.)

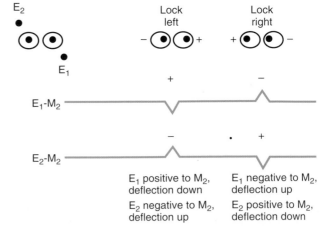

below the left outer canthus and for E2 is 1 cm above the right outer canthus (Fig. 29.10).[1] Because the electrodes are offset horizontally and vertically, eye movements in any direction will result in out-of-phase deflection (Fig. 29.11). Choice B is incorrect because this would require both electrodes be placed in the same location relative to each eye. Choice C is incorrect because this would reflect electrode placement in which each lead is placed lateral to and below the outer canthus

• **Figure 29.11** Schematic showing deflections in E1-M2 and E2-M2 from eye movements. (From Berry RB. Sleep stages and basic sleep monitoring. In: Goolsby J, Pritchard J, eds. *Fundamentals of Sleep Medicine.* Philadelphia, PA: Saunders Elsevier; 2012:1–11.)

of the respective eye. This is an alternate and acceptable, but not the recommended, placement of EOG leads. Choice D is wrong because this would reflect placement of both leads lateral to only one eye with one lead above and one lead below the eye.

2. **The correct answer is C. F3, F4, C3, C4, O1, O2.**

These leads represent frontal (F3, F4), central (C3, C4), and occipital (O1, O2) derivations, which are required and optimal to stage sleep (Fig. 29.12). K-complexes and slow wave activity are best seen in the frontal leads, sleep spindles are best seen in the central leads, and the alpha rhythm (posterior dominant rhythm) is best seen in the occipital leads. The recommended EEG derivations are F4-M1, C4-M1, and O2-M1, with backup electrodes placed at F3, C3, O1, and M2 to allow for display of F3-M2, C3-M2, and O1-M2 if the primary electrodes malfunction. An acceptable alternative to the recommended

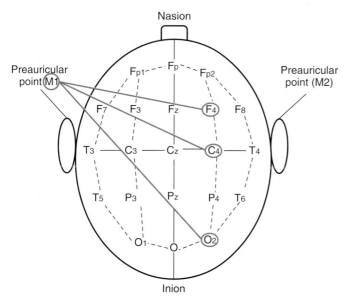

Nasion

Inion

• **Figure 29.12** Electrode placement in the 10–20 EEG system. Measurements are made at 10% and 20% from nasion to inion, between the preauricular points, and around the circumference of the head. Measurements from the nasion, inion, and bilateral preauricular points to the closest electrode are 10%, as are measurements from Fp to Fp1 and Fp2 and O to O1 and O2. All other measurements are 20%. The recommended derivations for polysomnography recording are F4-M1, C4-M1, and O2-M1, as indicated in red. (From Watson NF. Genetics of electroencephalography during wakefulness and sleep. *Sleep Med Clin*. 2011;6[2]: 155–169.)

EEG derivation is Fz-Cz, Cz-Oz, and C4-M1, with backup electrodes at Fpz, C3, O1, and M2 to allow for substitution of Fpz for Fz, C3 for Cz or C4, O1 for Oz, and M2 for M1 if the primary electrodes malfunction.[1] Temporal and parietal electrodes are not used in either the recommended or acceptable positions for electrode placement, so choices A, B, D, and E are incorrect.

3. **The correct answer is D.**

Greater than or equal to 20% of the epoch must consist of the characteristic waveform. The stage of sleep represented is stage N3 sleep, which typically comprises 10%–15% of TST and is predominantly seen during the first half of the night. This stage of sleep is also referred to as slow wave sleep, deep sleep, or delta sleep. In order to score an epoch as stage N3 sleep, at least 20% of the epoch must consist of slow wave activity, defined as waves of frequency 0.5–2 Hz with peak-to-peak amplitude greater than 75 µV, measured over the frontal regions.[1] Choice A is incorrect because, although sleep spindles are characteristic of stage N2 sleep, these may persist in stage N3 sleep. Choice B is incorrect because the previously used Rechtschaffen and Kales nomenclature of stage 4 sleep required greater than 50% of the epoch to consist of delta waves, but this scoring criteria is obsolete.[2] Choice C is incorrect because slow wave activity is best seen over the frontal leads. Choice E describes sawtooth waves, seen in REM sleep, and is therefore incorrect.

4. **The correct answer is C, 30.**

The patient described has clinical features of narcolepsy. One of the objective features of narcolepsy is early onset REM sleep, and a REM latency of less than 15 min on PSG is considered a SOREMP for diagnostic purposes (Fig. 29.13),[3] making it important to correctly identify REM latency on the PSG. REM sleep (stage R sleep) is characterized by the presence of REMs at any position within the epoch, low chin EMG tone, and low-amplitude, mixed-frequency (LAMF) EEG activity without K-complexes or sleep spindles. In the previous example, all of these features are present in epoch 32, so this epoch is considered definite stage R. However, preceding and contiguous epochs of sleep can also be considered as stage R if all of the following are present: the EEG shows LAMF without K-complexes or sleep spindles, the chin EMG tone is low at stage R level, there is no intervening arousal, and there is an absence of slow eye movements following an arousal or stage W.[1] Epochs 30 and 31 both meet these criteria, and since epoch 30 is the earliest epoch to meet these criteria, this is the correct answer. This means the REM latency is 14.5 min, meeting criteria for a SOREMP. Epoch 28 is stage

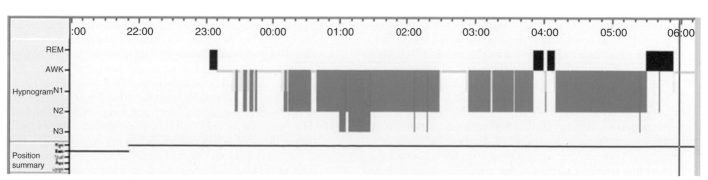

• **Figure 29.13** An example of a sleep onset rapid eye movement (REM) period on the hypnogram of a patient's polysomnogram. *AWK*, Awake.

N2 sleep because of a K complex in the first half of the epoch and a subsequent sleep spindle, and epoch 29 is also stage N2 sleep because of a K complex the second half of the epoch. If the K complex in epoch 29 were in the first half of the epoch, this epoch would be scored stage R.

5. **The correct answer is B.**
Nasal pressure transducer. Although the oronasal thermal airflow sensor is the recommended sensor for detecting apneas, when this is either not functioning or not reliable, the nasal pressure transducer is a recommended alternative for scoring apneas. The same criteria apply for scoring apneas in this situation, as when using the oronasal thermal airflow sensor: there must be a drop in peak signal excursion by ≥90% of pre-event baseline, and the duration of the drop in signal excursion must be ≥10 sec. Additional alternative measures that can be used in this situation include RIP sum or flow, or polyvinylidene fluoride (PVDF) sum.[1] Choice A is incorrect because esophageal manometry is used to monitor respiratory effort, not airflow or lack thereof. Choice C is incorrect because transcutaneous CO_2 is used to detect CO_2 levels in suspected hypoventilation. Choice D is incorrect because apneas can still be scored in this situation using one of the alternative measures detailed previously.

6. **The correct answer is A.**
Check her medication list for benzodiazepines. Beyond identifying electrographic seizure activity and allowing for staging of sleep, features seen on the EEG can provide insight into other aspects of a patient's clinical history. This EEG demonstrates excess beta activity, which is a well-known effect of benzodiazepine and barbiturate medications.[4] Correct identification of excess beta activity and distinction from epileptiform abnormalities has diagnostic and treatment implications. Choice B is incorrect because no specific EEG finding is associated with Chiari malformation. Choice C is incorrect because the excess beta activity pictured does not represent seizure activity. Choice D is incorrect because this EEG does not demonstrate triphasic waves, which can be seen in various encephalopathies including hepatic encephalopathy, in which case liver function tests would be warranted.

7. **The correct answer is E.**
Apply a notch filter. This is an example of 60-Hz artifact. Electrical outlets in the United States are at a 60-Hz frequency, and this frequency can intrude into PSG recording. Causes of this type of artifact include a bad ground, a broken or disconnected wire, poor electrode contact with high impedance levels, and interference from external equipment. Applying a notch filter can often eliminate this artifact and would be the appropriate next step.[5] Choice A is unnecessary at this time because this is not a problem with the computer and there are simpler options to try first. Choice B is incorrect because this would be a consideration if mu waves were present, which is not the case here. Mu waves occur in the 8–13-Hz alpha frequency, are typically recorded from central electrodes over the motor cortex, and are suppressed with voluntary movement.[4] Choice C is incorrect because this artifact will persist until other measures are taken. Choice D can be considered if the artifact persists despite application of a notch filter. If the artifact is only present in specific leads, those leads should be reapplied. If the artifact is only present in leads connected to a particular reference electrode, that reference electrode should be reapplied. If the artifact is present in all leads, multiple or all leads may need to be reapplied.

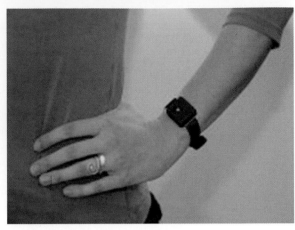

• **Figure 29.14** One example of an actigraph unit. Actigraphs are small, lightweight recorders worn on the wrist of the nondominant hand that record movement-induced accelerations to document rest-activity cycles. (From Wirz-Justice A, Bromundt V, Cajochen C. Circadian disruption and psychiatric disorders: the importance of entrainment. *Sleep Med Clin.* 2009;4[2]:273–284.)

8. **The correct answer is B.**
Sleep logs for at least 7 days that include school days and free days. This patient meets multiple diagnostic criteria for DSWPD, including complaints of an inability to fall asleep and difficulty awakening at a desired clock time, presence of symptoms for at least 3 months, improvement in sleep when allowed to sleep according to his delayed sleep preference on the weekends, and the absence of other disorders to explain his sleep disturbance. According to the ICSD-3, the only additional criteria necessary to confirm a diagnosis of DSWPD is sleep logs for at least 7 days (preferably 14 days) that demonstrate a delay in his sleep timing. This must include both school/work days and free days. Actigraphy (Fig. 29.14) is preferable whenever possible but is not mandatory.[6,7] Choice A is incorrect because although individuals with DSWPD may have increased rates of mood disorders, the presence of such is not necessary for diagnosis. Choice C is incorrect because a response to treatment is not necessary for diagnosis. Choices D and E are incorrect because although scoring as an evening type on the MEQ and demonstrating a delay in DLMO are helpful in confirming a diagnosis, they are not necessary.

9. **The correct answer is C, 14.**
This figure is representative of non-24-hour sleep-wake rhythm disorder (N24SWD), also referred to as free-running disorder. This may be seen in those with dementia or developmental disabilities, but most individuals with this disorder are totally blind, with loss of functional circadian photoreception. Their circadian pacemaker is not entrained to the solar day-night cycle, and their non-24-hour period is typically longer than 24 hours. According to current ICSD-3 diagnostic criteria, sleep logs *and* actigraphy must be done for at least 14 days to demonstrate a pattern of sleep and wake times that typically delay each day in N24SWD. In blind persons, recording for longer than 14 days is preferable but not required. Choice B is incorrect because the minimum recording duration is 7 days in delayed and advanced sleep-wake phase disorders as well as irregular sleep-wake rhythm disorder, although 14 days is preferred; in these conditions, actigraphy is not required in

addition to sleep logs. Shift work disorder requires sleep logs for a minimum of 14 days with concurrent actigraphy whenever possible.[8] Choices A, D, and E are incorrect because 5, 21, and 28 days are not the recommended minimum duration for actigraphy to confirm a diagnosis of N24SWD.

10. **The correct answer is D.**
Significant underestimation of TST reported by the patient compared with PSG recording of TST. This is a characteristic presentation for a patient with paradoxical insomnia, a subtype of chronic insomnia previously called "sleep state misperception." Despite severe subjective sleep disturbances, these patients have no objective evidence of sleep disturbance and perceive being awake much of the time they are actually asleep.[9] Choice A is incorrect because these patients typically overestimate their sleep onset latency and may underestimate their TST by at least 50% when compared with PSG measurements.[10] Choice B is incorrect. In normal sleep, the first REM period is typically the shortest, with subsequent REM periods progressively longer in duration; reversal of this pattern may be seen in depression but not specifically in insomnia disorders. Choice C is incorrect because sleep-onset REM sleep is a feature of narcolepsy and not paradoxical insomnia.

11. **The correct answer is E.**
CSF hypocretin-1 levels. This patient has clinical features of narcolepsy type 1 (previously narcolepsy with cataplexy). Narcolepsy type 1 is caused by hypocretin deficiency, defined as CSF levels ≤110 pg/mL or less than 1/3 of mean control values, and this is highly specific and sensitive for narcolepsy type 1. Although MSLT is routinely performed to diagnose narcolepsy, medications that influence sleep, including REM-suppressing antidepressant medications, must be discontinued for at least 14 days (or at least 5 times the half-life of the drug) to get reliable results. If this is not possible CSF hypocretin-1 testing is appropriate.[3] HLA DQB1*0602, not HLA DQB1*0601, is associated with narcolepsy type 1, so choice A is incorrect. In fact HLA DQB1*0601 is protective in the setting of HLA DQB1*0602.[11] Narcolepsy is not associated with serum ferritin levels, so choice B is incorrect. Choice C is incorrect because even if cataplexy is reported, an MSLT or CSF hypocretin-1 testing is necessary to confirm the diagnosis. RWA is a feature of REM sleep behavior disorder (RBD), and although this is seen in increased frequency in narcolepsy type 1, it is not necessary for diagnosis, so choice D is incorrect.

12. **The correct answer is B.**
A REM latency of 10 min. In testing for both narcolepsy type 1 (with cataplexy) and narcolepsy type 2 (without cataplexy), SOREMPs are an important objective finding. Two or more SOREMPs are required, in addition to a mean sleep latency ≤8 min on MSLT, to establish a diagnosis of narcolepsy. Although previous diagnostic criteria only considered SOREMP during the MSLT, updated criteria in the ICSD-3 allow for a SOREMP (within 15 min of sleep onset) on the preceding nocturnal polysomnogram to replace one of the SOREMPs on the MSLT.[3] This is based on data suggesting that a short REM latency (≤15 min) on PSG has a greater than 99% specificity for narcolepsy, but the sensitivity for this finding is low.[12] Therefore choice B is correct, and choice D is incorrect. Choice A is incorrect because there is no specific requirement in the diagnosis of narcolepsy regarding REM sleep duration. RBD is seen in increased frequency in narcolepsy, but it is not part of

the diagnostic criteria, so choice C is incorrect. Choice E is incorrect for two reasons: although short sleep latency on PSG is typical in narcolepsy, it is not part of the diagnostic criteria; and although a REM latency of 45 min is shorter than normal, it does not meet diagnostic criteria for a SOREMP as defined previously.

13. **The correct answer is A.**
The patient must be free of drugs that influence sleep for at least 14 days prior to the MSLT. Factors that can impact the results of the MSLT include, but are not limited to, insufficient sleep, sedating or stimulating medications/substances, drugs that suppress REM sleep (most antidepressants, antipsychotics, some antiepileptics, first-generation antihistamines, beta blockers, benzodiazepines, barbiturates), irregular and/or variable sleep schedules, circadian factors, and other sleep disorders (i.e., SDB, PLMD). To obtain reliable MSLT results, these confounding factors must be eliminated or ruled out. The patient must be free of drugs that influence sleep for at least 14 days, or at least 5 times the half-life of the drug and longer-acting metabolite, confirmed by a urine drug screen. This includes stimulants, stimulant-like medications, and REM-suppressing medications. Nocturnal PSG should be performed the night immediately preceding the MSLT to exclude other sleep disorders and also to ensure adequate sleep time with a goal of at least 6 hours of sleep, so choices B and D are incorrect. The sleep-wake schedule must be standardized to a minimum of 7 hours in bed each night for at least seven days before the PSG and MSLT, so choice C is incorrect. The sleep schedule should be documented by sleep log, preferably with concurrent actigraphy.[3,13]

14. **The correct answer is C, 8 min.**
This patient has typical clinical features of idiopathic hypersomnia (IH), including EDS for at least 3 months, the absence of cataplexy, long unrefreshing naps, and prolonged nighttime sleep. Patients with IH typically have high sleep efficiency on PSG, with a normal REM latency and normal proportions of nonrapid eye movement (NREM) and REM sleep. Objective findings to confirm a diagnosis of IH include a mean sleep latency of ≤8 min on MSLT and/or a total 24-hour sleep time (including nighttime sleep and daytime naps) of ≥660 minutes. This total 24-hour sleep time can be confirmed by 24-hour PSG monitoring or actigraphy in association with a sleep log over 7 or more days of unrestricted sleep.[14] When calculating the mean sleep latency on MSLT, the sleep latency is reported as 20 min for a nap opportunity without recorded sleep.[13] Her sleep latencies are therefore 3, 20, 8, 3, and 6 min, which totals 40 min. This is then divided by 5 to give the correct mean sleep latency of 8 min. Choice A is incorrect because the mean sleep latency can be calculated even in the absence of sleep during one or more nap opportunities. Choice B is incorrect because it assigns a sleep latency of 0 min (instead of 20 min) to nap 2. Choices D and E are incorrect because they do not give the accurate mean sleep latency for this patient.

15. **The correct answer is E.**
Two weeks of sleep logs and actigraphy. The most likely diagnosis is behaviorally induced insufficient sleep syndrome (BIISS). She is only getting at most 6 hours of sleep a night and as a result is chronically sleep deprived. Features of BIISS include daytime sleepiness, insufficient sleep most days for at least 3 months, the use of an alarm clock or other measures to limit sleep time, and extension of sleep time when these

measures are not used. Objective data from actigraphy combined with sleep logs help establish the diagnosis. The duration of actigraphy and sleep logs should be at least 2 weeks to capture both work/school days and days off, and these data will reflect longer sleep time on days when sleep is not limited by external factors. Extended sleep only on the weekends is not sufficient to alleviate symptoms. However, extension of TST on a consistent basis will result in elimination of daytime sleepiness in BIISS.[15] If sleepiness persists despite adequate sleep time, other causes should then be considered. Choice A is incorrect, as this patient does not have risk factors for or symptoms of SDB to suggest the need for PSG. Choice B is incorrect because her TST would need to be normalized before a reliable MSLT could be performed. CSF hypocretin deficiency is seen in narcolepsy type 1. Aside from daytime sleepiness, no other symptoms of narcolepsy (i.e., sleep paralysis, hypnagogic hallucinations, cataplexy) are reported to indicate the need for further testing for such at this time, so choice C is incorrect. Choice D is incorrect because the clinical history does not clearly suggest a circadian rhythm sleep-wake disorder, for which salivary DLMO may provide additional information but is not a typical component of standard clinical care.

16. **The correct answer is D.**
MWT. The MWT is a validated objective measure of the ability to stay awake for a defined time and is used in association with the clinical history to assess the ability to maintain wakefulness. It can be used when a patient's ability to remain awake constitutes a public or personal safety issue (i.e., pilots and commercial truck drivers) and can also be used to assess the efficacy of treatment for hypersomnia.[16] The recommended protocol is to perform four 40-min trials at 2-hour intervals, with the first trial to start 1.5–3 hours after wake-up time. PSG the night prior is optional, as are sleep logs. Drug screening is usually performed the morning of the MWT to ensure the results are not influenced by sedating or stimulating medications/substances. Trials are ended after unequivocal sleep (three consecutive epochs of stage N1 sleep or one epoch of any other stage of sleep), or after 40 min if no sleep occurs. Mean sleep latency less than 8 min is considered abnormal. Values of 8–40 min are considered normal, but these results must be considered in the clinical context and should not be used in isolation.[13] Choice A is incorrect because the MSLT measures sleepiness and not the ability to stay awake. Choice B is incorrect because actigraphy does not provide objective data regarding the patient's ability to stay awake. Choice C is incorrect because the sleep onset latency on nocturnal PSG does not correlate with the ability to maintain wakefulness and/or alertness during the day.

17. **The correct answer is B.**
PAP device download showing usage over a specified time period. Current PAP devices allow for data to be downloaded that provide information regarding compliance (number of nights used in a defined time period, percent of nights used for ≥4 hours, average hourly usage per night), mask leak, and AHI. Fig. 29.15 shows examples of two PAP downloads showing device usage; Panel A shows many nights with suboptimal or absent usage, whereas Panel B shows nightly PAP for approximately 8–10 hours a night. Current Federal Aviation Administration guidelines require that pilots with diagnosed OSA must be compliant with PAP therapy on a cumulative annual PAP device report, with compliance defined

as device usage for at least 75% of sleep periods for a minimum average of 6 hours per sleep period. The results and interpretive report of the patient's most recent sleep study, and a signed Airman Compliance with Treatment form must also be provided.[17] Expert panel recommendations to the Federal Motor Carrier Safety Administration regarding OSA and commercial truck drivers include PAP compliance defined as device usage at least 4 hours per night on at least 70% of the nights for a minimum of 1 week. The same expert panel also recommended that commercial truck drivers with diagnosed moderate-to-severe OSA be referred to a clinician with sleep expertise, have adequate PAP therapy verified through either an in-laboratory titration study or an auto-titration system, and demonstrate resolution of excessive sleepiness when driving. No specific recommendations were made regarding how to demonstrate the resolution of excessive sleepiness when driving in these patients.[18] Choices A, C, and D are incorrect because objective compliance data is required/recommended in these situations. A patient's subjective report, even when supported by other's observations or sleep logs, is insufficient.

18. **The correct answer is D.**
Sustained muscle activity in REM sleep in the chin EMG. This patient has a clinical history suggestive of RBD. RBD is the only parasomnia for which PSG is required to establish a diagnosis. In addition to the abnormal behaviors noted in sleep, PSG recording must demonstrate RWA per ICSD-3 diagnostic criteria.[19] RWA consists of either or both of the following: sustained muscle activity in REM sleep in the chin EMG or excessive transient muscle activity during REM in the chin or limb EMG. Sustained muscle activity is defined as an epoch of REM sleep, during which at least 50% of the epoch duration shows chin EMG amplitude greater than the minimum amplitude demonstrated in NREM sleep.[1] To identify excessive transient muscle activity in REM sleep, a 30-sec epoch of REM must be divided into 10 sequential 3-sec mini-epochs, and at least 5 (50%) of these must contain bursts of transient muscle activity 0.1–5.0 sec in duration and at least 4 times as high in amplitude as the background EMG activity. This activity can be identified in the upper and/or lower extremities; when RBD is suspected, limb EMG tone should be recorded at the bilateral anterior tibialis muscles, as well as the bilateral flexor digitorum superficialis muscles.[1] Choice A is incorrect because an increased periodic limb movement index in the appropriate clinical context (distinct from the one described) would support a diagnosis of PLMD. Choice B is incorrect because spike-and-wave activity in the frontal EEG leads would suggest frontal lobe seizures. Although frontal lobe seizures are associated with unusual sleep-related behaviors, the seizure activity typically occurs in stages N1 and N2 sleep without association to REM sleep or RBD. Choice C is incorrect because signs of autonomic arousal are more common in sleep terrors than in RBD; even if present in this patient, these findings would not be fully diagnostic for RBD. Choice E is incorrect because shortened REM latency with increased REM duration and increased REM density are seen in patients with depression and are not diagnostic of RBD.[20]

19. **The correct answer is A.**
Parkinson's disease. Fig. 29.6 is an epoch of REM sleep demonstrating sustained muscle activity in the chin EMG characteristic of RWA. This finding in combination with the behavior observed during the video recording confirms the

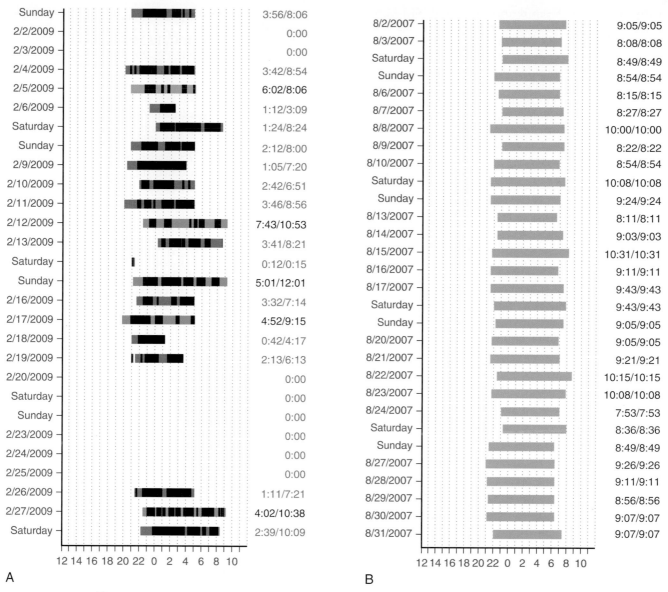

• Figure 29.15 Continuous positive airway pressure data downloads showing usage from two patients. Image A shows usage from a noncompliant patient, and image B is from a compliant patient. (Modified from King MS, Xanthopoulous MS, Marcus CL. Improving positive airway pressure adherence in children. *Sleep Med Clin.* 2014;9[2]:219–234.)

diagnosis of RBD.[19] Patients with idiopathic RBD (iRBD) are at risk to develop alpha-synucleinopathies, such as Parkinson's disease or dementia with Lewy bodies. iRBD may represent a prodromal phase of these disorders, often preceding more definite motor symptoms of these disorders by more than a decade.[21] Recent studies suggest that most patients (>80%) diagnosed with iRBD will develop a defined neurodegenerative syndrome over time, a much higher number than originally thought. The mean time from IRBD onset to neurodegenerative disease onset is a little more than 14 years.[22] Choice B is incorrect because although iRBD is associated with risk for some dementias like dementia with Lewy bodies, it is not associated with vascular dementia or cardiovascular disease. Choice C is incorrect, because although sleep disorders like RLS, insomnia, and SDB are more common in those with multiple sclerosis than the general

population, RBD is very rare. When RBD does occur, it can be an initial sign of multiple sclerosis related to brainstem lesions,[23,24] but the likelihood of RBD being associated with multiple sclerosis is much lower than the clearly defined association with alpha-synucleinopathies. Choice D is incorrect because there is no reported association of RBD with myasthenia gravis. Choice E is incorrect. It is recognized that patients with amyotrophic lateral sclerosis are at an increased risk for SDB, including nocturnal hypoventilation due to diaphragmatic weakness, but they also experience other sleep-related disorders, including RBD.[25,26] However, this association is much less than that of RBD with Parkinson's disease.

20. **The correct answer is E.**
No testing is indicated at this time. This presentation is typical of sleep terrors, also referred to as night terrors or

pavor nocturnus. Sleep terrors, a type of NREM-related parasomnia, are a disorder of arousal from stage N3 sleep most prevalent in children younger than 5 years of age. Sleep terrors typically occur during the first third to first half of the sleep period when stage N3 sleep is most prevalent. During episodes patients usually scream or cry, appear panicked, and demonstrate signs of autonomic activation including mydriasis, tachycardia, tachypnea, flushing of the skin, and diaphoresis. Patients are often found sitting in bed with their eyes open, and may thus appear awake. However, patients are unresponsive during episodes and may become more agitated when efforts are made to console them. Patients have partial or complete amnesia for the episodes, which usually last 1–10 min. For patients with sleep terrors in whom other sleep or medical disorders are not suspected, no further testing is indicated, and reassurance for the parents is appropriate as these behaviors resolve spontaneously in most children.[27,28] Choice A is incorrect because the clinical history is not characteristic of seizures and EEG is not indicated for evaluation of sleep terrors. Choice B is also incorrect, as the patient does not suggest symptoms of another sleep disorder to necessitate PSG. If PSG is done in patients with disorders of arousal, common findings include an increased number of arousals out of stage N3 sleep and increased cyclic alternating pattern rate, which is a measure of NREM instability. Choice C is incorrect as iron deficiency correlates with RLS but not NREM-related parasomnias. HLA-DQB1*0602 is associated with narcolepsy type 1 and not with sleep terrors, so choice D is incorrect.

21. **The correct answer is D.**
Serum iron studies. This woman meets diagnostic criteria for RLS, also known as Willis-Ekbom disease (WED), a neurological sensorimotor disease. The five essential diagnostic criteria for RLS/WED are: (1) an urge to move the legs usually accompanied by or thought to be caused by uncomfortable and unpleasant sensations in the legs; (2) these symptoms begin or worsen during periods of rest or inactivity, such as lying down or sitting; (3) these symptoms are partially or totally relieved by movement, such as walking or stretching, at least as long as the activity continues; (4) these symptoms only occur or are worse in the evening or night rather than during the day; and (5) these symptoms are not solely accounted for as symptoms primary to another medical or behavioral condition (e.g., leg cramps, myalgia, venous stasis, leg edema, arthritis, positional discomfort, habitual foot tapping). The diagnosis is based purely on clinical symptoms and no confirmatory testing is necessary, although the presence of PLMS on PSG is supportive of the diagnosis. Precipitating factors for RLS/WED include iron deficiency, certain medications, pregnancy, chronic renal failure, and prolonged immobility, with iron deficiency being the best characterized precipitating factor. Iron is a cofactor for the synthesis of tyrosine hydroxylase, which is the rate-limiting step in the synthesis of dopamine. Brain iron deficiency is the most consistent finding in studies of RLS/WED pathology. Central nervous system dopaminergic system involvement is suspected based on the clinical efficacy of dopaminergic drugs in treating RLS/WED, but the exact association remains unclear. Serum ferritin levels below 50 ng/mL have been associated with an increased severity of RLS/WED, and iron replacement to levels above 50–75 ng/mL can diminish RLS/WED symptoms.[29,30] Choices A, B, and C are incorrect, because these tests have no identified role in the evaluation of patients with RLS/WED.

22. **The correct answer is C, PLMS.**
PLMS are prominent in Fig. 29.7 and are evident in both the left and right anterior tibialis muscles. PLMS typically involve extension of the big toe along with flexion of the ankle, knee, and occasionally hip. An individual leg movement lasts 0.5–10 sec, with at least an 8-μV increase in EMG above the resting baseline. To be classified as PLMS, there must be a minimum of four consecutive such movements with a period length of 5–90 sec. If leg movements occur in different legs within 5 sec of each other, they are counted as a single leg movement.[1] PLMS frequently occur in children and adults with RLS/WED, with estimates between 70% and 90% in such patients.[31] In children, RLS/WED is often attributed to "growing pains," as noted in this case. Choice A is incorrect, as the arrows are pointing to PLMS and not to any respiratory abnormalities. Choice B is incorrect. Bruxism is tooth grinding and consists of brief or sustained elevations of chin EMG activity at least twice the background EMG amplitude. There are either three such elevations of 0.25–2-sec duration occurring in regular sequence, or sustained elevation longer than 2 sec.[1] In the example, there is a clear increase in chin EMG, but this is related to a PLM arousal. Choice D is incorrect because the arousals displayed appear related to the preceding PLMS.

23. **The correct answer is B.**
A drop in peak signal excursion by ≥90%. The respiratory events seen here are obstructive apneas. There are two criteria to score a respiratory event as an apnea on HSAT: there must be a drop in peak signal excursion by ≥90% of the pre-event baseline using a recommended or alternative airflow sensor, and the duration of the ≥90% drop in sensor signal must be ≥10 sec. Recommended sensors include oronasal thermal airflow sensors and nasal pressure transducers; alternative sensors include RIP sum or flow and PVDF sum. If the apnea is associated with continued or increased inspiratory effort throughout the entire period of absent airflow, the event is scored as an obstructive apnea. If there is absent inspiratory effort throughout the entire period of absent airflow, the event is scored as a central apnea, and if there is absent inspiratory effort in the initial portion of the event followed by resumption of inspiratory effort in the second portion of the event, the event is scored as a mixed apnea.[1] Choice A is incorrect because there is no desaturation requirement to score apneas. Choice C is incorrect because this is referring to the scoring criteria for hypopneas, in which there must be a drop in peak signal excursion by ≥30% of pre-event baseline using a recommended or alternative sensor. This drop in signal excursion must last ≥10 sec and be associated with greater than 3% oxygen desaturation from pre-event baseline. Choice D is incorrect, because in order to score any respiratory event in adults, it must have a duration of ≥10 sec.

24. **The correct answer is A.**
Pursue in-laboratory PSG. HSAT (Fig. 29.16) is increasingly utilized, driven by increasing evidence of its utility, economic pressures, long wait times for in-lab testing, and evolving insurance policies.[32] Clinical guidelines from the Portable Monitoring Task Force of the AASM state that this testing may be used for the diagnosis of OSA in patients, with a high pretest probability of moderate to severe OSA. These same guidelines also indicate that negative or technically inadequate HSAT in this population should prompt in-laboratory PSG.

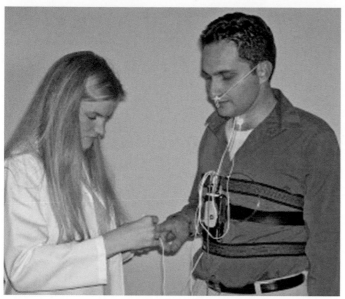

• **Figure 29.16** An illustration of a home sleep apnea testing device that measures airflow, respiratory effort, oxygen saturation, and heart rate. (From Patel MR, Davidson TM. Home sleep testing in the diagnosis and treatment of sleep disordered breathing. *Otolaryngol Clin North Am.* 2007;40[4]:761–784.)

Choice B is incorrect, as false negative rates in HSAT may be as high as 17%, indicating the need for further testing in a patient with high pretest probability of OSA and negative HSAT.[33] Potential causes of false negative HSAT include technical failure of the equipment, potential discrepancy between recording time and actual sleep time, and night-to-night variability in sleep-related breathing. Choice C is incorrect, as current guidelines do not recommend repeat HSAT but rather to proceed with in-lab testing. Choice D is incorrect, as serial overnight oximetry is not an accepted diagnostic modality for OSA; even if overnight oximetry results are abnormal, in-laboratory testing would then be indicated based on current guidelines. Choice E is incorrect, because even in patients with a high pretest probability of OSA, objective confirmation of the diagnosis is appropriate before initiating therapy.

25. **The correct answer is D.**

Esophageal pressure manometry. Esophageal pressure (Pes) manometry is a recommended method and is actually the current gold standard for monitoring respiratory effort. Its clinical use is limited because of its invasive nature and concerns about the possibility that the Pes probe could modify pharyngeal dynamics, so noninvasive thoracoabdominal plethysmography is used routinely in clinical practice. Pes manometry involves the use of air-filled balloon-tip catheters, fluid-filled catheters, and solid-state pressure sensors in the esophagus to measure changes in esophageal pressure. Changes in Pes reflect pleural pressure changes generated by respiratory muscle force and transmitted to the esophagus and other organs within the thoracic cavity during obstructive respiratory events. Choice C is incorrect because CO_2 monitoring is a measure of ventilation and not respiratory effort. The remaining choices (choices A, B, and E) are alternative techniques for monitoring respiratory effort, but have not been validated against esophageal manometry and are therefore not currently recommended.

Intercostal EMG (choice A) involves placement of standard surface electrodes in the right anterior chest intercostal space. Comparative studies show good correspondence with diaphragmatic EMG and esophageal manometry, but comparative studies with intercostal EMG and Pes manometry are not available. Suprasternal pressure monitoring (choice B) involves placement of a pressure transducer over the trachea in the sternal notch, with changes in intrathoracic pressure during obstructive events converted to a signal of respiratory effort. Limited data suggest very good concordance with Pes manometry, but this is currently not recommended by the AASM. Midsagittal jaw movement analysis (choice E) involves measurement of the change in distance between sensors on the forehead and below the lower lip on the mandible using magnetometry. Magnetometers are sensors used to sense magnetic fields. Each sensor is composed of two coupled resonant circuits, which are connected to an electronic circuit that converts the distance between the two sensors into voltage, as output voltage is a cubic function of distance. The signal can then be displayed either in absolute value (mm) or in normalized value (percentage of mouth opening). During obstructive respiratory events, the mandible is lowered during inspiration in proportion to the inspiratory effort, possibly due to caudal traction on the central airways.[34]

26. **The correct answer is C.**

A duration of ≥2 breaths. Three criteria are required to score a respiratory event as a hypopnea in children. First, the peak signal excursion must drop by ≥30% of the pre-event baseline using nasal pressure or an alternative hypopnea sensor. This is the same scoring criteria as adults, and choice A is therefore incorrect. Second, whereas in adults hypopneas need to be at least 10 sec in duration to be scored, in children the duration needs to be that of at least two breaths during baseline breathing, so choice C is correct. Third, there must be either a ≥3% oxygen desaturation from pre-event baseline, or the event must be associated with an arousal, so choice B is incorrect.[1] Choices D and E are incorrect, because although these are features of obstructive hypopneas that can help differentiate between obstructive and central hypopneas, they are not necessary criteria for scoring these events.

27. **The correct answer is E.**

Congestive heart failure. This is a classic example of Cheyne-Stokes breathing (CSB) that can be seen as one type of central sleep apnea (CSA), in which case it is classified as CSA with CSB (CSA-CSB). In CSA-CSB three or more consecutive central apneas and/or central hypopneas are separated by a crescendo and decrescendo change in breathing amplitude. The cycle length, defined as the time from the beginning of one central apnea to the start of the next apnea, is ≥40 sec, which helps distinguish CSA-CSB from other forms of CSA with a shorter cycle length. There are ≥5 central apneas and/or central hypopneas per hour over at least 2 hours of monitoring with the CSA-CSB pattern.[1] A delay in the nadir of the associated desaturation is often seen. Arousals in CSA-CSB typically occur at the zenith of the respiratory effort, as opposed to at the resumption of respiratory effort, as is typically seen with obstructive respiratory events. The majority of patients with CSA-CSB have congestive heart failure. Among those with congestive heart failure, risk factors for CSA-CSB include male sex, age older than 60 years, concurrent atrial fibrillation, and daytime hypocapnia.[35] Choice A is incorrect, because although patients on high-dose opioid pain medication are at increased risk for CSA, the respiratory pattern is typically ataxic; periodic breathing, if it occurs, has a cycle length shorter than 40 sec and lacks the crescendo-decrescendo respiratory pattern of CSA-CSB. Choices B and D are incorrect, as these are seen with increased prevalence in OSA and are not associated with CSA-CSB. Choice C is incorrect because patients with multiple system atrophy may experience OSA and laryngeal stridor, but not CSA-CSB. These patients also have a high prevalence of RBD.

28. **The correct answer is B.**

ABG with a partial $PaCO_2$ greater than 45 mmHg. Current diagnostic criteria for OHS requires the presence of hypoventilation while awake ($PaCO_2$ >45 mmHg) among persons with obesity (BMI >30 kg/m^2) in the absence of other causes of hypoventilation.[36] In addition to an awake $PaCO_2$ level, end-tidal PCO_2 or transcutaneous PCO_2 during sleep can be measured, in which case an increase in PCO_2 during sleep greater than 10 mmHg is consistent with hypoventilation. Choice A is incorrect, because although 80%–90% of patients with OHS will also have OSA with an AHI ≥5 per hour, the presence of comorbid OSA is not necessary to diagnose OHS. Choices C and D are both incorrect, because although overnight oximetry with baseline SaO_2 of 87% and serum bicarbonate greater than 27 mEq/L are suggestive of OHS, they are not diagnostic for the disorder. Chronic hypercapnia can lead to metabolic compensation, as reflected by elevated serum bicarbonate; a serum bicarbonate level greater than 27 mEq/L has been shown to have a high sensitivity of 92%, but a low specificity of 50% to identify OHS.[37] Choice E is incorrect. Polycythemia is common in OHS but is not necessary for the diagnosis.

29. **The correct answer is C.**

PHOX2B gene mutation. The patient described has congenital central alveolar hypoventilation syndrome (CCHS), also known as Ondine's curse. CCHS is a rare syndrome of autonomic dysfunction, with the most notable feature being failure of automatic respiratory control. The prominent finding is hypoventilation during sleep; in severe cases, hypoventilation during wakefulness will also be present. Both hypoxemia and hypercapnia will be present if PSG is performed. Contrary to other types of SDB in children, hypoxemia and hypercapnia may be more severe in NREM sleep compared with REM sleep. Infants with CCHS usually present with hypoventilation at birth and may have other problems including cyanosis, feeding difficulties, hypotonia, and/or central apneas. Most infants require mechanically assisted ventilation during sleep, but some require continuous ventilatory support. CCHS is due to a mutation of the PHOX2B gene leading to polyalanine repeat abnormalities on chromosome 4p12.[38,39] Choice A is incorrect because HLA-DQB1*0602 positivity is associated with narcolepsy with cataplexy, although it can often be seen in normal subjects. Choice B is incorrect because low ferritin levels have been associated with RLS but not CCHS. Choice D is incorrect because the D178N PRNP gene mutation is seen in fatal familial insomnia.

Suggested Reading

Berry RB, Brooks R, Gamaldo CE, et al. *The AASM Manual for the Scoring of Sleep and Associated Events: Rules, Terminology and Technical Specifications, Version 2.3*. Darien, IL: American Academy of Sleep Medicine; 2015. www.aasmnet.org.

Collop NA, Anderson WM, Boehlecke B, et al. Clinical guidelines for the use of unattended portable monitors in the diagnosis of obstructive sleep apnea in adult patients. Portable Monitoring Task Force of the American Academy of Sleep Medicine. *J Clin Sleep Med.* 2007;3(7):737-747.

The International Classification of Sleep Disorders. 3rd ed. Darien, IL: American Academy of Sleep Medicine; 2014. Multiple chapters referenced.

Littner MR, Kushida C, Wise M, et al. Practice parameters for clinical use of the Multiple Sleep Latency Test and the Maintenance of Wakefulness Test: an American Academy of Sleep Medicine Report. *Sleep.* 2005;28(1):113-121.

Vendrame M, Kothare SV. Recognizing normal, abnormal, and benign nonepileptiform electroencephalographic activity and patterns in polysomnographic recordings. *Sleep Med Clin.* 2012;7(1):23-38.

30

Practice Examination—Pediatric Sleep Disorders

TIMOTHY F. HOBAN

Questions

1. A 2-week-old infant girl is referred for evaluation of episodic cyanosis and shallow, irregular respiration during sleep. Cyanosis resolves and normal respiration resumes only when the child is stimulated and arouses from sleep. The parents report no snoring and no concerning respiratory symptoms during wakefulness. The child was born at term and is otherwise healthy. Physical examination is unremarkable. Polysomnography demonstrates baseline SpO_2 levels during sleep ranging from 75% to 90% and baseline transcutaneous CO_2 levels during sleep averaging 65 mm Hg in the absence of significant obstructive sleep apnea (OSA) or central sleep apnea (CSA). Which of the following represents the most likely cause of the child's symptoms and polysomnographic findings?
   A. Trisomy 21
   B. Duchenne muscular dystrophy
   C. *PHOX2B* mutation
   D. Gastroesophageal reflux disease (GERD)
   E. Laryngotracheomalacia
2. Which of the following pediatric conditions is most consistently associated with the sleep stage illustrated in Fig. 30.1?
   A. Nightmares
   B. Sleep terrors
   C. Nocturnal seizures
   D. Sleep-related rhythmic movement disorder
   E. Bruxism
3. Which of the following statements best characterizes the relationship between snoring and OSA in children?
   A. The likelihood of OSA increases in direct proportion to the severity of snoring.
   B. The absence of snoring excludes the possibility of OSA.
   C. The frequency rather than volume of snoring correlates with the presence and severity of OSA.
   D. There is no relationship between the volume of snoring and the presence or severity of OSA.
4. A 15-year-old high school freshman with poorly controlled diabetes is referred by her pediatrician for evaluation of chronic insomnia. For the last 3 years, she reports that it takes up to 4 hours for her to fall asleep after she goes to bed. On school days, she typically retires at 10:00 PM and is usually unable to fall asleep until well after midnight. During this time, she reports that she feels "wide awake" but denies rumination or leg discomfort. Once she falls asleep, she sleeps soundly until 7:00 AM, when she struggles to awaken in time to prepare for school. On weekends and nonschool days with later bedtimes, she falls asleep more quickly, as detailed in the sleep diary outlined in Fig. 30.2. Based on this history, which of the following treatments is most likely to be effective in treating this teenager's insomnia?
   A. Trazodone 50 mg 1 hour prior to bedtime on school nights
   B. Light therapy 10,000 lux for 20 minutes upon morning waking
   C. Melatonin 10 mg 1 hour before bedtime
   D. Referral for cognitive behavioral therapy (CBT)
   E. Zolpidem 10 mg at bedtime
5. Which of the following sleep disorders is equally prevalent in preadolescent boys and girls?
   A. OSA
   B. Kleine-Levin syndrome (KLS)
   C. Sleep enuresis
   D. Sleep-related hypoventilation secondary to Duchenne muscular dystrophy
6. A 30-second epoch of sleep for a 2-week-old term infant is illustrated in Fig. 30.3. Which of the following statements is true regarding the polysomnographic findings illustrated in this epoch?
   A. The respiratory pause near the center of the epoch can be scored as an apneic event.
   B. The paradoxical abdominal and thoracic movement is abnormal for age.
   C. The epoch demonstrates normal quiet (non-REM) sleep.
   D. The epoch demonstrates normal active (REM) sleep.
7. A 2-year-old child with Down syndrome is referred for evaluation of loud snoring and gasping respiration during sleep. Examination is significant for obesity, hypotonia, macroglossia, and 2+ tonsillar hypertrophy. A polysomnogram identifies

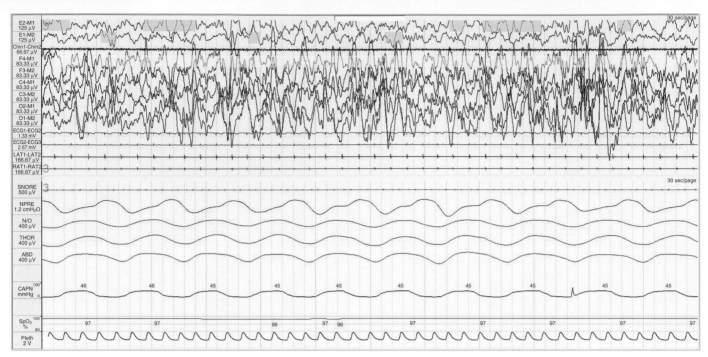

• **Figure 30.1** Thirty-second epoch of sleep. Channel legends as follows: *ABD*, Abdominal effort; *AT*, anterior tibialis electromyogram; *C*, central; *CAPN*, capnogram; *Chin*, chin electromyogram; *E*, eye; *F*, frontal; *N/O*, nasal-oral flow; *NPRE*, nasal pressure signal; *O*, occipital; *THOR*, thoracic effort.

TWO WEEK SLEEP DIARY

Instructions:
1. Write the date, day of the week, and type of day: Work, school, day off, or vacation.
2. Put the letter "C" in the box when you have coffee,cola or tea. Put "M" when you take any medicine. Put "A" when you drink alcohol. Put "E" when you exercise.
3. Put a line (I) to show when you go to bed. Shade in the box that shows when you think you fell asleep.
4. Shade in all the boxes that show when you are asleep at night or when you take a nap during the day.
5. Leave boxes unshaded to show when you wake up at night and when you are awake during the day.

Sample entry below: On a monday when i worked, i jogged on my lunch break at 1 PM, had a glass of wine with dinner at 6 PM, fell asleep watching TV from 7 to 8 PM, went to bed at 10:30 PM, fell asleep around midnight, woke up and couldn't get back to sleep at about 4 AM, went back to sleep from 5 to 7 AM, and had coffee and medicine at 7:00 in the morning.

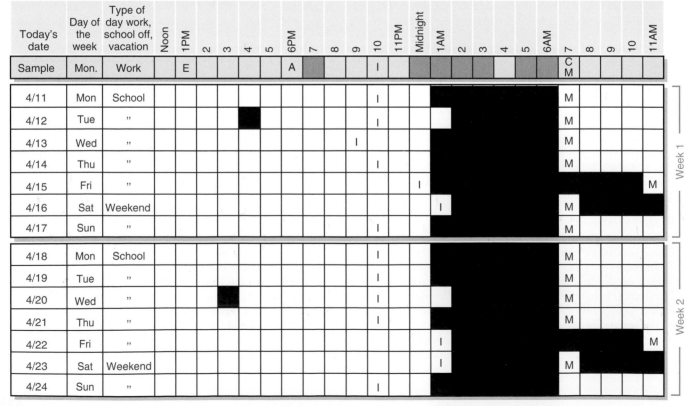

• **Figure 30.2** Sleep diary for a 15-year-old girl.

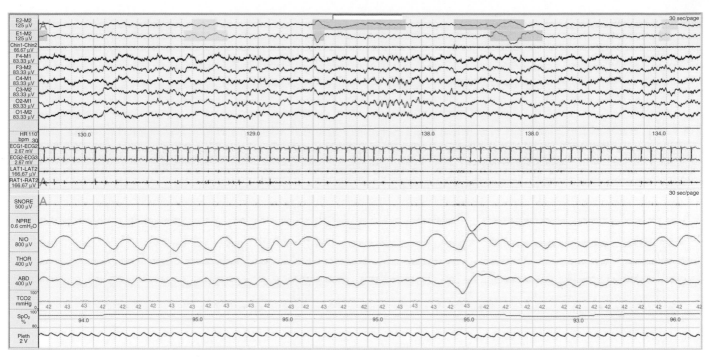

• **Figure 30.3** Thirty-second epoch of sleep in a 2-week-old term infant.

severe OSA characterized by frequent obstructive apneas and hypopneas associated with desaturations of SpO₂ to nadir levels of 75%–85%. Which of the following statements is true regarding potential treatments for this child's sleep-disordered breathing (SDB)?

A. CPAP can be started empirically at a pressure setting of 5 cm of water until the family can return to the sleep lab for a titration study.

B. The child can be empirically treated using supplemental oxygen by nasal cannula at 0.25 lpm during sleep.

C. The child may be at increased risk for respiratory complications if treated with adenotonsillectomy.

D. The child can be effectively treated using positional therapy and budesonide nasal spray administered at bedtime.

8. If polysomnograms were performed for each of the following patients, which study is likely to exhibit the highest proportion of REM (stage R) sleep compared with other stages?

A. 16-year-old boy with narcolepsy treated with modafinil

B. 7-year-old boy with no medical or sleep problems

C. 13-year-old girl with depression treated with fluoxetine

D. 7-year-old boy with untreated OSA

E. 1-month-old girl with no medical or sleep problems

9. Which of the following interventions is thought to be primarily responsible for a significant reduction in the incidence of sudden infant death syndrome (SIDS) in the United States over the last 30 years?

A. Prone sleeping position in the crib

B. Increasing use of home apnea monitors

C. Supine sleeping position in the crib

D. Increasing use of polysomnography for assessment of high-risk infants

10. A 2-minute epoch of stage N3 sleep is illustrated in Fig. 30.4. Which statement best characterizes the major polysomnographic findings during this epoch?

A. Limb movements associated with arousals

B. Subtle hypopneas associated with arousals

C. Subtle hypopneas associated with tachycardia

D. Limb movements associated with tachycardia

11. Which of the following statements is true regarding primary sleep enuresis?

A. Operant conditioning represents an effective treatment.

B. Concurrent OSA is present in the majority of cases.

C. The condition is more common in girls than boys.

D. The condition affects about one-third of 5-year-olds.

E. Enuresis occurs primarily during stage N3 sleep.

12. Which of the following treatments has been labeled by the US Food and Drug Administration (FDA) for the treatment of narcolepsy in children?

A. Modafinil

B. Armodafinil

C. Sodium oxybate

D. None of the above

13. Which of the following sleep disturbances in children is most consistently associated with the sleep stage illustrated in Fig. 30.5?

A. Somnambulism

B. Seizures

C. Enuresis

D. Night terrors

E. Bruxism

14. Which of the following statements most accurately characterizes childhood OSA?

A. OSA in children is more likely to be associated with daytime somnolence compared with adults.

B. OSA in children seldom persists or recurs following treatment with adenotonsillectomy.

C. OSA in children is more likely to be characterized by partial airway obstruction compared with adults.

D. OSA in children is more commonly associated with obesity compared with adults.

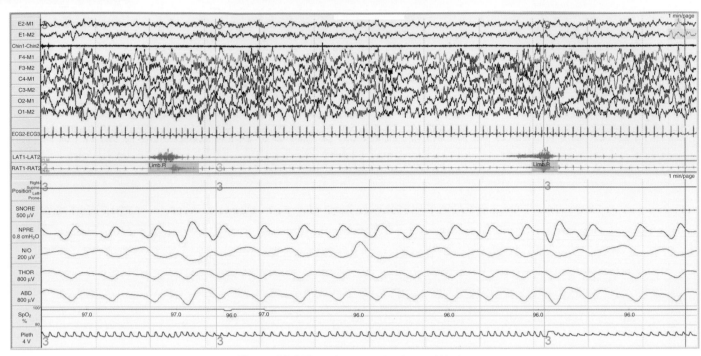

• **Figure 30.4** Two-minute epoch of stage N3 sleep.

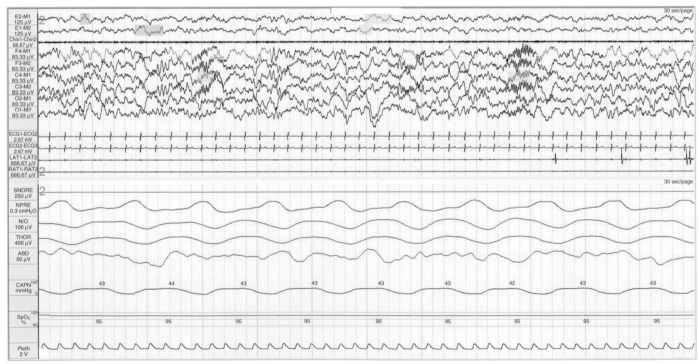

• **Figure 30.5** Thirty-second epoch of sleep from a 4-year-old child.

15. A 14-year-old boy is referred to the sleep clinic for evaluation of pervasive daytime sleepiness that has been present for 2 years. He reports falling asleep in class and during sedentary activities on weekdays despite receiving a minimum of 8 hours of nighttime sleep. Sleepiness and napping do not improve on weekends or during school vacations, when nighttime sleep is lengthened to at least 9 hours. Family members report no snoring, restlessness, or obstructive symptoms during nighttime sleep. The patient reports no cataplexy or sleep paralysis. A nocturnal polysomnogram demonstrates normal respiratory findings. Nighttime sleep architecture is normal, including total sleep time of 480 minutes, sleep efficiency of 91%, and REM latency of 100 minutes. Results of a multiple sleep latency test performed the day after the polysomnogram are summarized in Table 30.1. Based on the history and findings presented, which of the following represents the most likely diagnosis?

TABLE 30.1	Multiple Sleep Latency Test Findings in a 14-Year-Old Male					
Results	Nap 1	Nap 2	Nap 3	Nap 4	Nap 5	Mean
Time test began	8:34	10:28	12:36	14:29	16:32	
Time in bed (min.)	16.5	16.5	17	15.5	16	
Latencies to (min.)						
First sleep epoch	.5	.5	1	.5	1	0.7
REM sleep	1.5	1	1	2	1.5	

Number of REM periods = 5

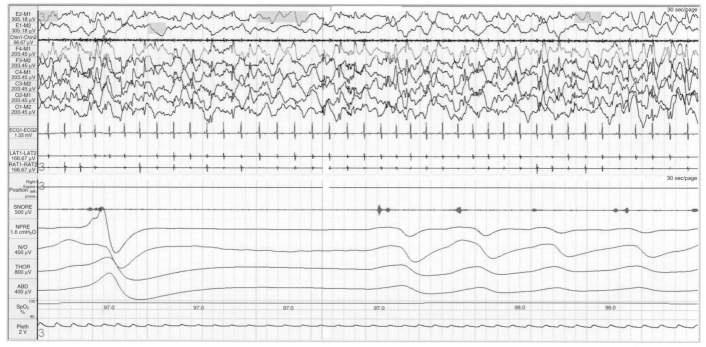

• **Figure 30.6** Thirty-second epoch of sleep from a 3-year-old boy.

A. Narcolepsy Type 1

B. Narcolepsy Type 2

C. Insufficient Sleep Syndrome

D. KLS

16. A 3-year-old boy with a history of cerebral palsy, Chiari I malformation, shunted hydrocephalus, and mixed apnea is referred to the sleep lab for a polysomnogram. Which of the following statements most appropriately characterizes the finding(s) demonstrated in the 30-sec epoch illustrated in Fig. 30.6?

A. Ten-second central apnea associated with arousal from sleep

B. Electrocardiogram (EKG) artifact within the electroencephalogram (EEG) tracing

C. Second-degree heart block, Mobitz type I

D. Stage R sleep

E. Spike discharges within the EEG tracing

17. A 17-year-old boy is referred for evaluation of excessive daytime sleepiness. During the previous year, he experienced several 2-week periods of extreme somnolence, where he would sleep for almost 20 hours per day, waking only for brief periods during the daytime. When awake during these episodes, the family reported increased appetite, decreased memory, and several instances of inappropriate sexual behavior. Outside of these episodes, the patient sleeps an average of 9 hours nightly, with no daytime sleepiness or napping and no concerning behavioral symptoms. A nocturnal polysomnogram performed midway through a typical episode demonstrates increased total sleep time of 670 minutes with sleep efficiency of 80% and no evidence of SDB. If a multiple sleep latency test is performed following the polysomnogram, which of the following findings is most likely?

A. Mean sleep latency of 7 min with no sleep-onset REM periods (SOREMPs)

B. Mean sleep latency of 3 min with two SOREMPs

C. Mean sleep latency of 18 min with no SOREMPs

D. Mean sleep latency of 10 min with two SOREMPs

18. Which of the following findings is least likely to be present in a 6-year-old boy with restless legs syndrome (RLS)?

A. Periodic limb movement index exceeding 5 per hour of sleep

B. Growing pains

C. Excessive daytime napping

D. Symptoms of attention deficit hyperactivity disorder
E. Family history of RLS

19. A nocturnal polysomnogram is performed for an 8-year-old girl who presents with a history of snoring, labored respiration during sleep, and inattention in school. The study demonstrates 4.2 obstructive hypopneas, 0.5 obstructive apneas, and 3.0 central apneas per hour of sleep. Central and obstructive events are associated with occasional, brief desaturations of SpO_2 to nadir levels of 85%–90%. End-tidal carbon dioxide ($ETCO_2$) levels during sustained sleep range from 45–53 mm Hg, with 20% of sleep time spent with $ETCO_2$ levels exceeding 50 mm Hg. Which of the following statements is true with respect to interpretation of the clinical and polysomnographic findings?
    A. Findings meet ICSD-3 criteria for the diagnosis of OSA and primary CSA.
    B. Findings meet ICSD-3 criteria for the diagnosis of OSA, obstructive hypoventilation, and primary CSA.
    C. Findings meet ICSD-3 criteria for the diagnosis of OSA and sleep-related hypoxemia.
    D. Findings meet ICSD-3 criteria for the diagnosis of OSA.

20. Which of the following conditions is most likely to be associated with excessive daytime somnolence when neither SDB nor disrupted nighttime sleep is present?
    A. Autism spectrum disorders
    B. Prader-Willi syndrome
    C. Trisomy 21
    D. Duchenne muscular dystrophy

21. A 10-year-old boy is referred to the sleep clinic for evaluation of sleepwalking. During typical episodes, the boy walks quietly to different parts of the house, usually encountering his parents, who recognize that he is not fully awake and gently redirect him to bed. On a single occasion, he left the house while sleepwalking and was found in the front yard. Episodes occur at variable times of the night, but most typically 1 or 2 hours after the child falls asleep. Events occur once monthly on average, sometimes coinciding with intercurrent illness or sleep deprivation. The family reports no snoring, restlessness, or other concerning symptoms during sleep. Sleepwalking also affected the child's father and older brother at a similar age. Which of the following represents the most appropriate initial recommendation for this family?
    A. Polysomnography to screen for OSA as a trigger for sleepwalking
    B. Clonazepam 0.1 mg at bedtime each evening
    C. Use of locks or alarms on exterior doors
    D. Anticipatory awakening nightly 20 min after sleep onset

22. A 60-sec epoch of REM sleep is illustrated in Fig. 30.7. Which of the following conditions is associated with increased risk for the respiratory disturbances illustrated in this epoch?
    A. Chiari malformation
    B. Down syndrome
    C. Duchenne muscular dystrophy
    D. KLS

23. Which of the following statements most accurately characterizes sleep architecture in infants compared with adolescents?

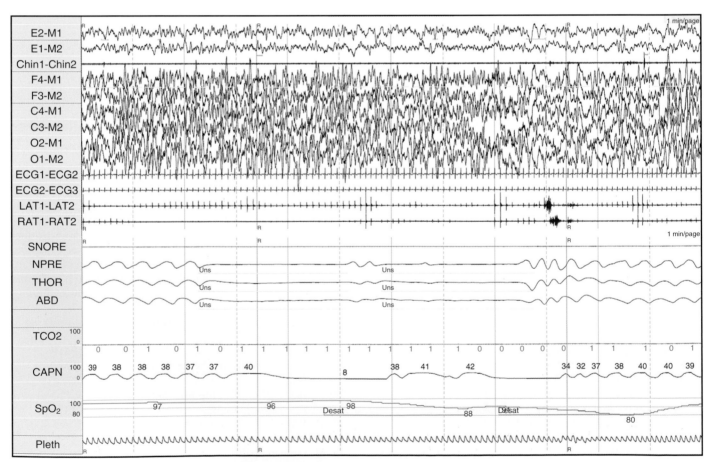

• **Figure 30.7** Sixty-second epoch of stage R sleep.

A. Infants have more REM sleep and longer sleep cycle duration compared with adolescents.

B. Infants have less REM sleep and longer sleep cycle duration compared with adolescents.

C. Infants have more REM sleep and shorter sleep cycle duration compared with adolescents.

D. Infants have less REM sleep and shorter sleep cycle duration compared adolescents.

24. A 3-year-old boy is referred to the sleep clinic for evaluation of long-standing insomnia. He is placed in bed at 8:00 PM following a bedtime routine consisting of brushing the teeth, changing into pajamas, and reading several stories. His parents then tuck him into bed, turn out the bedroom light, and leave him alone in his bedroom to fall asleep. On most nights, however, the boy will repeatedly leave the room and seek out his parents, stating calmly that he is scared and wants to sleep with them. The child's parents initially respond by giving the boy a hug and returning him to his bedroom, but the boy repeatedly leaves his room voicing the same request, eventually becoming upset that he is not being allowed to sleep close to his parents. At this point, the parents usually allow the boy to enter their bed and lay next to them, where he quickly settles and falls asleep within 10 min, staying in their bed for the remainder of the night until morning waking at 7:00 AM. The parents report that their son is developmentally normal and has had no other problems with anxiety or problematic behavior. No snoring, leg discomfort, or restlessness associated with sleep are reported. Which of the following measures represent the most appropriate first step in this case?

A. Initiation of melatonin 1 mg 1 hour prior to bedtime

B. Referral to a pediatric psychologist for evaluation and treatment of anxiety

C. Laboratory testing including complete blood count (CBC), iron profile, and ferritin level

D. Counseling parents regarding limit setting and sleep associations

E. Polysomnography

25. A 60-sec epoch of stage R sleep is illustrated in Fig. 30.8. Which condition or conditions are thought to be associated with increased risk for the variety of respiratory disturbance exhibited in this epoch?

A. Down syndrome

B. Prematurity

C. Maxillary hypoplasia

D. Down syndrome and maxillary hypoplasia

E. Down syndrome, prematurity, and maxillary hypoplasia

26. Which of the following represents the most optimal duration of nighttime sleep for healthy teenagers?

A. 6.5–7.5 hours

B. 7.5–8.5 hours

C. 8.5–9.5 hours

D. 9.5–10.5 hours

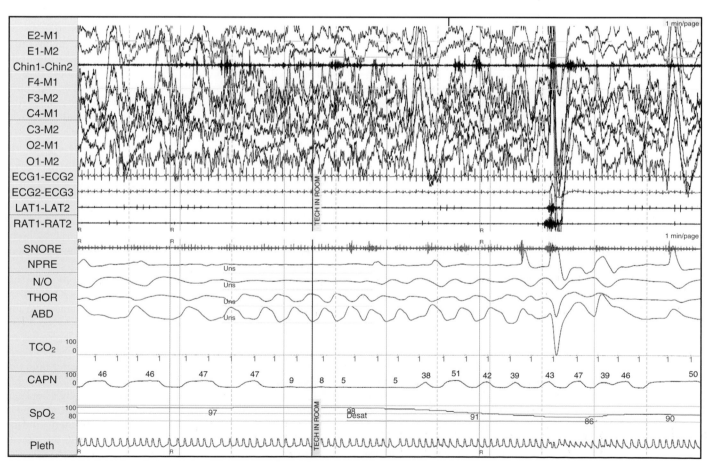

• **Figure 30.8** Sixty-second epoch of stage R sleep.

TABLE 30.2	Multiple Sleep Latency Test Findings in a 15-Year-Old Girl					
Results	Nap 1	Nap 2	Nap 3	Nap 4	Nap 5	Mean
Time test began	7:45	9:46	11:44	13:44	15:44	
Time in bed (min.)	20.0	18.5	20.0	22.0	22.5	
Latencies to (min.) First sleep epoch REM sleep	4.0 —	2.5 —	7.5 —	6.0 —	3.0 —	4.6

Number of REM periods = 0

27. A 15-year-old girl presents to the sleep clinic for evaluation of pervasive daytime sleepiness spanning several years' time. Daytime sleepiness is reported on a daily basis in spite of 10–11 hours of sleep on most nights. The patient naps for several hours each day, often falling asleep during sedentary activities, but awakens unrefreshed. The patient has never experienced sleep paralysis or cataplexy. No snoring or obstructive symptoms are reported during sleep. Previous screening for anemia, iron deficiency, hypothyroidism, substance abuse, autoimmune disease, and depression is reported to be negative. A nocturnal polysomnogram records 590 min of total sleep time, with latency to sleep of 5 min, sleep efficiency of 96%, and no evidence of significant respiratory disturbances. Findings for a multiple sleep latency test performed the next day are presented in Table 30.2. Based on the clinical history and test findings, which of the following represents the most likely diagnosis?
    A. Narcolepsy type 1
    B. Narcolepsy type 2
    C. KLS
    D. Idiopathic hypersomnia
    E. Insufficient sleep syndrome

28. Which of the following conditions is not associated with increased risk for sleep-related hypoventilation in children?
    A. Chiari malformation
    B. Rett syndrome
    C. *PHOX2B* mutation
    D. Myotonic dystrophy

29. Which of the following are considered first-line treatments for OSA in children?
    A. Adenotonsillectomy
    B. Budesonide nasal spray
    C. CPAP
    D. Adenotonsillectomy and CPAP
    E. Adenotonsillectomy, budesonide nasal spray, and CPAP

30. A 12-year-old boy in foster care is referred for polysomnographic evaluation of prominent leg kicking associated with sleep. The foster family reports recurrent kicking movements of one or both legs occurring in clusters lasting 5–20 sec without involvement of the face, arms, or trunk. Episodes are occasionally observed as the boy falls asleep and at scattered intervals during nighttime sleep, but are never observed during sustained wakefulness. Kicking movements are loud enough to disturb the sleep of other family members. Although the foster parents are uncertain to what extent the movements disturb the sleep of the child himself, they report that he often appears "tired and wired" while awake. The patient himself does not endorse evening time leg discomfort or restlessness. The boy is otherwise

healthy and takes no medications. There is no known family history of RLS, sleep disorders, or epilepsy. Physical examination is normal. A typical event is recorded during polysomnography, as illustrated in Fig. 30.9. Based on the history and polysomnographic findings, which of the following diagnoses is most likely?
    A. RLS
    B. Periodic limb movement disorder
    C. Sleep-related rhythmic movement disorder
    D. REM sleep behavior disorder

Answers

1. **Answer C. *PHOX2B* mutation.**
   Mutations of the homeobox gene *PHOX2B* represent the most common cause of *congenital central hypoventilation syndrome* (CCHS) in children.[1] This dominantly inherited condition is characterized by defective central regulation of respiration during sleep resulting in persistent hypercapnia and/or hypoxemia, which has the potential to be life-threatening unless promptly identified and treated. The condition is also associated with increased risk for Hirschsprung disease and neural crest tumors.

   The other listed conditions are unlikely to cause nonobstructive sleep-related hypoventilation during infancy. Down syndrome and laryngotracheomalacia are primarily associated with increased risk for OSA. GERD is more commonly associated with increased risk for CSA during infancy. Although older children with Duchenne muscular dystrophy can develop sleep-related hypoventilation, this X-linked disorder primarily affects boys.

2. **Answer B. Sleep terrors.** The 30-sec epoch of sleep illustrated in Fig. 30.1 illustrates stage N3 sleep, characterized by high-amplitude slow activity on EEG, deep and regular respiration, and paucity of eye movements.

   Among the listed conditions, *sleep terrors* are most consistently associated with deep non-REM sleep. Sleep terrors are clinically characterized by episodes of inconsolable agitation arising from sleep, usually during the first third of the night, for which the child is subsequently amnestic.[2] Episodes are caused by incomplete or aberrant arousal from stage N3 sleep, which is preferentially distributed during the early hours of nighttime sleep.

   None of the other listed conditions are closely associated with stage N3 sleep. Nightmares are associated exclusively with REM sleep. Sleep-related seizures occur primarily during stage NI and N2 sleep. Sleep-related rhythmic movement disorder occurs primarily at wake–sleep transition. Bruxism is not strongly associated with any single sleep stage.

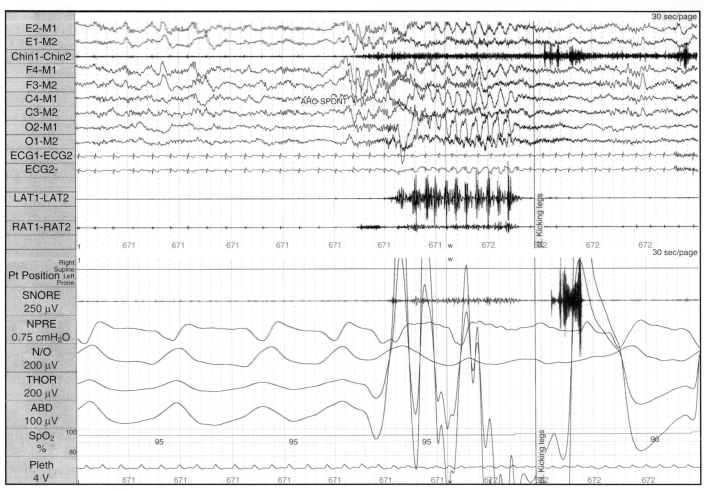

• **Figure 30.9** Thirty-second epoch of sleep from a 12-year-old boy. (Adapted with permission from Hoban TF. Pediatric polysomnography. In: Chokroverty S, Thomas R, Bhatt M, eds. *Atlas of Sleep Medicine*. 2nd ed. Philadelphia, PA: 2013.)

3. **Answer D. There is no relationship between the volume of snoring and the presence or severity of OSA.**

Although snoring is a symptom commonly associated with OSA in children, up to 12% of children may exhibit habitual snoring during nighttime sleep whereas only 1%–4% of children are estimated to suffer from OSA.[3,4] Many children with snoring do not have OSA, and snoring in children who do have OSA may be intermittent or variable in severity.

Neither clinical history nor analysis of audio recordings was found to be reliable in distinguishing primary snoring from OSA in children.[5,6]

4. **Answer B. Light therapy 10,000 lux for 20 min upon morning waking.**

The clinical history and sleep diary are most suggestive of *delayed sleep–wake phase disorder* (*delayed sleep phase syndrome*), a circadian rhythm disorder in which the brain's circadian sleep phase is substantially delayed compared with the sleep schedule appropriate for age.[7] Consistent sleep onset between 1:00 and 2:00 AM irrespective of bedtime and consistently late morning waking time on days when the patient is not forcibly awakened for school are more consistent with delayed sleep phase as opposed to other causes of insomnia in teenagers. Psychophysiological insomnia is unlikely in this case given

the lack of rumination near bedtime. RLS, sometimes observed in diabetics, is also unlikely due to the lack of leg discomfort near bedtime.

Among the listed treatments, morning time light therapy represents the treatment most appropriate for delayed sleep phase syndrome in a teenager.[8] Morning time exposure to bright light often helps advance the circadian sleep phase earlier, reducing insomnia at sleep onset and increasing overall nighttime sleep duration. Sedative medication near bedtime is usually ineffective or only transiently effective in the treatment of delayed sleep phase syndrome. CBT represents an appropriate treatment for psychophysiological insomnia, but is of limited benefit in circadian rhythm disorders.

Other potential treatments for delayed sleep phase syndrome include low-dose melatonin 5–5.5 hours prior to the desired time of sleep onset, avoidance of evening time exposure to bright light, and chronotherapy, a technique where bedtime and waking time are progressively delayed by 3 hours on successive days until the desired sleep schedule is attained.

5. **Answer A. Obstructive sleep apnea.**

OSA is equally prevalent in preadolescent boys and girls, in contrast to the significantly higher prevalence of OSA in males during adulthood.

Among the other listed conditions, KLS (recurrent hyper-somnia) typically affects adolescent and young adult males. Sleep enuresis is common in preadolescent children, but more frequently affects boys than girls. Sleep-related hypoventilation secondary to Duchenne muscular dystrophy affects boys almost exclusively due to the X-linked nature of this genetic disorder.

6. **Answer D. The epoch demonstrates normal active (REM) sleep.**

Active sleep in infants is characterized by rapid eye movements, mixed-frequency EEG activity, and irregular respiratory rate and effort, findings that are all apparent within this epoch. Quiet sleep can be distinguished by lack of rapid eye movements, high-amplitude EEG background, and deep, regular respiration.

The other choices listed do not represent abnormal findings for a child of this age. Brief central pauses in respiration during active sleep are common during infancy and do not meet criteria for scoring as central apneas unless they are prolonged (exceeding 20 sec) or unless they last at least the duration of two respiratory cycles and are additionally associated with arousal or ≥3% desaturation of SpO_2 from baseline.[9] Paradoxical respiratory effort represents a normal finding during active sleep in younger infants, thought to be secondary to high chest wall compliance at this age.

7. **Answer C. The child may be at increased risk for respiratory complications if treated with adenotonsillectomy.**

Adenotonsillectomy represents the most commonly administered treatment for OSA in children. Children under age 3, and children with underlying genetic, craniofacial, or neuro-muscular disorders represent populations associated with increased risk for respiratory complications following adenotonsillectomy.[10,11] Children having these risk factors require careful cardiorespiratory monitoring on an inpatient basis following adenotonsillectomy.

The other choices listed represent treatments that are less effective or less feasible for a child of this age. Nasal CPAP is commonly used to treat OSA in older children, but can be difficult to use safely and effectively for a 2-year-old child without lengthy advance preparation and desensitization as well as in-lab CPAP titration to establish optimal treatment settings. Use of supplemental oxygen by nasal cannula can reduce the frequency and severity of SpO_2 desaturation in children with OSA although upper airway obstruction persists. Similar to CPAP, titration of supplemental oxygen during polysomnography is recommended to assess its effectiveness and verify optimal treatment settings. Positional therapy and nasal steroids represent alternative treatments sometimes used for mild sleep apnea, but these are insufficient as primary treatment for severe OSA.

8. **Answer E. 1-month-old girl with no medical or sleep problems.**

Healthy infants spend approximately half of their total sleep time in active (REM) sleep, with the proportion of REM sleep gradually declining throughout childhood.[12] It is postulated that the high proportion of REM sleep during infancy may play an important but incompletely understood role in early brain maturation and development.[13]

The other listed choices are not associated with increased proportions of REM sleep. Narcolepsy may be associated with reduced latency to REM sleep during polysomnography without significant increases in the overall proportion of REM sleep. Treatment of depression with selective serotonin reuptake

inhibitor medication may be associated with reduced REM sleep. OSA is sometimes associated with reduced REM sleep, particularly in those cases where obstruction is significantly worse during stage R sleep.

9. **Answer C. Supine sleeping position in the crib.**

The most prominent decline in the incidence of SIDS in the United States coincided with the Back to Sleep public health campaign, which began in the early 1990s and educated parents and caregivers regarding the importance of placing infants on their backs for sleep.[14]

Among the other listed choices, use of home apnea monitors and use of polysomnography for high-risk infants may mitigate risk of SIDS in individual cases, but neither of these interventions is used widely enough to have impacted the incidence of SIDS as much as the Back to Sleep campaign.

Prone sleeping position in the crib is thought to be associated with increased risk for SIDS. Other risk factors are thought to include prematurity, maternal smoking, and other environmental influences.

10. **Answer D. Limb movements associated with tachycardia.**

This epoch demonstrates multiple episodes of limb movement associated with tachycardia without scorable arousal from sleep. Arousals cannot be formally scored due to the lack of clear-cut EEG state change, although it is postulated that event-associated tachycardia may represent a variety of "subcortical arousal" in children.[15]

No scorable respiratory events are demonstrated within this epoch. Clear decrement of flow for at least two breaths associated with either arousal or desaturation of SpO_2 from baseline would be required for scoring of hypopneas.[9]

11. **Answer A. Operant conditioning represents an effective treatment.**

Use of an enuresis alarm system for operant conditioning represents one of the most common and effective treatment strategies for childhood sleep enuresis.[16] A moisture sensor activates an audible alarm at the onset of enuresis, and the child is trained by the parent or caregiver to get up and use the toilet when this occurs. When applied consistently, the child gradually begins to awaken earlier during nocturnal voiding and eventually awakens to use the bathroom when the bladder is full but before voiding commences. Other potential treatments include desmopressin, anticholinergic agents, and limitation of late-day fluid intake.

None of the other listed statements are true. Although OSA represents one risk factor for persistent sleep enuresis, these conditions coincide in only a minority of cases. Sleep enuresis is more common in boys compared with girls and affects only about 15%–20% of 5-year-old children.[7] Although other common childhood parasomnias such as sleepwalking and night terrors occur primarily during stage N3 sleep, enuresis may occur during any sleep stage.

12. **Answer D. None of the above.**

There are currently no nonstimulant medications labeled by the FDA for treatment of narcolepsy in children. Modafinil, armodafinil, and sodium oxybate are labeled for treatment of narcolepsy in adults but have not been approved for pediatric indications.

Pharmacologic treatment of childhood narcolepsy usually consists of cautious off-label use of nonstimulant agents approved by the FDA for treatment of adults with narcolepsy, or use of stimulant agents such as methylphenidate or dextroamphetamine, which have been labeled for pediatric use.

13. **Answer B. Seizures.**
This 30-sec epoch demonstrates stage N2 sleep in a 4-year-old boy. The frequent sleep spindles apparent in the frontal and central leads are most consistent with stage N2. The amount of high-amplitude slow activity is insufficient to meet criteria for scoring the epoch as stage N3.

Among the conditions listed, nocturnal seizures are most closely correlated with this stage. Sleep-related seizures arise most commonly from stage N2 sleep, followed by stage N1.[17] Somnambulism (sleepwalking) and night terrors arise primarily from stage N3 sleep. Enuresis and bruxism may be observed in all sleep stages.

14. **Answer C. OSA in children is more likely to be characterized by partial airway obstruction compared with adults.**
The fact that partial airway obstruction is more common than complete obstruction in childhood OSA represents one factor that makes the condition more challenging for parents and medical providers to recognize, because children seldom exhibit the long, dramatic pauses in respiration commonly observed in affected adults.

The other statements listed do not accurately characterize pediatric sleep apnea. Children with OSA more commonly present with daytime symptoms of inattention, hyperactivity, and mood disturbance compared with overt daytime somnolence. Although adenotonsillectomy represents the most commonly administered treatment for childhood OSA, at least 20% of children fail to achieve complete resolution of SDB following this procedure.[18] Obesity represents a risk factor for OSA at all ages, but the association is more frequent for adults compared with children.

15. **Answer B. Narcolepsy Type 2.**
This patient meets ICSD-3 criteria for the diagnosis of Narcolepsy Type 2, also known as narcolepsy without cataplexy.[7] The patient presents with daily, pervasive sleepiness and napping without cataplexy. The multiple sleep latency test documents REM sleep during all five nap opportunities, with markedly reduced mean sleep latency of 0.7 minutes, both necessary for the diagnosis of narcolepsy.

The other listed diagnoses are not compatible with the case as described. The patient does not meet criteria for the diagnosis of Narcolepsy Type 1 due to the lack of associated cataplexy. Although the length of nighttime sleep is mildly insufficient for age on weekdays, the fact that sleepiness does not improve when sleep duration is lengthened on weekends and during school vacations makes insufficient sleep syndrome unlikely. KLS is characterized by recurrent, discrete episodes of hypersomnia as opposed to the pervasive sleepiness described in this case.

16. **Answer E. Spike discharges within the EEG tracing.**
Careful examination of the EEG tracing identifies apparent spike discharges that stand out from the electrographic background during this 30-sec epoch of non-REM sleep. These discharges do not coincide with the QRS complex, making EKG artifact unlikely as a cause. EEG discharges of this type are not uncommon in children with underlying neurological disorders, even in the absence of clear-cut clinical epilepsy.

The other listed choices do not accurately describe the findings within this epoch. The 10-sec central pause in airflow and respiratory effort cannot be scored as a central apnea due to lack of arousal or desaturation of SpO_2. EKG artifact is evident only on the EMG tracings, not the EEG tracings. The EKG tracing demonstrates mild sinus arrhythmia without alteration of the PR interval or other evidence of second-degree

heart block. The electrographic background during this epoch is inconsistent with stage R sleep, where low-amplitude mixed frequencies should predominate.

17. **Answer A. Mean sleep latency of 7 min with no SOREMPs.**
The clinical history is strongly suggestive of KLS, a variety of recurrent hypersomnia which primarily affects adolescent and young adult males. The pathophysiology of the condition is poorly understood, although underlying hypothalamic dysfunction has been hypothesized.[19]

When multiple sleep latency testing is performed during symptomatic periods, the testing usually identifies reduced mean sleep latency (below 8 min) without SOREMPs, consistent only with choice A.

18. **Answer C. Excessive daytime napping.**
Most children with RLS do not exhibit obvious daytime somnolence, as is also the case for the majority of children with OSA. In contrast, problems with inattention, impulsivity, and hyperactivity have frequently been reported in children with RLS.[20]

Among the other listed choices, excessive period limb movements of sleep and positive family history of RLS are common in childhood RLS and are considered supportive criteria for diagnosis of the condition in children.[21] Growing pains are also thought to be highly prevalent among children with RLS.[22]

19. **Answer D. Findings meet ICSD-3 criteria for the diagnosis of OSA.**
The findings in this case meet ICSD-3 criteria only for the diagnosis of pediatric OSA due to the presence of requisite clinical symptoms (obstructive symptoms during sleep plus daytime inattention) and the presence of more than one obstructive hypopnea or obstructive apnea per hour of sleep.[7]

The findings do not meet ICSD-3 criteria for the diagnosis of CSA, obstructive hypoventilation, or sleep-related hypoxemia. Diagnosis of primary CSA requires demonstration of at least five central apneas and/or central hypopneas per hour of sleep. Diagnosis of obstructive hypoventilation in children requires that hypercapnia ($PaCO_2$ exceeding 50 mm Hg) be present for more than 25% of total sleep time. Diagnosis of sleep-related hypoxemia in children requires demonstration of low SpO_2 levels ($\leq$90%) for at least 5 min during sleep.

20. **Answer B. Prader-Willi syndrome.**
Prader-Willi syndrome is a genetic disorder characterized by hypotonia, developmental disability, and hyperphagia, which most often results from microdeletion or uniparental disomy affecting the paternally derived regions of chromosome 15q11–13. The condition is frequently associated with excessive daytime somnolence, even in the absence of SDB.[23]

The other listed choices are associated with excessive sleepiness primarily when SDB is present (trisomy 21 and Duchenne muscular dystrophy) or when significant disruption of nocturnal sleep is present (autism spectrum disorders).

21. **Answer C. Use of locks or alarms on exterior doors.**
For children with occasional sleepwalking, maintaining a safe sleep environment represents the single most important aspect of treatment. Although the risk of serious injury during sleepwalking is thought to be low for patients within their own households, risk escalates considerably if a sleepwalker exits the home or has an episode while sleeping away from home in an unfamiliar environment. Judicious use of alarms or locks to limit egress to the unprotected exterior environment is essential for maintaining safety.

The other listed choices are less appropriate for a child with occasional sleepwalking and no other concerning sleep-related symptoms. Although OSA can sometimes represent a trigger for parasomnias, polysomnography is most appropriate when sleepwalking is excessive or when other symptoms concerning for OSA are present. Nightly use of clonazepam is effective and appropriate for children with highly frequent parasomnias, but seldom necessary for children who sleepwalk only occasionally. Anticipatory awakenings from sleep shortly prior to the time that a child's parasomnia usually occurs may be useful in children whose parasomnias occur frequently at a predictable time of night, but are of uncertain benefit for children whose parasomnias occur occasionally and at varied times of the night.

22. **Answer A. Chiari malformation.**
This 60-sec epoch of REM sleep demonstrates several central apneas associated with desaturation of SpO_2. Central apneas sometimes occur in the presence of underlying brainstem pathology, as can occur in type I Chiari malformation (ectopia of the cerebellar tonsils compressing the cervical medullary junction) or type II Chiari malformation (dysplasia and displacement of the lower brainstem associated with myelomeningocele).[24] Patients with these conditions often have concurrent OSA or hypoventilation as well.

Among the other listed choices, none are associated with significantly increased risk for primary CSA. Down syndrome is associated with significantly increased risk for OSA. Duchenne muscular dystrophy is associated primarily with increased risk for sleep-related hypoventilation. KLS is not typically associated with respiratory disturbances during sleep.

23. **Answer C. Infants have more REM sleep and shorter sleep cycle duration compared with adolescents.**
Infants spend approximately half of their total sleep time in REM (active) sleep, compared with about 20%–25% for healthy adolescents. It is thought that the higher proportion of REM sleep for infants may play an important but incompletely understood role in early childhood development and learning. Sleep cycle duration for infants is typically 50–60 min, compared with 90–100 min for adolescents and adults.[25]

24. **Answer D. Counseling parents regarding limit setting and sleep associations**.
Difficulty with falling asleep in young children is often the result of inconsistent limit setting at bedtime and/or suboptimal sleep onset associations, previously termed *behavioral insomnia of childhood*. These factors are both present in this case, because the parents initially try to redirect their son back to bed when he exits the bedroom but then stop enforcing this limit when he becomes upset. Allowing the boy to sleep with them results in him falling asleep relatively quickly but reinforces the suboptimal sleep association of dependence upon parental presence for comfortable sleep.

Optimal treatments for this variety of insomnia consist of behavioral strategies addressing limit setting and sleep associations.[26-28]

The other listed choices are all less appropriate for the given circumstances. Melatonin and other pharmacologic treatments are often only transiently effective in the treatment of childhood insomnia unless coupled with appropriate behavioral interventions. Formal psychological evaluation is usually necessary only if anxiety is extreme or apparent under other circumstances in addition to bedtime. Laboratory assessment of iron status is not indicated in the absence of symptoms suggestive of RLS or periodic limb movement disorder. Polysomnography is usually not required in children with clear-cut behavioral insomnia unless other symptoms of medical sleep disturbance are present or unless insomnia fails to improve with appropriate behavioral interventions.

25. **Answer E. Down syndrome, prematurity, and maxillary hypoplasia.**
This 60-sec epoch of REM sleep demonstrates obstructive apnea followed by partial airway obstruction and arousal from sleep. Airway obstruction is associated with paradoxical respiratory effort on the thoracic and abdominal channels as well as progressive desaturation of SpO_2 to a nadir of 86%.

Down syndrome, prematurity, and maxillary hypoplasia are all associated with increased risk for obstructive respiratory disturbances during sleep in children. Other common risk factors include adenotonsillar hypertrophy, obesity, and surgical repair of cleft palate.

26. **Answer C. 8.5–9.5 hours.**
Although most teenagers report average sleep durations of 6.5–7.5 hours, 8–10 hours is recommended by the National Sleep Foundation as being optimal for this age group.[29] In clinical practice, careful review of how a teenager's level of daytime function is impacted by changes in sleep duration—including examination of sleep diaries logging school days, weekends, and vacation times—sometimes permits identification of optimal sleep duration for individual patients.

27. **Answer D. Idiopathic hypersomnia.**
This patient's clinical presentation and study findings meet ICSD-3 criteria for the diagnosis of idiopathic hypersomnia.[30] Patients with idiopathic hypersomnia present with pervasive daytime sleepiness despite sufficient or even lengthy nighttime sleep. Naps are typically unrefreshing, in contrast to patients with narcolepsy. The multiple sleep latency test demonstrates findings typical for this condition, including sleep during all five nap opportunities, reduced mean sleep latency of 4.6 min, and lack of SOREMPs.

The other listed diagnoses are inconsistent with the patient's clinical presentation and test findings. The presence of at least two SOREMPs in addition to low mean sleep latency is required for the diagnosis of narcolepsy. KLS typically affects adolescent and young adult males and is associated with recurrent rather than pervasive hypersomnia. Insufficient sleep syndrome is unlikely in a teenager receiving 10 or more hours of sleep per night.

28. **Answer B. Rett syndrome.**
Because sleep-related hypoventilation may occur in the absence of snoring or obvious obstructive symptoms, clinicians must be cognizant of the medical conditions that predispose to nocturnal hypercapnia.

Chiari malformation (type 1 and 2), *PHOX2B* mutation (congenital central alveolar hypoventilation syndrome), and many muscular dystrophies are associated with increased risk for sleep-related hypoventilation. Girls affected by Rett syndrome exhibit episodic hyperventilation while awake, with normal respiration during sleep.

29. **Answer D. Adenotonsillectomy and CPAP.**
Adenotonsillectomy represents the most commonly administered treatment for OSA in children, however not every child is an appropriate candidate for the surgery and a proportion of the children who undergo the procedure will continue to

have persistent OSA.[31] CPAP is also considered a first-line treatment for childhood OSA. Although positive pressure therapy is thought to be effective and safe for use in children, acclimation and adherence to use can be challenging, particularly for younger or developmentally disabled children.[32]

Nasal steroids and leukotriene antagonists represent promising alternative treatments for childhood OSA in cases where first-line treatment is ineffective, poorly tolerated, or not feasible.[33,34]

30. **Answer C. Sleep-related rhythmic movement disorder.** Sleep-related rhythmic movement disorder is a parasomnia characterized by repetitive, stereotyped, body or limb movements that occur during drowsiness or sleep.[35] The 30-sec epoch of sleep illustrated in Fig. 30.9 demonstrates a spontaneous arousal from stage N1 sleep followed by a rhythmic 2-Hz movement artifact seen in the EEG leads and on the left anterior tibialis electromyography (EMG) lead.

The other listed choices are inconsistent with the clinical presentation and polysomnographic findings. RLS is excluded by the lack of subjectively reported dysesthesias or restlessness in the evening time. The rapid 2-Hz cluster of leg movements is inconsistent with periodic limb movements of sleep, which more typically occur at intervals of 20–40 sec. REM sleep behavior disorder, which is rare in children, is excluded because the movements do not arise from REM sleep.

Suggested Reading

Hoban TF. Sleep disorders in children. *Ann N Y Acad Sci*. 2010;1184:1-14.

Marcus CL, Moore RH, Rosen CL, et al. A randomized trial of adenotonsillectomy for childhood sleep apnea. *N Engl J Med*. 2013;368:2366-2376.

Mindell JA, Kuhn B, Lewin DS, et al. Behavioral treatment of bedtime problems and night wakings in infants and young children. *Sleep*. 2006;29:1263-1276.

Picchietti DL, Bruni O, de Weerd A, et al. Pediatric restless legs syndrome diagnostic criteria: an update by the International Restless Legs Syndrome Study Group. *Sleep Med*. 2013;14:1253-1259.

Schechter MS, Section on Pediatric Pulmonology SoOSAS. Technical report: diagnosis and management of childhood obstructive sleep apnea syndrome. *Pediatrics*. 2002;109:e69.

31
Cardiology in Sleep Medicine

ROBERT THOMAS, MELANIE POGACH

Questions

1. A 45-year-old woman with hypertension, managed with single agent therapy, and obese body mass index (BMI) (45 kg/m^2) is undergoing evaluation for dyspnea. She also has a history of loud snoring and witnessed apneas during sleep. She was diagnosed 5 years ago with rapid eye movement (REM)-dominant obstructive sleep apnea (OSA) (apnea-hypopnea index [AHI] 4%, 20 events/hour, oxygen saturation [O$_2$] nadir 80%) but declined continuous positive airway pressure (CPAP) therapy at that time. A transthoracic echocardiogram (TTE) is performed and shows symmetric left ventricular hypertrophy (LVH) and pulmonary hypertension of moderate severity. Which of the following will you tell her about the relationship between OSA and pulmonary hypertension?
   A. Pulmonary arterial pressures can be lowered by CPAP treatment in OSA.
   B. Severe pulmonary hypertension is a common consequence of untreated OSA.
   C. Untreated OSA causes mild pulmonary hypertension only when chronic obstructive pulmonary disease (COPD) and/or daytime hypoxemia are also present.
   D. Hypocapnia is one mechanism behind the development of pulmonary hypertension due to OSA.

2. A 50-year-old obese man is referred to your clinic for management of recently diagnosed sleep apnea (AHI 4% 35 events/hour, O$_2$ nadir 70%). His sleep study was ordered because he is excessively sleepy (Epworth Sleepiness Score = 15/24) and his bed partner is bothered by his loud snoring. He has a background of hypertension and chronic systolic heart failure (left ventricular ejection fraction, LVEF 35%). Clinically he appears euvolemic. You start treatment with autotitrating CPAP (APAP) 6–15 cm H$_2$O. At clinic follow-up, he reports poor treatment tolerance despite several mask fittings. He feels as though he is "suffocating" when he attempts to use the APAP device and he frequently removes his PAP mask in his sleep. You review his machine data. The device detects a residual AHI of 20 events/hour. The breath-to-breath waveform data from his device is shown in Fig. 31.1. What is your next recommendation?
   A. Prescribe a wake promoting medication, such as modafinil.
   B. Refer him for an attended titration study evaluating adaptive ventilation.
   C. Refer him for an attended titration study evaluating CPAP and rebreathing space.
   D. Refer him to a sleep dentist to pursue a mandibular advancement device to treat his sleep apnea.

3. A 60-year-old man has a history of hypertension (on an ace inhibitor, diuretic, and beta-blocker, all of which he takes in the morning), depression (on a selective serotonin reuptake inhibitor (SSRI), which he takes at bedtime), and newly diagnosed severe OSA (AHI 4% 40 events/hour, respiratory disturbance index (RDI) 60 events/hour, O$_2$ nadir 70% in supine REM), which is not yet treated. His risk of sudden cardiac death is:
   A. Highest at 8:00 PM, because his antihypertensive medication effect would have worn off.
   B. Highest in the morning hours of 6:00–11:00 AM.
   C. Highest during the hours of 10:00 PM–6:00 AM.
   D. Highest after exercise, regardless of the time of day.
   E. Increases with higher dose of SSRI.

4. What is the primary mechanism linking congestive heart failure and the type of sleep apnea shown in the polysomnogram snapshot in Fig. 31.2.
   A. Hyperventilation and increased CO$_2$-based chemoreflex sensitivity
   B. Blunted peripheral chemoreflex response
   C. Increased upper airway edema from volume shifts.
   D. Hypercapnia
   E. Increased delta end tidal carbon dioxide pressure (PCO$_2$) (between eupnea and threshold, Δpet CO$_2$)

5. Knowledge about sympathetic activity during wake and sleep has been generated through multiunit nerve recordings in animals (rats and cats) and humans. Which statement about muscle sympathetic nerve activity (MSNA) is correct?
   A. Patients with sleep apnea have increased MSNA during sleep compared with nonsleep apneics.
   B. Sleep apnea is associated with decreased MSNA during wakefulness compared with nonsleep apneics.
   C. In healthy humans, MSNA is increased in non-REM (NREM) and decreased in REM sleep.
   D. CPAP treatment in sleep apneics has no effect on MSNA.

6. A 45-year-old woman with obesity, impaired glucose tolerance, and refractory hypertension is referred to your clinic after she is found, on a home sleep apnea test (HSAT), to have severe sleep apnea with AHI 4% of 50 events/hour and O$_2$ nadir of 62%. Across the study, she spent 88 minutes with a SpO$_2$ less than or equal to 88%. What statement is correct regarding her blood pressure?
   A. Nocturnal oxygen therapy has been shown to reduce systolic, but not diastolic blood pressure.

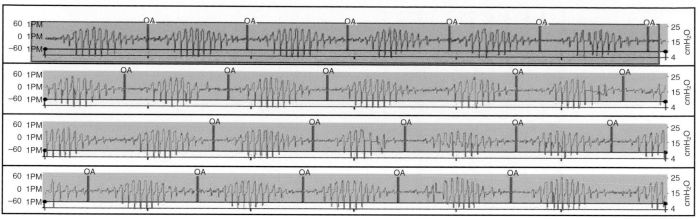

• **Figure 31.1** Continuous positive airway pressure machine waveform (airflow) data.

B. CPAP reduces mean arterial blood pressure (MAP).

C. Nocturnal oxygen therapy reduces both systolic and diastolic blood pressure.

D. CPAP has no significant effect on blood pressure.

7. Which statement below is correct regarding the respiratory pattern depicted in the polysomnogram snapshot below in Fig. 31.3 and your patient—a 55-year-old man with systolic heart failure (LVEF 25%).

A. Nocturnal oxygen therapy will reduce his mortality.

B. Adaptive-servo ventilation is associated with reduced cardiovascular mortality.

C. CPAP will eliminate this respiratory pattern.

D. The pattern shown in Fig. 31.3 may predict worse prognosis in heart failure.

8. Which is true regarding normal sleep (as compared with wake) and the cardiovascular system?

A. Metabolic rate is increased in REM sleep compared with wake state.

B. Blood pressure is decreased in sleep compared with wake state.

C. Cardiac vagal tone is decreased during sleep compared with wake state.

D. Sympathetic nervous system activity increases in sleep compared with wake state.

9. What is true regarding OSA and risk of myocardial ischemia and infarct?

A. Observational studies show that OSA patients treated with CPAP have a higher risk of nonfatal MI compared with non-OSA controls.

B. In patients with CAD, having OSA is associated with higher restenosis rates after PTCA versus controls without OSA.

C. Severe sleep apnea is not associated with increased risk of myocardial infarction (MI).

D. Vascular remodeling from OSA is one mechanism thought to lead to a decreased infarct area after MI.

10. A 65-year-old man with diabetes and long-standing hypertension recently developed atrial fibrillation with rapid ventricular response. A TTE shows normal left ventricular (LV) systolic function and no valvular abnormalities. He is rate controlled with sotalol, started on anticoagulation, and then undergoes direct current cardioversion (DCCV). Within 3 weeks of the procedure, he develops recurrence of atrial fibrillation. What do you recommend next?

A. He should be referred for a pacemaker.

B. His anti-arrhythmic medication should be switched to amiodarone.

C. He should be sent for a sleep study.

D. He should be sent for circumferential pulmonary vein ablation.

11. For the past 3 years, you have followed a now 49-year-old woman with obesity (BMI 40 kg/m^2), arthritis, diabetes mellitus, and hypertension. At the time of her initial presentation she reported loud snoring, apneas, daytime sleepiness, and desaturations witnessed during a hospitalization for uterine artery embolization. Under your supervision, she was diagnosed with severe OSA (AHI 4% 40, O$_2$ nadir 72%, no sleep hypoventilation by CO$_2$ monitoring) and has since been treated with APAP 12–16 cm with excellent clinical response. One year ago she underwent sleeve gastrectomy bariatric surgery. She has lost 100 pounds, and her BMI is now 33 kg/m^2. She returns for clinic follow-up reporting increased daytime sleepiness, despite continued CPAP use, and frequent unconscious mask removals. You repeat a polysomnogram and see the following pattern (Fig. 31.4). In regards to this clinical scenario, which of the following is most likely?

A. She has developed acute heart failure.

B. She now has treatment-emergent complex apnea because weight loss has improved degree of obstruction and "uncovered" heightened chemosensitivity.

C. She needs expiratory pressure relief.

D. The titration is suboptimal and higher CPAP pressure is needed to resolve the ongoing respiratory events.

12. A 25-year-old man of normal BMI and in general good health is being evaluated for syncope. His family history is notable for having several relatives (four in the past three generations, all under 50 years of age) who have died suddenly in their sleep. Which is true about the syndrome he has and sleep apnea? (The typical ECG in this syndrome is shown in Fig. 31.5.)

A. Patients with the suggested condition who have normal BMI do not have a higher prevalence of OSA compared with the general population.

B. In this syndrome, the majority of ECG changes in sleep occur in REM or shortly after arousal.

C. Beta blockade is an effective treatment.

D. Sudden death in this syndrome occurs near-exclusively during NREM sleep.

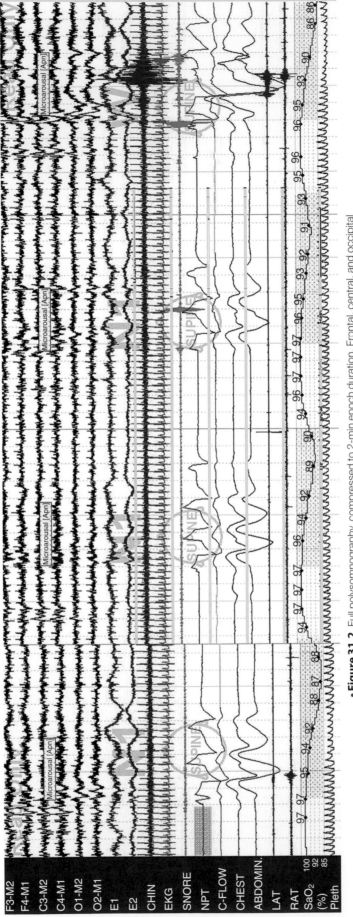

•**Figure 31.2** Full polysomnography, compressed to 2-min epoch duration. Frontal, central, and occipital EEG (F3-M2, F4-M1, C3-M2, C4-M1, O1-M2, O2-M1); electrooculogram, EOG (E1-M2, E2-M1); sub-mental and anterior tibialis electromyography, EMG (chin, LAT, RAT); electrocardiogram, ECG (EKG); snoring microphone (snore); thoracic and abdominal respiratory effort by inductive plethysmography (Chest, Abd), Nasal/Oral airflow with a thermistor (therm); nasal pressure transducer (NPT), CPAP flow transducer (C-flow), oxyhemoglobin saturation by pulse oximetry (SAT%) with plethesmography signal (plethe); end-tidal CO2 (EtCO2), as indicated including end-tidal plateau (waveform).

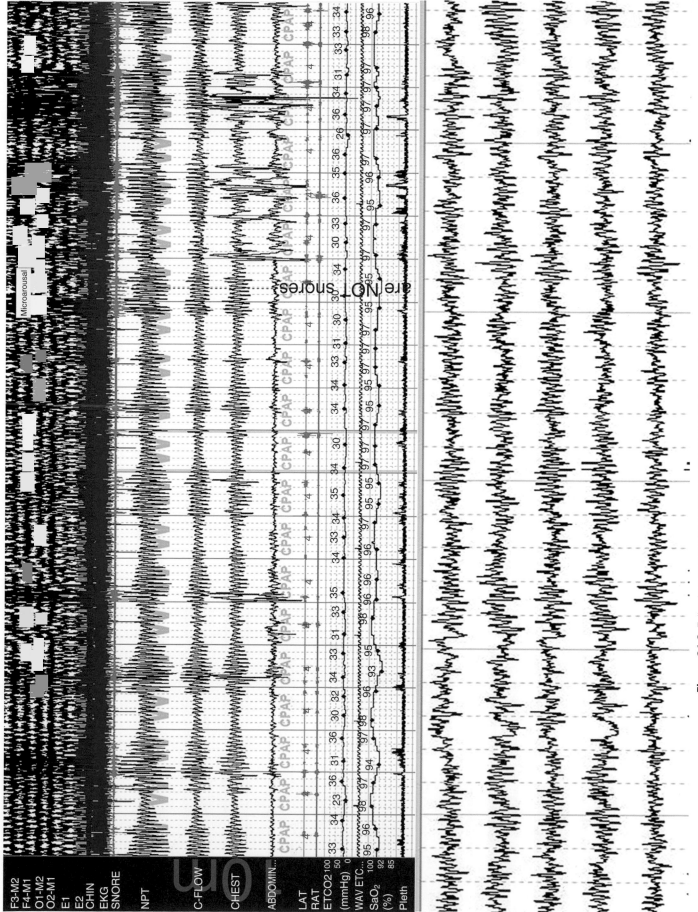

• **Figure 31.3** Full polysomnography, compressed to 10 min. Bottom portion is expanded for EEG stage. Please see Fig. 31.2 for key.

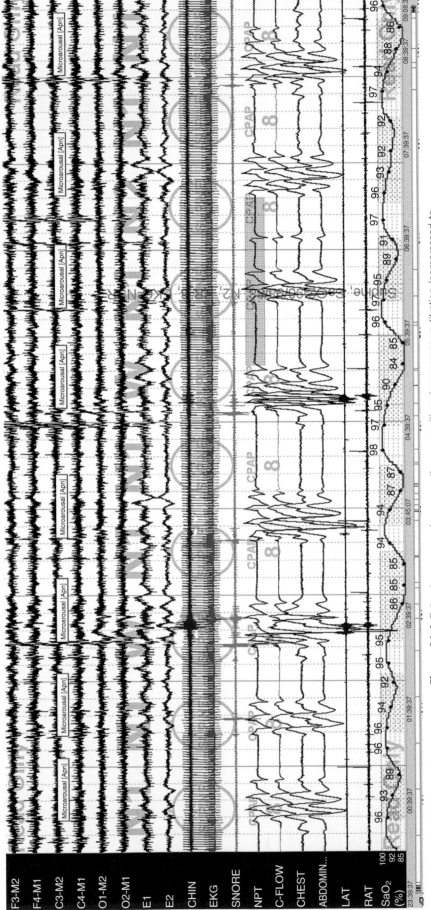

• **Figure 31.4** Full polysomnography, on continuous positive airway pressure titration (compressed to 5-min epoch duration), focus on respiratory and effort channels. Please see Fig. 31.2 for key.

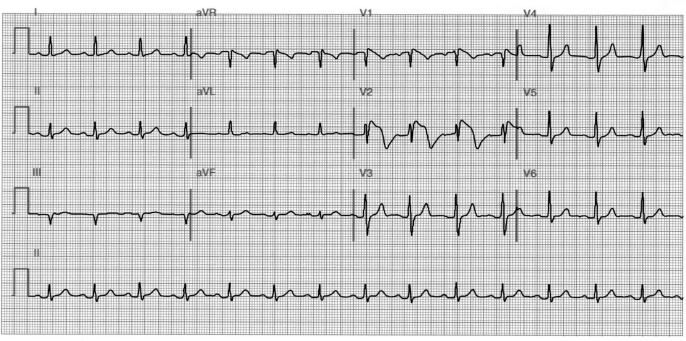

• **Figure 31.5** Note the coved ST-elevation in the right precordial leads and the right bundle branch pattern. (From Nathanson LA, McClennen S, Safran C, and Goldberger AL. ECG Wave-Maven: Self-Assessment Program for Students and Clinicians, *Proc AMIA Symp.* 2001:488–492.)

13. A 68-year-old man with hypertension, impaired glucose tolerance, overweight BMI, COPD, and active tobacco use disorder (30 pack-year history) presents to the emergency department with acute onset of right-sided facial droop, facial tingling, slurred speech, and confusion. A noncontrast head CT (NCHCT) reveals an acute ischemic stroke. He receives tissue plasminogen activator (TPA) and is admitted to the neuro-ICU. Which of the following is true regarding sleep apnea and stroke?
    A. Central sleep apnea (CSA) is a major risk factor for ischemic stroke.
    B. The risk of stroke attributed to OSA is mediated by important confounders including hypertension, diabetes, and atrial fibrillation.
    C. OSA is an independent risk factor for stroke.
    D. CPAP does not lower the risk of recurrent stroke.

14. What arrhythmia is most commonly associated with the pathology seen on this polysomnogram snapshot (Fig. 31.6)?
    A. Atrial fibrillation
    B. Sinus tachycardia
    C. Bradycardia and asystole
    D. Supraventricular tachycardia

15. The cardiovascular phenomenon shown in Fig. 31.7 typically occurs during which of the following?
    A. Healthy NREM sleep
    B. OSA
    C. CSA
    D. Wakefulness in a patient with hypertension

16. The polysomnogram snapshot in Fig. 31.8 is most likely to be from which of the following clinical scenarios?
    A. A 50-year-old man with systolic heart failure, LVEF 35%, and chronic atrial fibrillation.

B. A 45-year-old woman with morbid obesity (BMI 55 kg/m²) and loud snoring, but no known cardiac history.
    C. A 20-year-old college student who is healthy and presents with sleep initiation insomnia.
    D. A 60-year-old man with advanced amyotrophic lateral sclerosis (ALS).

17. A 35-year-old man with BMI of 40 kg/m² has dyslipidemia for which he takes a statin, hypertension, and chronic nasal congestion. He snores. For his nasal issues he uses chronic oxymetazoline (Afrin) nasal spray. He recently participated in a research study on obesity for which a TTE was performed that showed LVH. Which of the following is likely?
    A. He has developed Afrin-induced hypertension.
    B. He has sleep apnea.
    C. There was an artifact in the TTE.
    D. He hypoventilates.

18. Data from epidemiologic and experimental studies supports an association between shift work and adverse cardiometabolic outcomes. A variety of mechanisms have been implicated including stress, inflammation, obesity, chronic sleep deprivation, circadian misalignment, and depression. Which of the following statements is true?
    A. A reversal of normal cortisol rhythm is seen in simulated shift work.
    B. Shift workers have reduced leukocyte counts.
    C. Shift workers have lower risk of malignancy compared with nonshift workers.
    D. Cardiovascular risk is negligible, as long as shift workers achieve adequate sleep duration.

19. A 49-year-old man with long-standing hypertension is referred to your clinic due to complaints of snoring, apneas witnessed by his bed partner, and excessive daytime fatigue. A recent

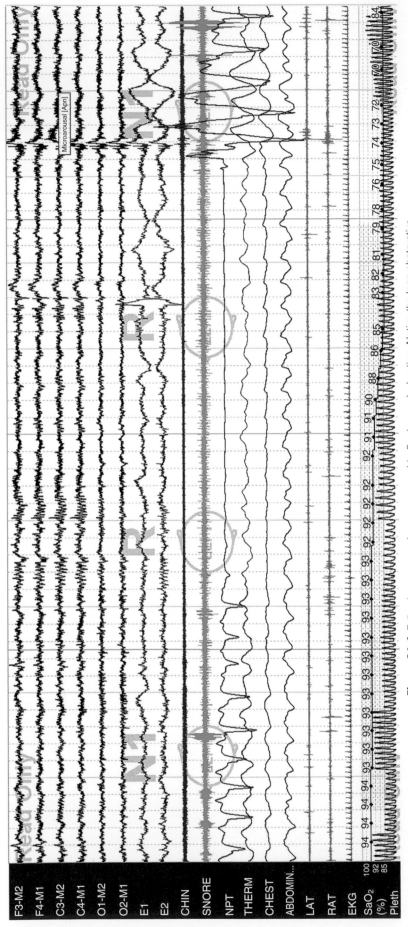

• **Figure 31.6** Full polysomnography, compressed to 2-min epoch duration. Notice the long obstructive apnea with associated hypoxia. Please see Fig. 31.2 for key.

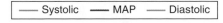

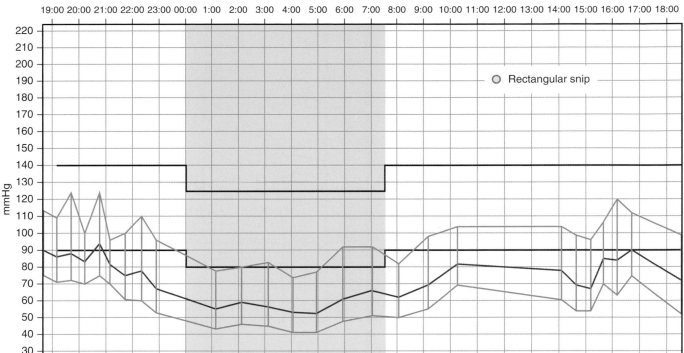

• **Figure 31.7** Legend: Ambulatory blood pressure recording. Notice the nocturnal pattern.

TTE revealed reduced LV systolic function. He is referred for an HSAT which shows severe OSA (AHI 4% 35 events/hour and O_2 nadir 80%). He is subsequently started on auto-titrating CPAP. What is correct regarding sleep apnea and his TTE findings?

A. CPAP use has been shown to improve LV function after 1 month of therapy.

B. The benefit of CPAP on LV function appears transient, and is not sustained with continued CPAP use.

C. CPAP only improves LV systolic function in central, not OSA.

D. CPAP does not impact LV systolic function, but will improve this patient's cardiac mortality risk.

20. A 65-year-old man presents to your clinic. He has chronic congestive heart failure with an LVEF of 30%. He reports chronic dyspnea, unrefreshing and disrupted sleep, and daytime fatigue. Fig. 31.8 is a snapshot from his diagnostic polysomnography (PSG). He is scheduled for a CPAP titration. Prospective randomized trials have shown mortality benefit from which treatment?

A. CPAP

B. Adaptive ventilation

C. Nocturnal oxygen

D. Acetazolamide

E. None of the above

21. A 50-year-old woman works the night shift as a security agent and has done so for the past 15 years. Her BMI is 34 kg/m². Her background medical history also includes hypertension diagnosed 4 years ago, controlled with an angiotensin converting enzyme (ACE) inhibitor, and an elevated fasting glucose of

130 mg/dL. She endorses loud snoring, insomnia, and excessive daytime sleepiness and admits to rare episodes of driving drowsy after working the evening shift. On nonwork days she sleeps overnight and much of the next day. After work shifts, she has difficulty sleeping for more than a few hours during the daytime. She is referred to the sleep clinic for evaluation. What do you tell her regarding her cardiovascular risk?

A. Sleep apnea is contributing substantially to her cardiovascular risk.

B. Shift work does not contribute significantly to cardiovascular pathology.

C. The ACE inhibitor should be changed to a β-blocker for improved cardioprotective effects.

D. Her shift work schedule may be contributing to her risk for obesity, diabetes, and hypertension.

22. A 52-year-old with refractory depression and well-treated OSA has persistent sleepiness despite perfect use of CPAP. He had no benefit from armodafinil, and was transitioned to dextroamphetamine (up to 100 mg/day), with substantial benefit. However, he developed worsening of hypertension (otherwise stable on two drugs), with blood pressures as high as 170–110 mmHg. The amphetamine was discontinued; the blood pressure returned to normal and was tracked several times a day by the patient, who graphed it. Severe sleepiness (ESS 15–18) returned, and a reinitiation of armodafinil only marginally helped the patient. He has no cardiovascular disease or other risk factors, but BMI is 32 kg/m². A positive pressure-titration showed no need to change pressures. He has never had angina, stroke, transient ischemic attack (TIA), migraine, or drug abuse. He has received electroconvulsive therapy

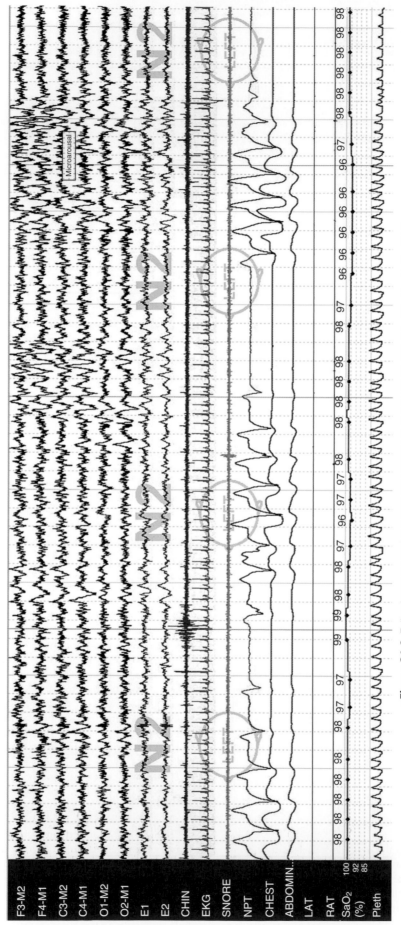

• **Figure 31.8** Full polysomnography, compressed image to 2-min epoch duration. Please see Fig. 31.2 for key.

(ECT) for depression in the past, but it caused substantial memory impairment. There is no seasonal sensitivity (winter depression). Transcranial magnetic stimulation provided only a transient benefit. He has consistently noted amphetamines as being the only drug that clearly improved his mood. Baseline antidepressant drugs are Fluoxetine, Aripiprazole, and Lamotrigine. Which of the following options is the NEXT BEST approach?

A. Amphetamines cannot be used.
B. Sodium oxybate
C. Perform ambulatory BP, and if normal, initiate amphetamines and track with ambulatory BP measurements.
D. Bright light therapy
E. Enroll him in a trial for deep brain stimulation.

23. A 32-year-old woman develops gestational hypertension (GH) during her second trimester. Fetal ultrasound and heart rate evaluation are within normal range and the woman has no proteinuria. In addition to initiation of antihypertensive medication, you should recommend which of the following?

A. Polysomnogram
B. Salt restriction
C. Weight loss
D. Initiation of steroids in preparation for urgent induction of labor
E. Ambulatory blood pressure monitoring

24. A 33-year-old male presents with a 5-year history of progressively worsening insomnia. Though he maintains a regular bed and wake time (11:00 PM–6:00 AM), sleep is persistently unrefreshing, sleep onset is delayed for at least 30 minutes, there are numerous awakenings, and daytime fatigue. Occasional use of zolpidem improves sleep quality and daytime fatigue. Cognitive behavioral therapy provides no benefit. A polysomnogram reveals a central AHI of 32 per hour of sleep, and an obstructive AHI of 14 per hour of sleep; the respiratory events are virtually all in NREM sleep. He returns for a positive pressure titration, which does not resolve the central disease. Resting end-tidal CO_2 measured at the start of the study is 36 mm Hg. He returns to the sleep clinic and asks what long-term risks he may have with his disease, now labeled idiopathic CSA. The risk of which of the following is increased?

A. Congestive heart failure
B. Atrial fibrillation
C. Stroke
D. Hypertension
E. Ventricular tachycardia

Answers

1. **Answer A. PA pressure can be lowered by CPAP treatment.**
Effective treatment for OSA can eliminate the impact of nocturnal pulmonary arterial hypertension (PAH). Older studies have demonstrated this effect after tracheostomy,[1] whereas more recent studies have found improvement in PA pressures with compliant use of effective CPAP.[2,3] The prevalence of pulmonary hypertension in OSA has been estimated between 15% and 70%.[4] Although mild PAH can be seen in OSA without the coexistence of underlying COPD and/or daytime hypoxemia, coexistent COPD and daytime hypoxemia is far more common when severe PAH is present.[4] Several mechanisms have been identified that contribute to the development of nocturnal PAH including: changes in cardiac output, lung volumes, LV diastolic function, and pulmonary circulation compliance and factors resulting in pulmonary arteriole vasoconstriction such as alveolar hypoxemia and hypercapnia.

2. **Answer C. Refer him for an attended titration study evaluating CPAP and rebreathing space.**
The breath-to-breath waveform data in Fig. 31.1 demonstrates periodic breathing (PB) and it is most likely due to central breathing events. This patient has developed CSA on positive pressure (also known as treatment emergent or complex apnea with respiratory instability). This patient is symptomatic from his sleep apnea with excessive sleepiness and thus treatment is warranted. Respiratory instability can be reduced by approaches to minimize hypocapnia during sleep or CO_2 modulation, including use of a nonvented mask or rebreathing space as an adjunct to positive pressure therapy. An attended titration of CPAP with application of rebreathing space (to modulate CO_2) would be appropriate of the choices offered. Adaptive servo-ventilation (ASV) is contraindicated in this scenario; Serve HF, a randomized study of 1325 patients with systolic congestive heart failure (CHF; ejection fraction 45% or less) and predominantly CSA (AHI 15 or more) that evaluated the effect of ASV compared with best medical care for heart failure, found an increase in all-cause mortality, a 34% increase in risk of cardiovascular death, and no improvement in heart failure symptoms or quality of life in systolic heart failure patients with predominantly CSA treated with ASV.[5] Because the patient is symptomatic from sleepiness, use of a wake-promoting medication could be considered, but is typically reserved for residual sleepiness after sleep apnea is treated. Although an MAD is an alternative to CPAP, it is usually reserved for mild to moderate disease, not severe as in this case. MAD treats only the obstructive portion and does not help with breathing control.

3. **Answer C. Highest during the hours of 10:00 PM– 6:00 AM.**
SCD is more likely to occur during usual sleep hours (10:00 PM and 6:00 AM) in individuals with OSA, whereas SCD is least likely to occur during those times in individuals without OSA and in the general population for whom the risk of SCD is greatest between 6:00 and 11:00 AM.[6,7] Hemodynamic changes related to surges in sympathetic activity, absence of blood pressure dipping, and relationship with arrhythmias in OSA are implicated to contribute to this association.[8,9]

4. **Answer A. Hyperventilation and increased CO_2-based chemoreflex sensitivity.**
Fig. 31.2 demonstrates Cheyne–Stokes respiration (CSR) also referred to as PB. CSR is a cyclic or waxing and waning/ crescendo and decrescendo pattern of repeated apneas and hypopneas alternating with hyperpneas, and is the classic form of CSA seen in patients with heart failure, occurring in between 30% and 40% of such patients. Patients with heart failure have a prolonged circulatory time. The cycle length in PB is inversely proportional to cardiac output, usually greater than 45 seconds duration, whereas short cycle PB (<45 seconds) is commonly seen at high altitude). The mechanism underlying CSR is heightened central and peripheral (carotid) respiratory chemoreflexes with a hyperventilatory state, resulting in hypocapnia in both sleep and wake. The $PaCO_2$ drops below the apnea threshold resulting in a central apnea after which the $PaCO_2$ again rises and the cycle continues. Therefore, in CSA, the central and peripheral chemoreflexes are not blunted,

but rather are hypersensitive to fluctuations in carbon dioxide and oxygen, stimulating ongoing hyperventilation. In addition to hyperventilation, PB is determined by the difference between the eupneic $PaCO_2$ and the apnea threshold PCO_2.[10] When the difference is narrowed, because the $PaCO_2$ is closer to the apnea threshold, PB ensues. Thus a narrowed, not increased, $\Delta pet\ CO_2$ predisposes to PB in CSA. Small studies have shown that the AHI can be lowered by the use of compression stockings worn by those with chronic venous insufficiency (CVI), thus suggesting that redistribution of fluid from the lower extremities to the neck at night may contribute to OSA in those with CVI.[11] These changes have not been implicated in PB/central apnea.

5. **Answer A. Patients with sleep apnea have increased MSNA during sleep compared with nonsleep apneics.**
Sleep apnea is associated with increased MSNA during wakefulness with further increases during sleep. Increased MSNA is a known precursor for hypertension and increased cardiovascular mortality. Although the mechanism for this increased MSNA in sleep apnea has not been fully elicited, experimental studies in humans show that intermittent hypoxia and sleep deprivation contribute. Two independent studies of 24-hour total sleep deprivation in humans demonstrated increased diastolic blood pressure and decreased sympathetic activity (determined by MSNA),[12,13] suggesting that either a peripheral mechanism contributing to altered vascular tone, or a central component resulting in resetting of the baroreflex, explain the change in diastolic blood pressure. In healthy humans, sleep is associated with specific MSNA profiles—a decrease in MSNA is seen in NREM and an increase in REM.[14] Studies of sleep apneics, including heart failure patients, treated with CPAP demonstrate reductions in MSNA.[15–18]

6. **Answer B. CPAP reduces mean arterial pressure.**
A total of 318 patients with known cardiovascular disease or multiple cardiovascular risk factors and sleep apnea (established by HSAT, those with AHI 15–50 events/hour included) were recruited from cardiology clinics and randomized to receive either sleep hygiene and healthy lifestyle education (control group), education plus CPAP, or education plus nocturnal supplemental oxygen. CPAP treatment, but not nocturnal supplemental oxygen, resulted in a significant reduction in 24-hour MAP after 12 weeks, compared with baseline.[19]

7. **Answer D. The pattern shown in Fig. 31.3 may predict a worse prognosis in heart failure.**
Fig. 31.3 demonstrates PB/CSR characterized by alternating periods of crescendo and decrescendo respiration followed by central apnea. In CSA, the use of supplemental oxygen eliminates sleep hypoxemia and lowers the AHI, shown in several randomized trials.[20] The proposed mechanism for the improvement in AHI with O_2 is that O_2 reduces chemoreceptor sensitivity or increases cerebral pCO_2 level. Neither O_2 nor CPAP has shown a mortality benefit in CSA. ASV, while previously recommended for CSA, is now contraindicated. The Serve HF, a randomized trial of 1325 patients with systolic CHF (ejection fraction 45% or less) and predominantly CSA (AHI 15 or more) that evaluated the effect of ASV compared with the best medical care for heart failure, found an increase in all-cause mortality, a 34% increase in risk of cardiovascular death, and no improvement in heart failure symptoms or quality of life in those treated with ASV.[5] CSR is felt to be a marker of heart failure and may be indicative of poor prognosis and clinical deterioration, especially if it occurs during wakefulness.[21,22]

8. **Answer B. Blood pressure is decreased in sleep compared with wake state.**
There are well-documented cardiovascular effects of normal sleep and wake states. The phenomenon of blood pressure dipping during sleep is associated with healthy cardiovascular physiology, while the absence of blood pressure dipping has been linked to increased cardiovascular risk.[23] The absence of blood pressure dipping is seen in sleep apnea, diabetes, stroke and myocardial infarction, as well as obesity.[24,25] Similarly, sympathetic nerve activity decreases in healthy, normal sleep as compared with wake, whereas sympathetic activity is increased in diseased sleep (sleep apnea, hypertension). There is an increase, not decrease, in cardiac vagal tone in healthy sleep. This is modulated by the parasympathetic nervous system and characterized by decreased heart rate in sleep and increased in heart rate variability. Normal heart rate variability is a sign of cardiac health, whereas loss of heart rate variability is a marker of cardiac risk.[26] Metabolic rate decreases by 15% in sleep compared with wake. During sleep, metabolic rate and glucose utilization is lowest in NREM and intermediate in REM (compared with wakefulness).[27]

9. **Answer B. In patients with CAD, having OSA is associated with higher restenosis rates after percutaneous transluminal coronary angioplasty (PTCA) versus controls without OSA.**
In patients with CAD undergoing elective percutaneous coronary intervention (PTCA), late lumen loss, a marker of vascular remodeling and restenosis, was increased in sleep apnea patients (defined here by AHI > 10). There may be some benefit to CPAP therapy.[28] Prior studies have also shown OSA to be a risk factor for increased cardiac death after percutaneous intervention.[29] Sleep apnea is considered an independent risk factor for cardiovascular disease, including coronary artery disease and myocardial infarction. Marin and colleagues showed in a prospective observational study that untreated severe sleep apneics had more fatal and nonfatal MIs compared with controls, whereas there was no difference between controls and those sleep apneics who used their CPAP.[30] Prospective observational studies have shown that patients with OSA (AHI > 15) who suffered a first acute MI had larger infarcts, lower final EF and less myocardial salvage compared with those without OSA.[31]

10. **Answer C. He should be sent for a sleep study.**
OSA is highly prevalent in patients with atrial fibrillation (ranging from 21%–80%).[32] The disorders share common risk factors including age, male sex, hypertension, congestive heart failure, and coronary artery disease. There are several proposed mechanisms by which sleep apnea might contribute to atrial fibrillation. Studies assessing heart rate variability suggest that nocturnal atrial fibrillation occurs during periods of increased vagal nerve activity.[33] Intermittent hypoxia and repeated arousals with recurrent exposure to sympathoexcitation and blood pressure surges leading to atrial distention and impacting stretch receptors have also been implicated. Studies demonstrate a higher recurrence of atrial fibrillation in untreated OSA patients compared with OSA patients treated with CPAP.[34–36] A study of 174 patients undergoing circumferential pulmonary vein ablation found the presence of severe OSA to be an independent predictor of ablation failure (1 year arrhythmia-free probability after ablation was 48.5% in those low risk for OSA, less than 30.4% in non-severe OSA [AHI 10–30], and 14.3% in the group with severe OSA [AHI ≥ 30]).[37]

11. **Answer B. She now has treatment-emergent complex apnea because weight loss has improved the degree of obstruction and "uncovered" heightened chemosensitivity.**

Fig. 31.4 shows frequent central apneas induced by positive pressure ventilation titration. Many patients have mixed features to their sleep apnea, with patterns of both obstructive and central physiology. In this case, prior to weight loss, obstruction was the most pronounced physiology. However, following significant weight loss, central features become more dramatic, amplified by the pressures previously needed to maintain airway patency and attenuate obstruction. This patient is also diabetic and has atrial fibrillation, additional risk factors for CSA.

12. **Answer B. In this syndrome, the majority of ECG changes in sleep occur in REM or shortly after arousal.**

Brugada syndrome (BS), an autosomal dominant syndrome that is a cause of SCD including nocturnal, in otherwise apparently healthy individuals.[38–40] The typical ECG pattern seen in patients with BS is characterized by ST segment elevation in the right precordial leads (V1–V3) and an incomplete or complete right bundle branch block (as is shown in Fig. 31.5). BS is implicated as the cause of 4%–12% of all SCD and up to 20% of SCD in those without structural heart disease. Its prevalence is estimated to be 1–5 per 10,000 inhabitants worldwide, though less frequent in Western countries and more (>5 per 10,000) in Southeast Asia, especially in Thailand and the Philippines. Mutations in the *SCN5A* gene are found in 18%–30% of patients; other mutations are also causative. Up to 20% of patients in Western countries and up to 30% in Japan have concomitant supraventricular tachycardias, most frequently atrial fibrillation. Three ECG repolarization patterns are currently recognized: Type I is diagnostic, coved ST-segment elevation ≥2 mm (0.2 mV) followed by a negative or flat T wave; the Type II ECG repolarization pattern is characterized by ST-segment elevation, which has a "saddleback" appearance with a high takeoff ST-segment elevation of ≥2 mm and either positive or biphasic T wave; Type III has either a saddleback or coved appearance with an ST-segment elevation of less than 1 mm. SCD is caused by polymorphic ventricular tachycardia (VT) and/or ventricular fibrillation. In BS, patients die from VT or fibrillation. Studies have shown that spontaneous changes in the ST segment, a risk for SCD, predominantly occur during REM or after arousal (not exclusively in NREM).[41] Sleep apnea is common in patients with BS (with Macedo et al. finding its coexistence in 45%–63% of those with BS, despite normal BMI).[41]

13. **Answer C. OSA is an independent risk factor for stroke.**

OSA is a risk factor for stoke, independent of confounders such as hypertension, obesity, diabetes, and atrial fibrillation.[42] A recent meta-analysis found that sleep apnea, primarily obstructive, is present in up to 72% of patients with ischemic and hemorrhagic stroke and TIAs. Male patients, those with recurrent stroke or strokes of unknown etiology were more likely, and those with cardioembolic stroke less likely to have sleep apnea.[43] The severity of OSA may worsen post stroke, in particular if there is involvement of the brainstem or nerves that control upper airway muscle tone.[44] CSA is very common post stroke, but typically resolves within months and is felt to be a consequence of the stroke rather than a risk factor for stroke. CPAP treatment in OSA has been shown to reduce stroke risk and risk for recurrent stroke, though some data is conflicted.[45] CPAP improves cognitive functioning of stroke patients with OSA.[46]

14. **Answer C. Bradycardia and asystole.**

The polysomnogram snapshot in Fig. 31.6 is an example of OSA, with an apnea and associated desaturation occurring in REM sleep. Bradycardia and asystole are the most common arrhythmias observed in OSA.[47,48] The mechanism may be related to increased parasympathetic activity and increased vagal tone. The frequency of these arrhythmias is significantly reduced by treatment of OSA with CPAP ventilation.[48] The frequency of atrial fibrillation in OSA is relatively low, though it is higher than in the general population and in patients with atrial fibrillation, the prevalence of OSA is high, with estimate ranges of 20%–80%.[32] OSA should be strongly considered in patients with recurrent or treatment refractory atrial fibrillation.[49] The prevalence of sinus tachycardia and SVT has not been well defined in OSA.

15. **Answer A. Healthy NREM sleep.**

Fig. 31.7 is a graphical display of an ambulatory blood pressure recording, notable for a "blood pressure dipping pattern" during the early morning hours. In healthy NREM sleep there is relative autonomic stability characterized by decrease in sympathetic activity with decrease in heart rate, blood pressure, stroke volume, cardiac output, and systemic vascular resistance. Cardiovascular autonomic control parallels the changes in the respiratory system and heart rate fluctuations couple with respiratory activity, called "normal respiratory sinus arrhythmia." Normal respiratory sinus arrhythmia is characterized by accelerated heart rate with inspiration and slowing heart rate with expiration.[26] This normal heart rate variability is a sign of cardiac health, whereas loss of heart rate variability is a marker of cardiac risk.[76] Blood pressure dipping is also associated with healthy cardiovascular physiology, whereas the absence of blood pressure dipping has been linked to increased cardiovascular risk.[23] The absence of blood pressure dipping is seen in sleep apnea, diabetes, stroke and myocardial infarction, and obesity.[24,25]

16. **Answer A. A 50-year-old man with systolic heart failure, LVEF 35%, and chronic atrial fibrillation.**

This polysomnogram snapshot in Fig. 31.8 demonstrates PB. Systolic heart failure and atrial fibrillation are strong risk factors for secondary CSA. The prevalence of CSA in heart failure patients is estimated to be between 30% and 40%.[50] (Estimates may underestimate true prevalence, due to referral biases, and many studies report prevalence for both obstructive and central disease in heart failure.) In an obese patient with loud snoring but no cardiac disease, REM-dominant OSA would be more likely. In a healthy 20-year-old student with sleep onset insomnia, a normal respiratory pattern with suggestion of circadian phase delay on hypnogram would be expected. In a patient with advanced ALS, sleep hypoxia and hypoventilation would be likely, though many patients with ALS also have pathophysiologic airflow features of OSA.

17. **Answer B. He has sleep apnea.**

Long-standing hypertension may be the primary etiology of his LV hypertrophy, but sleep apnea may contribute to hypertension, reduced systolic function, and LV hypertrophy. Cross-sectional and prospective studies have observed cardiac structural and functional abnormalities in patients with sleep apnea, more so with increasing degree of sleep apnea severity.[51,52] In the Wisconsin Sleep Cohort, participants underwent baseline polysomnography followed for a mean of 18 years (3.7 SD) by TTE. Investigators found OSA independently associated with depressed LV and RV systolic function.

Though confounded by obesity in their multivariate regression models, TTE measures of adverse cardiac remodeling were associated with sleep apnea and oxygen desaturation indices were independently associated with abnormal LV mass and wall thickness ($P < .03$).[51] In a cross-sectional study, 235 sleep clinic patients were evaluated with PSG, TTE, and B-type natriuretic peptide (BNP) levels. An increased frequency of cardiac structural abnormalities were observed with increased OSA severity.[52] Cloward et al. identified 25 patients with PSG-determined severe OSA and conducted TTE at baseline and then 1 and 6 months after initiation of CPAP. They found that LV hypertrophy was frequent (88%) in those with severe OSA and resolved after 6 months of CPAP treatment.[53]

18. **Answer A. Reversal of cortisol rhythm is seen in simulated shift work.**

    Shift work has been associated with a variety of adverse cardiovascular outcomes.[54–57] Several mechanisms have been implicated including stress, sleep deprivation, depression, and circadian misalignment. Chronic derangements in the body's time-keeping mechanisms, which are active in the cardiovascular system, may contribute to the increase in cardiovascular pathology observed in the shift-working population. A simulated shift-work forced desynchrony study in healthy humans found a 3% increase in MAP and a complete reversal of the cortisol rhythm during circadian misalignment when subjects ate and slept 12 hours out of phase from their habitual times.[58] Studies have reported increases in obesity,[59] diabetes,[60] cancer (breast and prostate)[61–63] and inflammation.[64] In a large cross-sectional European study comparing 877 day workers with 474 rotating shift workers, shift workers not only had higher BMI, waist circumference, diastolic blood pressure, and homeostatic model assessment (HOMA) index, but were also found to have increased leukocyte counts, independent of their age and smoking history.[64] A meta-analysis of 34 observational studies (total inclusion of over 2 million people), found significant links between shift work and myocardial infarction (risk ratio [RR] 1.2) and ischemic stroke (RR 1.05).[61]

19. **Answer A. CPAP use has been shown to improve LV function after 6 months of therapy.**

    Although this patient's long-standing hypertension may be the primary cause of his LV dysfunction, sleep apnea can contribute to both the hypertension and reduced systolic function. In a canine model of severe sleep apnea, subjects were exposed to repeated apnea during sleep. LV dysfunction developed in the dogs within 1–2 months of exposure.[65] In humans, the prevalence of LV dysfunction is high in those with OSA, and the prevalence of OSA is high in patients with heart failure. For example, in the Sleep Heart Health Study involving more than 6000 patients, the likelihood of having heart failure increased by an odds ratio of 2.5 when OSA was present.[66] Several treatment studies demonstrate improvement in LV function, typically by 6 months after CPAP treatment, providing additional evidence in support of causality between sleep apnea and LV dysfunction.[53,67–69]

20. **Answer E. None of the above.**

    The polysomnogram snapshot in Fig. 31.8 shows a PB pattern. In heart failure, improved survival with any sleep-apnea therapy has not yet been shown in a randomized prospective placebo-controlled trial. The Serve HF study, a randomized controlled trial of heart failure patients treated with best usual care versus ASV demonstrated an increase in cardiovascular and all-cause mortality.[5] CPAP, oxygen, nor acetazolamide have demonstrated reduced mortality in this population. It will likely be extremely difficult to show a mortality benefit in heart failure patients as heart failure management continues to improve. Alternative outcomes/end points, such as recurrent hospitalizations, respiratory failure, and quality of life indices should be considered.

21. **Answer D. Her shift work schedule may be contributing to her risk for obesity, diabetes, and hypertension.**

    Shift work has been associated with adverse cardiovascular outcomes.[54–57] Cardiomyocytes demonstrate robust circadian time-keeping systems.[70] Mice with genetic ablation of the important circadian clock gene *BMAL1* display premature aging and a prothrombotic phenotype.[71] Misalignments between the internal clock system and homeostatic sleep constitute risk factors for a variety of cardiometabolic disorders, including obesity,[59] diabetes mellitus,[60] and metabolic syndrome.[72] Evidence suggests that abnormal circadian function contributes to essential hypertension. A simulated shift-work forced desynchrony study in healthy humans found a 3% increase in MAP and complete reversal of the cortisol rhythm during circadian misalignment, when subjects ate and slept 12 hours out of phase from their habitual times.[58] Although this patient clearly has risk factors and signs/symptoms for sleep apnea, including obesity, hypertension, snoring, and excessive sleepiness, answer A, that sleep apnea is contributing substantially to cardiovascular risk, cannot be substantiated because we are not provided definite information regarding a sleep study. There is no data to support answer C, that the ACE inhibitor should be changed to a β-blocker for improved cardio protection.

22. **Answer C. Perform ambulatory BP, and if normal, initiate amphetamines and track with ambulatory BP.**

    It is clear that amphetamines are uniquely beneficial in this difficult-to-treat patient. Lower doses should be initiated and tracked by patient and by device. If BP does indeed rise, an antihypertensive drug can be added or increased, but clinical judgment is key. Sodium oxybate should be avoided. This is not even idiopathic hypersomnia, and the risk of suicidal overdose is real. Bright light therapy can be a useful adjunct even for nonseasonal depression, but it not likely to be enough in someone who is as refractory as this patient. Deep brain stimulation is likely to be a real option in the future, but until predictors of success are developed, it will largely remain investigational.

23. **Answer A. Polysomnogram.**

    Sleep apnea has been implicated as a risk factor for complications of pregnancy and labor and for adverse fetal outcomes.[73,74] Weight gain during pregnancy may put women at increased risk of developing or worsening preexisting OSA during pregnancy, especially with an obesity epidemic leading to more obese woman of gestational age.[75] It remains unclear whether there is a cause and effect versus a coexistence between sleep apnea and GH and/or preeclampsia (PEC). Sleep apnea results in a variety of systemic pathophysiologic effects including endothelial dysfunction, sympathetic stimulation, oxidative stress, and inflammation, mechanisms believed to contribute to PEC and GH. Small studies show that sleep apnea is more common in pregnant women with GH than in those with normotensive pregnancies.[76] Small studies have shown improvement in BP in PEC with use of CPAP.[77]

24. **Answer B. Atrial fibrillation.**

A link between atrial fibrillation and sleep apnea is supported by several reports. Although longitudinal data are sparse, OSA seems to increase the risk of atrial fibrillation and recurrence after treatment.[78] However, the association between CSA and atrial fibrillation is even more striking,[79,80] especially in those with idiopathic CSA. In a study of 60 consecutive patients with idiopathic CSA compared with equal numbers with equally severe and clinically matched obstructive apnea and healthy control, the prevalence of atrial fibrillation was 27%, 1.7%, and 3.3%, respectively.[79] Thus persistent respiratory chemoreflex driving of sympathetic tone may increase the risk of this arrhythmia, or there are common substrates for both disorders. Epidemiological data supports the increased risk of atrial fibrillation in those with CSA.[81] There is no evidence that the risk of any of the other conditions is increased by CSA, though there is little data due to the rarity of the condition.

Suggested Reading

Cowie MR, Woehrle H, Wegscheider K, et al. Adaptive servo-ventilation for central sleep apnea in systolic heart failure. *N Engl J Med.* 2015;373(12):1095-1105.

Digby GC, Baranchuk A. Sleep apnea and atrial fibrillation; 2012 update. *Curr Cardiol Rev.* 2012;8(4):265-272.

Gami AS, Howard DE, Olson EJ, Somers VK. Day-night pattern of sudden death in obstructive sleep apnea. *N Engl J Med.* 2005;352(12):1206-1214.

Gami AS, Olson EJ, Shen WK, et al. Obstructive sleep apnea and the risk of sudden cardiac death: a longitudinal study of 10,701 adults. *J Am Coll Cardiol.* 2013;62(7):610-616.

Scheer FA, Hilton MF, Mantzoros CS, Shea SA. Adverse metabolic and cardiovascular consequences of circadian misalignment. *Proc Natl Acad Sci USA.* 2009;106(11):4453-4458.

32

Pulmonary Sleep Clinical Case Studies

ILENE M. ROSEN, NALAKA GOONERATNE, GRACE W. PIEN

Questions

1. A 52-year-old patient with diabetes mellitus (DM) and hypertension (HTN) is diagnosed with obstructive sleep apnea (OSA, apnea-hypopnea index [AHI] = 16 events/hour). The patient undergoes an in-lab continuous positive airway pressure (CPAP) titration study. Representative respiratory events from the later portion of the night are noted in the 4-min tracing shown in Fig. 32.1 (note variable positive airway pressure [VPAP], abdominal [Abd], chest channels). A recent echocardiogram showed an ejection fraction (EF) of 70%. Based on the hypnogram depicted in Fig. 32.2, which of the following is the most reasonable first step in management of this patient's sleep-disordered breathing (SDB)?
   A. Proceed with positive airway pressure (PAP) therapy and prescribe oxygen at 2 L/min
   B. Proceed with PAP therapy and start furosemide at 40 mg daily
   C. CPAP therapy with a settings of 10 cm of water
   D. Adaptive-servo-ventilation (ASV) with settings of minimum expiratory positive airway pressure (EPAP) = 10, maximum IPAP = 25, PS = 8, and backup rate set to auto.
2. Which of the following is associated with untreated OSA?
   A. Ruptured thoracic aortic aneurysm
   B. Subarachnoid hemorrhage
   C. Left ventricular thrombus
   D. Myocardial infarction
3. A patient presents with atrial fibrillation that is recurrent despite several trials with antiarrhythmic drug therapy. Catheter ablation therapy is being considered. Which of the following sleep-related parameters increases the risk of recurrent atrial fibrillation after ablation?
   A. Untreated OSA
   B. Periodic limb movements of sleep (PLMS)
   C. Decreased time in rapid eye movement (REM) sleep
   D. Increased time in REM sleep
4. A 55-year-old woman with HTN, DM type 2 and chronic kidney disease (CKD) with glomerular filtration rate (GFR) = 45 mL/min per 1.73 m² and creatinine 1.3 presents complaining of trouble sleeping. She wakes up several times per night

to urinate. Her husband has moved out of the bedroom because she snores so loudly. Her current medications include amlodipine and metformin. She smokes cigarettes—approximately 2 packs per day. In the last 5 years since she went through menopause, she estimates that she has gained about 30 pounds. Her current body mass index (BMI) is 31 kg/m². Her neck circumference is 16 inches. Her other vital signs are within normal limits. Her physical examination is within normal limits except for a modified Mallampati class IV airway. Which of the following is true about her risk factors for OSA?
   A. Because she is a postmenopausal female, her risk of OSA is higher than a male who is the same age.
   B. Because she is a current smoker, her risk of OSA is higher than that of a nonsmoker.
   C. Type 2 DM is protective against OSA.
   D. Because she does not have end stage renal disease requiring dialysis, CKD is an unlikely risk factor for OSA.
5. Which of the following is true regarding alcohol consumption in relation to OSA?
   A. Consumption is safe in patients with primary snoring.
   B. Consumption worsens the duration but not the frequency of SDB events.
   C. Even daytime consumption can worsen OSA by contributing to obesity.
   D. Consumption worsens snoring but not the degree of oxyhemoglobin saturation.
6. A 63-year-old man undergoes an overnight sleep study. He is found to have an AHI of 18 events/h with an oxyhemoglobin desaturation nadir of 81% and an oxygen desaturation index (ODI) of 18 events/h. Which of the following statements is true?
   A. Nocturnal oxygen treatment increases apnea duration in patients with OSA.
   B. Intermittent hypoxia increases parasympathetic activity.
   C. The sequelae of OSA is more strongly linked to the AHI than ODI.
   D. Nocturnal oxygen treatment improves sleepiness more than CPAP in patients with OSA.
7. A 72-year-old man with ischemic cardiomyopathy and HTN complains of snoring and daytime sleepiness. He is scheduled for an overnight sleep study. The following pattern is noted throughout his sleep study (Fig. 32.3). Which of the following statements is true about this type of breathing?
   A. It is typically more pronounced during REM sleep.
   B. It is associated with higher resting arterial carbon dioxide tensions (PaCO₂).
   C. There is an increased ventilatory response to PaCO₂.

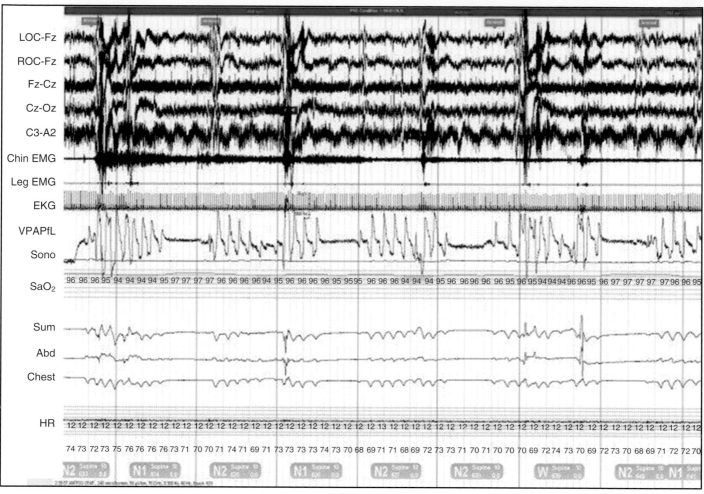

• **Figure 32.1** A 4-min excerpt from an overnight CPAP titration recording. *Abd,* Abdominal respiratory effort; *Chest,* thoracic respiratory effort; *Chin EMG,* chin electromyogram; *Cz-Oz,* occipital EEG lead; *C3-A2,* central EEG lead; *EKG,* electrocardiogram; *Fz-Cz,* frontal electroencephalographic (EEG) lead; *Leg EMG,* leg electromyogram; *LOC-Fz,* left eye; *ROC-Fz,* right eye; *SaO₂,* oxyhemoglobin saturation; *sono,* snore channel; *Sum,* combined representation of thoracoabdominal effort; *VPAPfL,* positive airway pressure flow.

D. This pattern is typically seen in patients with severe respiratory acidosis.

8. A 59-year-old male with HTN, DM, and chronic obstructive pulmonary disease (COPD) undergoes a sleep study and is found to have OSA. He is reluctant to initiate CPAP because he feels is "already on a lot of medications and changing many things in his life to improve his health." Which of the following statements should be considered when counseling this patient?
   A. Having coexistent OSA and COPD is protective against development of pulmonary HTN.
   B. Having coexistent OSA and COPD is associated with decreased hospitalizations due to COPD exacerbations.
   C. Treatment of coexistent OSA and COPD decreases the chances of developing lung cancer.
   D. Treatment of coexistent OSA and COPD improves all-cause mortality.

9. Which of the following is true about sleep in idiopathic pulmonary fibrosis (IPF)?
   A. Patients with IPF have increased REM sleep.
   B. Patients with IPF are more likely to have central sleep apnea (CSA).

C. Patients with IPF are more likely to have OSA.
   D. Patients with IPF are more likely to have REM behavior disorder (RBD).
   E. Patients with IPF have decreased respiratory frequency during sleep.

10. A 50-year-old female with a history of multiple sclerosis presents with excessive daytime sleepiness (Epworth Sleepiness Scale = 18 out of 24). In addition to her hypersomnolence, she reports diffuse muscle and lower back pain, which requires a fentanyl 75-mcg patch and hydromorphone, 8 mg three times daily. Which of the following statements is true about patients with chronic opioid use, as relating to sleep physiology?
    A. The risk of SDB increases because of an up regulation of mu-receptors.
    B. Chronic use of narcotics reduces the risk of SDB.
    C. Narcotics increase central apneas during REM sleep.
    D. Prevalence of central apnea positively correlates with opioid dose.

11. The following sleep study tracing (Fig. 32.4) is most likely to be observed while monitoring which of the following patients?

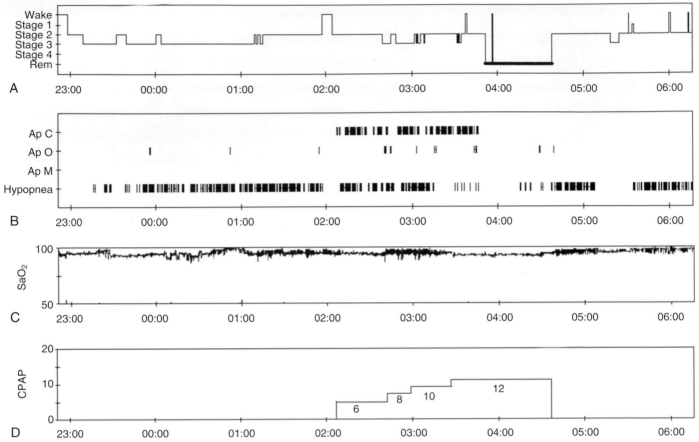

• **Figure 32.2** Hypnogram from Full Night Continuous Positive Airway Pressure Titration Study from the Same Patient. **A,** Shows sleep staging across the night. Wake = stage W, Stage 1 = stage N1, Stage 2 = stage N2, Stage 3 = stage N3, stage 4 = stage N3, REM = stage REM. **B,** Shows respiratory events across the night. *Ap C,* Central apneas; *Ap O,* obstructive apneas; *Ap M,* mixed apneas; *Hypopnea,* obstructive hypopneas. **C,** Shows pulse oximetry results across the night. *SaO2,* Oxyhemoglobin saturation. **D,** Shows continuous positive airway pressure levels increasing from 5 to 12 cm of water between 2 AM and 4 AM. *CPAP,* Continuous positive airway pressure.

A. A 55-year-old obese woman with HTN who reports loud snoring, witnessed apneas, and daytime sleepiness

B. A 30-year-old woman from San Diego (sea level) who has traveled to Manitou Springs, Colorado (altitude 2382 m/6358 feet), to compete in the Pike's Peak marathon (peak altitude 4302 m/14,111 feet)

C. A 68-year-old man with history of myocardial infarction and dilated cardiomyopathy who complains of witnessed apneas and daytime fatigue

D. A 42-year-old man with a history of heroin abuse now in a methadone maintenance program, who complains of daytime somnolence

12. A 38-year-old woman with HTN, prediabetes, and severe sleep apnea (AHI 50 events/h) treated with CPAP 9 cm H_2O undergoes gastric bypass surgery (BMI 48 kg/m^2). When she presents to your office 6 months after surgery for follow-up, she has lost significant weight (BMI now 33 kg/m^2), with resolution of HTN and prediabetes. She no longer uses CPAP regularly, noting that her energy level has improved, and she does not feel much different whether or not she used CPAP the prior night. Her bed partner notes that the patient's snoring (off CPAP) has improved. What do you recommend as the most appropriate next step in management?

A. Reduce the patient's CPAP setting to 7 cm H_2O.

B. Perform a CPAP titration study to determine a new therapeutic pressure.

C. Perform a baseline sleep study to assess whether the patient still has sleep apnea.

D. Discontinue CPAP therapy.

13. Which of the following statements about OSA in women is true?

A. Postmenopausal women are at reduced risk for OSA compared with premenopausal women.

B. Women with polycystic ovarian syndrome (PCOS) are at increased risk for OSA.

C. Women with endometriosis are at increased risk for OSA.

D. Nonpregnant women are at higher risk for OSA compared with pregnant women.

14. A 64-year-old obese man (BMI 47 kg/m^2) with a history of HTN presents with disruptive snoring and excessive daytime sleepiness. His wife accompanies him and reports he frequently awakens from sleep with gasping and choking. He notes multiple episodes of nocturia overnight, and he frequently struggles to stay awake at his job at a law firm. He takes amlodipine 10 mg daily for blood pressure (BP) control. On physical exam, the patient's BP is 142/88, his heart rate is 85,

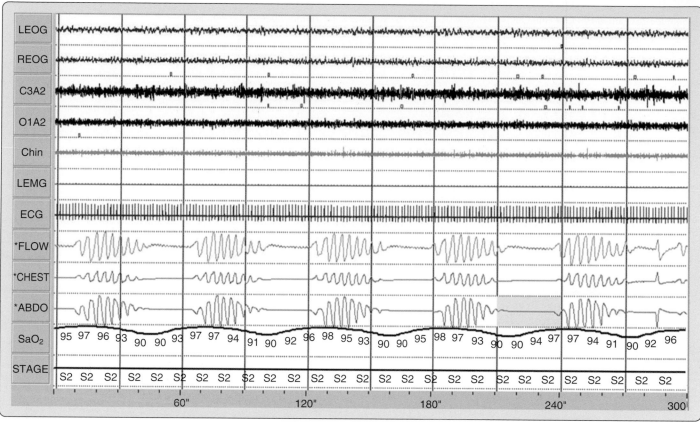

• **Figure 32.3** A 5-min Excerpt from an Overnight Sleep Study. The tracing shows crescendo-decrescendo pattern of breathing best seen in the FLOW channel. Note that the cycle length (i.e., start of central apnea to end of hyperpnea is ≥40 sec). *ABDO,* Abdominal respiratory effort; *C3-A2,* central electroencephalographic (EEG) lead; *CHEST,* thoracic respiratory effort; *Chin,* chin electromyogram; *ECG,* electrocardiogram; *FLOW,* nasal pressure airflow; *LEMG,* left leg electromyogram; *LEOG,* left eye lead; *O1-A2,* occipital EEG lead; *REOG,* right eye lead; *SaO₂,* oxyhemoglobin saturation; *STAGE,* sleep stage. (From Kryger MS. *Atlas of Clinical Sleep Medicine.* 2nd ed. Philadelphia, PA: Saunders; 2014.)

and his respiratory rate is 18. You note that the patient appears sleepy, has macroglossia and a large neck (48 cm, or 19 inches), with normal lung exam, distant heart sounds, and 1+ lower extremity edema bilaterally. As you review his medical record, you note his primary care provider performed blood work last month. Which of the following laboratory values is highly predictive of obesity hypoventilation syndrome (OHS)?

A. HCO_3 24
B. HCO_3 28
C. Hemoglobin 11.0
D. Hemoglobin 16.0

15. A 35-year-old woman is referred for evaluation of excessive daytime somnolence. She has a history of sickle cell disease, depression, and chronic pain. Her boyfriend reports that she snores intermittently, and he has noticed some episodes where she seems to stop breathing for "a long time." Although she reports getting 8–9 hours of sleep overnight, she struggles to stay awake during the day and frequently falls asleep while watching her children when they return home from school. She reports her depressive symptoms are well controlled at present. Her medications include oxycodone CR (80 mg twice daily) and citalopram (20 mg once daily). On exam, her BP is 120/77, heart rate 72, weight 135 lbs, BMI 22.5 kg/m². She undergoes an overnight sleep study, which reveals an AHI

of 32 events/hour with predominantly central apneas (central apnea index 24 events/hour, obstructive apnea index 3 events/hour, hypopnea index 5 events/hour). Although oxygen saturation was normal before sleep (SaO₂ 96%), she has persistent hypoxemia after sleep, with 55% of time asleep with SaO₂ less than 90% and nadir oxygen saturation of 81%. Which of the following therapies is *least* likely to effectively treat this patient's SDB?

A. Initiation of CPAP
B. Initiation of bilevel PAP (BPAP) with use of a backup rate
C. Initiation of ASV
D. Reduction in dose of opioid medications

16. A 34-year-old overweight (BMI 29.5 kg/m²) woman with HTN and a history of temporomandibular joint disorder complains of loud snoring and daytime fatigue. She has an overnight sleep study and is diagnosed with mild OSA (AHI 14 events/hour). At her follow-up visit, she states that she does not want to try CPAP therapy and asks about whether she would be a good candidate for oral appliance therapy. Which of the following statements about oral appliance therapy is most correct?

A. The patient should try CPAP first, since oral appliance therapy is recommended as an alternative OSA therapy only for patients who are unable to tolerate CPAP therapy.

Montage: PSG limbs-PFLOW Hifh Cut: 15 Hz Low Cut: 1.00 Hz Sensitivity: 10 µV/mm Speed: 120 s/page

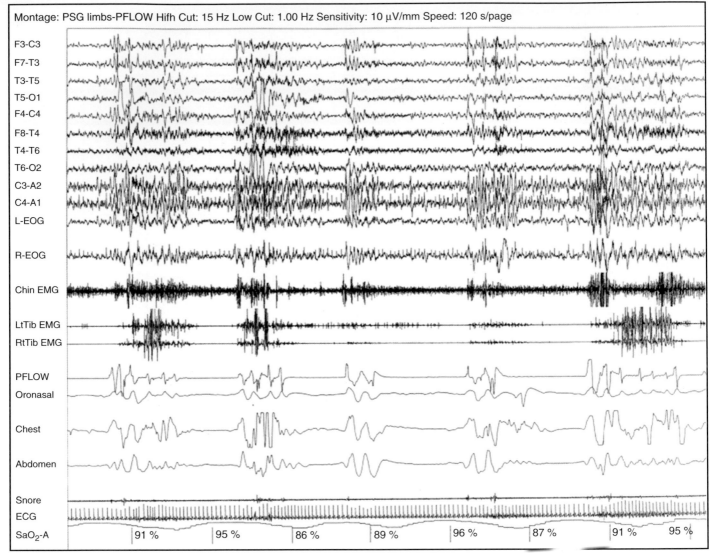

• **Figure 32.4** A 120-sec excerpt from an overnight polysomnographic recording. *C4-A1*, Central lead; *C3-A2*, central lead; *F3-C3*, fronto-central lead; *F7-T3*, fronto-temporal lead; *F4-C4*, fronto-central lead; *F8-T4*, fronto-temporal lead; *L-EOG*, left eye lead; *LtTib EMG*, left tibial lead; *Oronasal*, oronasal thermistor; *PFLOW*, nasal pressure transducer; *R-EOG*, right eye lead; *RtTib EMG*, right tibeal lead; *SaO2-A*, oxyhemoglobin saturation; *T3-T5*, temporal lead; *T5-O1*, temporo-occipital lead; *T4-T6*, temporal lead; *T6-O2*, temporo-occipital lead. (From Chokroverty S, Bhat S, Provini F. Sleep dysfunction and sleep-disordered breathing in miscellaneous neurological disorders. In *Atlas of Sleep Medicine.* 2nd ed. 2014.)

B. The patient's history of HTN makes her a poor candidate for oral appliance therapy because use of oral appliances does not improve BP.

C. The patient's temporomandibular joint disorder may worsen or recur with oral appliance use, and is a common contraindication for oral appliance therapy.

D. Patients with mild or moderate OSA are less likely to achieve successful treatment of OSA with an oral appliance compared with patients with severe OSA.

17. In which of the following patients is home sleep apnea testing (HSAT) most appropriate?

A. A 37-year-old obese woman with snoring, whose bed partner reports witnessed apneas and frequent kicking by the patient during sleep

B. A 62-year-old man with moderate COPD with snoring and witnessed apneas

C. A 55-year-old man with snoring, witnessed apneas, and unrefreshing sleep

D. A 68-year-old woman with history of myocardial infarction and dilated cardiomyopathy whose bed partner reports snoring and witnessed apneas

18. A 32-year-old woman at 28 weeks of gestation presents for evaluation of snoring and daytime fatigue. She began snoring in the first trimester of pregnancy and now snores loudly every night. She awakens multiple times nightly, mostly due to nocturia and sometimes with gasping or choking. She describes mild daytime somnolence despite 7 hours sleep each night and a 1-hour nap in the afternoon. Her pregnancy has been otherwise uneventful. She is overweight (5 feet, 3 inches; 165 lbs prepregnancy weight with BMI 29 kg/m²; 30 lb gestational weight gain, current BMI 34 kg/m²). Before agreeing to undergo a sleep study, she wants to know more about the

effects of OSA on pregnancy and its treatment. Which of the following statements regarding OSA in pregnant women and its treatment is true?

A. The risk for pulmonary embolism is reduced among pregnant women with OSA.

B. The risk for gestational HTN and preeclampsia is increased among pregnant women with OSA.

C. Oral appliances are a recommended treatment for pregnancy-associated OSA.

D. For treatment of OSA in pregnant women, BPAP is more effective and better tolerated than CPAP.

19. A 59-year-old woman who was referred for sleep apnea evaluation presents for initial consultation in your office, accompanied by her husband. Her past medical history is significant for obesity (BMI 33 kg/m^2), prediabetes, and HTN. She denies excessive daytime somnolence. Her physical exam reveals a modified Mallampati class 4 airway and macroglossia with tongue ridging. Her Epworth Sleepiness Score is 9. How should you approach risk assessment for drowsy driving in this patient?

A. Assessment for drowsy driving is unnecessary, since the patient does not endorse daytime somnolence and her Epworth Sleepiness Score is normal.

B. The patient's husband should be asked about whether he has observed any drowsy driving episodes when riding with the patient.

C. Assessment for drowsy driving should be deferred until 1 month after the patient initiates treatment for OSA with CPAP or another treatment modality.

D. Assessment for drowsy driving should be performed during this visit and should include explicit questions about whether the patient has experienced drowsy driving or had any near-miss incidents or actual crashes related to sleepiness.

20. A 42-year-old man with HTN and hyperlipidemia presents for evaluation of snoring and excessive daytime sleepiness. He reports that his wife has noted episodes where he stops breathing, and he has awakened with gasping and choking, especially if he sleeps supine or has a few beers after work. He usually gets 7–8 hours of sleep, but is often drowsy after eating lunch, and also has noted drowsiness with driving on a couple of occasions during his 35-min commute home. Once he "tapped" the bumper of the car in front of him at a traffic light. On another occasion, the patient dozed off with his foot on the brake at a red light and was awakened by the driver behind him honking. He takes hydrochlorothiazide, lisinopril, and atorvastatin. On exam, he is obese (BMI 36 kg/m^2) with a modified Mallampati class 3 airway and macroglossia. You order expedited overnight sleep testing for the patient. He notes he needs to drive to get to work and asks how he can reduce the likelihood of a drowsy driving crash before he initiates treatment for sleep apnea. How should you advise him?

A. He should pull over and take a brief nap if he becomes sleepy while driving.

B. He should drive with the air conditioning on to keep him alert.

C. He should play loud music if he becomes sleepy while he drives.

D. He should use a hands-free device to talk on his mobile phone while he drives.

21. A 52-year-old female patient presented earlier to your clinic with witnessed apneas and loud snoring. She is a caregiver for her elderly father, and requested that as much of the evaluation as possible be performed at home, since it would be difficult for her to arrange home care while she is at an in-laboratory sleep study. Her diagnostic home sleep study showed an AHI of 24 events/hour, consistent with moderate sleep apnea. She is willing to try PAP therapy, and you order an auto-titrating CPAP unit (ACPAP) for use at home. She used the unit for 4 weeks at home; the average pressure was 7.5 cm H$_2$O, the median pressure was 8.2 cm H$_2$O, the 90% pressure was 10.1 cm H$_2$O, and the maximum pressure was 14 cm H$_2$O. What fixed CPAP setting would you recommend based on the available data?

A. 5 cm H$_2$O

B. 7 cm H$_2$O

C. 10 cm H$_2$O

D. 14 cm H$_2$O

E. 16 cm H$_2$O

22. A 42-year-old male is evaluated in the sleep disorders clinic prior to bariatric surgery. His initial sleep study showed an AHI of 54 events/hour and CPAP 14 cm H$_2$O was recommended after a titration sleep study; he was started on CPAP therapy prior to surgery. He returns to you for follow-up after 1 month, during which he able to successfully lose 20 lbs. He has been successfully following his diet and anticipates losing further weight. He returns to you for follow-up. What changes would you recommend for his CPAP therapy?

A. He can stop CPAP, as his sleep apnea will likely resolve

B. Continue CPAP 14 cm H$_2$O

C. Convert to CPAP 12 cm H$_2$O

D. Convert to autotitrating mode with a minimum PS of 5 and a maximum of 15 cm H$_2$O

E. Convert to autotitrating mode with a minimum PS of 5 and a maximum of 12 cm H$_2$O

23. A 32-year-old male patient returns for a 6-week follow-up visit after starting CPAP therapy for moderate sleep apnea. He initially underwent a split-night sleep study that showed an AHI of 42 events/hour, with effective treatment at CPAP 10 cm H$_2$O. He wore an oronasal mask during the study based on his mask preference. He appeared to tolerate CPAP well during the sleep study and was willing to use it at home. He was then placed on a device with the following settings for use at home: CPAP 10 cm H$_2$O with ramp time at 20 min, expiratory pressure release (EPR) of 0, oronasal mask. At his follow-up visit, he reports that it has been difficult to use his CPAP. He has several complaints, including excessive pressure and mask discomfort. Which of the following options would you try next to improve his adherence?

A. Enable EPR feature

B. Increase humidifier setting

C. Switch to a nasal mask

D. Switch to a different oronasal mask

E. Refer him for cognitive-behavioral therapy for insomnia (CBT-I)

24. In which of the following clinical scenarios should BPAP not be used?

A. A trial of bilevel-autotitrating mode for a patient with severe OSA who was not effectively treated with CPAP during an in-lab titration study, but does not want to return for a second in-lab titration study

B. A patient newly diagnosed with sleep apnea who is concerned about having too much air pressure from the mask

C. A patient with moderate COPD and newly diagnosed sleep apnea

D. A patient who has been on CPAP PS 16 cm H_2O, but is having difficulty tolerating the pressure

E. A patient whose autotitrating PAP unit shows that she persistently reaches the 20 cm H_2O upper limit

25. A 53-year-old female patient with newly diagnosed sleep apnea presents for follow-up to discuss the results of her sleep study and treatment options. She is interested in learning more about CPAP and auto-setting PAP (APAP) therapies. Which of the following statements is true?
    A. APAP users have a higher sleep efficiency than CPAP users.
    B. APAP has a higher rate of adherence than CPAP.
    C. CPAP users spend more time in slow-wave sleep than APAP users.
    D. APAP leads to more effective BP reduction than CPAP.
    E. Daytime sleepiness is improved more with CPAP than with APAP.

26. A 72-year-old female with newly diagnosed sleep apnea (AHI 24 events/hour and oxyhemoglobin desaturation less than 88% for 6.5% of the night) and Alzheimer's dementia comes with her son for a second opinion regarding sleep apnea management with CPAP. The son's primary concern is related to progression of cognitive impairment. He notes that she tends to sleep for 8 hours a night and rarely has insomnia. Which of the following could you tell the patient and her son?
    A. Patients with Alzheimer's dementia can delay their cognitive decline when using CPAP.
    B. Total sleep time is associated with risk of cognitive impairment.
    C. Treating sleep apnea in patients with dementia will not improve daytime sleepiness.
    D. In terms of predicting cognitive impairment, having nocturnal hypoxia is more important than the presence of sleep apnea per se.
    E. Older adults with cognitive impairment cannot use CPAP.

27. A 32-year-old male with sleep apnea on CPAP therapy presents for follow-up. He complains of significant difficulty falling asleep, as well as difficulty staying asleep. He is using his CPAP machine only intermittently at this point, due to his insomnia. Which of the following would you recommend?
    A. Zaleplon 10 mg at bedtime and more consistent use of CPAP
    B. Refer for CBT-I
    C. Zolpidem 5 mg at bedtime and more consistent use of CPAP
    D. Eszopiclone 1 mg at bedtime and more consistent use of CPAP

28. A 56-year-old female with moderate sleep apnea presents with difficulty using an oronasal mask. She has a history of mouth breathing and nasal congestion, which led to an initial trial with an oronasal mask. Her CPAP is set to a pressure support of 12 cm H_2O. What would you advise her at this time?
    A. Mouth breathing is a contraindication to using a nasal mask.
    B. Her high CPAP pressure will make it difficult to use a nasal pillow mask relative to a nasal mask.
    C. A trial of an alpha-adrenergic agonist nasal decongestant, such as oxymetazoline
    D. A trial of a steroid nasal decongestant, such as fluticasone

E. Otorhinolaryngology consultation for rhinoplasty evaluation

29. A 25-year-old female with severe sleep apnea presents for a routine follow-up visit. Her CPAP unit is set to 10 cm H_2O, and her CPAP data is downloaded as part of the visit. She reports feeling more rested in the daytime, with no recurrence of the daytime sleepiness complaints she experienced prior to starting CPAP. There is minimal mask leak noted. In which of the following scenarios, as obtained from the CPAP data download, would you recommend increasing the CPAP setting to 12 cm H_2O?
    A. Residual AHI of 7.5 events/hour
    B. Residual AHI of 14.3 events/hour
    C. Residual AHI of 25 events/hour
    D. Residual AHI of 3 events/hour

30. A nephrology colleague is interested in the effects of CPAP treatment on BP in patients with HTN. He is interested in the average BP reduction in patients on CPAP. Which of the following is the correct answer?
    A. Systolic BP: −10 mmHg; diastolic BP: −5 mmHg
    B. Systolic BP: −5 mmHg; diastolic BP: −2.5 mmHg
    C. Systolic BP: −2.5 mmHg; diastolic BP: −1.5 mmHg
    D. CPAP treatment does not lead to a statistically significant reduction in BP

Answers

1. **Answer C.** This patient has treatment-emergent CSA. Note that in the hypnogram depicted in Fig. 32.2, most of the obstructive events are treated on CPAP at 12 cm of water, although many central apneas still remain (Fig. 32.5). In some observational studies, central apneas resolve in 50%–75% of patients after 2–3 months of CPAP therapy. Given this, a trial of CPAP therapy initially is reasonable. A repeat sleep study with CPAP should be performed after several months of treatment. For those patients who do not improve, options include changing the mode of PAP treatment with consideration of ASV therapy or BPAP with a backup rate. Due to expense and limited studies, modes of PAP therapy such as ASV are typically considered after a trial of CPAP. Although oxygen therapy can be considered as a first-line treatment option for patients with CSA in the setting of congestive heart failure (CHF), this patient has a normal EF. Additionally, while close assessment looking for symptomatic heart failure (HF) and signs of volume overload should be performed, a trial of diuretics would not be an appropriate first line therapy.[1–8]

2. **Answer D.** Untreated OSA of significant severity appears to be associated with an increased risk of fatal and nonfatal cardiovascular events, including myocardial infarction and stroke. This increased risk is likely related to increased activation of the sympathetic nervous system and chemoreceptor stimulation that occurs in response to repetitive respiratory disturbances in patients with OSA (Fig. 32.6). The increased risk is independent of obesity, HTN, and diabetes. It has been noted that higher AHI, as well as a greater percentage of sleep time with less than 90% oxygen saturation, are associated with high-sensitivity troponin levels, suggesting that OSA is associated with low-grade myocardial injury. Moreover, individuals with moderate to severe OSA had an increased incidence of sudden cardiac death, which may be related to increased cardiac vagal activation that occurs in response to intermittent nocturnal

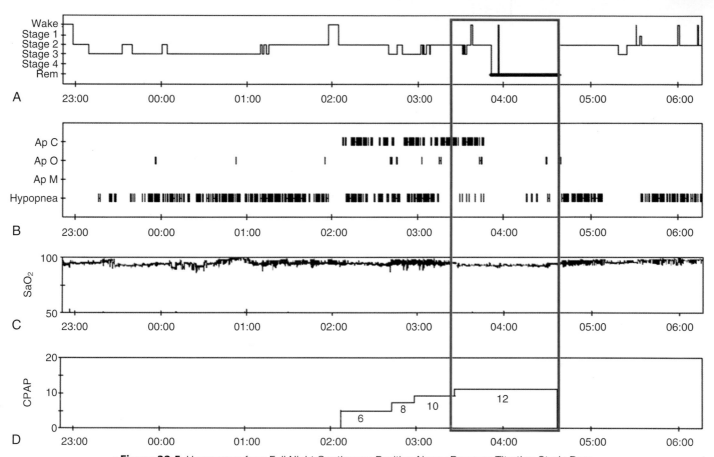

• **Figure 32.5** Hypnogram from Full Night Continuous Positive Airway Pressure Titration Study Demonstrating Continuous Positive Airway Pressure-Emergent Central Sleep Apnea. *Red rectangle* identifies the response to continuous positive airway pressure (CPAP) of 12 cm of water. Note that the patient has a reduction in obstructive events compared with other pressures. Central apneas resolve during rapid eye movement (REM) sleep but are still very much present during non-REM sleep at this pressure. Selection of positive airway pressure settings associated with maximal reduction of obstructive events without significant worsening of central events is a reasonable treatment option in patients with CPAP-emergent central apneas. **A,** Shows sleep staging across the night. Wake = stage W, Stage 1 = stage N1, Stage 2 = stage N2, Stage 3 = stage N3, stage 4 = stage N3, REM = stage REM. **B,** Shows respiratory events across the night. *Ap C,* Central apneas; *Ap O,* obstructive apneas; *Ap M,* mixed apneas; *Hypopnea,* obstructive hypopneas. **C,** Shows pulse oximetry results across the night. *SaO₂,* Oxyhemoglobin saturation. **D,** Shows CPAP levels increasing from 5 to 12 cm of water between 2 AM and 4 AM.

hypoxia, acidosis, and hypercarbia (see Fig. 32.6). While individuals with OSA have increased coronary artery calcification, there is no evidence of an increased risk of thoracic aortic aneurysm rupture. Lastly, although OSA may be a risk factor for venous thromboembolic disease, there is no known association with left ventricular thrombus.[9–11]

3. **Answer A.** Individuals with OSA have an increased cumulative risk of developing atrial fibrillation as compared with individuals without OSA (Fig. 32.7). This risk is a direct result of sleep fragmentation, hypoxia-reoxygenation episodes, and changes in intrathoracic pressures seen in OSA (Fig. 32.8). Moreover, untreated OSA is a predictor of recurrent atrial fibrillation after catheter ablation. Treatment of OSA reduces this risk. Patients undergoing cardiac ablation should have an evaluation for OSA and should be treated with CPAP prior to ablation. While REM sleep is conducive to arrhythmias due to reduced parasympathetic tone in the setting of surges

of sympathetic activity, there is no evidence that the recurrence of atrial fibrillation after ablation is related to REM sleep amounts. There is no known link between PLMS and atrial fibrillation.[12–14]

4. **Answer B.** Current smokers are at greater risk (approximately a threefold increase) for SDB than former smokers or those who have never smoked. Hypothesized mechanisms include airway inflammation due to smoking and tobacco-related lung disease. The effect of microwithdrawal from nicotine overnight affecting sleep stability has also been postulated. Although postmenopausal women are three times more likely to have at least moderate OSA than premenopausal women, the prevalence of OSA is still less than men of the same age. Insulin resistance and the metabolic syndrome are common consequences of untreated OSA. In one study of more than 300 participants, more than 80% of individuals with type 2 diabetes and obesity had at least mild OSA. It has been well

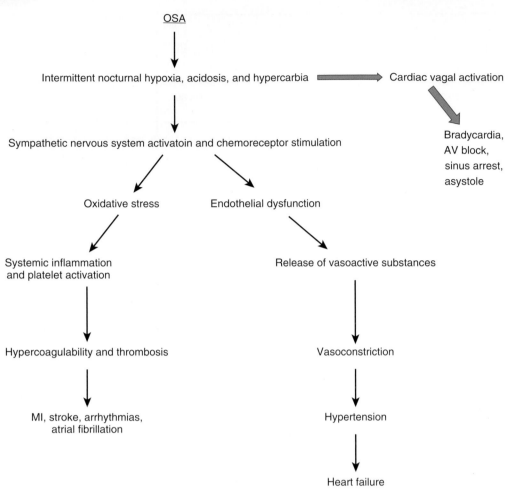

• **Figure 32.6** Physiologic effects of obstructive sleep apnea and the effects on the cardiovascular system. *AV,* Atrioventricular; *OSA,* obstructive sleep apnea; *MI,* myocardial infarction. (From Kar S. Cardiovascular implications of obstructive sleep apnea associated with the presence of a patent foramen ovale. *Sleep Med Rev.* 2014;18[5]:399–404.)

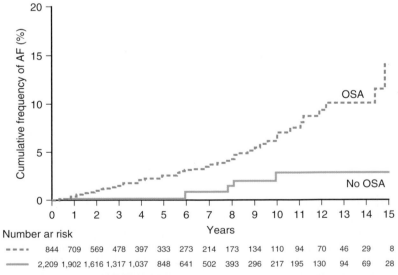

• **Figure 32.7** Incidence of atrial fibrillation based on presence or absence of OSA. Cumulative frequency curves for incident atrial fibrillation (AF) for subjects less than 65 years of age with and without obstructive sleep apnea (OSA) during an average 4.7 years of follow-up. *P* = .002. (From Gami AS, Hodge DO, Herges, RM, et al. Obstructive sleep apnea, obesity, and the risk of incident atrial fibrillation. *J Am Coll Cardiol.* 2007;49[5]:565–571.)

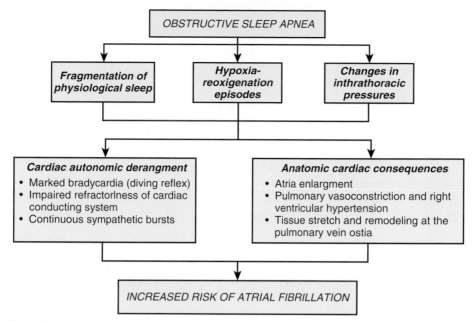

• **Figure 32.8** Obstructive sleep apnea (OSA) is one of the most common types of sleep-disordered breathing. OSA is characterized by repetitive episodes of upper airways collapse, which lead to sleep fragmentation, alteration of blood gases exchange, and significant changes in intrathoracic pressures. These mechanisms, through an important autonomic derangement and changes in cardiac anatomy, are responsible for an increased risk of atrial fibrillation in OSA patients. (From Tobaldini E, Costantino G, Solbiati M, et al. Sleep, sleep deprivation, autonomic nervous system and cardiovascular diseases. *Neurosci Biobehav Rev.* 2017;74:321–329.)

established that individuals with end stage renal disease requiring peritoneal dialysis or hemodialysis are significantly more likely to have OSA. More recently, recognition of the increased prevalence of OSA in patients with CKD has been appreciated. Notably, symptoms of daytime sleepiness, unrefreshing sleep, snoring, and nocturnal choking tend to be less predictive of the presence or absence of SDB in this population. Given that nocturnal hypoxia can lead to progression of renal function, objective testing for sleep-disordered should be considered in this population.[15–19]

5. **Answer C.** Patients with OSA should avoid even daytime alcohol consumption, as intake can contribute to weight gain and obesity. Additionally, nasal obstruction is increased and sensory processing to respiratory stimuli is altered with daytime alcohol consumption, which may persist during sleep. Alcohol has been shown to increase both the frequency and duration of respiratory events when ingested prior to bedtime. In addition, the degree of oxyhemoglobin desaturation is more pronounced. Alcohol ingestion is associated with an increase in the prevalence and severity of snoring. Moreover, patients with simple snoring can develop OSA after acute ingestion of alcohol prior to bedtime.[20–22]

6. **Answer A.** A recent meta-analysis looking at oxygen therapy in OSA showed that while nocturnal oxygen improves oxygen saturation in patients with OSA, there was an increase in duration of respiratory events. Intermittent hypoxemia is associated with increased sympathetic activity and norepinephrine levels that contribute to HTN. It is the degree and the duration of oxygen desaturation that is most strongly linked to the sequelae of OSA, as compared with the AHI or arousals during sleep. In one study, oxygen was less effective

than CPAP in the improvement of daytime sleepiness; another study showed no significant difference in improvement among CPAP, oxygen, and placebo.[23–25]

7. **Answer C.** Fig. 32.3 depicts the Cheyne-Stokes respiratory (CSR) pattern of breathing. The tracing shows crescendo-decrescendo pattern of breathing best seen in the FLOW channel. Note that the cycle length (i.e., start of central apnea to end of hyperpnea is ≥40 sec). Note the recurrent hypoxia/reoxygenation as a result of CSA. This develops due to a combination of factors that may be exacerbated in patients with HF. Individuals who have HF and CSR often have lower resting arterial carbon dioxide tensions. In response to this hypocapnia, a hypersensitive respiratory control center initiates an apnea. Due to some circulatory delay related to the presence of HF itself, the time to detect the rising $PaCO_2$ (as a result of the apnea) is prolonged. This leads to an overshooting of the $PaCO_2$, and hypercapnia exists by the time the respiratory control center terminates the apnea. Subsequently, a highly sensitive ventilatory control center responds to this hypercapnia with an exaggerated breathing response (i.e., hyperpnea). This exaggerated ventilatory response is the main contributor to the high loop gain seen in these patients (Fig. 32.9). It should be noted that the periodic cycle inclusive of apnea and hyperpnea is prolonged to 60 sec or more, compared with shorter durations in patients with idiopathic CSA or high-altitude breathing without HF (Fig. 32.10). CSR occurs more frequently during non-REM (NREM) sleep, as compared with wakefulness and REM sleep. Ventilation during NREM sleep is primarily under metabolic control such that alterations in $PaCO_2$ significantly affect breathing. This is in contrast with REM sleep, where ventilation is relatively insensitive to changes in $PaCO_2$, as

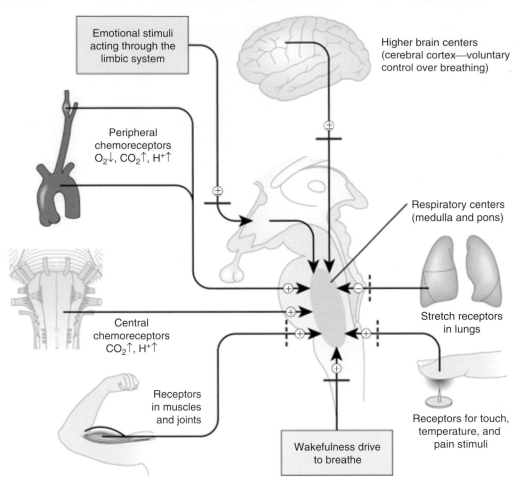

• **Figure 32.9** This figure depicts the loop-gain concept for control of breathing and initiation, and maintenance of Cheyne-Stokes Respiration. This schematic shows the multiple inputs that are capable of regulating breathing. During sleep, many of these inputs are either substantially diminished *(dashed red lines)* or absent *(solid red lines)*. Thus the predominant inputs to breathing during sleep are the chemoreceptors, which themselves also are downregulated and affected by state. Note: For simplicity, voluntary control of breathing is shown to act by way of the respiratory centers. Whether this is in fact the case or whether voluntary control acts directly on the respiratory motoneurons, however, has not been established. Refer to text for further details. (Modified from Eckert DJ, Roca D, Yim-Yeh S, Malhotra A. Control of breathing. In: Kryger M, ed. *Atlas of Clinical Sleep Medicine*. vol. 2. 2nd ed. Philadelphia, PA: Saunders; 2014:45–52).

arousability to chemical respiratory stimuli is diminished compared with NREM sleep (reducing hyperpnea). Additionally, respiratory drive and muscle activity are reduced in REM sleep so that $PaCO_2$ rises above the apnea threshold (reducing apnea). CSR is typically seen in patients with HF, who have a respiratory alkalosis.[26-30]

8. **Answer D.** The coexistence of COPD and OSA is denoted as "overlap syndrome." In a prospective cohort study involving more than 600 patients, individuals with the overlap syndrome had an increased risk of death from any cause, as well as an increased risk of hospitalization with a COPD exacerbation. Using CPAP in these patients improved survival and COPD related hospitalizations. Interestingly, there was no difference in cancer-related mortality in patients with overlap syndrome, where they were treated with CPAP or not, and patients with COPD alone. Patients with COPD should be assessed for any red flags that might suggest the presence of concurrent

OSA such as obesity, snoring, excessive daytime sleepiness, morning headaches or hypercapnia, or pulmonary HTN out of proportion to the pulmonary function test (PFT) abnormalities. After COPD is optimized, a polysomnography should be performed. Treatment considerations are shown in Fig. 32.11.[31,32]

9. **Answer C.** Over the last decade, it has been noted that patients with IPF have an increased incidence of OSA. This association is so strong that the 2011 IPF guidelines report OSA as a comorbid disease frequently associated with IPF. Pathophysiologic changes of IPF may contribute to OSA (Fig. 32.12). Patients with IPF have abnormal sleep architecture with loss of REM sleep, increased stage N1 sleep, and marked sleep fragmentation compared with age- and sex-matched controls. There is no evidence that patients with IPF are at increased risk of CSA or REM sleep behavior disorder (RBD). However, there is evidence for increased incidence of PLMS, as well as

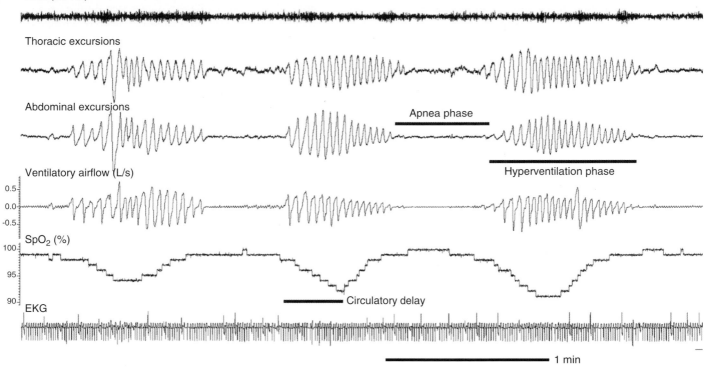

• Figure 32.10 This figure is a 4-min tracing from an overnight sleep study of a patient with Cheyne-Stokes respiratory breathing pattern. *EKG,* Electrocardiogram; *SpO₂,* oxyhemoglobin saturation. (From Sands S, Owens RL. Congestive heart failure and central sleep apnea. *Crit Care Clin.* 2015;31[3]: 473–495.)

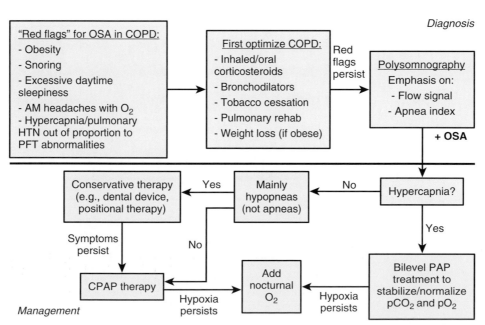

• Figure 32.11 It demonstrates the management algorithm for patients with chronic obstructive pulmonary disease (COPD) and consideration for those patients who might be at risk for obstructive sleep apnea (OSA). *CPAP,* Continuous positive airway pressure; *HTN,* hypertension; *PAP,* positive airway pressure; *PFT,* pulmonary function test. (From Dudley K, Owens, R, Malhotra A. Pulmonary overlap syndromes, with a focus on COPD and ILD. *Sleep Med Clin.* 2014;9[3]:365–379.)

increased complaints of insomnia. In addition, these patients have increased respiratory frequency during sleep.[33-35]

10. **Answer D.** In patients taking chronic opioids, the prevalence of central apnea positively correlates with opioid dose. In addition, there is also a dose-response relationship between opioid dose and obstructive apneas and hypopneas, as well as AHIs. There has been a dramatic increase in the usage of opioids for chronic malignant pain, partially related to the recognition that long-term use was associated with increased tolerance and decreased sedation and respiratory depression.

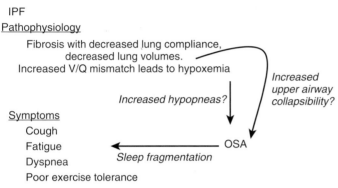

• **Figure 32.12** This figure demonstrates the pathophysiology implicated in the association between idiopathic pulmonary fibrosis and obstructive sleep apnea, as well as symptoms that can be attributed to each of this comorbidities. *IPF,* Idiopathic pulmonary fibrosis; *OSA,* obstructive sleep apnea. (From Dudley K, Owens RL, Malhotra A. *Sleep Med Clin.* 2014;9[3]: 365–379.)

However, the reduced respiratory effects are mainly seen in wakefulness, and significant SDB is seen during sleep. These respiratory effects are seen almost exclusively during NREM sleep, as seen in Figs. 32.13 and 32.14. The clinically available opioids stimulate mu-opioid receptors that are expressed on both respiratory and pain neurons. However, chronic opioid use is typically associated with downregulation of these receptors, and it is likely that mu-opioid receptors affect sleep related respiration by depression of the ventilatory hypoxic drive, as well as decreasing the discharge properties of cranial motoneurons controlling the patency of the upper airway and reducing pulmonary compliance via reduced chest and abdominal wall activity. Cessation of opioid use is associated with improvement in SDB (Fig. 32.15).[36-38]

11. **Answer D.** The sleep study tracing (see Fig. 32.4) shows Biot's breathing (a.k.a. ataxic breathing), which is characterized by significant variability in respiratory rate, rhythm, and depth with or without brief respiratory pauses less than 10 sec, or a repeating pattern of several breaths. In a study of taking opiate medications for long-term use, Biot's breathing was observed in 70% of patients, versus 5% of patients not taking opioids. In the same study, central apneas were much more common than in patients not taking opioids, and a dose-response relationship was observed between morphine dose equivalent and AHI. It should be recognized that despite the greater frequency of central apneas in long-term opioid users, obstructive apneas and hypopnea events are also common during sleep in these patients, and in fact often comprise a larger overall proportion of SDB events than central apneas. Nocturnal hypoxemia out of proportion with the degree of

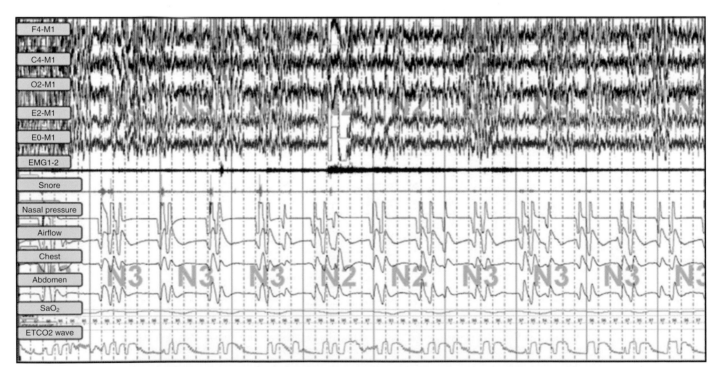

• **Figure 32.13** This is a 5-min tracing from an overnight polysomnogram. It shows central apneic events seen during stage N2 and stage N3. *C4-M1,* Central lead; *E0-M1,* left eye; *EMG1-2,* chin electromyogram; *E2-M1,* right eye; *ETCO₂,* end-tidal CO2; *F4-M1,* frontal lead; *O2-M1,* occipital lead; *snore,* snore microphone; *SaO₂,* oxyhemoglobin saturation. (From Tovar-Torres MP, Bodkin C, Sigua NL. A 44-year-old woman with excessive sleepiness. *Chest.* 2014;146[6]:e204–e207.)

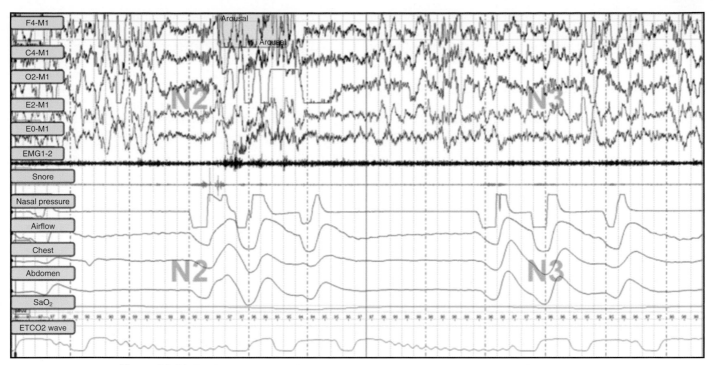

• **Figure 32.14** This is a 1-min tracing from an overnight polysomnogram. It shows central apneic events seen during stage N2 and stage N3. *C4-M1*, Central lead; *E0-M1*, left eye; *EMG1-2*, chin electromyogram; *E2-M1*, right eye; *ETCO₂*, end-tidal CO2; *F4-M1*, frontal lead; *O2-M1*, occipital lead; *snore*, snore microphone; *SaO₂*, oxyhemoglobin saturation. (From Tovar-Torres MP, Bodkin C, Sigua NL. A 44-year-old woman with excessive sleepiness. *Chest.* 2014;146[6]:e204–e207.)

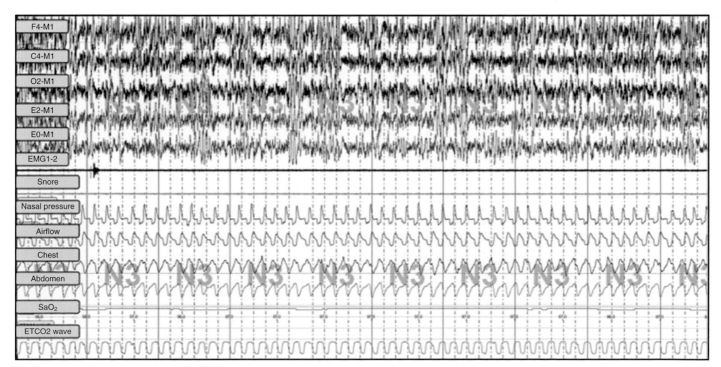

• **Figure 32.15** This is 9.5 min excerpt (300 sec/page) from an overnight polysomnogram. It shows complete resolution of central sleep apnea with opioid cessation. *C4-M1*, Central lead; *E0-M1*, left eye; *EMG1-2*, chin electromyogram; *E2-M1*, right eye; *ETCO₂*, end-tidal CO2; *F4-M1*, frontal lead; *O2-M1*, occipital lead; *snore*, snore microphone; *SaO₂*, oxyhemoglobin saturation. (From Tovar-Torres MP, Bodkin C, Sigua NL. A 44-year-old woman with excessive sleepiness. *Chest.* 2014;146[6]:e204–e207.)

sleep apnea has also been observed in long-term opioid users.[36,39,40]

12. **Answer C.** The patient has lost a substantial amount of weight, with a decrease in BMI from 48 to 33 kg/m². A recent systematic review reported that seven randomized controlled trials showed that weight reduction was associated with a decrease in AHI. Weight loss of 10%–16% reduced AHI by 20%–50% in three randomized controlled trials; three other uncontrolled studies reported that weight loss of 13%–30% reduced AHI by 10%–50%. Nevertheless, weight loss was often insufficient to normalize OSA parameters. Among bariatric patients with OSA, long-term adherence to CPAP therapy has been reported to be poor. However, nonadherence has recently been observed to be associated with weight gain. When sleep studies are performed after bariatric surgery, patients are often found to have persistent OSA for which treatment may be indicated. Thus especially in the setting of severe OSA prior to the patient's dramatic weight loss, a sleep study should be repeated to determine whether she still has OSA.[41–44]

13. **Answer B.** Women with PCOS have been observed to have rates of OSA at much higher rates compared with reproductively normal women. The increased risk for OSA has been attributed to testosterone excess and to higher rates of obesity among women with PCOS, though higher rates of OSA were observed even when control subjects were matched for age and BMI. Postmenopausal women are at two- to threefold greater risk for OSA compared with postmenopausal women, a finding observed in several large community-based cohort studies. Although reduced risk for OSA has been reported among users of hormone replacement therapy compared with postmenopausal women not taking hormone therapy, recent work suggests that this observation may have been due largely to healthy user bias rather than a real effect. During pregnancy, women are also at risk for developing SDB, which can increase the likelihood of adverse maternal fetal outcomes including gestational HTN, preeclampsia, and gestational diabetes. A relationship between endometriosis and OSA has not been hypothesized or assessed.[45–50]

14. **Answer B.** Patients with OHS, previously known as Pickwickian syndrome, are obese (BMI >30 kg/m²) and exhibit daytime hypercapnia (pCO₂ >45 mmHg) in the absence of other known causes of alveolar hypoventilation. OHS has been estimated to occur in 10%–20% of patients with OSA but frequently goes unrecognized, despite increased risk for morbidity and mortality. The prevalence of OHS is thought to be increasing, given the increase in prevalence of obesity, especially morbid obesity, in the United States. Although secondary polycythemia is frequently cited as a feature of OHS and has been observed to improve with treatment, hemoglobin levels have not been shown to be a predictor of OHS. Several recent studies have examined potential predictors of OHS and have found that serum bicarbonate (HCO_3) of 27 mEq/L or higher has a sensitivity of 86%–90% and specificity of 50%–90% for predicting OHS. Clinically, $HCO_3 \geq 27$ should prompt further investigation to determine if the patient has OHS, such as obtaining a daytime arterial blood gas to demonstrate daytime hypercapnia and/or performing transcutaneous CO_2 monitoring during the diagnostic sleep study (if available), and exclusion of other potential causes of chronic respiratory failure.[51,52]

15. **Answer A.** This patient has CSA associated with chronic use of opioid medications, which appears to be increasingly common, as prescription opioid use for chronic pain has increased dramatically in recent years. Patients chronically taking opioids frequently report daytime sleepiness and fatigue. Both obstructive and central apneas appear to be common with the long-term use of opioids, with CSA occurring much more frequently than among non-opioid users. Studies examining SDB in chronic opioid users suggest that risk factors differ from traditional risk factors for OSA, and include daily opioid dose greater than 200 mg morphine (or equivalent) and low to low-normal BMI, and in some studies, concomitant use of benzodiazepines and antidepressant medications. While CPAP therapy can eliminate obstructive events in patients with opioid-induced sleep apnea, it has minimal effect on ataxic breathing and hypoxemia, and can worsen central apnea associated with opioid use. Similarly, although BPAP augments tidal volume, central apneas can persist when BPAP is utilized without a backup rate. Thus BPAP should generally be used with a backup rate in patients with central apneas associated with chronic opioid use, to treat the central apnea component and provide ventilatory assistance. ASV has also been used successfully to treat opioid-induced SDB. In recent comparisons of either BPAP with a backup rate or CPAP with ASV, ASV was significantly more effective for treatment of CSA associated with chronic opioid use. Of note, given recently published results from the Treatment of Sleep-Disordered Breathing With Predominant Central Sleep Apnea by Adaptive Servo Ventilation in Patients With HF (SERVE-HF) study showing significantly higher all cause and cardiovascular mortality among patients using ASV, ASV should be avoided in patients with coexisting HF with decreased EF (<45%). Oxygen alone without PAP therapy is not adequate therapy for treatment of opioid-induced/associated sleep-disordered breathing, although it may be added to PAP therapies to maintain sleep-related hypoxemia.[53–57]

16. **Answer C.** While most physicians consider CPAP to be first-line therapy for patients with OSA, clinical guidelines recommend patient education regarding treatment options. Oral appliances are appropriate therapy for patients with mild to moderate OSA who express a preference for oral appliance therapy, or who are nonadherent or nonresponsive to PAP therapy. Although even patients with severe OSA may be treated effectively with an oral appliance, the proportion of patients with moderate and severe OSA who achieve successful treatment is lower using oral appliances compared with CPAP therapy. Younger age, lower BMI, and positional OSA have been observed in some studies to predict better outcomes with use of an oral appliance. Temporomandibular joint disease is the most common contraindication for oral appliances. Other contraindications include severe symptoms (e.g., history of drowsy driving or active cardiovascular issues), severe OSA-related oxyhemoglobin saturation, and inadequate dentition to support the use of an oral appliance. Oral appliance use is associated with modest reductions in systolic, diastolic, and mean BP, which appear to be nearly equivalent compared with CPAP. Thus the presence of HTN should not preclude the use of oral appliances.[58–60]

17. **Answer C.** Attended, in-laboratory polysomnography has long been the study of choice for establishing the diagnosis of OSA. However, in recent years, long wait times and high costs for these studies have led to intense interest in less costly HSAT and out-of-laboratory algorithms for diagnosing and treating

sleep apnea. Key to maximizing the diagnostic utility of HSAT is appropriate patient selection. Guidelines for the use of HSAT have been developed by organizations, including the American Academy of Sleep Medicine and Canadian Sleep Society/Canadian Thoracic Society. These guidelines state that HSAT is appropriate for patients who have a high pretest probability of moderate to severe OSA. However, they are not appropriate tests for patients with significant comorbidities that may limit the accuracy of HSAT (e.g., CHF, pulmonary disease, neuromuscular disease); patients with other suspected sleep disorders (e.g., CSA, periodic limb movement disorder, circadian rhythm disorders, insomnia); or for routine OSA screening in asymptomatic patients.[61,62]

18. **Answer B.** Multiple studies have described increased risk among pregnant women with OSA for adverse maternal-fetal outcomes, including gestational HTN, preeclampsia, and gestational diabetes, including a recent National Institutes of Health–funded prospective cohort study of more than 3700 mothers-to-be. One cross-sectional retrospective study of maternal hospital discharges has suggested that pregnancy-associated OSA may also be associated with an increased, not decreased, risk for pulmonary embolism. As CPAP can be initiated quickly, adjusted as OSA severity changes during pregnancy (e.g., using an auto-titrating device), and its effectiveness assessed with relative ease, it is generally recommended as initial treatment for pregnancy-associated OSA. In contrast, while oral appliances are an alternative first-line therapy for OSA in the general population, the time needed after initial OSA diagnosis to assess the patient's suitability for oral appliance therapy, manufacture the device, achieve the target treatment protrusion, and assess the device's effectiveness is generally longer and likely to preclude routine use of oral appliances for pregnancy-associated OSA. Studies comparing CPAP and BPAP for treatment of OSA in pregnant women have not been performed. However, OSA in pregnant women tends to be mild and is likely to be effectively treated with lower levels of PAP.[50,63,64]

19. **Answer D.** During the initial evaluation for suspected or confirmed OSA, all patients should be asked about daytime sleepiness and recent unintended motor vehicle crashes or near misses attributable to sleepiness, fatigue, or inattention—that is, characteristics of drivers at high risk for drowsy driving crashes. While the patient's Epworth score, reports from family, and self-reported sleepiness can provide additional clinical information, they are also subject to interpretation and bias. Thus clinicians should question patients directly to identify high risk drivers. Reassessment of driving risk should be performed in those identified as high risk after initiation of any treatment for OSA. Several studies have demonstrated that individuals with higher levels of sleepiness, objectively measured using the multiple sleep latency test (MSLT) or maintenance of wakefulness test (MWT), are more likely to perform poorly in tests of driving simulation. Nevertheless, associations between MSLT/MWT results and simulated or real driving performance are generally low to moderate, and the ability of these tests to predict future crashes has not been established. Thus in clinical practice the MSLT and MWT are generally not performed to assess drowsy driving risk.[65–67]

20. **Answer A.** Risk for motor vehicle crashes is increased by two to three times among patients with untreated OSA. Although prediction of crash risk in individual patients is imprecise, a high-risk driver is defined as one with moderate to severe daytime sleepiness and a recent unintended crash or near miss incident attributable to sleepiness, fatigue, or inattention. Drowsy driving crashes are more likely to involve a single vehicle, with no evidence of braking or attempts to avoid the crash; they are thus associated with higher rates of serious injury and mortality than nondrowsy driving crashes. Patients who are at high risk for drowsy driving crashes should receive timely diagnostic evaluation and treatment. However, at present, there is a lack of compelling evidence for the initiation of empiric CPAP therapy or the use of stimulant medication solely to reduce driving risk. If possible, high-risk drivers should refrain from driving until they can be diagnosed and treated. Otherwise, a nap break—that is, a 15-to-20-min sleep period—is suggested to be one of the most effective countermeasures against sleepiness and can improve simulated driving performance levels. Alternative countermeasures include stopping at the roadside to rest until the driver feels refreshed and ready to drive again, swapping drivers, and consuming caffeine. Opening the car window, running the air conditioner, and listening to loud music have not been found to be effective countermeasures against drowsy driving. Use of mobile phones is associated with increased crash or near-crash risk among both novice and experienced drivers, and should not be recommended.[65,68–72]

21. **Answer C.** The use of auto-titrating CPAP devices has increased over the years, in part due to the accumulating body of evidence showing efficacy, patient preferences for at-home evaluation, and because they allow for more rapid initiation of therapy without delays associated with titration studies.[73,74] ACPAPs adjust the pressure throughout the night using proprietary algorithms unique to each device manufacturer. Current technology uses a variety of methods to titrate the pressure, including flow-based sensors that assess the inspiratory flow waveform for flattening, or use of a forced oscillation technique to distinguish central from obstructive apneas that are implemented using real-time microprocessor analysis.[75] The initial settings generally include an upper and lower bound pressure range, with devices starting at the lower pressure value and performing further adjustments based on their algorithm. If the patient changes position, or enters a stage of sleep that may require reduced pressure support, the unit can adjust pressure downward to compensate.

The auto-titrating CPAP devices report a broad range of data statistics. In terms of adjusting pressure, the most commonly used are the P90 and P95 (90% pressure and 95% pressure, respectively) values. For example, the P90 value indicates the pressure at which the unit was effectively able to ablate apnea or hypopnea events for 90% of the night; thus for only 10% of the night did the unit have to exceed the P90 value. While some have noted that the P90 value is ideal,[76] others have suggested that the P95 value is more appropriate.[77] In part, the choice of using P90 or P95 is based on the calibration properties of the device algorithm, and manufacturers will generally report one or the other on their data sheets.

22. **Answer D.** Obesity is considered one of the major risk factors for sleep apnea. Correspondingly, weight loss is expected to reduce sleep apnea severity. One meta-analysis evaluating change in AHI in bariatric surgery patients noted that in the available pool of studies (which included follow-up ranging from 4 weeks to 24 months), the average BMI reduction was 2.3 kg/m^2 when comparing bariatric patients to controls in randomized trials, and sleep apnea severity decreased by an

average of 6 events/hour in the bariatric surgery patients.[42] This reduction in sleep apnea severity could theoretically lead to a reduction in CPAP pressure support settings. One study that followed patients postbariatric surgery noted an overall reduction in CPAP pressure of 18%. This led the authors to conclude that autotitrating PAP units may have a role, given the reduced CPAP pressure needs as patients lose weight.[78]

When considering the various possible answers, it is unlikely that the patient will have complete resolution of their sleep apnea after 1 month. While he can continue CPAP therapy at PS 14, it is likely that with his continued weight loss, he may need a lower pressure (choice B is possible, but not the best choice). A pressure such as CPAP PS 12 may work, but there is no well-defined correlation between weight change and CPAP PS need; therefore an empiric decrease to PS 12 is not necessarily correct. Autotitrating mode is the best option, and the remaining two choices provide different pressure ranges. A range of 5–15 is reasonable because it includes the pressure of 14 cm H_2O, which had previously been proven to be effective (choice D is correct). A range of 5–12 may be too low, since it does not include the setting of 14 cm H_2O.

23. **Answer C.** This patient is presenting with CPAP nonadherence due to a combination of mask and pressure discomfort. It can often be difficult to determine the exact etiology in these cases. EPR is a device feature that reduces the airway pressure during the initial exhalation phase, instead of maintaining the pressure at a constant value as is usually the case.[79] It differs from BPAP in that BPAP reduces the pressure to a preset value, the EPAP, while the EPR pressure varies depending on the exhalation flow rate from the patient. The specific algorithm that determines the EPR pressure depends on the device manufacturer. EPR settings refer to the degree of EPR correction provided by the device, and generally do not refer to a fixed pressure value. Thus an EPR of 2 does not necessarily mean that the EPR pressure will drop by 2 cm H_2O, but instead that it is a midvalue setting if the device has EPR options of 1, 2, and 3. EPR has not been shown to consistently lead to improved adherence,[80] and while it can benefit individual patients, it is not the recommended initial step.

Increasing the moisture content of the air via humidification can be beneficial, especially in cases where patients complain of oral or nasal dryness. While not all studies have shown a benefit from this intervention, it is generally considered consistent with good clinical practice.[81] Since this patient did not complain of dryness per se, it is unlikely that humidification alone will improve his adherence.

The patient is reporting that the mask is uncomfortable; thus a reasonable option would be to consider switching to a nasal mask. Several studies have shown that an oronasal mask (which covers both the mouth and nose) is associated with a higher rate of nonadherence,[82] with one prospective study observing an odds ratio of 2.0 for nonadherence when using an oronasal mask.[83] There are several possible reasons for this. First, the oronasal mask is larger than either a nasal mask or nasal pillows, thus potentially increasing patient perceptions of discomfort. Second, the oronasal mask, by delivering an increased pressure to the oral cavity, may lead to posterior displacement of the tongue, which in turn can narrow or occlude the upper airway.[82] Residual AHI is thus often higher when using an oronasal mask, and some patients may need higher CPAP pressures.[84] For these reasons, switching the patient to a different mask type, such as a nasal mask (choice

C is correct), is a better option than switching to a different oronasal mask. This patient is not complaining primarily of insomnia symptoms. Thus CBT-I is unlikely to have a major benefit.

24. **Answer B.** BPAP therapy was first developed by Sanders and Kern as a means of delivering two levels of PAP, an IPAP and a lower EPAP, which can help reduce perceived difficulty exhaling against PAP.[85] Several studies have been conducted examining the potential use of BPAP, with one recent retrospective study describing patterns of use in 2513 veteran patients.[86] The authors noted that BPAP tended to be used in patients with comorbid conditions, such as CHF, COPD or neurologic conditions, and that BPAP adherence was higher than CPAP. BPAP, when used in an autotitrating mode (bilevel-auto), can be effective in treating patients who continue to have respiratory events on CPAP, or have demonstrated intolerance to CPAP.[87] For patients with uncomplicated sleep apnea who are starting PAP treatment for the first time, though, BPAP is not recommended as a first-line treatment due to the paucity of evidence available to clarify the role of BPAP in newly diagnosed patients with uncomplicated sleep apnea.[88] While this patient is concerned about excessive pressure, one reasonable option would be to initiate therapy with an autotitrating PAP unit, as opposed to the more expensive BPAP units. A review of BPAP studies found no evidence of improved overall adherence with BPAP compared with CPAP.[80] One specific initial treatment scenario where BPAP can be useful is when patients have hypoventilation syndromes, such as COPD, because the pressure difference between the IPAP and EPAP mode can provide ventilatory support by increasing the tidal volume.[79] In addition, BPAP machines can deliver pressures that are greater than 20 cm H_2O, the usual upper limit for most CPAP or autotitrating PAP units. If a patient is consistently reaching the maximum pressure of 20 cm H_2O, a trial of using a BPAP unit is warranted.

25. **Answer B.** Several randomized trials have compared APAP and CPAP use on a variety of metrics, including adherence, sleep characteristics, and BP. A sufficient number of studies have been conducted so that meta-analyses of the results can now be performed. One recent meta-analysis by Ip et al. provides important pooled results from 24 randomized trials that can help guide clinicians when making management decisions related to APAP and CPAP.[89] In general, APAP was not associated with an increase in sleep efficiency when compared with CPAP, although this parameter was only reported by three of the studies. However, APAP did have a small but statistically significant increase in minutes of use in pooled analysis, with an average increase in adherence of 11 minutes (95% CI, 0.05–0.31 min; choice B is correct). The authors noted that this increased adherence was not influenced by baseline AHI severity. Several studies also examined the effects of APAP and CPAP on sleep architecture in terms of slow wave sleep and REM sleep: in general, there were no significant improvements with APAP as compared with CPAP. BP changes were reported in three trials, of which two showed no change, while a third suggested that systolic and diastolic BP decreased more with CPAP than with APAP (systolic by approximately 6 mmHg and diastolic by 8 mmHg).[90] Oxygen desaturation was also improved in CPAP relative to APAP (1.3% improvement in the oxygen desaturation nadir with CPAP; 95% CI, 2.2%–0.4%).[89] In regard to daytime sleepiness, there was a small but statistically significant improvement in

the Epworth Sleepiness Score in APAP users as compared with CPAP users of 0.48 (95% CI, −0.81 to −0.15); however, this was predominantly due to a large improvement noted in only two of the 22 trials; the other 20 trials showed no difference between APAP and CPAP.[89]

26. **Answer A.** With an estimated 43 million older adults in the United States in 2012 expected to increase to 72 million by 2030, and given the age-related increase in the development of cognitive impairment, many older adults may be interested in the role of sleep apnea in relationship to cognitive impairment. Several research studies have examined this. One of the largest studies was a prospective observational study in older females noting that the odds ratio for developing cognitive impairment (mild cognitive impairment or dementia) in study participants with an AHI index greater than 15 events/hour, over an average 4.7-year follow-up, was 2.36 in adjusted analyses that controlled for baseline cognitive function.[91] When considering other measures, such as whether oxygen saturation less than 90% occurred for greater than 1% of sleep time, they did not find an association, and total sleep time was also not associated, in adjusted analysis, with risk of cognitive impairment. Several studies have noted a delay in cognitive decline with CPAP treatment,[92,93] with one nonrandomized, single-blinded CPAP intervention study in patients with Alzheimer's dementia, noting a statistically significant reduction in the level of progressive cognitive impairment over a 3-year follow-up (choice A is correct).[94] A randomized study comparing patients with mild to moderate Alzheimer's dementia over a 3-week period found that the Epworth Sleepiness Score improved by 2.3 in the CPAP group, compared with 0.7 in the sham-CPAP group, confirming that CPAP can improve daytime sleepiness complaints in patients with dementia.[95] These studies have noted effective CPAP compliance in patients with cognitive impairment who had access to caregiver assistance, suggesting that cognitive impairment per se does not make CPAP use impossible.

27. **Answer B.** Insomnia symptoms are very common in patients with sleep apnea, with one review noting an average prevalence of 20%–35%[96]. This could be due to a variety of factors, such as the intermittent arousals caused by repetitive upper airway obstruction from sleep apnea, or increased adrenergic tone noted in patients with sleep apnea.[97] Some research suggests that sleep maintenance forms of insomnia are more closely linked to sleep apnea than sleep initiation insomnia.[98] It is also important to note that many patients who present with chronic insomnia may have undiagnosed sleep apnea that contributes to their persistent insomnia, with one retrospective case series noting that 71% of patients on long-term insomnia pharmacotherapy had undiagnosed sleep apnea.[99] Management of these patients with comorbid sleep apnea and insomnia can be challenging, in large part due to concerns regarding the possibility that sedative-hypnotics may increase sleep apnea severity. A particular concern is that a patient may take a sedative-hypnotic and then fail to use their CPAP, thus creating a situation where their sleep apnea is worse than usual due to the potential effects of the sedative-hypnotic on upper airway muscle tone. However, neglecting the insomnia complaints of sleep apnea patients may in turn increase the risk of nonadherence to CPAP.

In this context, recent research has evaluated several treatment options. The most promising of these is CBT-I. Several studies have evaluated CBT-I in the context of sleep apnea and shown that it can be safely administered and can improve insomnia symptoms (choice B is correct).[100,101] Zaleplon and zolpidem have not been effective in improving CPAP adherence.[102,103] Ramelteon improved objective sleep time, but not subjective symptoms in older adults with comorbid insomnia and sleep apnea on APAP.[104] Trazodone, which is commonly used for the treatment of insomnia (not US Food and Drug Administration approved indication), has been shown to improve sleep apnea severity in a crossover randomized study of 15 subjects.[105] Eszopiclone has also been used and found to improve CPAP adherence in one study; however, since CBT-I has fewer side effects, it is the preferred initial option.[106]

28. **Answer D.** Mouth breathing is a common complaint for patients with sleep apnea that often leads providers and support staff to initiate therapy using an oronasal mask. However, research suggests that even with a nasal mask, mouth breathing is decreased in sleep apnea patients. One study observed, for example, that the number of mouth-breathing episodes per hour during sleep decreased from 35.2 events/hour pretreatment to 5.0 events/hour when using a nasal mask and CPAP.[107] For this reason, mouth breathing per se is not a contraindication to using a nasal mask. Due to the smaller airflow opening on a nasal pillow mask, there is a concern that higher CPAP pressures may be difficult to tolerate, as compared with a standard nasal mask. However, research comparing a nasal pillow and nasal mask in patients requiring pressures greater than 12 cm H_2O found comparable efficacy and adherence.[108] Amelioration of nasal obstruction can improve mouth breathing. Use of oxymetazolone can provide short-term benefit, but is associated with rebound vasocongestion that may result in worsening of the nasal obstruction. Nasal steroids can be effective and are relatively well tolerated for short-term use (choice D is correct). Otorhinology evaluation for possible nasal surgery is a reasonable choice, after confirming that nasal steroids or other pharmacotherapy was ineffective, and would not be appropriate as an initial step.

29. **Answer C.** The residual AHI provided by the internal sensor of the CPAP unit is an important tool in sleep apnea chronic disease management. While often used interchangeably with the AHI derived from an overnight sleep study, it is important to note that the residual AHI derived from the CPAP sensor is usually based on a single sensor and thus a proxy for the AHI as derived on a sleep study. In this context, the criteria for a target residual AHI can differ from the criteria when performing an in-lab titration study. A recent American Thoracic Society subcommittee on CPAP Adherence Tracking Systems provided guidance regarding residual AHI values and adjustment of CPAP. The residual AHI recommendations were as follows: AHI less than 10 events/hour: no adjustment needed if there is no significant mask leak; AHI between 10 to 20 events/hour: clinical correlation, with further adjustment if the patient has residual symptoms; AHI greater than 20 events/hour: increase pressure and check for mask leak.[109] Since this patient does not have any residual symptoms and is thus having a good clinical response, the normal AHI presented in choice A is not a concern and the elevated residual AHI presented in choice B is not a major concern. However, the residual AHI of 25 events/hour is too high, even in the setting of a good clinical response, and thus choice C is correct.

30. **Answer C.** Several studies have evaluated the effects of CPAP therapy on BP. These results were pooled in a meta-analysis of sleep apnea and BP, which found that the average systolic

BP reduction, in those on CPAP therapy compared with the control group, was −2.22 mmHg in MAP, −2.46 mmHg in systolic BP, and −1.83 mmHg in diastolic BP (choice C is correct).[110] Of note, BP improvement in hypertensive patients with CPAP treatment may be most prominent in patients with daytime sleepiness symptoms, and in those who have longer nightly average durations of CPAP use.[79]

Suggested Reading

Ahmed O, Parthasarathy S. APAP and alternative titration methods. *Sleep Med Clin.* 2010;5(3):361-368.

Donovan LM, Boeder S, Malhotra A, Patel SR. New developments in the use of positive airway pressure for obstructive sleep apnea. *J Thorac Dis.* 2015;7(8):1323-1342.

Schwab RJ, Badr SM, Epstein LJ, et al. An official American Thoracic Society statement: continuous positive airway pressure adherence tracking systems. The optimal monitoring strategies and outcome measures in adults. *Am J Respir Crit Care Med.* 2013;188(5):613-620.

Wickwire EM, Lettieri CJ, Cairns AA, Collop NA. Maximizing positive airway pressure adherence in adults: a common-sense approach. *Chest.* 2013;144(2):680-693.

Xu T, Li T, Wei D, et al. Effect of automatic versus fixed continuous positive airway pressure for the treatment of obstructive sleep apnea: an up-to-date meta-analysis. *Sleep Breath.* 2012;16(4):1017-1026.

33

Psychiatry Clinical Case Studies

DAVID T. PLANTE

Questions

1. A 7-year-old boy presents with his mother to the sleep clinic for assessment of insomnia. The child has been diagnosed with autism spectrum disorder (ASD). His mother provides the full history, telling you that the patient lacks the capacity to use or understand language in any meaningful way. The mother notes that her son has significant difficulties with sleep initiation at the beginning of the night, but once asleep, generally sleeps until the morning. They have a regular bedtime routine, and go to bed around the same time every night. Which of the following is the best option for treatment of the child's insomnia?
   A. Cognitive therapy to address maladaptive beliefs about insomnia
   B. Zolpidem 2.5 mg 30 min prior to bedtime
   C. Melatonin 3 mg 30 min prior to bedtime
   D. Olanzapine 2.5 mg 30 min prior to bedtime
   E. Clonazepam 0.5 mg 30 min prior to bedtime

2. A 70-year-old woman presents to her primary care physician's office complaining of depression that has worsened in the context of several life stressors. The patient reports she had been on a medication for depression several years earlier, but cannot recall its name. She is reluctant to pursue psychotherapy and requests a medication for her depression. One month after starting the medication that was prescribed by her physician, she returns to the office complaining of new-onset restlessness of both legs that is worse at night, but transiently relieved by movement. Which medication has she most likely been taking for her depression?
   A. Clonazepam
   B. Clonidine
   C. Paroxetine
   D. Sertraline
   E. Mirtazapine

3. A 45-year-old woman was referred for overnight polysomnography (PSG) to assess for sleep disordered breathing due to loud snoring and witnessed apneas. Past medical history was significant for obesity and panic disorder (PD). She reported using alprazolam 0.5 mg as needed for panic attacks, requiring the medication roughly once a month. She endorsed being on sertraline for her anxiety disorder about 6 months previously, but discontinued it due to intolerable side effects. A representative 30-sec epoch observed during the sleep study is presented in Fig. 33.1.

   The most likely explanation of this observed finding is:
   A. Withdrawal from alprazolam
   B. Normal variant
   C. Medication effect of sertraline
   D. Perimenopausal phenomenon
   E. Polysomnographic recording artifact

4. Extended EEGmontage polysomnogram is performed on a 37-year-old man with a history of schizophrenia. Compared with persons without schizophrenia, which of the following is most likely to be observed during the sleep study?
   A. Increased total sleep time
   B. Increased slow wave sleep
   C. Increased rapid eye movement (REM) sleep latency
   D. Reduced sleep spindles
   E. Decreased sleep onset latency

5. A 27-year-old woman presents with depressed mood, anhedonia, impaired concentration, daytime fatigue, and suicidal ideation, without intent or plan to harm herself. She denies a history of symptoms consistent with mania or psychosis. She is not currently taking any medications, and is in good physical health. PSG would most likely reveal which of the following alterations in sleep architecture?
   A. Reduced REM latency
   B. Reduced percentage of REM sleep relative to total sleep time
   C. Reduced sleep onset latency
   D. Reduced wake after sleep onset
   E. Increased sleep efficiency

6. The police bring a 22-year-old man with bipolar disorder into the emergency department for bizarre behavior. When questioned, he indicates a subjective decreased need for sleep, a feeling of euphoria, and increased goal-directed activity, which have been ongoing for the last 2 weeks. He is also noted to be grandiose and have pressured speech at the time of exam. If PSG were to be obtained in this individual, his sleep architecture would most likely demonstrate:
   A. Decreased sleep onset latency
   B. Increased N1 sleep
   C. Increased slow wave sleep
   D. Normal to prolonged REM latency
   E. Decreased wake after sleep onset

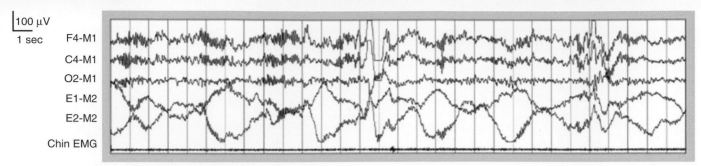

• **Figure 33.1** Representative 30-sec epoch from patient's polysomnogram. *EMG,* Electromyogram. (Modified from Berry RB. Biocalibration, artifacts, and common variants of sleep. In: *Fundamentals of Sleep Medicine.* Philadelphia, PA: Elsevier Saunders; 2012:49–64.)

7. A 30-year-old war veteran presents to the clinic seeking help for frequent nightmares that occur on a near nightly basis. The patient also notes being easily startled, and having flashbacks to combat encounters he had several years ago. The medication most likely to help improve his nightmares is:
   A. Clonazepam
   B. Prazosin
   C. Venlafaxine
   D. Nefazadone
   E. Carbamazepine

8. A 40-year-old woman without a history of posttraumatic stress disorder (PTSD) presents seeking help with recurrent nightmares. She is adamant that she does not want to take medication and prefers nonpharmacologic approaches. The type of psychotherapy most likely to help with her nightmares is:
   A. Eye-movement desensitization and reprocessing
   B. Exposure therapy
   C. Psychodynamic psychotherapy
   D. Hypnothcrapy
   E. Image rehearsal therapy (IRT)

9. A 55-year-old man presents with severe insomnia that has been ongoing for several years. He states he has to consume alcohol to fall asleep at night, and also admits to drinking approximately 12 beers per day on average. He feels the need to cut down on his drinking, but states every time he tries to abstain from alcohol, his insomnia becomes so severe that he relapses. What would be the best pharmacologic option to help the patient with his insomnia?
   A. Clonazepam
   B. Chloradiazepoxide
   C. Gabapentin
   D. Pramipexole
   E. Zolpidem

10. A 22-year-old woman with narcolepsy type 2 presents for follow-up in sleep medicine clinic. She has been taking an extended release preparation of methylphenidate for excessive daytime sleepiness; however, she finds she is still quite sleepy during the day. More pressing to her is the onset of worsening depressive symptoms that have occurred in the last 2 months. You decide to add an additional medication to her regimen to help with both sleepiness and depression. Which of the following medications would you choose?
    A. Sertraline
    B. Protriptyline
    C. Fluoxetine
    D. Mirtazapine
    E. Venlafaxine

11. A 24-year-old man with a history of a substance use disorder is referred for PSG to evaluate witnessed apneas. He states he has been able to refrain from substance use for the last 6 months, which he attributes to counseling and a medication he started taking a few months ago. A 5-min sample from his polysomnogram is displayed in Fig. 33.2.
    Which of the following medications is the patient most likely taking to treat his substance use disorder?
    A. Acamprosate
    B. Naltrexone
    C. Buprenorphine
    D. Disulfiram
    E. Oxycodone

12. A 55-year-old woman presents to sleep clinic with a chief complaint of very severe restlessness in her legs and an urge to move her legs at night. She reports the sensations are often accompanied by a "creepy-crawly" feeling in her legs and are only tcmporarily rclicvcd by movcmcnt. Shc statcs hcr ability to fall asleep is quite disrupted, and as a result, she feels fatigued during the day. She notes depressed mood, which she rates as mild. She endorses impaired concentration, which she attributes to her difficulty sleeping at night. She states this has been worse over the last year. She is not able to point to any precipitating factors. She takes simvastatin for hypercholesterolemia. Physical exam is largely unremarkable except for a body mass index (BMI) of 32 kg/m^2. Laboratory values are significant for a serum ferritin of 102 µg/mL. The next best step in management would be:
    A. Pramipexole trial
    B. Bupropion trial
    C. Gabapentin enacarbil trial
    D. Begin iron supplements
    E. Clonazepam trial

13. A 25-year-old woman with a history of unipolar major depressive disorder complains of significant excessive daytime sleepiness (Epworth Sleepiness Scale score = 14/24), occurring in concert with her psychiatric disorder. Among psychiatric patients with a complaint of excessive daytime sleepiness, approximately what percentage will demonstrate mean sleep latency below 8 min on the multiple sleep latency test (MSLT)?
    A. 0%
    B. 10%
    C. 25%
    D. 50%
    E. 75%

5 min epoch

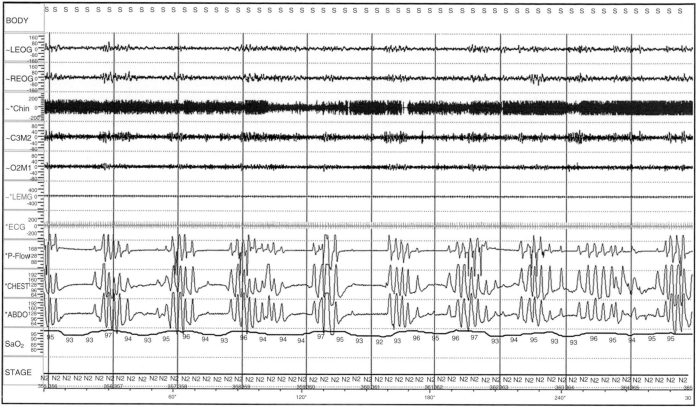

• **Figure 33.2** Five-minute epoch from the patient's polysomnogram. *ECG,* Electrocardiogram. (Modified from Javaheri S, Randerath WJ. Opioid-induced central sleep apnea: mechanisms and therapies. *Sleep Med Clin.* 2014;9:49–56.)

14. A 45-year old man presents complaining of insomnia, primarily difficulty falling asleep at the beginning of the night. He denies snoring or witnessed apneas, but endorses daytime fatigue he relates to his difficulty sleeping. Past medical history is significant for mild chronic obstructive pulmonary disease (COPD), likely due to a 40 pack per year smoking history. Additionally, he reports a history of alcohol dependence, but has maintained sobriety for the last year. The best pharmacologic option to treat the patient's insomnia would be:
    A. Lorazepam
    B. Eszopiclone
    C. Amitriptyline
    D. Trazodone
    E. Ramelteon

15. A 32-year old woman with a history of severe childhood maltreatment is referred for evaluation due to unwanted behaviors during sleep. She reports that she awakens in the morning with severe scratches on her forearms and legs, without recollection for how she received the injury, although she notes frequent nightmares about past abuse occurring on a near nightly basis. She informs you that she has a number of "alters" who have different personalities, and that she is in psychotherapy for this issue. She is not taking any medications, and her physical exam is unremarkable. She is referred for PSG, and an episode of self-injury is captured in the laboratory that occurs during a prolonged period of wakefulness. In the morning, the patient reports no recollection for the episode

of self-injury. The treatment most likely to help with her symptoms is:
    A. Clonazepam
    B. Pramipexole
    C. Melatonin
    D. Zolpidem
    E. Psychotherapy

16. A 30-year-old woman is referred to sleep medicine clinic for evaluation of eating excessive quantities of food at night. She reports that for the last 3 years, she will binge eat large amounts of food in the late evening and during middle of the night awakenings. She has recall of her eating episodes, but feels that she cannot stop herself from compulsively eating. She denies inappropriate compensatory behavior such as self-induced vomiting or use of diuretics/laxatives. Her BMI is 35 kg/m², and she has gained roughly 50 lbs since the onset of her symptoms. The most likely diagnosis is:
    A. Sleep-related eating disorder
    B. Night eating syndrome (NES)
    C. Bulimia nervosa
    D. Anorexia nervosa
    E. Rumination disorder

17. A 15-year-old boy is brought to a child psychiatrist for concern for possible attention-deficit hyperactivity disorder. The patient's mother reports that teachers have complained about inattention, which has prompted evaluation. He frequently "zones out" in class and puts his head down on the desk. His grades have

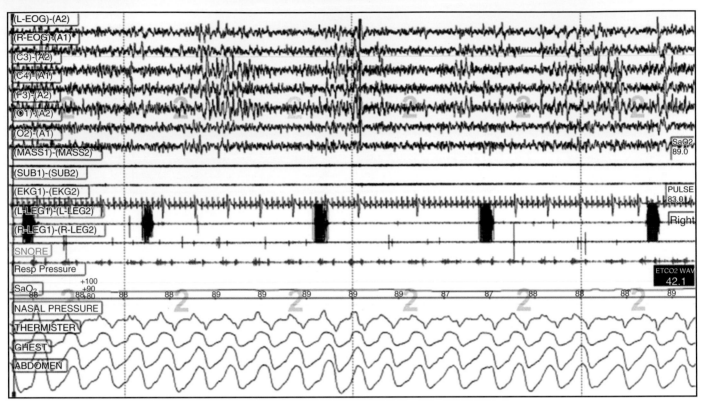

• **Figure 33.3** Representative 2-min epoch from patient's polysomnogram. (Modified from Rama AN, Zachariah R, Kushida CA. Differentiating nocturnal movements: leg movements, parasomnias, and seizures. *Sleep Med Clin.* 2009;4:361–372.)

gone down considerably, particularly in classes he takes prior to his lunch period. His BMI is 25 kg/m². The mother reports no snoring or witnessed apneas. The next most appropriate step in management would be:

A. Referral to otolaryngology for assessment of adenotonsillar hypertrophy
B. Start methylphenidate for attention deficit hyperactivity disorder
C. Obtain longitudinal assessment of sleep wake patterns with sleep logs/actigraphy
D. Refer for cognitive behavioral therapy
E. Begin guanfacine for attention deficit hyperactivity disorder

18. A 40-year-old woman with a history of depression and anxiety is referred for PSG. Her past medical history is significant for diabetes, hypertension, and obesity. Two minutes of her polysomnogram are displayed in Fig. 33.3. Which of her following medications is most likely to cause the observed polysomnographic finding?

A. Bupropion
B. Lorazepam
C. Fluoxetine
D. Clonidine
E. Metformin

19. A 30-year-old woman presents to the sleep clinic with complaints of frequent nightmares, nocturnal gasping, and severe difficulty initiating and maintaining sleep. She does not have a bed partner, and she is not sure if she snores. She reports she is frequently anxious, and will startle easily when she hears loud noises. She is referred for nocturnal PSG, and results are as follows:

• Time in bed: 440 min
• Total sleep time: 420 min
• Sleep onset latency: 5 min
• Wake after sleep onset: 15 min
• Sleep efficiency: 95%
• REM latency: 92 min
• Apnea/hypopnea index: 0.7/hour
• Periodic limb movement index: 1.2/hour

Upon awakening, the patient estimates she slept approximately 7 hours, and that her subjective sleep quality was much better in the laboratory than at home. The most likely diagnosis is:

A. Major depressive disorder
B. PTSD
C. Bipolar disorder
D. Paradoxical insomnia
E. Generalized anxiety disorder

20. A 70-year-old man without prior neuropsychiatric symptoms presents with his wife to a geriatric psychiatrist for consultation. His wife notes the patient has been having visual hallucinations for the last 6 months, as well as worsening memory to the point that he is easily confused and severely impaired. The patient's parents did not have a history of neurodegenerative disorder, and each lived into their eighth decade of life. The patient's wife also notes he frequently thrashes about

in his dreams, as if he is acting them out. The most likely diagnosis is:

A. Alzheimer's disease
B. Frontotemporal dementia
C. Dementia with Lewy bodies
D. Pseudodementia due to depression
E. Huntington's disease

21. A 37-year-old man with a history of heroin dependence presents to the emergency room complaining of an inner sense of restlessness in his legs. He states this problem started within the last 24 hours, but he has had similar symptoms at other times in the past. He also endorses loose stools and nausea. The patient reports taking fluoxetine for depression, but denies other medications. The most likely diagnosis is:

A. Neuroleptic-induced akathisia
B. Opioid withdrawal
C. Restless legs syndrome (RLS) secondary to antidepressant use
D. Periodic limb movement disorder
E. Nocturnal leg cramps

22. A 7-year-old girl is referred for evaluation in sleep clinic due to loud snoring and pauses in breathing. Her parents note she is inattentive and has been having behavioral problems at school. Also, the parents inform you that she recently underwent neuropsychological testing with a psychologist. On physical exam, she is noted to have 4+ tonsils. You inform her parents that you would recommend PSG to evaluate for sleep-disordered breathing, and likely referral to otolaryngology for possible adenotonsillectomy (AT) if sleep apnea is diagnosed. The parents ask whether her problems with inattention and behavioral disruption will improve if she ultimately gets a tonsillectomy. The best evidence-based response would be:

A. It is highly unlikely that either behavior problems or inattentiveness will improve with AT.
B. Attention and executive function that were assessed with neuropsychological testing will likely demonstrate improvement after AT.
C. Data suggest there is no relationship between AT and inattention/behavioral problems.
D. There is no randomized data to know whether tonsillectomy helps these problems in children with obstructive sleep apnea.
E. It is likely that the parents and teachers may perceive improvement in her symptoms, but less likely that neuropsychological testing will change.

23. A 57-year-old woman with a history of morbid obesity, diabetes mellitus, and obstructive sleep apnea presents for routine follow-up. She reports she has become increasingly depressed in the last several months, with symptoms of anhedonia, fatigue, and impaired concentration. She endorses passive thoughts of being dead, but denies active intent or plan to harm herself. Her continuous positive airway pressure (CPAP) device is in working order, with downloaded information that suggests excellent control of sleep apnea, without residual events detected by the machine. You decide to prescribe a medication for her depressive symptoms. Which of the following would be most potentially problematic, given her comorbidities?

A. Fluoxetine
B. Fluvoxamine
C. Sertraline
D. Paroxetine
E. Mirtazapine

24. A 27-year-old woman presents with a primary complaint of "seeing things that aren't there." She states that she frequently sees a man standing beside her bed when she wakes up at night. By the time she turns on the light, the man is gone. She states she often gets anxious as a result of these visions, and has trouble getting back to sleep. She denies having similar experiences during daytime hours and denies daytime sleepiness. She is noted to be euthymic on mental status exam. The next best step in management would be:

A. Prescribe antipsychotic medication for likely schizophrenia
B. Provide reassurance
C. Refer for PSG and multiple sleep latency testing
D. Refer for sleep-deprived EEG
E. Prescribe benzodiazepine medication

25. A 55-year-old woman presents with a chief complaint of depression and sleep disturbance, including difficulty falling and staying asleep. She reports she has been experiencing these symptoms for approximately 2 years, but she is unable to cite any clear precipitants. Her family history is notable for a younger sister who died of malignant melanoma 5 years earlier. The patient reports she is anxious about developing melanoma as well, since she spent a fair amount of time in the sun with her sister when she was younger. The patient currently applies sunblock three times per day and tries to avoid going outdoors whenever possible. She reports consuming animal products (eggs, meats) in her diet, but she is highly lactose intolerant and thus strictly avoids dairy. Her past medical history and physical exam are otherwise unremarkable. The next best step in management would be:

A. Check serum B12 level
B. Check methylmalonic acid level
C. Check thyroid-stimulating hormone
D. Check 25-hydroxy vitamin D level
E. Check complete blood count

26. A 29-year-old man with a history of bipolar disorder presents with a chief complaint of insomnia. He reports longstanding difficulty initiating and maintaining sleep, and an estimated total sleep time of about 5.5–6 hours nightly. His current medications include lithium carbonate, carbamazepine, and clonazepam. He reports he is not interested in taking pharmacologic agents for his insomnia, as he already feels he takes too many medications. On mental status exam, he is euthymic at the time of assessment. Which of the following components of cognitive-behavioral therapy could potentially be the most problematic for this patient if implemented?

A. Sleep hygiene
B. Sleep restriction therapy
C. Relaxation training
D. Cognitive therapy
E. Stimulus control therapy

27. A 30-year-old man with a 3-year history of depression is referred for PSG and MSLT due to longstanding daytime sleepiness, the onset of which preceded his depressive symptoms. He denies cataplexy, but does note rare sleep paralysis. At the time of evaluation, he is taking escitalopram 20 mg daily. The patient denies a history of suicidal ideation, and feels he would be able to safely taper off of this medication for his sleep tests. He is referred for PSG and MSLT, and is instructed to carefully begin tapering his antidepressant medication so he will have stopped this medication 2 weeks prior to sleep testing. The patient states he would like to be scheduled for these studies

as soon as possible, "so I can get to the bottom of these symptoms."

One week prior to his scheduled studies, another patient cancels his PSG/MSLT, and there is now an opening in your sleep laboratory. Your lab manager asks whether your patient could be rescheduled, so he does not have to wait until next week. The most accurate response would be:

A. His study should not be rescheduled, as doing so may affect the number of sleep-onset REM periods observed during MSLT.

B. His study should not be rescheduled, because doing so may affect the amount of slow wave sleep he attains.

C. His study should not be rescheduled, because doing so may affect the apnea/hypopnea index.

D. His study should be rescheduled so he can get his testing done as quickly as possible.

E. It does not matter whether testing is rescheduled to an earlier date.

28. A 45-year-old man with a history of Trisomy 21 is brought to the sleep clinic for assessment of sleep-disordered breathing by his social worker. The patient lives in a group home and has had increasing difficulty caring for himself, as his memory has gotten worse from his baseline over the last 2 years. He has been told by staff at his home that he snores loudly and also stops breathing in his sleep. Past surgical history is significant for tonsillectomy performed at age 7, as well as repair of a ventricular septal defect as a child. The next best step in management would be:

A. Order portable monitoring study to assess for sleep disordered breathing

B. Refer to otolaryngology for evaluation

C. Begin montelukast

D. Refer for neuropsychiatric testing

E. Order in-laboratory PSG

29. A 17-year-old male is referred for PSG and multiple sleep latency testing, due to increasing sleepiness and lethargy for the last 6 months. There is no report of cataplexy, sleep paralysis, or hypnopompic/hypnagogic imagery. The following results are obtained from his sleep studies:

PSG:

Time in bed: 400 min
Total sleep time: 330 min
Sleep onset latency: 10 min
Wake after sleep onset: 20 min
Sleep efficiency: 92.5%
REM latency: 72 min
Apnea/hypopnea index: 0.3/hour
Periodic limb movement index: 2.3/hour

MSLT:

Nap#1: Sleep onset latency 5.5 min; REM latency 3 min
Nap#2: Sleep onset latency 8.0 min; no REM sleep
Nap#3: Sleep onset latency 8.5 min; no REM sleep
Nap#4: Sleep onset latency 6.0 min; REM latency 12 min
Nap#5: Sleep onset latency 8.0 min; no REM sleep

In the technician note, it is described that the teenager asked the sleep technician for food, complained of dry mouth, and had injected conjunctivae on the night of their study. The next appropriate step in management would be:

A. Begin a trial of methylphenidate

B. Begin a trial of modafinil

C. Order urine toxicology screen

D. Repeat polysomnogram and MSLT

E. Order actigraphy

30. A 33-year old woman presents to the sleep clinic with a complaint of waking up gasping during the middle of the night. She states that during these episodes, she awakens with dyspnea and tachycardia, as well as feeling diaphoretic. Her husband notes she snores on occasion. Past medical history is significant for a diagnosis of PD. Her physical exam is significant for a crowded oropharynx and BMI of 37 kg/m². She is referred for PSG that demonstrates the following:

Time in bed: 420 min
Total sleep time: 330 min
Sleep onset latency: 37 min
Wake after sleep onset: 53 min
Sleep efficiency: 78.6%
REM latency: 88 min
Apnea/hypopnea index: 1.6/hour
Periodic limb movement index: 3.2/hour

The next appropriate step in management would be:

A. Begin a trial of autotitrating positive airway pressure

B. Referral for PAP titration

C. Trial of pramipexole

D. Referral for IRT

E. Trial of sertraline

Answers

1. **Answer C.** Melatonin supplementation (typically given at doses of 1–3 mg) has demonstrated efficacy at improving sleep initiation with minimal reports of adverse events in children with ASD.[1] Although behavioral approaches (choice A) may be helpful, a child without capacity to understand language would not likely benefit from cognitive approaches in the treatment of insomnia. There is not sufficient evidence to warrant treatment with zolpidem, olanzapine, or clonazepam (choices B, D, E), and in fact, the risks of these medications in the treatment of this patient's insomnia likely outweigh potential benefits.

2. **Answer E.** The patient is experiencing medication-induced RLS. Although there are several agents that can precipitate restless legs, mirtazapine has been associated with particularly high rates of incident RLS compared with other antidepressants, possibly due to its serotonergic and antihistamine properties.[2] Both paroxetine and sertraline (choices C and D) are specific serotonin reuptake inhibitors (SSRIs), both of which have been associated with incident RLS, but at rates roughly three- to fivefold lower than mirtazapine.[2] Although AASM practice parameters do not support the use of benzodiazepines (such as clonazepam; choice A) as the sole treatment for RLS, they are not associated with worsening or incident RLS.[3] Clonidine (choice B) has some limited data in support of its use in RLS.[3]

3. **Answer C.** The listed epoch presents oculomotor activity during N2 sleep that is frequently caused by SSRIs. Slow eye movements (SEMs) can be observed during periods of eyes closed drowsiness and wakefulness, as well as stage N1 sleep. However, these eye movements typically resolve and are not observed in stage N2 or N3 sleep. SSRIs can cause a mixture of slow and

more rapid eye movements that can be observed throughout non-REM (NREM) sleep (so-called "Prozac or SSRI eyes"). Notably, such oculomotor activity can be observed for months or longer after these medications are discontinued,[4,5] as is the case here.

4. **Answer D.** Reductions in sleep spindles, particularly centro-parietal spindles, have been demonstrated in persons with schizophrenia in several studies.[6–8] Patients with schizophrenia typically demonstrate difficulties with sleep initiation and maintenance, such as increased sleep onset latency and decreased total sleep duration.[9] Some studies have suggested patients with schizophrenia have reduced slow wave sleep and reduced latency to REM sleep; however, this has not borne out in meta-analyses.[9]

5. **Answer A.** Meta-analyses have demonstrated affective disorders, particularly depression, are associated with reduced REM latency, reduced sleep efficiency (including increased sleep onset latency and wake after sleep onset), and increased percentage of REM sleep relative to total sleep time.[10] One can remember that REM latency is reduced in depression by recognizing that SSRIs have the opposite effect and prolong REM latency.

6. **Answer B.** The patient presents with symptoms classical for a manic episode. PSG performed in patients with bipolar disorder experiencing a manic episode have demonstrated very similar sleep architecture to patients with unipolar major depression, including disturbed sleep continuity (reductions in sleep efficiency, increased number of awakenings), increased stage 1 sleep, reductions in total sleep time, and reduced REM latency relative to healthy controls.[11]

7. **Answer B.** The patient has PTSD. Prazosin, an alpha-1 receptor blocker, is recommended by the AASM for the treatment of PTSD associated nightmares.[12] Venlafaxine (choice C), a serotonin-norepinephrine reuptake inhibitor (SNRI), has not demonstrated improvements in nightmares in PTSD, but may improve other symptoms of the disorder. Nefazodone (choice D), an older antidepressant that is a potent 5-HT2A receptor antagonist, is not recommended due to its risk of hepatotoxicity. There is not sufficient data to suggest clonazepam (a benzodiazepine) or carbamazepine (an antiepileptic medication; choices A and E) may improve PTSD-related nightmares.

8. **Answer E.** IRT involves recalling the nightmare, writing it down, changing the theme and narrative to a more positive one, and rehearsing the rewritten dream scenario. Of behavioral approaches, it has the highest level of evidence supporting its use in the treatment of nightmares.[12] Exposure therapy (choice B) involves exposing a patient to a feared object of context in the absence of danger, to help overcome anxiety, and has been used to treat generalized anxiety disorder, specific phobias, and PTSD. Eye-movement desensitization and reprocessing (choice A; EMDR) is a psychological therapy that has been used to treat PTSD and emphasizes disturbing memories as a cause of psychopathology and uses various techniques to develop more adaptive coping mechanisms. Although both exposure therapy and EMDR might help with PTSD symptoms, including nightmares, they are less optimal choices here, as the patient has no history of PTSD. Psychodynamic psychotherapy (choice C) is a long-term treatment that focuses on revealing unconscious content in an effort to alleviate psychic tension that is not clearly indicated for sleep disorders. Hypnotherapy (choice D) involves creating subconscious change

in a patient through suggestion during hypnosis, a period of focused attention and reduced peripheral awareness. Hypnotherapy is sometimes used to treat NREM parasomnias such as sleepwalking, but not typically used to treat nightmares.

9. **Answer C.** The patient has alcohol dependence, which is frequently associated with insomnia, particularly during periods of abstinence, which may contribute to relapse. A recent randomized-controlled trial has demonstrated gabapentin may reduce the risk of relapse and improve insomnia.[13] Because alcohol enacts its effects in the central nervous system by potentiating the GABA-A receptor, agents that also have similar pharmacologic effects are generally not recommended in this patient population due to risks of synergistic effects and dependence. Lorazepam and chloradiazepoxide (choices A and B) are benzodiazepines that act on the GABA-A receptor and would not be advised in patients with alcohol use disorders. Zolpidem (choice E) is a benzodiazepine receptor agonist sedative-hypnotic that also potentiates the GABA-A receptor and is similarly not advised for use in this patient. Pramipexole (choice D) is a dopamine agonist used to treat RLS, and is unlikely to provide benefit as a sedative hypnotic.

10. **Answer B.** Of the antidepressants listed, protriptyline would be the agent most likely to also improve the patient's complaint of continued sleepiness. Protripytline is a tricyclic antidepressant that tends to be energizing, rather than sedating. Sertraline and fluoxetine (choices A and C; specific-serotonin reuptake inhibitors) and venlafaxine (choice E; SNRI), which are all approved to treat major depressive disorder, are less likely to improve vigilance. Mirtazapine (choice D) is an atypical antidepressant with noradrenergic and serotonergic activity, is commonly associated with sedation and weight gain, and would not be an optimal choice compared with protriptyline in this instance.

11. **Answer C.** The patient has central sleep apnea induced by buprenorphine. It has long been appreciated that classical opioids can induce central sleep apnea. Recent evidence has demonstrated that buprenorphine, a partial agonist opioid receptor molecule frequently used to treat opioid addiction, can also cause central sleep apnea.[14] Although oxycodone (choice E), a common opioid medication used to treat pain, can induce central sleep apnea, it is not approved for the treatment of opioid dependence. Acamprosate (choice A), naltrexone (choice B), and disulfiram (choice D) are agents used to treat alcohol dependence, and are not associated with central sleep apnea.

12. **Answer A.** The patient presents with symptoms consistent with severe RLS with mild depressive symptoms. In such instances, treating RLS first is generally recommended.[15] Bupropion (choice B), an antidepressant without significant serotonergic activity, would be a good choice if RLS was mild and depressive symptoms more significant. Iron supplementation (choice D) would not be indicated, as her serum ferritin is higher than 50–75 μg/mL. Benzodiazepines such as clonazepam (choice E) are not recommended as first-line agents for RLS. Although both dopamine agonists (such as pramipexole) and $\alpha_2\delta$ ligands (such as gabapentin enacarbil; choice C) may be beneficial in RLS, dopamine receptor agonists are generally preferred for initial therapy in patients with very severe symptoms, obesity, and comorbid depression, as is the case here.[16] Common reasons to select an $\alpha_2\delta$ agent as initial therapy include comorbid pain, anxiety, insomnia, addiction, or impulse control disorder.[17]

13. **Answer C.** Meta-analyses have demonstrated psychiatric patients with a complaint of excessive daytime sleepiness and have mean sleep latency values on the MSLT that are comparable to normative values in the general population, which means roughly 20%–25% of these patients will demonstrate a mean sleep latency below 8 min on the MSLT.[18]

14. **Answer E.** Ramelteon is a melatonin type (MT) 1 and 2 receptor agonist approved for the treatment of insomnia. It has a short half-life, and is best suited for difficulties with sleep initiation. It has a low likelihood of abuse, which is important in this case, given the patient's history of alcohol dependence, which would make agents that potentiate the GABA-A receptor (such as lorazepam or eszopiclone, choices A and B) potentially problematic for this patient. Ramelteon appears to have minimal effects on SpO_2 in patients with mild to moderate COPD, and thus would be reasonable in this instance.[19] Benzodiazepines such as lorazepam may compromise respiratory function in COPD.[19] Sedating antidepressants such as amitriptyline (choice C) and trazodone (choice D) are commonly used in the treatment of insomnia, and typically do not exacerbate respiratory function, but have less evidence in support of their use as a sedative-hypnotic compared with ramelteon.[19,20]

15. **Answer E.** The patient meets criteria for sleep-related dissociative disorder (SRDD). This disorder is a sleep-related variant of dissociative disorders such as dissociative identity disorder (formerly called multiple personality disorder) and dissociative fugue.[21] In this disorder, patients may carry out a number of behaviors during the sleep period that are consistent with symptoms of their daytime dissociative disorders. In addition, patients may enact other problematic behaviors such as reenactments of past trauma, self-mutilation, and even violence.[22] An important distinction between SRDD and other parasomnias is that the behavior occurs during EEG-defined wake. Psychotherapy is the treatment of choice for SRDD.

16. **Answer B.** The patient has symptoms consistent with NES, which is characterized by excessive eating between dinner and bedtime and during full awakenings during the sleep period.[21] What distinguishes NES from sleep related eating disorder (SRED; choice A), a specific form of sleep walking, which is a disorder or arousal (or a NREM parasomnia), is the level of awareness of the binge eating. The patient would not qualify for a diagnosis of bulimia nervosa (choice C), a disorder characterized by binge eating with compensatory behaviors such as induced vomiting, laxative/diuretic abuse. Similarly, rumination disorder (choice E), a disorder that typically affects young children, in which the patient brings back up and rechews partially digested food that has already been swallowed, would not be consistent with the patient's symptoms. Nor would she meet criteria for anorexia nervosa (choice D), a disorder associated with food restriction and significant weight loss, particularly given her above normal BMI.

17. **Answer C.** This adolescent is displaying signs of excessive daytime sleepiness, particularly in the morning, which should prompt assessment for a delayed sleep phase. Such patients are frequently misdiagnosed as having attention deficit hyperactivity disorder. In addition to obtaining a more comprehensive sleep history, sleep logs and actigraphy would help confirm the diagnosis of a delayed sleep phase circadian rhythm sleep disorder. On actigraphy, patients with a delayed sleep phase who do not have to wake at prescribed times to attend school or work frequently demonstrate chronically delayed bedtime and waketimes, often by several hours. However, when forced to awaken during the work week for school, as in this case, a common pattern observed among these patients is short total sleep times during the work week (due to delayed sleep onset times with enforced awakening), with prolonged sleep times (often into the late mornings or afternoons) on weekends, when school obligations do not require a prescribed wake time (Fig. 33.4). Starting medications for attention-deficit hyperactivity disorder (choices B, E) would be inappropriate in this context. Without snoring or witnessed apneas, referral to otolaryngology (choice A) would not be indicated at this juncture. Referral for cognitive behavioral therapy (choice D) would not be appropriate without attempting to clarify the diagnosis first.

18. **Answer C.** The figure depicts periodic limb movements of sleep (PLMS). It has been established that serotonergic antidepressants are associated with increases in PLMS.[23] Bupropion is an antidepressant not associated with increased PLMS, likely because it has little serotonergic activity. Other medications listed have not been associated with PLMS.

19. **Answer B.** The patient's symptoms of insomnia and nightmares, coupled with heightened startle response, are suggestive PTSD. It is not uncommon for patients with PTSD to sleep far better when observed in the sleep laboratory than at home, possibly due to a heightened sense of safety in the sleep lab. Because the patient accurately estimated her sleep duration, and acknowledged it was better than typical, paradoxical insomnia (choice D), which is characterized by a subjective insomnia complaint that is disproportionate and not congruent with EEG-measured sleep, would be unlikely. Disorders such as major depressive disorder, bipolar disorder, and generalized anxiety disorder (choices A, C, and E) are all commonly associated with sleep initiation and/or maintenance insomnia; however, nightmares and hypervigilance are not part of the diagnostic criteria for these disorders.

20. **Answer C.** The patient presents with visual hallucinations and memory impairments, along with likely REM sleep behavior disorder (RBD). This constellation of symptoms, along with parkinsonism, is common in dementia with Lewy bodies. Although RBD can occasionally be seen in other neurodegenerative disorders, it is by far most commonly associated with α-synucleinopathies (such as Parkinson's disease, dementia with Lewy bodies, and multisystem atrophy) that are characterized by abnormal deposition fibrillary aggregates of alpha-synuclein protein in selective populations of neurons and glia. None of the other neurodegenerative disorders listed are α-synucleinopathies. Huntington's disease (choice E) is not likely, given the absence of a family history (autosomal dominant inheritance pattern). Pseudodementia (choice D) refers to severe cognitive impairment mimicking dementia that can occur in the severely depressed elderly; however, this is less likely, given the absence of a history of a mood disorder. Frontotemporal dementia (choice B) results from progressive neuronal loss primarily involving the frontal or temporal lobes that commonly presents with noticeable changes in social/personal behavior, blunting of emotions, apathy, and deficits in expressive and receptive language. Alzheimer's dementia (choice A) is the most common form of dementia, characterized by deposition of amyloid plaques and neurofibrillary tangles, not excessive alpha-synuclein protein.

21. **Answer B.** The patient is most likely experiencing opioid withdrawal, the symptoms of which can include akathisia (a

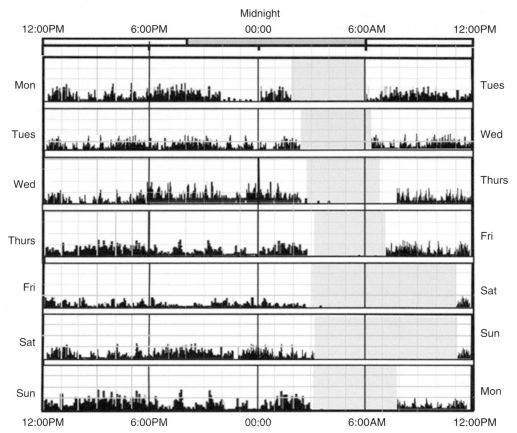

• **Figure 33.4** One-week actigraphic recording for a typical patient with delayed sleep phase forced to awaken for school/work, similar to that described in question 17. Note stable, but delayed sleep onset time around 02:00–03:00 with minimal movement detected during sleep intervals. Wake times around 06:00–07:00 during the school or work week result in sleep restriction. Wake time is notably delayed until 11:00 on weekends, a common pattern seen in these patients. (Modified from Circadian rhythm sleep-wake disorders. In: Berry RB, Wagner MH. *Sleep Medicine Pearls.* 3rd ed. Philadelphia, PA: Elsevier Saunders; 2015:626–634.)

state of agitation, distress, and restlessness), nausea/vomiting, and diarrhea. The patient is not taking a neuroleptic (antipsychotic) medication, so neuroleptic-induced akathisia (choice A) is not likely. Although RLS secondary to his antidepressant use (choice C) and nocturnal leg cramps (choice E) can be included in the differential diagnosis, the vignette would not support their diagnosis over opioid withdrawal. Nocturnal leg cramps are characterized by painful muscular contraction during the night, often interfering with or causing awakening from sleep. Periodic limb movement disorder (choice D) cannot be diagnosed without polysomnographic evidence of PLMS.

22. **Answer E.** This question refers to the results of the CHAT study (childhood AT trial), the largest randomized trial of AT in children with sleep apnea.[24] This study did not demonstrate the significant benefit of AT in the primary outcome measure of neuropsychological assessment of attention and executive function, but did demonstrate improvements in some secondary outcomes of behavior and quality of life assessed by teachers and caregivers.

23. **Answer E.** Mirtazapine is an antidepressant with effects on a wide array of neurotransmitter systems. Compared with SSRIs, mirtazapine is significantly more likely to induce weight gain,[25] which would be particularly problematic in this patient, given her history of morbid obesity, sleep apnea, and diabetes mellitus.

Fluoxetine, fluvoxamine, sertraline, and paroxetine (choices A, B, C, and D) are all SSRIs, which share a common side effect profile that can include headache, gastrointestinal disturbance, sexual side effects (including erectile dysfunction and/or anorgasmia), insomnia, and/or drowsiness.

24. **Answer B.** The patient is reporting hypnopompic hallucinations, which are a common normal variant in the population. Hallucinations isolated to sleep onset (hypnagogic) and/or offset (hypnopompic) are not consistent with a primary psychotic disorder such as schizophrenia (choice A). Although visual hallucinations can occur in schizophrenia, auditory hallucinations are the most common form of hallucination experienced by patients with schizophrenia. She does not describe excessive daytime sleepiness, and thus referral for PSG and multiple sleep latency testing (choice C) would not be indicated. Her symptoms are unlikely to be related to seizures, and thus EEG would not be indicated (choice D). There is no indication for a benzodiazepine (choice E) based on the vignette.

25. **Answer D.** The patient presents with depression and sleep disturbance, both of which may be associated with hypovitaminosis D.[26,27] Her avoidance of the sun and dairy products (which are frequently fortified by vitamin D) increase her risk of hypovitaminosis D. Vitamin B12 and methylmalonic acid levels (choices A, B) are less likely, given a diet that contains

animal products. Although hypothyroidism can be associated with hypersomnolence and depressive symptoms, there is nothing else in the vignette that would suggest hypothyroidism (choice C). Checking a complete blood count (choice E) might be reasonable if anemia were suspected to cause her symptoms, but again, there is nothing in the vignette that points specifically toward anemia.

26. **Answer B.** Cognitive-behavioral therapy for insomnia (CBT-I) is well established as an efficacious psychotherapy for insomnia, including those comorbid with mental illness. There are several potential components of CBT-I, and in patients with bipolar disorder already reporting low habitual sleep duration, sleep restriction could potentially be problematic due increased risk of affective switching.[28] Although sleep restriction therapy is not absolutely contraindicated, it does have the greatest potential for negative outcomes in these patients, and caution should be exercised if implemented. None of the other CBT-I techniques/practices are associated with increased risks of manic switching. Sleep hygiene (choice A) is a set of habits/practices conducive to sleeping. Relaxation training (choice C) involves several methods that help patients increase calmness, which can be conducive of sleep. Cognitive therapy (choice D) involves changing maladaptive thoughts, problematic behaviors, and distressing emotions related to sleep. Stimulus control therapy (choice E) involves a set of instructions designed to break negative associations between the bed/bedroom and difficulty sleeping.

27. **Answer A.** The patient is on a specific serotonin reuptake inhibitor. These agents are well known to suppress REM sleep and prolong REM sleep latency. In addition, discontinuing these agents too close to PSG and MSLT can result in rebound of REM sleep, increasing both the volume of REM sleep and sleep onset REM periods.[29] This is why the AASM recommends such medications should ideally be stopped at least 2 weeks prior to MSLT (or at least five times the half-life of the drug and longer-acting metabolite), ideally confirmed by a urine drug screen, so they have minimal effect on the interpretation of the study.[30] Notably, this period may need to be even longer in the case of fluoxetine, which has a very long half-life. Since the patient has only been off the medication for 1 week at this point, the most prudent step is to not reschedule his sleep study.

28. **Answer E.** This patient with Trisomy 21 most likely has obstructive sleep apnea, and further diagnostic testing is indicated. Patients with Trisomy 21 are at increased risk for sleep apnea, due to several factors, including midface and mandibular hypoplasia, macroglossia, medially displaced tonsils, contracted nasopharynx, and hypotonia of the airway. In-laboratory testing would be indicated, as the patient's memory impairment and medical conditions would make obtaining an accurate portable monitoring study (choice A) unlikely.[31] Referral to otolaryngology (choice B) at this juncture would

not be indicated, as diagnostic testing should be performed first, and the patient has a history of tonsillectomy as a child. Montelukast (choice C), a leukotriene receptor antagonist (LTRA) that is most commonly used to treat asthma, has demonstrated some efficacy for OSA in pediatric populations by reducing adenoidal tissue, but has not been shown to be specifically helpful for adults with Trisomy 21.[32] Neuropsychiatric testing (choice D) may help verify the patient's memory impairment, but would not be immediately indicated over polysomnographic testing.

29. **Answer C.** The patient exhibits clinical signs of cannabis intoxication as documented in the technician notes. Cannabis use could certainly explain his clinical complaints, and may also lead to false positive MSLT findings in teenagers.[33] Beginning a trial of a wake-promoting agent such as methylphenidate or modafinil (choices A, B) would not be indicated without clarifying the diagnosis. There is no indication based on the vignette for immediately repeating the sleep tests (choice D). Actigraphy (choice E) could be useful to document sleep duration and patterns prior to sleep testing, but ordering actigraphy at this juncture would not be as helpful from a diagnostic standpoint.

30. **Answer E.** The patient's complaints are most likely due to nocturnal panic attacks, which are not uncommon in patients with PD.[34] PAP therapy (choices A, B) would not be indicated, as PSG demonstrated no clinically significant sleep disordered breathing. Similarly, in the absence of a complaint of restless legs and no clinically significant PLMS observed on PSG, pramipexole (choice C) would not be indicated here. IRT (choice D) would be indicated if a nightmare disorder was diagnosed; however, there is no complaint of unwanted dream mentation in the vignette, making this unlikely. SSRIs are first-line agents in the treatment of PD, and nocturnal panic attacks may respond better to SSRIs than benzodiazepines.[34]

Suggested Reading

Aurora RN, Zak RS, Auerbach SH, et al. Best practice guide for the treatment of nightmare disorder in adults. *J Clin Sleep Med.* 2010;6:389-401.

Collop NA, Anderson WM, Boehlecke B, et al. Clinical guidelines for the use of unattended portable monitors in the diagnosis of obstructive sleep apnea in adult patients. Portable Monitoring Task Force of the American Academy of Sleep Medicine. *J Clin Sleep Med.* 2007;3:737-747.

Littner MR, Kushida C, Wise M, et al. Practice parameters for clinical use of the multiple sleep latency test and the maintenance of wakefulness test. *Sleep.* 2005;28:113-121.

Schutte-Rodin S, Broch L, Buysse D, et al. Clinical guideline for the evaluation and management of chronic insomnia in adults. *J Clin Sleep Med.* 2008;4:487-504.

Winkelman JW, Plante DT, eds. *Foundations of Psychiatric Sleep Medicine.* Cambridge, UK: Cambridge University Press; 2010.

34

Insomnia Clinical Pearls

DEIRDRE A. CONROY, LESLIE M. SWANSON

Questions, 509

Answers, 516

Suggested Reading, 520

Questions

1. A 45-year-old female presents with a 2-year history of difficulty initiating and maintaining sleep. During the day, she has increased anxiety about sleep and focuses on her insomnia. When she gets into bed, she feels tension in her body and her thoughts race about the fact that she is not sleeping. She does not have a history of a mental disorder. When she sleeps away from home, she reports that she sleeps "like a rock." To her surprise, she falls asleep quickly while riding on the bus, but cannot initiate sleep in her bed. Which one of the following diagnoses would best reflect the patient's sleep disorder?
   A. Insomnia due to a medical disorder
   B. Psychophysiological insomnia
   C. Idiopathic insomnia
   D. Insomnia due to a mental disorder

2. An 85-year-old female presents with the complaint "I don't sleep at night." She explains that she lies in bed for 8 hours each night and can hear all of the noises in the house all night long. She has no history of formally diagnosed psychiatric disorder (including bipolar disorder). Actigraphy completed in the week prior to the study show periods of activity separated by activity quiescence between 12 AM and 7 AM every night. A nocturnal polysomnogram (PSG) captures 420 minutes of sleep. Sleep onset latency is 20 minutes, N1 = 10%, N2 = 60%, N3 = 10%, and rapid eye movement (REM) sleep% = 20. On a morning questionnaire, she estimated that she slept 2 hours during the night. Which one of the following diagnoses best reflects the patient's sleep problem?
   A. Insomnia due to a mental disorder
   B. Idiopathic insomnia
   C. Paradoxical insomnia
   D. Psychophysiological insomnia

3. A 55-year-old female takes zolpidem 5 mg 3–4 nights per week. If she does not take it, she reports that it will take her "hours" to fall asleep. On those occasions, she gets in bed early and watches TV. She awakens several times during the night in the presence or absence of zolpidem. During the night, she has racing thoughts and ruminates about the upcoming day. She denies symptoms of generalized anxiety (but endorses focus on sleep) and has no history of depression or anxiety disorder. She would like treatment for her insomnia, and she specifically states that she would prefer to not take medication for insomnia "for much longer." Which one of the following treatment options best suits this patient?
   A. Switch to a longer-acting benzodiazepine receptor agonist to help her stay asleep.
   B. Advise her to increase the dose of zolpidem to 10 mg.
   C. Advise her to switch to an over-the-counter (OTC) sleep aid, as they are safer than prescription sleep aids.
   D. Advise cognitive behavioral therapy for insomnia (CBT-I)

4. A 55-year-old female presents with depression and insomnia. She has been taking zolpidem 10 mg every night for the last several years and would like to discontinue the medication. You agree to work with her to aid in the discontinuation process. Which one of the following strategies should you consider adding to her medication taper schedule?
   A. Add nothing; withdraw the medication as quickly as possible.
   B. Add diphenhydramine to the tapering schedule.
   C. Add CBT-I.
   D. Withdraw the medication every other night.

5. A 49-year-old female presents with chronic insomnia for the past 30 years. She reports that her life "revolves around sleep." She believes she needs 8 hours of sleep to function the next day. She worries about how she will function the next day and is certain she will be fired from her job. What component of CBT-I might be especially helpful for this patient?
   A. Sleep hygiene
   B. Benzodiazepine therapy
   C. Cognitive therapy
   D. Diagnostic PSG

6. A 23-year-old male graduate student reports that his sleep patterns are erratic and that he goes to bed and gets up at various times across the 24-hour day. The duration of the sleep episode is normal for the patient's age. The sleep episodes may occur during the patient's class time and if he is not able to manage his sleep, he may need to withdraw from school. You ask the patient to complete sleep diaries. Which one of the following assessment methods would be useful adjunct to evaluate the patient's sleep complaint?
   A. A diagnostic PSG
   B. Multiple sleep latency test (MSLT)

C. Actigraphy

D. Urine drug screen

7. A 53-year-old female comes in reporting a persistent early morning awakening at 4 AM for the past several years. One year ago, she was admitted to the psychiatric emergency room for a depressive episode. She has not been seen by any psychiatric provider since that time. She endorses low mood, loss of interest, low energy, difficulty concentrating, and a loss of appetite. When asked, she states that she feels she may be depressed. The best course of action might be:

A. Referral for a diagnostic PSG to analyze her sleep architecture

B. Referral back to psychiatric for further psychiatric management

C. Recommend the patient initiate continuous positive airway pressure (CPAP) therapy

D. CBT-I

8. A 23-year-old male typically falls asleep every night at 4 AM. He was just prescribed zolpidem 10 mg by his primary care physician, who told him that he should take the medication at a "reasonable time" at 11 PM. He takes zolpidem for several nights at 11 PM, reports that "it doesn't work," and asks to try a stronger medication. Which of the following is the best explanation for the medication "not working" for the patient?

A. The patient is taking the medication at a circadian time that promotes wakefulness and therefore may interfere with the perceived efficacy of the medication.

B. Ambien should be substituted with temazepam.

C. The patient is too young for zolpidem to be effective.

D. He has to take zolpidem with food.

9. A 56-year-old female presents with a history of bipolar disorder and insomnia. She reports that her bipolar is largely managed with medications, but she continues to struggle at times with sleeping. She reports that on some nights she does not sleep at all. You provide her with an actigraph, and she wears it for 7 days (Fig. 34.1). Which of the following descriptions best describes the sleep/wake pattern?

A. The actogram shows sleep episodes are uniform in length and occur at the same time each night. This is not consistent with the patient's complaint.

B. The actogram shows a delayed circadian sleep phase and is consistent with the patient's complaint.

C. The actogram shows a gradual reduction in sleep time and two full nights without sleep on 9/7/2014 and 9/8/2014. This is consistent with the patient's report of going nights without sleep.

D. The actogram shows the patient did not meet the appropriate number of steps to ensure a regular sleep pattern. This does not support the patient's complaint.

10. You are treating a 53-year-old female patient with a history of psychophysiological insomnia. She has tried numerous trials of sleep aids and would prefer a nontherapeutic sleep approach. You ask her maintain a sleep diary, and in the 2-week baseline period, you calculate that her average nightly total sleep time (TST) is found to be 6.5 hours. Which of the following directions should be given as part of her sleep restriction plan?

A. Begin at the average time that the patient wakes up and count forward 6.5 hours; this is the patient's assigned wake time.

B. Add 3 hours to the patient's time in bed (TIB) and adjust bedtimes and wake-up times to include at least that duration of time.

C. Set the patient's bedtime for 6.5 hours after they wake up in the morning.

D. Set bedtimes and wake-up times to approximate the mean TST, with the goal of achieving greater than 85% sleep efficiency (TST/TIB × 100%) over a 7-day period.

11. A 25-year-old woman complains to her primary care physician of difficulty falling asleep for more than 1 year. She lies in bed awake for up to 2 hours every night. During that time she worries about not getting her work done the next day and that her tiredness will result in her getting fired from her job. Although she is awake, she feels that she must stay in bed "because at least I'm getting some rest." She is frustrated by her inability to fall asleep and finds herself checking the time on her phone throughout the night, which leads to even more tension and distress about being awake. Which of the following strategies included in CBT-I would *not* be considered in this case?

A. Cognitive therapy for insomnia

B. Systematic desensitization

C. Stimulus control

D. Relaxation therapy

12. You have been working with a 72-year-old female on her insomnia for six sessions of CBT-I. She has not made any progress in therapy, and you suspect other factors may be at play. She carries a diagnosis of major depression and complains of a chronic low mood, anhedonia, and daytime sleepiness. You refer her for a diagnostic PSG to assess for other occult sleep pathology. Which characteristic in Table 34.1 is *not* consistent with PSG abnormalities in depression?

A. The high sleep efficiency of 89%

B. Abbreviated REM latency of 25 minutes

C. The absence of N3 sleep

D. Prolonged sleep onset latency of 60 minutes

TABLE 34.1	**Polysomnography Report**			
Lights Out/On (Clock Times)	22:36:05/06:52:06		Min	% of TST
Total recording time (TRT, min/h)	496.0/8:16.0	Wake after sleep onset	19.0	
Total sleep time (TST, min)	477.0	Stage N1 sleep	43.0	9.0
Latency to sleep (min)	60.00	Stage N2 sleep	285.0	59.7
REM latency (min)	25.0	Stage N3 sleep	0.0	0.0
Stage shifts (#)	150	Stage R sleep	68.5	14.4
Arousals (#)	0	Sleep efficiency		90%

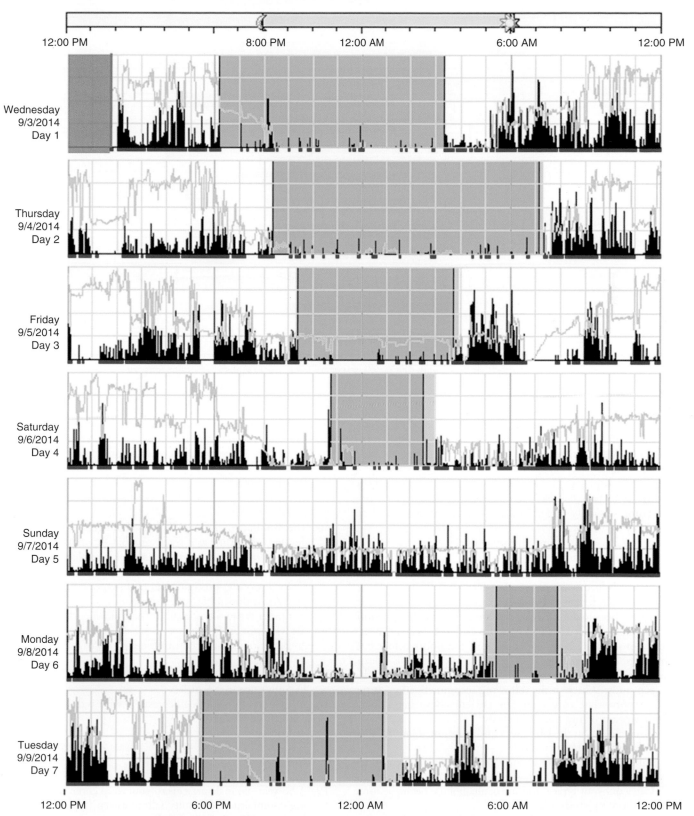

• **Figure 34.1** Actogram of 56-year-old female with bipolar disorder and insomnia.

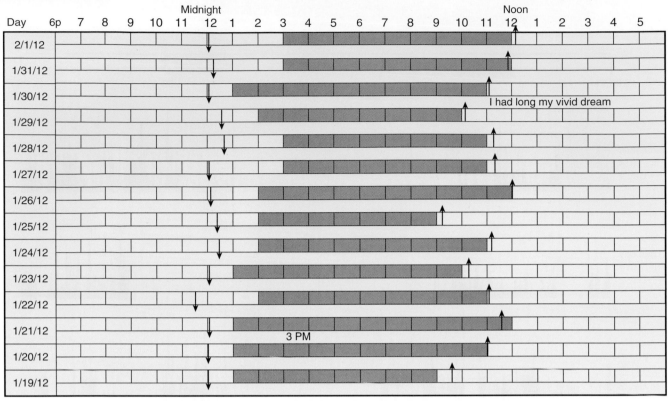

• **Figure 34.2** Sleep log of a 16-year-old female with depression and difficulty falling asleep.

13. A 16-year-old female presents with a 5-year history of depression and difficulty falling asleep. While lying in bed trying to fall asleep, she denies increased anxiety about sleep; she states that she "just doesn't feel tired." To gain a better understanding of her sleep complaint, you provide her with a sleep log and she returns it to you 2 weeks later. The patient is currently not attending school (see Fig. 34.2). What diagnosis is the sleep log most suggestive of?
    A. Irregular sleep-wake rhythm disorder
    B. Idiopathic insomnia
    C. Non-24-hour sleep-wake rhythm disorder
    D. Delayed sleep-wake phase disorder (DSWPD)
14. A 24-year-old female is brought in to the sleep center by her boyfriend because he is concerned about her drinking alcohol every night to fall asleep. Over the past few years, she has been consuming about 2–3 drinks in the hours before bed for sleep. The boyfriend tells you that once she falls asleep, she snores loudly, and this is disturbing his sleep. You order a sleep study. Which of the following recommendations is the most appropriate to give to the patient about her alcohol consumption before the sleep study?
    A. Bring alcohol to the laboratory and consume it immediately before lights are turned out.
    B. Take zolpidem 10 mg to substitute for evening alcohol for the sleep study night.
    C. Carry out your typical routine of alcohol use before bedtime on the sleep study night.
    D. Abruptly discontinue drinking alcohol at least 2 days before a sleep study can take place.
15. The currently recommended approach for nonpharmacological treatment of chronic insomnia is CBT-I. This is a multicomponent therapy that includes behavioral and cognitive strategies to improve sleep quality and daytime functioning. What percentage of people with insomnia does CBT-I help?
    A. 10%–20%
    B. 20%–30%
    C. 50%–60%
    D. 70%–80%
16. The multifactorial model of insomnia suggests that insomnia develops over time as a result of what three factors?
    A. Sleep restriction, stimulus control, and sleep hygiene
    B. Anxiety, depression, and psychoses
    C. Predisposing, precipitating, and perpetuating
    D. GABA, dopamine, and adenosine
17. Insomnia is prevalent in all of the following disorders except for which one?
    A. Behaviorally induced insufficient sleep syndrome (BIISS)
    B. Psychiatric disorders
    C. Sleep disorders
    D. Substance use disorders
18. After successfully treating depression, what is the most common residual symptom?
    A. Difficulty concentrating
    B. Guilt
    C. Fatigue
    D. Sleep disturbance
19. A 56-year-old male presents to your sleep clinic with a presenting complaint of difficulty falling asleep (typical sleep onset latency of 60 minutes) and difficulty with sleep maintenance (characterized by frequent awakenings, and on some nights he spends up to 2 hours awake during the middle of the night). He reports that he has had difficulty falling asleep for

the last 20 years; his difficulty with sleep maintenance began about 5 years ago. His bed partner reports that he snores loudly, and she often observes him inadvertently falling asleep when he is watching TV during the day. Which of the following statements describes the best next step in evaluating and treating this patient?

A. Prescribe nightly eszopiclone

B. Begin CBT-I

C. Perform actigraphy to evaluate for insomnia

D. Polysomnography to evaluate sleep-disordered breathing (SDB)

20. Which of the following is a common consequence of sleep restriction therapy for insomnia?

A. Conditioned arousal

B. REM sleep behavior disorder (RBD)

C. Slowed reaction time

D. There are no consequences of sleep restriction therapy for insomnia.

21. Which of the following is an effective stand-alone therapy for chronic insomnia?

A. Cognitive restructuring

B. Imagery training

C. Sleep hygiene

D. Stimulus control

22. You are planning to begin CBT-I for a 30-year-old male with chronic psychophysiological insomnia who is employed as a long-haul truck driver. Which of the following components of CBT-I is contraindicated for this patient?

A. Cognitive therapy

B. Sleep restriction

C. Sleep hygiene

D. Relaxation training

23. A 40-year-old female presents to your sleep clinic with a primary complaint of difficulty falling asleep for the last 15 years. She reports that she maintains a consistent TIB (11 PM–6 AM) 7 days per week, and she has good sleep hygiene. She describes that she feels very sleepy in her living room before she goes to bed, yet when she gets into bed, she feels wide awake, physically tense, and unable to fall asleep. When trying to fall asleep, she reports that she "is consumed with anxious thoughts" about all of the bad things that will happen the next day if she does not fall asleep right away. Which of the following factors is most likely perpetuating her insomnia?

A. Circadian rhythm dysregulation

B. Conditioned arousal

C. Excessive TIB

D. Female sex

24. A 40-year-old male presents to your sleep clinic with a complaint of early morning awakenings (waking around 3 AM and unable to return to sleep), which began 2 months ago, following the unexpected death of his wife. Which of the following medication is most appropriate for this patient, considering the nature of the patient's insomnia and the medication half-life?

A. Eszopiclone

B. Trazodone

C. Zaleplon

D. Zolpidem

25. Which of the following numbers most closely represents the risk ratio for insomnia in females versus males?

A. 0.5

B. 0.75

C. 1.4

D. 8.2

26. A 28-year-old female presents to your sleep clinic with a primary complaint of unrefreshing sleep and excessive daytime sleepiness, including dozing off at work meetings, over the past 4 months. She describes that her sleep is more refreshing on the weekends. You ask her to maintain a daily sleep-wake diary, and she returns to your office with the diary shown in Fig. 34.3. She reports that this week of diary is typical of her usual sleep pattern. Which of the following is the best diagnosis given her symptoms and diary data?

A. Insomnia

B. Insufficient sleep syndrome

C. Kleine-Levin syndrome

D. Sleep apnea

27. A 50-year female presents to your sleep clinic with complaints of difficulty falling asleep and maintaining sleep, which she has experienced for the past 15 years, around the time that she developed chronic back pain. She continues to report chronic back pain, despite receiving current treatment. Which of the following represents the best treatment option for this patient's sleep?

A. CBT-I

B. Sleep hygiene

C. Melatonin

D. Referral to a new pain management specialist

28. A 60-year-old female presents to your sleep clinic with a primary complaint of difficulty falling asleep. She reports that her insomnia began when her husband died 1 year ago. She notes that she feels tense and anxious in bed when unable to sleep, and gets out of bed 2 hours later on the weekends relative to her wake time during the week. You diagnose her with chronic insomnia. Which of the following represents the precipitating factor for this patient's chronic insomnia?

A. The death of her husband

B. Conditioned arousal

C. Female sex

D. Sleeping later on the weekend

29. An 81-year-old male presents to your sleep clinic with a primary complaint of early morning awakenings and difficulty returning to sleep when he awakes. He reports that he is very sleepy starting around 7 PM, and sometimes dozes off in his recliner when watching television in the evenings. He has completed a 1-week sleep diary (Fig. 34.4). Based on his primary complaint and sleep diary, which treatment is most appropriate for this patient?

A. CBT-I

B. Bright therapy administered in the evening

C. Bright therapy administered in the morning

D. Melatonin administered in the late afternoon

30. A 48-year-old male presents to your sleep clinic with a primary complaint of difficulty maintaining sleep; he reports that he spends up to 90 minutes attempting to return to sleep when he wakes during the night. His Epworth Sleepiness Scale score is 15. You have previously diagnosed him with obstructive sleep apnea, but he has been noncompliant with CPAP, using it for only 1–2 hours per night. Which of the following is the best next step in this patient's treatment plan?

A. Prescribe modafinil

B. Referral to a specialist for motivational enhancement for CPAP

C. Sleep restriction

D. Stimulus control

31. The parents of a 21-month-old child present to your sleep clinic, with a primary complaint that their daughter wakes

Today's date	4/5/08	2/8/16 Monday	2/9/16 Tuesday	2/10/16 Wednesday	2/11/16 Thursday	2/12/16 Friday	2/13/16 Saturday	2/14/16 Sunday
1. What time did you get into bed?	10:15 PM	1:30 AM	1:00 AM	12:30 AM	2:00 AM	12:45 AM	1:00 AM	1:15 AM
2. What time did you try to go to sleep?	11:30 PM	1:40 AM	1:20 AM	1:00 AM	2:10 AM	1:00 AM	1:20 AM	1:30 AM
3. How long did it take you to fall asleep?	55 min.	10 min.	5 min.	20 min.	5 min.	10 min.	20 min	15 min.
4. How many times did you wake up, not counting your final awakening?	3 times	2 times	3 times	1 time	0 time	2 times	1 time	2 times
5. In total, how long did these awakenings last?	1 hour 10 min.	10 min.	15 min.	5 min.	0 min.	15 min.	10 min.	5 min.
6. What time was your final awakening?	6:35 AM	6:00 AM	6:00 AM	6:15 AM	6:10 AM	9:00 AM	9:30 AM	6:00 AM
7. What time did you get out of bed for the day?	7:20 AM	6:00 AM	6:15 AM	6:30 AM	6:15 AM	9:00 AM	9:00 AM	6:15 AM
8. How would you rate the quality of your sleep?	☐ Very poor ☑ Poor ☐ Fair ☐ Good ☐ Very good	☐ Very poor X Poor ☐ Fair ☐ Good ☐ Very good	☐ Very poor X Poor ☐ Fair ☐ Good ☐ Very good	☐ Very poor ☐ Poor X Fair ☐ Good ☐ Very good	☐ Very poor X Poor ☐ Fair ☐ Good ☐ Very good	☐ Very poor ☐ Poor ☐ Fair X Good ☐ Very good	☐ Very poor ☐ Poor ☐ Fair ☐ Good X Very good	☐ Very poor X Poor ☐ Fair ☐ Good ☐ Very good
9. Comments (if applicable)	I have a cold							

• **Figure 34.3** Sleep diary of a 28-year-old female with unrefreshing sleep and excessive daytime sleepiness.

frequently during the night and cries for her parents; she is unable to fall back asleep until her father comes into her room and sits next to the bed. The parents report that the child's father is responsible for putting the child to bed every night, and he remains in her room until she falls asleep. Which of the following is the best diagnosis for this child?
A. Behavioral insomnia of childhood, limit-setting type
B. Behavioral insomnia of childhood, sleep-onset association type
C. Nightmare disorder
D. Sleep terrors

32. The parents of a 4-year-old child present to your sleep clinic. They report that their son refuses to go to bed, and as a result, he does not fall asleep until an hour after his bedtime. They describe that the child will refuse to change into his pajamas, and once he is in bed, he will ask his parents for repeated requests, including water, reading another story, and hugs after the lights are turned out. The parents note that they typically indulge the child's refusal to put on his pajamas by allowing him to watch television for another 30 minutes, and they also fulfill his requests after lights out in an effort to appease him. However, once he falls asleep, he is able to maintain

sleep throughout the night without signaling for his parents. Which of the following is the best diagnosis for this child?
A. Behavioral insomnia of childhood, limit-setting type
B. Behavioral insomnia of childhood, sleep-onset association type
C. Nightmare disorder
D. Sleep terrors

33. A 60-year-old male presents to your sleep clinic with a complaint of difficulty falling asleep and maintaining sleep. He recently completed an overnight sleep study. Which of the following diagnoses is most appropriate based on the patient's symptoms and the hypnogram and overnight oximetry shown in Fig. 34.5?
A. Insomnia
B. Insomnia and comorbid obstructive sleep apnea
C. Obstructive sleep apnea
D. Periodic limb movement disorder

34. Which of the following diagnosis and treatment combination is most likely to result in the hypnogram in Fig. 34.6?
A. Insomnia and comorbid anxiety treated with clonazepam
B. Insomnia and comorbid depression treated with an antidepressant
C. Insomnia and comorbid depression treated with zolpidem

Today's date	4/5/08	11/2/15 Monday	11/3/15 Tuesday	11/4/15 Wednesday	11/5/15 Thursday	11/6/15 Friday	11/7/15 Saturday	11/8/15 Saturday
1. What time did you get into bed?	10:15 PM	8:30 PM	7:30 PM	8:00 PM	9:00 PM	7:30 PM	8:00 PM	8:30 PM
2. What time did you try to go to sleep?	11:30 PM	8:30 PM	8:00 PM	8:30 PM	9:00 PM	8:00 PM	8:30 PM	8:30 PM
3. How long did it take you to fall asleep?	55 min.	10 min.	20 min.	5 min.	5 min.	10 min.	5 min.	10 min.
4. How many times did you wake up, not counting your final awakening?	3 times	2	3	4	2	2	3	2
5. In total, how long did these awakenings last?	1 hour 10 min.	10 min.	30 min.	20 min.	10 min.	10 min.	15 min.	10 min.
6. What time was your final awakening?	6:35 AM	4:00 AM	3:30 AM	3:00 AM	4:30 AM	5:00 AM	4:30 AM	4:30 AM
7. What time did you get out of bed for the day?	7:20 AM	6:00 AM	5:00 AM	5:30 AM	6:00 AM	6:00 AM	5:00 AM	5:30 AM
8. How would you rate the quality of your sleep?	☐ Very poor ☑ Poor ☐ Fair ☐ Good ☐ Very good	☐ Very poor ✗ Poor ☐ Fair ☐ Good ☐ Very good	☐ Very poor ✗ Poor ☐ Fair ☐ Good ☐ Very good	☐ Very poor ☐ Poor ✗ Fair ☐ Good ☐ Very good	☐ Very poor ✗ Poor ☐ Fair ☐ Good ☐ Very good	☐ Very poor ✗ Poor ☐ Fair ☐ Good ☐ Very good	☐ Very poor ☐ Poor ✗ Fair ☐ Good ☐ Very good	☐ Very poor ✗ Poor ☐ Fair ☐ Good ☐ Very good

• **Figure 34.4** Sleep diary of an 81-year old male with early morning awakenings.

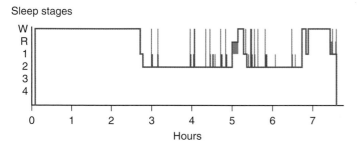

Sleep stages

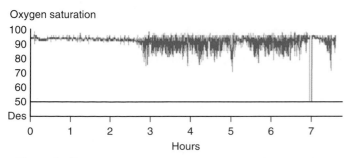

Oxygen saturation

• **Figure 34.5** Hypnogram and overnight oximetry. (From Edinger JD, Kryger MH, Roth T, eds. *Insomnia*. 2nd ed. Philadelphia, PA: Elsevier; 2014 and Kryger M, ed. *Atlas of Clinical Sleep Medicine*. 2nd ed. Philadelphia, PA: Saunders; 2013:156.)

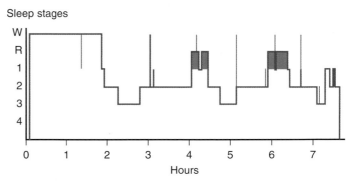

Sleep stages

• **Figure 34.6** Hypnogram. (From Edinger JD, Kryger MH, Roth T, eds. *Insomnia*. 2nd ed. Philadelphia, PA: Elsevier; 2014 and Kryger M, ed. *Atlas of Clinical Sleep Medicine*. 2nd ed. Philadelphia, PA: Saunders; 2013:155.)

D. Nightmares and posttraumatic stress disorder treated with prazosin

35. A 22-year-old male presents to your sleep clinic with a 3-year history of difficulty staying asleep. During the evaluation, he reports that he leaves the television in his bedroom on throughout his entire sleep period. Which of the following diagnoses best reflects the patient's sleep problem?

A. Idiopathic insomnia

B. Inadequate sleep hygiene

C. Obstructive sleep apnea

D. Paradoxical insomnia

Answers

1. This question describes a patient with psychophysiological insomnia. **Response B is correct** because psychophysiological insomnia is characterized by anxiety and rumination about sleep.[1-3] Response A is incorrect, as there is no mention of a medical problem causing or exacerbating the insomnia. Response C is incorrect, as the onset of the insomnia began 2 years ago and has not been present since childhood. Response D is incorrect, as there is no history of a mental disorder.

2. This question describes a patient with paradoxical insomnia. **Response C is correct** because the patient misperceived the TST compared with an objective measure of sleep.[4,5] Response A is not correct, as she has no history of formally diagnosed psychiatric disorders, including bipolar disorder. Bipolar disorder is specifically mentioned, as patients with this disorder may experience several nights without sleep in the manic phase. Response B is incorrect: It can be considered as a differential diagnosis, but the information provided does not suggest the onset of insomnia was in childhood. Response D is incorrect: It can be considered a differential diagnosis; however, patients with paradoxical insomnia are more likely to report little to no sleep and may engage in fewer activities incompatible with sleep.

3. This question describes a patient who may be a good candidate for CBT-I to aid in the process of medication discontinuation. **Response D is correct.** In a study that compared older adults who received CBT-I alone with those who received temazepam 7.5–30 mg and those that received a combination for 8 weeks, CBT-I alone had the most durable benefits to sleep after 2 years.[6] Response A is incorrect: While this option may be beneficial, in this case there are at least two reasons to consider CBT-I first: (1) the patient is already demonstrating inadequate sleep hygiene (e.g., she gets in bed early and watches TV when she cannot sleep), suggesting that a behavioral approach may be more beneficial, and (2) she specifically states that she prefers to not take medications for insomnia for much longer. Option B is incorrect: It has been found that higher morning zolpidem blood levels were highly associated with impaired driving skills, especially for women. On January 10, 2013, the US Food and Drug Administration announced the following: Reduce the night dose of zolpidem for women by 50% so as to avoid morning sleepiness (recommending 5 mg instead of 10 mg; http://www.fda.gov/Drugs/DrugSafety/ucm334033.htm). Response C is incorrect: Patients frequently use OTC sleep aids to improve sleep, but there may be anticholinergic side effects that can affect cognitive functioning. Although herbal supplements are considered "natural," they may also carry side effects. Moreover, studies show that OTC medications are not associated with significant improvements in sleep. When 184 mild insomniacs received 28 days of valerian-hops (versus placebo) or 14 days of diphenhydramine versus (placebo), there were no differences in sleep onset latency.[7]

4. This question describes a treatment option for a patient with comorbid depression and insomnia. **Response C is correct.** CBT-I has been shown to improve sleep in patients with both depression and insomnia.[8] In addition, a meta-analysis of studies of benzodiazepine discontinuation found that systematic tapering along with adjunctive cognitive behavioral therapy was superior to systematic tapering alone.[9,10] Response A is incorrect, as withdrawing the medication quickly may result in worsening of insomnia symptoms. Response B is incorrect, as diphenhydramine is an OTC medication that may be associated with next-day drowsiness, and no current data support its use when added to a discontinuation scheduling. Response D is incorrect, as withdrawing the medication every other night may result in worsening of the insomnia on the nights without the medication.

5. The question describes a patient with psychophysiological insomnia with a strong cognitive component. **Response C is correct.** While behavioral components of CBT-I help improve cognitions, cognitive therapy has been shown to be particularly helpful in lowering dysfunctional beliefs below a level considered clinically significant at posttreatment and 12-month follow-up.[11] Response A is incorrect, as sleep hygiene has been found to not be effective as a stand-alone treatment.[12] Response B is not correct. Studies suggest that while medications may be effective for short-term relief of insomnia, sleep improvements are more durable even after 2 years in patients who undergo CBT-I.[13] Response D is not correct, as polysomnography is not indicated for routine evaluation of insomnia in the absence of symptoms such as snoring, apneic spells, and nocturnal leg jerks.[14]

6. The question describes a patient with a possible circadian rhythm sleep disorder. **Response C is correct.** Actigraphy is a method used to evaluate sleep/wake patterns by assessing movement. Patients wear a wristwatch device on their non-dominant hand for several days. This method provides the clinician information about rest/activity patterns to help with the diagnosis.[15] Response A is incorrect, as polysomnography is not indicated to evaluate rest/activity patterns. Response B is incorrect, as an MSLT is administered following a PSG to document level of daytime sleepiness. Response D is incorrect: While a urine drug screen may provide helpful information, it is not would not be as useful as the multiday assessment that actigraphy provides.

7. **Response B is correct.**
   The patient's history suggests her depression is not well managed, and therefore referral back to psychiatry will likely be the best course of action for this patient. Although studies have shown that CBT-I can improve both sleep and mood in depressed patients,[16] the depressive symptoms when unmanaged may interfere with the patient's ability to engage in and benefit from therapy.

8. **The correct response is A.**
   The case describes a situation in which the patient is taking zolpidem at a time when the circadian system is promoting wakefulness and may contribute to the perception that zolpidem "doesn't work."[17] Response B is not correct. Similar to zolpidem, the influence of the circadian system might also affect temazepam in a similar way.[18] Response C is incorrect. The patient is considered an adult, and there is no indication that zolpidem would not be effective in a male in this age group. Response D is incorrect, as the effect of zolpidem tablets may be slowed by ingestion with or immediately after a meal.

9. This actogram was collected from a patient with bipolar disorder. Bipolar patients are known to have erratic sleep/wake patterns,

even in periods of euthymia.[19] **The correct response is C.** The sleep episodes (in blue) are quite long in the first part of the week, but then begin to become abbreviated on 9/5/2014 and 9/6/2014. During this time, the patient may have experienced a decreased need for sleep characteristic of a manic episode. By 9/6/2014, there is consistent motor activity that persists throughout the night of 9/7/2014 and 9/8/2014. Response A is not correct. The actogram shows irregular sleep bouts of variable duration. Response B is not correct. An actogram showing a delayed circadian sleep phase sleep may show a prolonged TIB awake prior to the onset of sleep. Response D is incorrect. Activity based measurement from actigraphy detects a threshold of movement per minute and does not require a minimum number of "steps" to establish a regular sleep pattern.

10. **Response D is correct.**
    The procedure for sleep restriction is to assign the amount of time sleeping, as assessed by a 1–2-week sleep diary, to the TIB.[20] Response A is incorrect. While establishing a consistent wake time with the patient is an important step of sleep restriction, this response would have the patient awakening 6.5 hours later than their typical wake time. Response B is incorrect. Once the patient's sleep efficiency is greater than 85%, time can be added to the TIB, typically 15–30 minutes, not 3 hours.

11. **The correct response is B.**
    Systematic desensitization is a technique used to treat certain phobias and other extreme or erroneous fears based on principles of behavior modification. The patient is not noted to have any specific phobias, and it is not a core component of CBT-I and would not be the first line in this case. Cognitive therapy for insomnia and stimulus control are two strategies that are Included in CBT-I and can be helpful in this patient because they target her maladaptive thoughts and behaviors around sleep, respectively. In the practice of stimulus control therapy (choice C), the patient is asked to leave the bed after lying awake for approximately 15–20 minutes.[21] The patient's habit of lying in bed awake for up to 2 hours every night believing that resting is as good as sleep is an example of sleep effort. Over time, the patient learns (through classical conditioning) that the bed is a cue to be awake rather than to be asleep. Cognitive therapy for insomnia (choice A) will help address her frustration when not falling asleep and her fears about losing her job as a result of her insomnia.[22] Relaxation therapy (response D) can help address physiological arousal and may be helpful to reduce the patient's tension while awake.[23] Stimulus control alone will help the patient learn to avoid spending excessive TIB, but many not address the maladaptive thoughts about sleep such as the fear of losing her job as a result of her insomnia.

12. **The correct response is A.**
    Key polysomnographic sleep disturbances during sleep include: sleep continuity disturbances, slow wave sleep (SWS) deficits, and REM sleep abnormalities.[24] Depressed patients may show difficulties with sleep continuity reflected in low sleep efficiencies. The abbreviated REM latency, absence of SWS (N3), and a prolonged sleep onset latency are characteristic of depression.[25]

13. **The correct response is D, delayed sleep-wake phase disorder (DSWPD).**
    The sleep log shows a significant delay in the phase of the major sleep episode in relation to the desired sleep time.

Studies have shown a higher rate of DSWPD in adolescents with depression.[26] Response A is incorrect, as irregular sleep-wake rhythm would show irregular sleep and wake episodes throughout the 24-hour period and at least three sleep bouts across the 24-hour period. The sleep episodes illustrated in Fig. 34.2 show rather consistent sleep bouts. Response B is incorrect, as idiopathic insomnia is a long-standing insomnia, with onset often occurring in early childhood. The patient's insomnia began 5 years ago. Response C is incorrect, as a non-24-hour sleep-wake disorder might be characterized by sleep logs that show sleep and wake times that delay each day, with a circadian period longer than 24 hours.

14. **The correct answer is C.**
    Ask the patient to continue her typical routine of alcohol use before bed. The purpose of the PSG is to understand the patient's sleep physiology in their typical conditions. If the patient has obstructive sleep apnea, it may be exacerbated by alcohol use, and this would be captured in the sleep study. Response A is incorrect because alcohol has a biphasic effect on sleep, such that there is an initial stimulating effect and then a sedating effect.[27] Alcohol consumption before bedtime might prolong sleep latency and compromise sleep study findings.[28] Response B is incorrect, as prescribing a new medication on the night of the sleep study might change the patient's typical sleep patterns. Response D is incorrect, as discontinuing alcohol 2 days before the study may induce sleep onset insomnia. A study[29] showed that 2 days without alcohol at bedtime in chronic users was associated with prolonged sleep latency.

15. **Response D is correct.**
    CBT-I helps 70%–80% of patients with insomnia; its benefits last longer than those of medications. CBT-I is a treatment that is recommended by the American College of Physicians as a first-line treatment for chronic insomnia.[30] This therapy combines four main components: stimulus control, sleep restriction, sleep hygiene education, and cognitive therapy.[12–14,31,32] In the practice of stimulus control therapy, the patient is asked to leave the bed after lying awake for approximately 15–20 minutes.[21] The procedure for sleep restriction is to assign the amount of time sleeping, as assessed by a 1–2 week sleep diary, to the TIB.[20] Sleep hygiene provides the patient education about proper sleep habits.[23] Cognitive therapy addresses maladaptive thoughts or beliefs about sleep.[22]

16. **The correct response is C.**
    Often referred to as the "3 P Model," the three factors that contribute to insomnia include predisposing, precipitating, and perpetuating factors.[33] Predisposing factors are the factors the increase the vulnerability towards insomnia such as age or sex. A precipitating factor is often a trigger for the onset of the insomnia. Perpetuating factors are those behavioral or cognitive factors that keep the insomnia going over time. Response A is incorrect. Sleep restriction, stimulus control, and sleep hygiene are treatment strategies in CBT-I. Response B is incorrect. Anxiety, depression, and psychoses may play reflect symptoms that predispose or perpetuate insomnia; they do not reflect the three main factors in the multifactorial model of insomnia. Response D is incorrect. GABA, dopamine, and adenosine are neurotransmitters involved in sleep regulation.

17. **Response A is correct.**

    BIISS is the result of limiting time and opportunity for sleep and does not reflect insomnia. Responses B through D list many of the common disorders in which insomnia is common.[34,35]

18. **The correct response is D, sleep disturbance.**

    Responses A–C are other common residual symptoms of depression, but rates of these symptoms were not as high as sleep disturbance in patients treated openly with fluoxetine 20 mg/day for 8 weeks.[36]

19. **Response D is correct, polysomnography to evaluate sleep-disordered breathing.**

    This patient's symptoms are suggestive of SDB comorbid with insomnia, which requires polysomnography for diagnosis.[37] Hypnotic medications (response A) are contraindicated in untreated patients with suspected SDB, as they may exacerbate breathing issues. Although CBT-I (response B) may improve the patient's sleep onset latency, given that he is experiencing excessive daytime sleepiness in the context of suspicion for SDB, the next step should be to evaluate and treat the SDB before proceeding with insomnia treatment, as some of the treatment components in CBT-I may increase daytime sleepiness. Response C (perform actigraphy to diagnose insomnia) is incorrect, as insomnia is diagnosed by self-report and diagnosis does not require objective monitoring such as actigraphy.

20. **Response C is correct, slowed reaction time.**

    A 2014 study by Kyle et al. showed sleep restriction, when used to treat insomnia, leads to a reduction in psychomotor vigilance (response C)[38] Conditioned arousal (response A) describes the phenomenon that occurs when the bed becomes a stimulus for wakefulness through repeated pairings of the bed with wakeful activities. RBD (response C) is a REM parasomnia that is characterized by a loss of normal voluntary muscle atonia associated with dream enactment behavior during REM sleep, and is not associated with sleep restriction therapy.

21. **The correct response is D, Stimulus control.**

    In the 2006 practice parameters paper for the psychological and behavioral treatment of insomnia,[39] only response D (stimulus control) is categorized as an effective stand-alone therapy for insomnia. Stimulus control is a behavioral therapy designed to recondition the bed and bedroom as strong cues for sleep, with demonstrated efficacy as a single-component therapy for insomnia in numerous randomized controlled trials. Responses A (cognitive restructuring), B (imagery training), and C (sleep hygiene) are often used as components of CBT-I, but do not have demonstrated efficacy as stand-alone treatments.

22. **The correct response is B, sleep restriction.**

    This patient's occupation, long-haul truck driving, requires optimal alertness and vigilance. Thus any therapy components that may lead to sleep loss and affect daytime functioning are contraindicated for this patient. Response B, sleep restriction, is contraindicated in patients who are employed in occupations that require a high level of vigilance (e.g., transportation, heavy machinery operation, assembly line work, and air traffic control), as the technique may increase risk for accidents due to sleep loss.[38] Cognitive therapy (response A) involves identifying and restructuring negative thoughts about sleep, which would not lead to significant sleep loss. Sleep hygiene (response C) refers to education

TABLE 34.2	Half-Life for Commonly Used Benzodiazepine Receptor Agonists
Generic Name	**Elimination Half-Life (h)**
Eszopiclone	6
Zaleplon	1
Zolpidem	1.5–2.4
Zolpidem extended release	1.6–4.5

regarding healthy sleep habits, and is not associated with sleep loss/sleep deprivation. Relaxation training (response D) is not associated with reductions in TST.

23. **The correct response is B, conditioned arousal.**

    This patient is describing symptoms suggestive of conditioned arousal, which is one of the factors believed to perpetuate insomnia. Conditioned arousal occurs when the bed is repeatedly paired with wakefulness (such as "trying" to sleep and ruminative worry); over time, the bed becomes a stimulus for wakefulness.[40] A patient who describes feeling sleepy in situations other than their bed (e.g., on the couch, in the other room) and wide awake when they get into bed is likely experiencing conditioned arousal. Although many patients with insomnia spend long periods of TIB, in this case, the patient is only spending 7 hours in bed, which would not be considered excessive. There is no evidence to suggest that she is experiencing a circadian rhythm disorder. Female sex is an established predisposing, not perpetuating, factor for insomnia.[41]

24. **The correct response is C, zaleplon.**

    Zaleplon has the shortest half-life of the response options and can be taken by a patient who has less than a 7–8 hour sleep opportunity (see Table 34.2 for the half-life for commonly used benzodiazepine receptor agonists). It has been shown to improve sleep when administered in the middle of the night (e.g., with less than 5 hours sleep opportunity remaining) without residual effects the next morning.[42] Eszopiclone (response A) has a 6-hour half-life. Trazodone (response B) has a half-life of 10–12 hours. Response D, zolpidem, has a half-life of 1.5–2.4 hours, which although shorter than the others, is still long enough to require a 7–8 hour sleep opportunity.

25. **The correct response is C, 1.4.**

    Overall, insomnia is more prevalent in females than in males, with many studies showing that women are 1.3–1.8 times as likely to experience insomnia relative to males. Thus the risk ratio for females to males is greater than 1, which makes responses A and B incorrect, but not higher than 2, which makes response D incorrect. The correct response, C (1.4), represents the risk ratio for insomnia in females versus males as estimated in a large meta-analysis of epidemiologic studies.[41]

26. **The correct response is B.**

    Insufficient sleep syndrome. The patient's sleep diary shows that she is spending less than 5 hours in bed on weeknights, and spending approximately 8 hours in bed on weekends. She is able to fall asleep quickly and maintain sleep without significant time spent awake during the night. According to the *International Classification of Sleep Disorders*, 3rd edition, insufficient sleep syndrome (response B) is characterized by an "irrepressible need" to sleep, a sleep time that is shorter than would be expected given age on workdays, longer sleep times on days off or weekends, and a reprieve of symptoms on days when sleep is of longer duration.[43] Insomnia (response A) cannot be diagnosed when the sleep complaints can be explained by inadequate sleep opportunity. Response C, Kleine-Levin syndrome, characterized by recurrent episodes of excessive sleepiness and sleep duration, lasting between 2 days and 5 weeks, is not correct, as the patient is not reporting excessive sleep duration. Sleep apnea (response D) is unlikely, given her age, sex, and that her sleep is refreshing on the weekends.

27. **The correct response is A.**

Recent studies have shown that CBT-I (response A) is an effective treatment for insomnia in patients with chronic pain.[44] Sleep hygiene (response B) does not have evidence to support its efficacy in treatment of insomnia.[45] Research studies have shown that response C, melatonin, has small effects on sleep onset latency, with little effect on sleep maintenance; thus it would not be a good treatment option for a patient with chronic insomnia.[45] Response D, referral to a new pain management specialist, is not the best first-line treatment response for this patient's insomnia, as she is already receiving treatment for her chronic pain, and she may see significant benefit from CBT-I.

28. **The correct response is A, the death of her husband.**

The multifactorial model of chronic insomnia[40] identifies three factors (predisposing, precipitating, and perpetuating) that produce chronic insomnia over time. In this mode, precipitating factors are triggers for insomnia; these are typically life changes or stressors. Response A, the death of her husband, is the only item on the list that represents a life stressor. Conditioned arousal (response B) is a perpetuating factor for insomnia. Response C, female sex, would be considered a predisposing factor (or risk factor) for the development of insomnia. Sleeping later on the weekend (response D) characterizes variability in the sleep-wake schedule, which is a perpetuating factor for insomnia.

29. **The correct response is B.**

Light therapy. This patient's presenting complaint and sleep diary are suggestive of an advanced phase circadian rhythm disorder. Early sleep onset and sleep offset, with adequate sleep duration, in the absence of difficulty falling asleep in an older adult are most consistent with a circadian rhythm disorder, and not suggestive of insomnia. Thus response A is incorrect, as the patient is not experiencing insomnia. Response B, light therapy, is an evidence-based therapy for circadian rhythm disorders.[46] To treat an advanced circadian phase, bright light therapy should be administered in the evening (response B). Administration of bright light therapy in the morning (response C) is indicated for delayed phase circadian rhythm disorder, and it may further advance the patient's circadian rhythm. Melatonin administered in the late afternoon (response D) is another treatment option for delayed phase circadian rhythm disorder, and may also exacerbate the patient's sleep problem.

30. **The correct response is B, referral to a specialist for CPAP desensitization.**

As many as half of patients prescribed CPAP are considered nonadherent to the therapy. Motivational enhancement (response B) has been shown to increase CPAP usage,[47] and may be helpful for this patient. Response A, to prescribe modafinil, is contraindicated, as practice guidelines state that stimulant therapies (such as modafinil) are recommended only in cases where excessive daytime sleepiness persists despite adequate treatment of apnea. As this patient is not adequately using CPAP, he is not a candidate for stimulant therapies. Response C (sleep restriction) is contraindicated, given the patient's excessive daytime sleepiness. Response D (stimulus control) is contraindicated as the next step, as his primary complaint (difficulty with sleep maintenance) may be addressed with adequate CPAP usage. Stimulus control and/or sleep restriction should be considered if the patient's insomnia persists despite optimal treatment of his apnea.

31. **The correct response is B, behavioral insomnia of childhood, sleep-onset association type.**

This toddler's symptoms are most consistent with response B, behavioral insomnia of childhood, sleep-onset association type. This disorder is common in infants and toddlers, and is characterized by night wakings that require a parent to intervene for the child to fall back asleep. The child has developed sleep associations (specific conditions that are typically present at bedtime, often parental presence) that must be present when the child wakes during the night in order for the child to return to sleep. Children are generally able to fall asleep quickly when the required conditions are present. In contrast, response A (behavioral insomnia of childhood, limit-setting type) is characterized by bedtime refusal or the child stalling with frequent requests before they will go to bed, and sleep onset is often delayed. There is no evidence of the child waking due to disturbing dreams (response C, nightmare disorder) or the dramatic arousal (e.g., extreme agitation or fright) associated with response D, night terrors.[43]

32. **The correct response is A, behavioral insomnia of childhood, limit-setting type.**

This child's parents have not set adequate bedtime limits, and the child's refusal of bedtime and stalling (such as demands for water and parental attention) is likely a consequence of these inadequate bedtime limits. This child's sleep problems are therefore most consistent with response A (behavioral insomnia of childhood, limit-setting type). Response B (behavioral insomnia of childhood, sleep-onset association type) is characterized by night wakings that require parental intervention for the child to return to sleep, such as a child who wakes in the night and cries for his parent until they come to rock him back to sleep. As the child is able to maintain sleep through the night, responses C (nightmare disorder) and D (sleep terrors) are not correct.[43]

33. **The correct answer is B, insomnia and comorbid obstructive sleep apnea.**

This patient's hypnogram shows a prolonged sleep onset latency, and a long awakening in the morning, consistent with his complaints of difficulty falling asleep and maintaining sleep. These features are suggestive of insomnia. This patient's overnight oximetry shows features of obstructive sleep apnea, specifically significant variability in his oxygen saturation levels, associated with arousals on his hypnogram.[48] Therefore response B, insomnia and comorbid obstructive sleep apnea, is the best-fitting diagnosis for this patient. Response D, periodic limb movement disorder, cannot be diagnosed from the information presented.

34. **The correct response is B, insomnia and comorbid depression treated with an antidepressant.**

    The hypnogram shows a patient with prolonged sleep onset latency, suggestive of insomnia, and a significantly prolonged REM latency, with reduced time spent in REM across the night. These features are most suggestive of response C, insomnia and comorbid depression treated with an antidepressant. Antidepressant medications are known to significantly increase REM latency and reduce the amount of time spent in REM. The medications in response A (insomnia and comorbid anxiety treated with clonazepam) and response C (insomnia and comorbid depression treated with zolpidem) are benzodiazepines, which have a very mild effect on REM sleep. Nightmares and posttraumatic stress disorder treated with prazosin (response D) would likely result in increased total REM and longer REM periods.[49,50]

35. **The correct response is B.**

    Inadequate sleep hygiene. Inadequate sleep hygiene (response B) is characterized by maladaptive sleep habits. In this case, leaving the television in the bedroom on the entire night would be the most likely cause of the patient's difficulty staying asleep. Idiopathic insomnia (response A) must begin in childhood and persist into adulthood without an identifiable cause. There is nothing in the patient's presentation to suggest obstructive sleep apnea (response C). As no objective sleep monitoring has been completed with this patient, response D, paradoxical insomnia, is incorrect.[48]

Suggested Reading

Bonnet M, Burton G, Arand D. Physiological and medical findings in insomnia: implications for diagnosis and care. *Sleep Med Rev.* 2014;18(2):111-122.

Buysse D. Insomnia. *JAMA.* 2013;309(7):706-716.

Manber R, Buysse DJ, Edinger J, et al. Efficacy of cognitive-behavioral therapy for insomnia combined with antidepressant pharmacotherapy in patients with comorbid depression and insomnia: a randomized controlled trial. *J Clin Psychiatry.* 2016;77(10):e1316-e1323.

Morin C, Beaulieu-Bonneau S, Belanger L, et al. Cognitive-behavior therapy singly and combined with medication for persistent insomnia: impact on psychological and daytime functioning. *Behav Res Ther.* 2016;87:109-116.

Winkelman J. Clinical practice. Insomnia disorder. *NEJM.* 2015;373(15): 1437-1444.

35

Neurology in Sleep Medicine: Polysomnography and Case-Based Assessment

RAMAN K. MALHOTRA, SHALINI PARUTHI

Questions

1. A 20-year-old female reports spells during sleep of violent kicking of the legs and movements of the arms. These spells occur exclusively during sleep and last less than a minute. She typically wakes up and is almost immediately back to baseline. She reports a family history of similar spells in her father and his siblings. Electroencephalogram (EEG) is performed (Fig. 35.1). Based upon the history and the findings in Fig. 35.1, what is the most likely diagnosis?
   A. Frontal lobe epilepsy
   B. Vasovagal syncope
   C. Confusional arousal
   D. Juvenile myoclonic epilepsy (JME)
   E. Absence seizures

2. A 63-year-old man presented to clinic with his wife of 30 years. They have been sleeping in separate bedrooms for the last 3 years because he has injured her several times during sleep the last 5 years. For example, she described he has punched her in his sleep; he claimed he was just defending himself from a home intruder in his dream. They present now because 2 weeks ago, he leapt out of bed and injured himself on the dresser corner, breaking his right arm. He was dreaming that he was running from a man with a machete. With each of these episodes, he quickly awakens and becomes fully alert of his surroundings. It is often between 3 AM and 6 AM. He can almost always describe a violent dream that he was having immediately prior to awakening. He has no excessive daytime sleepiness or snoring. He has a normal neurological exam including: cranial nerves I–XII are all intact, strength is 5/5 in all extremities, intact heat/cold, pressure sensation, 2+ reflexes. The rest of his physical exam is also normal. He undergoes in-lab polysomnography. This shows an apnea-hypopnea index (AHI) of 2 and minimum oxygen saturation

of 91% (Fig. 35.2). His diagnosis is associated with an increased risk of which of the following:
   A. Myasthenia gravis
   B. Myoclonic epilepsy with ragged-red fibers (MERRF)
   C. Parkinson's disease
   D. Primary progressive aphasia
   E. Charcot-Marie tooth disease type 2

3. A patient was diagnosed with idiopathic rapid eye movement (REM) sleep behavior disorder by history and polysomnography findings of REM sleep without atonia (Fig. 35.3). He is initially prescribed clonazepam 1 mg with excellent response for the first 2 months. Then, slowly, the dream enactment resumed to nearly nightly, despite increasing the dose up to 2 mg at bedtime. Which of the following would be the next best treatment?
   A. Deep brain stimulation of the subthalamic nucleus
   B. Electroconvulsive therapy
   C. Melatonin
   D. Venlafaxine
   E. Suvorexant

4. A 16-year-old boy presents with what appears to be a generalized seizure with loss of consciousness. Parents report a 3-year history of weekly sudden, brief, bilateral jerks of his arms that occur in the early morning from sleep or sometimes out of wakefulness. He is otherwise healthy and has a normal neurological examination. EEG findings are shown in Fig. 35.4. Given the history and EEG findings, which of the following is the likely prognosis for this child?
   A. Seizures will not likely return in his lifetime.
   B. He will require long-term therapy with antiepileptic medication.
   C. He will have progressive deterioration of cognitive function in young adulthood.
   D. Epilepsy surgery is likely to provide a cure for his seizures.

5. A 10-year-old boy undergoes in-lab, attended polysomnography to look for possible obstructive sleep apnea (OSA). He also has a history of waking up with drooling and twitching of his lower face several times a year (Fig. 35.5). What is the most likely diagnosis?

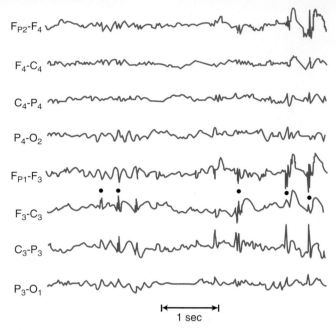

• **Figure 35.1** Electroencephalogram fragment in bipolar montage. **Channel Key:** Fp2-F4: right frontal region, F4-C4: right frontocentral region, C4-P4: right centroparietal region, P4-O2: right parieto-occipital region, FP1-F3: left frontal region, F3-C3: left frontocentral region, C3-P3: left centroparietal region, P3-O1: left parieto-occipital region. (From Kaufman DM, Milstein MJ. *Kaufman's Clinical Neurology for Psychiatrists*. Philadelphia: Saunders; 2013:201–237.)

A. Frontal lobe epilepsy
B. Benign occipital lobe epilepsy
C. Hypnic jerks
D. Benign epilepsy with centrotemporal spikes (BECTS)
E. JME

6. A 65-year-old female with a history of Parkinson's disease presents to clinic with excessive daytime sleepiness and occasional snoring. Past medical history is also significant for hypertension and diabetes. Home medications include ropinirole, lisinopril, and metformin. Overnight, in-lab attended polysomnography is performed demonstrating an apnea-hypopnea index of 3.4 and a minimum oxygen saturation of 94%. Chin and limb electromyogram (EMG) tone during REM sleep was within normal limits. Which of the following is the most likely etiology for this patient's excessive daytime sleepiness, given the sleep study findings and the provided medical history?
A. Central sleep apnea (CSA)
B. OSA
C. REM sleep behavior disorder (RBD)
D. Ropinirole

7. A 68-year-old male with a history of Parkinson's disease for 5 years presents to your office with difficulties of sleep maintenance insomnia for the last 6 months. It takes him 15 minutes to fall asleep, but he wakes up every 2 hours and then cannot get back to sleep for at least an hour. He gets up to go to the restroom twice a night, which takes him longer than expected, due to his slow gait. In addition, he has difficulties getting comfortable in bed and changing position. He is currently

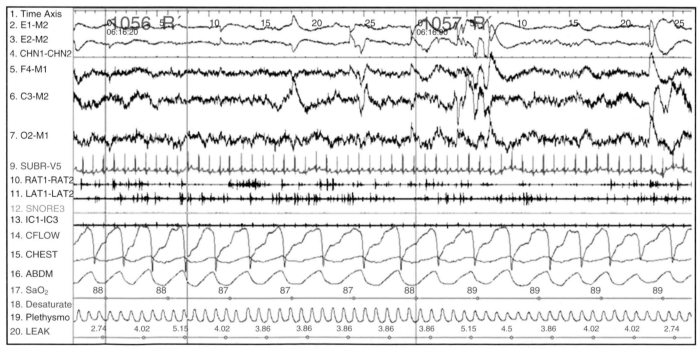

• **Figure 35.2** 60-second polysomnographic fragment. **Channel Key:** Time axis: seconds within epoch, E1-M2: left oculogram, E2-M2: right oculogram, CHN1-CHN: chin electromyogram, F4-M1: right frontal electroencephalogram, C3-M2: left central electroencephalogram, O2-M1: right occipital electroencephalogram, SUBR-V5: electrocardiogram, RAT1-RAT2: right anterior tibialis, LAT1-LAT2: left anterior tibialis, SNORE3: snore microphone, IC1-IC3: intercostal electromyogram, CFLOW: continuous positive airway pressure device flow, CHEST: chest respiratory effort, ABDM: abdominal respiratory effort, SaO₂: oximetry, Desaturate: channel marked for >3% oxygen desaturations, Plethysmography: oxygen saturation plethysmography signal, LEAK: leak from positive airway pressure mask.

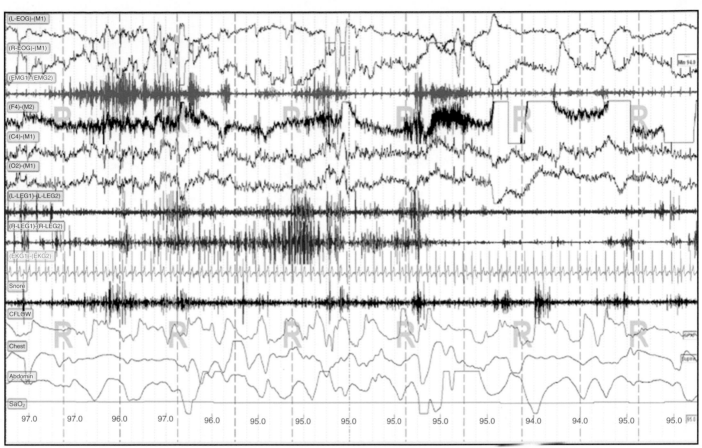

• **Figure 35.3** Sixty-second polysomnography fragment. **Channel Key:** L-EOG-M1: left oculogram, R-EOG-M1: right oculogram, EMG1-EMG2: chin electromyogram, F4-M2: right frontal electroencephalogram, C4-M1: right central electroencephalogram, O2-M1: right occipital electroencephalogram, L-LEG1-L-LEG2: left anterior tibialis, R-LEG1-R-LEG2: right anterior tibialis, EKG1-EKG2: electrocardiogram, Snore: Snore microphone, CFLOW: continuous positive airway pressure device flow, Chest: chest respiratory effort, Abdomen: abdominal respiratory effort, SaO₂: oximetry.

taking carbidopa/levodopa 25/350 mg once in the morning, at lunch, and before dinner. In-lab polysomnogram (PSG) is performed and demonstrates an apnea-hypopnea index of 3.4 and a minimum oxygen saturation of 90%. Periodic leg movement index is 1/hour. What is the best option to help improve this patient's insomnia?

A. Carbidopa/levodopa extended release at bedtime
B. Clonazepam at bedtime
C. Quetiapine fumarate at bedtime
D. Ramelteon at bedtime

8. A 53-year-old woman presented to sleep clinic for recurrent awakenings from sleep accompanied by headaches. These headaches are often bilateral, usually last 20 minutes, and are not associated with conjunctival injection, lacrimation, nasal congestion, rhinorrhea, forehead and facial sweating, miosis, ptosis, or eyelid edema. She notes they usually occur about the same time every night between midnight and 2 AM, and usually just once a night when she has them. She does not get headaches during the day when she is awake. What is the most likely diagnosis?

A. Chronic paroxysmal hemicrania
B. Cluster headaches
C. Headache due to sinusitis
D. Hypnic headache
E. Common migraine headache

9. To make the diagnosis of hypnic headaches, episodes must occur with a frequency of (headaches per month):

A. <1
B. 1–4
C. 5–9
D. 10–14
E. >15

10. A 20-year-old female presents with severe excessive daytime sleepiness for 3 years. She also complains of generalized muscle weakness, muscle spasms, and contractions in her hands that have been occurring for even longer. She is undergoing evaluation of her neuromuscular complaints. She undergoes overnight, in-lab attended polysomnography, as well as a multiple sleep latency test (MSLT) with the following results: AHI 3.2, minimum oxygen saturation 92%; total sleep time is 411 minutes on the overnight study. On the MSLT, she had a mean sleep latency of 4.5 minutes with two sleep-onset REM periods (SOREMPs). What is the most likely neuromuscular disorder that would produce these polysomnography and MSLT findings?

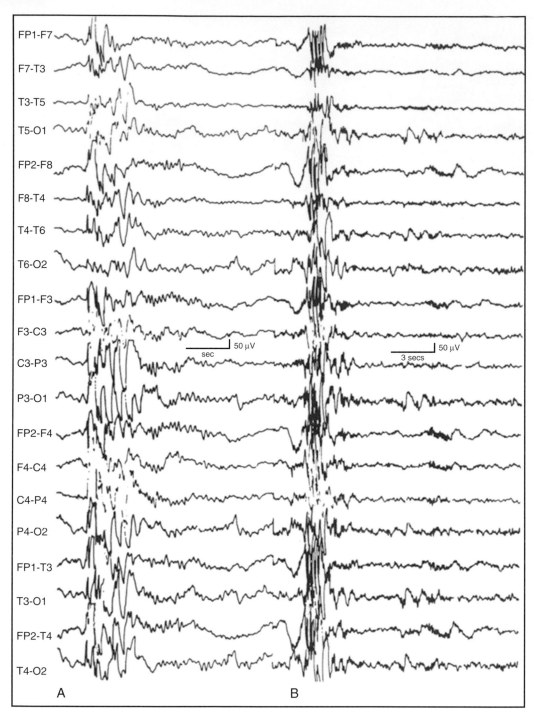

• **Figure 35.4** The electroencephalogram (EEG) recording is at 30 mm/sec (10-second epoch, conventional EEG speed) on the left (**A**) and at 10 mm/sec (30-second epoch, conventional polysomnogram speed) on the right (**B**). **Channel Key:** FP1-F7: left frontal region, F7-T3: left frontotemporal region, T3-T5: left temporal region, T5-O1: left temporo-occipital region, FP2-F8: right frontal region, F8-T4: right frontotemporal region, T4-T6: right temporal region, T6-O2: right temporo-occipital region, FP1-F3: left frontal region, F3-C3: left fronto-central region, C3-P3: left centroparietal region, P3-O1: left parieto-occipital region, FP2-F4: right frontal region, F4-C4: right fronto-central region, C4-P4: right centroparietal region, P4-O2: right parieto-occipital region, FP1-T3: left frontotemporal region, T3-O1: left temporo-occipital region, FP2-T4: right frontotemporal region, T4-O2: right temporo-occipital region. (From Chokroverty S, Montagna P. Sleep and epilepsy. In: Chokroverty S, ed. *Sleep Disorders Medicine: Basic Science, Technical Considerations, and Clinical Aspects.* 3rd ed. Philadelphia: Saunders/Elsevier; 2009:49–529.)

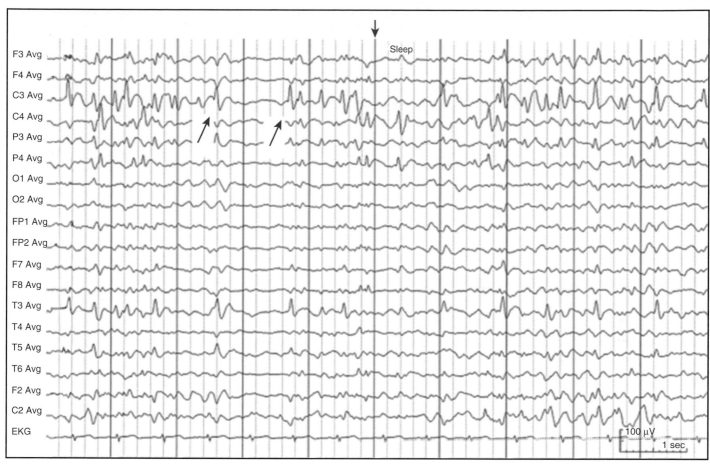

• **Figure 35.5** 16 channel electroencephalogram. **Channel Key:** F3-AVG: left frontal, F4-AVG: right frontal, C3-AVG: left central, C4-AVG: right central, P3-AVG: left parietal, P4-AVG: right parietal, O1-AVG: left occipital, O2-AVG: right occipital, FP1-AVG: left frontal pole, FP2-AVG: right frontal pole, F7-AVG: left frontal, F8-AVG: right frontal, T3-AVG: left temporal, T4-AVG: right temporal, T5-AVG: left temporal, T6-AVG: right temporal, PZ-AVG: centro-parietal, CZ-AVG: central, EKG: electrocardiogram. (From Kryger M, Roth T, Dement W, eds. *Principles and Practice of Sleep Medicine.* 6th ed. Philadelphia: Elsevier; 2016.)

A. Motor neuron disease
B. Myasthenia gravis
C. Myotonic dystrophy
D. Peripheral neuropathy

11. A 54-year-old man was recently diagnosed with the motor neuron disease amyotrophic lateral sclerosis (ALS). He has generalized weakness, along with involvement of bulbar muscles. His astute neurologist recommended a polysomnographic evaluation as he reported daytime sleepiness. He was diagnosed with sleep-related hypoventilation on the PSG. Findings of hypoventilation include:
   A. Sleep end-tidal CO_2 ranging 51–54 mm Hg for 8 consecutive minutes
   B. Sleep end-tidal CO_2 ranging 56–58 mm Hg for 16 consecutive minutes
   C. Wake end-tidal CO_2 ranging 41–44 mm Hg for 25 consecutive minutes
   D. Wake end-tidal CO_2 of 41 mm Hg and sleep end-tidal CO_2 of 51 mm Hg for 8 consecutive minutes
   E. Wake end-tidal CO_2 of 44 mm Hg and sleep end-tidal CO_2 of 51 mm Hg for 15 consecutive minutes

12. A 78-year-old woman suffered an ischemic stroke. She began to have witnessed pauses in breathing in the intensive care unit. The following is a 60-second fragment from her PSG (Fig. 35.6). What is the diagnosis?
   A. OSA
   B. Sleep-related hypoventilation
   C. CSA
   D. Sleep-related hypoxemia
   E. Late-onset central hypoventilation with hypothalamic dysfunction

13. A 36-year-old female with multiple sclerosis presents to clinic with complaints of disrupted sleep and daytime fatigue for the last 8 months. She reports rare snoring, but no apneas. She denies any leg discomfort before going to sleep or in middle of the night. She falls asleep within 30 minutes at about 11 PM and wakes up at 6:30 AM. She has frequent awakenings during sleep that are less than 5 minutes each. Overnight PSG is performed with an AHI of 2.3, minimum oxygen saturation of 92%, and a total sleep time of 411 minutes. Polysomnography fragment is shown in Fig. 35.7. What is the most likely diagnosis in this patient?

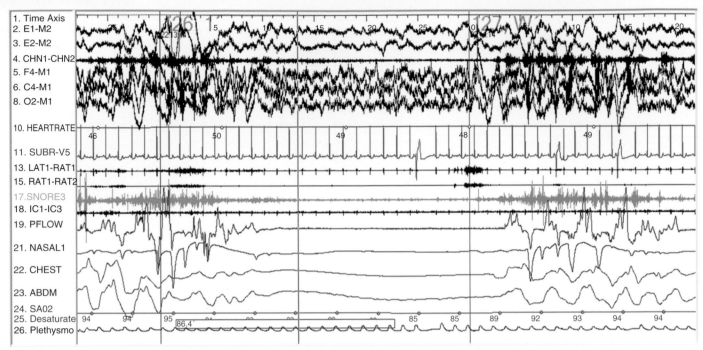

• Figure 35.6 Sixty-second epoch on polysomnogram showing a drop in the peak signal excursion by ≥90% of prevent baseline using an oronasal thermal sensor for greater than 10 seconds, associated with absent inspiratory throughout the entire period of absent airflow. **Channel Key:** Time axis: seconds within epoch, E1-M2: left oculogram, E2-M2: right oculogram, CHN1-CHN: chin electromyogram, F4-M1: right frontal electroencephalogram, C4-M1: right central electroencephalogram, O2-M1: right occipital electro-encephalogram, HEARTRA: heart rate, SUBR-V5: electrocardiogram, LAT1-RAT1: left anterior tibialis, RAT1-RAT2: right anterior tibialis, SNORE3: snore microphone, IC1-IC3: intercostal electromyogram, PFLOW: nasal pressure, NASAL1: oronasal thermal sensor, CHEST: chest respiratory effort, ABDM: abdominal respiratory effort, SaO₂: oximetry, Desaturate: channel marked for >3% oxygen desaturations, Plethysmo: oxygen saturation plethysmography signal.

A. CSA
B. OSA
C. Periodic limb movement disorder
D. Seizure disorder

14. A 44-year-old male with history of spinal cord injury reports daytime sleepiness and disrupted sleep. Overnight PSG is performed with findings as noted on PSG fragment in Fig. 35.8. What is the most likely diagnosis?
A. Sleep-related hypoventilation
B. OSA
C. Periodic limb movement disorder
D. Cheyne stokes periodic breathing

15. A 48-year-old male presents to clinic with dream enactment behaviors. His wife reports he kicks and screams while sleeping. Many times he will remember dream content related to the activity. He has no other medical history besides diabetes and OSA. He wears continuous positive airway pressure (CPAP) of 8 cm of water. Objective download shows adherence at 90% over 4 hours per night. His last titration occurred 4 years ago. Cardiopulmonary and neurological examination is within normal limits. He undergoes overnight, in-lab polysomnography (Fig. 35.9). What is the most likely diagnosis?
A. RBD
B. Pseudo-RBD
C. Confusional arousal
D. Seizure

16. A 28-year-old female reports severe daytime sleepiness for the last year. One year ago, she was injured in a car crash, which resulted in traumatic brain injury. She suffers from chronic headaches as well as daytime sleepiness ever since the car crash. She sleeps at least 8–9 hours per day. She denies cataplexy or sleep-related hallucinations, but has had sleep paralysis once. She underwent polysomnography and an MSLT the next morning. Overnight in-lab polysomnography showed a normal respiratory disturbance index of 3, no periodic leg movements, and a total sleep time of 406 minutes. The MSLT showed a mean sleep latency of 6.5 minutes with one sleep-onset REM period. Magnetic resonance imaging (MRI) of the brain is in Fig. 35.10. Per the history, findings, and imaging noted previously, what is the most likely diagnosis?
A. Idiopathic hypersomnia
B. Hypersomnia due to a medical disorder
C. Narcolepsy type 1
D. Narcolepsy type 2

17. A 62-year-old man is admitted to the hospital because of rapidly worsening symptomatology characterized by decreased cognition and mental status, gait difficulty, involuntary jerking especially upon startle, and insomnia. He has agitation and visual hallucinations that have appeared over the last couple of months. On clinical examination the patient appears to be severely demented. A cerebellar syndrome with dysarthria, upbeat nystagmus, and multifocal myoclonus is also observed.

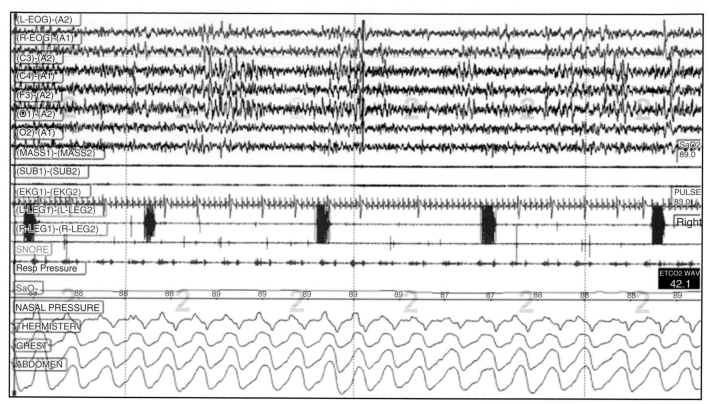

• **Figure 35.7** This 90-second polysomnography epoch demonstrates repetitive limb movements seen in the left leg electromyogram lead (L-LEG1-L-LEG2). At least four repetitive leg movements are required to score a series of periodic limb movements. **Channel Key:** L-EOG-A2: left electro-oculogram, R-EOG-A1: right electro-oculogram, C3-A2: left central region, C4-A1: right central region, F3-A2: left frontal region, O1-A2: left occipital region, O2-A1: right occipital region, MASS1-MASS2: masseter electromyograph, EKG1-EKG2: electrocardiogram, L-LEG1-L-LEG2: left anterior tibialis electromyograph, R-LEG1-R-LEG2: right anterior tibialis electromyograph, SNORE: snore microphone: nasal pressure: nasal pressure transducer, SaO2: oximetry, Thermister, Chest, Abdomen. (From Rama AN, Zachariah R, Kushida CA. Differentiating nocturnal movements: leg movements, parasomnias, and seizures. *Sleep Med Clin.* 2009;4[3]361–372.)

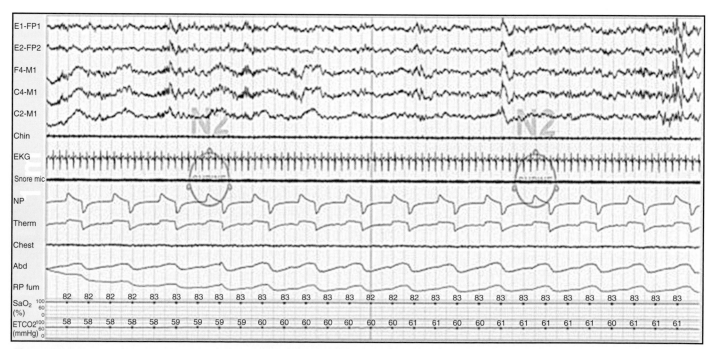

• **Figure 35.8** 60-second epoch of polysomnography. **Channel Key:** E1-FPz: left electrooculogram, E2-FPz: right electrooculogram, F4-M1: right frontal region, C4-M1: right central region, O2-M1: right occipital region, Chin: chin electromyogram, EKG: electrocardiogram, Snore Mic: snore microphone, NP: nasal pressure transducer, Therm: oronasal thermistor, Chest: chest respiratory effort, Abd: abdominal respiratory effort, RIP-sum: respiratory inductance plethysmography sum channel, SaO2: oximetry, TcCO2: transcutaneous carbon dioxide. (From Grigg-Damberger MM, Wagner LK, Brown LK. Sleep hypoventilation in patients with neuromuscular diseases. *Sleep Med Clin.* 2012;7[4]:667–687.)

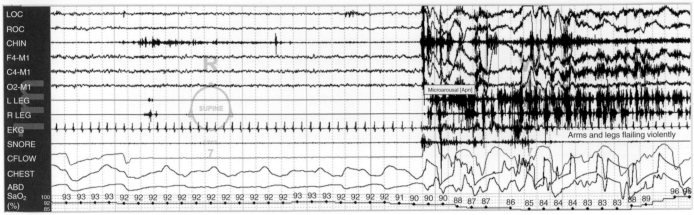

• **Figure 35.9** Sixty-second polysomnography epoch. **Channel Key:** LOC: left electrooculogram, ROC: right electrooculogram, CHIN: chin electromyogram, F4-M1: right frontal region, C4-M1: right central region, O2-M1: right occipital region, L Leg; left anterior tibialis electromyogram, R Leg: right anterior tibialis electromyogram, EKG: electrocardiogram, SNORE: snore microphone, CFLOW: positive airway pressure device flow, CHEST: chest respiratory effort, ADB: abdominal respiratory effort, SaO2 (%): oximetry (Copyright Alon Y. Avidan, MD, MPH).

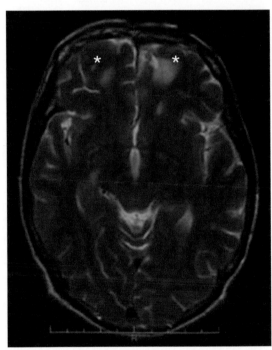

• **Figure 35.10** Brain magnetic resonance imaging (T2 image) axial image. *Lesions seen on brain MRI. (From Bassetti C. Primary and secondary neurogenic hypersomnias. *Sleep Med Clin*. 2012;7[2]:249–261.)

Brain MRI shows hyperintensities in the basal ganglia, EEG shows generalized slowing without periodic and triphasic waves, and cerebrospinal fluid (CSF) examination documents the presence of 14-3-3 protein. Autopsy 1 month later confirmed the diagnosis of Creutzfeldt-Jakob disease (CJD). What finding on the PSG is characteristic of patients with CJD or prion disease late in the course of the disease?

A. Loss of sleep spindles
B. Increased REM sleep
C. Increased stage N3 sleep
D. Alpha intrusion

18. A 36-year-old female presents to clinic with spells of loss of muscle tone for the last month. She loses muscle tone in her legs and sometimes her whole body. The spells last 30 seconds to a minute, and afterward, she gradually regains muscle strength in less than a minute. She retains memory and consciousness during the spells. The spells occur in relation to excitement or hearing something humorous. She has no other known medical history, but admits to having loss of vision in one eye years ago, as well as other unexplained neurological symptoms that she never sought evaluation for. An MRI of the brain is performed and is consistent with demyelinating lesions of multiple sclerosis in the periventricular white matter, brainstem, and hypothalamus. She does report hypersomnia. Overnight polysomnography was within normal limits with a total sleep time of 415 minutes. MSLT demonstrates a mean sleep latency of 3 minutes and three sleep onset REM periods. What is the most likely diagnosis?

A. Idiopathic hypersomnia
B. Narcolepsy type 1 due to a medical/neurological condition
C. Narcolepsy type 2
D. Sleep terrors

19. A 56-year-old woman was diagnosed with multiple system atrophy-cerebellar type (MSA-C) after her dysphagia worsened despite dopaminergic medication for the last 3 years. In addition, she has begun to "act out her dreams" in the last 4 months, per her husband of 31 years. She also makes a high-pitched sound with inspiration during sleep. Her neurologist sends her for a PSG and consultation with a sleep physician. Treatment with which of the following will most likely improve her median survival time?

A. Carbidopa/levodopa
B. Continuous positive airway pressure
C. Deep brain stimulation
D. Intravenous immunoglobulin
E. Oxybutynin

20. A 21-year-old woman presents with headache, especially when laughing, coughing, or with exertion. She also notes neck pain and vertigo at times. Upon further questioning, she also reports awakenings at night, snoring, witnessed apneas, and awakenings

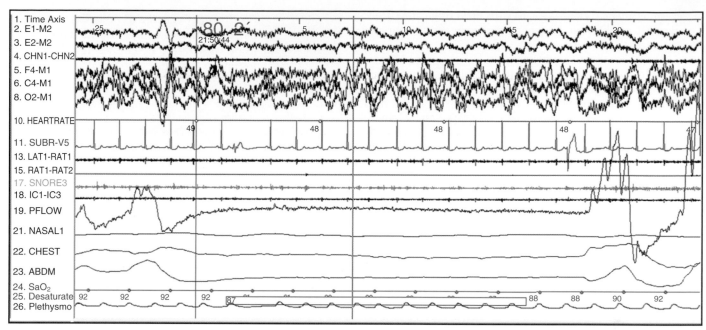

- **Figure 35.11** This is a 30-second epoch of sleep. **Channel Key:** Time axis: seconds within epoch, E1-M2: left oculogram, E2-M2: right oculogram, CHN1-CHN: chin electromyogram, F4-M1: right frontal electroencephalogram, C4-M1: right central electroencephalogram, O2-M1: right occipital electroencephalogram, HEART RATE: heart rate, SUBR-V5: electrocardiogram, LAT1-RAT1: left anterior tibialis, RAT1-RAT2: right anterior tibialis, SNORE3: snore microphone, IC1-IC3: intercostal electromyogram, PFLOW: nasal pressure, NASAL1: oronasal thermal sensor, CHEST: chest respiratory effort, ABDM: abdominal respiratory effort, SaO₂: oximetry, Desaturate: channel marked for >3% oxygen desaturations, Plethysmo: oxygen saturation plethysmography signal.

with shortness of breath. She also has excessive daytime sleepiness. An arterial blood gas during the day showed PCO₂ of 46 mm Hg. A sleep study showed the following (Fig. 35.11): What is the diagnosis?

A. CSA with Cheyne-Stokes breathing

B. Central apnea due to a medical disorder without Cheyne-Stokes breathing

C. Primary CSA

D. Late-onset central hypoventilation with hypothalamic dysfunction

E. Idiopathic central alveolar hypoventilation

21. Which of the following tests are diagnostic for a disorder that causes CSA?

A. Cerebrospinal fluid culture

B. Cerebrospinal hypocretin level

C. Ictal single-photon emission computed tomography

D. Lumbar puncture opening pressure

E. Magnetic resonance imaging of brain

22. A 68-year-old male with late-stage Alzheimer's dementia presents to clinic for loud snoring. Polysomnography is performed demonstrating a normal apnea-hypopnea index of 4.3 and minimum oxygen saturation of 90%. What is the most likely finding from the polysomnography that you would expect in a patient with late Alzheimer's dementia?

A. Prolonged REM sleep latency

B. Increased stage N3 sleep

C. Poorly formed sleep spindles

D. Increased REM density

23. A 72-year-old female with early Alzheimer's dementia presents to clinic with insomnia. Her daughter, who mainly takes care of her, reports that she has a difficult time going to sleep at

night and staying asleep. Many times, she is confused, anxious, and sometimes agitated before bed. During the day, it is unusual for her to have these symptoms. She typically wakes up at 3 AM or 4 AM and cannot fall back asleep. It is not uncommon to find her asleep in the late evening time on the couch. What is the most likely treatment below to help with this patient's sleep symptoms?

A. Morning light

B. Evening light

C. Fluoxetine

D. Morning melatonin

Answers

1. **The correct answer is A.**

The most likely diagnosis is nocturnal frontal lobe epilepsy (NFLE). Seizures in patients with NFLE involve violent movements of the extremities, sometimes twisting, or dystonic movements. Movements are stereotypical. They can present in clusters and occur mainly out of sleep, though they can also appear out of wakefulness. Consciousness may be preserved during the seizure, and there may be very short to no post-ictal confusion or mental status change. NFLE can be familial with autosomal dominant transmission, though there are sporadic cases. EEG may show frontal lobe sharp waves or spike waves, but many times are normal (or obscured by muscle artifact), even during a seizure. In this case, Fig. 35.1, on at least five occasions (marked by dots), sharp waves and spikes, in phase reversal, appear to point toward each other. These sharp waves and spikes originate from the common electrode, F3, situated over the left frontal lobe. Seizures usually arise from nonrapid eye movement (NREM) sleep, with 70% originating from stage N1 or N2 sleep. Carbamazepine is an effective antiepileptic for NFLE.[1,2]

The spells are not consistent with vasovagal syncope (Answer B) by history and due to the abnormal EEG findings in Fig. 35.1. Confusional arousals (Answer C) are not likely, as they also do not demonstrate EEG abnormalities seen in Fig. 35.1 and are not typically characterized by stereotyped motor activity. In addition, patients with confusional arousals do not typically remember events and do not return to baseline quickly. Confusional arousals are NREM sleep parasomnias arising out of NREM sleep (usually stage N3) characterized by mental confusion with an absence of terror or ambulation out of the bed.[3] JME (Answer D) is a generalized epilepsy and has motor activity mainly occurring in the morning time with brief myoclonic jerks. EEG typically shows generalized spike or poly-spike and wave, which were not noted on this patient's EEG. Absence seizures (Answer E) mainly present with staring and do not have an abundance of motor activity. EEG in absence seizures demonstrate 3 Hz generalized spike and wave discharges.[2]

2. **The correct answer is C. Parkinson's disease.**
The case describes classic findings for RBD. This disorder is most commonly observed in men, older than age 50 years, characterized by repeated episodes of sleep-related vocalization and/or complex motor behaviors, documented on in-lab polysomnography showing REM sleep without atonia, and is not better explained by another sleep disorder, mental health disorder, medication, or substance use. RBD is often associated with a delayed emergence of a neurodegenerative disorder, most often a synucleinopathy, such as Parkinson's disease, multiple system atrophy, or dementia with Lewy bodies. Studies have reported up to 81%–90% of patients with idiopathic RBD will develop neurodegenerative disorders, including parkinsonism, dementia, or mild cognitive impairment.[3,4]

Fig. 35.2 is of a 60-second PSG fragment that shows excessive transient muscle activity (phasic activity) in REM sleep. REM sleep without atonia may be scored as sustained muscle activity (tonic activity) in REM sleep; this is seen as an epoch of REM sleep with at least 50% of the duration of the epoch having a chin EMG amplitude greater than the minimum amplitude demonstrated in NREM sleep. REM sleep without atonia may also be scored as excessive transient muscle activity in REM sleep in the chin or limb EMG leads. In a 30-second epoch of REM sleep divided into 10 sequential 3-second mini-epochs, at least 50% of the mini-epochs contain bursts of transient muscle activity. In RBD, excessive transient muscle activity bursts are 0.1–5.0 seconds in duration and at least 4 times as high in amplitude as the background EMG activity.[5] Table 35.1 reviews findings seen in patients with RBD who will go on to develop a synucleinopathy. Answers B and D are not correct, as there are no associated higher rates of RBD in MERRF or primary progressive aphasia. Answers A and E are not correct, as patients with RBD are not at increased risk to develop myasthenia gravis or Charcot-Marie tooth disease type 2.[3]

3. **The correct answer is C. Melatonin.**
Studies show that clonazepam and melatonin have similar treatment efficacy, with melatonin having less potential side effects. Melatonin may reestablish the atonia of REM sleep when taken at doses of 6–15 mg. Most patients respond well to clonazepam at low doses 0.5–1 mg at bedtime. Clonazepam may be problematic in elderly patients prone to falls, may

TABLE 35.1	Prodromal Features of Fully Expressed Synucleinopathies in Patients with Idiopathic Rapid Eye Movement Sleep Behavior Disorder

Physiologic Abnormalities

- Reduced olfaction
- Reduced color vision
- Autonomic dysfunction (symptoms, cardiovascular tests, ^{123}I-MIBG myocardial scintigraphy)
- Motor dysfunction
- Cognitive dysfunction
- Electroencephalogram power abnormalities

Imaging Abnormalities

- Midbrain—transcranial sonography
- Striatal dopamine transporters—single-photon emission computed tomography (SPECT) scans
- Putaminal volume—magnetic resonance imaging (MRI) scans
- Parkinson's disease–related covariance pattern—positron emission tomography and SPECT scans
- Hyper- and hypoperfusion of various brain regions—SPECT scans
- Pons and midbrain abnormalities—MRI diffusion tensor imaging
- Hippocampal gray matter—voxel-based morphometry
- Cerebellum and pontine tegmentum—voxel-based morphometry

From Kryger M, Roth T, Dement W, eds. *Principles and Practice of Sleep Medicine*. 6th ed. Philadelphia: Elsevier; 2016.

cause morning grogginess after awakening, or patients may develop tolerance.[4]

It is also important to ensure comorbid sleep disorders such as OSA and periodic limb movement disorder are treated. Treatment of periodic limb movements of sleep with pramipexole has been shown to reduce movements at night.[4]

Answer A is incorrect as deep brain stimulation of the subthalamic nucleus may improve subjective sleep, but has not been shown to decrease dream enactment behaviors or reestablish REM sleep atonia. Answers B and E are incorrect as electroconvulsive therapy and suvorexant have not been associated with treatment for RBD.[4] Venlafaxine is not a treatment for RBD, and can, at times, cause secondary RBD and REM sleep without atonia. Thus Answer D is incorrect. Fig. 35.3 shows increased chin tone EMG found in patients with RBD.

4. **The correct answer is B. The most likely diagnosis is JME.**
JME is a form of generalized epilepsy with a strong genetic component characterized by myoclonic jerks that are most frequent in the early morning. Generalized tonic-clonic seizures are also observed. Age of onset is typically 8–24 years of age, with a peak at 12–18 years of age.[2] Myoclonic jerks, mainly of the upper extremities, can occur in the early morning, or during the daytime, sometimes causing the patient to drop or throw objects, or even fall to the ground. Consciousness is retained during the myoclonic jerks. The patients eventually develop generalized tonic-clonic seizures, and may develop absence seizures.[6] Drugs, alcohol, stress, sleep deprivation, and photic stimulation can trigger seizures. Intelligence is not affected; therefore Answer C is incorrect. EEG typically demonstrates inter-ictal 3–6 Hz generalized spike or poly-spike and wave discharges, as noted in Fig. 35.4. Seizures respond well to treatment with valproic acid, lamotrigine, topiramate,

or zonisamide. Although antiepileptic medications are usually successful in treating seizures, patients require therapy long term, as relapse is high when antiepileptics are withdrawn; therefore Answer A is incorrect.[6] Epilepsy surgery is not performed for generalized epilepsy, so Answer D is incorrect.

5. **The correct answer is D. The most likely diagnosis is BECTS, also known as benign rolandic epilepsy.**

   BECTS is the most common partial epilepsy in childhood. The typical seizure occurs upon awakening, involving motor activity of the lower face, drooling, or dysarthria. The seizures respond well to therapy in childhood, and typically remit in adolescence.[2,6] EEG shows characteristic central and temporal spikes bilaterally (channels C3-T3-C4-T4) but independent, which is what is noted on Fig. 35.5. Answers A and B are incorrect, as the case is not consistent with occipital or frontal lobe epilepsy given the EEG findings demonstrating epileptiform activity in the central and temporal regions. Answer C is incorrect, as hypnic jerks would not involve solely the face and would not have the EEG findings in Fig. 35.5. Hypnic jerks, or sleep starts, are sudden, brief muscle contractions of the body or body segment occurring during sleep onset. The hypnic jerk may be associated with a sensory component or a feeling of falling. Hypnic jerks are not associated with epileptiform activity, and when captured on polysomnography, demonstrate increased EMG activity or possibly a vertex wave.[3] Answer E is incorrect, as JME is a generalized epilepsy that can cause myoclonic jerking upon awakening, but usually in the extremities and not the face. In addition, EEG in this condition shows generalized spike and wave or poly-spike and wave.

6. **The correct answer is D. Ropinirole, a dopamine agonist commonly used to treat Parkinson's disease, can cause excessive daytime sleepiness as a side effect.**

   Other medications commonly used to treat Parkinson's disease such as carbidopa/levodopa and pramipexole, other dopamine agonists, also can cause hypersomnia as a side effect.[7] Answers A and B are incorrect, as though OSA and CSA can be seen in patients with Parkinson's disease, the overnight PSG had an apnea-hypopnea index below 5 and was not consistent with these diagnoses. Parkinson's disease patients are at higher risk for developing sleep apnea as compared with age-matched controls in some studies.[8] Parkinson's disease patients are also at higher risk for restless legs syndrome and periodic leg movements of sleep in some studies. Answer C is incorrect. Parkinson's patients have a much higher rate of RBD. However, in this case, neither the history provided nor the polysomnography was consistent with this diagnosis, as there was no history of dream enactment behavior and normal, expected low tone on EMG was observed during REM sleep on the sleep study.[3] A subset of Parkinson's patients have severe excessive daytime sleepiness and have similar findings that are seen in narcolepsy.[9] MSLTs in these patients demonstrate hypersomnia, along with the presence of sleep-onset REM periods. Although hypocretin levels in the cerebrospinal fluid are normal, there are studies demonstrating damage to hypocretin neurons in some Parkinson's patients (Table 35.2).

7. **The correct answer is A. Carbidopa/levodopa extended release.**

   It is common for patients with Parkinson's disease to have insomnia. Insomnia is multifactorial, as Parkinson's patients can suffer from OSA, restless legs syndrome, or circadian rhythm disturbances. Insomnia can be due to underlying mood disorders, or as a side effect to some antiparkinsonian

TABLE 35.2 Comparison Between Parkinson's Disease and Narcolepsy with Cataplexy

	Narcolepsy With Cataplexy	Parkinson's Disease
Excessive daytime sleepiness	+	+
Sleep attacks	+	+
Cataplexy	+	−
Hallucinations	+	+
Sleep paralysis	+	−
REM sleep behavior disorder	+	+
HLA DQB1*0602	>90%	30%
Sleep-onset REM periods in the Multiple Sleep Latency Test	+	+/−
Absent hypocretin in cerebrospinal fluid	+	−
Loss of hypocretinergic cells in the hypothalamus	90%	23%–62%

HLA, Human leukocyte antigen; *REM*, rapid eye movement.
From Iranzo A. Sleep and neurodegenerative diseases. *Sleep Med Clin.* 2016;11(1):1–18.

medications. One other common cause of insomnia is worsening motor symptoms at night, as many patients do not have their medication prescribed before bedtime. Common motor difficulties that can occur during the day, such as bradykinesia, muscle stiffness, and difficulties in moving, can occur during the night when patients try to use the restroom or change positions in bed, causing insomnia.[7] Satin sheets can ease movements in bed.[2] See Fig. 35.12, demonstrating a tremor noted during polysomnography in a patient with Parkinson's disease. Carbidopa/levodopa extended release at bedtime will help with these motor symptoms in this patient (walking to the restroom and getting comfortable in bed). Answer B, clonazepam, is not the best option, because in this population, benzodiazepines should be used with caution as they can cause a higher risk of falls and can worsen sleep-disordered breathing. Clonazepam can be helpful in cases of RBD and restless legs syndrome, but this is not described in this case. Periodic leg movement index was also noted to be within normal limits on the PSG. Answer C is incorrect, as quetiapine fumarate, an atypical antipsychotic, though sedating, could worsen parkinsonian symptoms, since it is a dopamine antagonist. Answer D is incorrect, as ramelteon is mainly used to help with sleep onset and not sleep maintenance insomnia.

8. **The correct answer is D. The clinical history best helps the clinician characterize the headache.**

   Here this patient is clear that the headaches occur only at night; thus this is hypnic headache. Hypnic headaches only occur during sleep. Hypnic headaches are uncommon, but can often be distinguished from other types of headaches that may occur in sleep and/or during the day. The other Answers A, B, and E are incorrect, as other primary headaches such as migraines, cluster headaches, and chronic paroxysmal hemicranias occur during the day and may occur at night.

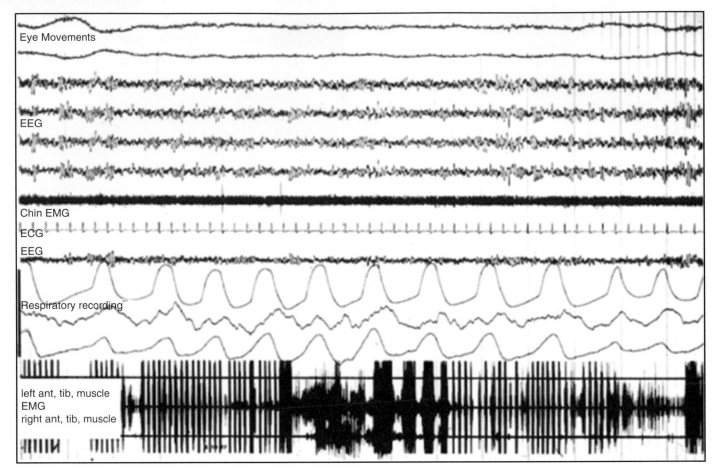

• **Figure 35.12** Sixty-second polysomnogram fragment in a patient with Parkinson's disease and nocturnal rest tremor of the left leg occurring between wakefulness and stage N1 sleep. The regular unilateral rest tremor is interrupted by bilateral motor activity. **Channel Key:** eye movements: electro-oculograms, EEG: electroencephalogram, Chin EMG: submentalis muscle electromyography, ECG: electrocardiogram, respiratory recording: airflow, chest and abdominal effort, left ant tib muscle: left anterior tibialis muscle, right ant tib muscle: right anterior tibialis muscle. (From Kryger M, Roth T, Dement W, eds. *Principles and Practice of Sleep Medicine.* 6th ed. Philadelphia: Elsevier; 2016, Table 92.1.)

Secondary headaches may also occur due to other medical, neurological, psychiatric, or sleep disorders, such as hypertension, brain tumors, arteriovenous malformation, cerebral venous thrombosis, trauma, depression, or OSA, among others. These headaches may occur during sleep, present upon awakening from sleep, or develop later in the day. Migraines commonly last between 4 and 72 hours, with unilateral, pulsating pain, and are often associated with nausea, photophobia, or phonophobia. Approximately 50% of migraines start between 4 AM and 9 AM, and can arise from any stage of sleep. Migraines may be preceded by an aura (i.e., visual field defects or scotomas) if the patient is awake. Patients may also experience unilateral paresthesias, weakness, aphasia, vertigo, tinnitus, dysarthria, decreased hearing, diplopia, or ataxia. Cluster headaches are often severe, unilateral, periorbital, or temporal, and peak within 10–15 minutes. These headaches may occur at the same hour each day, daily in cluster periods, often with one to three attacks per day over a period of 1–2 months, and then remit. Most patients have one cluster period per year. Approximately 75% of cluster episodes occur between 9 PM and 10 AM. They are often associated with cranial autonomic features, including ipsilateral conjunctival injection,

lacrimation, nasal congestion, rhinorrhea, forehead and facial sweating, miosis (a constricted pupil), ptosis (a weak, droopy eyelid), or eyelid edema, of which this patient has none. Cluster headaches are strongly associated with REM sleep. Chronic paroxysmal hemicrania headaches are similar to cluster headaches, but occur far more frequently, most often more than five per day, and are also strongly associated with REM sleep. Answer C is also incorrect as headaches due to other medical conditions such as sinusitis are likely to occur at night or during the day, along with other clinical symptoms such as nasal congestion or rhinorrhea.[3]

9. **The correct answer is E. Hypnic headaches are an uncommon type of headache, usually lasting at least 15 minutes, with a frequency of at least 15 times per month.**
Patients are usually 50 years or older and report often a bilateral headache, that is not severe, without cranial autonomic features (ipsilateral conjunctival injection, lacrimation, nasal congestion, rhinorrhea, forehead and facial sweating, miosis, ptosis, or eyelid edema), occurring 1–3 times per night, often at the same time each night. The patient may experience isolated nausea, photophobia, or phonophobia. Hypnic headaches typically occur in REM sleep and have been described in stage

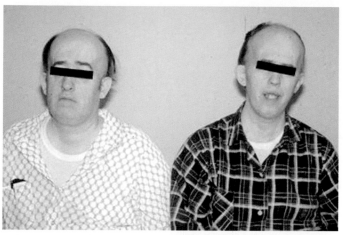

• **Figure 35.13** Two brothers who have myotonic dystrophy show the characteristic facies with temporalis muscle wasting, fish mouth, and thin neck. Frontal alopecia is also prominent. (From Culebras A. Sleep-disordered breathing in neuromuscular disease. *Sleep Med Clin.* 2008;3[3]: 377–386.)

N3 sleep. Answers A, B, C, and D are incorrect, as a frequency of greater than 15 headaches per month is required for the diagnosis.[3]

10. **The correct answer is C. Myotonic dystrophy is the most common type of muscular dystrophy in adults and is characterized by progressive myopathy, myotonia, and multiorgan involvement.**

Patients suffering from myotonic dystrophy have a characteristic phenotype, including temporal wasting and frontal balding (Fig. 35.13). Two genetically distinct entities have been identified: myotonic dystrophy type 1 (DM1 or Steinert's disease) and myotonic dystrophy type 2 (DM2). Myotonic dystrophies are strongly associated with sleep dysfunction.[10] Sleep-disordered breathing in the form of OSA and CSA, as well as sleep-related hypoventilation, is frequently seen in patients with myotonic dystrophy (Fig. 35.14). In addition to sleep-disordered breathing, some patients with DM1 have been noted to have severe hypersomnia with REM sleep dysregulation, similar to findings seen in patients with narcolepsy. Low levels of cerebrospinal fluid hypocretin have been found in these patients, along with MSLT results consistent with narcolepsy (mean sleep latency ≤8 minutes and two or more sleep onset REM periods).[3] Loss of 5-hydroxytryptamine (serotonin) neurons of the dorsal raphe nucleus and the superior central nucleus have also been suggested as possible pathophysiology for these findings.[11] Answers A and B are incorrect, as although sleep-disordered breathing and hypersomnia are noted in higher rates in patients with myasthenia gravis and motor neuron disease, there has not been any evidence of a hypocretin deficiency or REM sleep dysregulation phenomena consistent with narcolepsy. Answer D is also not correct, as peripheral neuropathy does not put patients at higher risk of hypersomnia or narcolepsy, though it can be associated with higher rates of restless legs syndrome.

11. **The correct answer is B.**
Hypoventilation in adults is defined on polysomnography as (1) an increase in the arterial PCO_2 (or surrogate) to a value greater than 55 mm Hg for ≥10 minutes or (2) there is a ≥10 mm Hg increase in arterial PCO_2 (or surrogate) during sleep (in comparison to an awake supine value) to a value exceeding 50 mm Hg for ≥10 minutes.[3,5]

In addition, it is important to recognize that hypoventilation may occur in REM sleep or NREM sleep, though is likely to be more severe in REM sleep. In most people, muscle tone is lowest during REM sleep, and there is critical dependence on diaphragmatic contraction to maintain adequate ventilation. Given the diaphragmatic dysfunction and loss of muscle tone in accessory muscles in patients with ALS, significant hypoventilation and hypoxia can occur.[3,12]

Home oximetry testing or home sleep apnea testing does not provide information regarding sleep stages. A marked reduction in REM sleep duration has been associated with reduced survival. Mortality is reduced when patients are adequately ventilated.[12]

Patients should be started on noninvasive positive pressure ventilation (bilevel positive airway pressure [BPAP]) due to the improved tolerability of BPAP once bulbar symptoms occur. In addition, a trial of BPAP can be considered when $PaCO_2$ is greater than 45 mm Hg, maximum inspiratory pressure (MIP) is less than 60% predicted, forced vital capacity (FVC) is less than 50% predicted, SpO_2 is ≤88% for at least 5 consecutive minutes during sleep, sniff nasal pressure (SNP) is less than 40% predicted, or the clinical symptom of orthopnea appears.[12]

Pressures should be started low and titrated to patient tolerance, with goal of normalization of awake gas exchange and relief of symptoms. In one study, frequent adjustments were required: 50% of ALS patients required at least one adjustment in the first 6 months and 20% of patients required three or more adjustments in the first 12 months. Patients monitored by modem (attached to the BPAP machine) had fewer outpatient visits, emergency room visits, and inpatient admissions.[12]

Answers A, C, D, and E are all incorrect, as they do not meet the definition for hypoventilation.

12. **The correct answer is C.**
Central sleep apnea is a cessation of airflow accompanied by lack of respiratory effort, usually associated with oxygen desaturation.[2,3,5] CSA may be seen in up to 26% of patients after a stroke and may improve.[2] CSA may occur in patients with anterior circulation lesions or larger strokes. The presence of CSA after stroke is associated with a poorer prognosis compared with patients without CSA. Treatment of CSA after stroke includes PAP therapy and possibly adaptive servo-ventilation (ASV).[2]

Answer A is incorrect, as the PSG fragment clearly shows central apnea. However, OSA is observed more often in patients with a history of stroke or transient ischemic attack, with estimates as high as 72% for AHI > 5/hour, and 38% for AHI > 20/hour. The American Heart Association recommends screening for OSA for stroke prevention. Patients who have atrial fibrillation and OSA develop stroke more often than patients with atrial fibrillation without OSA.[2]

Answer B is incorrect, as sleep related hypoventilation in adults is defined on polysomnography as (1) an increase in the arterial PCO_2 (or surrogate) to a value greater than 55 mm Hg for ≥10 minutes or (2) there is a ≥10 mm Hg increase in arterial PCO_2 (or surrogate) during sleep (in comparison to an awake supine value) to a value exceeding 50 mm Hg for ≥10 minutes.[5] Answer D is incorrect, as sleep-related hypoxia is the presence of arterial oxygen saturation during

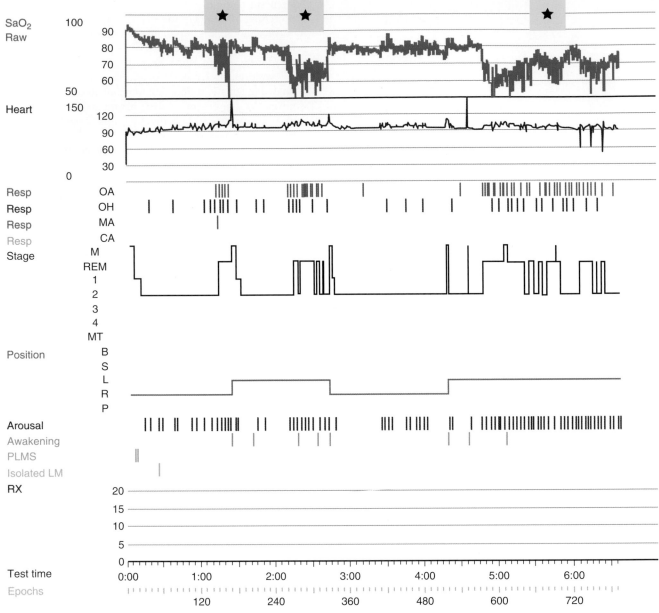

• **Figure 35.14** A hypnogram characteristic of patients with myotonic dystrophy. Rapid eye movement (REM)-related hypoventilation is noted *(stars)* and is associated with severe oxygen desaturations and arousals during REM sleep. **Channel Key:** SaO_2 Raw: oximetry, Heart: heart rate, OA: obstructive apnea, OH: obstructive hypopnea, MA: mixed apnea, CA: central apnea, M: wake, REM: Rapid eye movement sleep, 1: stage N1, 2: stage N2, 3: Stage N3, 4: stage 4, MT: movement time, B: back, S: supine, L; left, R: right, P: prone, Arousal: arousal, Awakening: awakenings, PLMS: periodic limb movements during sleep, Isolated LM: isolated leg movement, RX: positive airway pressure setting, Test time: time in hours from lights out, Epochs: epochs. (From Culebras A. Sleep-disordered breathing in neuromuscular disease. *Sleep Med Clin.* 2008;3:377–386.)

sleep of ≤88% in adults for ≥ 5 minutes.[5] Answer E is incorrect, as late-onset central hypoventilation with hypothalamic dysfunction (LOCHHD) symptoms begin in early childhood, are not associated with stroke, and although central apneas may be present, hypoventilation with decreased tidal volume and respiratory rate are more common. In addition, these patients with LOCHHD will have at least two of the following: obesity, endocrine abnormalities of hypothalamic origin, severe emotional or behavioral disturbances, or tumor of neural origin.[3]

13. **The correct answer is C.**
The PSG fragment in Fig. 35.7 demonstrates periodic limb movements of sleep. Patients with multiple sclerosis (MS) have more sleep complaints than the general population (Fig. 35.15). One of the more common symptoms in MS is fatigue. MS patients are at higher risk of having periodic limb movements of sleep and periodic limb movement disorder. RBD and narcolepsy are also seen more often in multiple sclerosis as well. Hypothalamic lesions involving the tuberomammillary nucleus or hypocretin/orexin production can cause sleepiness

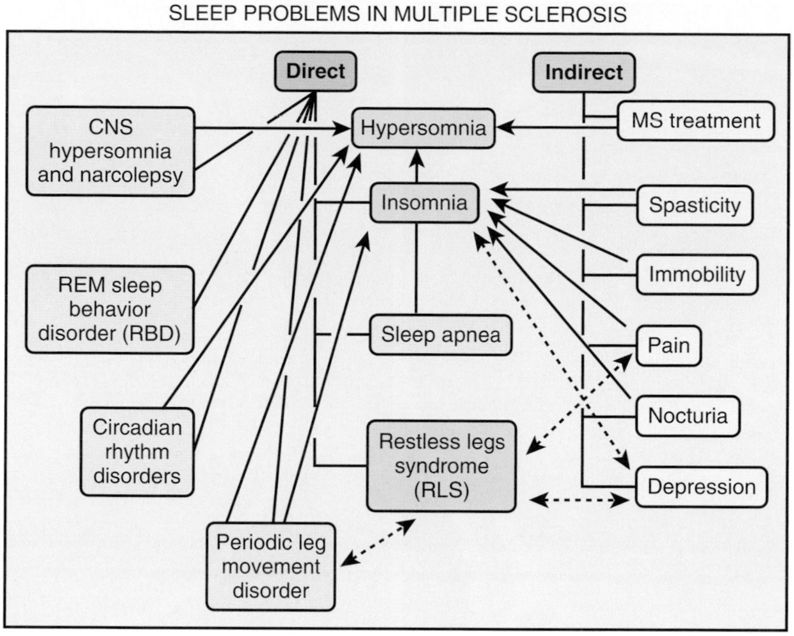

SLEEP PROBLEMS IN MULTIPLE SCLEROSIS

• **Figure 35.15** Sleep and its disorders, Bradley's Neurology in Clinical Practice. *CNS*, Central nervous system. (From Braley T, Avidan A. Sleep in Multiple Sclerosis. In: Geisser B [Ed.] Primer on Multiple Sclerosis. Cambridge; 2011.)

from secondary narcolepsy. Pontine lesions involving areas such as the sublaterodorsal tegmental nucleus can precipitate RBD (Fig. 35.16). Muscle spasms, pain, mood disorders, and medication side effects can cause sleep disruption in multiple sclerosis patients.[13] Sleep-disordered breathing (central sleep apnea and OSA) are more common in multiple sclerosis patients, but the findings on polysomnography in this patient did not demonstrate this, so Answers A and B are incorrect. No epileptiform abnormalities were noted on the PSG fragment in Fig. 35.7, and there is no clinical history suggestive of seizures, so Answer D is incorrect.

14. **The correct answer is A.**
The PSG fragment in Fig. 35.8 demonstrates sleep-related hypoventilation. Hypoventilation in adults is defined per the American Academy of Sleep Medicine (AASM) Scoring Manual as an increase in the arterial PCO_2 (or surrogate) to a value greater than 55 mm Hg for ≥10 minutes, or a ≥10 mm Hg increase in arterial PCO_2 (or surrogate) during sleep (in comparison to an awake supine value) to a value exceeding 50 mm Hg for ≥10 minutes.[5] Hypoventilation is typically seen in REM sleep or worse in REM sleep.[3] Sleep-related hypoventilation is found frequently in patients with spinal cord disease, especially if muscles of respiration are affected (cervical or thoracic spinal cord injury).[14] Although patients with spinal cord injury are at risk for OSA or CSA, this was not noted on the PSG fragment; thus Answers B and D are incorrect. Answer C is also incorrect, as periodic limb movements are not observed on the PSG fragment.

15. **The correct answer is B.**
This PSG fragment demonstrates an obstructive apnea during REM sleep that leads to an arousal and subsequent motor activity. This is not idiopathic RBD, given the motor activity occurs secondary to OSA. In this case, this patient had partially treated OSA, and likely needed a higher positive airway pressure setting to treat his obstructive events. A patient with idiopathic

RBD will have REM sleep without atonia (increased chin and limb EMG tone) on PSG but in the absence of respiratory events.[3] Therefore Answer A is not correct. Answer C is not correct, as the history and the PSG fragment are not consistent with confusional arousal, which is an NREM sleep parasomnia that typically occurs from stage N3 sleep. In addition, as the PSG demonstrates REM sleep, and the patient recalls dream content related to the activity; this is not characteristic of a confusional arousal. Answer D is also unlikely, given the lack of any epileptiform activity on the PSG.

16. **The correct answer is B. Hypersomnia due to a medical disorder.**
Per the International Classification of Sleep Disorders, 3rd Edition (ICSD-3), the patient must have daytime sleepiness for at least 3 months, must have a neurologic or medical condition that can explain the sleepiness, and an MSLT demonstrating a mean sleep latency of ≤8 minutes and less than 2 sleep onset REM periods. The sleepiness cannot be better explained by another underlying sleep disorder, medication, or psychiatric disorder.[3] The traumatic brain injury that this patient suffered at the onset of symptoms is a condition that commonly causes hypersomnia. Other medical or neurological conditions that have been shown to cause hypersomnia include metabolic encephalopathy, stroke, brain tumors, brain infections, systemic inflammation (e.g., chronic infections, rheumatologic disorders, cancer), genetic disorders, and neurodegenerative diseases. Patients suffering brain injury are at higher risk of not only hypersomnia but also narcolepsy secondary to the brain injury.[15] Sleep is commonly affected in patients suffering from traumatic brain injury (Fig. 35.17). Traumatic brain injury can cause both OSA or CSA and difficulties with insomnia and circadian rhythm disorders. Some studies have reported decreased production of melatonin immediately after a brain injury that is typically transient and improves as the patient heals from the injury.[16] These sleep

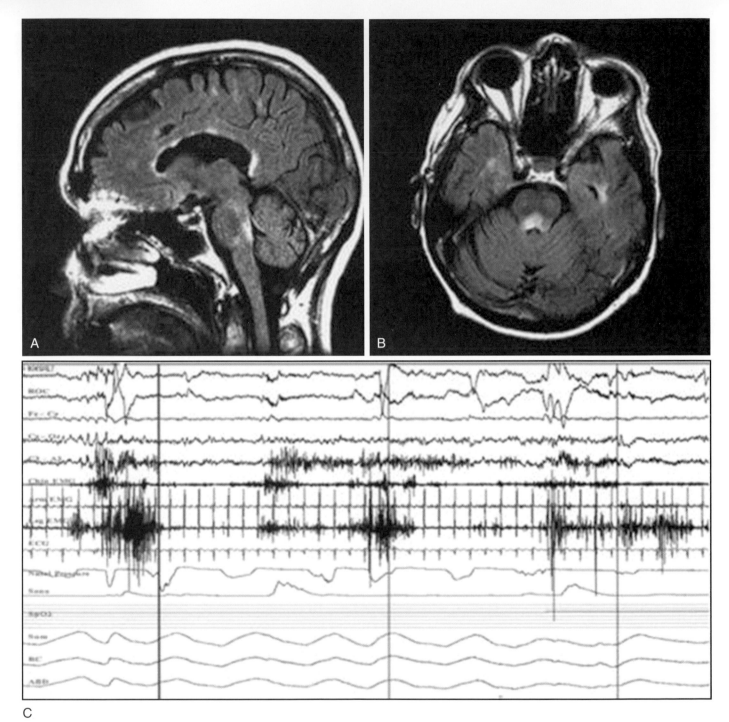

• **Figure 35.16** (A) Sagittal and (B) axial fluid-attenuated inversion-recovery magnetic resonance images, showing the demyelinating lesion in the dorsal pons. Additional demyelinating lesions were present in the white matter of both cerebral hemispheres, and in the splenium corporis callosi. (C) 30-second PSG Fragment of REM sleep. **Channel Legend:** LOC/ROC: eye leads applied to left and right outer canthus, referenced to Fpz (frontopolar midline electrode), Fz-Cz: frontal midline to central midline electrode, C3-A2: left parasagittal to right ear electrode, Cz-Oz: central midline to occipital midline electrode, chin, arm, leg EMG: electromyography channels; SpO$_2$: oxygen saturation, SUM: sum of rib cage and abdominal respiratory bands, RC: rib cage respiratory band; ABD: abdominal respiratory band. (From Brass SD, Duquette P, Proulx-Therrien J, Auerbach S. Sleep disorders in patients with multiple sclerosis. *Sleep Med Rev.* 2010;14[2]:121–129. Figure 2.)

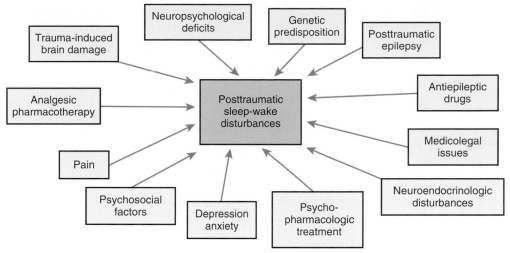

• **Figure 35.17** (From Kryger M, Roth T, Dement W, eds. *Principles and Practice of Sleep Medicine.* 6th ed. Philadelphia: Elsevier; 2016, Table 99.2.)

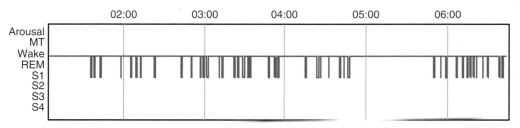

• **Figure 35.18** Hypnogram from a patient with Creutzfeldt-Jakob disease, showing severe insomnia. **Channel Key:** Arousal: arousals, MT: movement time, Wake: wake, REM: Stage Rapid Eye Movement, S1: stage N1, S2: stage N2, S3: stage N3, S4: stage N4.

disorders may occur in both mild or severe brain injury. Answer A, idiopathic hypersomnia, is not the correct answer, as there is history of traumatic brain injury at the onset of symptoms. Answers C and D are not correct, as there was no history of cataplexy and the MSLT did not demonstrate two or more sleep-onset REM periods.

17. **The correct answer is A.**
Patients with prion disease, such as CJD or fatal familial insomnia, typically have loss of sleep spindles, slow wave sleep, and REM sleep, late in the course of the condition, likely due to severe damage to sleep controlling portions of the brain.[2] Fig. 35.18 is a hypnogram from a patient with CJD. CJD is a prion-related transmissible spongiform encephalopathy causing extensive neuronal degeneration and pathologic changes, especially in the cortex, resulting in myoclonic jerks and rapidly evolving dementia, leading to death. The mean survival duration is 4–8 months. Most patients with CJD will have frequent awakenings and insomnia at the late stages of the disease before death. In some patients, insomnia is the prodromal or early symptom of the condition. Frequent seizures may also be seen with periodic sharp waves on EEG.[2] Answers B and C are incorrect because increases in stage N3 or REM sleep are not seen late in prion disease. Similarly, Answer D is incorrect, as alpha intrusion has not been reported to be seen in prion disease. Alpha intrusion has been observed on PSG in patients with fibromyalgia, chronic pain, and other primary sleep disorders.

18. **The correct answer is B.**
This patient has narcolepsy type 1 secondary to neurological disease (in this case, multiple sclerosis). The patient was diagnosed with multiple sclerosis based upon the history of past neurological deficits (or attacks) along with brain imaging showing demyelinating lesions, including a lesion in the hypothalamus. MSLT is consistent with narcolepsy with a mean sleep latency less than or equal to 8 minutes and two or more sleep-onset REM periods.[3] The spells described seem consistent with cataplexy; thus Answer C is incorrect. Narcolepsy type 2 is without cataplexy. Patients with multiple sclerosis are at higher risk of developing narcolepsy or hypersomnia. This is due to demyelinating lesions affecting hypothalamic function and possibly due to both conditions showing genetic susceptibility coded by genes within or close to the human leukocyte antigen (HLA) DR-DQ subregion. Answer A is incorrect, as this case is not consistent with idiopathic hypersomnia, given the presence of cataplexy, as well as the presence of sleep-onset REM periods. This case also could not be considered idiopathic, given the presence of lesions in the central nervous system that could cause sleep symptoms. The spells described are not consistent with sleep terrors (Answer D), as sleep terrors occur out of sleep (NREM sleep) with abrupt terror, typically beginning with an alarming vocalization such as a frightening scream. There is intense fear and signs of autonomic arousal, including mydriasis, tachycardia, tachypnea, and diaphoresis during an episode.

19. **The correct answer is B. CPAP.**

Stridor is a life-threatening condition. It is a harsh, high-pitched inspiratory noise caused by partial obstruction of the larynx. Stridor can be observed in up to 42% of patients with MSA.[2,17,18] Nighttime stridor can be treated effectively with nasal CPAP. CPAP can improve quality of life and improve median survival time.[17,18] The other Answers of A, C, D, and E are incorrect, as the other treatment options have not been shown to improve median survival time. For example, parkinsonism symptoms in MSA may respond to levodopa in 60% of patients. Deep brain stimulation surgery, intravenous immunoglobulin, and oxybutynin will not improve median survival time.[2,17,18]

20. **The correct answer is B. Central apnea due to a medical disorder.**

This patient has a Chiari malformation. CSA and OSA can be seen on polysomnography in patients with central nervous system lesions. It is important to remember that a diagnosis of CSA does not exclude a diagnosis of OSA.[3]

The diagnostic criteria for CSA with Cheyne-Stokes breathing (CSA-CSB), CSA without CSB, and primary CSA all include at least one of the following: sleepiness, difficulty initiating sleep, difficulty maintaining sleep, frequent awakenings, nonrestorative sleep, awakening short of breath, snoring, witnessed apneas. In addition, the PSG must include five or more central apneas and/or central hypopneas per hour of sleep, and the total number of central apnea and/or central hypopneas is greater than 50% of the total number of apneas and hypopneas.[3]

Specific to CSA due to medical disorder without CSB, as in this patient, the diagnostic criteria include the absence of CSB, and the disorder occurs as a consequence of a medical or neurological condition, but is not due to medication use or substance use. It may be seen in patients with brainstem lesions of developmental, vascular, neoplastic, degenerative, demyelinating, or traumatic origin. The CSA is thought to occur due to dysfunction or impairment of the ventilatory control centers in the brainstem.[3]

Answer B is incorrect, as Cheyne-Stokes breathing is not seen on the PSG fragment. Specific to CSA-CSB, the diagnostic criteria include the presence of one or more of the following: atrial fibrillation, atrial flutter, congestive heart failure, or a neurological disorder, and the PSG should show the pattern of ventilation criteria for CSB. In addition, the longer cycle length (>40 seconds; typically, 45–60 seconds) distinguishes CSB from other CSA types. The cycle length is longer in patients with systolic heart failure than in patients with diastolic heart failure. In patients with CSA-CSB, the arousal from sleep tends to occur at the highest point of respiratory effort between contiguous central apneas or hypopneas. In general, CSA-CSB is seen in patients greater than 60 years of age, with chronic congestive heart failure, stroke, and possibly renal failure.[3]

Answer C is incorrect, as primary CSA is differentiated from that noted previously, as there is absence of CSB, absence of daytime or nocturnal hypoventilation, and no known cause is identified. People with primary CSA may have low normal arterial $PaCO_2$ during wake (<40 mm Hg). In primary CSA, there are usually no more than 4–5 breaths between apneas.[3]

Answer D and E are incorrect, as this fragment does not show hypoventilation. LOCHHD is also known as rapid-onset obesity with hypothalamic dysfunction, hypoventilation, and autonomic dysregulation (ROHHAD). Sleep-related hypoventilation must be present, and the patient must have at least two of the following: obesity, endocrine abnormalities of hypothalamic origin, severe emotional or behavioral disturbances, or tumor of neural origin. In addition, the PHOX2B gene is not present and the disorder is not better explained by another sleep, medical or neurological disorder, medication use, or substance use.[3]

In idiopathic central alveolar hypoventilation, sleep-related hypoventilation must be present and is not due to lung parenchymal or airway disease, pulmonary vascular pathology, chest wall disorder, medication use, neurologic disorder, muscle weakness, or obesity or congenital hypoventilation syndromes.[3]

21. **The correct answer is E. MRI of the brain.**

CSA is usually observed in disorders such as lesions of the central nervous system, congestive heart failure, and stroke. CSA can also be observed in patients on opioid mediations, or in high altitudes. An MRI of the brain can identify central nervous system lesions. An echocardiogram will assist in identification of cardiac dysfunction if present. Answer A is incorrect, as cerebrospinal fluid culture is necessary to identify a bacterial cause of meningitis. Answer B is incorrect, as (CSF) hypocretin ≤110 pg/mL, or less than one-third the mean values obtained in normal subjects on the same standardized assay, is diagnostic for narcolepsy type 1. Answer C is incorrect, as ictal single photon emission computed tomography is used in the presurgical evaluation of refractory partial seizures. Lastly, Answer D is incorrect, as lumbar puncture opening pressure may be diagnostic in disorders of intracranial pressures.[3]

22. **The correct answer is C.**

Patients with Alzheimer's dementia (late stage) frequently have poorly formed sleep spindles and K complexes.[19] Answer B is incorrect, as these patients will likely have decreased or absent stage N3 sleep. Although there may be decreases in REM sleep percentage, REM sleep latency and REM density typically remain unchanged in late-stage Alzheimer disease patients, so Answers A and D are incorrect. In addition to these changes, patients with Alzheimer's dementia may have a slower dominant rhythm.

23. **The correct answer is B.**

This patient with a history of dementia is having sundowning. Sundowning is a delirium-like state that occurs in the elderly or cognitively impaired in the late evening or nighttime. Symptoms include worsening confusion, agitation, and aggression. Although both occur at night in the elderly, there are significant differences between sundowning and RBD. RBD is dream enactment that occurs from sleep, mainly during the second half of the night. Sundowning is typically noted in the evening or early portion of sleep period. Patients may have recall of the dream content related to the motor activity in RBD. Sundowning may occur due to impairment in the biological clock or suprachiasmatic nucleus.[2] As people age, secretion of many hormones, including melatonin, can be reduced and can be even more disrupted in Alzheimer's dementia patients. Dementia patients typically have an advanced sleep-wake phase disorder, where there is an advance (early timing) in the phase of major sleep episode in relation to the desired or required sleep time and wake-up time.[3] This circadian rhythm disorder can be improved with evening light to help delay the circadian clock and bedtime to later at night. Answer A is incorrect, as morning light would likely worsen sundowning. Morning light is typically used to treat delayed sleep-wake phase disorder, which is typically seen in younger populations. Answer C is incorrect, as fluoxetine can be activating and may worsen insomnia. It is typically used to help with depression. Answer D is incorrect, as morning melatonin would not assist nighttime symptoms of sundowning, and may actually cause sleepiness during the day.

Suggested Reading

Iranzo A. Sleep and neurodegenerative diseases. *Sleep Med Clin.* 2016;11(1):1-18.

Kataria L, Vaughn BV. Sleep and epilepsy. *Sleep Med Clin.* 2016;11(1):25-38.

Mims KN, Kirsch D. Sleep and stroke. *Sleep Med Clin.* 2016;11(1):39-51.

Rama AN, Zachariah R, Kushida CA. Differentiating nocturnal movements: leg movements, parasomnias, and seizures. *Sleep Med Clin.* 2009;4(3):361-372.

Watson NF, Viola-Saltzman M. Sleep and comorbid neurologic disorders. *Continuum (Minneap Minn).* 2013;19(1 Sleep Disorders):148-169.

36

Hypersomnia Case Studies

CHAD M. RUOFF, VIKAS JAIN, TODD SWICK

Questions

Questions 1–14 Refer to Patient A

Patient A: You are evaluating a 13-year-old girl who presents to the sleep clinic for evaluation. She has been having difficulties staying awake in school since she was approximately 10 years of age and has been napping on weekends at home and on vacation. She denies seeing strangers in her room when transitioning to sleep at bedtime or when falling back asleep during the night. She reports frequent awakenings during the night and reports that she has had moments where she feels "frozen for a few seconds" upon awakening. She reports getting about 8–9 hours of total sleep each night. Upon further questioning, her parents report they have noticed her jaw sagging open and tongue thrusting on occasion particularly when laughing over the past year. The patient reports that her knees have given out a few times in the last year when playing and laughing with her sister and friends. Her vital signs and general physical and neurologic exams are unremarkable.

1. Which of the following is considered the most common symptom of narcolepsy?
   A. Excessive daytime sleepiness (EDS)
   B. Hypnogogic and hypnopompic hallucinations
   C. Disrupted nighttime sleep
   D. Sleep paralysis
   E. Cataplexy

2. Which of the following findings would confirm your suspicion for cataplexy in this patient, if the patient had an episode during your evaluation?
   A. The patient reports that an episode lasts for 10 minutes or more.
   B. The patient reports a loss of consciousness during the episode.
   C. There is a transient reversible loss of deep tendon reflexes during an episode.
   D. The episodes are triggered when she is feeling sad.
   E. She reports feeling short of breath during the episodes.

3. Which of the following human leukocyte antigen (HLA) markers would best support your suspicion for narcolepsy type 1 in this patient?
   A. HLA DQB1*05:01
   B. HLA DRB1*15:01
   C. HLA DQB1*03:01
   D. HLA DQB1*06:02
   E. HLA DQB1*06:01

4. Patient A's parents are concerned about the risk of their other children also having narcolepsy. What is the risk of developing narcolepsy type 1 in first-degree relatives?
   A. 0.01%–0.05%
   B. 1%–2%
   C. 5%–10%
   D. 10%–20%
   E. 20%–40%

5. The *first* step in objectively evaluating Patient A's symptoms is to order:
   A. Polysomnography
   B. Multiple Sleep Latency Test (MSLT)
   C. Maintenance of Wakefulness Test (MWT)
   D. Actigraphy with sleep log
   E. HLA typing

6. The parents mention that Patient A started taking an antidepressant for "depression" after visiting a physician a few months ago. The parents do not think their daughter is depressed, but they were desperate to find a solution so they agreed to the trial of the antidepressant. They have not noticed any change in her mood since starting the medication.
   Patient A is then scheduled for a polysomnography (PSG) and MSLT. For the correct interpretation of the MSLT, what should the physician, in consultation with the prescriber of the antidepressant, recommend with regard to the antidepressant she is taking?
   A. Stop the antidepressant for at least 14 days prior to testing (or at least 5 times the half-life of the drug and longer-acting metabolite).
   B. Stop the antidepressant for at least 7 days prior to testing (or at least 5 times the half-life of the drug and longer-acting metabolite).
   C. Decrease the dose of the antidepressant.
   D. Increase the dose of the antidepressant.
   E. Stop the antidepressant the day prior to testing.

7. One of the most concerning side effects of abrupt withdrawal of an antidepressant in a patient with type 1 narcolepsy, in addition to changes in mood, is worsening of which of the following symptoms?
   A. EDS
   B. Hypnogogic/hypnopompic hallucinations
   C. Disrupted nighttime sleep
   D. Sleep paralysis
   E. Cataplexy

Patient A eventually undergoes overnight nocturnal polysomnography (NPSG) followed by a MSLT, and the results from the first nap of the MSLT are shown as follows.

Epoch	Stage	Comments
10	W	Lights out
11	W	
12	W	
13	W	
14	W	
15	W	
16	W	
17	W	
18	N1	
19	W	
20	N1	
21	N1	
22	N1	
23	N2	
24	W	
25	REM	

8. What is the sleep onset latency for nap 1?
   A. 8 minutes
   B. 4 minutes
   C. 4.5 minutes
   D. 6 minutes
   E. 6.5 minutes
9. What is the rapid eye movement (REM) latency for nap 1?
   A. 3.5 minutes
   B. 2.5 minutes
   C. 30 seconds
   D. 1 minute
   E. 7 minutes
10. What epoch should nap 1 be terminated on?
    A. 50
    B. 58
    C. 53
    D. 48
    E. 55

Polysomnography followed by a MSLT is performed and results are shown as follows. Other appropriately ordered objective tests were unremarkable.

Polysomnogram	Result
Total sleep time	425 min
Sleep latency	7 min
Rapid eye movement sleep latency	8 min
N1 sleep %	14%
N2 sleep %	44%
N3 sleep %	22%
Rapid eye movement sleep %	20%
Respiratory disturbance index (RDI)	0.2 events per hour
Minimum oxygen saturation	94%

Multiple Sleep Latency Test	Sleep Onset Latency	Rapid Eye Movement Sleep Observed
Nap 1	4	Yes
Nap 2	8	None
Nap 3	12	None
Nap 4	6	None
Nap 5	5	None

11. The calculated mean sleep latency for the MSLT results noted previously is 7 minutes. If Patient A had no sleep on the fifth nap, what would the calculated mean sleep latency for the five naps be for this MSLT, assuming all results remained the same?
    A. 6
    B. 12
    C. 10
    D. 8
    E. 20
12. According to the 3rd edition of the International Classification of Sleep Disorders (ICSD-3), the polysomnogram and MSLT results, in addition to the clinical history, are consistent with which of the following?
    A. Secondary narcolepsy
    B. Narcolepsy type 1
    C. Idiopathic hypersomnia (IH)
    D. Insufficient sleep syndrome
    E. Kleine-Levin syndrome (KLS)
13. Which of the following drugs has the US Food and Drug Administration (FDA) approved for the treatment of cataplexy in adults?
    A. Protriptyline
    B. Duloxetine
    C. Venlafaxine
    D. Fluoxetine
    E. Sodium oxybate
14. Which of the following drugs has been given a standard level of recommendation by the American Academy of Sleep

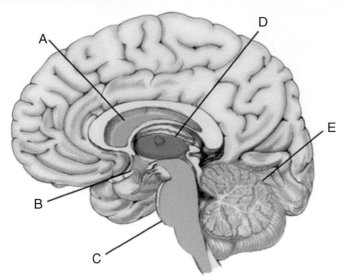

• **Figure 36.1** A, Basal Ganglia; B, Hypothalamus; C, Brainstem; D, Thalamus; E, Cerebellum. (Modified from Norden A, Blumenfeld H. The role of subcortical structures in human epilepsy. *Epilepsy Behav.* 2002;3[3]: 219–231.)

Medicine (AASM) for the treatment of EDS in adult patients with narcolepsy (PWN)?
A. Modafinil
B. Dextroamphetamine
C. Selegiline
D. Methylphenidate
E. Ritanserin

15. Narcolepsy type 1 is associated with a loss of cells located in which part of the brain?
Please select the following brain regions (Fig. 36.1):
A, B, C, D, or E

16. Which of the following predisposing and precipitating factors has been associated with narcolepsy patients?
A. Staphylococcus aureus antibodies
B. Exposure to second-hand smoke
C. Vaccination against H1N1 (Pandemrix)
D. HLA B27 positivity
E. Exposure to pesticides

17. Which of the following is the most likely finding in human narcolepsy?
A. Preprohypocretin mutation
B. Loss of hypocretin neurons
C. Hypocretin 2 receptor mutation
D. Hypocretin 1 receptor mutation
E. Loss of cells in the substantia nigra

Questions 18–20 Refer to Patient B

Patient B: A 38-year-old gentleman who is a commercial truck driver presents for a follow-up visit to the sleep clinic for an evaluation requested by his employer to ensure that his EDS has been adequately addressed after being diagnosed and subsequently treated for moderate obstructive sleep apnea (OSA) with a continuous positive airway pressure (CPAP) device. CPAP settings were based upon an in-laboratory CPAP titration that clearly documented

resolution of his OSA at the prescribed pressures. Prior to treatment with CPAP, his Epworth Sleepiness Scale was 14, but it has since decreased to 7. He reports he is compliant with his CPAP machine. Download of his PAP device demonstrates that he is 100% compliant with a residual apnea-hypopnea index (AHI) of 1 event/hour at the prescribed CPAP pressure. His employer has specifically requested a statement on his ability to stay awake and continue to be employed as a commercial trucker.

18. Which of the following is true regarding the MWT?
A. It consists of five trials, each lasting 20 minutes, separated by 2-hour intervals.
B. It is used for the diagnosis of narcolepsy and other hypersomnias.
C. The predictive value of the MWT mean sleep latency for assessing accident risk and safety in real world circumstances is not established.
D. Performance of a PSG prior to the MWT is required to objectively document adequate sleep the night prior to MWT.
E. Documentation that an individual is able to stay awake during all trials of a MWT guarantees that the subject will not experience sleepiness in the work environment.

During the First Trial of the MWT, the Following Results Are Obtained

Epoch	Stage	Comments
1	W	First epoch of trial
2	W	
3	N1	
4	W	
5	W	
6	N1	
7	N1	
8	N1	
9	W	
10	N2	

19. The trial should be terminated at the beginning of which epoch?
A. At epoch 3
B. At epoch 6
C. At epoch 7
D. At epoch 9
E. At epoch 10

Patient B follows up in the sleep clinic a few weeks later to review the results of his MWT. The MWT demonstrated a mean sleep latency of 5 minutes. After discussing these results, he admits that he is still suffering from EDS. Today, he admits that his Epworth Sleepiness Scale is 11. Download of his CPAP machine data card demonstrates that he remains very compliant with treatment and his residual AHI remains at 1 event/hour.

20. Which of the following medications is US FDA approved to improve wakefulness in adult patients with persistence of EDS in spite of adequate treatment of OSA?
    A. Modafinil
    B. Acetazolamide
    C. Sodium oxybate
    D. Methylphenidate
    E. Protriptyline

Questions 21–22 Refer to Patient C

Patient C: A 34-year-old gentleman who presents to the sleep clinic for evaluation. He states that he has woken up in the middle of the night with a deep sense of terror and feels paralyzed. He feels tired during the day. He admits he has been under increased stress at work lately. His sleep schedule for the last several years consists of going to bed around 1:00 AM and getting out of bed around 7:00 AM on weekdays. On weekends, he will sleep in until around 10:00 AM. Review of systems is otherwise negative. His bed partner specifically denies hearing snoring or witnessing respiratory pauses. The patient is otherwise healthy with unremarkable vital signs and physical exam findings. The Epworth Sleepiness Scale is 10/24. He has read about narcolepsy type 2 on the Internet and is concerned that he may suffer from this condition.

21. The most appropriate next step for this patient is to:
    A. Order an overnight polysomnogram followed by a MSLT and treat appropriately
    B. Prescribe an antidepressant
    C. Prescribe a stimulant or wake-promoting agent
    D. Prescribe a hypnotic
    E. Provide reassurance and encourage sleep extension

Patient C returns to clinic a month later and reports that his daytime sleepiness and feelings of paralysis during the night have resolved after following your recommendation(s). His Epworth Sleepiness Scale is now 5.

22. The most likely diagnosis at this time is which of the following?
    A. Recurrent isolated sleep paralysis
    B. OSA
    C. IH
    D. Narcolepsy type 2
    E. Insufficient sleep syndrome

Questions 23–25 Refer to Patient D

Patient D: A 40-year-old women with a long-standing history of EDS presents to the sleep clinic. She denies any history of sleep-related hallucinations, cataplexy, and disrupted nighttime sleep but has experienced several episodes of sleep paralysis in her lifetime. She does occasionally experience irritability. She presents with completed sleep logs she has filled out, documenting a bedtime around 10:00 PM and wake time around 9:00 AM on weekdays and 10:00 AM on weekends. She has tried extending her total sleep time to upwards of 12 hours each night for weeks on end without relief of her daytime sleepiness. She takes a nap for up to an hour most days of the week. She underwent her second set of sleep tests about a year ago (see results later). Both sets of sleep tests yielded very similar results. Her current Epworth Sleepiness Scale is 15/24. Her vital signs and physical exam are unremarkable. She denies any medications including recreational drug use. She states she just wants some answers.

Polysomnogram	Result
Lights out time	22:00
Lights on time	08:00
Total sleep time	532 min
Sleep efficiency	95%
Sleep latency	4 min
Rapid eye movement sleep latency	130 min
N1 sleep %	12%
N2 sleep %	39%
N3 sleep %	25%
Rapid eye movement sleep %	24%
Respiratory disturbance index (RDI)	3 events per hour
Minimum oxygen saturation	93%

Multiple Sleep Latency Test	Sleep Onset Latency	REM Sleep Observed
Nap 1	8	None
Nap 2	6	None
Nap 3	12	None
Nap 4	9	None
Nap 5	10	None

23. The next best step to confirm the diagnosis is:
    A. At least 7 consecutive days of wrist actigraphy with sleep logs
    B. HLA DQB1*06:02 testing
    C. Repeat overnight sleep testing following day MSLT
    D. 24-hour PSG if available
    E. MWT

*Patient D returns to the clinic 2 weeks later to review the results of the recommended testing. In addition, she found some past reports showing HLA DQB1*06:02 positivity and cerebrospinal fluid (CSF) hypocretin value of 240 pg/mL.*

24. The most likely diagnosis is which of the following?
    A. IH
    B. Narcolepsy type 1
    C. Narcolepsy type 2
    D. KLS
    E. Long sleeper

25. Spectral analysis has shown that patients with this diagnosis had a reduction in which polysomnographic parameter?
    A. Stage W
    B. Stage N1
    C. Stage N2
    D. Stage N3
    E. Stage REM

Questions 26–29 Refer to Patient E

Patient E: A 14-year-old male presents to the sleep clinic due to recurrence of an episode of abrupt EDS. His parents report that he had an episode about 6 months previously; however, the EDS seemed to correct itself within a week. His parents report that he has maintained good grades in school, and they have not had issues waking him up in the past. Over the past 2 weeks, his parents report that he has been increasingly difficult to arouse in the morning. He missed school for the past week because of difficulty awakening in the morning and for sleeping for long periods of time throughout the day. When he is awake, they have found him somewhat confused and masturbating on several occasions. His vital signs and physical exam were unremarkable. He also denies the use of any medications including recreational drug use. He undergoes appropriately ordered sleep testing with results from PSG and MSLT as follows.

Polysomnogram	Result
Lights out time	21:00
Lights on time	09:00
Total sleep time	698 min
Sleep efficiency	97%
Sleep latency	3 min
Rapid eye movement sleep latency	133 min
N1 sleep %	14%
N2 sleep %	49%
N3 sleep %	15%
Rapid eye movement sleep %	22%
Respiratory disturbance index (RDI)	2.8 events per hour
Minimum oxygen saturation	94%

Multiple Sleep Latency Test	Sleep Onset Latency	Rapid Eye Movement Sleep Observed
Nap 1	6	Yes
Nap 2	4	None
Nap 3	13	Yes
Nap 4	8	None
Nap 5	11	Yes

26. Which of the following is the most likely diagnosis?
    A. IH
    B. Narcolepsy type 1
    C. Narcolepsy type 2
    D. KLS
    E. Klüver-Bucy syndrome
27. When an identifiable trigger is present, what is the most commonly reported precipitating factor?
    A. Alcohol use
    B. Sleep deprivation
    C. Stress
    D. Infection
    E. Physical exertion
28. During the follow-up visit in the sleep clinic, the parents mention they found a private clinic to perform a single-photon emission computed tomography test during a symptomatic period. You reassure the parents that structural imaging studies are often normal. However, functional imaging studies have demonstrated which of the following findings during a symptomatic period in KLS?
    A. Hyperperfusion of the substantia nigra
    B. Hypoperfusion in the thalamus
    C. Hyperperfusion in the hypothalamus
    D. Hypoperfusion in the pineal gland
    E. Hyperperfusion in the ventrolateral preoptic nucleus
29. Which medication has been reported to aid in terminating a hypersomnia episode in these patients?
    A. Lithium
    B. Amantadine
    C. Modafinil
    D. Valproate
    E. Amphetamine

Questions 30–32 Refer to Patient F

Patient F: A 35-year-old male presents to the sleep clinic for an evaluation. His chief complaint is one of EDS, particularly after his employer found him napping in the break room over lunch. He feels his sleep is nonrefreshing and feels he has developed a nightly fear of getting into bed and trying to sleep.

He naps at home in the early afternoon on vacations and weekends. His Epworth Sleepiness Scale is 14.

On further questioning he complains of uncomfortable and almost painful sensations in his legs when he first sits down for dinner in the evening that are relieved with walking and movement. The symptoms started at age 30 but have been worsening over the past 2 years. As soon as he sits back down or gets into bed, the symptoms return. He describes increasing difficulty falling asleep because of the constant need to move his legs and/or the need to get up and walk around. When he finally falls asleep, his wife reports that he is constantly kicking and/or jerking his legs, which has impacted her ability to sleep, and as such she has moved out of the bedroom.

He denies any medical or surgical past history. He is on no prescription medication. He reports worsening of leg symptoms when he tried an over-the-counter sleep aid (diphenhydramine) with no improvement in his ability to fall or stay asleep. He reports that his mother had similar symptoms but was never diagnosed or treated. He has no siblings. His general physical and neurologic exams were normal. In particular, there was no evidence of a motor or sensory neuropathy based on detailed examination.

30. What is the most likely sleep diagnosis that explains his constellation of symptoms?
    A. Myotonic dystrophy
    B. Psychophysiologic insomnia
    C. Restless legs syndrome (RLS)
    D. Periodic limb movement disorder
    E. IH
31. What diagnostic evaluation would you carry out?
    A. PSG and MSLT
    B. HLA DQB1*06:02 testing
    C. Serum Ferritin level

D. Glucose tolerance test
E. Nerve biopsy
32. What treatment regimen should be instituted?
A. Cognitive behavioral therapy for insomnia (CBT-I)
B. Hypnotic medication
C. Dopamine agonist therapy
D. Stimulant/wake-promoting agent
E. Long-acting opiate therapy

Answers

1. **Answer A. EDS.**
EDS is the cardinal symptom of narcolepsy and central disorders of hypersomnolence. EDS is usually the first symptom to present in PWN. They often experience repeated episodes of uncontrollable episodes of sleep but may report a feeling of pervasive sleepiness throughout the day. Frequently PWNs feel "refreshed" after a short period of sleep (15–30 minutes); however, the powerful urge to sleep may return within hours. Hypnogogic/hypnopompic hallucinations (B) and sleep paralysis (D) are present in approximately 33% and 50% of narcoleptic patients, respectively. Sleep paralysis and hallucinations are reported in approximately 6%–20% of the general population, respectively. The clinician should carefully differentiate sleep paralysis from a strong desire not to move. Disrupted nighttime sleep (C) is present in up to 95% of patients. Although cataplexy can cause the complete loss of muscle tone, the cataplexy phenotype can vary widely, and many patients may only have partial cataplexy attacks. Cataplexy (E) is present in only 40%–70% of narcolepsy cases. The onset of cataplexy, when it occurs, may follow EDS by weeks to months, but can be delayed for 3–5 years or for as long as several decades.[1-6]

2. **Answer C. There is a transient reversible loss of deep tendon reflexes during an episode.**
Cataplexy is a phenomenon that is unique to PWN (Fig. 36.2). It is characterized by a sudden partial or complete loss of muscle tone, typically but not necessarily bilateral, and is triggered by strong emotions (usually a positive emotion such as laughter and excitement but less frequent triggers may include anger, surprise, or embarrassment; D). Cataplexy episodes are typically brief (less than 2 minutes; A), respiration is undisturbed (E), and patients retain consciousness throughout the episode (B). The degree of muscle tone lost can be variable, impacting various muscle groups. Although rare to witness an attack during a sleep evaluation, the loss of deep tendon reflexes during an episode is a strong diagnostic finding.

3. **Answer D. HLA DQB1*06:02.**
Narcolepsy type 1 has been closely associated with the HLA subtypes DRB1*15:01 (B) and DQB1*06:02 (Fig. 36.3). Almost all patients who have narcolepsy type 1 are positive for HLA DQB1*06:02 (D). Subtypes such as HLA*DQB1 03:01 (C) may increase an individual's susceptibility to contracting narcolepsy. HLA*DBQ1 05:01 (A) and HLA DQB1*06:01 (E) are protective when positive along with HLA DQB1*06:02.
In routine cases of narcolepsy with typical cataplexy and corroborative PSG and MSLT findings, it is not necessary to check for the HLA DQB1*06:02 marker. One must bear in mind that 12%–35% of the general population (depending on the population and geographic locale) have this marker and do not have narcolepsy. For example, nearly 40% of African Americans and 25% of Caucasians demonstrate HLA DQB1*06:02 positivity. In more challenging cases such as

patients with atypical cataplexy or when MSLT interpretation is confounded by other comorbidities and/or medications, it might be useful to check for the HLA DQB1*06:02 marker. Almost all cases of narcolepsy type 1 will be positive for HLA DQB1*06:02, except for in certain neurologic conditions/CNS lesions (Fig. 36.4); therefore screening for the HLA DQB1*06:02 marker is indicated before considering a lumbar puncture for CSF hypocretin measurement. If the diagnosis of narcolepsy, specifically type 1 narcolepsy, remains uncertain, then performing a lumbar puncture for CSF hypocretin measurement, if available, may be indicated.

4. **Answer B. 1%–2%.**
There has been a low prevalence of familial cases of narcolepsy type 1. The risk of first-degree relatives of affected individuals also having narcolepsy type 1 is 1%–2%. The incidence of narcolepsy with cataplexy in identical twins is approximately 30%. The population prevalence of narcolepsy type 1 is about 50 in 100,000 or 0.05%.

5. **Answer D. Actigraphy with sleep log.**
Prior to evaluating hypersomnia with a polysomnography (A) and multiple sleep latency test (B), it is recommended that patients demonstrate that they are getting on average of greater than 6 hours of nightly sleep for at least 1 week prior to the sleep testing. This can be done using actigraphy, but if actigraphy is not available, sleep logs can be an acceptable substitute. The use of actigraphy/sleep diaries may bring circadian sleep disorders to light, as well as exclude other causes of EDS, such as insufficient sleep. Maintenance of wakefulness testing would also not be appropriate as an initial step in the workup of this patient (C). According to the ICSD-3, HLA typing is not part of the routine workup for narcolepsy (E).[7]

6. **Answer A. Stop the antidepressant for at least 14 days prior to testing (or at least 5 times the half-life of the drug and longer-acting metabolite).**
According to the ICSD-3, for the correct interpretation of PSG and MSLT findings, the patient must be free of drugs that influence sleep for at least 14 days (or at least 5 times the half-life of the drug and longer-acting metabolite), not for at least 7 days (B), and not only the day prior to testing (E). Antidepressants and other drugs can suppress REM sleep; therefore a decrease or increase in the dose of the antidepressant is not the correct decision (C and D). Additionally, the abrupt discontinuation of an antidepressant can theoretically lead to REM rebound, so abruptly stopping the antidepressant the day prior to testing could theoretically lead to an increase in REM sleep. Therefore the drugs in question should be stopped according to ICSD-3 recommendations. It is recommended to consult with the patient's treating psychiatrist when considering adjustment or a short drug holiday to allow for appropriate testing.

7. **Answer E. Cataplexy.**
Sudden withdrawal of an antidepressant may lead to rebound cataplexy. "Status cataplecticus" may occur during which long-lasting cataplectic attacks may persist virtually continuously and sometimes end with sleep which can be misdiagnosed as a "seizure." This can also occur when an antidepressant medication is changed, or doses missed.[8,9]

8. **Answer B. 4 minutes.**
The sleep onset latency is determined by the time from lights out to the first epoch of any stage of sleep, including stage N1 sleep. In this example, sleep onset occurs on epoch 18 and lights out was on epoch 10. When calculating sleep onset

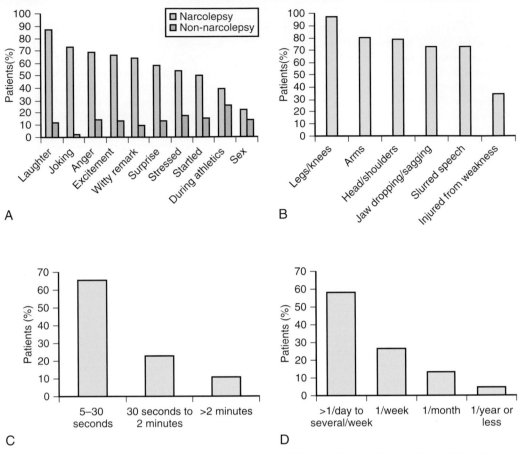

• **Figure 36.2** Characterization of Cataplexy: Emotional Triggers, Muscles Groups Affected, Duration, and Frequency. **A,** Comparison of emotional triggers for typical cataplexy and cataplexy-like episodes (e.g., physiological muscle weakness) in narcoleptics (*n* = 63) and non-narcoleptic subjects (*n* = 416/909). Surprisingly, cataplexy-like symptoms were endorsed by 46% of the non-narcolepsy subjects. Cataplexy is best differentiated from other types of muscle weakness when triggered by only three typical situations: "when hearing or telling a joke," "while laughing," or "when angry."* **B,** Muscle groups affected in typical cataplexy. The most commonly affected muscle group is the legs and knees. A typical attack, oftentimes indiscernible from normal behavior by an observer, results in the knees buckling, arms dropping to the sides, slurred speech, and/or a slight dropping of the jaw.** **C,** Duration of cataplexy attacks. Cataplexy typically lasts from seconds to less than 30 sec.** **D,** Frequency of cataplexy attacks in narcolepsy cases. Attacks typically occur at least once per day to several times per week.** (From Kryger M, Avidan AY, Berry R. *Atlas of Clinical Sleep Medicine*, originally adapted from *Anic-Labat S, Guilleminault C, Kraemer HC, Meehan J, Arrigoni J, Mignot E. Validation of a cataplexy questionnaire in 983 sleep-disordered patients. *Sleep*. 1999;22[1]:77–87. **Adapted from Okun M, Lin L, Pelin Z, Hong S, Mignot E. Clinical aspects of narcolepsy-cataplexy across ethnic groups. *Sleep*. 2002;25[1]:27–35. All subjects [*n* = 351] were HLA DQB1*06:02 positive.)

latency one must be mindful that each epoch is defined as 0.5 minutes. Therefore the sleep onset latency is 4 minutes.

9. **Answer A. 3.5 minutes.**
REM latency is taken as the time of the first epoch of sleep to the beginning of the first epoch of REM sleep regardless of the intervening stages of sleep or wakefulness. In this example, sleep onset occurs on epoch 18 and REM sleep occurs on epoch 25. Therefore the calculated REM latency is 3.5 minutes.

10. **Answer D. 48.**
The clinical MSLT continues for 15 minutes from after the first epoch of sleep. The duration of 15 minutes is determined by "clock time," and is not determined by a sleep time of 15 minutes. In this example, sleep onset occurs on epoch 18.

Therefore the nap should continue for a total of 15 minutes (i.e., 30 epochs) after epoch 18. Therefore the nap should be terminated on epoch 48.

11. **Answer C. 10.**
A nap session is terminated after 20 minutes if sleep does not occur. The absence of sleep on a nap opportunity is recorded as a sleep latency of 20 minutes. Therefore this would result in a calculated sleep latency of 10 minutes (i.e., 4 + 8 + 12 + 6 + 20 minutes = 50; 50 minutes/5 nap opportunities = 10 minutes).

12. **Answer B. Narcolepsy type 1.**
According to ICSD-3 criteria, a diagnosis of narcolepsy is defined as a mean sleep latency ≤8 minutes on the MSLT and at least two sleep-onset rapid eye movement periods (SOREMPs)

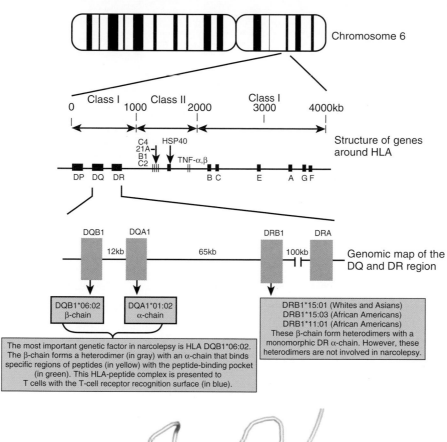

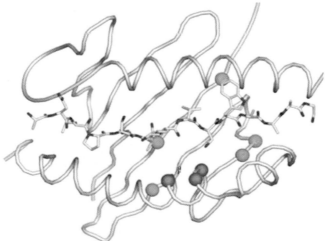

• **Figure 36.3** Human leukocyte antigens (HLA) involved in narcolepsy susceptibility. The HLA genes are located on chromosome 6 and are distributed over more than 4000 kilobases (kb). Antigen-presenting cells, macrophages, and dendritic cells have HLA class I (A, B, and C) and II (DQ, DR, and DP) protein; the locations of genes enclosing these proteins are shown. The HLA gene family is divided into two classes and is located in major histocompatibility complex (MHC) class I (A, B, and C) and class II (DQ, DR, and DP) regions. Close to the HLA genes in the MHC class III region are genes that encode complements 2 and 4, tumor necrosis factor (TNF), and heat shock protein (HSP40). The HLA DR and DQ genes are located very close to each other. HLA class II DR and DQ genes are heterodimers encoded by two genes each: one generates an α-chain, and the other a β-chain. All these genes are located within a small genetic distance, leading to extremely high linkage disequilibrium. DRA is monomorphic and does not contribute significantly to HLA diversity, in contrast with DQA1, DQB1, and DRB1, which have several hundred possible alleles. The most important genetic factor in narcolepsy is HLA DQB1*06:02. In whites and Asians, the associated DR2 subtype DRB1*15:01 is typically observed with DQB1*06:02 (and DQA1*01:02) in narcoleptic patients. In African Americans, either DRB1*15:03, a DNA-based subtype of DR2, or DRB1*11:01, a DNA-based subtype of DR5, is observed most frequently, together with DQB1*06:02—the most specific marker for narcolepsy across all ethnic groups. DQB1*06:02 forms a heterodimer *(in gray)* with an α-chain that binds specific regions of peptides with the peptide-binding pocket *(in green)*. This HLA-peptide complex is presented to T cells with the T-cell receptor recognition surface *(in blue)*. (From Kryger M, Avidan AY, Berry R. *Atlas of Clinical Sleep Medicine*, originally modified from Nishino S, Mignot E. Narcolepsy and cataplexy. *Handb Clin Neurol*. 2011;99:783–814; and Jones EY, Fugger L, Strominger JL, Siebold C. MHC class II proteins and disease: a structural perspective. *Nat Rev Immunol*. 2006;6:271–282.)

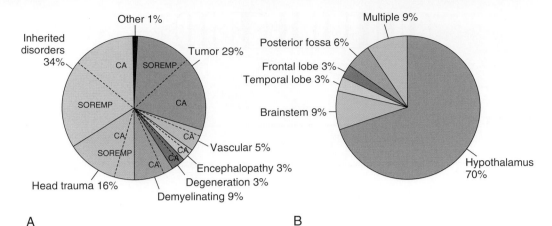

• **Figure 36.4** Neurologic Diseases and Location of Brain Lesions in 113 Cases of Secondary Narcolepsy. **A,** Neurologic diseases by category reported as secondary narcolepsy. Tumors, inherited disorders, and head trauma are the three most frequent causes. The percentage of cataplexy (CA) or sleep-onset rapid eye movement periods (SOREMPs) is denoted in each category with a dashed line. **B,** Location of brain lesions in symptomatic cases with narcolepsy associated with brain tumor; lesions in the hypothalamus and adjacent structures are the most common location. Included are 113 symptomatic cases of narcolepsy. (From Kryger M, Avidan AY, Berry R. *Atlas of Clinical Sleep Medicine*, originally modified from Kanbayashi T, Sagawa T, Takemura F, et al. The pathophysiologic basis of secondary narcolepsy and hypersomnia. *Curr Neurol Neurosci Rep*. 2011;11[2]:235–241.)

on the PSG and MSLT. A SOREMP on either the PSG or MSLT is defined as a REM latency of ≤15 minutes. The overnight PSG also demonstrated a REM latency of ≤15 minutes. The MSLT demonstrated a mean sleep latency of 7 minutes and one SOREMP. As such, the PSG and MSLT results are consistent with a diagnosis of narcolepsy based on ICSD-3 criteria. In addition, the clinical history is consistent with cataplexy. Therefore the history and sleep testing results are diagnostic for narcolepsy type 1. On the other hand, according to the prior version of the International Classification of Sleep Disorders (ICSD-2), the PSG and MSLT results would have been consistent with IH (C), since a SOREMP on the preceding nocturnal PSG was not included in the total number of SOREMPs. The patient reported an adequate amount of sleep by history prior to the administration of the PSG and MSLT, and all other appropriately ordered objective tests were unremarkable (D). There is no evidence of periodic hypersomnia in this case, so this rules out the diagnosis of KLS (E). Secondary narcolepsy is unlikely given the clinical history, normal neurologic exam, and unremarkable objective tests. Secondary narcolepsy can be seen in certain neurologic diseases/CNS lesions.

13. **Answer E. Sodium oxybate.**
When treating PWN with cataplexy, there are a variety of pharmacologic agents that can be of benefit to patients. Antidepressants, which increase aminergic signaling, can help suppress cataplexy. Protriptyline, a tricyclic antidepressant, is effective at reducing cataplexy attacks (A). The use of tricycle antidepressants in the treatment of cataplexy is often hampered by their side effect profile. Duloxetine (B) and venlafaxine (C), which inhibit norepinephrine and serotonin reuptake, are effective anticataplectic medications with a more favorable side-effect profile than tricyclic antidepressants. Fluoxetine (D), a serotonin reuptake inhibitor, is also an effective anticataplectic medication. Sodium oxybate, which currently has

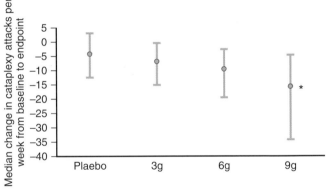

• **Figure 36.5** Median change in weekly cataplexy attacks at the end of the 4-week trial period (* denotes *P* = .0008). For placebo, 3, 6, and 9 g groups, the median changes in the frequency of cataplexy attacks were –4.3, –7.0, –9.9, and –16.1, respectively. This change was significant across doses (*P* = .0021), indicating a dose-related effect. (Modified from The US Xyrem Multicenter Study Group. A randomized, double blind, placebo-controlled multicenter trial comparing the effects of three doses of orally administered sodium oxybate with placebo for the treatment of narcolepsy. *Sleep*. 2002;25:42–49.)

an unknown mechanism of action upon cataplexy, has been shown to effectively reduce cataplectic episodes, as well as improve daytime alertness (Fig. 36.5). Currently sodium oxybate is the only medication that is FDA approved for the treatment of cataplexy in adults. A systematic review and meta-analysis found that sodium oxybate significantly reduced mean weekly cataplexy attacks by 8.5 events compared with placebo. The other listed medications described previously have been used "off label" for the treatment of cataplexy. There are no FDA-approved medications for the treatment of cataplexy in children.[10,11]

14. **Answer A. Modafinil.**

Modafinil, armodafinil, sodium oxybate, methylphenidate, and dextroamphetamine are all FDA approved for the treatment of EDS in adults with narcolepsy (Table 36.1). According to the 2007 AASM "Practice Parameters for the Treatment of Narcolepsy and Other Hypersomnias of Central Origin," only modafinil, armodafinil, and sodium oxybate have been given a "standard" level of recommendation. Older agents such as methylphenidate and dextroamphetamine (B and D) have been relegated to second line agents, due to abuse potential and side effect profiles, and have a "guideline" level of recommendation. Of note there are no FDA-approved medications for the treatment of IH to date in either children or adults. Selegiline (C) and ritanserin (E) both carry an "option" level of recommendation. Selegiline is a monoamine oxidase inhibitor (which can raise concern for drug-drug interactions) that has shown improvement in daytime sleep episodes in PWN. Ritanserin, which is not currently available for use in the United States, has limited data to support an improvement in subjective daytime sleepiness.

15. **Answer B. Posterior hypothalamus.**

Narcolepsy type 1 is due to a deficiency/loss of hypocretin/orexin neurons that are confined to the postero-lateral aspect of the hypothalamus. On average, up to 90% of hypocretin/orexin cells are typically lost in PWN (Fig. 36.6). The other letters refer to (A) basal ganglia, (C) brain stem, (D) thalamus, and (E) cerebellum.

16. **Answer C. Vaccination against H1N1 (Pandemrix).**

Several studies have found associations that suggest that narcolepsy/cataplexy occurs as an autoimmune phenomenon. An increase in antistreptolysin O (ASO) antibodies, a marker of infection with Streptococcus pyogenes, not Staphylococcus aureus (A), has been found in PWN close to the onset of the illness (Fig. 36.7). More recently, both H1N1 infection and H1N1 vaccination (specifically with the vaccine Pandemrix) have been shown to be associated with increased risk of the contracting the disease (Fig. 36.8). Almost all patients who have narcolepsy type 1 are positive for HLA DQB1 06:02, not HLA B27 (D). There has not been an association between narcolepsy and either second-hand smoke exposure (B) or exposure to pesticides (E).[12]

17. **Answer B. Loss of hypocretin neurons.**

An autoimmune process, which leads to the loss of hypocretin neurons, is the most likely pathophysiological mechanism in most cases of human narcolepsy type 1 (Fig. 36.9). Only one patient to date has been reported to have narcolepsy due to a single peptide mutation of the preprohypocretin gene (A). This patient had a young age of onset (6 months), severe cataplexy, HLADQB1*06:02 negativity, and undetectable cerebrospinal fluid levels of hypocretin-1. Canine narcolepsy was first described in the 1970s. The cause of autosomal recessive canine narcolepsy is a mutation in the hypocretin receptor 2, causing complete dysfunction of the receptor (C). Rodent models lacking (i.e., knockout models) either the hypocretin receptor 1 or hypocretin receptor 2 are available (D). Parkinson's disease is due to the loss of dopamine neurons in the substantia nigra (E).[1]

18. **Answer C. The predictive value of the MWT mean sleep latency for assessing accident risk and safety in real world circumstances is not established.**

The four-trial MWT 40-minute protocol is recommended. The MWT consists of four trials performed at 2-hour intervals, with the first trial beginning about 1.5–3 hours after the patient's usual wake-up time. The MSLT, on the other hand, consists of five trials, each lasting 20 minutes, separated by 2-hour intervals (A). The predictive value of the MWT mean sleep latency for assessing accident risk and safety in real world circumstances has not been systematically studied; documentation that an individual is able to stay awake during all trials of a MWT does not guarantee that the subject will not experience sleepiness in the work environment (E). Performance of a PSG prior to the MWT is left to the discretion of the clinician based upon clinical circumstances (D). The ability to remain awake in the work environment on a daily basis is influenced by several variables. The results of the MWT are only part of the assessment in determining the ability of an individual to maintain wakefulness in the work environment. It is not currently used to establish a diagnosis of narcolepsy or other hypersomnias (B).

19. **Answer D. At Epoch 9.**

The AASM Practice Parameters recommend a 40-minute MWT protocol. The MWT consists of four trials that are performed at 2-hour intervals. The first trial should be initiated 1.5–3 hours after the patient's usual wake time. Each nap trial is ended either after 40 minutes if no sleep occurs, or after the first epoch of unequivocal sleep. Unequivocal sleep is defined as three consecutive epochs of stage 1 sleep or one epoch of any other stage of sleep. In the previous results, the first epoch of unequivocal sleep would be Epoch 8. Therefore the nap should be terminated at the beginning of epoch 9.

20. **Answer A. Modafinil.**

Currently only modafinil and armodafinil are FDA approved to improve wakefulness in adult patients with excessive sleepiness associated with OSA. Recent meta-analyses continue to find significant improvements in both subjective and objective measures of daytime sleepiness with both drugs. For example, the Epworth Sleepiness Scale significantly improved in the modafinil (weighted mean difference [WMD], −2.96) and armodafinil group (WMD, −2.63). Sleep latency, as measured on the MWT, was significantly prolonged in the modafinil (WMD, 2.51) and armodafinil group (WMD, 2.71). Sodium oxybate and methylphenidate (C and D) are not FDA approved for the treatment of excessive daytime due to OSA. However, these medications can improve symptoms of daytime sleepiness and are often used in the treatment of hypersomnia syndromes. Acetazolamide (B) has been shown to have a beneficial effect in mild cases of OSA believed to be due to augmentation of central respiratory drive, as well as having a stabilizing effect on ventilatory control. Protriptyline (E) is a tricyclic antidepressant that inhibits both noradrenergic and serotoninergic reuptake and also has anticholinergic effects. Although subjects in several trials reported improvement in subjective sleepiness, its use is limited as there has been insufficient evidence that shows improvement in the Apnea-Hypopnea Index in OSA patients.[13]

21. **Answer E. Provide reassurance and encourage sleep extension.**

Sleep paralysis is described as the inability to move while transitioning into and/or out of sleep. Patients may describe complete awareness of their surroundings and frequently will describe a feeling of falling, impending doom or being in imminent danger. Episodes typically can last for up to a few minutes. Although sleep paralysis is often seen in PWN, it also occurs in normal individuals as well as patients with IH.

TABLE 36.1 | **Pharmacologic Agents for Central Nervous System Hypersomnias**

Compound (Class)	Pharmacologic Properties	Usual Daily Dose	Other Considerations and Common/Serious Side Effects
Stimulants			
Modafinil	Mode of action controversial, but likely involves relatively selective DA reuptake inhibition Minimal, if any, addiction potential Less effective than amphetamine-based stimulants	Modafinil, 100–400 mg in the morning or as divided doses R-modafinil, 50–250 mg in the morning	Headaches are possible but minimized by starting at lower doses and slow uptitration May decrease efficacy of oral contraceptives Monitor blood pressure and heart rate Possible allergic effects (e.g., rash); monitor especially in children R-enantiomer of modafinil (R-modafinil) has a longer half-life and is approximately 2 times more potent once steady state is achieved
Methylphenidate	Blocks monoamine uptake No effect on reverse efflux or VMAT Potential for addiction, especially for immediate-release compounds More effective than modafinil	10–60 mg daily or as divided doses	Low cost Various preparations and formulas can have different interindividual effects Monitor blood pressure and heart rate Immediate release (5–10 mg) can be helpful on an as-needed basis to counter gaps in alertness during the daytime (e.g., sleep inertia or after a meal) in hypersomniacs
D-amphetamine sulfate	Increases monoamine release Primary effects of usual dosages due to reverse efflux of dopamine through the dopamine transporter as well as inhibition of monoamine storage via the VMAT	5–60 mg daily or as divided doses	Use similar to methylphenidate Monitor blood pressure and heart rate Preference given to longer lasting formulations Can be more effective than methylphenidate in some patients At higher doses may partially treat cataplexy due to adrenergic effects
Antidepressants*			
Clomipramine (tricyclic)	Monoamine uptake blocker Anticholinergic effects Desmethylclomipramine is an active metabolite	10–150 mg	Side effects (e.g., dry mouth, blurred vision, orthostatic hypotension, anorexia, sweating, constipation, and drowsiness) tend to limit use, but cost is low Contraindicated in patients with cardiovascular conduction abnormalities and in those with open-angle glaucoma
Fluoxetine (SSRI)	Specific serotonin reuptake blocker Active metabolite norfluoxetine has more adrenergic effects	20–60 mg	Less potent than clomipramine but lacks anticholinergic and antihistaminergic effects Very long half-life, so more stable effect on cataplexy Useful with concomitant anxiety disorder
Venlafaxine (SNRI)	Specific serotonin and adrenergic reuptake blocker Short half-life; extended-release formulation preferred Mild stimulant effect	37.5–150 mg, max 300 mg/day	Side effects include gastrointestinal upset (main reason for discontinuation) and transient constipation Potential withdrawal side effects on abrupt cessation (e.g., sudden electric shock–like feelings)
Atomoxetine (NRI)	Specific adrenergic reuptake blocker (norepinephrine) Mild stimulant effect	10–60 mg, usually as divided doses, max 80 mg/day	Side effects include urinary retention and reduced appetite Monitor pulse and blood pressure Short half-life Indicated for attention deficit hyperactivity
Other			
Sodium oxybate	Debatable mechanism but probably involves dopamine release and may act on γ-aminobutyric acid or specific γ-hydroxybutyrate receptors Treats all aspects of narcolepsy, including disrupted nocturnal sleep, excessive daytime sleepiness, cataplexy, and other REM-related phenomena	4.5–9 g (at a minimum divided into bi-nightly doses)	Side effects include nausea, weight loss, parasomnia, enuresis, and psychiatric complications Use with caution in presence of hypoventilation or significant sleep apnea Decreasing dosage may be helpful with parasomnia-like behavior or enuresis Uptitration and/or trinightly divided dosing can be helpful with disrupted nocturnal sleep and/or inadequate sleep time Immediate effects on disrupted nocturnal sleep Complete effects on cataplexy and daytime sleepiness may take several weeks Only FDA-indicated treatment for cataplexy

*All antidepressants are immediately effective on cataplexy. Abrupt discontinuation of antidepressant(s) may lead to rebound cataplexy.
FDA, Food and Drug Administration; *NRI*, norepinephrine reuptake inhibitor; *REM*, rapid eye movement; *SNRI*, serotonin–norepinephrine reuptake inhibitor; *SSRI*, selective serotonin reuptake inhibitor.
From Kryger M, Avidan AY, Berry R, eds. *Atlas of Clinical Sleep Medicine.* 2nd ed. Philadelphia: Saunders; 2014.

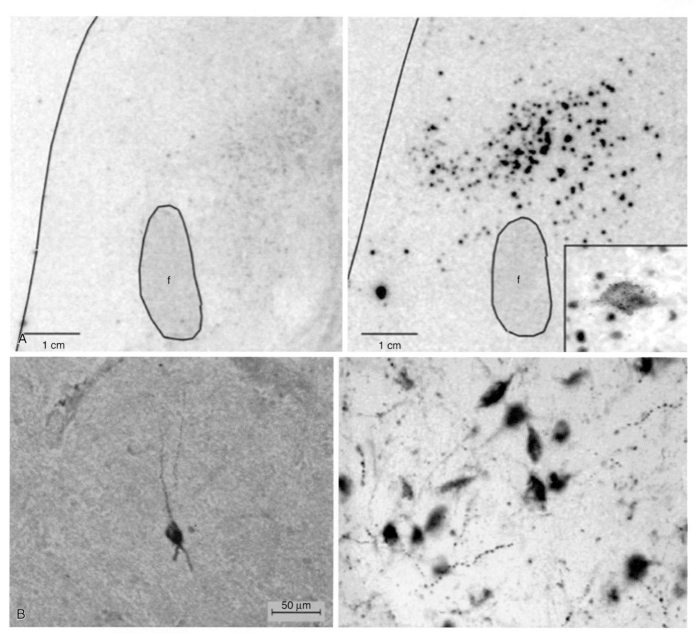

• **Figure 36.6** Hypocretin Peptides and Neurons in the Lateral Hypothalamus of Narcoleptics Versus Controls. **A,** Significant reduction of hypocretin mRNA expression in the lateral hypothalamus in a narcoleptic *(left)* versus a control brain *(right)*. **B,** Significant reduction of hypocretin-stained peptides in hypocretin cells (in the lateral hypothalamus) in a narcoleptic *(left)* versus a control brain *(right)*. Narcoleptics have an 85% to 95% reduction in the number of hypocretin neurons. (From Kryger M, Avidan AY, Berry R. *Atlas of Clinical Sleep Medicine*, originally modified from Peyron C, Faraco J, Rogers W, et al. A mutation in a case of early onset narcolepsy and a generalized absence of hypocretin peptides in human narcoleptic brains. *Nat Med.* 2000;6:991–997. **B,** modified from Thannickal TC, Moore RY, Nienjuis R, et al. Reduced number of hypocretin neurons in human narcolepsy. Neuron 2000;27[3]:469–474.)

It can be precipitated by stress, irregular sleep-wake schedules, or ingestion of alcohol. Although it can be alarming, sleep paralysis can occur in 5%–40% of the normal population, depending upon the study, and in the absence of other significant signs/symptoms, the management is typically reassurance that this is a normal phenomenon. According to the ICSD-3, recurrent isolated sleep paralysis is classified as a REM parasomnia. If behavioral therapy and reassurance fail to relieve the patient, then a trial of a medication may be warranted, but only after carefully weighing the risks and benefits of such an intervention. According to the 2007 AASM "Practice Parameters for the Treatment of Narcolepsy and Other Hypersomnias of Central Origin," tricyclic antidepressants, selective serotonin reuptake inhibitors (SSRIs), and venlafaxine have been given an "option" level of recommendation.

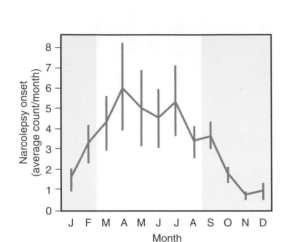

A

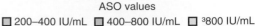

Anti-streptolysin O antibodies in patients
with narcolepsy and matched controls

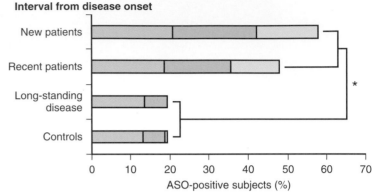

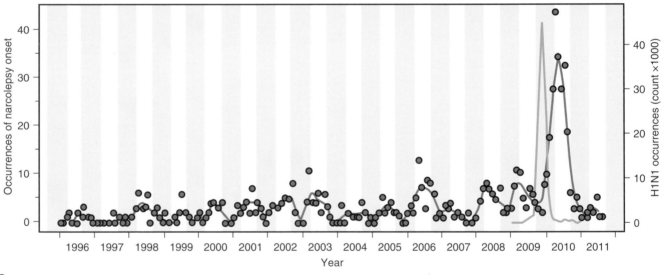

New patients - less than 1 year from first symptom (n = 19)
Recent patients - symptoms began 1–3 years before the test (n = 48)
Long-standing - more than 10 years from first symptom (n = 67)
Controls - age and season matched to above patients (n = 134)
*P < .001(ASO positivity in patients with new and recent onset vs
patients with long-standing disease or controls)

B

C

• **Figure 36.7** Environmental Triggers and Genetic Factors in Narcolepsy. **A,** Seasonality and the incidence of narcolepsy in China. Data as mean ± standard error of the mean of monthly occurrences, corrected by the number of days per month and leap years, in percentage of 12 months across the year (mean of 15-year data). Onset of disease is approximately sixfold to sevenfold more frequent in the late spring and early summer versus late fall or early winter *(shaded areas).* **B,** Antistreptolysin O (ASO) antibodies in patients with narcolepsy with hypocretin deficiency (n = 200) and age-matched controls (n = 200). Higher ASO titers were seen in narcoleptics, particularly closer to disease onset, compared with controls. This suggests that streptococcal infections are probably a significant environmental trigger for narcolepsy. **C,** The 2009 H1N1 pandemic in China was associated with a threefold increase in narcolepsy onset. Monthly counts of onset occurrences over a 15-year period (raw data) with a 3-month moving average trend line are depicted in red (n = 629 diagnosed with narcolepsy/hypocretin deficiency at People's Hospital, Beijing University, China). Note the clear seasonal fluctuations of the trend line with lower onset counts in fall and winter *(shaded areas)* and higher onset counts in spring and summer. The number of H1N1 infections documented by governmental statistics is depicted in green. The peak of infections was followed by a large increase in incident narcolepsy cases in 2010, which was largely independent of H1N1 vaccination (only 8 of 142 patients recalled receiving the vaccination), followed by an abrupt decline in 2011. (From Kryger M, Avidan AY, Berry R. *Atlas of Clinical Sleep Medicine*, originally modified Adapted from Han F, Lin L, Warby SC, et al. Narcolepsy onset is seasonal and increased following the 2009 H1N1 pandemic in China. *Ann Neurol.* 2011;70[3]:410–417; Aran A, Lin L, Nevsimalova S, et al. Elevated anti-streptococcal antibodies in patients with recent narcolepsy onset. *Sleep.* 2009;32[8];979–983.)

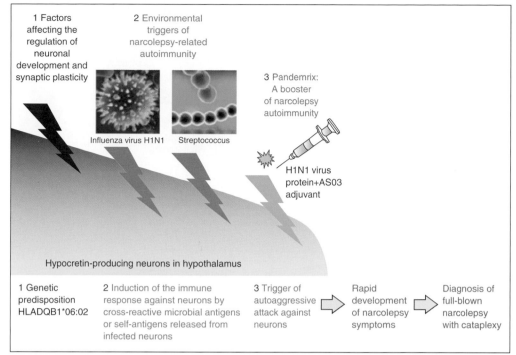

1 Factors affecting the regulation of neuronal development and synaptic plasticity

2 Environmental triggers of narcolepsy-related autoimmunity

Influenza virus H1N1

Streptococcus

3 Pandemrix: A booster of narcolepsy autoimmunity

H1N1 virus protein+AS03 adjuvant

Hypocretin-producing neurons in hypothalamus

1 Genetic predisposition HLADQB1*06:02

2 Induction of the immune response against neurons by cross-reactive microbial antigens or self-antigens released from infected neurons

3 Trigger of autoaggressive attack against neurons

Rapid development of narcolepsy symptoms

Diagnosis of full-blown narcolepsy with cataplexy

• **Figure 36.8** The development of narcolepsy after AS03 adjuvanted H1N1 vaccination in an individual with genetic predisposition. Several hits are probably needed for development of full-blown narcolepsy. The first hit is associated with the neuronal development, the second induces the narcolepsy-related autoimmunity (e.g., influenza virus or streptococcal infection), and the final trigger (i.e., Pandemrix vaccine) activates the underlying autoimmunity leading to the rapid development of the symptoms of narcolepsy. (Modified from Partinen M, Kornum B, Plazzi G, Jennum P, Julkunen I, Vaarala O. Narcolepsy as an autoimmune disease: the role of H1N1 infection and vaccination. *Lancet Neurol.* 2014;13:1072–1073.)

22. **Answer E. Insufficient sleep syndrome.**

According to the ICSD-3, to diagnose recurrent isolated sleep paralysis (A), IH (C), or narcolepsy (D), the condition must not be better explained by another sleep disorder, mental disorder, medical condition, medication, or substance use. Specifically, the ICSD-3 criterion requires that the patient must have a behavioral complaint attributable to sleepiness. The patient's sleep time is shorter than what would be expected for their age, and the sleep pattern has been present for at least 3 months. The patient may report sleeping in later on weekends or using alarms to curtail sleep time. Extending sleep time typically results in resolution of the symptoms of sleepiness. The patient was appropriately counseled to extend his sleep times. During a follow-up visit he reported his symptoms of daytime sleepiness and sleep paralysis resolved. The diagnosis is most consistent with insufficient sleep syndrome. There was no evidence in the history to suggest OSA (B).

23. **Answer D. 24-hour PSG if available.**

The history seems consistent with IH. According to the ICSD-3, a diagnosis of IH in this patient in light of previous testing relies upon documentation of either total sleep times of ≥660 minutes on 24-hour polysomnographic monitoring or by wrist actigraphy with a sleep log. The use of 24-hour PSG, but not wrist actigraphy (A), has been validated against controls for IH; therefore 24-hour PSG is the next best step to confirm the diagnosis if available. In the setting of two negative MSLTs for narcolepsy and no history of cataplexy, there is no diagnostic value in repeating PSG and MSLT (C),

obtaining HLA DQB1*06:02 genotyping (B), or performing a MWT (E).

24. **Answer A. IH.**

Two past PSG and MSLTs were not diagnostic for narcolepsy, so this makes the diagnosis of narcolepsy type 1 or 2 far less likely (B and C). In addition, CSF hypocretin measurement documented normal hypocretin values, which definitively rules out narcolepsy type 1. A CSF hypocretin value below 110 pg/mL or a third of mean normal control values is the biological definition of narcolepsy type 1. HLA DQB1*06:02 status in this case, particularly in the setting of documented normal CSF hypocretin level, is of no diagnostic utility. HLA DQB1*06:02 positivity can be seen in 12%–35% of normal individuals depending upon ethnicity. There is no evidence of periodic hypersomnia (D). In spite of significant sleep extension up to 12 hours per day, she continues to experience daytime sleepiness, so this rules out long sleep time (E).

25. **Answer D. Stage N3.**

Sforza and colleagues performed spectral analysis on 10 patients with IH compared with controls. Spectral analysis is the process by which an electroencephalography signal is decomposed into its constituent frequency components (e.g., delta, theta, alpha, and beta frequency bands). Polygraphic data revealed that there was no statistical significant difference in stage W, specifically wake after sleep onset (A), stage N1 (B), and N2 parameters (C). However, stage N3 was significantly reduced, and stage REM was significantly increased (E). These data would lend themselves toward the hypothesis that patients with IH have a decrease in their homeostatic sleep drives, and

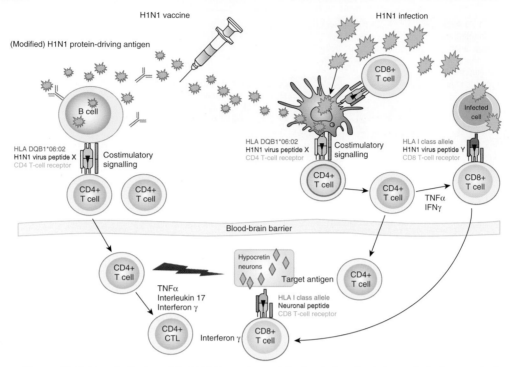

• **Figure 36.9** Hypothetical model of H1N1 vaccine or infection-induced autoimmunity in the onset of narcolepsy. The role of H1N1 virus proteins and the HLA DQB1*06:02 allele in the development of type 1 narcolepsy is supported by epidemiological studies showing increased incidence of narcolepsy after H1N1 vaccination (Pandemrix) in individuals with HLA DQB1*06:02 genotype, and by the possible cross-reactivity of hypocretin-specific CD4+ T cells with H1N1 virus protein in patients with narcolepsy. Increase in narcolepsy incidence has also been reported after H1N1 infection. In our model an H1N1 peptide X is presented in the complex of HLA DQB1*06:02 molecule to CD4+ T cells by antigen-presenting cells, such as dendritic cells or B cells. Because the risk of narcolepsy is seemingly associated only with Pandemrix and not with other adjuvanted or unadjuvanted H1N1 vaccines, an H1N1 viral antigen modified in the manufacturing process of Pandemrix might be presented as peptide X. Viral peptide X-specific CD4 T cells further activate CD8 cells, which recognize H1N1 viral peptide Y. Activated CD4 and CD8 cells cross the blood–brain barrier and infiltrate the hypothalamus, where hypocretin neurons are located. The destruction of hypocretin neurons can be mediated by inflammatory cytokines (e.g., TNFα, interferon γ, and interleukin 17) secreted by CD4 cells or DC4 cells, which acquire cytotoxic phenotype, or by cytotoxic CD8 cells. The neuronal autoantigen might show molecular mimicry with the H1N1 viral peptides X or Y, or the role of viral peptide X might be that of driving antigen of the narcolepsy-related autoimmunity. *APC*, Antigen presenting cell; *CTL*, cytotoxic T lymphocyte; *TNFα*, tumor necrosis factor α. (Modified from Partinen M, Kornum B, Plazzi G, Jennum P, Julkunen I, Vaarala O. Narcolepsy as an autoimmune disease: the role of H1N1 infection and vaccination. *Lancet Neurol*. 2014;13:1072–1073.)

perhaps the increased tendency toward greater sleep times may be an attempt to catch up on the lost SWS.

26. **Answer D. KLS.**

The periodicity that the parents report along with the patient's age is most consistent with KLS. KLS is a rare condition that affects adolescent males to females in a ratio of 2:1. Most patients are teenagers during KLS onset, but KLS cases with onset as early as 9 years of age and as old as 35 years of age have been reported. Jewish heritage is a possible risk factor for developing the syndrome, though it should be emphasized that no genetic link has clearly been demonstrated. Birth or development problems are reported by a third of patients. Familial cases of KLA are found in 5% of patients.

The clinical picture of KLS has been recently revised to include hypersomnia, cognitive, psychiatric, and behavioral disturbances. Hypersexuality and hyperphagia were part of the original descriptions; large series now show a somewhat different constellation of signs and symptoms including

derealization (striking feeling of unreality), confusion and apathy (disinhibited behavior is less frequent). PSG and MSLT data may be helpful; however, data has not been consistent and sleep parameters can vary depending on if the patient is studied during the first or second half of the symptomatic episode. Although narcolepsy and IH should be a part of the differential diagnosis (A, B, C), these disorders are typically accompanied by complaints of daily sleepiness rather than periodic episodes of hypersomnia. Although patients with Klüver-Bucy syndrome may also present with similar symptoms of hyperphagia and hypersexuality, these patients can typically be differentiated from KLS due to the presence of brain lesions (typically bilateral lesions affecting the medial temporal lobe; E).

27. **Answer D. Infection.**

Although many patients with KLS do not have an identifiable trigger for their episodes, it is important to question patients about events surrounding symptom onset. Reviews of case studies in patients with KLS have shown that the most common reported symptom is infection, followed by alcohol use (A), sleep deprivation (B), stress (C), and physical exertion (E). Types of infections reported include a flu-like illness, an infection of the upper airway, or a gastroenteritis. Infectious etiologies are rarely identified, but reports have included Epstein-Barr virus, varicella virus, Asian influenza virus, enterovirus, H1N1 virus, and streptococcus.

28. **Answer B. Hypoperfusion in the thalamus.**
Several areas of hypoperfusion during symptomatic episodes have been reported, and include the thalamus, hypothalamus, as well as the temporal, frontal, and sometimes the parietal and occipital areas (Fig. 36.10). These areas typically lessen during asymptomatic periods in half of patients.

29. **Answer B. Amantadine.**
KLS is a difficult disorder to treat, as many medications have shown limited benefit in these patients. The natural history of KLS makes it rather challenging to evaluate the effectiveness of medication(s) as well. For example, episodes last, on average, 13 days, but short episodes limited to only a day or two and as long as 3–4 months have been reported. The mean interval between episodes is approximately 6 months. On average,

patients have 19 episodes, and the duration of the disease lasts approximately 14 years. In general, it is commonly reported that the disease disappears in most cases after the age of 30–35 years of age.

Amantadine, an antiviral that may direct and indirect effects on dopaminergic neurons, has been reported to help terminate the hypersomnia episode, but there have been no corroborative studies to recommend the routine use of amantadine in KLS. Stimulants such as modafinil and amphetamines (C and E) have not shown significant benefit in these patients. Lithium and valproate (A and D) may be useful in helping prevent further episodes of hypersomnia. A recent open-label, controlled study suggested that the benefit/risk ratio is good for KLS. The authors concluded that lithium therapy led to approximately 1 month less in episodes per year. Although nearly 50% of patients treated with lithium experienced at least one adverse event (e.g., tremor, polyuria-polydipsia, diarrhea, TSH increase, weight increase), no serious adverse events were documented.[14]

30. **Answer C. RLS.**
The history is consistent with moderate-severe primary RLS as the cause of insufficient sleep leading to his daytime

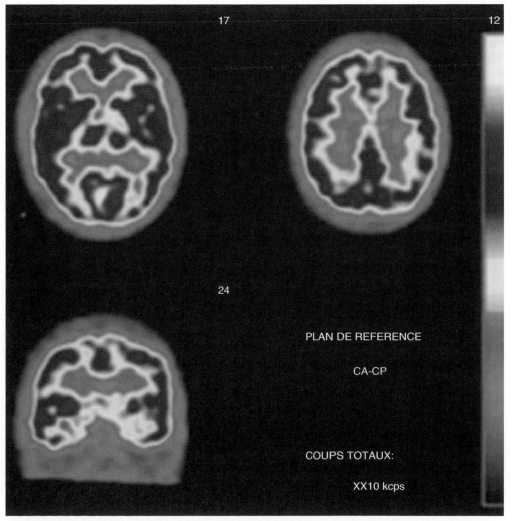

• **Figure 36.10** Brain scintigraphy during a Kleine-Levin syndrome episode in a boy. (Modified from Arnulf I. Kleine-Levin syndrome. *Sleep Med Clin*. 2015;10:151–161.)

hypersomnia. The patient clearly describes an urge to move his legs associated with uncomfortable or unpleasant sensations in his legs; the symptoms start when he is resting or inactive, starting at generally the same time each day (early evening). The urge to move and the unpleasant sensations are relieved by movement but recur when the movement stops. There is presumably a positive family history. He has developed "insomnia" with fear of bedtime, because he knows that he will be extremely uncomfortable and unable to fall asleep or stay asleep (B). The worsening of the symptoms with the central acting antihistamine also is consistent with RLS. There is no evidence of a concomitant neuropathy. Periodic limb movements of sleep are commonly associated with RLS; however, the underlying mechanisms that are responsible for this patient's symptoms clearly relate to RLS (D). The unremarkable neurologic exam makes a diagnosis of myotonic dystrophy very unlikely (A). It should be noted that myotonic dystrophy may present with EDS and demonstrate sleep testing consistent with narcolepsy type 2 (i.e., narcolepsy type 2 due to a medical condition). The net result of his RLS symptoms has resulted in the diagnosis of hypersomnia due to a medical disorder (ICD-10-CM code G47.14) rather than IH (E).

31. **Answer C. Serum ferritin.**

Reduced brain iron has been associated with RLS; in particular it has been shown that low serum ferritin in spite of normal serum iron and a normal hemogram contributes to the pathophysiology of the RLS symptoms. When such clear-cut RLS symptoms are present, it is not necessary to do sleep studies (even if periodic limb movements are part of the differential diagnosis) or HLA testing (A and B). Diabetes and other neuropathic conditions as the cause of a sensory/motor neuropathy can be associated with RLS; however, there are no signs or symptoms

of hyperglycemia (polyuria, polyphagia, or weight loss) or any other neuropathy, so a glucose tolerance test or even a nerve biopsy (D and E) might be carried out if all other conditions are excluded.

32. **Answer C. Dopamine agonist therapy.**

The AASM in 2012 updated their recommendations for treatment of RLS and include as a "standard" level of treatment: pramipexole, ropinirole. Therapies with a "guideline" level of recommendation include levodopa with dopa decarboxylase inhibitor, opioids (E), gabapentin enacarbil, and cabergoline. Therapies with an "option" level of recommendation include gabapentin, pregabalin, carbamazepine, clonidine, and supplemental iron. CBT-I could be used in conjunction with the DA therapy if sleep does not improve with the treatment of the primary sleep disorder (A). Hypnotics and wake promoting agents were not included in the guideline recommendations (B and D).

Suggested Reading

Berry RB, Brooks R, Gamaldo CE, et al. *The AASM Manual for the Scoring of Sleep and Associated Events: Rules, Terminology and Technical Specifications, Version 2.2*; 2015. www.aasmnet.org. Darien, IL: American Academy of Sleep Medicine.

Littner MR, Kushida C, Wise M, et al. Practice parameters for clinical use of the multiple sleep latency test and the maintenance of wakefulness test. *Sleep.* 2005;28(1):113-121.

Morgenthaler TI, Kapur VK, Brown TM, et al. Practice parameters for the treatment of narcolepsy and other hypersomnias of central origin. *Sleep.* 2007;30(12):1705-1711.

Nishino S, Mignot E. Narcolepsy and cataplexy. *Handb Clin Neurol.* 2011;99:783-814.

Thorpy MJ. Update on therapy for narcolepsy. *Curr Treat Options Neurol.* 2015;17(5):347.

37

Clinical Cases: Circadian Rhythm Sleep-Wake Disorders

CATHY GOLDSTEIN

Questions

1. A 17-year-old male notes that over the past few months he has had difficulty falling asleep prior to 1:00 AM. His mother has to awaken him in the morning as he sleeps through his 7:15 AM alarm and she notes he is groggy at this time. He is often late to school and is sleepy during the day, particularly while in his first two classes. During summer vacation, he slept well from around 2:00 AM to 11:00 AM and was not sleepy during the day. What physiological change most likely resulted in his symptoms?
   A. Lengthening of the intrinsic circadian period
   B. Mutation of the *hPer2* gene
   C. More rapid accumulation of homeostatic sleep drive after puberty
   D. Enhancement of the phase advance portion of the PRC to bright light

2. A daughter brings her 68-year-old mother to sleep clinic for the evaluation of excessive sleepiness. The patient is on an extended stay at her daughter's home. Excessive sleepiness, to the extent that the patient is nodding off after dinner (around 8 PM), has been witnessed. To appease her daughter's family, she tried to sleep in so she could stay up later at night but could not sleep later than 5 AM. On further inquiry the mother reports that she was feeling just fine prior to her trip to her daughter's home. At home, she was going to bed by 7:30–8:00 PM and awakening no later than 4:00 AM. On this schedule she had no problems with tiredness. What would you expect to find in this patient's diagnostic evaluation?
   A. Overnight polysomnogram (PSG) conducted at a conventional time would show prolonged sleep onset latency and increased rapid eye movement (REM) onset latency.
   B. Dim-light melatonin onset (DLMO) would be expected at 10:00 PM.

   C. Horne Ostberg morningness-eveningness questionnaire (MEQ) is likely to demonstrate a score below 41.
   D. Actigraphy would demonstrate a stable advance in sleep onset and offset.

3. A 37-year-old female plans a 14-day trip to London (British Summer Time [BST] = Greenwich Mean Time [GMT]+1). She will be departing from Detroit (Eastern Daylight Time [EDT] = BST-5). She typically sleeps well at home, from 11:00 PM to 7:00 AM. However, last time she was in Europe she had a difficult time falling asleep at night and had trouble awakening when desired in the morning.
   She arrives at Heathrow airport at 11:15 AM. What should you recommend after arriving in London to reduce her symptoms of jet lag?
   A. Avoid bright light upon arrival in London by wearing dark sunglasses for the rest of the afternoon.
   B. Seek bright light upon arrival and throughout the afternoon and take melatonin 3 mg at bedtime (11:00 PM).
   C. Take melatonin 3 mg at 4 PM and attempt sleep at 11:00 PM.
   D. Take melatonin 0.5 mg upon arriving and avoid bright light by wearing dark sunglasses for the rest of the afternoon.

4. Which of the following is true in regard to sleep duration in shift workers?
   A. Although circadian misalignment is present, sleep duration is similar in night shift workers and permanent day workers.
   B. Sleep duration is on average 120 min shorter in shift workers with shift work disorder compared with permanent day workers.
   C. Rotating shift workers have longer sleep duration than evening shift workers.
   D. Rotating shift workers have shorter sleep duration than evening shift workers.

5. A 28-year-old female presents to her physician with the report of being unable to sleep after starting a new job that required her to awaken at 6:30 AM. Prior to this, she was a graduate student and had a great deal of flexibility in regard to her work hours. At that time, she would typically arrive to work around noon and had no problems falling asleep around 3:00 AM. Currently, she gets in bed at 11:00 PM and tosses and turns for what seems like 2 or 3 hours. She hits the snooze button on her alarm multiple times and is exhausted during

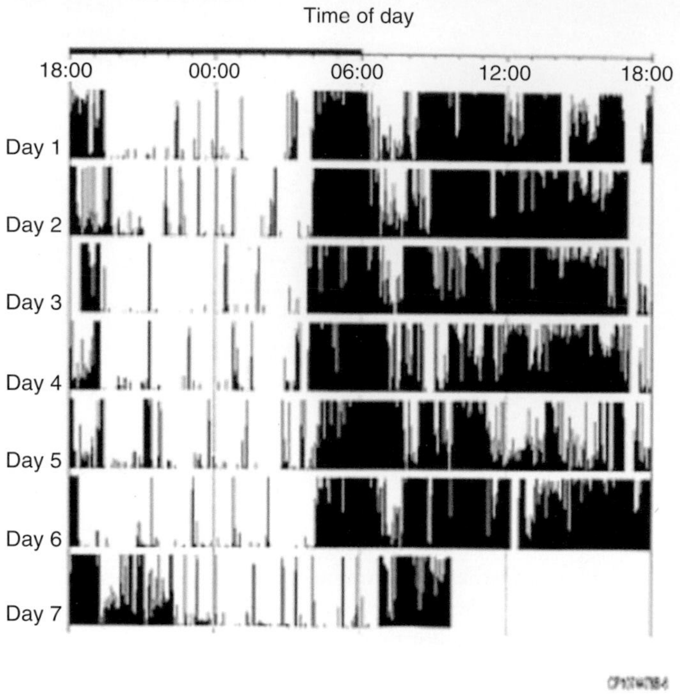

Time of day

• **Figure 37.1** Actigraphy. (Used with permission from Auger R. Advance-related sleep complaints and advanced sleep phase disorder. *Sleep Med Clin.* 2009;4[2]:219r–227r.)

the day, frequently falling asleep during meetings. On the weekends she "goes back to her old ways" of sleeping and does not have difficulty falling asleep or maintaining alertness during the day. Her other medical conditions include type I diabetes complicated by mild hypertension (recently started on enalapril), anxiety, and depression. Which of the following accurately represents the interaction between her comorbidities and her current sleep complaints?

A. Circadian disruption has resulted in the metabolic dysfunction underlying her type I diabetes.

B. Her difficulty with sleep onset is most likely secondary to cognitive and somatic hyperarousal due to anxiety.

C. More than 50% of individuals with her sleep disorder have symptoms of depression.

D. Enalapril may cause interruption of the signaling pathways responsible for melatonin secretion and resulted in her difficulty falling asleep.

6. Actigraphy is recorded on a 53-year-old female (Fig. 37.1) who notes pronounced evening sleepiness that interferes with business dinner meetings and awakening at least 2 hours before her 7:00 AM alarm, even on the weekends. Which of the following is true regarding the epidemiology of this disorder?

A. There is a 2 : 1 female to male preponderance.

B. A familial form of this condition has been reported.

C. Prevalence is approximately 10%.

D. There is a bimodal distribution of symptom onset with the first peak in adolescence and the second peak in the thirties.

7. A 20-year-old male presents to a sleep medicine clinic with excessive daytime sleepiness. On further inquiry you determine that he is only getting around 6 hours of sleep, as he has marked difficulty falling asleep before 4:00 AM and he sets

an alarm for 10:00 AM. His sleepiness is most pronounced in the morning and did not develop until he began taking classes with start times before 11:00 AM this semester. When he sleeps 8–9 hours, he typically feels well rested. Which statement is correct in regard to hypothetical findings in this patient?

A. MEQ is likely to demonstrate a score below 41.

B. Salivary DLMO would be expected at approximately 10:00 PM.

C. Overnight PSG conducted at the patient's preferred sleep times is likely to demonstrate short sleep duration.

D. Actigraphy would estimate total sleep time with approximately 75% sensitivity and 90% specificity (compared with gold standard PSG).

8. Ramelteon, administered 30 minutes before bedtime, has demonstrated the ability to help re-entrain circadian phase in response to simulated travel of five time zones eastward. How is this achieved?

A. A phase advance elicited due to lower affinity for MT1 and MT2 receptors than melatonin

B. A phase advance elicited by action on MT1 and MT2 receptors at high doses

C. A phase advance elicited by action on MT1 and MT2 receptors at low doses

D. A phase delay elicited by action on MT1 and MT2 receptors at low doses

9. Familial forms of advanced sleep-wake phase disorder (ASWPD) have been associated with the following genetic abnormality:

A. Deletion of *hPer2*

B. Missense mutation of *hPer2*

C. Variable number tandem repeat (VNTR) in *hPer3*

D. Duplication of *CKIδ*

10. Which of the following most accurately describes the sleep-wake pattern in sighted individuals with non-24-hour sleep-wake disorder (N24SWD)?

A. In those attempting to adhere to a day wake, night sleep schedule a stable delay of 1 hour per day is always seen.

B. The average circadian period is 24.18 hours.

C. In more than 50%, when the endogenous propensity for sleep onset has delayed to the morning hours, delay phase "jumps" occur.

D. At least three sleep bouts are dispersed through a 24-hour day.

11. Which statement best describes treatment of irregular sleep-wake rhythm disorder (ISWRD) in children and adolescents?

A. Melatonin is contraindicated when ISWRD is comorbid with autism.

B. Melatonin the hour before bedtime may be considered for treatment of ISWRD in children and adolescents with neurological disorders.

C. Melatonin may be considered for treatment of ISWRD in children and adolescents with neurological disorders; however, this is only in the context of multimodal therapy with bright light.

D. Melatonin improves sleep ratings by caregivers but not objectively recorded total sleep time.

12. Which of the following is correct regarding the relationship of night shift work with breast cancer?

A. Individuals carrying the four repeat variant of the *hPer3* VNTR are more likely to develop breast cancer with exposure to night shift work.

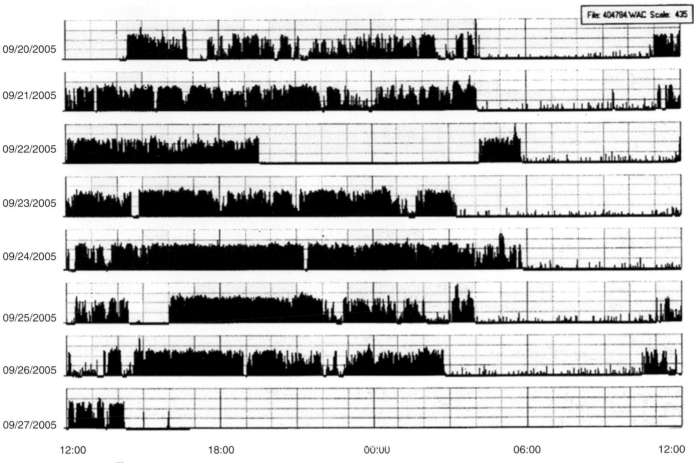

09/20/2005
09/21/2005
09/22/2005
09/23/2005
09/24/2005
09/25/2005
09/26/2005
09/27/2005

12:00   18:00   00:00   06:00   12:00

File: 404784.WAC Scale: 435

• **Figure 37.2** Actigraphy. One 24-hour period plotted on each horizontal line. Black lines represent activity.

B. Short sleep duration underlies the pathogenesis of increased breast cancer risk in night shift workers.

C. Although night shift work is associated with increased breast cancer risk, a dose response relationship has not been found.

D. Night shift work may increase the risk of breast cancer due to the suppression of melatonin by light at night.

13. A 42-year-old female executive from Denver (mountain daylight time [MDT]) is flying to Dubai (Gulf Standard Time [GST] =MDT+10). She has an extremely demanding schedule and cannot make any changes to her 11:00 PM–6:00 AM sleep schedule prior to departure. Once in Dubai, she will have meetings where important financial decisions will be made, so she would like to "reset" her clock as quickly as she can after arriving.

    She departs Denver International Airport at 05:45 AM (MDT) and arrives in Dubai at 06:45 AM (GST). What do you recommend to facilitate her entrainment to GST?

    A. Seek a lot of morning and early afternoon light in Dubai and avoid late afternoon/evening bright light.

    B. Avoid morning/early afternoon light in Dubai; use a 10,000 lux broad spectrum light box for 2 hours at 6 PM daily.

    C. Avoid early morning bright light in Dubai; seek afternoon bright light, and take melatonin 1 mg 2 hours before bedtime.

    D. To avoid inappropriate light exposure in flight, use zolpidem 10 mg after cruising altitude has been reached.

14. You have obtained actigraphy on a 35-year-old patient with a suspected circadian rhythm sleep-wake disorder. Based on this recording (Fig. 37.2) and the patient's desire to sleep from approximately 12:00 AM to 8:00 AM to attend to family and occupational responsibilities, which of the following treatment strategies is most appropriate?

    A. Tasimelteon 20 mg at bedtime, 2 hours of bright white, broad spectrum light of 4000 lux at 11:00 AM

    B. Tasimelteon 20 mg at bedtime without light therapy

    C. Melatonin 3 mg at 9 PM–11 PM

    D. 2 hours of bright white, broad spectrum light of 4000 lux at 7 AM

15. A 29-year-old female presents with difficulty falling asleep and daytime sleepiness. After working on her online blog on a desktop computer, she gets into bed at 11:30 PM and sets an alarm for 7:00 AM. She tosses and turns for about 2 hours during the weeknights. However, she sleeps great on the weekends when she gets into bed at 1:00 AM–2:00 AM and has no problem falling asleep during naps. Which is true about the impact of light from her nighttime computer use on her disorder?

    A. Long wavelength light may exacerbate her difficulty sleeping, as the peak sensitivity of melanopsin is 650 nm.

    B. Retinal ganglion cells are required for transmission of bright light to the circadian timing system.

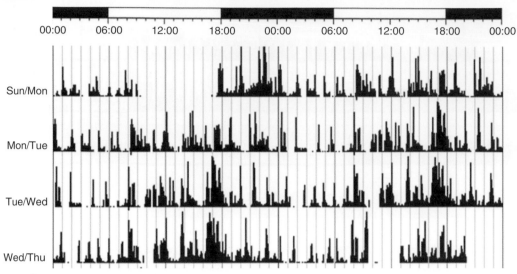

• **Figure 37.3** Actigraphy. Two days are plotted on each horizontal line (with the second day repeated as the first on the next day). Black lines represent activity. (Used with permission from Abbott SM, Zee PC. Irregular sleep-wake rhythm disorder. *Sleep Med Clin.* 2015;10[4]:517–522.)

C. Both retinal ganglion cells and rods and cones are required for transmission of bright light to the circadian timing system.

D. The phase resetting properties of bright light are linear.

16. Which of the following is true in regard to the use of melatonin in children and adolescents with delayed sleep-wake phase disorder (DSWPD)?
    A. Melatonin should be avoided in children who also have attention deficit hyperactivity disorder (ADHD) but may be used in children without comorbidities.
    B. Melatonin may improve subjective sleep quality but is not expected to reduce sleep onset latency.
    C. Melatonin may be considered at a dose of 0.15 mg/kg 2 hours before bedtime for the treatment of DSWPD.
    D. Melatonin may be considered at a dose of 0.15 mg/kg during nighttime awakenings for the treatment of DSWPD.

17. Which of the following mechanisms has been demonstrated to underlie the pathophysiology of familial advanced sleep-wake phase disorder (FASWPD)?
    A. Shortened endogenous circadian period
    B. Reduced response to photic entrainment
    C. More rapid accumulation of homeostatic sleep drive
    D. More rapid dissipation of homeostatic sleep drive

18. A 68-year-old widowed male falls asleep easily around 7:30 PM and awakens feeling refreshed by 4:00 AM. This schedule has not been problematic for him in the past; however, he has started dating and feels very sleepy during dinners beginning after 6:00 PM. Despite pushing himself to remain awake later, he still awakens at 4:00 AM. Which treatment option is most likely to be beneficial for this individual?
    A. Melatonin 0.5 mg at 4:00 AM, awakening with return to sleep
    B. Melatonin 3 mg approximately 3 hours prior to estimated DLMO (estimated at 5:30 PM)
    C. Full spectrum bright light exposure for approximately 2 hours beginning at 6:00 PM
    D. A progressive 3-hour delay in sleep-wake times every 2 days until desired sleep-wake time has been achieved

19. A 78-year-old man with Alzheimer's dementia is brought to sleep clinic by his 24-hour per day caregiver. She notes that the patient is very sleepy during the day, and she often finds him sleeping in the recliner for 2 hours at a time, multiple times per day. Despite this degree of tiredness he seems to have a difficult time staying asleep at night, as he is often up in the middle of the night watching TV. The caregiver has enforced strict habits to improve sleep, such as no TV in the bedroom, no caffeine after 1:00 PM, no heavy meals or exercise within 4 hours of bedtime, but nothing seems to help. The sleep physician obtains actigraphy (Fig. 37.3) and diagnoses this patient with ISWRD. Which of the following confirms the diagnosis ISWRD?
    A. The presence of excessive sleepiness
    B. The presence of insomnia
    C. Actigraphy showing a progressive delay of the sleep-wake period
    D. Actigraphy demonstrating least 3 sleep bouts per 24-hour period

20. In regard to the previous patient, which of the following treatment options should be considered?
    A. White broad spectrum light therapy at 4000 lux for 2 hours at 09:00 AM
    B. Doxepin 3 mg at bedtime
    C. Melatonin, 1 mg 2 hours before habitual bedtime
    D. Melatonin, 1 mg 5 hours prior to habitual bedtime in conjunction with white spectrum light therapy of 4000 lux

21. An art professor who typically sleeps well from 10:00 PM to 6:00 AM is flying from New York (EDT) to California (Pacific Daylight Time [PDT] = EDT-5). Without targeted treatment, in what direction and with what magnitude will his endogenous circadian rhythm adjust to destination time?
    A. Advance, 60 min/day
    B. Delay, 60 min/day
    C. Advance, 90 min/day
    D. Delay 90 min/day

22. The same individual in the question noted previously is giving a lecture from 6:00 PM to 8:00 PM the first day he arrives

in California. He is concerned he will be sleepy during this lecture and would like to make some modifications prior to departure. Which is the best intervention to assist with appropriately shifting his sleep-wake schedule?

A. Melatonin 1 mg 3 hours before estimated DLMO for 3 days prior to departure

B. Avoidance of bright light after 7:00 PM, including use of blue spectrum blocking lenses and full spectrum 4000 lux light therapy from 06:00 AM to 07:00 AM for 3 days prior to departure

C. Melatonin 0.5 mg at 06:00 AM the day before departure

D. Bright light therapy from 08:00 PM to 10:00 PM daily for 2–3 days prior to departure, and avoidance of bright light upon awakening with blue spectrum blocking lenses

23. Which of the following accurately describes the sleep-wake disturbances in dementia?

A. Although the sleep-wake rhythm is disrupted, melatonin rhythms remain normal.

B. Increased fragmentation of the rest activity pattern correlates with degree of cognitive impairment.

C. The circadian rest activity amplitude is increased.

D. Circadian clock gene expression remains synchronized throughout the brain.

24. A 20-year-old female presents to sleep clinic with intermittent insomnia and sleepiness beginning 3 years ago. She would sleep well for around 3 days at a time and then have difficulty falling asleep with subsequent daytime sleepiness. She had such severe sleepiness during the school day at times that she withdrew from high school and was home schooled by her mother, who lets her "sleep when she wants," which is sometimes during the day but other times at night. She is healthy with the exception of depression. She would like to go to college one day and does not think she can on this schedule. You obtain actigraphy to evaluate the patient's sleep-wake symptoms (Fig. 37.4). Which of the following is true regarding the patient's presentation?

A. Psychiatric comorbidity is common in this group.

B. This disorder is more often seen in females.

C. Sleep duration is often shorter than age adjusted normative values.

D. Overnight PSG in this patient would demonstrate increased sleep onset latency and reduced sleep efficiency during the first half of the night.

25. What is the most likely underlying pathophysiology of the previously noted case?

A. Shortened endogenous circadian period

B. Impaired ability to phase shift in response to bright light

C. Enhanced accumulation of homeostatic sleep pressure

D. Alteration of the normal phase angle between the endogenous circadian phase and actual sleep-wake timing

26. A 20-year-old athlete flies from Mexico City (central daylight time [CDT]) to Calgary (MDT = CDT-1) to compete in a track and field event. He notes decreased appetite and stomach upset, fatigue, and impaired performance during practice the day of his arrival. Which of the following statements is accurate regarding his symptoms?

A. Impaired performance would not be expected from jet lag.

B. His gastrointestinal symptoms are thought to be secondary to food consumption out of alignment with the circadian timing system.

C. His symptoms are likely secondary to travel fatigue.

D. His symptoms will resolve with appropriately timed light and melatonin to entrain circadian phase to destination time.

27. A 42-year-old male who has been totally blind since birth notes that he has episodes of difficulty falling asleep and severe daytime sleepiness; however, sometimes sleep is not a problem for him at all, and he falls asleep and stays asleep well with good daytime alertness. He notes that sometimes he is even a "great sleeper and is out by 8 PM." You obtain sleep logs and plot the patient's sleep-wake times (Fig. 37.5). What is the most likely underlying pathophysiology of his sleep-wake disorder?

A. Degeneration of suprachiasmatic nucleus cells

B. Complete loss of rod and cone visual photoreceptors

C. Absence of light input to the circadian timing system

D. Missense mutation of the *CK1δ* gene

28. In regard to the previously noted case, which therapy is most likely to effectively entrain the circadian phase?

A. Morning full spectrum light of 4000 lux beginning on March 1st

B. Melatonin 0.5 mg at 9:00 PM beginning on March 1st

C. Melatonin 0.5 mg at 9:00 PM beginning on February 15th

D. Melatonin 10 mg at 9:00 PM beginning on February 15th

29. A 37-year-old male reports insomnia and is falling asleep at work. This has developed in the context of a change in his shift as a respiratory therapist from 7 AM–5 PM to 9 PM–7 AM.

His bedtime is 8:30 AM. He typically takes 15–30 minutes to fall asleep and sleeps well for around 4 hours. His sleep then becomes light and fragmented. At 2–3 PM he usually gives up and gets out of bed. He feels exhausted at work and will often doze off if he is not involved in direct patient care. This is facilitated by the dim lighting in his office. He looks forward to his 3 days off where he can finally "sleep like a normal person," which for him, is about 11:00 PM–7:00 AM. He always slept well prior to his change to night shift and hopes to improve his symptoms.

Which of the following is accurate in regard to this patient's disorder?

A. This disorder is present in nearly 50% of individuals working nonconventional shifts.

B. This disorder is due to low circadian alerting signal during the time allotted for sleep.

C. This disorder is due to buildup of homeostatic sleep drive, coinciding with the start of the daytime sleep bout.

D. This disorder is due to a desynchrony between the internal circadian timing system and the externally imposed sleep-wake schedule.

30. What do you recommend in the individual in the previous case to maximize *both* circadian alignment and alertness with night shift work?

A. Modafinil 200 mg 1 hour before the shift

B. Melatonin 3 mg prior to the daytime sleep bout

C. Bright light exposure during his shift and sunglasses on the commute home

D. Napping in conjunction with caffeine

Answers

1. **The correct answer is A.**

This adolescent has difficulty falling asleep and waking up at the desired conventional times with resultant sleepiness that

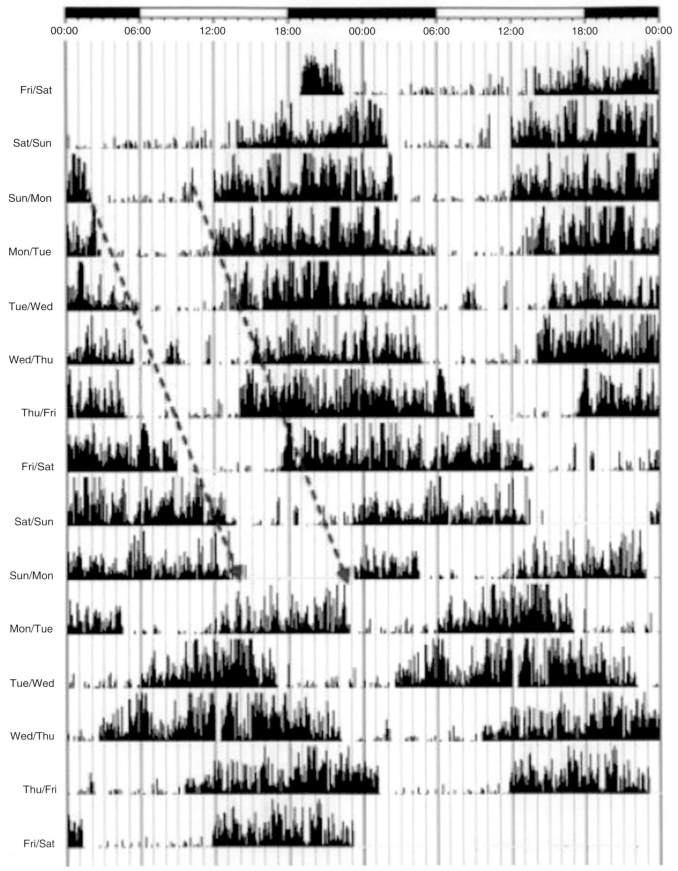

• **Figure 37.4** Actigraphy. Two days are plotted on each horizontal line (with the second day repeated as the first on the next line). *Black* lines represent activity. (Used with permission from Endara-Bravo AS, Thammasitboon S, Thomas D. Free-running disorder in a sighted adolescent. *J Pediatr.* 2012;160[5]:877.)

case 1

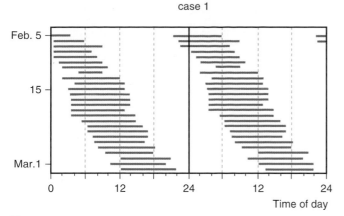

• **Figure 37.5** *Green* Rectangles Represent Sleep Times. Two days are plotted on each horizontal line (with the second day repeated as the first on the next line).

is particularly pronounced during the morning. Although he has insomnia at sleep onset, chronic insomnia does not explain his symptoms, as he slept well during the summer at his self-selected, later sleep times. This is not a central hypersomnia, as when his sleep duration is adequate, he is not sleepy. The patient's presentation is consistent with the circadian rhythm sleep-wake disorder, DSWPD.[1]

Sleep-wake patterns are well known to delay in adolescents. Although initially felt to be primarily behavioral, physiological changes of the homeostatic and circadian regulation of sleep may explain the shift to evening preference.[2,3] In particular, the circadian period may become longer in adolescence[3] resulting in a later circadian phase due to the greater the amount of adjustment required to entrain the internal clock to the 24-hour light-dark cycle.[4,5]

A mutation of the *hPer2* gene has been described in ASWPD, not DSWPD.[6] A slower accumulation of process S during wake has been seen in mature adolescents compared with pre- or early pubertal adolescents.[7] Increased accumulation of homeostatic sleep drive would facilitate sleep onset. Enhancement of the advance portion of the PRC to bright light would theoretically result in a tendency to advance as opposed to delay circadian phase (Fig. 37.6).[8–10]

2. **The correct answer is D.**
This patient has evening sleepiness and early morning awakenings in the context of adhering to a conventional schedule but sleeps well and feels alert when keeping her own desired, early sleep-wake times of 7:30 PM–4 AM. This presentation is consistent with ASWPD.[1] Actigraphy, at minimum for 7 days but preferably 14 days, would demonstrate a stable advance of the habitual sleep period.[1]

Polysomnography is not indicated in the evaluation of circadian rhythm sleep-wake disorders unless another sleep disorder (particularly, a sleep related breathing disorder) is suspected. However, if conducted at conventional laboratory times, shortened sleep onset latency and shortened REM latency may be seen.[11,12] DLMO is early in ASWPD,[12–14] and in this patient would be expected around 6:00 PM. Individuals with ASWPD would be expected to score as morning types (59 and above) on the MEQ (see Appendix 4).[15]

3. **The correct answer is B.**
Assuming a normal phase relationship between sleep-wake times and endogenous circadian timing, this individual's core body temperature minimum (CBT_{min}) is around 4:00–5:00 AM EDT, and DLMO is around 9:00 PM EDT (Fig. 37.7). Because circadian phase does not change instantaneously with the abrupt change in the external light-dark cycle secondary to jet travel, CBT_{min} and DLMO will correspond with BST of 9:00–10:00 AM and 2:00 AM, respectively (see Fig. 37.7). Therefore this individual will be delayed in respect to BST, and a phase advance is required to align with local time. Based on the PRCs to bright light and melatonin (see Fig. 37.6), bright light exposure after arrival at 11:15 AM BST and melatonin at bedtime around 11:00 PM will correspond with the phase advance portions of both the PRCs to bright light and melatonin (see Fig. 37.7). A systematic review of 12 placebo-controlled trials of melatonin, mostly in the context of eastward travel, found that melatonin strengths 0.5–10 mg both prior to and after arrival in destination demonstrated an improvement in jet lag symptoms.[16] Sleep duration and quality improved with melatonin and objective measures of circadian phase demonstrated faster entrainment to destination time.[16] Appropriately timed light exposure has demonstrated improvement in jet lag symptoms and sleep in simulated studies of eastward travel[17–21] and real life travel situations.[22,23]

Avoiding bright light after arrival in London at 11:15 will result in avoidance of bright light during the phase advance portion of the PRC to bright light. To produce a phase advance while at origin location (Detroit), taking melatonin as early as 4:00 PM would be beneficial; however, melatonin at 4:00 PM destination time (immediately after arrival) will fall into the phase delay portion of the melatonin PRC.[24] Taking melatonin at 11:15 AM will also fall into the phase delay portion of the melatonin PRC.[24] Since aligning to local time (and thus reducing jet lag symptoms) requires a phase advance, none of the other answer choices are appropriate.

4. **The correct answer is D.**
Shift workers sleep on average 30–60 minutes less than day workers,[25–27] and individuals who meet criteria for shift work disorder sleep almost 1.5 hours shorter on average than day workers without sleep complaints.[28] Evening shift work may be the most advantageous, as evening shift workers have significantly longer sleep duration on average than rotating shift workers, permanent night shift workers, and permanent day shift workers.[27]

Night shift workers have shorter sleep duration than day shift workers, as noted previously. Individuals with shift work disorder sleep less than day workers but that difference is closer to 90 minutes.[28]

5. **The correct answer is C.**
This individual has difficulty falling asleep and waking at conventional times but slept well when able to self-select a later schedule on weekends and prior to taking this job. She has developed both insomnia of sleep onset and daytime sleepiness due to her inability to adhere to an earlier sleep-wake schedule. These symptoms are suggestive of the circadian rhythm sleep-wake disorder DSWPD.[1]

In a group of 205 patients with DSWPD, more than 50% reported a history of depression. In another cohort, 64% of DSWPD patients were in a moderate to severely depressed state.[29,30]

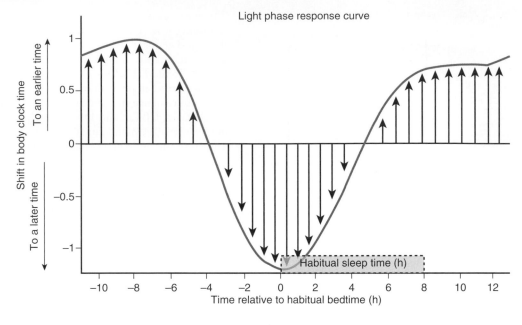

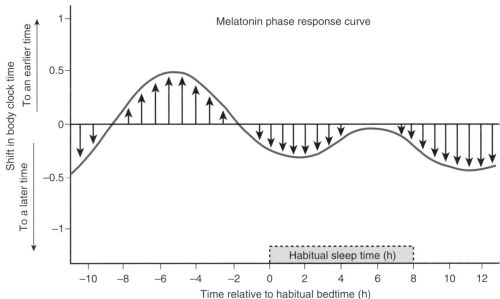

• **Figure 37.6** Phase Response Curves (PRCs) to Bright Light and Melatonin. The *x*-axis depicts time in hours from the start of habitual sleep time (zero is equivalent to habitual sleep onset). The magnitude of circadian shift is depicted on the *y*-axis, with phase advances denoted by positive numbers and phase delays denoted by negative numbers. PRCs predict the response of the circadian timing system to stimuli delivered at different times. PRCs provide estimates only, and may differ by the strength of the stimuli as well as the testing protocol. The PRCs in this figure were derived from a 1-hour pulse of full spectrum bright light and 3 days of 0.5 mg melatonin (scaled appropriately here to demonstrate one time dosing). (Used with permission from Emens JS, Burgess HJ. Effect of light and melatonin and other melatonin receptor agonists on human circadian physiology. *Sleep Med Clin.* 2015;10[4]:435–453.)

Circadian disruption has been implicated in impaired glucose metabolism but not destruction of insulin producing beta-cells.[31] Although there is a subtype of insomnia due to mental disorder and anxiety has a bidirectional relationship with insomnia,[32] her insomnia resolves with sleeping at selected times so is attributable to DSWPD.[1] Beta-1-blockers, not ACE inhibitors, interrupt sympathetic signaling to the pineal gland, which results in decreased secretion of melatonin (Fig. 37.8).[33–35]

6. **The correct answer is B.**
The actigraphy of this patient shows sleep onset typically by 8:00 PM and sleep offset at 4:00 AM. These findings in the context of sleepiness in the evening and awakening before desired when attempting to adhere to conventional sleep-wake times is consistent with ASWPD. Multiple familial cases with an autosomal mode of inheritance of the disorder have been identified.[12–14,36]

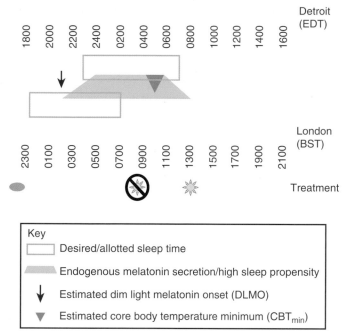

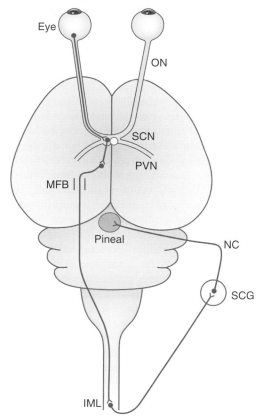

• **Figure 37.7** Relationship of estimated endogenous circadian rhythm in relation to habitual sleep bout at location of origin (Eastern Daylight Time [EDT]) and desired sleep bout at destination (British Summer Time [BST]). Melatonin and light avoidance/exposure is timed strategically at the destination to produce phase advance, such that the endogenous circadian rhythm aligns with local time.

There does not appear to be a gender predilection of this disorder. Prevalence is uncertain and likely rare,[37] but in one group of middle aged individuals the prevalence was around 1%.[38] ASWPD is more frequent with advancing age.[1]

7. **The correct answer is A.**
This patient presents with difficulty falling asleep prior to 4:00 AM, resulting in sleep loss and excessive daytime sleep when he needs to awaken in the morning to attend class. When he sleeps adequate hours, he has normal levels of alertness; therefore his presentation is most consistent with the circadian rhythm sleep-wake disorder, DSWPD. Individuals with DSWPD typically score as evening types on the MEQ, a validated tool to assess time of day preference or chronotype.[15] Scores of 41 and below indicate "evening types," scores of 59 and above indicate "morning types," and scores between 42 and 58 indicate "intermediate types."[15]

Although not typically used in a clinical setting, DLMO, the time of initial endogenous melatonin secretion in dim light, is the most reliable marker of circadian timing.[39] DLMO is approximately 2–3 hours before habitual bedtime,[40] so in this individual it would be expected around 1:00–2:00 AM. Sleep duration is typically normal for age[41] in individuals with DSWPD; therefore, if PSG was conducted at the patients' preferred sleep times, sleep duration should not be decreased. However, if PSG was conducted during conventional sleep laboratory times, sleep onset may be prolonged.

Actigraphy is a wrist worn device that uses accelerometry to measure movement. Actigraphy is an accurate way to estimate sleep-wake patterns and would be an appropriate test to evaluate this individual with a suspected circadian rhythm sleep-wake disorder[1]; however, actigraphy has greater sensitivity for sleep (>90%) and lower specificity (approximately 30%–50%).[42–44]

• **Figure 37.8** The suprachiasmatic nucleus (SCN) sends projections to the paraventricular nucleus of the hypothalamus (PVN). During the day, the SCN inhibits the PVN, but during the night, inhibition is released. Excitatory projections from the PVN travel via the medial forebrain bundle (MFB) to the sympathetic preganglionic neurons in the intermediolateral cell column (IML). The IML sends cholinergic projections to the superior cervical ganglion (SCG). From the SCG, postganglionic sympathetic neurons send noradrenergic projections to the alpha and beta receptors in the pineal gland resulting in the production of melatonin. (Used with permission from Moore RY. Neural control of the pineal gland. *Behav Brain Res.* 1996;73[1–2]:125–130.)

8. **The correct answer is C.**
Ramelteon is an MT1 and MT2 receptor agonist that is capable of shifting circadian phase in both humans and animals. Although the complete ramelteon PRC unknown, it appears to shift the circadian rhythm in a similar manner to melatonin.[45,46] After an abrupt advance in the light-dark cycle by 5 hours (comparable to eastward travel of five time zones), 1, 2, and 4 mg doses of ramelteon resulted in significant advances of dim light melatonin offset.[45]

Ramelteon has a higher affinity for MT1/MT2 receptors than melatonin.[47] A higher dose of ramelteon of (8 mg) did not produce a significant phase advance, potentially due to active drug or metabolites spilling later into the night and producing a phase delay as is possible with melatonin.[45] A phase advance as opposed to phase delay is needed to entrain to simulated eastward travel.

9. **The correct answer is B.**
In familial forms of ASWPD, genetic alterations have been identified. These include a missense mutation in the casein kinase I epsilon (CKIε) binding region of *hPer2* in one family[48] and a missense mutation of the *CK1δ* gene in another.[49] These mutations both affected circadian period.

The mutation of *hPer2* and *CK1δ* are described previously. VNTRs polymorphisms of *hPer3* have been associated with diurnal preference and response to sleep deprivation but not familial ASWPD.[50]

10. **The correct answer is C.**

In sighted individuals with N24SWD, the steady delay of sleep-wake patterns is typically seen in the absence of social constraints that interfere with daytime sleep. As most individuals will continue attempts to adhere to a day wake, night sleep schedule, the classic free running appearance is seen only when the high propensity for sleep onset coincides with night/early morning. However, when the high propensity for sleep onset delays to a mid or late morning clock time, sleep episodes are extremely disrupted as the individual attempts to remain awake to adhere to everyday obligations. During this time, more than 50% of individuals will demonstrate phase "jumps" where the sleep-wake cycle delays more rapidly.[51] This finding is likely secondary to daylight, coinciding with the delay portion of the PRC to bright light.[51,52]

A stable progressive delay of sleep-wake times (the classic 'free running' pattern) is typically seen when individuals do not have social constraints that require daytime wakefulness.[52] Individuals with N24SWD have a longer than normal circadian period; 24.18 is the approximate 'normal' circadian period.[53] A sleep pattern with multiple sleep bouts (at least 3) dispersed through the 24-hour day is suggestive of ISWRD, not N24SWD.

11. **The correct answer is B.**

Melatonin given the hour before bedtime has demonstrated improvement in both parental reported total sleep time[54] and actigraphically recorded total sleep time[55] in children with both ISWRD and neurological disorders including autism.[56] Therefore the American Academy of Sleep Medicine (AASM) recommends this treatment option for children and adolescents with neurological disorders and ISWRD.

Melatonin has been studied in children/adolescents with ISWRD, and autism and benefit was demonstrated and no serious adverse events were seen.[56] Melatonin may be used as a stand-alone treatment without bright light.[56] Both objective and subjective improvement in sleep have been reported, as noted previously.

12. **The correct answer is D.**

Shift work has been associated with multiple health conditions including gastrointestinal disorders,[28,57,58] mood disturbances,[28] obesity,[59] diabetes,[59] cardiovascular disease,[60] reproductive dysfunction,[61] and cancer.[62,63] Shift work has been associated with breast cancer, and meta-analyses have estimated increased risk of up to 20%.[62] The suppression of endogenous melatonin secretion by light at night is thought to underlie this relationship, as melatonin may serve a protective benefit against neoplastic processes such as mutagenesis, oxidative damage, DNA abnormalities, and impaired immunity.[63]

Period3 (*hPer3*) is one of the core components of the molecular circadian clock. This gene contains a VNTR polymorphism in which a 54-nucleotide coding-region segment is repeated 4 or 5 times. Polymorphisms of the *hPer3* VNTR are implicated in circadian preference and response to sleep loss in reference to circadian timing.[50] Individuals with shift work disorder who carry the five repeat variant of the *hPer3* VNTR are more likely to manifest sleepiness than those with the four repeat variant who report insomnia as the predominant

symptom.[64] *hPer3* plays is involved in tumor suppression and mixed results have been found regarding the role of the five repeat variant of the *hPer3*VNTR in conferring an increased risk of breast cancer.[65–67] Recent meta-analyses found that short sleep duration does not confer an increased risk of breast cancer in shift workers 0.96 (95% CI 0.86–1.06); therefore it is unlikely to be the sole factor responsible for this association. A dose response relationship has been found with increased incidence of breast cancer with longer years of shift work.[63]

13. **The correct answer is A.**

The internal timing system typically undergoes a phase delay to align with destination time during westward travel and phase advance to entrain to local time after eastward travel. However, with travel of eight or more time zones eastward, the circadian rhythm may delay as opposed to advance.[68–70] This phenomenon is known as antidromic shifting and is due to exposure of the delay portion of the light PRC to a time of day when bright light is ample. Although the magnitude of phase shift required is larger in the phase delay direction (Fig. 37.9), this shift may be easier because of both light availability and the predilection for the circadian clock to delay, as opposed to advance due to a circadian tau greater than 24 hours.[53] This is particularly important in an individual who cannot shift their sleep-wake schedule prior to departure. In the individual described previously, his estimated CBT_{min} will be around 4:00 AM MDT, which coincides with 2:00 PM GST (see Fig. 37.9). Bright light is readily available in the hours leading up to 2:00 PM and easy to avoid thereafter, facilitating a phase delay.

Avoidance of daytime bright light in Dubai and exposure to bright light in the evening with a light box will produce a phase advance which may be both more difficult to achieve and impractical with travel. Melatonin 3 mg 1–2 hours before bedtime in Dubai will likely have a soporific effect as it is not being produced endogenously[71]; however, the phase shifting effect is less clear at this time, as it nears the crossover point from delay to advance.[24,72,73] Additionally, this answer choice also recommends a light avoidance/exposure regimen to achieve a phase advance, which is more difficult to achieve than a phase delay in this setting. Studies of eastward travel have demonstrated improvement in sleep and jet lag symptoms with zolpidem.[74,75] However, hypnotics must be used with care in jet lag, due to potential side effects. The US Food and Drug Administration (FDA) has issued a safety warning that recommends 5 mg as the starting of dose of zolpidem in women. This reduction in starting dose was prompted by the finding that next day blood levels of zolpidem are high enough to negatively impact alertness and driving performance.[76]

14. **The correct answer is C.**

The actigraphy recording on this individual demonstrates sleep onset around 3:00 AM–6:00 AM and sleep offset between 11:00 AM and 12:00 PM, placing estimated DLMO between 12 AM and 4 AM (2–3 hours before habitual sleep onset).[40] Strategically timed melatonin is recommended for the treatment of DSWPD.[56] Evidence suggests the phase advancing (movement of the circadian rhythm earlier) effects of melatonin are greatest when given prior to DLMO (see Fig. 37.6),[24,72,73,77] with greater phase advances produced with earlier dosing.[77,78] Melatonin is typically well tolerated; however, caution must be exercised, as melatonin is a dietary supplement and not regulated by the FDA.

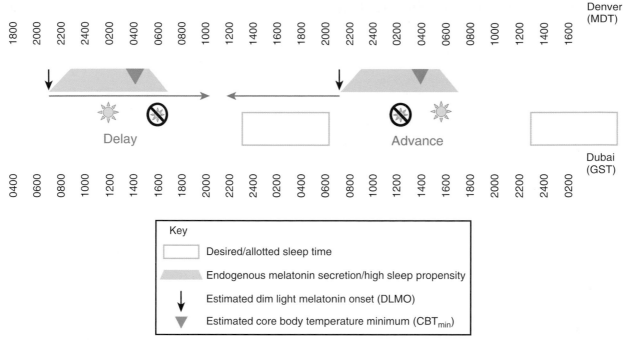

• **Figure 37.9** Relationship of estimated endogenous circadian rhythm in relation to desired sleep-wake timing with eastward travel of 10 time zones. Times are double plotted. A shorter number of hours is required if endogenous circadian phase advances (10 hours) to align with local time than if endogenous circadian phase delays (14 hours). However, estimated core body temperature minimum immediately after travel is positioned such that bright light is ample prior to core body temperature minimum and less available after core body temperature minimum. CBT_{min}, Core body temperature minimum; *DLMO*, dim light melatonin onset; *GST*, gulf standard time; *MDT*, mountain daylight time.

Tasimelteon is used and is currently approved by the FDA for the management of circadian rhythm sleep-wake disorder and non-24-hour sleep-wake rhythm disorder.[79] The crossover point from light producing a phase delay to phase advance is approximately 3 hours prior to habitual wake time[8–10] around the time of the minimum of core body temperature (see Fig. 37.6), such that in this patient, bright light prior to 8:00–9:00 AM could result in a phase delay, and bright light after that time would result in a phase advance.

15. **The correct answer is B.**
The patient in this case has difficulty falling asleep at conventional hours but not during self-selected, later times on free days. This is consistent with the DSWPD.[1]

The primary zeitgeber, or time giver, synchronizing the internal circadian timing system to the 24-hour day is bright light.[80] Light is transmitted to the suprachiasmatic nucleus by a subset of melanopsin containing retinal ganglion cells,[81] which give rise to the retinohypothalamic tract.[82] The retinohypothalamic tract is required for photic entrainment of the circadian timing system.[83]

The circadian timing system is most sensitive to blue and short-wavelength green light, as the peak sensitivity of melanopsin is 450–500 nm.[84,85] Rods and cones are not necessary for transmission of light to the circadian timing system,[80] as demonstrated by the preserved retinohypothalamic pathway in some individuals with blindness.[86] The phase shifting effect of bright light is nonlinear; 100 lux (1%) is responsible for half of the resetting properties of a 10,000 lux light stimulus.[87]

16. **The correct answer is C.**
Exogenous melatonin has the ability to shift circadian phase. Melatonin given a few hours prior to DLMO is capable of producing a phase advance based on the melatonin PRC (see Fig. 37.6).[24,72,73,77] Specifically, in children and adolescents with DSWPD, melatonin has been demonstrated to significantly advance sleep onset time,[88–90] reduce sleep latency,[88] and advance circadian phase as measured by DLMO.[89,90] Doses either based on weight (0.05–0.15 mg/kg)[88] or absolute doses of 3–5 mg[89,90] have been used 1.5–2 hours before bedtime[88] or at 06:00–07:00 PM[89,90] in randomized controlled trials with success.

Melatonin has demonstrated efficacy in children/adolescents with DSWPD comorbid with ADHD and other psychiatric disorders.[89,90] Sleep onset latency decreases of around 40 min have been demonstrated with the use of melatonin in DSWPD.[88] Melatonin should be strategically timed based on the PRC to melatonin, and is expected to produce the greatest benefit when administered prior to DLMO; therefore giving during an awakening from sleep is not likely to be beneficial.

17. **The correct answer is A.**
An individual with FASWPD as well as an individual with nonfamilial ASWPD have demonstrated endogenous circadian period or Tau shorter than 24 hours.[12,91]

Interestingly, in the case of shortened circadian tau in FASWPD, a serine to glycine mutation within the casein kinase I epsilon (CKIε) binding region of *hPer2* was identified. This mutation causes hypophosphorylation by CKIε in vitro, which alters the circadian period.[48] In another family with FASWPD, although circadian period was not determined, a mutation of $CK1\delta$ was found, and shortened circadian period was observed in the presence of this mutation in transgenic mice.[49]

The average intrinsic period of the circadian pacemaker is just longer than 24 hours.[53] Shortening of the endogenous circadian period would be expected to result in an earlier onset of sleep relative to the 24-hour environmental light-dark cycle.[92]

FASWPD disordered patients have not been demonstrated to have a reduced response to photic entrainment. Additionally, in an individual with ASWPD (nonfamilial), the responsiveness to photic entrainment was intact and even somewhat enhanced.[91] Although more rapid accumulation and dissipation of homeostatic sleep drive could result in earlier sleep onset and offset, this has not been demonstrated in FASWPD.

18. **The correct answer is C.**
The patient described in this case has a stable advance of sleep-wake times with profound evening sleepiness and early morning awakenings when attempting to conform to a later schedule. These symptoms are consistent with ASWPD.[1]

Evening light therapy is recommended for treatment of ASWPD.[56] A parallel group study compared bright, 4000 lux white light to dim red light between 8:00 PM and 11:00 PM for 2 hours, ending before habitual bedtime in patients with ASWPD. The bright light group demonstrated a significant delay in circadian phase and increased total sleep time.[93] Therefore strategically timed light during the phase delay portion of the PRC to bright light (see Fig. 37.6) is the only therapy listed that would benefit ASWPD disorder. As per the PRC to bright light, positioning therapy at 6:00 PM is likely to result in a phase delay in this patient.

Although melatonin dosed at 4:00 AM would fall in the phase delay portion of the PRC to melatonin (see Fig. 37.6) melatonin is not indicated in ASWPD due to lack of evidence to use melatonin for this purpose.[56,94] Additionally, melatonin at this time would confer increased risk of side effects (e.g., excessive daytime sleepiness).[94] Melatonin dosed as described in answer B would produce a phase advance not delay. Chronotherapy with a progressive delay of sleep-wake times may be considered for DSWPD. Chronotherapy in the opposite direction, advancement of the sleep-wake schedule 3 hours every 2 days, has been described as effective in one individual with ASWPD.[56]

19. **The correct answer is D.**
ISWRD is a circadian rhythm sleep-wake disorder characterized by a chronic pattern of irregular sleep where sleep periods are dispersed throughout a 24-hour day resulting in the complaint of excessive sleepiness (napping) during the daytime and insomnia during the typical sleep period.[1] At least three sleep bouts during a 24-hour day are required for diagnosis. Multiple sleep bouts may be demonstrated by a sleep log or actigraphy (at least 7 days, but preferably 14 should be recorded).[1]

Excessive daytime sleepiness and insomnia are presenting symptoms of ISWRD; however, at least three sleep bouts per 24-hour period are required for the diagnosis.[1] A progressive delay of the sleep-wake period would be seen with non-24-hour sleep-wake rhythm disorder.[1]

20. **The correct answer is A.**
Bright light therapy tested at levels from 1000 to 8000 lux from 45 minutes to 2 hours has demonstrated benefits in

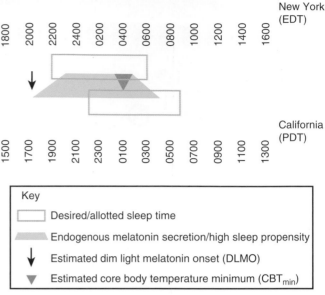

• **Figure 37.10** Relationship of estimated endogenous circadian rhythm in relation to habitual sleep bout at location of origin (Eastern Daylight Time [EDT]) and desired sleep bout at destination (Pacific Daylight Time [PDT].) CBT_{min}, Core body temperature minimum; *DLMO*, dim light melatonin onset.

behavior, cognition, and mood, and resulted in improved consolidation of rest and activity periods in elderly, demented individuals with ISWRD.[56] In particular, two randomized controlled trials of institutionalized elderly subjects used bright light from 2500 to 5000 lux for 1–2 hours between 9 and 11 AM.[95,96] Significant improvements in behavior were seen in the light therapy groups including decreased wandering, violent behavior, restlessness, and delirium.[95,96]

Due to the potential for adverse effects in this patient population, hypnotic medications are not indicated for ISWRD in older, demented individuals. Melatonin, alone[97] or in addition to bright light therapy,[96] has not demonstrated benefit in ISWRD. Due to the negative impact on mood and functioning and lack of benefit, melatonin is not recommended for ISWRD.[56]

21. **The correct answer is D.**
The endogenous circadian clock does not adjust immediately after jet travel; however, because light is the strongest entraining factor, re-entrainment of the circadian clock to the new light-dark cycle will occur over time. With eastward travel the circadian clock typically phase advances (see Fig. 37.7) to align with the new time zone and with westward travel, a phase delay is required (Fig. 37.10). Without targeted treatment, the circadian timing system will adjust to destination time by advancing roughly 1 hour per day after eastward travel and delaying 1.5 hours per day after westward travel.[98] The sleep-wake cycle is easier to delay than advance, as the average human circadian tau is just over 24 hours and therefore tends to drift later, even in the absence of any time cues.[53]

22. **The correct answer is D.**
A delay of the circadian timing system is required to align to destination time after westward travel. This may be achieved even before departure with appropriately timed light. Based on the PRC to light (see Fig. 37.6), bright light in the evening prior to CBT_{min} and avoidance of bright light in the morning

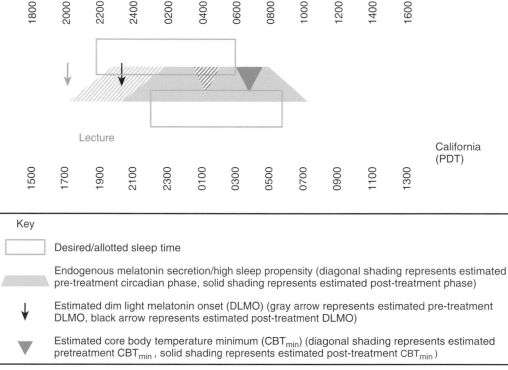

• **Figure 37.11** Relationship of estimated endogenous circadian rhythm in relation to habitual sleep bout at location of origin (Eastern Daylight Time [EDT]) and desired sleep bout at destination (Pacific Daylight Time [PDT]). After a pre travel phase delay, internal circadian timing aligns appropriately with desired sleep-wake times at destination.

after the CBT_{min} will produce a phase delay[8–10] such that his circadian phase is no longer advanced in respect to PDT after landing (Fig. 37.11), reducing the potential for sleepiness during his evening lecture.

Melatonin prior to DLMO will result in a phase advance which is the opposite of the desired effect. Avoidance of evening bright light and exposure to morning bright light will also produce a phase advance. Melatonin at 6:00 AM would fall into the delay portion of the melatonin PRC;[24,72,73,77] however, due to next day sedation, this is not a recommended method to shift circadian phase.

23. **The correct answer is B.**
An irregular sleep-wake pattern and reduced amplitude of the circadian rest activity pattern has been demonstrated frequently in elderly individuals with dementia.[99–101] Importantly, greater fragmentation of the rest activity was independently associated with lower levels of cognitive performance, even when total amounts of rest and activity were similar.[101]

In addition to abnormal sleep-wake patterns, objective markers of circadian phase are abnormal with increased melatonin levels during the daytime in demented patients.[102] The circadian rest activity amplitude is decreased, not increased. After death, circadian expression of clock genes was present in Alzheimer's patients but not synchronized across different brain regions.[103]

24. **The correct answer is A.**
This patient has episodic insomnia and excessive daytime sleepiness with intervening periods of normal sleep along with actigraphy demonstrating a progressive delay of sleep-wake

times. These findings are consistent with the circadian rhythm sleep-wake disorder non-24-hour sleep-wake disorder.[1] Individuals with this disorder demonstrate a sleep-wake cycle longer than 24 hours, with a steady delay of sleep-wake times typically by 1 hour per day but dependent on the endogenous circadian period.[1] Symptoms vary based on when sleep and waking are attempted in reference to the circadian propensity for sleep and wakefulness. For example the individual may have a few days without sleep complaints when the high propensity for sleep aligns with the environmental night, but as the time of high propensity for sleep drifts later (in relation to the 24-hour day) the patient will have insomnia of sleep onset and morning sleepiness. If continued attempts to sleep at night and wake during the day are made, the patient will begin to have marked difficulty achieving sleep, and night and daytime sleepiness will become more pronounced.[1] Although most common in individuals with total blindness (approximately two-thirds of totally blind patients will have the disorder), multiple case reports of non-24-hour sleep-wake rhythm in sighted individuals have been published,[52] including a case series of 57 individuals.[104] In this series, around 70% of patients were male and nearly 30% had comorbid psychiatric disorders.[104] Psychiatric disorders often precede the development of N24SWD and include schizophrenia, bipolar disorder, depression, obsessive-compulsive disorder, or schizoid personality.[52]

As noted previously, most individuals with this disorder are male. Sleep duration in individuals with non-24-hour sleep-wake rhythm is normal to long, with median sleep duration of 9 hours.[104] Findings on PSG would be dependent on when the PSG is conducted in reference to intrinsic circadian timing, and therefore would vary.[105]

25. **The correct answer is D.**

Bright light is the most potent stimuli to entrain circadian phase.[106] The effect of light on the circadian timing system is dependent on the time of exposure in reference to endogenous circadian phase. Bright light after the core body temperature nadir (in the early morning in normally entrained individuals) moves the circadian rhythm earlier (phase advance) and bright light prior to the core body temperature nadir (in the evening in normally entrained individuals) moves the circadian rhythm later (phase delay).[8-10] Bright light produces the largest magnitude phase shifts when delivered during the biological night, particularly when delivered close to the minimum of core body temperature (Fig. 37.6). Therefore the time the circadian system is most sensitive to bright light is masked by sleep, when individuals demonstrate a normal relationship between endogenous circadian phase and sleep-wake times. (Minimum core body temperature is positioned 4–6 hours after habitual sleep onset and 2–3 hours prior to habitual wake.)

In sighted individuals with non-24-hour sleep-wake disorder (N24SWD), the phase angle between endogenous circadian phase and sleep-wake timing is thought to be altered such that sleep is initiated at a later circadian phase.[107-109] Therefore more of the delay segment of the light PRC is exposed, and more of the advance segment of the light PRC remains during the sleep period. The cumulative effect of this abnormal phase angle is a perpetual phase delay.[52]

Lengthened as opposed to shortened, circadian tau has been demonstrated in individuals with N24SWD.[110] Although impaired ability of the circadian system to phase shift in response to bright light could theoretically be implicated in N24SWD in sighted individuals, only blunting of the ability of light to suppress melatonin has been demonstrated.[111,112] The alteration of phase angle may result from impaired ability of N24SWD patients to accumulate homeostatic sleep drive,[109] and has also been demonstrated in individuals with delayed sleep-wake phase disorder,[113] which may underlie the representation of these two disorders on a spectrum.

26. **The correct answer is C.**

This individual has symptoms of GI upset, impaired performance, and fatigue in the setting of travel that crosses only one time zone. A diagnosis of jet lag requires the presence of insomnia and/or excessive daytime sleepiness with impaired function, fatigue, or somatic complaints in the context of jet travel across at least two time zones.[1] Therefore the underlying cause of this patient's symptoms is not misalignment between endogenous circadian phase and destination time. His symptoms are most likely due to travel fatigue.[114] Travel fatigue is contributed to by disruption of normal sleep routine, dehydration, restricted space, and stress of travel, as opposed to circadian misalignment, and typically resolves with a good quality sleep period.[114]

Impairment of both cognitive and physical performance has been reported in jet lag.[114-116] Gastrointestinal disturbances are the most common somatic symptoms seen along with jet lag, and include decreased appetite and constipation.[114] These symptoms may be secondary to food consumption out of alignment with the circadian timing system;[117] however, this individual's symptoms are not due to jet lag, as he has not crossed at least two time zones.[1]

27. **The correct answer is C.**

This case depicts an individual completely blind from birth with insomnia and excessive daytime sleepiness alternating with days without sleep complaints and sleep logs demonstrating a progressive delay of sleep-wake times.[1] These findings are consistent with non-24-hour sleep-wake disorder (N24SWD).[1] Symptoms are dependent on the relationship of his endogenous circadian propensity for sleep with the external solar cycle.[1] When high propensity for sleep aligns with nighttime he has no sleep complaints; when high propensity for sleep onset occurs in the early morning hours there is prolonged sleep onset latency and excessive daytime sleepiness. When endogenous circadian phase has drifted (in respect to the 24-hour day) such that sleep onset is biologically timed in the early evening, the patient may notice particular ease falling asleep.

This disorder is thought to be present in up to two-thirds of totally blind individuals.[52] In totally blind individuals, light detection by the intrinsically photosensitive retinal ganglion cells is absent and therefore, the circadian timing system cannot be entrained to the 24-hour day as occurs in normal individuals upon daily exposure to morning bright light.[118] Sleep and wake occur based on the endogenous, non-24 hour circadian tau resulting in a cyclical sleep disturbance characterizing N24SWD.[52] Because the circadian tau is typically longer than 24 hours, this results in a sleep propensity that occurs at later clock times each day.

Degeneration of the suprachiasmatic nucleus would be expected to result in absence of a circadian rhythm as in irregular sleep-wake rhythm disorder. Rods and codes are responsible for visual photoreception but are not responsible for light detection for circadian entrainment. Intrinsically photosensitive retinal ganglion cells are responsible for light input to the circadian timing system via the retinohypothalamic tract.[119] Even if conscious vision is absent due to disruption of the rods and cones, if the retinal ganglion cells remain intact, light can be transmitted to the suprachiasmatic nucleus.[86,120-122] Missense mutation of the *CK1δ* gene has been implicated in advanced sleep-wake phase disorder, not N24SWD.[49] However, a single nucleotide polymorphism in the PER3 gene has been associated with N24SWD.[123]

28. **The correct answer is C.**

Melatonin has been shown to effectively entrain circadian phase in blind individuals.[118] The action of melatonin on the circadian timing system is approximately 180 degrees out of phase with bright light (see Fig. 37.6).[73] In normally entrained individuals, when dosed in the late afternoon/early evening, melatonin advances the circadian rhythm; when taken in the morning, it produces phase delays.[24,72,73,77] The phase shifting as well as sedative effects[71] of melatonin are greatest when it is not being secreted by the pineal gland. Therefore appropriately timed melatonin can oppose the perpetual delay of the sleep-wake cycle in N24SWD. Lower doses (0.5 mg) may be particularly effective,[124,125] and this may be due to the ability to correctly target the phase advance portion of the PRC to melatonin without crossing into the phase delay region,[72,126] which could be the case of higher doses that persistently elevate serum melatonin levels. In the case at hand, sleep onset on February 15th is between 2:00 AM and 4:00 AM (see Fig. 37.5); therefore, low-dose melatonin at 9:00 PM would be expected to produce a phase advance.

Even in individuals without conscious light perception, circadian entrainment may still occur with bright light (given

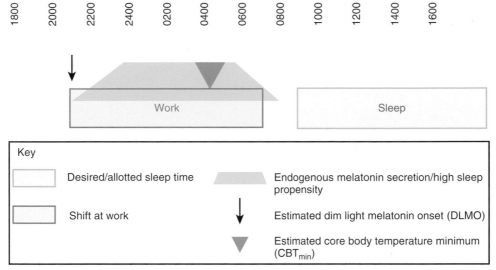

• **Figure 37.12** Relationship of estimated endogenous circadian rhythm in relation to night shift work. In an individual who has habitual sleep-wake times of 11:00 PM–7:00 AM, upon initiating night shift work, the high propensity for sleep and low circadian alerting signal coincide with work times. The nadir of alertness will occur near the end of the work shift. The allotted time for sleep will overlap with the time of high circadian alerting signal, and therefore sleep quality may be poor and sleep duration shorter.

the retinal ganglion cell layer is intact).[120] However, these individuals would not be expected to present with N24SWD, and further, morning bright light on March 1st would fall in the phase delay portion of the PRC to bright light (see Fig. 37.6). Melatonin given at 9 PM beginning on March 1st is unlikely to entrain circadian phase based on its timing in reference to endogenous phase (although would eventually be timed appropriately as the circadian phase delays in reference to the 24-hour day). Melatonin of 10 mg may be inferior to 0.5 mg for entrainment of circadian phase.

29. **The correct answer is D.**
This individual has excessive sleepiness during the work period and insomnia during the allotted time for sleep. His symptoms coincide with a switch from conventional day shifts to night shifts and are consistent with a diagnosis of shift work disorder.[1] Shift work disorder is secondary to the allotted time for sleep coinciding with a high circadian alerting signal resulting in sleep loss and excessive sleepiness. Additionally, the overlap of work time with a low circadian alerting signal further augments sleepiness and impaired performance during the shift (Fig. 37.12). This has been demonstrated in actual night shift workers. Night shift workers with melatonin rhythms that rise at night and are low during the day are at higher risk of shift work disorder.[127–131] Conversely, night shift workers with melatonin secretion that aligns with a day sleep period are less likely to manifest symptoms of shift work disorder (Fig. 37.13).[128,130,131]

The prevalence of shift work disorder among night and rotating shift workers is estimated around 10%.[28] Circadian alerting signal is thought to be high during the allotted time for sleep (daytime) in shift work disorder. Homeostatic sleep drive is likely high at the start of the daytime sleep period in shift work disorder, but this is not what results in symptoms of shift work disorder.

30. **The correct answer is C.**
Strategically timed bright light exposure can improve alertness[132–137] and promote circadian alignment with night shift

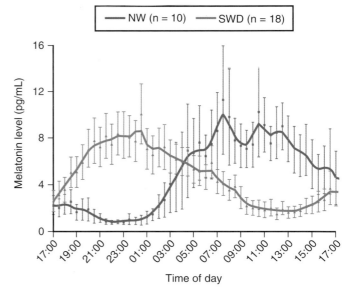

• **Figure 37.13** Salivary melatonin in night workers without symptoms of shift work disorder (NW) and night workers with shift work disorder (SWD). (Used with permission from Gumenyuk V, Howard R, Roth T, Korzyukov O, Drake CL. Sleep loss, circadian mismatch, and abnormalities in reorienting of attention in night workers with shift work disorder. *Sleep.* 2014;37[3]:545–556.)

work (Table 37.1).[133,138] In addition to the well-known ability of bright light to shift circadian phase through its action via the retinohypothalamic tract, bright light has direct alerting affects due at least in part to melatonin suppression and increase in body temperature.[139] In conjunction with bright light during the shift, light avoidance during phase advance portion of the light PRC (morning) promotes a phase delay. This strategy further augments circadian adaption and improves daytime sleep and nighttime alertness.[136,138]

TABLE 37.1

Investigation	Light Intervention	Light Avoidance in Morning	Alertness Improved	Circadian Phase Shift	Sleep Improvement
Costa et al. 1993	2350 lux Intermittent during shift	No	Yes	No	Yes
Budnick et al. 1995	6000–12,000 lux Greater than half of shift	No	Yes	Yes	Mixed
Stewart 1995	8800–10,670 lux First half of shift	No	Yes	NA	Yes
Boivin et al. 2002	2500 lux As much as allowed during shift	Yes	NA	Yes	NA
Yoon et al. 2002	4000–6000 lux 01:00–05:00 AM	Yes (one group)	Yes[a]	NA	Yes[a]
Lowden et al. 2004	2500 lux 20 min between 0300 and 0400	No	Yes	NA[b]	Yes
Bjorvatn et al. 1998	Bright light 30 min	No	Minimal	NA	Minimal

[a]Most pronounced benefits in sleep and alertness were seen in the group with the combined light exposure and post shift light avoidance; however, both intervention groups had improved symptoms in comparison with placebo.
[b]Phase was not assessed, but melatonin secretion was suppressed.
Investigations that assessed the impact of light exposure and avoidance in shift workers with shift work disorder.
NA, Not assessed.

Both modafinil and napping alone or in combination with caffeine improve alertness in shift work disorder.[16] However, neither of these interventions target circadian realignment.

Suggested Reading

Auger RR, Burgess HJ, Emens JS, et al. Clinical practice guideline for the treatment of intrinsic circadian rhythm sleep-wake disorders: advanced sleep-wake phase disorder (ASWPD), delayed sleep-wake phase disorder (DSWPD), non-24-hour sleep-wake rhythm disorder (N24SWD), and irregular sleep-wake rhythm disorder (ISWRD). An update for 2015: an American Academy of Sleep Medicine Clinical Practice Guideline. *J Clin Sleep Med*. 2015;11:1199-1236.

Lewy A. Clinical implications of the melatonin phase response curve. *J Clin Endocrinol Metab*. 2010;95:3158-3160.

Sack RL, Auckley D, Auger RR, et al. Circadian rhythm sleep disorders: part I, basic principles, shift work and jet lag disorders. An American Academy of Sleep Medicine review. *Sleep*. 2007;30:1460-1483.

St Hilaire MA, Gooley JJ, Khalsa SB, et al. Human phase response curve to a 1 h pulse of bright white light. *J Physiol*. 2012;590:3035-3045.

Uchiyama M, Lockley SW. Non-24-hour sleep-wake rhythm disorder in sighted and blind patients. *Sleep Med Clin*. 2015;10:495-516.

38

Rapid Eye Movement and Nonrapid Eye Movement Parasomnias

MICHAEL HOWELL

Questions, 573

Answers, 579

Suggested Reading, 586

Questions

1. A 4-year-old male presents with his parents who describe distressing nightly behaviors dating back for 1 year. After going to sleep at about 8 PM, he awakens at 11 PM, screaming. He is difficult to console. Attempting to calm him only results in more screaming. His mother describes that during these episodes he is "possessed by a demon."

   These events last approximately 30 minutes, and then he falls back asleep. In the morning he has no recollection of events. He was born at 34 weeks gestation but otherwise has had a normal medical history. On examination he is at the 30th percentile for height and the 5th percentile for weight.

   What is accurate about his condition?

   A. It is a consequence of his prematurity.

   B. It is a consequence of his weight.

   C. His condition is benign and he will most likely outgrow the behaviors.

   D. He needs a magnetic resonance imaging (MRI) of his brain and scalp electroencephalogram (EEG), as his condition may lead to developmental delay.

2. A 20-year-old college male presents to the sleep clinic after campus police found him confused in his (parked) car. His roommate describes that his sleepwalking behaviors have increased in the last month as he has approached end of the semester examinations.

   Prior to college, the patient had a history of sleepwalking dating back to early childhood that was benign and typically without consequence. For example, he would wake up in his brother's room or move a bicycle from the garage into the living room.

   Now, however, he is concerned about possibly operating a motor vehicle during one of his episodes. In addition, these events can be embarrassing since he once wondered through a common area in his dormitory wearing only his underwear. He is amnestic for the behaviors and does not recall any dreams. There is no history of snoring, and he describes himself as a "night owl."

He is busy. He plays baseball for his university and is taking a heavy course load, as he wants to go to medical school. Because of this he is usually falling asleep at about midnight and waking up at 7 AM on weekdays. When studying for finals, he has been "cramming" course material until 2–3 in the morning most nights. On the weekends when is not traveling for the baseball team, he will sleep in until noon. He has done well in school up until this semester, when his grades slipped in physics and organic chemistry.

On examination he has a BMI of 26.2 kg/m^2 and has a normal physical and neurological exam.

What is the most appropriate next step in his management?

A. Order an in-laboratory polysomnogram (PSG) with four-limb electromyographic (EMG) leads.

B. Order an in-laboratory PSG with extended electroencephalographic (EEG) montage.

C. Optimize the duration and circadian timing of his sleep.

D. Start oral clonazepam at bedtime.

3. In the *International Classification of Sleep Disorders*, 3rd Edition (2014), sleep-related eating disorder (SRED) is classified as a

   A. NREM-related parasomnia

   B. Sleep-related movement disorder

   C. REM-related parasomnia

   D. Other parasomnia

4. What parasomnia is most likely to be seen as a side effect of paroxetine?

   A. REM sleep behavior disorder

   B. SRED

   C. Exploding head syndrome

   D. Sleep terrors

5. Pressman's 3 P's model is the most commonly cited framework for understanding the processes that trigger disorders of arousal. Which of the following is *not* one of processes in Pressman's 3 P's model?

   A. Proximate

   B. Predisposing

   C. Precipitating

   D. Priming

6. A 54-year-old female presents with a 2-year history of enuresis (bed wetting). Approximately twice a week she will wake up realizing that she has urinated in her bed at night.

She did not have troubles with bedwetting as a child and is very embarrassed about these events. Her sleep is not refreshing and she frequently falls asleep in meetings at work and is terrified she is going to lose bladder control during the day. She knows that she snores but is unsure about apneas since she has been without a bed partner since her divorce 7 years ago.

She did not have enuresis during her in-laboratory PSG but she did have severe obstructive sleep apnea (OSA; AHI = 42) with near complete resolution on continuous positive airway pressure (CPAP) (AHI = 3).

What step is most appropriate *first step* that would likely to result in correction of her enuresis?

A. Clonazepam
B. Mandibular repositioning appliance
C. CPAP
D. Cognitive behavioral therapy

7. A 17-year-old male presents with a 9-month history of dream enactment behavior. He undergoes an in-laboratory PSG that confirms REM sleep without atonia in the absence of sleep disordered breathing (Fig. 38.1).

In addition, he has a history of excessive daytime sleepiness that he assumed was due to depressed mood. He also has had unusual spells where he will "suddenly get weak when laughing." These spells improved 2 months ago after he was started on venlafaxine for depression.

What is the most likely etiology of his REM sleep behavior disorder (RBD)?

A. Orexin (hypocretin) deficiency
B. Early alpha-synuclein neurodegeneration
C. Toxic effect related to venlafaxine
D. Mood disorder

8. When prescribing a medication, which neurotransmitter appears to modulate REM-related motor tone?

A. Dopamine
B. Norepinephrine
C. Serotonin
D. Histamine

9. Sleep terrors peak between which ages?

A. 0–6 years of age
B. 7–12 years of age
C. 13–19 years of age
D. Greater than 50 years of age

10. A 52-year-old male is brought to the clinic by his wife after numerous episodes of abnormal nighttime behavior. One example from last week, he suddenly awoke, sat up, and proclaimed, "I missed my bus!," even though it was 1 AM and his bus did not leave until 7 AM. The events vary in nature. On another occasion he sat up and frantically began looking in the bed linens for his house keys. They were downstairs hanging on a hook near the door. His wife estimates that the events typically last less than 2 minutes and occur 1–2 hours after falling asleep.

He is amnestic for these behaviors that now occur weekly. They have been increasing in frequency over the last 2 years. He snores, but his wife has not witnessed any apneas. In the last year he has been more tired at work and frequently falls asleep in meetings.

On examination he has a body mass index of 37 kg/m^2, BP of 142/96, HR 78, RR 20. Neck circumference was 41 cm (about 16 inches). The rest of his examination was normal.

What is the most appropriate next step?

A. Arrange for him to have a PSG with extended EEG montage looking closely for nocturnal seizures.
B. Arrange for him to have a standard PSG looking for sleep-disordered breathing.
C. No further investigation needed at this time. Advise him to increase his sleep intake and avoid sleep deprivation.

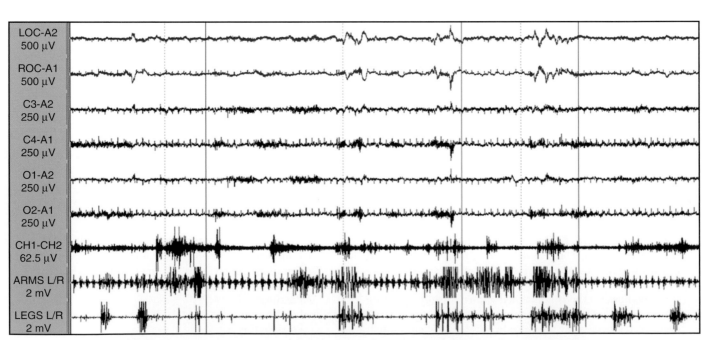

• **Figure 38.1** Ninety-second PSG epoch; Electromyogram: Arms L-left forearm, Arms R-right forearm, CH1-chin central, CH2-chin right, Legs L-left tibialis anterior, Legs R-right tibialis anterior; Electroencephalography (International 10-20 Electrode Placement System): C3-left central, C4-right central, O1-left occipital, O2-right occipital; Electrooculography: LOC-left outer canthus, ROC-right outer canthus.

D. Start clonazepam for the treatment of an NREM parasomnia.

11. A 9-year-old girl presents with her parents and describes terrifying nocturnal events for the last 3 months. At least weekly she has a vivid terrifying dream. She then wakes up and sees tormenting images of demons standing over her bed. She tries to cry out but she cannot. She is "frozen" and cannot move. It is difficult to determine how long the events last. They seem to last at most a minute or two, but for the patient they seem to stretch out for much longer. Once she awakens she runs into her parents' room to tell them that the "monsters are back."

The events typically happen about 5–6 hours after falling asleep. She is distressed for several minutes, and has an elevated respiratory and heart rate. She remembers the dreams clearly and is immediately consolable.

What is the diagnosis?

A. Sleep terrors
B. REM sleep behavior disorder
C. Confusional arousals
D. Nightmare disorder

12. A 57-year-old male presents with his wife who has been describing violent dream enactment for the last 4 years. Behaviors include thrashing, kicking, and punching while shouting expletives. His wife states that these events typically occur at about 4 o'clock in the morning and they can be readily halted if she firmly places a hand on his shoulder and says, "Honey, it's OK; you are having a dream."

However, one night when she was out of town, he leapt out of bed into a plate glass window. This resulted in lower extremity abrasions and lacerations (Fig. 38.2).

Polysomnography demonstrates REM sleep without atonia without sleep-disordered breathing (AHI = 4.2) or excessive periodic limb movements (PLM index = 9.0).

In addition to parkinsonian symptoms (tremor, bradykinesia), the presence (or absence) of what other historical feature

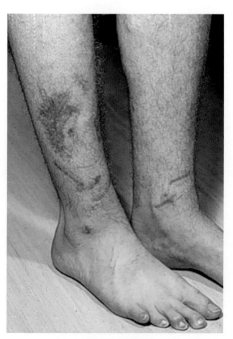

• **Figure 38.2**

could help stratify this patient's risk for developing a alpha-synuclein neurodegenerative condition?

A. Hyposmia
B. Loose stools
C. Alcoholism
D. Hypertension

13. A 64-year-old female presents with a 2-year history of dream enactment behavior confirmed to be REM sleep behavior disorder on polysomnography. Her review of systems was normal, except for a history of difficulty smelling and constipation.

Her past medical history was significant for posttraumatic stress disorder (PTSD) related to repeated sexual assault as teenager. Her PTSD symptoms had been under good control with prazosin and group psychological counseling. She is functioning well, has a career as an attorney, and claims that she has a loving supportive husband and family.

However, her dream enactments are often violent. She is frequently punching and kicking attackers. These often resulted in her husband becoming bruised and scratched.

Which of the following is true regarding the patient's dream enactment behaviors?

A. They are caused by her childhood traumas.
B. They are caused by a subconscious conflict with her husband.
C. They could be resolved with psychoanalysis.
D. They are unrelated to her PTSD.

14. A 72-year-old male with a history of REM sleep behavior disorder is initiated on oral clonazepam.

Which of the following is not a possible side effect of clonazepam?

A. Morning sedation
B. Gait impairment
C. Parkinsonism
D. Depressed mood

15. A 39-year-old female patient arrives in your clinic and claims that she has been a sleepwalker since she was a young child. According to her bed partner, she has near nightly (5 times a week) episodes where she will arise out of bed, typically in the first half of the night, and start walking. The emotional intensity of these events will vary, with a sizable minority of episodes being characterized by distress. One time she pounded on a window, breaking the glass. Afterward she will describe these episodes in detail and explain.

She has never left the house and is not on any medications.

Polysomnography included REM supine and did not demonstrate clinically significant sleep-disordered breathing (AHI = 2.1; PLM index of 4.2). She did have frequent spontaneous arousals during NREM sleep (arousal index was 24). She had an elevation of both tonic and phasic motor activity during REM sleep, and small movements in her hand consistent with dream enactment ("hand babbling").

What is this patient's diagnosis?

A. Sleepwalking
B. Sleep terrors
C. REM sleep behavior disorder (RBD)
D. Parasomnia overlap disorder

16. A 29-year-old developmentally delayed male, due to a viral encephalitis as a child, presents with nightly episodes for 5 years that have been very distressing to his family. He will roll prone in bed and start rhythmic pelvic thrusting while grunting and shouting incoherently. These events occur up to 20 times a night. All the events are nearly identical to each other.

What is the most appropriate next step?

A. Refer to a psychiatrist who performs psychoanalysis to see if he is suffering from repressed sexual abuse.

B. Start clonazepam for presumed REM sleep behavior disorder (RBD).

C. Arrange for an overnight PSG with four-limb leads to watch for RBD.

D. Arrange for an overnight PSG with extended EEG montage to watch for seizure activity.

17. After visiting with a sleep doctor and taking a prescribed medication, a patient has a 60-minute sleepwalking episode. This 55-year-old female ended up crashing her car on the road leading to work. What agent most likely induced this behavior?

A. Trazodone

B. Zolpidem

C. Modafinil

D. Amitryptaline

18. What condition or environmental exposure is not associated with an increased risk of developing REM sleep behavior disorder (RBD)?

A. Tobacco smoking

B. Pesticide exposure

C. Fewer years of education

D. Alcohol

19. A sleep-deprived 27-year-old female internal medicine resident awakens suddenly from a nap to a loud noise that went off inside her head. She immediately realizes it was an auditory hallucination and describes it as if someone had banged on a piano. This happened about 6 months ago when she was postcall.

What is the diagnosis?

A. Early schizophrenia

B. Hypnic jerk

C. Exploding head syndrome

D. Ruptured cerebral aneurysm

E. Hypnopompic hallucination

20. Sleepwalking peaks between which ages?

A. 0–6 years of age

B. 7–12 years of age

C. 13–18 years of age

D. 19–24 years of age

21. Which of the following can precipitate a disorder of arousal?

A. Noise

B. Sleep deprivation

C. Sedative hypnotic medication

D. Alcohol

22. What EEG activity typically precedes a disorder of arousal on polysomnography?

A. Burst in slow wave activity (SWA)

B. Saw tooth waves

C. K complex

D. Sleep spindle

23. A 64-year-old male presents with a 2-month history of dream enactment following a stroke. Otherwise, he has recovered from his stroke without impairment.

On examining his history, you find out that prior to his stroke he was a good sleeper, except for moderate OSA treated with CPAP. He can smell and does not have problems with constipation.

He has a PSG that does not demonstrate sleep disordered breathing on CPAP. However, in contrast to his previous PSG

(performed 3 years ago to establish a diagnosis of OSA), he now has increased tonic motor activity during REM sleep in the chin and limb leads (Figs. 38.3–38.5).

An MRI scan is most likely to demonstrate that the patient's stroke was in what region of the brain?

A. Occipital lobe

B. Medulla

C. Pons

D. Frontal lobe

24. A 72-year-old female RBD patient whose symptoms are well controlled on 0.25 mg of clonazepam arrives at the clinic with her family. They note that she has been getting lost lately and will frequently describe seeing nonexistent animals, such as her long dead cat and other cartoonish like creatures, in the room with her.

Her current troubles are most likely caused by

A. Clonazepam

B. Alzheimer's disease

C. Schizophrenia

D. Dementia with Lewy bodies (DLB)

25. What parasomnia is a common side effect of zolpidem?

A. REM sleep behavior disorder

B. SRED

C. Exploding head syndrome

D. Sleep terrors

26. Which behavior has been reported to increase sleepwalking in adolescents?

A. Evening caffeine

B. Cigarette smoking

C. Alcohol

D. Frequent television viewing

27. Which of the following survey tools are useful in assessing the presence and severity of disorders of arousal?

A. Epworth Sleepiness Scale (ESS)

B. Berlin Questionnaire

C. Paris Arousal Disorders Severity Scale (PADSS)

D. Pittsburgh Sleep Quality Index (PSQI)

28. Which of the following disorders is not strongly linked to REM sleep behavior disorder (RBD)?

A. Parkinson's disease

B. Progressive supranuclear palsy

C. Multiple system atrophy

D. DLB

29. A 72-year-old woman presents 3 months after a nearly fatal "fall" out of bed that resulted in a fracture of the second cervical vertebral body. She was dreaming that she was chasing after a grandchild who was running into a busy street. This resulted in the patient diving out of bed into her bedroom door (Fig. 38.6).

Prior to these events, she was unaware of any previous dream enactment behaviors. Her medical history is remarkable for hypertension, obesity (BMI = 32.4 kg/m²), diabetes, and recently diagnosed depression. Her medications include hydrochlorothiazide, lisinopril, metformin, and fluvoxamine.

Which of her medications decrease her risk of early conversion to Parkinson's disease?

A. Hydrochlorothiazide

B. Lisinopril

C. Metformin

D. Fluvoxamine

30. Which of the following is true about the mental health of patients with parasomnias?

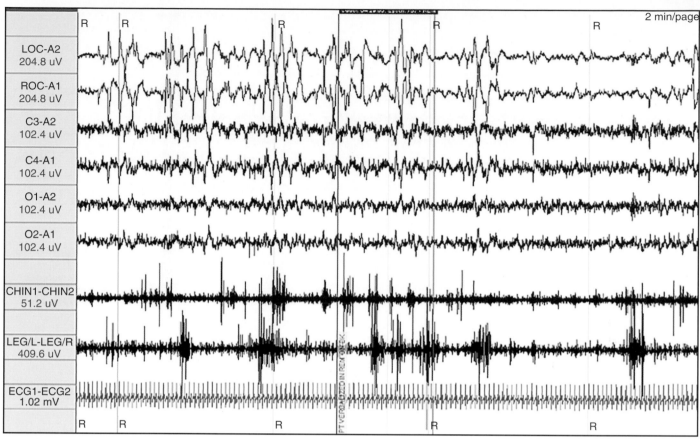

• **Figure 38.3** Sixty-second PSG epoch; Electroencephalography (International 10-20 Electrode Placement System): C3-left central, C4-right central, F3-left frontal, F4-right frontal, O1-left occipital, O2-right occipital; Electromyogram: Chin 1-chin central, Chin 2-chin right; Electrooculography: LOC-left outer canthus, ROC-right outer canthus, Rarm1-right forearm 1st lead, Rarm2-right forearm 2nd lead.

A. Adult patients who sleepwalk have a higher incidence of psychological conflict and psychotherapies improve their nocturnal behaviors.

B. Adult patients who have REM sleep behavior disorder have a higher incidence of psychological conflict and psychotherapies improve their nocturnal behaviors.

C. Children with sleep terrors have a higher incidence of psychological conflict and psychotherapies improve their nocturnal behaviors.

D. The vast majority of parasomnias do not represent an underlying psychological disorder.

31. A 52-year-old male patient with confusional arousal undergoes a PSG. The sleep study demonstrated moderate OSA (AHI = 26) with sleep-related hypoxemia (12 minutes spent with an oxygen saturation of less than 88%). No confusional arousals were noted during the study.

   What of the following is most likely to stop the patient's confusional arousals?

   A. Clonazepam at bedtime
   B. Auto-titration CPAP
   C. Supplemental oxygen
   D. Melatonin at bedtime

32. A 19-year-old female, who is not sleepy during the day and does not have a history of sleep fragmentation, presents with a 6 month history of recurrent episodes of waking up feeling paralyzed and unable to move.

   In addition to these episodes of sleep paralysis, what other phenomenon is she likely to experience?

   A. Hypnogogic hallucination
   B. Hypnopompic hallucination
   C. Cataplexy
   D. Orthostasis upon awakening

33. A 5-year-old girl wakes up at midnight screaming. Her parents find her inconsolable, tachycardic, and diaphoretic. These events started after the child began kindergarten.

   How would you advise the parents?

   A. Reassurance that the child is suffering a common condition that does not typically represent brain pathology
   B. Recommend the patient see a child psychiatrist
   C. MRI scan of the head
   D. Wait 1 year before starting kindergarten, as the child is not psychologically ready for school

34. Compared with Parkinson's disease patients without rapid eye movement sleep behavior disorder (RBD), Parkinson's patients with RBD have which of the following?

   A. More rapid cognitive decline
   B. More autonomic dysfunction
   C. Faster progression of motor impairment
   D. All of the above

35. Besides dream enactment, how do most patients with RBD describe their sleep?

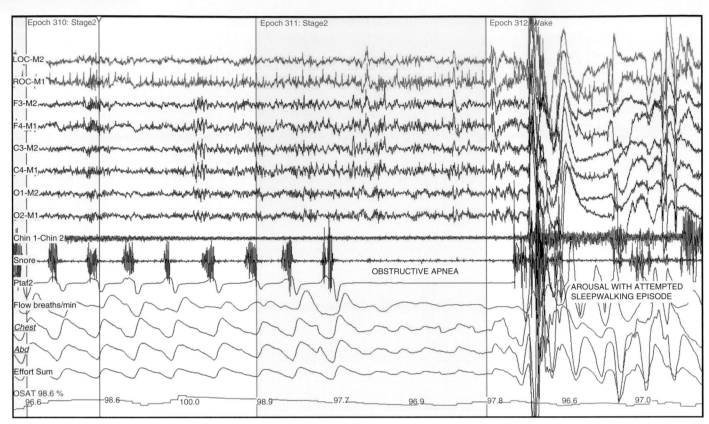

• **Figure 38.4** A 90-second PSG epoch; Electroencephalography (International 10-20 Electrode Placement System): C3-left central, C4-right central, F3-left frontal, F4-right frontal, O1-left occipital, O2-right occipital; Electromyogram: Chin 1-chin central, Chin 2-chin right; Electrooculography: LOC-left outer canthus, ROC-right outer canthus; Rarm1-right forearm 1st lead, Rarm2-right forearm 2nd lead.

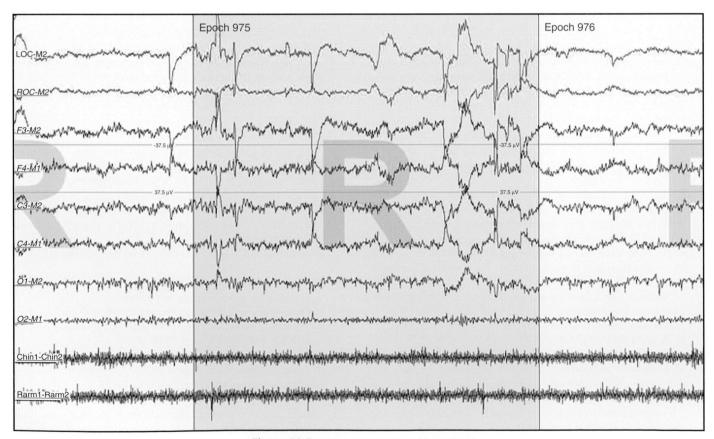

• **Figure 38.5** Increased Tonic REM Motor Tone.

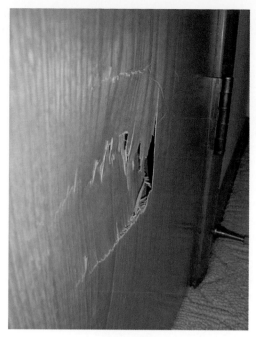

• **Figure 38.6**

A. Normal, restful sleep
B. Nonrestful due to sleep fragmentation
C. Nonrestful due to waking up feeling sore
D. Nonrestful due to sleep onset anxiety

36. What strategy could be used to induce a disorder of arousal while a patient is in a sleep laboratory?
   A. Sleep extension in the 2 weeks leading up to the sleep study
   B. Alcohol ingestion the evening of the sleep study
   C. 25 hours of sleep deprivation leading up to the sleep study, followed by a sudden noise while the patient is in deep NREM (N3) sleep
   D. 25 hours of sleep deprivation leading up to the sleep study, followed by a sudden noise while the patient is in light NREM (N2) sleep

37. Why do disorders of arousal such as sleepwalking typically occur in the first half of the night?
   A. Because N1 sleep is more predominant in the first half of the night
   B. Because N2 sleep is more predominant in the first half of the night
   C. Because N3 sleep is more predominant in the first half of the night
   D. Because REM sleep is more predominant in the first half of the night

38. Which of the following is the first and most appropriate goal of managing patients with the REM sleep behavior disorder (RBD)?
   A. Minimize alcohol intake prior to going to sleep
   B. Quantify the patients' REM atonia index
   C. Treat any co-morbid sleep disordered breathing
   D. Barricade sharp objects, and remove firearms and other dangerous weapons from the bedroom

39. A 74-year-old male with a 20-year history of polysomnographically confirmed RBD presents after a hip fracture suffered while he was ambulating to the bathroom in the morning after waking up. His dream enactment behavior has been well controlled on 0.5 mg of clonazepam; however, he has had increasing difficulty with morning fatigue and mental "cloudiness" that he attributes to the clonazepam. He tried to decrease the dose down to 0.25 mg but started to have breakthrough dream enactment.

Repeat polysomnography confirms REM sleep without atonia with only mild OSA (AHI = 11.4). He tried auto-titration CPAP, but quit after 1 month. He stated that it did not decrease his dream enactment behavior, and that he did not feel more refreshed in the morning.

What management step would most likely decrease his dream enactment behavior without substantial side effects?
   A. Switch the patient from autoCPAP to fixed CPAP.
   B. Discontinue clonazepam and start oral melatonin at bedtime 3–6 mg.
   C. Switch the patient from autoCPAP to a mandibular repositioning appliance.
   D. Increase his dose of clonazepam to 1.0 mg at bedtime.

40. A 42-year-old obese male presents with a 4-year history of amnestic nocturnal urination in bed. He is embarrassed to discuss these episodes and breaks down crying on numerous occasions during his interview. His bedwetting occurs at least 5 nights a week. Prior to 4 years ago, he had normal nocturnal urinary continence. He has never had any difficult with daytime continence.

What is this patient's diagnosis?
   A. Nocturnal epilepsy
   B. Diabetes mellitus
   C. Primary enuresis
   D. Secondary enuresis

41. A 39-year-old female presents with an 8-month history of amnestic nocturnal sexual behavior. She was told by her significant other that she has been initiating sexual intercourse with him, even though she does not recall it the morning. During wakefulness she describes a healthy sex life and libido.

She has been on the sedative hypnotic medication, eszopiclone, for the last 3 years with occasional (monthly) episodes of benign sleepwalking and amnestic nocturnal sleep eating (SRED). About 1 year ago, the dose was increased from 2 mg to 3 mg due to progressive lack of efficacy.

Understandably, she would like the amnestic behaviors to stop, and she is worried about the possibility of an unplanned pregnancy and would like to be fully aware of these behaviors.

What immediate strategy is most likely to resolve this patient's sexsomnia?
   A. Contact law enforcement to report a possible sexual assault with sodium oxybate.
   B. Have the patient undergo an in-lab PSG.
   C. Discontinue eszopiclone.
   D. Start clonazepam 0.5 mg at bedtime.

Answers

1. **The correct answer is C.**
His condition is benign, and he will most likely outgrow the behaviors. This child is suffering from sleep terrors. Sleep terrors occur primarily in preadolescent children and peak around the age of 3. They are characterized by a sudden awakening with a loud cry or scream early in the first half of the sleep period. Patients are unable to be consoled, which is often quite distressing to parents. Autonomic activation with increased sweating and tachycardia is often noted. It is not

unusual for parents to activate emergency medical services, as they are convinced their child is suffering a seizure or some other serious neurological event.

In the *International Classification of Sleep Disorders*, 3rd Edition (ICSD-3), night terrors are considered a disorder of arousal in the category of NREM parasomnias. They may represent an overlap in features of both NREM and REM sleep: the high arousal threshold from SWA of deep NREM (N3) sleep and the autonomic activation, as well as frightening mentation (possibly dream) from REM sleep. These features help distinguish sleep terrors from nightmares (Table 38.1).

Sleep terrors are treated like other disorders of arousal by correcting any underlying condition that increases homeostatic sleep pressure. These conditions include sleep deprivation, circadian misalignment, sleep disordered breathing, and sleep-related movement disorders. Additional sedating medications should be minimized or eliminated, if possible. Of note, many cases of sleep terrors occur after children lose a previously scheduled afternoon nap, such as when they change from daycare to preschool.

Answers A, B, and D are incorrect. There is no clear causal association between prematurity, weight, and sleep terrors. Despite his parents' concern, these events are not consistent with seizures, and a neurological evaluation is not necessary.[1,2]

2. **The correct answer is C. Optimize the duration and circadian timing of sleep.**
Between the sleep deprivation and environmental disruption (i.e., noise), college is often the perfect storm for disorders of arousal.

This individual is predisposed to sleepwalking; however, his behaviors are clearly primed by sleep deprivation. This has been exacerbated by a circadian delay and his volitional sleep restriction. It is important to explain to the patient the nature of arousal disorders and the critical need to unload the homeostatic sleep drive through sleep extension. In addition, in this patient's case, he would benefit from circadian alignment (morning sun or 10,000 lux light box exposure with low dose melatonin 4–6 hours prior to desired bedtime). However, it is worth noting that these behavioral changes are very difficult

for a college student. One motivating factor for this individual would be his desire to get into medical school. One could explain to him the benefits of sleep on academic performance and memory consolidation, especially since his grades have recently dropped.

He does not need a PSG at this time. He describes very typical sleepwalking behaviors exacerbated by sleep deprivation with no history of symptoms suggestive of sleep-disordered breathing. There is no history of dream enactment that would necessitate a PSG for RBD evaluation (A) and the behaviors are not stereotyped suggestive of nocturnal seizure (B).

While clonazepam has historically been cited as a treatment for sleepwalking, recent reviews have casted doubt on its effectiveness in NREM parasomnias (D). Further, the sedating nature of clonazepam has been reported to exacerbate sleepwalking behaviors. This is in contrast to RBD, where clonazepam still appears to demonstrate a clinical utility.[1,3,4]

3. **The answer is A. NREM parasomnia.**
Typically NREM parasomnias are also considered disorders of arousal (Answer B). The one exception is SRED. SRED is not currently classified as a disorder of arousal but is a NREM parasomnia. This is likely mere semantics, as many authors suggest that SRED is in fact a form of sleepwalking and should be considered a disorder of arousal; however, the ICSD has not yet recognized this.

Previously, in the ICSD-2 (2005), SRED was classified as an "other parasomnia" (Answer D) (Table 38.2). The amnestic

TABLE 38.1	Sleep Terrors and Nightmares	
	Sleep Terrors	**Nightmares**
Vocalization	Screaming common	Typically silent
Awareness	– – (Poor recall)	++ (Can describe dream mentation in detail)
Consolable	– – (Typically increases agitation)	++ (Can typically calm a patient down in moments)
Purported mechanism	Overlap between N3 and REM sleep	Overlap between REM sleep and wakefulness
Autonomic activation	–/+	++ (Tachycardia, tachypnea, sweating)
Age of resolution	Typically at adolescence	May persist into adulthood

REM, Rapid eye movement.

TABLE 38.2	Changes to the International Classification of Sleep Disorders Criteria for Parasomnias	
	ICSD-2 (2005)	**ICSD-3 (2014)**
NREM parasomnias	Confusional arousals Sleepwalking Sleep terrors	Disorders for arousal Confusional arousals Sleep walking Sleep terrors Sleep-related eating disorder
REM parasomnias	REM sleep behavior disorder Recurrent isolated sleep paralysis Nightmare disorder	REM sleep behavior disorder Recurrent isolated sleep paralysis Nightmare disorder
Other parasomnias	Sleep-related eating disorder Sleep-related dissociative disorder Sleep enuresis Sleep-related groaning (Catathrenia) Exploding head syndrome Sleep-related hallucinations	Sleep-related dissociative disorder Sleep enuresis Exploding head syndrome Sleep-related hallucinations
Isolated symptoms and normal variants		Sleep talking

ICSD, International Classification of Sleep Disorders; *NREM,* nonrapid eye movement; *REM,* rapid eye movement.

nocturnal eating of SRED is distinct from the wakeful nocturnal eating of night eating syndrome (Table 38.3).

SRED is not considered a REM-related parasomnia (Answer C).[2,5-7]

4. **The correct answer is A.**

Since the 1970s, antidepressant medications have been reported to induce vigorous dream enactment behavior. Later, paroxetine and other selective serotonin reuptake inhibitors have been noted to increase REM sleep motor activity and dream enactment. Thus paroxetine is the agent most likely to induce REM sleep behavior disorder (RBD; Answer A). It has been suggested that antidepressant medications are not truly inducing RBD in these cases, but instead unmasking RBD early, in patients who may be likely to exhibit the RBD phenotype later in life. Evidence for this theory includes the difficulties with smell (anosmia) and constipation also seen in these individuals. Both anosmia and constipation are frequently comorbid with RBD, and suggest that these individuals have a prodromal syndrome of alpha-synuclein neurodegeneration, placing them at risk of ultimately developing a parkinsonian disorder.

SRED (Answer B) is commonly induced with benzodiazepine receptor agonists such as zolpidem and eszopiclone. Neither exploding head syndrome (Answer C) nor sleep terrors (Answer D) have been commonly reported to be induced by paroxetine.[1,8]

5. **The correct answer is A. Proximate.**

Pressman's model was described in a 2007 *Sleep Medicine Review* article and nicely summarizes the processes that lead to disorders of arousal including sleepwalking, sleep terrors, and confusional arousals. Predisposing factors include a family history of sleepwalking and motor restlessness. The predisposed individual is then primed by processes that impair cortical arousal such as sedating medications, sleep deprivation, circadian

misalignment, and/or untreated sleep disorders. Precipitating factors include any suddenly alerting process that could trigger an arousal from deep slow-wave (N3) sleep. These include pathological processes such as OSA, arousals associated with periodic limb movements, or environmental sleep disruption (i.e., noise).

Proximate is not one of Pressman's 3 P's. However, John William Polidori (1795–1821), an English physician, wrote about somnambulism and its causes. He described three: the proximate, the remote, and the predisposing. In addition to these early insights, he also was an inspiration for his contemporary Mary Shelley, the author of *Frankenstein*.[9,10]

6. **The correct answer is C.**

Untreated OSA is the most common cause of secondary enuresis and its correction typically resolves the bedwetting. While mandibular repositioning devices (Answer B) are often effective at treating mild to moderate OSA, they are not first-line therapy in severe OSA, and considering the patients' treatment response during the PSG, CPAP would be the best initial management. Neither clonazepam (Answer A) nor cognitive behavioral therapy (Answer D) would be expected to correct this patient's enuresis.

Sleep enuresis is far more common in adults than typically perceived, with a prevalence of 2.1% among community dwelling older adults.[1,2]

7. **The correct answer is A.**

This patient has narcolepsy type 1 (narcolepsy with cataplexy, or hypocretin deficiency syndrome), a disorder that typically strikes in the teenager or young adult. It is caused by orexin (hypocretin) deficiency. RBD, as well as findings of REM sleep without atonia and periodic leg movements during REM sleep, are common in narcolepsy, and approximately 50% of patients with narcolepsy also have RBD symptoms.

The mechanism of RBD in narcolepsy is different from other forms of RBD, and related to the failure of orexin to stabilize REM sleep. RBD is commonly caused by alpha-synuclein neurodegeneration (Answer B) as well as antidepressant medications (Answer C); however, the clinical picture in this case is one of narcolepsy, and the patient's venlafaxine was started after the onset of dream enactment. Of note, venlafaxine, by suppressing REM sleep phenomena, does help treat cataplexy, as it did in this case. Mood disorders (Answer D) are not a cause of RBD.[11,12]

8. **The correct answer is C.**

Antidepressants frequently increase REM motor tone and induce REM sleep behavior disorder (RBD). These effects appear to be due to the effect of serotonin on REM-related neurons in the pons. Dopamine (Answer A), Norepinephrine (Answer B), and Histamine (Answer D) do not exhibit this effect on REM- associated motor tone.[13]

9. **The correct answer is A.**

Sleep terrors are more common among young children ages 0–6 years (Answer A). The incidence of sleepwalking peaks immediately prior to adolescence (Answer B) and occasionally persists into the teenage years (Answer C). The parasomnia that most typically presents after the age of 50 (Answer D) is REM sleep behavior disorder (Answer D).[2,14]

10. **The correct answer is B.**

The patient has confusional arousals with nonstereotyped behaviors. He should have a PSG looking for any priming and precipitating causes. Even with his wife denying nocturnal

TABLE 38.3	Sleep-Related Eating Disorder and Night Eating Syndrome	
	Sleep-Related Eating Disorder (SRED)	Night Eating Syndrome (NES)
Initial report	1991, Schenck	1955, Stunkard
Association with obesity	++	++
Purported mechanism	Breakdown in the physiology of the overnight fast	Circadian misalignment between appetite and sleep
Evening hyperphagia (excessive calories after dinner before bedtime)	–	++
Nocturnal eating (eating after an awakening from sleep)	++(amnestic)	+(Wakeful)
Morning anorexia	–/+	++
Associated conditions	RLS	Mood and anxiety disorders

RLS, Restless legs syndrome.

apneas, he has a high pretest probability of OSA with a STOP-BANG score of 7. The components of STOP-BANG include snoring, tiredness, observed apneas, elevated blood pressure, age greater than 50, neck circumference greater than 40 cm, and male gender. A score of 5 or higher places him at high risk of OSA. Correction of sleep-disordered breathing typically resolves the disorder of arousal.

Answer A is incorrect, as the patient's events are not typical of nocturnal seizures. They are not stereotyped, and their frequency is more typical of confusional arousals. Nocturnal frontal lobe epilepsy is often characterized by up to 20 stereotyped behaviors a night.

While it is always a good idea to optimize the duration and circadian timing of sleep, reassurance with sleep hygiene recommendations (Answer C) are not appropriate at this time, since the patient's disorder of arousal is most likely secondary to an untreated sleep disorder that has substantial cardiovascular consequences if left untreated.

While clonazepam has historically been cited as a treatment for disorders of arousal, recent reviews have casted doubt on its effectiveness (Answer D). Further, the sedating nature of clonazepam has been reported to exacerbate these disorders. This is in contrast to RBD where clonazepam still has clinical utility.[1,2,9]

11. **The correct answer is D. The patient has nightmare disorder.**

The disorder can be characterized as intermittent frightening dream mentation with a subsequent arousal. The mentation is clearly described by the patient, typically a preadolescent child. Unlike sleep terrors (Answer A), once the patient arouses from the dream they are consolable. In addition, patients often describe sleep paralysis and hypnopompic hallucinations. Nightmares are a REM-related parasomnia and may be understood as an overlap between REM sleep and wakefulness. The patients are awake in that their cerebral cortex is able to perceive the environment around them; however, they are still partially in REM sleep, as demonstrated by the persistent dream mentation (hypnopompic hallucinations) and REM atonia (sleep paralysis).

Nightmares are common in childhood but often occur in the setting of sleep deprivation. In this patient's case, she had recently started early morning gymnastic practice. Efforts were made to get the child to bed earlier. These measures improved but did not fully resolve the nightmares. Once the gymnastics season was over and she was able to sleep in on a daily basis, the events resolved.

Unlike REM sleep behavior disorder (Answer B), which is characterized by vigorous dream enactment, this patient has sleep paralysis.

The patient does not have a confusional arousal (Answer C), as she has clear mentation and is able to describe the dreams in vivid detail. Confusional arousals are not typically frightening.[1,2]

12. **The correct answer is A.**

When comorbid with RBD, difficulty with smell (hyposmia) increases a patient's risk for early conversion (<5 years) to Parkinson's disease or related conditions such as DLB or multiple system atrophy. Other concerning symptoms include constipation, orthostasis, and erectile dysfunction. Loose stools (Answer B), alcoholism (Answer C), and hypertension (Answer D) are not strongly linked to an increased risk of Parkinson's disease.[13,15,16]

13. **The correct answer is D.**

Prior to the discovery of RBD in 1986, many patients were mistakenly diagnosed with a mental health disorder or believed that dream enactment represented a subconscious psychological conflict. This assumption was mistaken in the overwhelming number of RBD cases. REM sleep in normal individuals is characterized by intense emotional mentation that can include violent, frightening, or sexual content.

This patient also had previously unexplained constipation, anosmia, and orthostasis, suggesting that her RBD was related to a disorder of alpha-synuclein degeneration. Thus her symptoms are not caused by childhood trauma (Answer A) or conflict with her husband (Answer B), nor would Freudian psychoanalysis (Answer C) be of any value.[16,17]

14. **The correct answer is C.**

While RBD patients are at high risk of developing alpha-synuclein neurodegeneration, there is no evidence to suggest that clonazepam increases the incidence of parkinsonism. Common side effects of clonazepam include morning sedation (Answer A), gait impairment (particularly when going to the bathroom in the middle of the night; Answer B), and depressed mood (Answer D).[1]

15. **The correct answer is D.**

While the patient's history is mostly consistent with sleepwalking (Answer A), she also has REM sleep without atonia on polysomnography to suggest RBD (Answer C). When patients meet criteria for both an NREM parasomnia and RBD, they have parasomnia overlap disorder (Answer D). Despite intermittent agitation, the patient does not have a history suggestive of sleep terrors (Answer B). Sleep terrors occur after a sudden scream or cry, and patients have tachycardia, tachypnea, diaphoresis, confusion during the event, and are amnestic for the episode the next morning.

Parasomnia overlap disorder is common. In one series, 28% of sleepwalking patients also had evidence on PSG of RBD, and thus were diagnosed with parasomnia overlap disorder.[2,18]

16. **The correct answer is D.**

The patient most likely has frontal lobe epilepsy based upon the recurrent, abnormal, stereotyped episodes. They are likely secondary to his history of viral encephalitis. Of note, the seizure focus is often in the deep frontal lobes and difficult to measure with scalp EEG; thus a low therapeutic threshold is warranted. In this case, the patient's EEG did not demonstrate seizures, but his events resolved with nightly oral carbamazepine.

Many patients with these seizures end up needlessly referred for various psychotherapies (Answer A). His events are too frequent and stereotyped to likely represent RBD (Answers B and C).[1,2]

17. **The correct answer is B.**

Of the listed medications, zolpidem, a commonly prescribed benzodiazepine receptor agonist, is most likely to induce sleepwalking. Zolpidem can suppress hippocampal memory function for several hours, and it is not unusual for patients to describe prolonged complicated amnestic behaviors such as driving, cooking, or sexual activity.

While both trazodone (Answer A) and amitryptaline (Answer B) are mildly sedating and both have been (rarely) associated with sleepwalking, they do not suppress hippocampal function to the same degree as zolpidem. Modafinil (Answer C) is a stimulant and would not be expected to induce sleepwalking.[1,19]

18. **The correct answer is D.**

Similar to Parkinson's disease, RBD is associated with various environmental exposures and behavioral risk factors. In particular, RBD patients are more likely to have a history of smoking (Answer A), traumatic brain injury, pesticide exposure (Answer B), and fewer years of education (Answer C). Alcohol (Answer D) is not linked to an increased risk of RBD.[20,21]

19. **The correct answer is C.**

The patient has exploding head syndrome, characterized by a sense of an explosion in the head typically at the transition between wakefulness to sleep. A flash of light, or myoclonic jerk often referred to as a hypnic jerk (Answer B), may simultaneously occur. These symptoms, if persistent, can be distressing and convince afflicted individuals that they have either an impending thought disorder such as schizophrenia (Answer A) or a ruptured cerebral aneurysm (Answer D). However, the course is benign and typically resolves if the underlying sleep concern, which in this case is sleep deprivation, is addressed.[2]

20. **The correct answer is B.**

The incidence of sleepwalking peaks prior to adolescence. This is related to the increased SWA (NREM sleep stage N3) at this age. Sleep terrors are more common among young children ages 0–6 (Answer A). While sleepwalking does persist after adolescence in some children ages 13–18 (Answer C), and may recur in college aged years 19–24 (Answer D) due to sleep deprivation, the frequency does not reach the same level as preadolescent children.[2,14]

21. **The correct answer is A.**

Disorders of arousal such as sleepwalking or confusional arousals occur when the cortex incompletely activates from deep NREM sleep (N3). Pressman's "3P model" suggests that *predisposed* patients are *primed* by conditions that impair normal arousal. Parasomnias are then subsequently precipitated by events that lead to sudden wakefulness. Priming (not precipitating) factors include sleep deprivation (Answer B) and sedative medications (Answer C). *Precipitators* can be internal pathologies (sleep-disordered breathing; see Fig. 38.3) or external factors (noise). There is no compelling evidence to suggest that alcohol (Answer D) precipitates sleepwalking behaviors.[9,22]

22. **The correct answer is A.**

A spike in SWA is often noted on EEG immediately preceding a disordered arousal. These findings are not noted among control subjects when they wake from sleep, nor are they seen when sleepwalkers have a normal, nondisoriented arousal from sleep. It has been speculated that cortical neurons, having received an internal stimulus, attempt to block the arousal by increasing the density of SWA. Ultimately, the internal stimulus partially overcomes the brain's attempt to maintain sleep, awakening the individual in a disoriented state and leading to sleepwalking. Sleepwalking is also associated with a rapid cyclic alternating pattern (CAP) rate. This EEG finding is a marker of NREM sleep instability.

Saw tooth waves (Answer B) are REM-related EEG activity. K complexes (Answer C) and sleep spindles (Answer D) are typically light N2 NREM activity and do not usually precede a disorder of arousal.[23]

23. **The correct answer is C.**

Occasionally lesions affecting the brainstem such as stroke, malignancies, aneurysms, or white matter disease will cause RBD, and these cases do not progress to neurodegeneration. Cortical lesions in the frontal (Answer D) or occipital (Answer A) lobes would not be expected to cause acute RBD. While medullary (Answer B) lesions can occasionally cause RBD, cranial imaging typically shows pontine pathology where the majority of REM modulating neurons are localized.[13]

24. **The correct answer is D.**

The combination of RBD, cognitive impairment particularly in visual-spatial domains, along with visual hallucinations is highly suggestive of DLB (Answer D). While clonazepam (Answer A) has a long half-life and can lead to morning confusion, she is on a low dose and the clinical syndrome is a classic DLB presentation. Alzheimer's disease (Answer B) does not present with visual hallucinations or RBD as frequently as DLB. Schizophrenia typically presents in young adulthood, and hallucinations are most typically auditory.[13]

25. **The correct answer is B.**

Several groups of investigators have reported the induction of sleep walking with eating, SRED, after starting zolpidem. This appears to be most common in the setting of patients with underlying RLS. Patients describe waking up in the morning with a distended abdomen and evidence of binge eating the night before. Typically high caloric foods, such as peanut butter and ice cream, are ingested. Occasionally patients with SRED will engage in stove top cooking and other dangerous food preparation. Discontinuing zolpidem and treating RLS, if present, resolves the parasomnia.

REM sleep behavior disorder (Answer A) can be induced by antidepressant medications but not zolpidem. Neither exploding head syndrome (Answer C) nor sleep terrors (Answer D) are commonly reported to be induced by zolpidem.[1,24]

26. **The correct answer is D.**

Teenagers who are frequent television viewers are four times more likely to report sleepwalking. While the rest of the answers, evening caffeine (Answer A), cigarette smoking (Answer B), and alcohol (Answer C), can lead to sleep difficulties, they have not been consistently demonstrated to increase the frequency of sleepwalking.[1,25]

27. **The correct answer is C.**

PADSS is a new scale for assessing the presence and severity of arousal disorders. Ranging from 0 to 50, a PADSS score higher than 13 suggests an active sleepwalking problem with a high risk for injury (sensitivity of 84% and a specificity of 88%). The Epworth Sleepiness Scale (Answer A) quantifies subjective sleepiness, the Berlin Questionnaire (Answer B) screens for OSA, and the PSQI (Answer D-the Pittsburg Sleep Quality Index) is a general assessment of sleep quality.[26]

28. **The correct answer is B.**

RBD is a prodromal syndrome of neurodegenerative disorders caused by alpha-synuclein pathology. Parkinson's disease (Answer A), multiple system atrophy (Answer C), and DLB (Answer D) are all alpha-synuclein disorders. RBD is not seen at higher rates among cases of progressive supranuclear palsy (Answer B), which is a disorder of hyperphosphorylated tau proteins.[13]

29. **The correct answer is D.**

Serotonergic antidepressants are linked to REM sleep without atonia and RBD. They appear to either induce RBD through a direct toxic effect on brainstem REM generating neurons, or may in fact unmask RBD among patients who would ultimately develop RBD later. Regardless, the presence of current antidepressant medication use decreases their likelihood of early conversion (<5 years) to Parkinson's disease. Hydrochlorothiazide (Answer A), lisinopril (Answer B), and metformin (Answer C) are not known to alter risk of neurodegeneration.[15,16]

30. **The correct answer is D.**

Many clinicians still mistakenly assume that parasomnias are the result of psychological disease. Because of this, patients with sleepwalking (Answer A), REM sleep behavior disorder (Answer B), and sleep terrors (Answer C) are sometimes advised to pursue expensive and meaningless psychotherapies.

Although studies have noted a higher degree of mood and anxiety symptoms among sleepwalkers compared with controls, the vast majority of sleepwalking patients do not report clinically significant levels of anxiety or depression. Further, the association may be accounted for by the increased exposure among these individuals to agents known to induce sleepwalking. Thus most subjects can be reassured that sleepwalking does not represent an underlying mental health disorder.[1,27]

31. **The correct answer is B.**

Treating conditions that suddenly fragment sleep, such as sleep-disordered breathing and bedroom noise (e.g., televisions, phones), are often effective at preventing disorders of arousal. Thus treating moderate OSA is the best step to take in order to treat the patient's confusional arousals. Supplemental oxygen (Answer C), while helpful in addressing the patient's hypoxemia, would not decrease the patient's sleep fragmentation.

Clonazepam (Answer A) and melatonin (Answer D) are often prescribed to treat REM sleep behavior disorder, but their efficacy in disorders of arousal is questionable. Further, clonazepam would be likely to exacerbate the patient's sleep disordered breathing.[1,3,4,28]

32. **The correct answer is B.**

Sleep paralysis occurs when there is persistence of REM sleep atonia into wakefulness. There is often a persistence of REM dream mentation as well, with frightening hypnopompic hallucinations (Answer B). Hypnogogic hallucinations (Answer C) are similar but appear as the patient is falling asleep, not waking up. While sleep paralysis and sleep-related hallucinations are often described in narcolepsy, they are not specific for an orexin disorder. They can intermittently occur in normal individuals who are sleep deprived or suffering from another sleep disorder. This patient is not sleepy and thus is unlikely to have narcolepsy with cataplexy (Answer C). Orthostasis (Answer D) is not typically described after an event of sleep paralysis.[1]

33. **The correct answer is A.**

The child is experiencing sleep terrors that are due to missing her afternoon nap since she is now in school. Sleep extension through some combination of going to bed earlier, sleeping in later, and/or taking weekend naps will likely address the problem. There is no need at this time for the child to see a mental health professional (Answer B), undergo neuroimaging (Answer C), or hold off on starting school (Answer D).[1]

34. **The correct answer is D.**

RBD in Parkinson's disease is associated with more rapid cognitive (Answer A) and motor (Answer C) decline, increased levodopa dosing, greater autonomic impairment (Answer B), and ocular abnormalities. Further, the presence of RBD in Parkinson's disease predicts faster motor progression and more extensive alpha-synuclein pathology on postmortem examination.[16,29]

35. **The correct answer is A.**

In the absence of injury, most RBD patients attribute only minimal daytime consequences, if any, to their condition. One recent study reported that 70% of patients reported good sleep quality. This is in contrast to their bed partners, however. Of note, nearly half of RBD patients are unaware of dream enactment until their bed partners tell them.[30] Thus the majority of RBD patients do not describe sleep fragmentation (Answer B), soreness (Answer C), or bedtime anxiety (Answer D).[30]

36. **The correct answer is C.**

History alone may be unable to distinguish sleepwalking from other nocturnal events, and further scrutiny is often needed to identify the predisposing, priming, and precipitating mechanisms underlying sleepwalking behaviors. Thus an objective evaluation using in-laboratory polysomnography may be necessary. Prior to polysomnography, a protocol of 25 hours of sleep deprivation, with forced awakenings during N3 not N2 (Answer D), increases the likelihood of inducing a parasomnia from slow-wave sleep (Figs. 38.7 and 38.8). However, even when abnormal behavior does not occur, polysomnography is often helpful by identifying or ruling out sleep-disordered breathing or periodic limb movement disorder as a precipitant of the nocturnal behaviors.

Sleep extension for 2 weeks leading up to a sleep study (Answer A) is a useful strategy for patients with a hypersomnolent syndrome. When used with wrist actigraphy, a sleep specialist can confirm that sleep restriction is the cause of the patient's symptoms prior to proceeding with an MSLT. There is no compelling evidence to suggest that alcohol (Answer B) precipitates sleepwalking behaviors.[9,22,31]

37. **The correct answer is C.**

Disorders of arousal typically emerge out of N3, not N1 (Answer A) or N2 (Answer B), which predominates the first half of the night. REM sleep (Answer D) is more predominant the second half of the night.[1]

38. **The correct answer is D.**

The first step in parasomnia management is always to improve bedroom safety. Weapons, in particular firearms, need to be removed from the bedroom in order to prevent accident injury or death. If the patient has violent dream enactment, then the bed partner should sleep separately. Quantifying REM atonia index (Answer B) is often helpful in establishing a diagnosis of RBD. In addition, identifying and treating comorbid sleep disordered breathing (Answer C) may decrease parasomnia behaviors. However, both of the strategies take time, and meanwhile the patient and bed partner are at risk of injury unless environmental changes are made. Minimizing alcohol intake (Answer A) is often a good decision to improve health and well-being; however, it is unlikely to improve parasomnias, as there is very little compelling evidence to suggest that alcohol (Answer D) precipitates sleepwalking behaviors.[1,22]

39. **The correct answer is B.**

Investigators have reported that melatonin is effective either in combination with clonazepam or as the sole therapy. A recent direct comparison study noted that melatonin was equal to clonazepam in treatment efficacy and superior in side effect profile. Patients on melatonin reported fewer adverse effects, in particular falls and injuries, compared with clonazepam. In the setting of neurodegenerative disease, melatonin is a particularly intriguing option, as it is only mildly sedating. Melatonin suppresses both phasic and tonic REM sleep motor

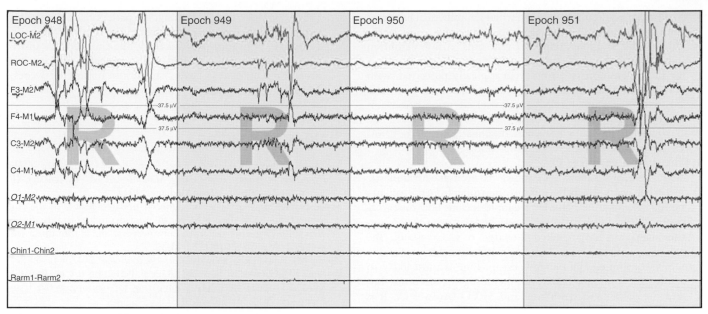

• **Figure 38.7** 120-second PSG epoch; Electroencephalography (International 10-20 Electrode Placement System): C3-left central, C4-right central, F3-left frontal, F4-right frontal, O1-left occipital, O2-right occipital; Electromyogram: Chin 1-chin central, Chin 2-chin right; Electrooculography: LOC-left outer canthus, ROC-right outer canthus; Respiratory channels: Abd-abdominal respiratory effort, Chest-thoracic respiratory effort, Effort Sum-summative respiratory effort, Flow-oronasal thermal airflow, OSAT-oxygen saturation, Ptaf2-Nasal pressure transducer.

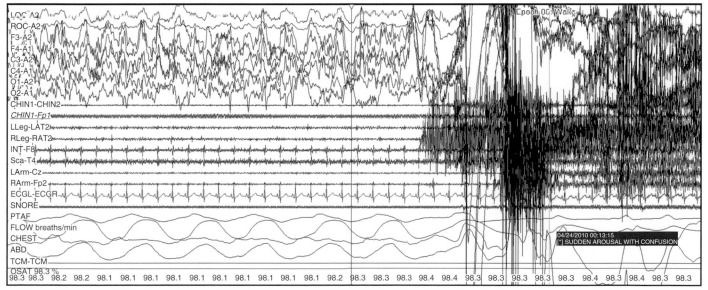

• **Figure 38.8** Confusional Arousal Precipitated by Sudden Noise.

activity, and its effect persists for weeks after the agent is discontinued.

Clonazepam should not be increased (Answer D) but instead discontinued if possible in this patient, as it is the most likely cause of his fall and melatonin alone may control his symptoms. While REM-related OSA can present as RBD, his AHI was within the standard distribution for his age according to the Sleep Heart Health Study. Further, as he was titrating down on his clonazepam, sleep apnea was unlikely to be the trigger of his dream enactment. Thus neither switching to fixed CPAP

(Answer A) or a mandibular repositioning appliance (Answer C) would likely address his dream enactment.[16,32]

40. **The correct answer is D.**
The patient has secondary enuresis, as he has troubles with recurrent involuntary voiding during sleep. The events occur at least twice a week, and it has been present for at least 3 months.

While nocturnal epilepsy (Answer A) and diabetes mellitus (Answer B) are recognized causes of secondary enuresis, these diagnosis have not yet been established in this patient.

Primary enuresis is diagnosed when an individual has never been consistently dry during sleep. Enuresis is common in children, with 15%–20% of 5-year-olds. Among children it is three times more common in boys. Sleep enuresis is far more common in adults than typically perceived, with 2.1% of community dwelling older adults. Many, such as this patient, do not bring it to clinical attention because of embarrassment.

This patient had a PSG that demonstrated severe OSA. Once treated, the patient's enuresis resolved.[2]

41. **The correct answer is C.**

Sexsomnia, or sleep sex, is a confusional arousal with amnestic sexual behaviors. The behaviors can often differ from the patient's typical wakeful sexual behavior. Examples include both masturbation and sexual activity initiated on a bed partner. On occasion these behaviors have resulted in charges of sexual assault. The prevalence of sexsomnia is likely underestimated.

Discontinuing the patient's eszopiclone is most likely to resolve the amnestic behaviors, including the sleep sex, but also the patient's sleepwalking and SRED (Answer C). It is important to always consider the possibility that the patient was sexually assaulted (Answer A); however, in this case eszopiclone is a more likely cause and more likely to immediately resolve the parasomnia. Besides snoring, the patient has a low pre-test probability of sleep-disordered breathing, and a PSG is not necessary at this time (Answer B). While clonazepam (Answer D) has historically been cited as a treatment for disorders of arousal recent, reviews have casted doubt on its effectiveness. Furthermore, the sedating nature of clonazepam has been reported to exacerbate these disorders.[1,2]

Suggested Reading

American Academy of Sleep Medicine. *International Classification of Sleep Disorders: Diagnostic and Coding Manual*. 3rd ed. Westchester, IL: American Academy of Sleep Medicine; 2014.

Boeve BF. REM sleep behavior disorder: updated review of the core features, the REM sleep behavior disorder-neurodegenerative disease association, evolving concepts, controversies, and future directions. *Ann N Y Acad Sci*. 2010;1184:15-54.

Howell MJ. Parasomnias: an updated review. *Neurother*. 2012;9(4):753-775.

Postuma RB, Gagnon JF, Bertrand JA, et al. Parkinson risk in idiopathic REM sleep behavior disorder: preparing for neuroprotective trials. *Neurology*. 2015;84:1104-1113.

Pressman MR. Factors that predispose, prime and precipitate NREM parasomnias in adults: clinical and forensic implications. *Sleep Med Rev*. 2007;11(1):5-30.

39

Seizures and Sleep

SILVIA NEME-MERCANTE, ZAHREDDIN ALSHEIKHTAHA, NANCY FOLDVARY-SCHAEFER

Questions

Questions 1–3 are based on Case 1:

Case 1: A 16-year-old Caucasian female with no known past medical history presents with a new onset of arm jerks for the past 2 months. The episodes are abrupt and brief and occur exclusively 1–2 hours after awakening. Her jerks can occur singly or in a series with increasing intensity, but without alteration of awareness. She admits to staying up later than usual (11 PM) for her upcoming Scholastic Aptitude Test (SAT). She has been drinking 4–5 cups of coffee to remain alert during the day. She does not snore, and her body mass index (BMI) is 22 kg/m². She denies a history of seizures, oral trauma, and incontinence. She has a cousin with epilepsy that is controlled with medication.

1. The correct diagnosis will be confirmed with which of the following?
   A. Periodic limb movement index of 15 on an overnight PSG
   B. Serum ferritin of 15 ng/mL
   C. Burst of generalized polyspikes and 4–6 Hz spike and wave complexes on a sleep-deprived EEG
   D. Mesial frontal meningioma on a brain MRI
   E. Independent right and left frontal spikes on a routine EEG

2. Medical treatment was initiated and the patient now reports worsening symptoms. Her legs are also jerking, resulting in falls, with no loss of awareness. Her total sleep time is 4 hours a day. Which of the following is the next most appropriate recommendation?
   A. PSG followed by a multiple sleep latency test (MSLT)
   B. Initiate treatment with a sedative hypnotic agent
   C. Long-term video-EEG monitoring
   D. Extend sleep duration
   E. Cognitive behavioral therapy for insomnia

3. All of the following epileptic syndromes typically manifest predominantly during sleep or after awakening, except

A. Lennox-Gastaut syndrome
B. Juvenile myoclonic epilepsy
C. Landau-Kleffner syndrome
D. Rasmussen's encephalitis
E. Continuous spike and wave during NREM sleep

Questions 4–7 are based on Case 2:

Case 2: A 48-year-old African American man with a 10-year history of drug-resistant focal epilepsy taking carbamazepine, lamotrigine, and clonazepam is being evaluated for excessive daytime sleepiness (EDS) of 7 year's duration. His wife reports snoring, breathing holding, and leg jerks in sleep. She also reports a recent onset of grunting and leg stiffening that occurs most nights and does not resemble his typical seizures. He scored 16 of 24 on the Epworth Sleepiness Scale (ESS) and has dozed off at work. His examination reveals a neck circumference of 18 inches, BMI of 32 kg/m², retrognathia, and a crowded posterior airway with a grade 3 Friedman tongue position.

4. What is the most likely sleep disorder diagnosis?
   A. Obstructive sleep apnea syndrome (OSAS)
   B. Bruxism
   C. Restless legs syndrome (RLS)
   D. Narcolepsy without cataplexy
   E. Periodic limb movement disorder (PLMD)

5. Which of the following will best confirm the diagnosis?
   A. Out-of-center sleep testing (home sleep testing)
   B. Electromyography (EMG)
   C. In-laboratory video PSG with expanded EEG
   D. Iron and ferritin levels
   E. MSLT

6. What would be the best initial treatment given the known history of epilepsy?
   A. Supplemental oxygen
   B. Mandibular advancement device
   C. Continuous positive airway pressure (CPAP)
   D. Dopamine agonist
   E. Clonazepam

7. The patient reports nightly seizures that wake him from sleep and are characterized by screaming with thrashing movements lasting 10–20 sec and associated with preserved awareness. A typical event was captured on EEG (Fig. 39.1). What can you conclude from the EEG?
   A. EEG reveals a seizure with EEG onset localized to the left frontal region.
   B. EEG is consistent with movement artifact suggesting a confusional arousal.

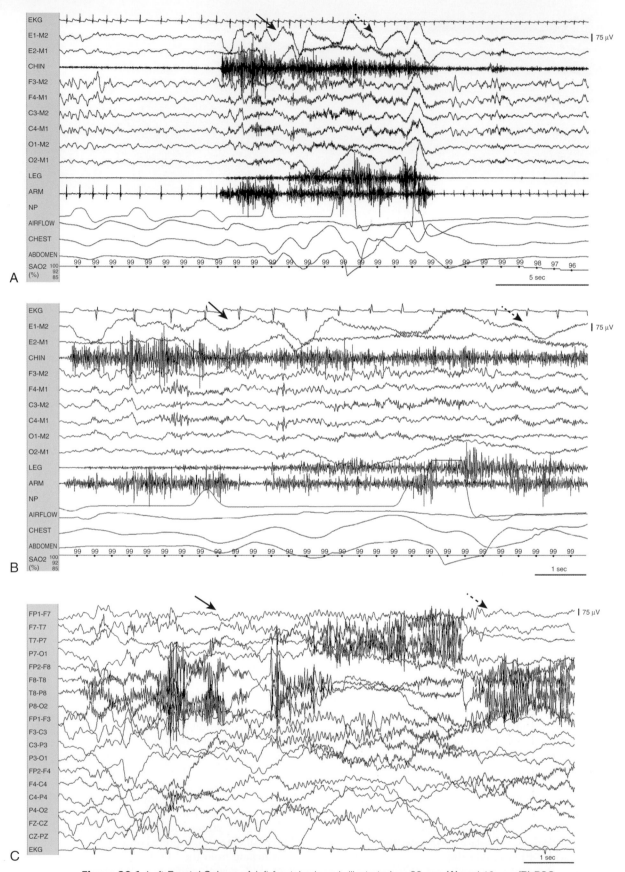

• **Figure 39.1** Left Frontal Seizure. A left frontal seizure is illustrated on 30-sec **(A)** and 10-sec **(B)** PSG montage and an 18-channel EEG montage **(C)**. EEG onset is characterized by rhythmic evolving beta activity maximal in the frontopolar region *(solid arrow)* that becomes diffuse 3 sec later. Clinical onset is depicted by the *dotted arrow*. Note the hypopnea during the clinical seizure.

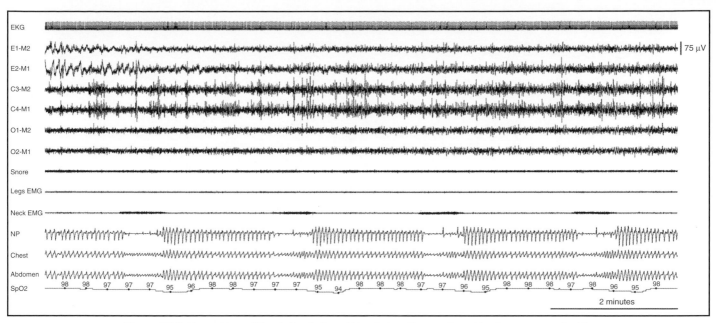

• **Figure 39.2** Vagus Nerve Stimulation-Induced Respiratory Events. Repetitive hypopneas coinciding with the activation of vagus nerve stimulation (VNS) are observed on this 2-minute epoch from a routine PSG tracing (note the cyclical appearance of VNS activation artifact recorded from the lateral neck electromyography electrode). Respiratory changes are seen precisely during VNS activation and terminate abruptly with the end of stimulation. Because of the nature of stimulation, this occurs in a seemingly periodic fashion.

C. EEG is obscured by muscle artifact suggesting a psychogenic nonepileptic seizure

D. EEG represents an arousal from N2 sleep.

E. This is a normal wake EEG.

Questions 8–11 are based on Case 3:

Case 3: A 46-year-old Caucasian woman with a 40-year history of drug resistant focal epilepsy treated with lamotrigine, phenytoin, and clorazepate presents to the sleep clinic for evaluation of daytime sleepiness of 3 month's duration. She underwent implantation of a vagus nerve stimulation (VNS) device 6 months prior and had experienced a 50% reduction in seizures. She has missed 3 days of work in the past month as a result of her severe morning sleepiness. She had a PSG 1 year ago that showed an apnea-hypopnea index (AHI) of 5.6. She declined a trial of CPAP therapy at that time. She sleeps alone and is not aware of snoring or respiratory disturbances in sleep. On examination, she has a BMI of 35 kg/m^2 (increased from 31 kg/m^2 1 year ago), retrognathia, and a grade 3 Friedman tongue position.

8. Given the patient's persistent daytime sleepiness, you recommend a repeat in-laboratory PSG that showed an AHI of 22. Fig. 39.2 shows a 10-minute epoch from the study. Which of the following best explains the increase in AHI?

A. Obstructive sleep apnea induced by antiepileptic drug polytherapy

B. Central sleep apnea induced by antiepileptic drug polytherapy

C. VNS-induced sleep-related breathing disorder

D. Sleep-related seizures causing central apnea

E. Benzodiazepine-induced sleep-related breathing disorder

9. Which of the following is the most appropriate initial treatment?

A. Adaptive servo ventilation (ASV)

B. Discontinue benzodiazepines

C. Positive airway pressure therapy

D. Adjust VNS settings

E. Start modafinil for wake promotion

10. Two months later, the patient returns reporting persistent daytime sleepiness. In addition, she reports an increase in seizure frequency. A repeat in-laboratory PSG shows an AHI of 45 (100% obstructive hypopneas). What is the next most reasonable step?

A. PAP titration study

B. Nasal expiratory airway pressure

C. Hypoglossal nerve stimulation therapy

D. ENT referral for upper airway surgery

E. Antiepileptic drug adjustment

11. As part of sleep and epilepsy counseling, you inform the patient of which of the following?

A. Adherence with CPAP therapy reduces seizure frequency by ≥50% in some cases.

B. Hypoglossal nerve stimulation decreases seizure frequency by ≥50%.

C. Avoidance of supine sleep reduces OSA and risk of SUDEP (sudden unexplained death in epilepsy).

D. A 10-lb weight loss will effectively cure the OSA and decrease seizure frequency.

E. Acetazolamide normalizes the AHI and decreases seizure frequency by ≥50%.

Questions 12–15 are based on Case 4:

Case 4: A 7-year-old girl with infrequent sleepwalking since the age of 4 presents with abnormal movements in sleep for the past 3 weeks. The episodes are characterized by twitching of the left side of the face that spreads to the left arm and leg, associated with drooling and grunting. Episodes occur every night soon after falling asleep. Birth and development were normal. Neurological examination and brain MRI are unremarkable.

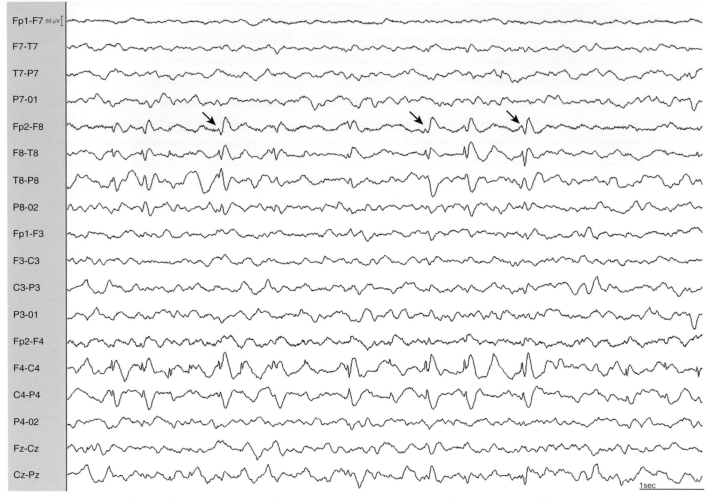

• **Figure 39.3** Centrotemporal Sharp Waves in Benign Rolandic Epilepsy. Interictal EEG tracing showing centrotemporal sharp waves *(arrows)* displayed on an 18-channel anterior-posterior bipolar montage on a 10-sec epoch. The morphology and distribution of the waveforms are characteristic of benign focal epileptic discharges (BFEDs) seen in benign rolandic epilepsy (also known as benign focal epilepsy of childhood). Sharp waves have a stereotyped morphology characterized by a small positivity followed by a prominent negativity and a subsequent negative slow wave that is always of lower amplitude than the sharp wave. BFEDs can be unilateral or bilateral; the latter is more typical in sleep.

12. You recommend a sleep deprived EEG as shown in Fig. 39.3. What abnormality is illustrated by the arrows?
    A. Vertex waves
    B. Bifrontal spikes
    C. Electrode artifact
    D. Centrotemporal sharp waves
    E. Generalized polyspikes

13. In this syndrome, the predominate epileptic abnormality is
    A. Unilateral
    B. Negative in the centrotemporal region and positive in the frontal region
    C. Predominately in REM sleep
    D. Limited to wakefulness
    E. Generalized

14. Based on the clinical history and EEG, what is the correct diagnosis?
    A. NREM parasomnia
    B. REM sleep behavior disorder
    C. Lennox-Gastaut syndrome
    D. Benign rolandic epilepsy (benign childhood epilepsy with centrotemporal spikes)
    E. Panayiotopoulos syndrome

15. Which of the following is the preferred initial therapy?
    A. Imipramine
    B. Clonazepam
    C. Carbamazepine
    D. Melatonin
    E. Vagal nerve stimulation therapy

Questions 16–20 are based on Case 5:

Case 5: A 78-year-old male with a history of focal epilepsy taking lamotrigine and topiramate has been seizure free for 7 years. Seizures in the past were described as an epigastric discomfort followed by reduced awareness and purposeless repetitive manual activity with lip smacking. The patient returns with a 2-month history of unexplained bruising in sleep. His wife describes uncharacteristic sleep-related behaviors, including shouting and swearing, kicking and thrashing of the arms, occurring 3 times per week, usually 1–2 hours after falling asleep.

His past medical history is remarkable for febrile seizures during childhood.

16. What is the most likely etiology of this patient's unexplained bruising?
    A. REM sleep behavior disorder
    B. Nocturnal panic attacks
    C. Psychogenic nonepileptic seizures
    D. Confusional arousals
    E. Sundowning
17. Which of the following will best confirm the diagnosis?
    A. In-laboratory video PSG with expanded EEG and EMG
    B. Out-of-center sleep testing (home sleep testing)
    C. Routine EEG
    D. Brain MRI
    E. Long-term video-EEG monitoring
18. Which of the following findings are likely to be seen on the diagnostic test?
    A. Generalized intermittent rhythmic delta activity maximal in the bifrontal regions
    B. Excessive phasic submental or limb EMG twitching and elevated submental EMG tone in REM sleep
    C. Right frontal sharp waves
    D. Normal brain anatomy
    E. Obstructive apneas and hypopneas with oxygen desaturation
19. Based on suspected diagnosis and PSG findings what would be the best initial treatment?
    A. Clonazepam
    B. Paroxetine
    C. Lacosamide
    D. Venlafaxine
    E. Light therapy
20. The diagnostic study captured epileptic discharges and one of the patient's typical seizures as shown in Fig. 39.4. Which of the following is the most likely epilepsy diagnosis based on the clinical history and EEG findings?
    A. Occipital lobe epilepsy
    B. Generalized epilepsy with febrile seizures
    C. Frontal lobe epilepsy
    D. Temporal lobe epilepsy
    E. Dravet syndrome

Questions 21–23 are based on Case 6:

Case 6: An 8-year-old boy with normal birth and development presents with a 3-month history of abnormal behavior in sleep and daytime fatigue. Episodes are described as brief, tonic contractions of the axial musculature occurring in clusters during sleep nearly every night. Two routine EEGs were reported as normal. The parents noticed that the patient's eyes were open but he was unresponsive. A paternal uncle and the patient's father had similar behavior during sleep in childhood, though milder and less frequent. His examination was unremarkable except for tonsillar hypertrophy.

21. Given the clinical presentation, what is the most likely diagnosis?
    A. REM sleep behavior disorder
    B. Confusional arousal
    C. Autosomal dominant nocturnal frontal lobe epilepsy (ADNFLE)
    D. PLMD
    E. Lennox-Gastaut syndrome
22. A tracing from the patient's sleep-deprived EEG is shown in Fig. 39.5. What does the EEG reveal?

A. Wicket spikes
B. Left frontal spike
C. Vertex wave
D. Asymmetric eye movements
E. Asymmetric sleep spindles

23. Which of the following features is more characteristic of nocturnal frontal lobe seizures than NREM disorders of arousal?
    A. Duration exceeding 3 minutes
    B. Spontaneous remission in the second or third decades of life
    C. Multiple episodes per night
    D. Lack of episode stereotypy
    E. Episodes arising from N3 sleep

Answers

Case 1

1. **The correct answer is C. Burst of generalized polyspikes and 4–6 Hz spike and wave complexes on a sleep-deprived EEG.**

    The patient's seizures semiology is consistent with juvenile myoclonic epilepsy (JME).

    JME is the prototypical form of idiopathic generalized epilepsy (IGE) that affects about 150,000 children and adolescents in the United States each year and accounts for 20%–27% of all patients with IGE.[1,2] The mean age of seizure onset is between 12 and 18 years.[1] Patients with JME have normal cognition, neurological examination, and neuroimaging. Other types of seizures include generalized tonic-clonic (GTC) seizures and absence seizures. Myoclonic and GTC seizures typically occur in the morning within 1–2 hours of awakening and can be dramatically activated by sleep deprivation.[3] Myoclonic seizures most commonly involve the arms but can involve any part of the body. Consciousness is typically preserved. GTC seizures frequently follow a series of myoclonic seizures of crescendo intensity.

    The EEG characteristically features generalized, spike, and wave complexes and/or polyspike and wave complexes at a frequency of 4–6 Hz maximal bifrontal (Fig. 39.6). Interictal discharges increase at sleep onset and on awakening, and are markedly attenuated in sleep. Therefore sleep deprivation prior to EEG is likely to increase the yield of recording epileptic discharges.

    Periodic limb movements (A) is incorrect, as arm jerks occurred exclusively 1–2 hours after awakening, not during sleep. Serum ferritin (B) and brain MRI (D) are normal in patients with JME. Independent right and left frontal spikes (E) would be observed in frontal lobe epilepsy and would not be an EEG manifestation of JME.

2. **The correct answer is D. Extend sleep duration.**

    Sleep deprivation, alcohol, and photic stimulation are the major seizure precipitants in patients with JME and other types of IGE. The mechanisms by which sleep deprivation activates epileptic discharges and seizures are unclear. A lowering of seizure threshold due to neuronal excitability has been hypothesized. Although lifelong treatment is typically required, the prognosis for seizure control is excellent.

    PSG followed by MSLT (A) is recommended in the evaluation of narcolepsy and other CNS hypersomnia disorders, and would not be useful in the management of epilepsy unless the patient presented with severe daytime sleepiness that persisted after extending sleep duration. Long-term video-EEG

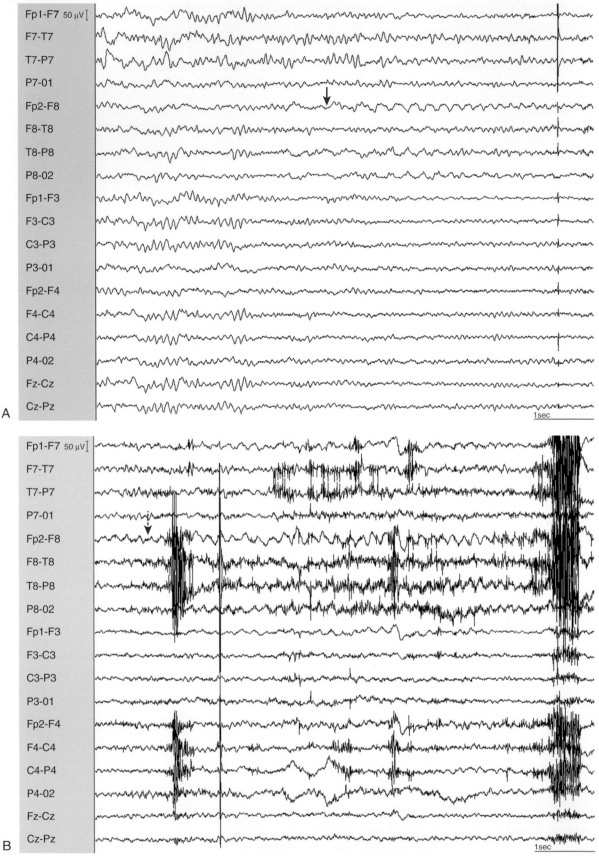

• **Figure 39.4** Temporal Seizure. Shown are consecutive 10-sec epochs of a right temporal seizure displayed on an 18-channel anterior-posterior bipolar montage. EEG onset (**A**, *solid arrow*) shows rhythmic activity evolving in the right temporal chain. Clinical onset (**B**, *dotted arrow*) begins after EEG onset and features oral automatisms that produce electromyography artifact in the frontotemporal regions bilaterally.

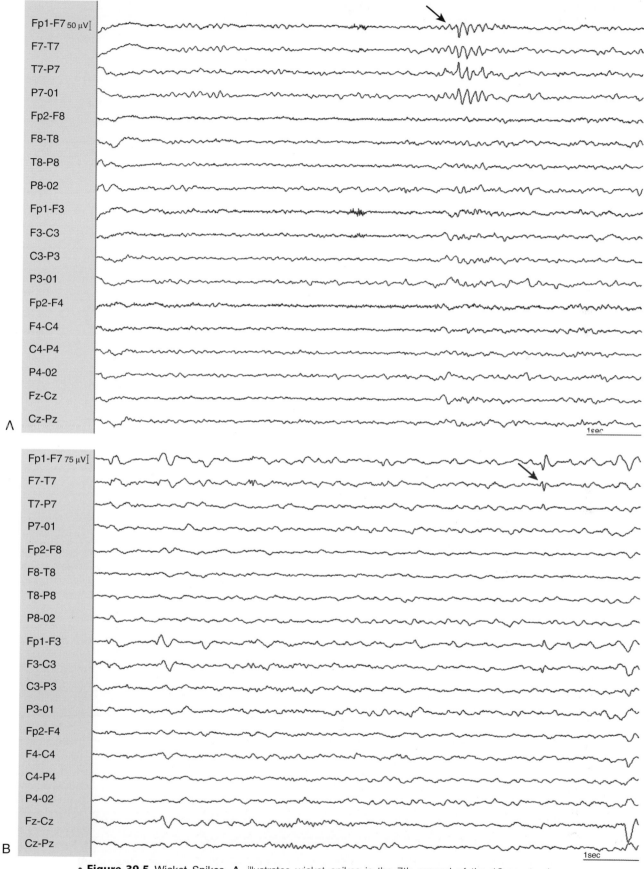

• **Figure 39.5** Wicket Spikes. **A,** illustrates wicket spikes in the 7th second of the 10-sec tracing recorded on an 18-channel anterior-posterior (A-P) bipolar montage. Wicket spikes have an arciform morphology without the after-coming slow wave and are present in the temporal regions. In contrast, **B** illustrates a left frontal spike in the 8th second of the 10-sec tracing recorded on an 18-channel A-P bipolar montage. A negative phase reversal is observed at F7, followed by F3. Irregular slowing is also observed in the left frontal region.

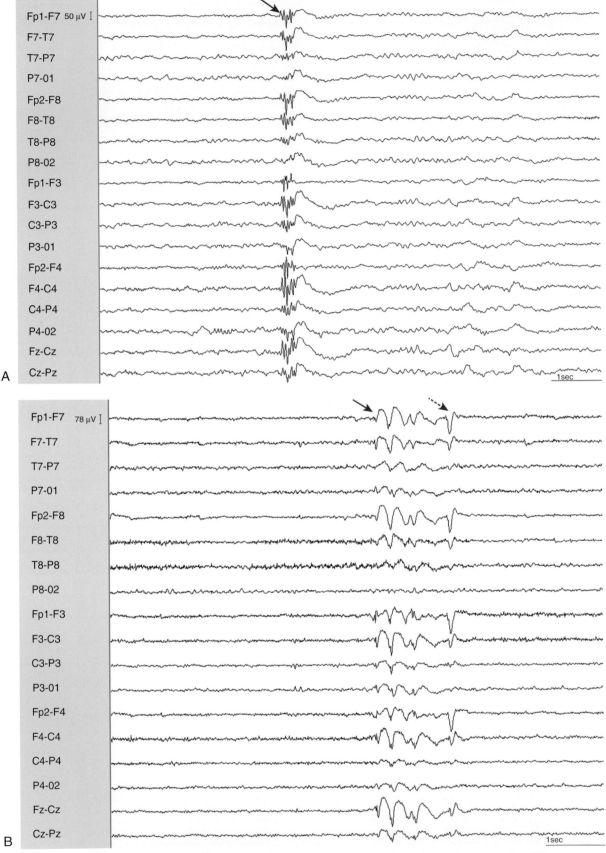

• **Figure 39.6** Generalized Polyspikes and Spike and Wave Complexes. Generalized polyspikes **(A)** and 3–4 Hz spike and wave complexes **(B)** in a 16 year-old female with juvenile myoclonic epilepsy illustrated on a 10-sec tracing featuring an 18-channel, anterior-posterior bipolar EEG montage (double banana). Note the bifrontal maximum amplitude of the epileptic discharges *(solid arrows)*. Eye blinks *(dotted arrows)* are seen in **(B)**.

monitoring (C) would be indicated if seizures fail to respond to appropriate medical therapy and/or if concern is raised regarding the correct diagnosis. Cognitive behavioral therapy (E) and sedative hypnotics (B) would be appropriate only if the short sleep was due to insomnia. In this case, it appears to be volitional.

3. **The correct answer is D. Rasmussen's encephalitis.**

Rasmussen encephalitis is a chronic, inflammatory neurological disorder characterized by intractable epilepsy, progressive hemiparesis, and unilateral hemispheric atrophy presenting in childhood.[4] Seizures are typically focal motor in type, often evolve to status epilepticus (epilepsia partialis continua), and are frequent, occurring during sleep and wakefulness. An autoimmune etiology is hypothesized.

Lennox-Gastaut syndrome (A), JME (B), Landau-Kleffner syndrome (C), and continuous spike and wave during NREM sleep (E) are incorrect, as they are all sleep-related epilepsies.

Case 2

4. **The correct answer is A. OSAS.**

The history of snoring, witnessed apnea, and EDS is highly suggestive of OSAS. The patient's sleep history does not describe features of RLS (C) or bruxism (B). While the patient does report significant EDS, narcolepsy (D) is incorrect, as this diagnosis would be considered only after treatment of OSAS. PLMD (E) should not be considered as the primary diagnosis until other sleep disorders are excluded and a PSG demonstrates periodic limb movements in sleep (PLMS) resulting in sleep disruption.

5. **The correct answer is C. In-laboratory video PSG with expanded EEG.**

A PSG is the most appropriate test to confirm the diagnosis of sleep apnea in the setting of abnormal motor activity or behaviors in sleep that raise concern for PLMs, seizures, or parasomnias. Additional EEG monitoring using electrode placements of the 10–20 International Electrode System is required for the evaluation of seizures and epileptic discharges when epilepsy is suspected. Nocturnal seizures can produce sleep fragmentation, EDS, central and obstructive respiratory events, hypoxia, and hypercapnia.

Out-of-center sleep testing (A) would not allow for the evaluation of the patient's abnormal motor activity in sleep. EMG (B), iron studies (D), and MSLT (E) would not help clarify the nature of his nocturnal symptoms.

6. **The correct answer is C. CPAP.**

CPAP is the first-line treatment for most patients with OSAS and has been shown to improve seizure control in many patients with epilepsy and comorbid sleep apnea.[5] Use of nocturnal oxygen (A) would be the incorrect answer, because it is not sufficient to prevent upper airway collapse in sleep. The efficacy and safety of a mandibular advancement device (B) in patients with epilepsy and OSAS has not been established. Dopamine agonists (D) are not indicated in OSAS. The use of benzodiazepines including clonazepam (E) is incorrect, as these may reduce upper airway tone, thereby contributing to OSAS.

7. **The correct answer is A. The EEG reveals a seizure with EEG onset localized to the left frontal region.**

The patient's history of nocturnal seizures having a hypermotor quality is suggestive of frontal lobe epilepsy.

Fig. 39.1 illustrates a seizure arising from the left frontal region. EEG onset is characterized by rhythmic evolving beta activity maximal in the frontopolar region (solid arrow) that becomes diffuse 3 sec later. Clinical onset is depicted by the dotted arrow. Note the hypopnea during the clinical seizure. An 18-channel EEG montage is shown in Fig. 39.1C. Electro-clinical correlation with high-resolution video would help rule out nonepileptic motor and behavioral activity.

The EEG changes associated with confusional arousals (B) and other NREM arousal disorders typically consist of hypersynchronous delta waves intermixed with faster frequencies that would not evolve considerably and would be generalized in distribution. Psychogenic nonepileptic seizures (C) typically arise during wakefulness and are characterized by normal waking background activity with superimposed muscle or movement artifact. An arousal pattern (D) consists of an abrupt shift of EEG frequency including alpha, theta, and/or frequencies greater than 16 Hz that last at least 3 sec and are not seen on the EEG. The normal wake EEG (E) in adults is characterized by an occipital dominant alpha rhythm admixed with fast activities that are enhanced with eye closure and in the relaxed state.

Case 3

8. **The correct answer is C. VNS-induced sleep-related breathing disorder.**

VNS was approved by the FDA in 1997 as adjunctive therapy for focal epilepsy in patients ≥12 years of age. Although the exact mechanism is unknown, VNS reduces the frequency and severity of seizures by delivering small pulses of electrical stimulation at preset regular intervals. A handheld magnet is used to activate the generator during a seizure, which can reduce the intensity or duration of the event.

In this case, the patient reports worsening of daytime sleepiness after VNS implantation. The emergence or worsening of apneas and hypopneas with VNS therapy has been reported in both adults and children.[6,7] One of the largest series investigated 16 adults with medically intractable epilepsy with PSG before and 3 months after VNS implantation.[7] Postimplantation, the AHI increased in 14 of 16 subjects, and all subjects had decreased airflow and diminished effort with or without tachypnea, coinciding with device activation. A pediatric series reported the emergence of sleep-related breathing disturbances in 8 of 9 children following VNS implantation, including one who developed severe OSA with an AHI of 37.[6] CPAP therapy normalized the AHI in all cases, and resolution of VNS-related apneas was observed after device deactivation.

Ictal and postictal central apneas (D) can occur in patients with nocturnal seizures. However, the answer is incorrect, since the history of worsening symptoms soon after VNS implantation are highly suggestive of a VNS-induced sleep-related breathing disorder, as shown in the figure, and seizures are not observed. Antiepileptic drug polytherapy does not produce obstructive (A) or central (B) apneas, and would not be expected to occur in a periodic fashion. As AED therapy had not been changed since the initial PSG, benzodiazepine therapy (E) would not likely explain the increase in AHI and presentation of severe EDS.

9. **The correct answer is D. Adjust VNS settings.**

In patients with VNS-induced sleep-related breathing disturbances, lowering the generator's stimulus frequency or prolonging the off-time can reduce respiratory events and their effects, including daytime sleepiness.[8] VNS adjustment should be attempted, particularly given the patient's good response to therapy. Due to reports of emergence or worsening of apneas and hypopneas with VNS therapy in both adults and children, the manufacturer of VNS added a warning statement to their product label stating that patients with OSA may have increased apneic events during stimulation. PSG should be considered in all patients prior to VNS implantation and careful follow up thereafter is warranted.

PAP therapy (C) would be considered if the patient remains symptomatic after adjusting VNS settings. ASV (A) is an advanced from of PAP therapy that is indicated for the treatment of central sleep apnea, not OSAS. Reduction or discontinuation of benzodiazepines (B) is unnecessary. Modafinil (E) might be considered for the treatment of residual daytime sleepiness only after OSAS is treated.[9]

10. **The correct answer is A. PAP titration study.**

Based on the patient's medical history and PSG, treatment of OSAS should be initiated and PAP therapy is the treatment of choice given the severity in this case. Alternative treatments for OSA might be considered if PAP therapy is not tolerated. Another approach, not offered as an option in this case, is discontinuation of VNS therapy if the risks of therapy outweigh the benefits. The effects of nasal expiratory airway pressure (B) and hypoglossal nerve stimulation therapy (C) have not been studied in patients with epilepsy. Because of the severity of OSAS, PAP therapy and not upper airway surgery (D) would be the most appropriate treatment. Antiepileptic drug adjustment (E) is unnecessary.

11. **The correct answer is A. Adherence with CPAP therapy reduces seizure frequency by ≥50% in some cases.**

CPAP has been shown to reduce seizures as well as epileptic discharges in adults with epilepsy and OSA.[5,10] Hypoglossal nerve stimulation (B), weight loss (D), and acetazolamide (E) have not been studied for the treatment of OSA in epilepsy.

SUDEP is the number one cause of epilepsy-related death in people with pharmaco-resistant epilepsy. The mechanisms underlying SUDEP are not well understood and may involve several pathophysiological mechanisms including cardiovascular and respiratory dysfunction. Consistent risk factors include poor AED compliance, early age of seizures onset, male gender, GTCs, and nocturnal seizures.[11] Avoidance of supine sleep reduces OSA and risk of SUDEP (A) is the incorrect answer because SUDEP has been associated with sleeping in the prone, not supine, position.[12]

Case 4

12. **The correct answer is D. Centrotemporal sharp waves.**

These sharp waves (arrows) are characterized by their morphology, distribution, and relationship to the sleep-wake cycle.

An electrode pop is caused by an abrupt impedance change between the electrode and the skin surface. Drying of the electrolyte gel/paste or inadequate application of the electrode causing poor contact with the skin produces an electrode pop. Cleaning and reapplication of the electrode can eliminate the artifact. Electrode artifacts have a variety of morphologies but are restricted to a single electrode and do not disturb the EEG background activity, making answer C incorrect.

Answer A is incorrect because vertex waves are normal manifestations of NREM sleep that are maximal in the frontocentral regions and symmetric in normal individuals. Bifrontal spikes (B) are typically seen in focal epilepsy arising from the frontal or vertex region. Generalized polyspikes (E) are bilaterally symmetric discharges seen in virtually all derivations but maximal in the frontal regions.

13. **The correct answer is B. Negative in the centrotemporal region and positive in the frontal region.**

Epileptic discharges in benign rolandic epilepsy (benign childhood epilepsy with centrotemporal spikes) have a stereotyped morphology characterized by a small positivity followed by a prominent negativity and a subsequent negative slow wave that is always of lower amplitude than the sharp wave in the temporal and central derivations. Discharges are usually bilateral and independent. Sharp waves are markedly activated by NREM sleep and appear exclusively in sleep in up to 80% of cases.[13]

On a bipolar montage, the localization of an epileptic discharge is determined by identifying the phase reversal. A negative phase reversal (pen deflections point toward each other) on a bipolar montage identifies the electrode of maximum negativity. On a referential montage, the stereotyped dipole field of these discharges has a negative polarity in the centrotemporal region and positive polarity anteriorly in the frontal region. This is due to the orientation of the generator that is tangential to the cortical surface in the lower rolandic region. Answers A, C, D, and E are therefore incorrect.

14. **The correct answer is D. Benign rolandic epilepsy (benign childhood epilepsy with centrotemporal spikes).**

The clinical history is suggestive of seizures in a child with benign rolandic epilepsy. This syndrome accounts for 15%–25% of childhood epilepsies and features seizures arising from the rolandic area in close proximity to motor cortex.[13] Seizures typically begin around the age of 3–13, with a peak around 8–9 years, and spontaneous remission occurs in most cases in the late teenage years. Patients with benign focal epilepsy of childhood have characteristic unilateral focal sensorimotor seizures, typically involving the face and arm, that frequently evolve into GTCs in sleep.

Answers A and B are incorrect, as twitching of the face with localized progression to the arm and leg are not features of NREM parasomnias or REM sleep behavior disorder.

Lennox-Gastaut syndrome (C) is incorrect, since this epilepsy syndrome is characterized by intractable seizures of multiple types (particularly tonic and atonic seizures), generalized slow spike wave on EEG, and intellectual impairment. Panayiotopoulos syndrome (E) occurs in otherwise normal children and manifests mainly with infrequent autonomic epileptic seizures and autonomic status epilepticus, which is not described in this case.

15. **The correct answer is C. Carbamazepine.**

A number of antiepileptic drugs are effective in children with benign focal epilepsy. However, carbamazepine is recommended as the first-line agent. Valproate, gabapentin, and levetiracetam have been found to be effective as well.[14] Antidepressants (A), benzodiazepines (B), melatonin (D), and vagal nerve stimulation therapy (E) are incorrect answers because they either would not be effective or, in the case of B and E, are not considered first-line treatments of focal epilepsy.

Case 5

16. **The correct answer is A. REM sleep behavior disorder.**

Rapid eye movement sleep behavior disorder (RBD) is a REM sleep parasomnia, first described in cats and later in humans. It is characterized by dream-enacting behavior associated with the loss of normal skeletal muscle atonia resulting in abnormal, excessive motor activity mirroring dream content during REM sleep. Symptoms range from minor limb twitches to more complex and violent movements, including talking, laughing, yelling, swearing, punching, kicking, jumping, and running, that can result in injuries, including dislocations, lacerations, fractures, and hematomas.[15]

Answers B and D are incorrect, as nocturnal panic attacks and confusional arousals do not include major, violent movements as part of the behavioral spectrum. Confusional arousals are in general present in early childhood and are longer in duration (several minutes) and less stereotyped. Psychogenic nonepileptic seizures (C) are typically seen in patients with psychiatric disorders and generally arise from wakefulness. Sundowning (E) is characterized by confusion, restlessness, and wandering that occurs in the evening or nighttime in patients with cognitive impairment or dementia, and is not described in this case.

17. **The correct answer is A. In-laboratory video PSG with expanded EEG and EMG.**

PSG with expanded EEG and additional EMG leads on the arms and legs is recommended for the diagnosis of RBD. Expanded EEG will help differentiate RBD from nocturnal seizures. Epileptic abnormalities are not observed in RBD.

Out-of-center sleep testing (B) would not provide EEG or EMG recording, and is not indicated when conditions other than OSAS are suspected.

While a routine EEG (C) and brain MRI (D) may be useful, neither would clarify the nature of the current episodes nor confirm the diagnosis of RBD. Long-term video EEG (E) would not be indicated unless routine and sleep-deprived EEGs and other appropriate outpatient testing fail to confirm a diagnosis and EEG characterization of spells is required.

18. **The correct answer is B. Excessive phasic submental or limb EMG twitching and elevated submental EMG tone in REM sleep.**

The polysomnographic characteristics of RBD include sustained muscle activity in REM sleep in the chin EMG and excessive transient muscle activity during REM in the chin or limb EMG.[16]

While brain MRI (D) is normal in the majority of RBD patients, neuroimaging is not required or helpful in confirming the diagnosis in most cases. Generalized intermittent rhythmic delta activity maximal in the bifrontal regions (A), right frontal sharp waves (C), and obstructive apneas and hypopneas with oxygen desaturation (E) are not features of RBD.

19. **The correct answer is A. Clonazepam.**

Clonazepam (A) is considered a first-line treatment for RBD, although clinical trials are lacking. Due to the risk of adverse effects, it should be used with caution in patients with dementia, gait disorders, and comorbid OSA. The effective dose is usually 0.25–2.0 mg prior to bedtime.

Lacosamide (C) and light therapy (E) are not treatments of RBD. Paroxetine (B) is a selective serotonin reuptake inhibitor and venlafaxine (D) is a serotonin-norepinephrine reuptake inhibitor, both of which have been implicated as triggers of RBD.

20. **The correct answer is D. Temporal lobe epilepsy.**

The figure illustrates a right temporal seizure an 18-channel A-P bipolar montage. Together with the clinical history of an epigastric discomfort, reduced awareness, and purposeless manual and oral automatisms, this would support the diagnosis of right temporal lobe epilepsy (TLE).

TLE is the most common focal epilepsy in adolescents and adults.[17] Seizures of temporal lobe origin typically begin with an aura of a rising epigastric sensation, fear, déjà vu (an illusion of familiarity), or depersonalization (a feeling of lack of reality in one's sense of self). Common ictal manifestations include behavioral arrest with staring and oral (lip smacking, chewing, or licking) or limb automatisms. Seizures typically occur in both wake and sleep. Mesial TLE is associated with febrile seizures occurring in the first decade of life.

Answers A, B, C, and E are incorrect. Seizure semiology in occipital lobe epilepsy (A) typically includes visual and oculomotor disturbances. Elementary visual hallucinations are common, and postictal headache occurs in more than half of patients.

Generalized epilepsy with febrile seizures (B) is an autosomal dominant disorder usually caused by mutations in SCN1A (a voltage-gated sodium channel). One-third of patients have febrile seizures only; two-thirds have a variety of epilepsy syndromes, both focal and generalized.

Frontal lobe seizures (C) typically feature hypermotor or asymmetric tonic posturing, usually brief (<30 sec) and occurring in clusters in sleep.

Dravet syndrome (E) is a pharmaco-resistant epilepsy that occurs in the first year of life in previously healthy children, manifested by prolonged generalized or unilateral seizures.

Case 6

21. **The correct answer is C. ADNFLE.**

The mostly likely diagnosis is ADNFLE, as suggested by the clinical and family histories. This was the first genetic epilepsy identified, associated with mutations in the CHRNA4 gene that encode for the neuronal nicotinic acetylcholine receptor α4 subunit.[18] The mean age of onset is approximately 12 years of age. Seizures are stereotyped, brief (<60 sec), hyperkinetic or tonic, and can appear violent due to the abrupt onset and offset of large, proximal body movements of high amplitude and velocity. Consciousness is often preserved. Brain imaging and EEG are often normal, as the epileptic generator is believed to be deep in the ventromesial frontal regions.

Lennox-Gastaut syndrome (E) features pharmaco-resistant seizures of multiple types in children with developmental impairment. RBD (A), confusional arousals (B), and periodic limb movements (D) do not produce repetitive axial tonic activity in sleep.

22. **The correct answer is A. Wicket spikes.**

Wicket spikes are considered a normal EEG variant characterized by trains of spike-like waveform having an arciform appearance and not accompanied by distortion of the background or an after-coming slow wave, as seen in epileptic discharges. Wicket spikes have a frequency of 6–11 Hz and an amplitude ranging from 60 to 200 mV and are present in the temporal regions mainly during drowsiness.

A left frontal spike (B) is shown in Fig. 39.5B. The figure illustrates a discharge with a phase reversal at F7 and slowing in the left frontal region. As shown, epileptic discharges stand out from the background and are commonly followed by an aftergoing slow wave. Discharges are typically differentiated by duration, with spikes lasting between 20 and 70 msec and sharp waves longer than 70 msec.

Answers C and E are incorrect. Vertex waves (C) are sharply contoured waves with a maximum amplitude in the central regions and duration less than 0.5 sec. The initial deflection is surface negative, and is followed by a low voltage positive wave with the same distribution. Vertex waves are most often seen during transition to stage N1 sleep but can occur in either N1 or N2 sleep. Spindles (E) are trains of 11–16 Hz waves ≥0.5 sec, maximal in amplitude in the central derivations. Vertex waves and spindles can be asymmetric in the setting of large structural lesions. The patient is in N2 sleep and no appreciable eye movements (D) are observed in the figure.

23. **The correct answer is C. Lack of episode stereotypy.**

Nocturnal frontal lobe seizures typically arise from light NREM sleep (N1 or N2), less often from N3. Seizures arising from REM sleep are exceptionally rare due to the lack of EEG synchronization and presence of muscle atonia. Seizures often occur multiple times per night and are stereotyped with similar, if not identical, clinical manifestations from one episode to another. Seizures are in general short (a few seconds to less than one minute) and begin in the first or second decade of life, although age of onset is highly variable. In contrast, the NREM arousal disorders, including confusional arousals, sleepwalking, and sleep terrors, in general present in early childhood with episodes of longer duration (A), that are not stereotyped (D) and less frequent and predominate in N3 sleep (E). Spontaneous remission in the second decade of life is common (B).

40

Sleep-Related Movement Disorders

DENISE SHARON, ARTHUR S. WALTERS, CINDY MACK

Questions

Questions 1 and 2 refer to patient 1:

Patient 1: A 55-year-old overweight, divorced, Caucasian woman reports that she "cannot sleep": she has difficulty falling asleep several nights per week. Once asleep she rarely wakes up, but when she does she has difficulty resuming sleep. She is very upset with her sleep problems. It all started the year before after she had coronary bypass surgery. Around the same time, she started drinking a glass of red wine with dinner "because it is good for the heart." The patient reports that she is so busy she cannot sit down until late night. Sometimes she is so exhausted that she falls asleep on the sofa. Her bedtime varies between 10 PM and midnight. Once in bed, she rubs her legs to help her sleep. She has always done this, and both her sister and her daughter do it. Occasionally, she may need to get up and go to the kitchen. She reports having difficulty waking up at her regular 6 AM and having a "slow start" after such nights. She usually does not have a problem taking a short nap in the afternoon. She denies excessive daytime sleepiness and reports no difficulty driving during the day. In the evening she needs to stop and stretch her legs or get out of the car after an hour-long drive, and this frustrates her. She is not sure about snoring.

1. The most likely pathophysiologic process and diagnosis in this patient are:
   A. Dopamine and restless legs syndrome (RLS)
   B. Gamma amino butyric acid (GABA) and chronic insomnia
   C. Leptin and obstructive sleep apnea (OSA)
   D. Serotonin and depressive disorder
2. What is the most appropriate course of action for patient 1?
   A. Check ferritin level; diagnostic polysomnography (PSG) and, if needed, therapeutic or combined (split) night; a selective serotonin reuptake inhibitor (SSRI)
   B. Manage with stimulus control; zolpidem 10 mg at bedtime; home sleep apnea testing (HSAT)
   C. Obtain serum iron stores; pramipexole 0.125 mg; eliminate red wine
   D. Request patient to complete sleep diaries; cognitive behavior therapy (CBT); sleep hygiene education

3. RLS is more common in:
   A. African American multipara women
   B. African American nullipara women
   C. Asian multipara women
   D. Asian nullipara women
   E. European and North American multipara women
   F. European and North American nullipara women
4. The best documented abnormality associated with RLS is:
   A. Brain dopamine deficiency
   B. Brain iron deficiency
   C. Decreased glutamate in the brain
   D. Loss of dopamine cells
5. Neuroimaging studies suggest that RLS involves the:
   A. Cerebellum, sensorimotor cortex, thalamus
   B. Cerebral cortex, hippocampus, corticospinal tract
   C. Pons, hypothalamus, amygdala
   D. Putamen, substantia nigra, medulla
6. Which of the following is mostly associated with increased risk of RLS?
   A. Child bearing history, anemia, and sleep bruxing
   B. Female gender, family history of RLS, and presence of periodic limb movements (PLMs)
   C. Hypnic jerks, stress, and brief myoclonic electromyographic (EMG) bursts (75–100 msec)
   D. Male gender, family history of Parkinson's disease, and presence of REM atonia
7. The main factor in the diagnosis of RLS is:
   A. How relief of symptoms is achieved
   B. How rest affects the symptoms
   C. The circadian predilection to occur in the evening
   D. The urge to move the legs
8. In order to diagnose RLS in a child:
   A. The child has to describe how he or she relieves the discomfort in his or her own words.
   B. The child has to describe the discomfort in his or her own words.
   C. The parent has to notice PLMs.
   D. The parent has to observe when the discomfort occurs.
9. Periodic limb movements of sleep (PLMS) are:
   A. Frequently associated with RLS
   B. Rarely observed with other sleep disorders
   C. To be treated when observed
   D. Very frequent in otherwise normal PSG in young adults
10. The term "mimics" of RLS refers to:
    A. Associated polysomnographic findings
    B. Comorbidities

C. Confounders

D. Risk factors

11. Classes of treatment options approved in the United States by the Food and Drug Administration (FDA) for the treatment of RLS include:

A. Dopamine agonists and an alpha 2 delta ligand

B. Dopamine agonists and benzodiazepines

C. Nonpharmacologic options and opioids

D. Opioids and benzodiazepines

12. Avoiding the following may improve RLS symptoms:

A. Alcohol, tannins, and caffeine

B. Exercise, yoga, and weight loss

C. Hot baths, compression stockings, and sexual activity

D. Massage, botulinum toxin type A, and enhanced external counter-pulsation (EECP)

13. The main considerations for choosing how to manage RLS include:

A. Age, gender, and interference with daily functioning

B. Family history, PLMS, and response to treatment

C. Frequency of symptoms, interference with daily functioning, and sleep

D. The presence of pain, family history, and PLMS

14. Once a dopamine agonist is prescribed, the following needs to be monitored at every encounter:

A. Ferritin level and hemoglobin

B. Quality of life and depression

C. Weight and blood pressure

D. Worsening of symptoms and impulse control disorders (ICD)

Question 15 refers to patient 2:

Patient 2: A 57-year-old female presents as a new patient to the clinic with a documented history of RLS. Initially, her symptoms would start at 9 PM and she was treated with ropinirole 1 mg at 8 PM. On this dose, she got good control of her symptoms for 3 months. Then she returns to the clinic with symptoms now beginning at 5 PM. Her physician added a second dose of ropinirole at 4 PM. She again got good control of symptoms for 3 months, after which she returns to the clinic with symptoms now beginning at 1 PM. Current symptoms seem to be more severe than initially, and her arms are also involved. Following a recent rib fracture, she was prescribed oxycodone that seemed to improve her RLS symptoms. Now she is out of oxycodone. The patient reports that she knows she is not anemic and thinks she had a normal ferritin level within the last 3 months.

15. Management of patient 2 includes:

A. Discontinue ropinirole

B. Increase the daily dose of ropinirole to 2 mg TID

C. Increase the evening dose of ropinirole from 1 to 2 mg

D. Prescribe oxycodone with the evening dose of ropinirole

16. Augmentation is characterized by all answers except:

A. An earlier appearance of the RLS symptoms during the day

B. A shorter duration of treatment efficacy and/or greater intensity of symptoms

C. A shorter latency period of the symptoms at rest

D. Symptoms appearing in the early morning

E. The symptoms spreading proximally to the legs, to the arms, and to other body parts

17. Patients with RLS:

A. Can deteriorate when they are hospitalized because of increased mobility

B. Can deteriorate when they are in the perioperative setting because of adverse effects of medications

C. Can improve when they are hospitalized because of increased opportunities to sleep

D. Can improve when they are hospitalized because their anemia is better monitored

Questions 18 and 19 refer to patient 3:

Patient 3: The parents of 4-year-old Tommy report that their child is easily distracted in the evening, becomes fidgety at bedtime, complains of pains and aches, scratches his legs, and refuses to go to bed. He frequently falls asleep on the floor after tucking his feet under his dog. Once asleep, he may kick his legs for a couple of hours then he sleeps throughout the night. It is hard to wake him up in the morning, but he has no complaints during the day and he is doing well in school. When asked, Tommy explains that he needs to walk around because he needs to get rid of "itzy bitzy spider climbing" on his legs. Upon further questioning the mother, who was diagnosed with attention deficit disorder (ADD), she remembers she needed frequent Epson salt baths to calm her legs when she was pregnant but this ceased after the delivery.

18. Your most likely diagnosis for Tommy is:

A. Attention deficit hyperactivity disorder (ADHD), because Tommy is so fidgety and easily distracted, which is supported by the family history

B. Growing pains because of Tommy's complaints of aches and pains at night with no daytime symptoms

C. Periodic limb movement disorder (PLMD) because of reported kicking during sleep

D. RLS because of Tommy's report of "itzy bitzy spider climbing" on his legs, supported by kicking and probably by family history

19. Your initial management plans for Tommy will include:

A. Diagnostic PSG, sleep diaries, rotigotine transdermal patch

B. Methylphenidate, relaxing bedtime routine, discontinue caffeinated sodas and chocolate

C. Serum iron stores, diagnostic PSG, regular sleep routine

D. Sleep hygiene, use of a heating pad, supplemental iron

20. In pregnant women, RLS frequently can:

A. Appear de novo

B. Cause OSA

C. Continue after delivery

D. Improve

21. The following treatments for refractory RLS might be considered during pregnancy and also during lactation:

A. Gabapentin

B. Iron

C. Pramipexole

D. Vitamin D

22. Ropinirole is considered the choice dopamine agonist to treat RLS in the following group of patients:

A. Breast-feeding

B. Hepatic disease

C. Pregnant

D. Renal disease, chronic

23. The diagnosis of RLS in the cognitively impaired elderly is supported by all following statements except:

A. Better sleep quality in daytime than at nighttime

B. Low ferritin level

C. Noticeable leg discomfort that may worsen during periods of inactivity

D. Use of restraints at night

E. Worse sleep quality in daytime than at nighttime

24. The causal relationship between RLS and psychiatric disorders is likely bidirectional and complicated by the treatment of both with psychoactive medications. Please match the following types of medications with their effect on RLS: exacerbating, partially exacerbating, or not. Please note that one or more groups of drugs can produce a similar effect.

I.	Bupropion	1.	Does not exacerbate
II.	Benzodiazepines	2.	Some can exacerbate
III.	Second generation antipsychotics	3.	Exacerbate
IV.	SSRIs		

    A. Do exacerbate: bupropion and SSRIs
    B. Do exacerbate: SSRIs and benzodiazepines
    C. Do not exacerbate: benzodiazepines and second-generation antipsychotics
    D. Do not exacerbate: bupropion and benzodiazepines
    E. Some can exacerbate: benzodiazepines and SSRIs

Question 25 refers to patient 4:

Patient 4: You are interpreting a diagnostic PSG of a 45-year-old male with a body mass index (BMI) of 31 kg/m^2. The PSG shows a sleep latency (SL) of 50 minutes. The apnea-hypopnea index (AHI) was 8. The AHI in rapid eye movements (REM) sleep was 15. Throughout the study, there were few oxyhemoglobin desaturations to a low of 89% and a periodic limb movement of sleep index (PLMSI) of 45, mostly in the first couple of hours.

25. What will be your first recommendation to the referring physician?
    A. Clinical evaluation for RLS or PLMD
    B. Obtain a continuous positive airway pressure (CPAP) titration
    C. Position training
    D. Weight loss
26. Periodic limb movements of sleep (PLMS) are:
    A. Always pathological
    B. Frequent during REM sleep
    C. Scored based on amplitude, duration, and frequency
    D. Scored based on duration, frequency, and arousability
27. All of the following are important when treating periodic limb movement disorder (PLMD) except:
    A. Assessing the iron stores
    B. The perceived impact on sleep and overall functioning
    C. The risk for cardiovascular disease, stroke, and mortality
    D. Unilateral versus bilateral leg movements

Question 28 refers to patient 5:

Patient 5: Charlie is 9 months old and started banging his leg forcefully, rhythmically every second and repeatedly every time he is put to bed, and this stereotyped behavior seems to interfere with his ability to fall asleep. These episodes seem to persist continuously up to approximately 20 minutes. Otherwise, his sleep and development is reportedly normal and age appropriate milestones were achieved.

28. The most probable diagnosis for Charlie is:
    A. Benign sleep myoclonus of infancy
    B. PLMD
    C. Propriospinal myoclonus at sleep onset
    D. Sleep-related rhythmic movement disorder
29. Morning headaches are a common symptom of:
    A. OSA
    B. OSA and sleep bruxism
    C. RLS and OSA
    D. Sleep bruxism and RLS
30. The prevalence of sleep bruxism is higher in:
    A. Adolescents
    B. Adults
    C. Children
    D. The elderly
31. The complaint of painful sensations in the leg occurring during or before sleep and relieved by forceful stretching is mostly associated with:
    A. Hypnic jerks
    B. PLMD
    C. RLS
    D. Sleep-related leg cramps
32. Diagnostic PSG is necessary to establish a diagnosis of:
    A. PLMD
    B. RLS
    C. Sleep bruxism
    D. Sleep-related leg cramps

Question 33 refers to Record 1 (Fig. 40.1):

33. This is a 2-minute PSG tracing. How would you score this tracing?
    A. Artifact
    B. Normal in some patients with the beginning of CPAP use
    C. Part of a spontaneous arousal
    D. PLMD

Questions 34 and 35 refer to patient 6, Record 2 (Fig. 40.2):

Patient 6: A 61-year-old woman presents for a diagnostic PSG for the evaluation of snoring and daytime sleepiness. Record 2 shows a fragment of her diagnostic PSG.

34. Based on current American Academy of Sleep Medicine (AASM) scoring criteria, how many PLMs are scorable in this 5 minute fragment?
    A. 0
    B. 2
    C. 4
    D. 8
    E. 16
35. This is a 5-minute PSG tracing. How would you characterize the events in this tracing?
    A. Artifact
    B. OSA and PLMD
    C. OSA with arousal
    D. PLMD

Answers

1. **The correct answer is A. Dopamine and RLS.**
This question addresses both the diagnosis of this patient and the possible underlying pathophysiology. The patient is concerned by sleep difficulties associated with an urge to move her legs (she cannot sit down, needs to go) that is relieved by movement (rubs her legs, gets up and goes, stretches her legs), triggered by rest (needs to stop after an hour drive). It is more prominent in the evening (evening drive, cannot sit down until late night, rubs her legs to sleep in the evening, but not in the afternoon). Box 40.1 lists the RLS diagnostic criteria based on the ICSD-3. The diagnosis of RLS is further supported by family history (sister and daughter)[1] triggered by blood loss during surgery possibly due to low iron stores[2] and tannins (red wine drinking).[3] In addition, the patient is a Caucasian female, a population group that has a higher incidence of RLS. The most likely pathophysiologic processes in RLS are iron deficiency and dopamine dysregulation.[2] (Answer A is correct.)

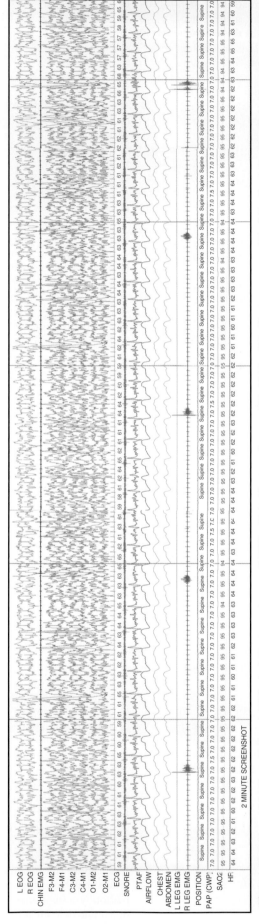

• **Figure 40.1 Record 1. Channel Key:** L-EOG—Left Electrooculogram; R-EOG—Right Electro-culogram; Chin EMG—Chin Electromyogram; F3-M2—Frontal Left to Right Mastoid (or Auricular); F4—M1—Frontal Right to Left Mastoid (or Auricular); EEG—C3/M2—Electroencephalogram: Left Central to Right Mastoid (or Auricular); EEG—C4/M1—Electroencephalogram: Right Central to Left Mastoid (or Auricular); EEG—O1/M2—Electroencephalogram: Left Occipital to Right Mastoid (or Auricular); EEG—O2/M1—Electroencephalogram: Right Occipital to Left Mastoid (or Auricular); EKG—Electrocardiogram; PTAF—Pressure Transducer Air Flow sensor cannula; L Leg EMG—Left Leg Electromyogram; R Leg EMG—Right Leg Electromyogram; PAP (CWP)—Positive Airway Pressure measured in centimeters of water pressure; SaO2—Oxyhemoglobin saturation; HR—Heart Rate.

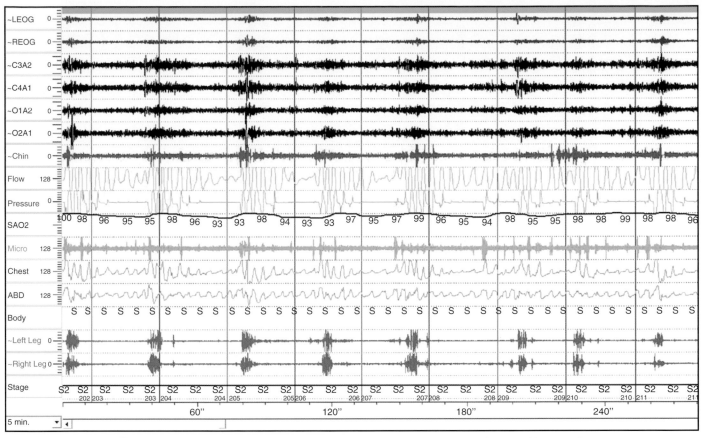

• **Figure 40.2** Record 2. **Channel Key:** L-EOG—Left Electrooculogram; R-EOG—Right Electrooculogram; EEG—C3A2 Electroencephalogram. Left Central to Right Auricular; EEG—C4A1—Electroencephalogram: Right Central to Left Auricular; EEG—O1A2—Electroencephalogram: Left Occipital to Right Auricular; EEG—O2/M1—Electroencephalogram: Right Occipital to Left Auricular; SAO2—Oxyhemoglobin saturation; Micro—Microphone; ABD—Abdominal breathing. (From Phillips B. Special conditions, disorders and clinical issues of SRMD. In: Kushida C, ed. *The Encyclopedia of Sleep*. 1st ed. Elsevier, 2013:109–113. Waltham, MA: Academic Press, with permission).

• **BOX 40.1** **Diagnostic Criteria for Restless Legs Syndrome (ICSD-3)**

A. An urge to move the legs usually accompanied by or thought to be caused by uncomfortable and unpleasant sensations in the legs. These symptoms must:
1. Begin or worsen during periods of rest or inactivity such as lying down or sitting
2. Be partially or totally relieved by movement, such as walking or stretching, at least as long as the activity continues
3. Occur exclusively or predominantly in the evening or night rather than during the day
B. These features are not solely accounted for as symptoms of another medical or behavioral condition
C. The symptoms of RLS cause concern, distress, sleep disturbance, or impairment in mental, physical, social, occupational, educational, behavioral, or other important areas of functioning.

RLS, Restless legs syndrome.

The patient describes difficulty initiating and maintaining sleep for over a year, which may suggest a diagnosis of chronic insomnia disorder that has been associated with GABA dysregulation.[4] However, her sleep difficulties occur only in association with her need to move, making the RLS diagnosis a more probable one. The role of GABA in RLS has not been thoroughly elucidated, although Winkelman et al. (2014) showed that GABA levels correlated with PLM indices and RLS severity.[5] (Answer B is incorrect.)

The patient is middle-aged and overweight, describes difficulty waking up in the morning, and is not sure about her snoring, providing limited support for a possible diagnosis of OSA, which is presumably associated with leptin dysregulation.[6] Her sleep difficulties seem to be better explained by a diagnosis of RLS than of OSA. (Answer C is incorrect.)

The patient reports being very upset about her sleep problems that started after major surgery. Major surgeries have been associated with depression and personality changes.[7] Serotonin dysregulation has been involved in depression.[8] However, other symptoms of depression such as depressed mood, hopelessness, and helplessness were not reported. The frequent association of RLS with pain and with depression points to a role for serotonin dysregulation in RLS as well. (Answer D is incorrect.)

2. **The correct answer is C. Obtain serum iron stores; pramipexole 0.125 mg; eliminate red wine.**
The assessment of the iron stores in RLS is strongly recommended.[9] Start treatment for RLS because the patient is highly symptomatic affecting her sleep and function. Published treatment guidelines[10] recommend starting at the lowest therapeutic dose and increasing gradually to control symptoms.[11] Commonly used RLS medications are listed in Table 40.1.

TABLE 40.1 **Commonly Used Pharmacologic Treatments for Restless Legs Syndrome**

Class	Medication and Generic Availability	Dosage for Restless Legs Syndrome	Half-life (h)	Metabolism/Excretion	Augmentation %	Specific Indications	Main SE	Use in Children (C) During Pregnancy (P) and Lactation (L)	Food and Drug Administration Status*	American Academy of Sleep Medicine Recommendation
Alpha-2-delta Ligands	Gabapentin (generic)	300–1200 mg up to 2700 mg/d po	5–7	Renal (unchanged)	None reported	Painful symptoms, sleep difficulties, Combined with DAs	Somnolence dizziness, fever, ataxia, nystagmus, weight gain, depression, increased suicidal thoughts	C: reduced symptoms and improved sleep P: impairment of synaptogenic process in mice L: 300–900 mg in the evening	Off label use	Option
	Gabapentin enacarbil (extended release gabapentin)	600–1200 mg/d po	5–6	Renal (unchanged)	None reported	Chronic, moderate to severe RLS, painful symptoms, sleep difficulties, augmentation	As noted previously, plus blurred vision, tremor, irritability, dry mouth, decreased sexual drive, hypersensitivity reactions, eosinophilia	No reports	Approved for 600 mg/d	Guideline
	Pregabalin	50–450 mg/d po	6	Renal	None reported	Chronic, painful symptoms, moderate to severe RLS	Angioedema, hypersensitivity reactions, infection, blurred vision, ataxia, dizziness, tremor, dry mouth, weight gain, vertigo, depression, suicidal thoughts	No reports	Off label use	Option
Benzodiazepines	Clonazepam (generic)	0.5–4 mg/d po	30–40		None reported	Sleep difficulties	Drowsiness, dizziness, ataxia, cough, depression, constipation, urinary retention, myalgia, hypersensitivity reaction	C: aggravates hyper-activity if comorbid with ADHD P: orofacial clefts early and sedation at term; if needed, 0.25–1 mg/d during trimester 2 and 3; not with anticonvulsants	Off label use	No recommendation unless to promote sleep
	Temazepam (generic)	15–30 mg/d po	10		None reported	Sleep difficulties	Insomnia, dizziness, lethargy, irritability, drowsiness constipation, urinary retention	P: increased fetal mortality if combined with diphenhydramine	Off label use	No recommendation unless to promote sleep

	Dose		Elimination			Side effects		Off label use	Guideline
Dopamine agonists									
Carbido Carbidopa/levodopa (generic) Carbidopa/levodopa sustained release	25 mg/100 mg po	1–2	Primarily renal	60–82	Intermittent use up to 2/wk (flights, long drives)	Dizziness, nausea, insomnia, augmentation, end of dose rebound	C: reportedly effective P: ER 20/100–50/200 L: inhibits milk production	Off label use	Standard (ER form not included)
Pramipexole (generic) Pramipexole ER	0.125 mg up to 2 mg po	8–12	Renal	33	Chronic Also with hepatic dysfunction	Drowsiness, insomnia, constipation, headaches, orthostatic hypotension, hallucinations, augmentation, ICD, dry mouth	C: reportedly effective	Approved (not ER)	Standard (ER form not included)
Ropinirole (generic) Ropinirole XL	0.25/0.5 mg up to 4 mg po	6	Primarily hepatic	24	Chronic Also with renal dysfunction	Syncope, nausea, headaches, dizziness, orthostatic hypotension, augmentation, insomnia, confusion, ICD	C: reportedly effective	Approved (not XL)	Standard (XL form not included)
Rotigotine	1–3 mg/24 h transdermal patch	Secreted continuously	Primarily renal with some hepatic	5	Chronic Also with symptoms throughout the day, or when oral treatment not possible	Insomnia, nausea, headaches orthostatic hypotension, augmentation, application side reactions	C: trial results awaited	Approved	Standard
Iron									
Oral—elemental iron (generic), i.e., ferrous sulfate 325 mg has 65 mg elemental iron	65 mg + Vit C/2–3/day	1–2	GI	None reported	Ferritin less than 75 ng/L	Nausea, constipation, anorexia, heartburn, vomiting, diarrhea, dark stools, stomach cramps	C: 3 mg/kg/d if ferritin less than 50 ng/L P: 65 mg 1–2/d if ferritin less than 75 ng/L L: oral iron if ferritin less than 75 ng/mL		Option
IV Sodium ferric gluconate (generic) Iron sucrose	1000 mg IV possible + subsequent 450 mg IV	6–8	GI	None reported	Ferritin less than 30 ng/L	Muscle cramps, blurred vision, nausea, vomiting, diarrhea, constipation, cough, joint pain, dizziness	P: if ferritin less than 30 ng/L during trimester 2 and 3 and postpartum		

Continued

TABLE 40.1 Commonly Used Pharmacologic Treatments for Restless Legs Syndrome—cont'd

Class	Medication and Generic Availability	Dosage for Restless Legs Syndrome	Half-life (h)	Metabolism/ Excretion	Augmentation %	Specific Indications	Main SE	Use in Children (C) During Pregnancy (P) and Lactation (L)	Food and Drug Administration Status*	American Academy of Sleep Medicine Recommendation
Opioids	Oxycodone (generic)	2.5–30 mg/d po	3–4		None	Chronic Refractory symptoms	Constipation, nausea, vomiting, drowsiness, pruritus, tolerance, respiratory depression, sedation	P: increased birth defects in trimester 1; 5–20 mg/d in trimester 2 and 3 in very severe RLS and not carriers of CYP2D6	Off label use	Guideline
	Methadone	5–30 mg/d po	15–30		None	Chronic Refractory symptoms	Anxiety, nervousness, dry mouth, diarrhea, constipation, loss of appetite, loss of sex drive, tolerance, respiratory depression, sedation	P: linked with SIDS	Off label use	Guideline
	Tramadol (generic)	50–200 mg	6–7		One study	Chronic Refractory symptoms	Pruritus, anxiety, tremor, hallucinations, diarrhea, constipation, tolerance	P and L: 50–100 mg/d cautiously	Off label use	Guideline
Adrenergic agonists	Clonidine (generic)	0.05–0.9 mg/d	12–16	Mainly hepatic	None	C: with ADHD (FDA approved)	Hypotension, orthostatic hypotension, sedation, drowsiness, dizziness, dry mouth, dry eyes, decreased total REM sleep and increased REM sleep latency	C: reportedly effective P: detrimental effect in animal studies L: passes in breast milk	Off label use	Option

*Indicates US Food & Drug Administration Approval as of June 2016.

Abbreviations: AASM, American Academy of Sleep Medicine; ADHD, attention deficit hyperactive disorder; DA, dopamine agonists; FDA, US Federal Drug Administration; IV, intravenous; mg, milligram; mg/d, milligram/day; po, oral administration; REM, rapid eye movement; RLS, restless legs syndrome also known as Willis-Ekbom disease; SE, side effects; SIDS, sudden infant death syndrome.

In addition, it might help to eliminate red wine to avoid alcohol and tannins.[12] (Answer C is correct.)

Answer A provides an incomplete assessment of the iron stores. It also adds a SSRI that may worsen RLS.[13] PSG is not indicated for the diagnosis of RLS. (Answer A is incorrect.)

Answer B refers to insomnia management (stimulus control and zolpidem 10 mg at bedtime). HSAT is not helpful in patients with RLS, since usually it does not include tibialis anterior channels, unless it is coupled with a limb movement activity-monitoring device such as PAM-RL[14] or similar. (Answer B is incorrect.)

Answer D concentrates on insomnia management. Although sleep diaries, CBT, and sleep hygiene education might be used in the management of RLS, this does not represent the most appropriate course of action. Alternately an RLS specific sleep diary might be used (Table 40.2). (Answer C is incorrect.)

3. **The correct answer is E. European and North American multipara women.**
The prevalence of RLS as defined by the ICSD-3 is twice as high in women than in men and higher in Europe and North America where it can reach 5%–10% for mild, intermittent RLS, and 1.5%–3% for clinically significant disease.[15] It has also been positively associated with pregnancy and parity number.[16] (Answer E is correct.)

One of the risk factors for RLS is pregnancy, and the odds increase with the parity number. (Answers B, D, and F are incorrect.)

The prevalence of RLS in Asia is approximately 2% compared with 15%–16% in Europe and North America.[17] (Answer C is incorrect.)

It is also lower in African American women than in women of European origin.[18] (Answer A is incorrect.)

4. **The correct answer is B. Brain iron deficiency.**
The brain iron deficiency in RLS patients has been confirmed by several laboratories in six studies using different methods.[2] Reduced iron was noted in the substantia nigra, the red nucleus, the putamen, the caudate, and the thalamus (Fig. 40.3). This reduction correlated with RLS severity.[19] Fig. 40.4 maps the basal ganglia. (Answer B is correct.)

Studies assessing the dopamine pathophysiology in RLS patients presented contradictory findings.[2] Positron emission tomography (PET) studies showed both a decrease in striatal

TABLE 40.2	Sample Restless Legs Syndrome Diary		
Day	**Period of Day**	**Symptoms**	**No Symptoms**
Day 1	AM		
	PM (before 6 PM)		
	Night (after 6 PM)		
	Sleep initiation		
	Sleep maintenance		
Day 2	AM		
	PM (before 6 PM)		
	Night (after 6 PM)		
	Sleep initiation		
	Sleep maintenance		
Day 3	AM		
	PM (before 6 PM)		
	Night (after 6 PM)		
	Sleep initiation		
	Sleep maintenance		
Day 4	AM		
	PM (before 6 PM)		
	Night (after 6 PM)		
	Sleep initiation		
	Sleep maintenance		
Day 5	AM		
	PM (before 6 PM)		
	Night (after 6 PM)		
	Sleep initiation		
	Sleep maintenance		
Day 6	AM		
	PM (before 6 PM)		
	Night (after 6 PM)		
	Sleep initiation		
	Sleep maintenance		
Day 7	AM		
	PM (before 6 PM)		
	Night (after 6 PM)		
	Sleep initiation		
	Sleep maintenance		

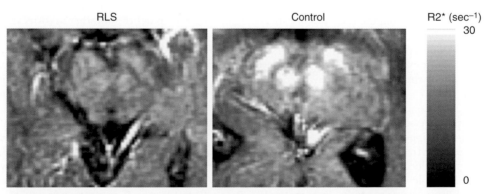

• **Figure 40.3** Magnetic Resonance Imaging Measurements of Brain Iron.[19] R2* images in a 70-year-old RLS patient and a 71-year-old control subject. Much lower R2* relaxation rates are apparent in the RLS case in both red nucleus and substantia nigra. *RLS*, Restless legs syndrome. (From Allen RP, Barker PB, Wehri FW, Song HK, Earley CJ. MRI measurement of brain iron in patients with restless legs syndrome. *Neurology*. 2001;56[2]:263–265, with permission.)

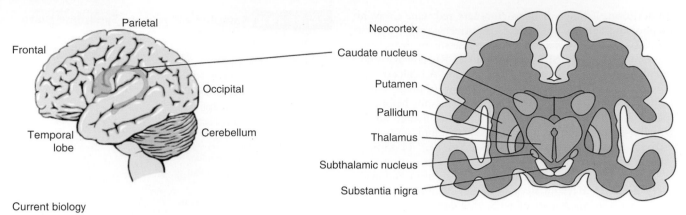

• **Figure 40.4** Schematic Depiction of the Basal Ganglia. The basic anatomy of the brain showing the major regions within the basal ganglia: the striatum *(blue)*, which is made up of the caudate nucleus and the putamen; the pallidum *(pink)*, which is made up of outer and inner segments; the subthalamic nucleus *(green)*; and the substantia nigra *(yellow)*. (From Graybiel AM. The basal ganglia. *Curr Biol.* 2000;10[14]:R509–R511.)

D2 receptors and an increase in receptor binding, with no change or reduction in dopamine transporter (DAT). (Answer A is incorrect.)

Proton magnetic resonance spectroscopy (H MRS) data suggest that although levels of glutamate were not different in RLS patients,[5] increased and not decreased glutamate in the thalamus might be associated with the sleep difficulties in RLS.[20] (Answer C is incorrect.)

There appears to be no loss of dopamine cells, as demonstrated by analyzing RLS autopsy brain tissue. On the other hand, it was shown that there is a down regulation of D2 receptors, implying that there is actually increased dopamine in the brain of RLS patients.[21] (Answer D is incorrect.)

5. **The correct answer is A. Cerebellum, sensorimotor cortex, thalamus.**
In a recent comprehensive literature review, Provini and Chiaro[22] concluded that both structural and functional neuroimaging studies showed RLS to be associated with changes in the thalamus, sensorimotor cortex, and cerebellum. Functional magnetic resonance imaging (fMRI) studies performed at night during periods of sensory leg discomfort showed a bilateral activation of the cerebellum and a contralateral activation of the thalamus, while associated PLMs produced an involvement of the motor cortex.[23] H-MRS studies detected abnormalities of aspartate, glutamate, and GABA in the thalamus of patients with RLS. (Answer A is correct.)

RLS is associated with decreased iron in the putamen and in the substantia nigra as demonstrated by MRI. No RLS-related changes were noted in the medulla. (Answer D is incorrect.)

Voxel-based morphometry MRI (VBM MRI) in RLS patients showed regional decreases in gray matter (GM) density in the cerebral cortex and hippocampus, but no RLS-related changes in the corticospinal tract. (Answer B is incorrect.)

Pontine lesions were described in patients with RLS secondary to stroke and to multiple sclerosis, but not in patients with primary RLS. Overactivation of the hypothalamic-pituitary-adrenal (HPA) system might contribute to the enhanced load of cardiovascular disease in RLS patients.[24] The amygdala is part of the basal ganglia motor circuit and may play a role in motor neuron hyperactivity as a result of dopamine loss. However, no RLS-related changes have been noted in the amygdala. (Answer C is incorrect.)

6. **The correct answer is B. Female gender, family history of RLS, and presence of PLMs.**
A positive family history of RLS and female sex confer increased risk for RLS. The presence of PLMs is supportive of RLS diagnosis, as defined in the ICSD-3. (Answer B is correct.)

The risk of RLS increases with the number of pregnancies.[25] Anemia is a risk factor for RLS. Lavigne and Montplaisir[26] found a 10% coexistence of sleep bruxism and RLS, implying a possible coexistence and common risk factors. (Answer A is incorrect because the question asks about the "mostly associated risk," making Answer B a better answer.)

Sleep starts or hypnic jerks are sudden, brief, simultaneous contractions of the body, or one or more body segments occurring at sleep onset as defined in the ICSD-3. Sleep starts are very common (60%–70% in the general population) and mostly benign, unless reaching abnormal proportions in frequency and amplitude that can interfere with sleep.[27] Hypnic jerks need to be differentiated from other sleep-related movement disorders (SRMD) such as RLS,[28] but were not associated with increased risk for RLS. Increased stress might be associated with sleep deprivation that in turn can trigger RLS, although stress per se was shown to be associated with PLMD and not with RLS.[29] On the other hand, anxiety disorder was shown to be associated with RLS.[30] Brief myoclonic EMG bursts or fragmentary myoclonus are nonperiodic, very brief (usually 75–150 msec), asymmetrical, asynchronous EMG potentials in various muscles of the face, trunk, arms, and legs, with varied amplitude from 50 to several hundred microvolts, at times associated with no visible movements or with small twitch-like movements at the corner of the mouth or the distal fingers. This polysomnographic finding with no known clinical consequence has not been associated with increased risk for RLS. (Answer C is incorrect.)

Although RLS can occur in males, male gender does not confer an increased risk for RLS. REM atonia was not associated with an increased risk for RLS. Therefore, despite possible increased prevalence of RLS in patients with Parkinson's disease,[31,32] and one RLS case with a family history of Parkinson's disease,[33] Answer D is incorrect.

7. **The correct answer is D. The urge to move the legs.**
RLS is a sensorimotor disorder characterized by a strong, nearly irresistible urge to move the legs as defined in the ICSD-3. (Answer D is correct.)

Answers A, B, and C refer to the necessary characteristics of the main symptom (the urge to move the legs) that are: worse at rest, better with movement, and predominantly in the evening or at night. Box 40.1 lists the ICSD-3 diagnostic criteria for RLS. (Answers A, B, and C are incorrect.)

8. **The correct answer is B. The child has to describe the discomfort in his or her own words.**
The diagnosis of RLS in children is challenging and therefore special considerations were added to the diagnostic criteria, including the description of the discomfort in the child's own words (ICSD-3). (Answer B is correct.)

The child's description of how she or he relieves the discomfort is important and contributes to the diagnosis, but is not necessary to make the diagnosis. (Answer A is incorrect.)

The parent's observations of PLMs and of the start of the discomfort further support the diagnosis of RLS, but are not necessary for making the diagnosis. (Answer C and D are incorrect.)

9. **The correct answer is A. Frequently associated with RLS.**
PLMS occur in approximately 85% of RLS patients.[34] (Answer A is correct.)

PLMS are observed in a considerable proportion of patients with various sleep disorders.[35] (Answer B is incorrect.)

PLMS require treatment based on the association with clinical findings.[36] (Answer C is incorrect.)

PLMS greater than 5 per hour are very uncommon in children and adults younger than 40 years, but increase with age, occurring in more than 45% of the elderly. (Answer D is incorrect.)

10. **The correct answer is C. Confounders.**
Hening et al.[37] coined the term "mimics" to describe the presence of confounders of RLS in a case-control study using a validated telephone diagnostic interview based on the four diagnostic criteria of RLS. Table 40.3 classifies and lists RLS confounders or "mimics."[38] (Answer C is correct.)

Although PLMS are frequently observed in RLS patients, there are no pathognomonic polysomnographic findings in RLS. (Answer A is incorrect.)

Comorbidities are conditions associated with RLS, not "mimicking" it (Table 40.4). Frequently, RLS can be diagnosed secondary to these conditions, or these conditions can be diagnosed during the workup for RLS.[38] These conditions may trigger or worsen RLS and affect treatment effectiveness. (Answer B is incorrect.)

Risk factors for RLS include any attribute, characteristic, exposure, or condition of an individual that increases the likelihood of developing RLS and not mimicking RLS. (Answer D is incorrect.)

11. **The correct answer is A. Dopamine agonists and an alpha 2 delta ligand.**
Since Akpinar's[39] and Sandyk et al.[40] reports on the effect of levodopa on RLS symptoms, there have been more than 400 reports studying the effects of dopamine agonists on RLS. Most these studies were performed in the last 20 years when more dopamine agonists (ropinirole, pramipexole, rotigotine) became available. Alpha 2 delta ligands starting with gabapentin[41-43] have been shown to successfully control RLS symptoms, and improve mood and quality of life.[44,45] Currently the FDA-approved dopamine agonists for treatment of RLS include ropinirole, pramipexole, and rotigotine. The only alpha-2-delta ligand approved by the FDA for treatment of RLS is gabapentin enacarbil. (Answer A is correct.)

Benzodiazepines are not FDA approved for the treatment of RLS. Opioids were the first pharmacologic treatment used by Willis[46] for symptoms of RLS, even before the disease was labeled. Opioids continue to be used successfully to treat RLS and treatment resistant symptoms,[47-49] and are approved for use in European countries. There are more than a hundred studies on the effects of opioids on RLS. (Answers B and D are incorrect.)

Among nonpharmacologic options, history accounts and old wives' tales suggest that massage might have been the first treatment for RLS, even before the disorder was recognized. To date, there are very few studies on the nonpharmacologic options for the treatment of RLS,[50] and only the sensory neuro-stimulation pad (Relaxis) is FDA approved. (Answer C is incorrect.)

TABLE 40.3	Conditions That Can Be Confused with Restless Legs Syndrome/Wed (Restless Legs Syndrome "Mimics")[38]			
Abnormal Restlessness	**Nocturnal Leg Discomfort/Pain**	**Hypermotor Activity and Leg Discomfort/Pain**	**Nocturnal Hypermotor Activity**
Akathisia: neuroleptic induced	Growing pains	Painful muscle cramps, including nocturnal leg cramps	Rhythmic movement disorder
Anxiety/agitated depression	Small fiber neuropathies	Intermittent claudication	Periodic limb movement disorder
Attention-deficit/hyperactivity disorder	Venous stasis-varicose veins		Hypnagogic foot tremor
Habitual foot tapping	Myalgias Arthritis Radiculopathies Delusional parasitosis		Alternative leg muscle activation Hypnic jerks Propriospinal myoclonus at sleep onset

(Adapted with permission from Chokroverty S. Differential diagnoses of restless legs syndrome/Willis-Ekbom disease. *Sleep Med Clin.* 2015;10[3]:249–262.)

TABLE 40.4 Restless Legs Syndrome Comorbidities[38]

Medical Disorders	Neurologic Disorders	Medications, Surgical, and Miscellaneous Conditions
Iron deficiency and anemia	Parkinson's disease	Tricyclic antidepressants
Renal failure	Multiple sclerosis	Neuroleptics
Rheumatologic disorders	Myelopathies	Dopamine antagonists
Diabetes mellitus	Polyneuropathies	Antihistamines (mostly H1 antagonists)
Thyroid dysfunction: hypo- and hyper-	Meralgia paresthetica	Nonsteroidal antiinflammatory drugs
Chronic obstructive pulmonary disease	Saphenous nerve entrapment	Lithium
Congestive heart failure	Cortical and subcortical infarctions	Antinausea agents (i.e., metoclopramide)
Thrombophlebitis	Lumbosacral radiculopathies	Gastric reduction
Magnesium deficiency	Isaac syndrome	Lung transplantation
Celiac disease	Stiff man syndrome	Blood donors
Crohn's disease	Spinocerebellar ataxia	Spinal anesthesia (transient RLS)
Sjögren's syndrome	Hyperekplexia	Attention Deficit/Hyperactivity Dis.
Obstructive sleep apnea		Growing pains
		Pregnancy

RLS, Restless legs syndrome.
(Adapted with permission from Chokroverty S. Differential diagnoses of restless legs syndrome/Willis-Ekbom disease. *Sleep Med Clin.* 2015;10[3]:249–262.)

12. **The correct answer is A. Alcohol, tannins, and caffeine.**
Aldrich and Shipley[51] demonstrated worsening of RLS symptoms and increase in PLMS in patients who drank two or more alcoholic beverages per day. Tannins were anecdotally reported to worsen RLS tentatively explained by possible interference with iron absorption, as it was shown in plants.[3] A few studies supported the association of caffeine with PLMD and with RLS. There are only a limited number of studies suggesting that avoiding alcohol, tannins, and caffeine may improve RLS symptoms.[50] (Answer A is correct.)

Among the other options listed, only weight gain and obesity[52] have been associated with an increased risk for RLS. All the other options have been associated scientifically or anecdotally, with improvement in RLS symptoms. (Answers B, C, and D are incorrect.)

13. **The correct answer is C. Frequency of symptoms and interference with daily functioning and sleep.**
A criterion (labeled C) addressing the clinical significance of RLS was added to the diagnostic criteria in the most recent revision of the ICSD (ICSD-3). Box 40.1 lists the diagnostic criteria for RLS. The European RLS Study Group[53] and the medical advisory board of the RLS Foundation[54] advise to consider if RLS symptoms are intermittent or continuous (daily) when recommending medications for RLS. Fig. 40.5 illustrates an algorithm for RLS management (Answer C is correct.)

Age but not gender is a consideration in the management of RLS. At present, the FDA has approved no medication for the treatment of RLS in children. (Answer A is incorrect.)

Response to treatment but not family history is a consideration in choosing how to manage RLS symptoms. In the absence of overt RLS symptoms, family history may play a role in family and genetic counseling. (Answer B is incorrect.)

The presence of pain is an important consideration for treatment once the frequency and the intensity of the symptoms, as well as the interference with daily functioning, are assessed. PLMS in the context of RLS are not an important consideration for treatment unless they interfere with the sleep of the patient or the bed partner. Therefore Answer C is a better answer and Answer D is incorrect.

14. **The correct answer is D. Worsening of symptoms and ICD.**
The purpose of pharmacologic treatment for RLS is to decrease severity of symptoms. Although used as initial treatment for RLS, dopamine agonists may later in the clinical course result in a worsening of RLS symptoms. In these cases it is important to differentiate between a progression of the disease that can occur with any treatment, and rebound and augmentation that are more specific to dopamine agonists. The appearance of de novo ICD has been documented in Parkinson's disease and in RLS patients treated with dopamine agonists. In RLS patients the most common ICD's include compulsive shopping, pathologic gambling, compulsive eating, hypersexuality, and punding.[55] (Answer D is correct.)

The assessment of iron stores is an important part of the RLS patient evaluation but does not need to be monitored at every encounter, unless there is reason to believe blood loss has occurred. (Answer A is incorrect.)

Once the symptoms of RLS are treated with a dopamine agonist, quality of life and depression may improve,[56] and it makes clinical sense to reassess them. However, there is no need to monitor them at every encounter. (Answer B is incorrect.)

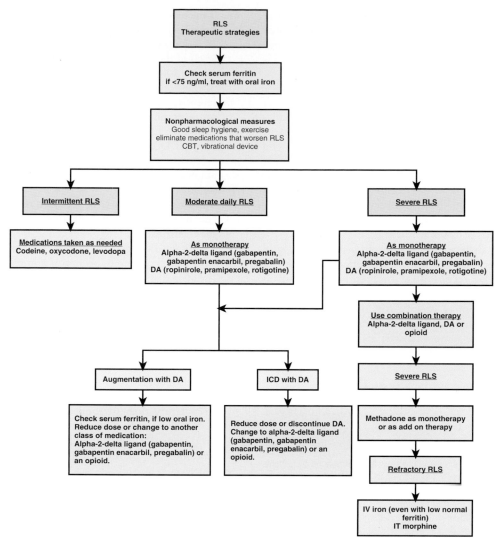

• **Figure 40.5** Algorithm for Restless Legs Syndrome Management. The restless legs syndrome (RLS) diagnosis is based on accepted criteria, including urge to move legs that is relieved by movement, is worse while relaxing, and worse in the evening or night, while mimics are excluded. Iron stores including ferritin, transferrin, IBC, and serum iron, but at least ferritin should be evaluated in all patients with a suspected or an established diagnosis of RLS. Iron replacement therapy is suggested for patients with iron deficiency or low to normal ferritin in an attempt to increase serum ferritin to greater than 75–100 µg/mL. Nonpharmacologic therapy options include avoidance of aggravating factors (sleep deprivation, early morning awakening), substances (caffeine, alcohol), and medications (selective serotonin reuptake inhibitors, antihistamines) and activities that reportedly could ameliorate symptoms. Such activities include maintaining adequate sleep hygiene, mental alerting activities, daytime exercise, leg and calf massage, applied heat, pressure, or vibrations. RLS symptoms are evaluated by their severity and their frequency. Symptoms can be mild, moderate, or severe, and their severity may not be constant. Symptoms can occur occasionally or intermittently (up to 2–3 evenings per week, daily, or regularly (almost daily for continuous periods of time), or starting earlier in the day, or being nonresponsive to treatment. Pharmacologic therapy for RLS reported in the literature, including American Academy of Sleep Medicine practice parameters, RLS Foundation Scientific and Medical Advisory Board, International RLS Study Group (see also Table 40.1) includes: (1) Dopamine agonists: carbidopa/levodopa (25/100 mg 1–2/d), pramipexole (0.125–2 mg/d), ropinirole (0.25–4 mg/d), rotigotine (1–3 mg/d); (2) Alpha-2 delta-ligands: gabapentin enacarbil (600–1200 mg/d), gabapentin (300–2700 mg/d), pregabalin (50–450 mg); (3) Low potency opioids: oxycodone (2.5–30 mg/d), methadone (5–30 mg/d); (4) Iron: oral (325 mg three per day), IV (1000 mg); (5) Medications to promote sleep might be added if needed such as clonazepam (0.5–2 mg). If augmentation occurs (see Box 40.2 for augmentation criteria): (1) Recheck iron stores, at least serum ferritin and depending on the severity of the symptoms. (2) Reduce dopamine agonists or change to long acting if mild symptoms or if severe discontinue for a couple of weeks, while counseling and supporting the patient regarding even worse symptoms initially. (3) Start or transition to an alpha-2-delta ligand such as gabapentin enacarbil for severe symptoms. (4) An opioid can be started or added, such as methadone for severe symptoms. (5) Reiterate nonpharmacological measures. (6) Add sleep promoting treatment if needed (cognitive behavior therapy, pharmacological). *ICD,* Impulse control disorders; *DA,* dopamine agonist.

The assessments of weight and blood pressure are part of the RLS patient evaluation but do not need to be monitored at every encounter, unless there is reason to believe a change has occurred that may have a clinical impact. (Answer C is incorrect.)

15. **The correct answer is A. Discontinue ropinirole.**
Patient 2 presents signs of augmentation: worsening of symptoms compared with prior to starting ropinirole, an earlier onset of symptoms, paradoxical response to treatment (worsening after dose increases), and spreading to the arms. Criteria for augmentation are presented in Box 40.2. The management of augmentation depends on the severity of the symptoms (severe in this case) and on the causing dopaminergic agent (short-acting ropinirole). It includes several options: change to longer-acting dopamine agonist, slowly withdraw the drug, or abruptly stop it. (Answer A is correct.)

Increasing the daily ropinirole dose to a total of 6 mg in three divided doses will probably not be effective in view of the failure of the recent dose increase. (Answer B is incorrect.)

Increasing the evening dose of ropinirole or prescribing oxycodone with the evening dose of ropinirole will probably not be effective since symptoms start at 1 PM, earlier than the evening dose. (Answers C and D are incorrect.)

> **• BOX 40.2 Criteria for Augmentation Based on Max-Plank-Institute Criteria**

Augmentation is a worsening of RLS symptom severity experienced by patients undergoing treatment for RLS. The RLS symptoms in general are more severe than those experienced at baseline.

A. Basic features (all of which need to be met)
1. The increase in symptom severity was experienced in 5 out of 7 days during the previous week.
2. The increase in symptom severity is not accounted by other factors, such as a change in medical status, lifestyle, or the natural progression of the disorder.
3. It is assumed that there has been a prior positive response to treatment.

In addition, B, C, or both have to be met:

B. Persisting (although not immediate) paradoxical response to treatment: RLS symptom severity increases some time after a dose increase, and improves some time after a dose decrease.

C. Earlier onset of symptoms:
1. An earlier onset by at least 4 hours
   or
   An earlier onset (between 2 and 4 hours) occurs with one of the following compared with symptom status before the treatment:
   a. Shorter latency to symptoms when at rest
   b. Spreading of symptoms to other body parts
   c. Intensity of symptoms is greater (or increase in periodic limb movements if measured by polysomnography or the suggested immobilization test)
   d. Duration of relief from treatment is shorter
   Augmentation requires criteria A and B, A and C, or A and B and C to be met.

RLS, Restless legs syndrome.
(Adapted with permission from García-Borreguero D, Allen RP, Kohnen R, et al. Diagnostic standards for dopaminergic augmentation of restless legs syndrome: report from a World Association of Sleep Medicine-International Restless Legs Syndrome Study Group consensus conference at the Max Planck Institute. Sleep Med. 2007;8[5]:520–530.)

16. **The correct answer is D. Symptoms appearing in the early morning.**
RLS symptoms reappearing in the early morning when plasma levels of the dopaminergics decline are mostly associated with rebound or end-of-dose effect that is related to the half-life of the dopaminergic used. Therefore it is important to differentiate between early morning hours and mid- or late morning hours when augmented symptoms can occur. No correlation has been found between rebound and augmentation. (Answer D is correct.)

Answers A, B, C, and E represent individual features of augmentation (Box 40.2). (Answers A, B, C, and E are incorrect.)

17. **The correct answer is B. Can deteriorate when they are in the perioperative setting because of adverse effect of medications.**
Hospitalization and the perioperative setting can trigger or worsen RLS symptoms because of immobility, sleep deprivation, circadian disruption, blood loss and subsequent iron deficiency, withdrawal from RLS therapy, and adverse effects of medications.[57] (Answer B is correct.)

Therefore hospitalized RLS patients may deteriorate because of decreased mobility, not increased mobility. (Answer A is incorrect.)

The sleep of hospitalized patients, including those with RLS, is fragmented, and the circadian rhythms are disrupted. Despite increased opportunities to sleep, it is less restful and sleep deprivation is frequent. (Answer C is incorrect.)

While anemia is better monitored, improvement in RLS symptoms does not immediately follow, and it may take a few months to rebuild the iron stores. (Answer D is incorrect.)

18. **The correct answer is D. RLS because of Tommy's report of "itzy bitsy spider climbing" on his legs, supported by kicking and by probable family history.**
Tommy reports the urge to move in his own words. The urge appears when he tries to sleep at nighttime and is relieved by movement. His kicking during sleep and the family history of possible RLS during his mother pregnancy supports the diagnosis of RLS. (Answer D is correct.)

Tommy does not seem to have daytime symptoms suggestive of ADHD. His restlessness is mainly in the evening and at night. (Answer A is incorrect.)

Tommy is at the age when growing pains may appear, and he complains of aches and pains. Therefore, despite the likelihood of RLS diagnosis, comorbidity with growing pains needs to be considered. Although growing pains need to be considered as a stand-alone diagnosis, the kicking movements in sleep most likely represent PLMS that have been more frequently reported with RLS. In addition, patients with growing pains do not move around to relieve their leg discomfort, as opposed to patients with RLS. Since there was no option for a combined diagnosis, Answer B is incorrect.

The diagnostic criteria for PLMD (Box 40.3) state that the PLMS and associated symptoms are not explained by another current sleep disorder, medical or neurological disorder, or mental disorder (Criterion D). Since in this case the PLMS might be explained by RLS, Answer C is incorrect.

19. **The correct answer is C. Serum iron stores, diagnostic PSG, regular sleep routine.**
The recommended diagnostic approach for children with RLS includes a thorough clinical history and examination, PSG to

---

• **BOX 40.3** **Diagnostic Criteria of Periodic Limb Movement Disorder (ICSD-3)**

Criteria A–D must be met

A. Polysomnography demonstrates PLMS, as defined in the most recent version of the AASM Manual for the Scoring of Sleep and Associated Events.

B. The frequency is greater than 5/h in children and greater than 15/h in adults.

C. The PLMS cause clinically significant sleep disturbance or impairment in mental, physical, social, occupational, educational, behavioral, or other important areas of functioning.

D. The PLMS and the symptoms are not better explained by another current sleep disorder, medical or neurological disorder, or mental disorder.

AASM, American Academy of Sleep Medicine; *PLMS*, periodic limb movements of sleep.

---

assess the presence of PLMS, and an iron profile. Management for children with RLS includes maintaining a regular sleep schedule, good sleep hygiene, avoidance of caffeine (alcohol and nicotine in older adolescents), and regular light exercise.[58] (Answer C is correct.)

Presently there are no high level evidence-based studies for the use of dopamine agonists in children.[59] Although dopamine agonists such as the rotigotine patch may be attempted as a therapy later in the clinical course, the initial management is usually more conservative, with iron replacement as needed. (Answer A is incorrect.)

Relaxing bedtime routine and discontinuation of caffeinated beverages are recommended in the treatment of children with RLS. Methylphenidate treatment can be considered for ADHD. (Answer B is incorrect.)

Improved sleep hygiene and the use of a heating pad can improve the symptoms of RLS. Supplemental iron is recommended only in cases where iron stores are depleted (i.e., ferritin less than 35 nanograms per milliliter).[60] (Answer D is incorrect.)

20. **The correct answer is A. Appear de novo.**
Pregnancy is one of the main risk factors for RLS, more so with subsequent pregnancies. RLS prevalence during pregnancy ranges between 11% and 29%, with a ratio of 3:1 to nonpregnant women. RLS can appear for the first time or worsen during pregnancy, with peak prevalence during the third trimester.[61,62] (Answer A is correct.)

The prevalence of OSA is high during pregnancy, mostly in the third trimester. Snoring correlates with RLS symptoms.[63] CPAP treatment for OSA leads to improvement in RLS symptoms, suggesting that sleep-related breathing disorders (SRBD) are a risk factor for RLS in pregnancy. (Answer B is incorrect.)

In most cases, symptoms of RLS tend to disappear after delivery.[62] (Answer C is incorrect.)

Symptoms of RLS do not improve in pregnancy. (Answer D is incorrect.)

21. **The correct answer is B. Iron.**
Oral iron might be considered for the treatment of RLS during pregnancy and lactation if serum ferritin level is less than 75 nanograms per milliliter. IV iron might be considered for the treatment of refractory RLS during the second or third trimester and postpartum if there is a failure of oral iron and serum ferritin level is less than 30 nanograms per milliliter.

Limited data indicate that breast milk iron levels are not increased after IV infusion.[62] (Answer B is correct.)

Gabapentin may be considered for the treatment of refractory RLS during lactation in doses of 300–900 mg in the evening or at night. There is insufficient evidence and therefore no consensus regarding the use of gabapentin during pregnancy. Very high doses were associated with impaired synaptogenesis in mice.[64] Gabapentin does enter breast milk, but the infant is estimated to receive only 1%–4% of the maternal weight-adjusted dose, and no adverse effects were observed in neonates.[62] (Answer A is incorrect.)

Dopaminergics are first-line medications for the treatment of nonpregnancy RLS. The use of carbidopa/levodopa for the treatment of refractory RLS may be considered during pregnancy (25/100–50/200 mg extended release in the evening or at night) based on a case series showing no adverse effects.[65] However, given the limited safety data on pramipexole and other dopaminergics, there is no consensus among the International Restless Legs Syndrome Study Group (IRLSSG) panel of experts in regard to the use of these medications in pregnancy.[62] (Answer C is incorrect.)

A single study[66] reported reduced vitamin D levels in female RLS patients. There is insufficient evidence for benefit from vitamin D in RLS, and there is some concern of causing harm in pregnancy at doses above the recommended daily allowance. (Answer D is incorrect.)

22. **The correct answer is D. Renal disease, chronic.**
Ropinirole is a nonergot D2 and D3 agonist that is extensively metabolized by the liver. Therefore no dose adjustment is necessary in patients with mild to moderate renal impairment (creatinine clearance 30–50 mL/min).[11] (Answer D is correct.)

The use of dopamine agonists, including ropinirole, was not sufficiently studied in pregnancy and postpartum (breast-feeding). Thus there is no consensus.[61] Since dopaminergics inhibit lactation, ropinirole is not the drug of choice for RLS during breast-feeding. (Answers A and C are incorrect.)

Ropinirole is metabolized by the liver and consequently is not the drug of choice in advanced liver disease. (Answer B is incorrect.)

23. **The correct answer is E. Worse sleep quality in daytime than at nighttime.**
RLS prevalence increases with age and with age-related risk factors and comorbidities.[67] The diagnosis of RLS is based on the clinical examination, challenging in the cognitively impaired. Special considerations for the assessment of RLS in the elderly have been proposed by the IRLSSG (Box 40.4).[68] In addition, the IRLSSG[68] proposed supportive criteria to be considered for the diagnosis of RLS or probable RLS in the cognitively impaired elderly (Box 40.5). Worse sleep quality during daytime than at nighttime is not suggestive of RLS. (Answer E is correct.)

Noticeable leg discomfort that may worsen during periods of inactivity is one of the features considered for the diagnosis of RLS in the cognitive impaired elderly. (Answer C is incorrect.)

Better sleep quality during daytime than at nighttime, low ferritin level, and the use of restraints at night are supportive criteria for the diagnosis of probable RLS in this population. (Answers A, B, and D are incorrect.)

24. **The correct answer is D. Do not exacerbate: bupropion and benzodiazepines.**

BOX 40.4 Diagnostic Considerations for the Diagnosis of Restless Legs Syndrome in the Cognitively Impaired Elderly[67]

Signs of legs discomfort: rubbing or kneading the legs and/or groaning while holding the lower extremities.

1. Excessive motor activity in the lower limbs: pacing, fidgeting, repetitive movements of legs, repetitive foot tapping, rubbing the feet together, and the inability to remain seated.
2. Signs of leg discomfort exclusively present or worse during periods of inactivity.
3. Signs of leg discomfort are diminished with activity.
4. Criteria 1 and 2 occur only in the evening or at night, or are worse at those times.

(Adapted with permission from Figorilli M, Puligheddu M, Ferri R. Restless legs syndrome/ Willis-Ekbom disease and periodic limb movements in sleep in the elderly with and without dementia. Sleep Med Clin. 2015;10[3]:331–342.)

BOX 40.5 Supportive Features for the Diagnosis of Probable Restless Legs Syndrome in the Cognitively Impaired Elderly[67]

1. Response to dopaminergic therapy
2. Patient's past history suggestive of RLS as reported by caregiver or family member
3. Positive family history of RLS
4. Observed PLMs or recorded by polysomnography or actigraphy
5. Significant sleep onset problems
6. Better sleep quality in the day than during the night
7. Use of restraints at night (for institutionalized patients)
8. Low serum ferritin level
9. End-stage renal disease
10. Diabetes mellitus

PLMs, Periodic limb movements; *RLS*, restless legs syndrome.
(Adapted with permission from Figorilli M, Puligheddu M, Ferri Raffaele. Restless legs syndrome/ Willis-Ekbom disease and periodic limb movements in sleep in the elderly with and without dementia. Sleep Med Clin 2015[10]:331–342)

Psychological distress and psychiatric disorders are frequently noted in RLS patients and may affect their response to RLS treatment.[69] This effect underlines the importance of treating these conditions, even if some of the medications may adversely impact the symptoms of RLS.[70] Table 40.5 lists psychoactive medications with their respective effect on RLS.[71] Bupropion, a norepinephrine dopamine reuptake inhibitor, does not seem to worsen RLS and may even improve it.[72] Benzodiazepines have been used to treat SRMD by themselves or in combination with other medications. (Answer D is correct.)

SSRIs and serotonin-norepinephrine reuptake inhibitors (SNRIs) have been associated with increased incidence and worsening of RLS.

Mirtazapine, a noradrenergic and serotonergic antidepressant, was associated with the highest frequency of RLS.[73] (Answers A, B, and E are incorrect.)

Among the second-generation antipsychotics, most are potential triggers for RLS. However, aripiprazole, an atypical antipsychotic with partial dopamine agonist activity, improved the symptoms of RLS in a small case series.[74] (Answer C is incorrect.)

25. **The correct answer is A. Clinical evaluation for RLS or PLMD.**
The PSG results are inconclusive and require corroboration with clinical data. The PSG demonstrates PLMS with a frequency of 45 per hour. If the patient has indeed difficulty initiating sleep, as suggested by his prolonged sleep onset latency of 50 minutes, and the PLMS could not be better explained by another disorder, a diagnosis of PLMD could be made. Box 40.3 lists diagnostic criteria for PLMD. PLMS are frequently seen in RLS patients that may also present with difficulty initiating sleep, as suggested by the prolonged sleep onset latency. RLS diagnosis is based on clinical evaluation. Box 40.1 lists the diagnostic criteria for RLS. It should be noted that difficulty initiating sleep and symptoms of RLS or PLMD could affect compliance with treatment for SRBD. (Answer A is correct.)

CPAP titration and position training are therapeutic options for OSA. In this case the diagnosis of OSA has to be corroborated with clinical data before treatment can be initiated. Box 40.6 lists the diagnostic criteria for OSA. (Answers B and C are incorrect.)

Weight gain has been associated with OSA and other sleep disorders. The effect of weight management in the treatment of sleep disorders is not yet fully understood. While achieving and maintaining an ideal weight is a valid recommendation in sleep medicine, answer A is better as first recommendation. (Answer D is incorrect.)

26. **The correct answer is C. Scored based on amplitude, duration, and frequency.**
PLMS are scored based on their amplitude, an 8-μV increase above resting EMG, their duration, 0.5–10 sec by AASM criteria, and their frequency, four or more limb movements at 5–90 sec intervals. Record 4 (Fig. 40.6) shows a recording of PLMS. (Answer C is correct.)

The prevalence of PLMS is estimated at approximately 8% of adults, with only about half of them reporting sleep disturbance. The prevalence of PLMS increases markedly in late adulthood, occurring in over 45% in the elderly without marked increase in sleep-related complaints. (Answer A is incorrect.)

PLMS are less frequent, their duration is shorter, and the intermovement interval is longer in REM.[75] (Answer B is incorrect.)

Some of the PLMS may result in arousals that are scored and a PLM Arousal Index is calculated. Since not all PLMS result in arousal, Answer D is incorrect.

27. **The correct answer is D. Unilateral versus bilateral leg movements.**
In most cases PLMS present as a combination of unilateral of each leg and bilateral movements. When treating PLMD no differences were noted based on the location of the movements. (Answer D is correct.)

The perceived PLMS impact on sleep and overall functioning, and the potential risk for cardiovascular disease, stroke, and mortality are important considerations in the treatment of PLMD.[76] (Answers B and C are incorrect.)

The availability of stored iron is a main consideration when choosing the treatment for PLMD. (Answer A is incorrect.)

28. **The correct answer is D. Sleep-related rhythmic movement disorder.**
Sleep-related rhythmic movement disorder is characterized by repetitive, stereotyped, and rhythmic motor behaviors that

TABLE 40.5 The Effect of Psychoactive Medications on Restless Legs Syndrome[71]

Medication Class	Examples	Typical Psychiatric Indication	Likelihood of Exacerbating Restless Legs Syndrome
Selective serotonin reuptake inhibitors	Fluoxetine, citalopram, sertraline, paroxetine	Depression, anxiety	++
Serotonin-norepinephrine reuptake inhibitors	Duloxetine, venlafaxine	Depression, anxiety	++
Norepinephrine dopamine reuptake inhibitor	Bupropion	Depression	−
Tricyclic antidepressants (except desipramine)	Nortriptyline, amitriptyline	Depression, anxiety	+
Tricyclic antidepressant	Desipramine	Depression, anxiety	0
Tetracyclic antidepressant (also noradrenergic and selective serotonergic)	Mirtazapine	Depression, anxiety, increased appetite	+++
Other	Trazodone	Insomnia, depression	+/−
Second-generation antipsychotics	Quetiapine, olanzapine, risperidone	Schizophrenia, bipolar disorder	++
Second-generation antipsychotic (partial dopamine agonist)	Aripiprazole	Schizophrenia, bipolar disorder	+/−
Antihistamines, first generation	Diphenhydramine, hydroxyzine	Insomnia, anxiety	+++
Dopamine agonists	Pramipexole, ropinirole	Depression	− − −
Alkali metal	Lithium	Bipolar disorder	+/0
Benzodiazepines	Lorazepam, clonazepam, alprazolam	Anxiety disorders, insomnia	−
Antiepileptics (except alpha-2-delta agents)	Topiramate, levetiracetam	Bipolar disorder	0
Antiepileptics (alpha-2-delta only)	Gabapentin, pregabalin	Bipolar disorder	− − −

(Adapted with permission from Mackie S, Winkelman JW. Restless legs syndrome and psychiatric disorders. *Sleep Med Clin.* 2015;10[3]:351–357.)

• BOX 40.6 Diagnostic Criteria for Obstructive Sleep Apnea, Adult (ICSD-3)

(A and B) or C satisfy the criteria:

A. The presence of one or more of the following:
1. The patient complaints of sleepiness, nonrestorative sleep, fatigue, or insomnia symptoms.
2. The patient wakes with breath holding, gasping, or choking.
3. The bed partner or other observer reports habitual snoring, breathing interruptions, or both during the patient's sleep.
4. The patient has been diagnosed with hypertension, a mood disorder, cognitive dysfunction, coronary artery disease, stroke, congestive heart failure, atrial fibrillation, or type 2 diabetes mellitus.

B. PSG or HSAT demonstrates:
5. Five or more predominantly obstructive respiratory events (obstructive and mixed apneas, hypopneas, or RERAs) per hour of sleep during a PSG or per hour of monitoring (HSAT).

OR

C. PSG or HSAT demonstrates:
6. Fifteen or more predominantly obstructive respiratory events (apneas, hypopneas, or RERAs) per hour of sleep during a PSG or per hour of monitoring (HSAT).

PSG, Polysomnography; *RERAs*, respiratory effort–related arousals.

• BOX 40.7 Diagnostic Criteria for Sleep-Related Rhythmic Movement Disorder (ICSD-3)

Criteria A–C must be met:

A. The patient exhibits repetitive, stereotyped, and rhythmic motor behaviors involving large muscle groups.
B. The movements are predominantly sleep related, occurring near nap or bedtime, or when the individual appears drowsy or sleepy.
C. The behaviors result in a significant complaint as manifested by at least one of the following:
1. Interference with normal sleep
2. Significant impairment in daytime function
3. Self-inflicted bodily injury or likelihood of injury if preventive measures are not used
D. The rhythmic movements are not better explained by another movement disorder or epilepsy.

Charlie exhibits a repetitive, stereotyped, and rhythmic motor behavior involving his leg that occurs at bedtime and interferes with his sleep. The behavior is not explained by another movement disorder, and there is no history of epilepsy. (Answer D is correct.)

Benign sleep myoclonus of infancy is characterized by brief clusters of repetitive myoclonic jerks separated by brief periods without movement. This pattern is different from the pattern in the sleep-related rhythmic movement disorder that is characterized by continuous repetitive movements that persist for several minutes. Benign sleep myoclonus of infancy occurs

occur predominantly during drowsiness or sleep and involve large muscle groups. It is most commonly characterized by head banging or body rocking, but may present with other types of stereotypic movements as in this case. Box 40.7 lists diagnostic criteria for sleep-related rhythmic movement disorder.

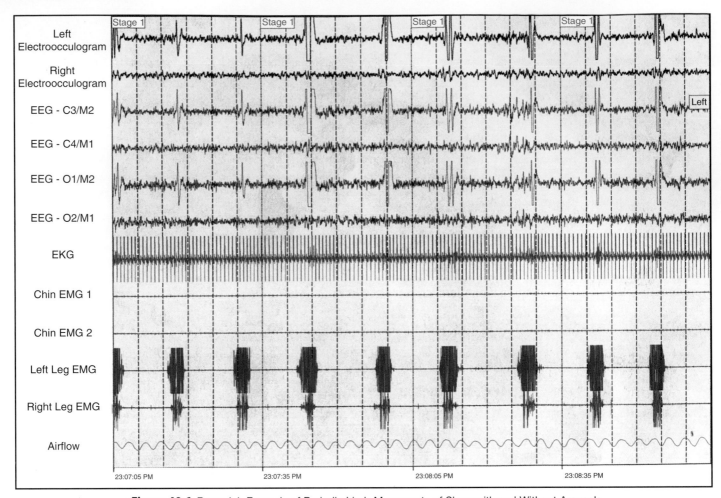

• **Figure 40.6** Record 4. Example of Periodic Limb Movements of Sleep with and Without Arousals. In this 2-minute, compressed polysomnography tracing, periodic limb movements are seen in the leg lead channels *(left leg, right leg)*. The limb movements are bilateral and, for the most part, very rhythmic. Their amplitude is fairly constant around 30–50 μV. Their duration is also constant between 2 and 4 sec. Based on this 2-minute tracing, the frequency would be 240 per hour. However, very rarely patients maintain this frequency throughout the night. Please note the potential arousability of these limb movements. Several are associated with a K complex and most with alpha activity, frequently longer than 3 sec, the minimum duration for scoring arousal. Although there is an EEG correlate to all of these leg movements, some of them do not meet the minimum duration of 3 seconds which is the AASM criterion to score arousal. **Channel Key:** EEG—C3/M2—Electroencephalogram: Left Central to Right Mastoid (or Auricular); EEG—C4/M1—Electroencephalogram: Right Central to Left Mastoid (or Auricular); EEG—O1/M2—Electroencephalogram: Left Occipital to Right Mastoid (or Auricular); EEG—O2/M1—Electroencephalogram: Right Occipital to Left Mastoid (or Auricular); EKG—Electrocardiogram; Chin EMG 1—Chin Electromyogram Left; Chin EMG 2—Chin Electromyogram Right; Left Leg EMG—Left Leg Electromyogram; Right Leg EMG—Right Leg Electromyogram.

in neonates and infants. It only happens during sleep and disappears immediately upon awakening, as opposed to sleep-related rhythmic movement disorder that occurs primarily during wakefulness prior to sleep onset, although occasionally it may persist during sleep. In benign sleep myoclonus of infancy there might be prolonged periods of quiescence and rocking the infant during sleep may precipitate the movements. Box 40.8 lists the ICSD-3 diagnostic criteria for benign sleep myoclonus of infancy. Charlie's movements are localized to his leg, occur prior to sleep, and he was 9 months old when this behavior started—older that the typical birth to 6 months age for benign sleep myoclonus of infancy. (Answer A is incorrect.)

• **BOX 40.8** **Diagnostic Criteria for Benign Sleep Myoclonus of Infancy (ICSD-3)**

Criteria A–E must be met:
A. Observation of repetitive myoclonic jerks that involve the limbs, trunk, or whole body
B. The movements occur in early infancy, typically from birth to 6 months of age.
C. The movements occur only during sleep
D. The movements stop abruptly and consistently when the infant is aroused.
E. The disorder is not better explained by another sleep disorder, medical or neurological disorder, or medication use.

> **• BOX 40.9 Diagnostic Criteria for Propriospinal Myoclonus at Sleep Onset (ICSD-3)**
>
> Criteria A–E must be met:
> A. The patient complains of sudden jerks, mainly in the abdomen, trunk, and neck.
> B. The jerks appear during relaxed wakefulness and drowsiness, as the patient attempts to fall asleep.
> C. The jerks disappear upon mental activation and with onset of a stable sleep stage.
> D. The jerks result in difficulty initiating sleep.
> E. The disorder is not better explained by another sleep disorder, medical or neurological disorder, mental disorder, medication use, or substance abuse.

> **• BOX 40.10 Diagnostic Criteria for Sleep-Related Leg Cramps (ICSD-3)**
>
> Criteria A–C must be met:
> A. A painful sensation in the leg or foot associated with sudden, involuntary muscle hardness or tightness, indicating a strong muscle contraction.
> B. The painful muscle contractions occur during the time in bed, although they may arise from either wakefulness or sleep.
> C. The pain is relieved by forceful stretching of the affected muscles, thus relaxing the contraction.

PLMD is uncommon in infants. It involves extension of the big toe, often in combination with partial flexion of the ankle, the knee, and sometimes the hip. Also the intervals between the movements in sleep-related rhythmic movement disorder are much shorter than the usual interval in PLMs (5–90 sec apart). The characteristic PLMs pattern was not noted in Charlie's case. See Box 40.3 for the diagnostic criteria of PLMD. (Answer B is incorrect.)

Propriospinal myoclonus at sleep onset is characterized by sudden myoclonic jerks occurring in the transition from wakefulness to sleep and rarely during intrasleep wakefulness or upon awakening in the morning (ICSD-3). It is a rare condition, affecting mostly males, and was not reported in children. In contradiction to this, sleep-related rhythmic movement disorder is a very common condition affecting up to 59% infants gradually declining to 5% by the age of 5 years and to approximately 50 cases reported in adolescents and adults. Box 40.9 lists the ICSD-3 diagnostic criteria for propriospinal myoclonus at sleep onset. (Answer C is incorrect.)

29. **The correct answer is B. OSA and sleep bruxism.**
OSA patients frequently report morning headaches that resolve shortly after awakening.[77] Patients with sleep-related bruxism, adults and children, also report frequent morning headaches. The sleep bruxism–related headaches involve the temporal regions and have the characteristics of tension headaches. In patients with wake bruxism, headaches are reported during the day. (Answer B is correct.)

OSA has been associated with morning headaches, but so is sleep bruxism. (Answer A is correct, but Answer B is a more comprehensive answer.)

RLS has not been associated with increased frequency of morning headaches. (Answers C and D are incorrect.)

30. **The correct answer is C. Children.**
The prevalence of sleep-related bruxism is highest in children, standing at 14%–17%. It decreases over the life span to 12% in adolescents and young adults, 8% in the middle-aged, and 3% in the elderly (ICSD-3). (Answer C is correct; Answers A, B, and D are incorrect.)

31. **The correct answer is D. Sleep-related leg cramps.**
Sleep-related leg cramps are common in adults, reportedly 16% and up to 50%–60% by some accounts. It is less frequent in children, approximately 8%.[78] These are painful sensations caused by sudden and intense involuntary contractions of muscles and muscle groups, during which there is muscle spasm and hardness for several seconds. The cramps can be relieved by strongly stretching the affected muscle and sometimes by massage, application of heat, and movement of the affected limb. The cramps are often visible because of the contracted strips of muscles. Polysomnographic studies may reveal nonperiodic bursts of gastrocnemius EMG activity.[79] Box 40.10 lists the ICSD-3 diagnostic criteria for sleep-related leg cramps. (Answer D is correct.)

Hypnic jerks are common, with a prevalence of 60%–70% affecting all ages and both sexes. These are sudden, brief, simultaneous contractions of the entire body or body segments occurring at sleep onset. The motor activity is often associated with a sensory component, often a sensation of falling. The course is usually benign, but when the jerks are frequent, it may lead to insomnia. Hypnic jerks are rarely associated with pain and are not relieved by forceful stretching. (Answer A is incorrect.)

PLMS, the pathognomonic feature of PLMD, are characterized by clusters of repetitive, periodic leg movements, are almost never painful, and may last for a couple of hours. (Answer B is incorrect.)

RLS sensations present with an urge to move the legs, are not all associated with pain, are relieved by any movement, usually of the legs, have a gradual onset, a circadian pattern, and may last for hours.[38] Table 40.6 differentiates RLS from nocturnal leg cramps. (Answer C is incorrect.)

32. **The correct answer is A. PLMD.**
The diagnostic criteria for PLMD include the demonstration of PLMS during diagnostic PSG (Box 40.3). The 2-minute compressed PSG tracing presented in Fig. 40.6 (Record 4) shows eight leg movements. The interval is approximately 15 sec. (Answer A is correct.)

RLS diagnosis is a clinical diagnosis. Even if PSG is not routinely performed, it can demonstrate significant objective abnormalities such as increased latency to sleep onset, higher arousal index, and presence of PLMS that are more prevalent in the first half of the night and can be associated with arousals. Box 40.1 lists the diagnostic criteria for RLS. (Answer B is incorrect.)

PSG is not required for the diagnosis of sleep-related bruxism. Box 40.11 lists the ICSD-3 diagnostic criteria for sleep-related bruxism. PSG might be indicated to demonstrate the disorder and to rule out other sleep-related disorders. If performed, PSG is ideally recorded with masseter muscle activity (rhythmic masticatory muscle activity; RMMA) and with audio-video signal to increase the diagnostic reliability.[80] Record 5 (Fig. 40.7) shows a recording of sleep-related bruxism. (Answer C is incorrect.)

PSG is not required for the diagnosis of sleep-related leg cramps. When performed, it revealed nonperiodic bursts of gastrocnemius EMG activity. (Answer D is incorrect.)

TABLE 40.6 **Differentiating Features of Restless Legs Syndrome/WED and Nocturnal Cramps**[38]

Characteristics	Restless Legs Syndrome/WED	Nocturnal Leg Cramps
An urge to move	+	+
Uncomfortable sensation	+ (Painful in up to 35%–40% of cases)	+ (Painful in 100% of cases)
Relief by	Any movement (usually of the legs)	Specific movement (e.g., dorsiflexion of the foot in case of calf cramps)
Onset	Gradual	Sudden
Circadian pattern of symptoms	+	Always nocturnal
Duration	Hours	Minutes
Distribution of symptoms	Usually in the legs but maybe in the arms also	Localized to the calf with palpable contracting muscle
Response to dopaminergic drug	+	–

(Adapted with permission from Chokroverty S. Differential diagnoses of restless legs syndrome/Willis-Ekbom disease. *Sleep Med Clin*. 2015;10[3]:249–262)

• **BOX 40.11** **Scoring Periodic Limb Movements in Sleep (American Academy of Sleep Medicine Scoring Manual)**

1. The following define a significant LM event:
   a. The minimum duration of a LM event is 0.5 sec.
   b. The maximum duration of a LM event is 10 sec.
   c. The minimum amplitude of a LM event is an 8-μV increase in EMG voltage above resting EMG (duration of at least 0.5 sec).
   d. The timing of the onset of a LM event is defined as the point at which there is an 8-μV increase in EMG voltage above resting EMG.
   e. The timing of the ending of a LM event is defined as the start of a period lasting at least 0.5 sec, during which the EMG does not exceed 2 μV above resting EMG.
2. The following define a PLM series:
   a. The minimum number of consecutive LM events needed to define a PLM series is 4 LMs.
   b. The period length between LMs (defined as the time between onsets of consecutive LMs) to include them as part of a PLM series is 5–90 sec.
   c. Leg movements on two different legs separated by less than 5 sec between movement onsets are counted as a single leg movement. The period length to the next LM following this group of LMs is measured from the onset of the first LM to the onset of the next.
3. An arousal and an LM that occur in a PLM series should be considered associated with each other if they occur simultaneously, overlap, or when there is less than 0.5 sec between the end of one event and the onset of the other event, regardless of which is first.
4. An LM should not be scored if it occurs during a period from 0.5 sec preceding an apnea, hypopnea, RERA, or sleep-disordered breathing event to 0.5 sec following the event.
5. When a period of wakefulness shorter than 90 sec separates a series of LMs, this does not prevent LMs, preceding the period of wake from being included with the subsequent LMs as part of a PLM series.

EMG, Electromyographic; *LM*, leg movement; *PLM*, periodic limb movement; *RERA*, respiratory effort–related arousal.

---

33. **The correct answer is B. Normal in some patients with the beginning of CPAP use.**

It is common to see limb movements in the beginning of CPAP titrations. As the patient adjusts to the CPAP pressure during the night, these typically fade away. (Answer B is correct.)

Artifact in PSG (Record 6, Fig. 40.8) refers to features in the recording that are not naturally present, but occur as a

result of the sleep study situation. PSG artifacts are rarely an isolated episode in the recording. Examples of common artifacts include 60 Hz, muscle artifact, movement, eye movement, sweat, respiratory, ECG, pulse, electrode popping, and reversed polarity. (Answer A is incorrect.)

Record 1 (Fig. 40.1) shows several leg movements during CPAP titration, but no clear spontaneous arousal. In a 2-minute tracing, it is hard to assess the contribution of one event to another. Since leg movements with or without arousals are frequently observed at the beginning of CPAP use, Answer B is a more comprehensive answer. (Answer C is incorrect.)

A PLM series consists of at least four leg movements at 5–90 sec intervals. However, for the diagnosis of PLMD, clinical evidence that the PLMS are causing significant sleep disturbance or impairment in mental, physical, social, occupational, educational, behavioral, or other important areas of functioning is needed (Box 40.3). (Answer D is incorrect.)

34. **The correct answer is A. 0.**

A 5-minute, compressed PSG tracing is presented in Record 2. Eight bilateral PLMs are seen in the leg lead channels, marked "left leg; right leg." However, these leg movements are part of the arousal response to obstructive respiratory events, seen clearly in the respiratory channels ("flow, pressure") and therefore cannot be scored as PLMs (less than 0.5 sec duration from the respiratory event). This is a common finding that highlights the importance of the clinical evaluation in the diagnosis of PLMD. The current AASM criteria for scoring PLMS are presented in Box 40.11. (Answer A is correct.)

Limb movements that are periodic are a common finding in most SRBD, narcolepsy, REM sleep behavior disorder, and can be seen in patients taking antidepressants, or in older males.[81] These LMs occur on two different legs almost simultaneously, less than 5 sec apart, and therefore are counted as one. (Answers B, C, and E are incorrect.) If these LMs had qualified as PLMs, there would have been eight PLMs (Answer D is incorrect).

35. **The correct answer is C. OSA with arousal.**

It is common to see limb movements (and whole body jerks) during respiratory event arousals. In this 5-minute, compressed PSG tracing, PLMs are seen in the leg lead channels ("left leg, right leg"). However, inspection reveals that these leg movements are part of the arousal response to obstructive respiratory events, seen clearly in the respiratory channel ("flow,

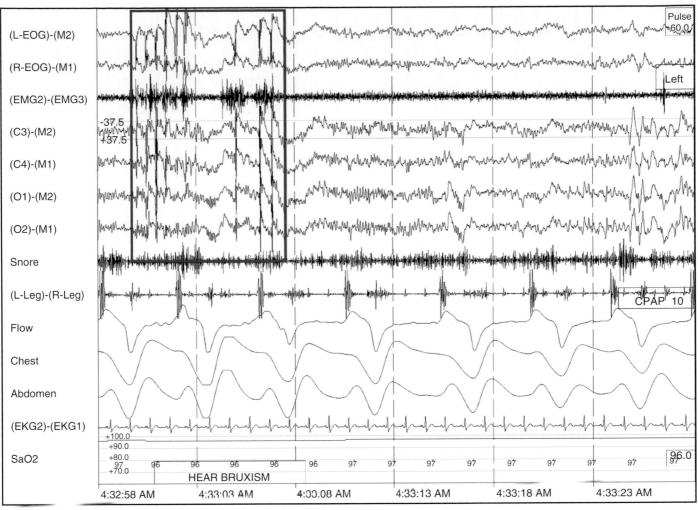

• **Figure 40.7** Record 5. Recording of Sleep Bruxism. In this 30-sec polysomnography, tracing bruxism events are seen in the chin electromyographic (within the *red quadrangle*) and are also reflected in the eye leads and in the EEG and EOG. There is also a tech note reporting that bruxism is heard and is also noted in the leg EMG. **Channel Key:** L-EOG—M2—Left Electrooculogram to Right Mastoid (or Auricular); R-EOG—M1—Right Electrooculogram to Left Mastoid (or Auricular); EMG2—EMG3—Right Chin EMG—Central Chin EMG; EEG—C3/M2—Electroencephalogram: Left Central to Right Mastoid (or Auricular); EEG—C4/M1—Electroencephalogram: Right Central to Left Mastoid (or Auricular); EEG—O1/M2—Electroencephalogram: Left Occipital to Right Mastoid (or Auricular); EEG—O2/M1—Electroencephalogram: Right Occipital to Left Mastoid (or Auricular); L-Leg—R-Leg—Left Leg and Right Leg Electromyogram; EKG—Electrocardiogram; SaO2—Oxyhemoglobin Saturation.

pressure"). This common finding likely accounts for many cases of "PLMD" and is a major reason why the diagnosis of PLMD should be made only after careful exclusion of sleep-disordered breathing, medication side effects, or other causes of movement.

Please see the answer to question 33 for the description of artifact. (Answer A is incorrect.) The PLMS in this case are associated with the respiratory events. In order to establish a diagnosis of PLMD, the PLMS need not be better explained by another sleep disorder (Criterion D, Box 40.3). (Answers B and D are incorrect.)

36. The correct answer is D. Twitches in REM sleep.

In this 300-sec PSG tracing, REM are noted in the EOG channels. Both leg channels show low amplitude frequent muscle twitches. Please note that there is no periodicity in the tracing noted previously, as opposed to what will be characteristic of PLMD. For the most part, the anterior tibialis signals have low amplitude. True PLMD is in general suppressed during REM sleep. Excessive fragmentary myoclonus, which is a NREM phenomenon mostly reported in adult males, is less common than REM twitches. (Answer D is correct.) Please see question 33 for the description of artifact. (Answer A is incorrect.)

Although it is hard to see in a 5-minute tracing, there is no EEG evidence of arousal. (Answer B is incorrect.)

The amplitude for most events is reportedly lower than 8 μV above the baseline, and there is no periodicity. (Answer C is incorrect.)

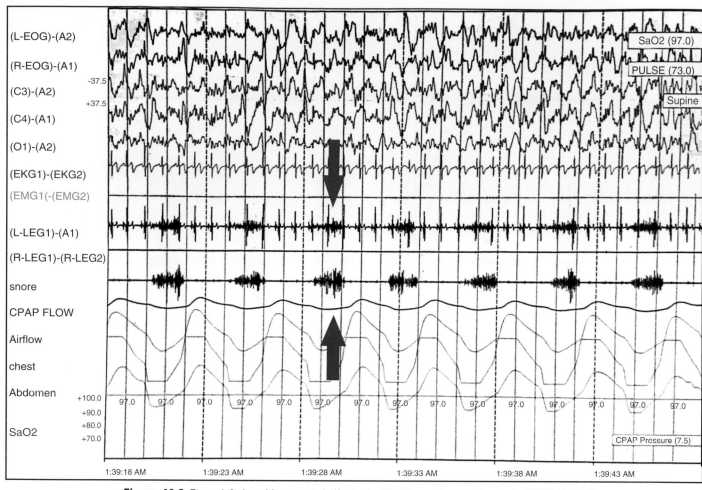

• **Figure 40.8** Record 6. Leg Movement Artifacts. In this 30 sec therapeutic study (CPAP titration) tracing there are two separate leg artifacts. The first is EKG artifact seen in the left leg. The second is also seen in the left leg (see arrows) and represents respiratory artifact. **Channel Key:** L-EOG—A2—Left Electrooculogram—Right Auricular; R-EOG—A1—Right Electrooculogram—Left Auricular; EEG—C3/ A2—Electroencephalogram: Left Central to Right Auricular; EEG—C4/A1—Electroencephalogram: Right Central to Left Auricular; EEG—O1/A2—Electroencephalogram: Left Occipital to Right Auricular; EKG1— EKG 2—Electrocardiogram; EMG 1—EMG 2—Left Chin Electromyogram—Right Chin Electromyogram; PTAF—Pressure Transducer Air Flow sensor cannula; L Leg EMG—Left Leg Electromyogram; R Leg EMG—Right Leg Electromyogram; CPAP Flow—Continuous Positive Airway Pressure flow; SaO2—Oxy-hemoglobin saturation; HR—Heart Rate.

Acknowledgments

The authors would like to thank Supat Thammasitboon, MD, Sleep Medicine Program Director, Tulane University School of Medicine, for his valuable comments and suggestions, and Alon Avidan, MD, Director Sleep Disorders Center, UCLA for his continuous support and extraordinary editorial assistance.

Suggested Reading

Allen RP, Picchietti DL, Garcia-Borreguero D, et al. Restless legs syndrome/Willis-Ekbom disease diagnostic criteria: updated International Restless Legs Syndrome Study Group (IRLSSG) consensus criteria—history, rationale, description, and significance. *Sleep Med.* 2014; 15(8):860-873.

American Academy of Sleep Medicine. *ICSD-3: International Classification of Sleep Disorders, 3rd ed: Diagnostic and Coding Manual.* Darien, IL: American Academy of Sleep Medicine; 2014.

American Academy of Sleep Medicine. *Version 2-2 of the AASM Manual for the Scoring of Sleep and Associated Events: The Definitive Reference for Standardized Sleep Monitoring and Scoring.* Darien, IL: American Academy of Sleep Medicine; 2015.

Chokroverty S, Allen RP, Walters AS, Montagna P, eds. Periodic limb movements in sleep. In: *Sleep and Movement Disorders.* 2nd ed. New York: Oxford University Press; 2013.

Ferini-Strambi L, Walters AS, Sica D. The relationship among restless legs syndrome (Willis-Ekbom Disease), hypertension, cardiovascular disease, and cerebrovascular disease. *J Neurol.* 2014;261(6): 1051-1068.

García-Borreguero D, Allen RP, Kohnen R, et al. Diagnostic standards for dopaminergic augmentation of restless legs syndrome: report from a World Association of Sleep Medicine-International Restless Legs Syndrome Study Group consensus conference at the Max Planck Institute. *Sleep Med.* 2007;8(5):520-530.

Garcia-Borreguero D, Kohnen R, Silber MH, et al. The long-term treatment of restless legs syndrome/Willis-Ekbom disease: evidence-based guidelines and clinical consensus best practice guidance: a report from the International Restless Legs Syndrome Study Group. *Sleep Med.* 2013;14(7):675-684.

Garcia-Borreguero D. Dopaminergic augmentation in restless legs syndrome/Willis Ekbom disease: identification and management. *Sleep Med Clin.* 2015;10(3):287-292.

Henning WA, Allen RP, Chokroverty S, Earley CJ, eds. Restless legs syndrome. In: *Sleep Medicine Clinics*. Philadelphia: Elsevier; 2009.

Picchietti DL, Hensley JG, Bainbridge JL, et al. Consensus clinical practice guidelines for the diagnosis and treatment of restless legs syndrome/ Willis-Ekbom disease during pregnancy and lactation. *Sleep Med Rev.* 2015;22:64-77.

Sharon D, Lee Chiong Jr, eds. Restless legs syndrome and sleep related movement disorders. In: *Sleep Medicine Clinics*. Philadelphia: Elsevier; 2015. 10(3).

Silber MH, Becker PM, Earley C, et al., Medical Advisory Board of the Willis-Ekbom Disease Foundation. Willis-Ekbom Disease Foundation revised consensus statement on the management of restless legs syndrome. *Mayo Clin Proc.* 2013;88(9):977-986.

Sleep in Medical Disorders and Special Populations

SCOTT RYALS, RICHARD B. BERRY

Questions

Endocrine

1. A 45-year-old man with daytime sleepiness, fatigue, and a recent diagnosis of acromegaly presents to your clinic on referral from his endocrinologist. He has severe snoring and endorses gasping at night. You send him for a diagnostic PSG, which yields a normal total sleep time, normal sleep efficiency, and an apnea-hypopnea index (AHI) of 25.6/hour. Review of respiratory events shows 30 obstructive apneas, 5 mixed apneas, 145 central apneas, and 20 hypopneas. What percent of patients with acromegaly have the type of sleep apnea found in this patient's PSG results?
   A. 5%
   B. 33%
   C. 50%
   D. 75%
   E. 90%

2. All of the following are *true* regarding sleep apnea in Acromegaly, *except*:
   A. Hypertension in acromegaly is strongly associated with sleep apnea.
   B. Increased ventilatory responsiveness and elevated GH and insulin-like growth factor—one (IGF-1) levels contribute to the pathogenesis of central sleep apnea in these patients.
   C. Circulating IGF-1, body mass index (BMI), male gender, age, and disease duration are all independently correlated with the presence of sleep apnea in patients with acromegaly.
   D. Polysomnography is recommended in the routine workup of acromegaly, even if acromegaly is in remission.
   E. In cases of treated acromegaly, sleep apnea typically resolves within 2–3 years of biochemical remission.

3. Refer to Fig. 41.1. Which of the following hormones is tied to the onset of the sleep stage shown in this 30-sec epoch from a full channel polysomnogram?
   A. Melatonin
   B. Ghrelin
   C. Growth hormone
   D. Leptin
   E. Testosterone

4. Sleep deprivation is associated with which of the following findings?
   A. Increased leptin
   B. Improved glucose tolerance
   C. Increased ghrelin
   D. Decreased cortisol secretion

HIV

5. All of the following are *true* regarding human immunodeficiency virus (HIV) infection, *except*:
   A. Fatigue increases as HIV infection worsens (CD4 count decreases).
   B. Sleep disturbance decreases as HIV infection worsens (CD4 count decreases).
   C. During early stages of HIV infection there is an increase in SWS that is more prevalent later in the night.
   D. Alpha-delta pattern may be observed in patients with HIV.

6. Vivid dreams have been associated with which one of the following treatments for HIV?
   A. Lamivudine
   B. Abacavir
   C. Efavirenz
   D. Ritonavir
   E. Enfuvirtide

GI

7. All of the following are *true* regarding sleep and gastroesophageal physiology, *except*:
   A. Upper esophageal sphincter tone decreases at sleep onset.
   B. Saliva production decreases significantly during sleep.
   C. Swallowing ceases during sleep, and occurs only during arousals.
   D. The main cause of gastroesophageal reflux (GER) during sleep is inadequate lower esophageal sphincter (LES) pressure.
   E. Esophageal acid clearance is prolonged during sleep.

8. All of the following are *true* regarding treatment of nocturnal GER, *except*:
   A. Patients should avoid eating for at least 2 hours before bedtime, and avoid GER-promoting foods such as chocolate, mint, and alcohol in general.

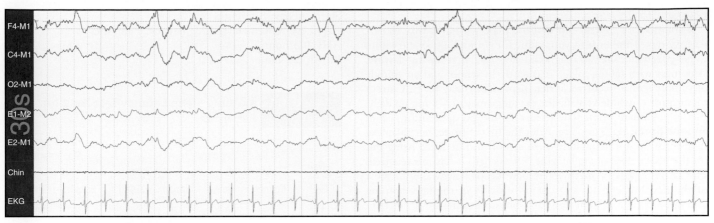

• **Figure 41.1** A 30-second epoch from a Full Channel PSG is shown. *C4-M1*, Central derivation; *Chin EMG*, chin electromyography; *EKG*, electrocardiogram; *E1-M2 & E2-M1*, electrooculographic (EOG) derivations; *F4-M1*, frontal derivation; *O2-M1*, occipital derivation. The *dotted lines* above and below the F4-M1 derivation are at −37.5 µV and +37.5 µV, respectively.

B. Dosing of GER-promoting medications such as bisphosphonates, prostaglandins, and calcium channel blockers should be avoided prior to sleep, if possible.

C. Smoking cessation helps treat nocturnal GER as smoking significantly decreases LES pressure.

D. The right lateral decubitus position is the best position for sleep-related GER.

E. Treating OSA in patients with OSA and nocturnal GER improves nocturnal GER symptom scores.

9. A patient reports that symptoms of reflux are disturbing sleep. The patient is currently taking 20 mg of omeprazole at bedtime. No snoring is reported. What alterations in proton pump inhibitor (PPI) treatment do you recommend for this patient?

A. Increased dose of omeprazole to 40 mg

B. Switch to another PPI

C. Add a histamine blocker such as ranitidine

D. Change the timing of PPI dose

Pregnancy

Questions 10–11 refer to patient A.

Patient A: A 24-year-old G2P1 female presents at 26 weeks' gestation. In recent months she has developed restless legs symptoms, which begin in the early evening and last until she falls asleep. These symptoms occur 4–5 nights a week, delay sleep latency more than an hour, and are increasingly bothersome. She does not snore. She does not smoke, does not drink caffeine, and takes no other medications. Vital signs and physical exam are normal. You send for iron panel with ferritin, which are all unremarkable.

10. The patient cannot tolerate these symptoms anymore and wishes to begin a medication for restless legs syndrome (RLS). Of the following, which is the best treatment choice for the patient?

A. Ropinirole

B. Pramipexole

C. Rotigotine transdermal

D. Gabapentin

E. Oxycodone IR (immediate release)

11. What is the typical natural course of RLS that develops during pregnancy, once delivery occurs?

A. Symptoms resolve shortly after delivery

B. Symptoms persist for 2–3 months and then resolve

C. Symptoms persist at the same level as they were during the third trimester

D. Symptoms worsen over the next few months

Questions 12–14 refer to patient B.

Patient B: A 34-year-old G4P3 female in the 24th week of pregnancy presents to your office. She has experienced disrupted sleep throughout the pregnancy, with symptoms including heartburn and musculoskeletal discomfort. In recent weeks she has had more instances of disrupted sleep, which now has been punctuated with fetal movement as well as nocturia.

12. Put in order the prevalence of disrupted sleep in pregnancy by trimester, from *most* disrupted to least.

A. 1st, 2nd, then 3rd

B. 1st, 3rd, then 2nd

C. 2nd, 3rd, then 1st

D. 3rd, 1st, then 2nd

E. 3rd, 2nd, then 1st

13. Shorter sleep duration in pregnancy is linked to which of the following?

A. Shorter labor duration and lower risk of cesarean deliveries

B. Longer labor duration and lower risk of cesarean deliveries

C. Shorter labor duration and higher risk of cesarean deliveries

D. Longer labor duration and higher risk of cesarean deliveries

14. Patient B presents 8 weeks later now with snoring and daytime sleepiness with an ESS of 14. She is now requiring a 1–2 hour nap most days. Diagnostic PSG is significant for an AHI of 12.5. Which of the following is the best treatment for this patient?

A. Advise the patient that her snoring is likely from weight gain in pregnancy and it should resolve postdelivery.

B. Advise the patient that snoring can be improved with sleeping in the lateral position.

C. Mild OSA that develops during pregnancy does not need to be treated.

D. Begin CPAP.

Questions 15–16 refer to patient C.

Patient C: A 23-year-old G0P0 female with a history of narcolepsy type 1 presents to your clinic for counseling, as she wishes to get pregnant. She was diagnosed at age 17 after having daytime sleepiness with falling asleep frequently in school and an episode of cataplexy that occurred at her surprise birthday party. Current medications include venlafaxine extended-release 75 mg po daily, methylphenidate immediate-release 10 mg po qam and q 1 pm, and she has an IUD in place. After the first episode, her cataplexy had occurred approximately once a month, but since being put on the above dose of venlafaxine 3 years ago, it has not recurred. Her current dose of methylphenidate keeps her awake for most of the day, but it tends to wear off quickly in the late morning and late afternoon. Vital signs and physical exam are normal.

15. Which of the following medication changes do you advise before the patient begins trying to get pregnant?
    A. Methylphenidate should be stopped but venlafaxine can be continued.
    B. Methylphenidate should be stopped, and venlafaxine should be slowly titrated to 37.5 mg po daily.
    C. Methylphenidate can be continued, but venlafaxine should be slowly titrated off to prevent rebound cataplexy.
    D. Methylphenidate should be stopped, and venlafaxine should be slowly titrated off to prevent rebound cataplexy.

16. Patient C comes to you a year later at 8 months' gestation. She has done well through her pregnancy and plans to breastfeed her child until 6 months of age. When can she resume her same medications and doses?
    A. Both medications can be restarted postdelivery, as neither will be transferred in breast milk.
    B. Both medications can be restarted only when the baby is done breast-feeding.
    C. Venlafaxine can be resumed postdelivery, but methylphenidate must wait until after breast-feeding is complete.
    D. Methylphenidate can be resumed post delivery, but resumption of venlafaxine must wait until after breast-feeding is complete.

Questions 17–18 refer to Patient D.

Patient D: A 23-year-old female presents with a chief complaint of daytime sleepiness since high school. She sleeps 8–9 hours a night and wakes up rested, but within a few hours of getting up, she is sleepy and has fallen asleep at the dinner table, in church, and on the toilet. Recently this has become more of a problem, as this past summer she fell asleep during an important meeting for a company where she was doing an internship. She has also fallen asleep during multiple classes for her current master's program. If she gets sleepy when driving, she has to pull over to take a 30–45 minute nap, which she wakes refreshed from. She reports visions when she is lying down, just prior to the wake to sleep transition. She wakes 2–3 times a week with sleep paralysis lasting 20–40 sec. She has had multiple instances where while laughing with her friends her neck became weak, her head pitched forward, and her face lost tone for approximately 1–2 minutes. She experienced no loss of consciousness, and these symptoms quickly resolve. Physical exam is normal. She is sexually active, and her only medication is hormonal birth control. You order an overnight PSG to be followed by multiple sleep latency test (MSLT). Diagnostic PSG results are listed. MSLT data are found in Table 41.1.

Diagnostic PSG
Total sleep time: 460 minutes
Sleep efficiency: 97%

Sleep latency: 8 minutes
Rapid eye movement (REM) latency: 7 minutes
AHI: 0.6/hour
PLMI: 2.2/hour

TABLE 41.1	Multiple Sleep Latency Test Data for Patient D					
Nap	**Lights out**		**Sleep Onset**		**Rapid Eye Movement Onset**	
—	**Epoch**	**Time**	**Epoch**	**Time**	**Epoch**	**Time**
1	20	08:32	28	08:36	34	08:39
2	92	10:38	94	10:39	104	10:44
3	144	12:41	145	12:41	—	—
4	188	16:31	196	14:35	—	—
5	240	16:31	247	16:34	253	16:37

17. What is your diagnosis according to the ISCD-3?
    A. Atypical depression
    B. Excessive daytime sleepiness
    C. Idiopathic hypersomnia
    D. Narcolepsy type 1
    E. Narcolepsy type 2

18. Which medication should be avoided in *Patient D* when treating her symptoms of daytime sleepiness?
    A. Dextroamphetamine/amphetamine
    B. Sodium oxybate
    C. Modafinil
    D. Venlafaxine
    E. Methylphenidate

Fibromyalgia

19. Which of the following is *not* true concerning the epidemiology and pathogenesis of fibromyalgia (FM)?
    A. FM is more common in men.
    B. FM patients often have a history of previous discrete pain syndromes.
    C. FM can be triggered by certain types of infections (Epstein-Barr virus, Lyme disease, Q fever, viral hepatitis).
    D. FM is present in 2%–8% of the population.
    E. Patients with FM often have comorbid psychiatric conditions (depression, anxiety, obsessive compulsive disorder, PTSD).

20. Which of the following is *not* a typical polysomnographic finding in patients with fibromyalgia?
    A. Decreased REM latency
    B. Decreased sleep efficiency
    C. Increased awakenings and wake after sleep onset
    D. Increased sleep latency and stage N1

21. Which of the following is *not* a core complaint in patients with fibromyalgia?
    A. Long sleep duration
    B. Nonrestorative sleep
    C. Musculoskeletal discomfort
    D. Fatigue
    E. Memory problems

22. Which of the following EEG findings are common in patients with FM?
    A. Increased sleep spindles
    B. Alpha sleep
    C. Decreased arousals
    D. Increased slow waves

23. Which of the following treatments for FM is *not* approved by the FDA?
    A. Pregabalin
    B. Amitriptyline
    C. Milnacipran
    D. Duloxetine

Chronic Fatigue Syndrome

24. Which of the following statements is *true* concerning sleep in chronic fatigue syndrome (CFS)?
    A. There are PSG findings that discriminate normal subjects and patients with CFS.
    B. Improvement of sleep has been shown to improve fatigue in CFS.
    C. A significant proportion of patients diagnosed with CFS meet criteria for FM.
    D. Diffuse muscular pain is uncommon in CFS.

25. An 18-year-old woman with symptomatic postural (orthostatic) tachycardia syndrome complained of unrefreshing sleep and extreme daytime fatigue. Her Epworth Sleepiness Scale was 11/24. The patient reported sleeping about 7–8 hours per night. She denied feeling depressed but was anxious about her condition. The patient denies cataplexy, and unless she has exertion, muscle tenderness is not prominent (although she feels "wiped out" after minimal exertion). A polysomnogram found a long sleep-onset latency of 35 minutes, but was otherwise unremarkable (near normal total sleep time and normal REM latency). A multiple sleep latency test (MSLT) shows a mean sleep latency of 16 minutes and only one sleep-onset REM period. What is the most likely diagnosis?
    A. Idiopathic hypersomnia
    B. Chronic fatigue syndrome
    C. Depression
    D. Narcolepsy without cataplexy

Renal

26. A 60-year-old man with chronic kidney disease (CKD) has not started hemodialysis. He complains of both snoring and insomnia. Which of the following is a *true* statement?
    A. From 10%–20% of dialysis patients complain of insomnia or daytime sleepiness.
    B. The prevalence of sleep disorders worsens with progression of renal disease based on CKD stages.
    C. The prevalence of sleep disorders in patients with CKD not on dialysis is greater than those on dialysis.
    D. There is no evidence that CKD can worsen OSA.

27. Which of the following is true about differences in symptoms and sleep study findings in OSA patients with and without end-stage renal disease (ESRD) with equivalent AHI?
    A. BMI is higher in OSA patients with ESRD.
    B. History of snoring is lower in OSA patients with ESRD.
    C. Central events per hour are lower in OSA patients with ESRD.

D. Witnessed apnea is higher in OSA patients with ESRD.
E. PLMS index is lower in OSA patients with ESRD.

28. Which of the following is *not* a true statement about patients with ESRD and RLS?
    A. Patients with ESRD and RLS are more likely to have insomnia than ESRD patients without RLS.
    B. The prevalence of RLS in ERD is at least twice that in the general population.
    C. Transplantation does *not* substantially improve RLS in dialysis patients.
    D. ESRD patients with RLS have an increased likelihood of cardio/cerebrovascular events and mortality.

Cancer

29. Which of the following symptoms are common problems in cancer patients?
    A. Excessive fatigue
    B. Insomnia
    C. Excessive sleepiness
    D. Restless legs
    E. All of the above

Answers

1. **The correct answer is B. 33%.**
   This patient has predominantly central sleep apnea (CSA), as defined by the ICSD-3, with the total number of central apneas being greater than 50% of the total number of apneas and hypopneas.[1] Grunstein et al. studied 53 consecutive patients with acromegaly. Snoring was present in nearly all of these patients, and hypertension in acromegaly was strongly associated with sleep apnea. Of the 53 patients, 81% had sleep apnea. CSA was the predominant type of apnea in 33% of those with sleep apnea, while obstructive sleep apnea was found in the other 67%.[2]

2. **The correct answer is E (the statement is false). Sleep apnea does NOT reliably resolve within 2 to 3 years of biochemical remission.**
   This answer is false. Davi et al. showed that sleep apnea syndrome can persist after recovery of acromegaly in a relatively high percentage of patients. They studied 36 patients, 18 of which had active disease and 18 of which had achieved biochemical remission. Sleep apnea syndrome was found in 47% of the overall group: 56% in the group with active disease and 39% in the biochemically controlled group.[3] The remaining answers are true. Grunstein et al. studied 53 consecutive patients with acromegaly. Of the 43 that had sleep apnea, 22 had hypertension. Of the 10 that did not have sleep apnea, all were normotensive. Those with hypertension had a significantly higher respiratory disturbance index and lower minimum oxygen desaturation compared with those who were normotensive (Answer A is true). Indeed, Grunstein et al. showed that higher levels of elevated growth hormone and IGF-1 were associated central sleep apnea in these patients.[2] Grunstein et al. found that increased ventilatory responsiveness as well as elevated measures of disease activity contributed to CSA in patients with acromegaly (Answer B is true).[4] Davi et al. found that IGF-1, BMI, male gender, age, and disease duration were all independently correlated with the disease (Answer C is true). Given the incidence of sleep apnea in this population, as well as the negative impact of sleep apnea if untreated, they

recommended that PSG be performed at least once in every acromegalic patient, whether they have active or controlled disease (Answer D is true).[3]

3. **The correct answer is C. Growth hormone.**

Fig. 41.1 shows an epoch of Stage N3 sleep. The American Academy of Sleep Medicine (AASM) Scoring Manual defines slow wave activity as waves with a frequency of 0.5 Hz–2 Hz and peak-to-peak amplitude greater than 75 μV, measured over the frontal regions referenced to the contralateral ear or mastoid. Slow wave activity must be present in ≥20% of the epoch to meet criteria as stage N3, as seen here.[5] Growth hormone secretion is tied to the start of stage N3 rather than the time of day, and indeed whether it is nocturnal or daytime sleep a burst of GH occurs with this sleep stage. The amount of GH secretion correlates to the duration of stage N3. Of note, in men the sleep-onset GH pulse usually accounts for the majority of GH secretion in a 24-hour span, whereas in women, although the sleep-associated GH pulse is still present, there can also be bursts of GH secretion throughout the day.[6] Van Cauter et al. studied a group of 102 healthy nonobese men, ages 18–83, and showed that the nocturnal increase in GH decreases with age in parallel with the amount of stage N3.[7] Melatonin, ghrelin, leptin, and testosterone are not tied to any sleep phase and are therefore incorrect.

4. **The correct answer is C. Increased ghrelin.**

Sleep deprivation is associated with increased Ghrelin (increased appetite). Ghrelin is a peptide released mainly by the stomach, and in humans it causes increased appetite and food intake. This may be one of the reasons that sleep restriction is associated with obesity (Answer C is correct). Sleep deprivation is associated with *decreased* leptin (Answer A is incorrect). Leptin is primarily secreted by adipose tissue and promotes satiety (decreased appetite).[8,8a] Spiegel et al. showed decreased glucose tolerance in those with sleep-debt compared with those who were fully rested (Answer B is incorrect). They also found that that sleep-debt leads to elevated evening cortisol concentrations and sympathetic nervous system activity (Answer D is incorrect).[8]

5. **The correct answer is B. Sleep disturbance decreases as HIV infection worsens (CD4 count decreases).**

This answer is false. Sleep disturbances have been found to *increase* (not decrease) in proportion to the severity of the disease. Darko et al. noted that sleep disturbance is a frequent symptom in patients with advanced HIV when compared with HIV negative comparison subjects.[9] Parish also noted that the severity of sleep complaints seems to be related to the stage of the disease, with mild symptoms of sleep disruption in early stages of infection (CD4 count >400) and severe insomnia and daytime fatigue in those with advanced stages (CD4 <200).[10] The remaining answers are true. Of note, Norman et al. did observe changes in sleep architecture in asymptomatic men in the early stages of HIV infection. The amount of SWS in these patients was found to be increased and was more prevalent later in the night compared with normal subjects.[11] Refer to Table 41.2 regarding symptoms and sleep study findings by varying stages of disease of HIV infection.[12]

6. **The correct answer is C. Efavirenz.**

Efavirenz is a nonnucleoside reverse transcriptase inhibitor (NNRTI) used in the treatment of HIV infection that has been well-documented as commonly *causing vivid dreams*.[13,14] Abers et al. note that within 2–4 weeks of initiating therapy,

TABLE 41.2	Symptoms and Sleep Study Findings by Varying Stages of Disease of Human Immunodeficiency Virus Infection

Stage of Disease	Symptoms	Sleep Study Findings
Early CD4 >400/mm³	Mild insomnia Mild daytime fatigue	Increased SWS Alpha intrusion may occur
400/mm³ > CD4 > 200	Significant insomnia Moderate daytime fatigue	Decreased SWS
CD4 <200/mm³	Severe insomnia Severe fatigue	Absent SWS Fragmented sleep architecture

SWS, Slow wave sleep (stage 3, 4 NREM sleep).
Reproduced from Berry RB, Harding SM. Sleep and medical disorders. *Med Clin N Am.* 2004;88:679–703.

patients may experience CNS toxicity symptoms. While the definition of "CNS toxicity" varies in the literature, they noted that in these patients, it can include vivid dreams, sleep disturbance, dizziness, lightheadedness, and nervousness. This typically resolves without dose alteration in the coming 6–8 weeks. These adverse effects may be related to certain CYP2B6 alleles that influence the clearance of efavirenz.[14] Kenedi et al. note that in approximately 2%–6% of patients, the drug must be discontinued due to persistent to severe neuropsychiatric side effects. Regarding these neuropsychiatric effects, Kenedi et al. note that "There is no clear evidence of a systematically increased risk of suicide or violent behaviors on efavirenz, However, convincing cases of psychiatric decompensation following initiation of efavirenz have been reported, and due clinical caution is required when initiating this agent" (pp. 1815).[15] The other medications listed have not been documented to cause vivid dreams and are therefore incorrect.

7. **The correct answer is D. The main cause of GER during sleep is inadequate LES pressure.**

This answer is false. It is commonly assumed that inadequate LES pressure is the cause of nighttime GER; however, *most patients with GER have normal LES pressure*.[12] The most common mechanism of sleep-related GER in normal subjects is actually due to transient LES relaxations (TLESR), rather than simply decreased LES pressure.[16] Dent et al. noted that during the night, episodes of TLESR and acid GE reflux occurred only during arousals or prolonged periods of wakefulness—never during actual sleep. In these cases the esophagus was typically cleared of refluxed contents by primary or secondary peristalsis, but in a few instances the subjects fell back asleep before the clearance was complete.[17] GER therefore occurs when sleep is interrupted by arousals, not during actual sleep, and is not simply due to lower LES pressure. Answers A, B, C, and E are all true and occur as a part of normal esophageal physiology. It is important to note that esophageal acid clearance is prolonged during sleep due to decreased saliva production and absent swallowing.

8. **The correct answer is D. The right lateral decubitus position is the best position for sleep-related GER.**

This answer is false. Khoury et al. studied 10 patients to evaluate sleeping positions and their effect on GER. A GER episode was defined in this study as a fall in esophageal pH to less than 4.0 for ≥15 sec, and the end of the episode when the esophageal pH returned to 4.0. Esophageal acid clearance time therefore is considered the amount of time it takes for the esophagus to clear its contents and bring the pH above 4.0. Khoury et al. found that the right lateral decubitus position actually worsens GER and is associated with a greater percent time, with pH less than 4 and longer esophageal acid clearance time compared with the left, supine, and prone positions. The *left lateral decubitus position is the preferred position to minimize sleep-related GER* and is associated with shorter esophageal clearance time.[18] The other statements are true—patients should avoid eating acid-promoting foods and medications before sleep (Answers A and B are true). Smoking worsens nocturnal reflux due to its effect of decreasing LES pressure; therefore smoking cessation can help with nocturnal GER[12] (Answer C is true). Green et al. studied 331 patients diagnosed with OSA. Of 331, 62% had nocturnal GER prior to treatment with nasal CPAP. Follow-up was obtained in 181 patients of the 204 started on CPAP; 165 (91%) were still using CPAP. Patients compliant with CPAP were found to have a 48% improvement in nocturnal GER. Additionally, higher pressures of nasal CPAP were associated with greater improvement in nocturnal GER[19] (Answer E is true).

9. **The correct answer is D. Change the timing of PPI dose.**
PPI medication should be given about 30 minutes before a meal for maximum efficacy. The standard recommendation is 30 minutes before breakfast (PPI effect is greatest after a period of fasting). If twice a day dosing is desired, then 30 minutes before breakfast and 30 minutes before the evening meal is another option. Most PPI medications have a coating to protect against acid degradation in the stomach. Once absorbed into the gastric mucosa, PPIs need to be activated in an acidic environment at the parietal cells. Food activates parietal cell acid secretion that is needed for PPIs to work. The need to achieve acid exposure in the parietal cell but not the stomach is why PPIs should be taken before meals. In a study of 100 patients taking PPI for GERD, compliance was determined using a questionnaire about dosing habits and timing. Only 46% dosed optimally. Among the 54% who were dosed suboptimally, 39% dosed more than 60 minutes before meals, 30% after meals, 28% at bedtime, and 4% as needed.[20] If proper timing of once daily dosing is verified before breakfast, increasing the frequency to twice a day (before breakfast and dinner) can be trialed, followed by increasing the dosage if necessary. Bedtime addition of a H_2-receptor antagonist (H_2RA) to the daily PPI therapy can then be considered in patients with nighttime reflux.[21] In contrast to other PPIs, the combination of omeprazole and sodium bicarbonate is an immediate release preparation, using bicarbonate to prevent acid degradation and to stimulate parietal cell secretion presumably by lower gastric pH. Use of this medication at bedtime has been shown to be effective at healing severe refractory reflux esophagitis. The FDA-approved prescribing information still recommends taking the combination on an empty stomach 1 hour before a meal once daily.[22]

10. **The correct answer is E. Oxycodone IR (immediate release).**
RLS is common in pregnancy, with a quarter of pregnant women meeting criteria for RLS. As in nonpregnant patients, habits that are known to trigger RLS, such as smoking or caffeine, should be eliminated in these patients. Any medications that contribute to these symptoms, such as histamine-1 receptor blockers, should be eliminated as well. Iron deficiency is commonly associated with RLS in pregnancy, and indeed iron requirements are increased during pregnancy. Adequate iron stores should be verified in pregnant women who present with these symptoms. Symptoms can improve with replenishment of iron stores; however, iron deficiency being responsible for the increased prevalence of RLS in pregnancy does not explain the quick improvement of symptoms after delivery.[23] The American Academy of Sleep Medicine updated practice parameters for the treatment of RLS in 2012; however, in those guidelines it was noted that pregnant women are a special population where there is insufficient evidence to make a recommendation.[24] Answers A–D are all listed as FDA pregnancy category C medications. Oxycodone IR is listed as pregnancy category B, so is the only possible correct answer. Oxycodone IR must of course be used in the lowest possible effective dose, and it is not recommended for use in patients immediately before or during labor given risk of respiratory depression in the newborn. Prolonged use of opioids during pregnancy can contribute to neonatal opioid withdrawal syndrome.[25]

11. **The correct answer is A. Symptoms resolve shortly after delivery.**
RLS that develops during pregnancy rapidly improves in the postpartum period (Answer A is correct).[23] Answers B–D are all incorrect statements. According to Prosperetti and Manconi, RLS is three times more prevalent in pregnant compared with nonpregnant women. Symptoms are more pronounced in strength and frequency during the third trimester, and disappear around delivery. If RLS is present before pregnancy, it tends to worsen during pregnancy. Women who experience RLS during pregnancy have a higher risk of symptoms in later pregnancies. They also have a higher risk of developing RLS later in life, compared with women free of symptoms during pregnancy.[26]

12. **The correct answer is D. 3rd, 1st, then 2nd.**
In the third trimester, women experience the most sleep disturbances. The majority of women in the third trimester experience multiple nocturnal awakenings as they approach the 40th week of pregnancy. This sleep disruption is mainly associated with the physical changes that occur with the growing uterus—urinary frequency, physical discomfort, reflux, and shortness of breath. Additionally, fetal movements, vivid dreams or nightmares, leg cramps, and even anxiety about labor and delivery (particularly in women in their first pregnancy) can interrupt sleep. Eventually, irregular uterine contractions may occur. In this trimester women get the least nocturnal sleep, but total sleep time may approach prepregnancy values when adding in naps during the day. The first trimester is the second-most interrupted trimester. Sleep disturbances in the first trimester are thought to be related to marked alterations in hormone levels compared with prepregnancy, which contribute to morning sickness, mood changes, physical discomforts including back pain and tender breasts, and fatigue and daytime sleepiness. The second semester tends to be the least disrupted, with most women reporting more energy and less fatigue, which is thought to be due to stabilization in hormone levels. Awakenings increase near the end of the second trimester as the woman transitions from the second to third trimesters (Table 41.3).[27]

13. **The correct answer is D. Longer labor duration and higher risk of cesarean deliveries.**

TABLE 41.3 **Sleep Pattern, Nocturnal Features, and Daytime Symptoms in Each Trimester and During Labor/Delivery[13]**

Characteristic	First Trimester	Second Trimester	Third Trimester	Labor/Delivery
Pattern	↑ TST ↑ Number of naps ↑ WASO ↓ SE ↓ SWS	↓ TST ↑ SE ↓ SWS ↓ WASO	↑ TST ↑ Number of naps ↑ WASO ↑ Stage 1 sleep ↓ SE ↓ SWS ↓ REM	↓TST ↓ SE ↓ NREM ↓ REM
Nocturnal features	Urinary frequency Physical discomforts—tender breasts/back pain	Onset of snoring, restless legs, irregular uterine contractions Dreams Back, neck, and joint pain	Urinary frequency Physical discomfort Irregular uterine contractions Muscle/leg cramps Shortness of breath Heartburn Dreams/nightmares Snoring Restless legs	Anxiety Forceful uterine contractions
Daytime symptoms	Fatigue Drowsiness Waking with nausea Mood changes	Nasal congestion	Fatigue Drowsiness Impaired vigilance Nasal congestion	Fatigue Anxiety Pain

NREM, Nonrapid eye movement; *REM,* rapid eye movement; *SE,* sleep efficiency; *SWS,* slow wave sleep; *TST,* total sleep time; *WASO,* wake (time) after sleep onset.
Reproduced from Kryger M, Roth T, Dement WC, eds. *Principles and Practice of Sleep Medicine.* 6th ed. Philadelphia: Elsevier; 2017.

Lee et al. studied 131 women in their ninth month of pregnancy with 48-hour actigraphy and sleep logs. When controlling for infant birth weight, women who *slept less than 6 hours* at night had longer labors and were 4.5 times *more likely to have cesarean deliveries.* Indeed, with even more disrupted sleep, longer labors were seen and these women were 5.2 times more likely to have cesarean deliveries. For this reason, Lee et al. recommend that providers include sleep quantity and quality in their prenatal assessments and that 8 hours of bedtime should be prescribed during pregnancy.[28] The remaining answers A–C are incorrect.

14. **The correct answer is D. Begin CPAP.**
There are many physiologic changes during pregnancy that contribute to decreased airway patency and likelihood of development of sleep-disordered breathing. These changes include upper airway edema, nasal congestion, and increased Mallampati score. Sleep-disordered breathing has been associated with negative pregnancy outcomes such as gestational hypertension and diabetes. It is unclear if treatment with CPAP can prevent these negative outcomes, but treatment of pregnant patients should be performed according to the same guidelines uses to treat the nonpregnant. In this case, the patient is symptomatic in the setting of mild OSA, and treatment with CPAP is indicated. (Answer D is correct.)[23] While pregnant patients commonly develop snoring due to increased nasal congestion and upper airway edema in sleep, the patient at hand does not have primary snoring. (Answer A is incorrect.) Similarly, while snoring can improve in the lateral position compared with supine, again the patient in this question does not have primary snoring but rather has symptomatic OSA, indicating treatment. (Answer B is incorrect.) Finally, Answer C is incorrect, as mild OSA that develops in pregnancy and is symptomatic should be treated.

15. **The correct answer is D. Methylphenidate should be stopped, and venlafaxine should be slowly titrated off to prevent rebound cataplexy.**
Methylphenidate is FDA approved for the treatment of excessive daytime sleepiness due to narcolepsy.[29] It is short acting, is effective for "as needed" dosing, and can be stopped abruptly without withdrawal symptoms. Methylphenidate is listed as FDA pregnancy risk category C and therefore should not be taken in pregnancy or in women who are trying to become pregnant.[30] The use of venlafaxine for the treatment of cataplexy is a guideline recommendation by the AASM practice parameters and recommendations for the treatment of cataplexy.[29] Venlafaxine is listed in the FDA pregnancy risk category C, and therefore also should not be used in this case.[25] Care must be taken, however, in stopping this medication, as rebound cataplexy—termed "status cataplecticus"—can occur with abrupt withdrawal with this medication, and even with skipped doses. Venlafaxine must be weaned slowly to avoid this unwanted effect.[31]

16. **The correct answer is B. Both medications can be restarted only when the baby is done breast-feeding.**
Both methylphenidate and venlafaxine are listed as FDA pregnancy category C. They are both excreted in human breast milk, and mothers breast-feeding their children must make a decision to either stop nursing or stop the medication.[25] Answer B therefore is the only correct answer.

17. **The correct answer is D. Narcolepsy type 1.**
This patient meets criteria A and B, as outlined in the *International Classification of Sleep Disorders,* 3rd Edition (ICSD-3), for narcolepsy type 1 (narcolepsy with cataplexy). Criterion A outlines that the patient must have had symptoms including the "irrepressible need to sleep or daytime lapses into sleep" for at least 3 months—the patient in this question

has had it for years. Criteria B includes the presence of at least one or both of the following labeled 1 and 2: "(1) Cataplexy (as defined under Essential Features) and a mean sleep latency of ≤8 minutes and two or more sleep onset REM periods (SOREMPs) on an MSLT performed according to standard techniques. A SOREMP (within 15 minutes of sleep onset) on the preceding nocturnal polysomnogram may replace one of the SOREMPs on the MSLT. (2) CSF hypocretin-1 concentration, measure by immunoreactivity, is either ≤110 pg/mL or less than 1/3 of mean values."[1] This patient has clear cataplexy as described in the stem. The nocturnal PSG for this patient yields a normal AHI, indicating no sleep-disordered breathing that would be contributing to her symptoms. It also includes 1 SOREMP, given that the REM latency was 7 minutes. As noted previously, the ICSD-3 now stipulates that a SOREMP on the overnight PSG preceding MSLT can count toward the two needed. The mean sleep latency (MSL) as calculated from the table is 2.6 minutes, and SOREMPS occurred on naps 1, 2, and 5. This patient's MSL is 2.6 minutes and there are a total of four SOREMPS (one overnight and three during the MSLT), which both meet the criteria of MSL ≤8 minutes, and two or more SOREMPs, respectively. Answers C and E are incorrect, as the patient does not meet diagnostic criteria for them. Answer B is incorrect, as excessive daytime sleepiness is not a diagnosis in the ISCD-3. Answer A is incorrect, as the stem does not describe atypical depression.

18. **The correct answer is C. Modafinil.**
Modafinil is metabolized in the liver by the cytochrome p-450 (CYP450) system and can induce CYP450 3A4, which can decrease the levels of drugs that are metabolized by this enzyme. Ethynyl estradiol is one such example of a drug metabolized by this enzyme, and the decreased levels that result from induction of the enzyme can make it less effective. Due to this, oral contraceptive pills (OCPs) can be less effective once modafinil is started and up to a month after it is stopped. Females of childbearing age should use an alternate (nonhormonal) form of birth control.[41a] Davies et al. reported pregnancies that have occurred in patients taking both modafinil and OCPs.[32] Modafinil should therefore be avoided in this patient, as she is of childbearing age and her only method of birth control is OCP. Answers A, B, D, and E can all be used to treat narcolepsy type 1.

19. **Answer A (FM is more common in men) is false.**
FM is more common in women (2:1 ratio).[33] The other answers are correct.

20. **Answer A (decreased REM latency) is false.**
A decreased REM latency has not been reported in FM.[34,35] Studies of sleep in patients with fibromyalgia have shown somewhat inconsistent results. Most studies were composed of relatively small numbers of patients and controls. In some of the studies, patients were taking antidepressants that can themselves affect sleep architecture. Some but not all studies have shown *decreased total sleep time, decreased stage R, and stage N3 sleep (corrected for age)*. Most studies have found decreased sleep efficiency (total sleep time X100/total recording time), and increased sleep latency (or increased latency to persistent sleep) and increased stage N1. Many studies have found an increased number of awakenings and sleep stage shifts.

21. **Answer A (long sleep duration) is false.**
Patients with FM usually complain of short and nonrestorative sleep. Although complaints of excessive sleepiness are sometimes confused with fatigue, patients with FM do not usually complain of difficulty remaining awake.[33] In a recent study by Diaz-Piedra, only 13 of 53 FM patients had an Epworth sleepiness scale greater than 10.[35] In contrast, FM patients usually complain of fatigue and low energy. Sleep complaints are nearly always present and often include a long sleep latency, short total sleep time, and nonrestorative sleep. MSLT of FM patients does *not* show a short mean sleep latency. A complaint of memory problems is also common in patients with FM.[33]

22. **The correct answer is B. Alpha sleep.**
Alpha intrusion (alpha sleep) is reportedly present in 70% of patients with FM.[36] Roizenblatt reported 50% of FM patients had a phasic alpha pattern (episodic alpha activity present when slow waves were present), and 20% had diffuse alpha pattern (alpha present throughout NREM sleep).[37] Alpha intrusion is neither sensitive nor specific for a diagnosis of FM. It may be seen in patients with other chronic pain syndromes, patients with psychiatric disorders, patients with medical disorders, and in normal individuals.[38] Patients with FM have *decreased spindles* and EEG power in the sigma band (12–14 Hz).[39] They have increased arousals and decreased amount of stage N3 sleep (corrected for age).[35] A recent study showed FM patients have a decreased delta/alpha frequency power.[40]

23. **The correct answer is B. Amitriptyline.**
The other three medications are FDA approved for treatment of FM.[33,41] Although studies have shown that amitriptyline is effective in FM, this sedating tricyclic antidepressant is not FDA approved for this indication. Amitriptyline is usually given in doses of 10–75 mg at bedtime. It has significant anticholinergic activity that may be minimized by using the lowest effective dose (the starting dose of 10 mg may be effective). Pregabalin binds to the $\alpha_2\delta$ subunit of voltage-gated calcium channels in the central nervous system. Although an analog of GABA, it does not bind GABA-A or GABA-B receptors. The dose for fibromyalgia is 150–225 mg po bid. The starting dose is 75 mg po bid that may be increased to 150 po bid in 1 week. The medication should be tapered if discontinued. Side effects of pregabalin include sleepiness, dizziness, blurry vision, weight gain, trouble concentrating, swelling of the hands and feet, and dry mouth. Allergic reactions, although rare, can occur. If daytime sleepiness is a problem, more of the pregabalin daily dose may be given at bedtime. Some patients may only tolerate a dose at bedtime. Although not FDA approved for FM, gabapentin has also been shown to be effective in FM. The drug binds the same receptors as pregabalin. A wide range of doses have been used, but 300–600 mg tid is typical. It should be started at 300 mg daily (e.g., 100 mg tid) and increased slowly. Common side effects are similar to those of pregabalin. Some patients will tolerate a higher dose of gabapentin at bedtime. Both pregabalin and gabapentin may improve sleep quality in some patients. Milnacipran (Savella) is a serotonin and norepinephrine reuptake inhibitor. The usual dose in 50 mg bid. The medication is started 12.5 mg X1 day, 25 mg po daily X4 days, and then 50 mg bid. The maximum dose is 200 mg per day. Side effects include nausea, constipation, dizziness, insomnia, excessive sweating, vomiting, palpitations or increased heart rate, dry mouth, and high blood pressure. Duloxetine (Cymbalta) also inhibits serotonin and norepinephrine reuptake, and is also FDA approved for FM as well as depression, diabetic neuropathic pain, and generalized anxiety disorder. For FM, the

recommended dose is 60 mg daily. Usually the starting dose is 30 mg for one week. Of note, some patients respond to the starting dose. A gradual taper is recommended if either milnacipran or duloxetine are to be discontinued. Cymbalta's side effects include nausea, dry mouth, sleepiness, constipation, decreased appetite, and increased sweating. Like some other antidepressants, Cymbalta may increase the risk of suicidal thinking and behavior in people who take the drug for depression. Some people with fibromyalgia also experience depression, and duloxetine may be effective for this comorbid problem. Of note, SSRIs like citalopram or escitalopram may be helpful for depression, but have not been effective treatments for FM. Other medications often used in FM include cyclobenzaprine, a centrally acting muscle relaxant, and tramadol. Cyclobenzaprine (Flexeril) can cause drowsiness and fatigue.[33,41] It may be effective in even low doses, and is often given at night. Tramadol is a μ-opioid receptor agonist but also blocks reuptake of serotonin and norepinephrine. Side effects include nausea, vomiting, constipation, and somnolence. More potent opioids have not been shown to be of benefit in FM. Sodium oxybate has been shown to be effective in FM[42] but was not approved by the FDA for FM treatment due to safety concerns.

24. **The correct answer is C. A significant proportion of patients diagnosed with CFS meet criteria for FM.**

A significant proportion of patients meeting diagnostic criteria for CFS meet criteria for FM. Diffuse muscular pain, fatigue, and sleep disturbances are part of the definitions of both CFS and FM. The current CDC Case Definition of CFS[43] (Table 41.4) is based on the 1994 publication by Fukuda et al.[44] The syndrome is also called myalgic encephalomyelitis. According to the CDC, "Conditions that exclude a diagnosis of CFS include: (1) Any active medical condition that may explain the presence of chronic fatigue, such as untreated hypothyroidism, sleep apnea, and narcolepsy, and iatrogenic conditions such as side effects of medication. (2) Some diagnosable illnesses may relapse or may not have completely resolved during treatment. If the persistence of such a condition could explain the presence of chronic fatigue, and if it cannot be clearly established that the original condition has completely resolved with treatment, then such patients should not be classified as having CFS. Examples of illnesses that can present such a picture include some types of cancers and chronic cases of hepatitis B or C virus infection. (3) Any past or current diagnosis of: major depressive disorder with psychotic major depressive disorder with psychotic or melancholic features, bipolar affective disorders, schizophrenia of any subtype, delusional disorders of any subtype, dementias of any subtype, anorexia nervosa, or bulimia nervosa. (4) Alcohol or other substance abuse, occurring within 2 years of the onset of chronic fatigue and any time afterwards. (5) Severe obesity is defined as having a body mass index equal to or greater than 45. The following conditions do NOT excluded CFS: (1) Any condition defined primarily by symptoms that cannot be confirmed by diagnostic laboratory tests, including fibromyalgia, anxiety disorders, somatoform disorders, nonpsychotic or melancholic depression, neurasthenia, and multiple chemical sensitivity disorder. (2) Any condition under specific treatment sufficient to alleviate all symptoms related to that condition and for which the adequacy of treatment has been documented. Such conditions include hypothyroidism for which the adequacy of replacement hormone has been verified by normal thyroid-stimulating hormone levels, or asthma in which the adequacy

TABLE 41.4	**Diagnostic Criteria for Chronic Fatigue Syndrome[43,44]**

CDC Diagnostic Criteria

Consider a diagnosis of chronic fatigue syndrome (CFS) if these three criteria are met:

1. The individual has severe chronic fatigue for 6 or more consecutive months that is not due to ongoing exertion or other medical conditions associated with fatigue (these other conditions need to be ruled out by a doctor after diagnostic tests have been conducted) and is not substantially relieved by rest.
2. The fatigue significantly interferes with daily activities and work.
3. The individual concurrently has four or more of the following eight symptoms that are either new or did not start before the onset of fatigue:
   - Postexertion malaise lasting more than 24 hours
   - Unrefreshing sleep
   - Significant impairment of short-term memory or concentration
   - Muscle pain
   - Multijoint pain without swelling or redness
   - Headaches of a new type, pattern, or severity
   - Tender cervical or axillary lymph nodes
   - A sore throat that is frequent or recurring

Institutes of Medicine (IOM) Diagnostic Criteria[45,46]

Diagnosis requires that the patient have the following three symptoms:

1. A substantial reduction or impairment in the ability to engage in pre-illness levels of occupational, educational, social, or personal activities, that persists for more than 6 months and is accompanied by fatigue, which is often profound, is of new or definite onset (not lifelong), is not the result of ongoing excessive exertion, and *is not substantially alleviated by rest*, and
2. Postexertional malaise[a]
3. Unrefreshing sleep[a]

At least one of the two following manifestations is also required:

1. Cognitive impairment[a]
2. Orthostatic intolerance

[a]Frequency and severity of symptoms should be assessed. The diagnosis of ME/CFS (SEID) should be questioned if patients do not have these symptoms at least half of the time with moderate, substantial, or severe intensity.

of treatment has been determined by pulmonary function and other testing. (3) Any condition, such as Lyme disease or syphilis that was treated with definitive therapy before development of chronic symptoms. (4) Any isolated and unexplained physical examination finding, or laboratory or imaging test abnormality that is not enough to strongly suggest the existence of an exclusionary condition. Such conditions include an elevated antinuclear antibody titer that is inadequate, without additional laboratory or clinical evidence, to strongly support a diagnosis of a discrete connective tissue disorder."

The Institutes of Medicine (IOM) has renamed the syndrome systemic exertion intolerance disease (SEID) and provided new diagnostic criteria.[45,46] The IOM criteria emphasize a reduction in the ability to engage in pre-illness levels of occupational, educational, social, or personal activities rather than diffuse muscle pain. The presence of sleep disturbance and postexertional malaise is also required. Patients may report muscle soreness after nonstrenuous activity while others feel mentally tired after minimal effort. Answer A is incorrect because there are no PSG findings that can discriminate normal subjects and patients with CFS. Sleep architecture findings also do not correlate well with the degree of sleep complaints. In CFS patients that *do not have FM*, alpha intrusion does not appear to be a common finding. Answer B is incorrect because improving sleep or treating comorbid sleep disorders does not reliably improve fatigue. Answer D is incorrect because diffuse muscular pain is *common* in CFS (overlap between FM and CFS), at least using CDC diagnostic criteria. The Diagnostic Criteria for CFS from the CDC and IOM are found in Table 41.4.

25. **The correct answer is B. Chronic fatigue syndrome.**
Chronic fatigue syndrome is associated with postural orthostatic tachycardia syndrome (POTS) in adolescents and young adults.[47] Patients are considered to have POTS if (i) heart rate at 2 minutes following standing was at least 30 bpm higher than the baseline value, (ii) there was no concurrent orthostatic hypotension, defined as a drop in systolic blood pressure of greater than 25 mm Hg or a drop in diastolic blood pressure of greater than 10 mm Hg, or (iii) the patient reported at least one qualitative symptom of orthostatic intolerance (OI), such as dizziness, tingling, light-headedness, or presyncope.[48] In an Australian cohort of 306 CFS cases, there were 33 cases (11%) identified as having comorbid POTS.[47] Polysomnographic findings in CFS are usually unremarkable, and the degree of daytime fatigue is often not correlated with objective sleepiness on MSLT. The polysomnography and MSLT findings provided in this question do not substantiate either narcolepsy without cataplexy or idiopathic hypersomnia. Depression is in the differential of chronic fatigue and sleep disturbance. However, sleep quality on the PSG was relatively normal except for the long sleep latency. Nevertheless, although CFS may be considered the most likely diagnosis given the presence of POTS, one cannot absolutely rule out depression.

26. **The correct answer is D. The prevalence of sleep disorders worsens with progression of renal disease based on CKD stages.**
There is evidence to suggest that the prevalence of sleep disorders worsens with progression of renal disease based on CKD stages. For example, most studies suggest that the prevalence of RLS[49,50] and OSA[51] increase with declining renal function.[51] In contrast, a recent study by Lee et al. did not find an increase in RLS in patients with CKD versus those with ESRD (on dialysis), although the prevalence of RLS in their study was very high in both groups (26%).[52] Answer A is incorrect because more than 50% of patients on dialysis (irrespective of type) report insomnia or daytime sleepiness.[53] Answer C is incorrect because the prevalence of sleep disorders is higher in patients on dialysis compared with CKD patients not yet requiring dialysis. Answer D is incorrect, as there is evidence that by causing fluid retention CKD can worsen upper airway edema and worsen OSA due to a nocturnal fluid shift[54] and nocturnal dialysis may improve sleep apnea.[55] Common sleep complaints and sleep disorders in patients with CKD are listed in Box 41.1.

27. **The correct answer is B. History of snoring is lower in OSA patients with ESRD.**
Patients with ESRD and OSA are less likely to have a history of snoring than OSA patients without ESRD (Box 41.2).[56] Answers A and D are incorrect, as patients with ESRD and OSA tend to have lower BMI and are less likely to have a history of witnessed apnea than OSA patients without ESRD. ESRD patients have a higher PLMS index; therefore answer E is incorrect. Of interest, patients with OSA and ESRD have

---

• BOX 41.1 Common Sleep Disturbances Among Chronic Kidney Disease Patients

Sleep Complaints
- Poor sleep quality
- Prolonged sleep latency
- Frequent awakenings
- Early awakenings
- Nonrestorative sleep

Sleep Disorders
- Insomnia
- Restless legs syndrome
- Periodic limb movements in sleep (with or without symptoms)
- Obstructive sleep apnea

From Canales M, Berry RB. Sleep disorders in chronic kidney disease. In: Kryger M, Avidan AY, Berry RB, eds. Atlas of Clinical Sleep Medicine. *Philadelphia: Elsevier; 2014:349–352.*

• BOX 41.2 Key Differences in Obstructive Sleep Apnea Patients with End-Stage Renal Disease Compared with Those with Normal Renal Function (Equivalent Apnea-Hypopnea Index)

BMI	Lower in ESRD
Neck circumference	Lower in ESRD
History of snoring	Lower in ESRD
History of apnea	Lower in ESRD
Total sleep time	Lower in ESRD
Central events/hour	Higher in ESRD
PLMS/hour	Higher in ESRD

ESRD, End stage renal disease.
Data from Beecroft JM, Pierratos A, Hanly PJ. Clinical presentation of obstructive sleep apnea in patients with end-stage renal disease. J Clin Sleep Med. 2009;5(2):115–121.
Table adapted from Canales M, Berry RB. Sleep disorders in chronic kidney disease. In: Kryger M, Avidan AY, Berry RB, eds. Atlas of Clinical Sleep Medicine. *Philadelphia: Elsevier; 2014: 349–352.*

---

a higher amount of central apnea compared with OSA patients without ESRD.

28. **Answer C (Transplantation does *not* substantially improve RLS in dialysis patients) is false.**
Patients with ESRD and RLS who undergo transplantation usually *do* have a significant improvement or resolution of RLS, as long as the transplant is functioning well.[57] Answer A is true, as patients with ESRD and RLS tend to be more likely to complain of insomnia than those with ESRD and no RLS.[58] Answer B is true, as the RLS is common in ESRD, affecting from 25%–62% of patients, which is substantially higher than the 5%–15% prevalence rate in the general population.[58] Answer D is true, as studies suggest that ESRD patients with RLS have an increased risk of cardio/cerebrovascular events and mortality.[59]

29. **The correct answer is E. All of the above.**
Davidson et al. surveyed 982 patients with varying types of cancer. The most prevalent problems reported in this survey were excessive fatigue in 44% of patients, leg restlessness in 41%, insomnia in 31%, and excessive sleepiness in 28%.[60]

Suggested Reading

Balserak BI, Lee KA. Chapter 156: Sleep and sleep disorders associated with pregnancy. In: Kryger M, Roth T, Dement WC, eds. *Principles and Practice of Sleep Medicine*. 6th ed. Philadelphia: Elsevier; 2017 Online:1525-1539.

Berry RB, Harding SM. Sleep and medical disorders. *Med Clin North Am*. 2004;88:679-703.

Clauw DJ. Fibromyalgia: a clinical review. *JAMA*. 2014;311(15):1547-1555.

Lee J, Nicholl DDM, Ahmed SB, et al. The prevalence of restless legs syndrome across the full spectrum of kidney disease. *J Clin Sleep Med*. 2013;9:455-459.

Parish JM. Sleep-related problems in common medical conditions. *Chest*. 2009;135(2):563-572.

42

Sleep Pharmacology

MATT T. BIANCHI

Questions

1. Benzodiazepines and the so-called z-drugs both are used to treat insomnia. Which of the following statements is most accurate regarding the distinctions between the classes?
   A. Z-drugs are shorter acting than all traditional benzodiazepines.
   B. Z-drugs have distinct GABA-A receptor subtype targets, which account for sleep-specific effects of z-drugs compared with benzodiazepines that also possess anticonvulsant, muscle relaxant, and antianxiety effects.
   C. Z-drugs act on GABA-B receptors, while benzodiazepines bind to GABA-A receptors, which accounts for the lower tolerance and addiction potential of z-drugs.
   D. Z-drugs and benzodiazepines both act on the same benzodiazepine receptors, but engage different cytochrome P450 pathways, which accounts for their distinct clinical uses in sleep versus anticonvulsant and anxiolytic and muscle relaxant actions.

2. You see a 27-year-old female for evaluation of worsening sleepiness, as well as hypnagogic hallucinations, but no cataplexy by history. Polysomnography (PSG) followed by multiple sleep latency test (MSLT) confirms the diagnosis of narcolepsy with fast latencies and three of the naps contained rapid eye movement (REM) sleep. You discuss treatment options for the patient. Which of the following is the most appropriate statement about initiating pharmacotherapy?
   A. Quetiapine to help improve sleep and reduce hallucinations
   B. Venlafaxine monotherapy for the hypnagogic hallucinations
   C. An amphetamine agent or modafinil, with instructions to monitor heart rate and blood pressure
   D. Sodium oxybate, in divided doses at night, titrating up to 9 g total, as monotherapy

3. A 38-year-old man has chronic insomnia not improved, despite numerous attempts at alternative remedies and a course of validated online cognitive behavioral therapy (CBT) therapy for insomnia. He is healthy but consumes nightly alcohol. He has researched the "z-drugs" and seeks your opinion about which is best for him. His problem is that he wakes up at about 2 AM and cannot get back to sleep before his alarm sounds at 6 AM to awaken for work. Which of the following is the most accurate statement about z-drugs?
   A. Zaleplon, zolpidem, or eszopiclone could be equally effective for this patient if taken at bedtime.
   B. A short-acting formulation is most appropriate, to avoid morning hangover if taken in the middle of the night.
   C. The US Food and Drug Administration (FDA) announced that men have slower metabolism of these drugs and thus morning hangover, prompting the FDA to recommend a lower dose for men.
   D. Eszopiclone is an option because the patient only has a short commute to work.

4. A postmenopausal 70-year-old woman who is otherwise healthy seeks your consultation regarding long-standing sleep onset insomnia. She has managed with relaxation techniques and various "nutraceuticals" for many years, but this is no longer effective for her. After declining first-line CBT for insomnia that you suggest, you review medication options for ideally short-term use. Which of the following medications would be a reasonable first choice?
   A. Diphenhydramine
   B. Clonazepam
   C. Ramelteon
   D. Quetiapine

5. Which of the following best describes the impact of nicotine on sleep?
   A. Most of the effects occur later in the sleep period due to the 4–6 hour half-life.
   B. Sleep fragmentation derives from interaction with adrenergic metabotropic receptors.
   C. Increased waking physiology occurs despite subjective reports of relaxation.
   D. The time spent in REM sleep is increased.

6. Adenosine has been widely studied for its involvement in the homeostatic aspects of sleep physiology. Which of the following statements is most accurate regarding adenosine?
   A. Caffeine enhances adenosine actions to facilitate wakefulness.

B. Human genetics have linked adenosine receptor polymorphisms to sleepiness and slow wave sleep physiology.

C. Only adenosine receptor AD1 is implicated in the sleep effects of adenosine.

D. Sedating antidepressants work in part for insomnia due to action on the adenosine system.

7. Melatonin is commonly used to treat sleep complaints in primary care and in sleep centers. Which of the following is most accurate regarding the melatonin system?

A. Melatonin may increase the INR in patients taking warfarin.

B. Ramelteon is a synthetic melatonin analog that targets the MT1 subset of receptors.

C. Melatonin dosing of 3 mg or higher is required to deliver endogenous physiological levels.

D. Light suppresses blood levels of melatonin, even from exogenous administration.

8. Which of the following is the most accurate statement regarding sodium oxybate?

A. It is a derivative of an endogenous neurosteroid.

B. The mechanism of action is via ionotropic GABA receptors.

C. Because of sedating effects, caution is needed if sleep disordered breathing is suspected.

D. Narcolepsy patients benefit from alerting effects, but cataplexy is not affected.

9. A 67-year-old woman presents to review a polysomnogram ordered by her primary care physician to evaluate her snoring. Although no obstructive sleep apnea (OSA) was seen, she did have elevated periodic limb movements of sleep. On further questioning, she does endorse sleep maintenance insomnia, which she attributed to her age and menopause but never spoke to a physician about it until now. Which of the following statements is true regarding insomnia medication choice in this setting?

A. Diphenhydramine is preferred due to a dual benefit of sedation and reducing congestion.

B. Mirtazapine is appropriate because it will not worsen her breathing during sleep.

C. Zolpidem 10 mg should not be used because it could induce further leg symptoms.

D. Treating her periodic limb movements of sleep (PLMS) with agents used for restless legs syndrome (RLS), such as iron or dopaminergic agents, may improve sleep, even though she has no RLS symptoms.

10. A 50-year-old woman presents with gradually worsening restless legs symptoms. She is quite risk-averse when it comes to prescriptions, and takes no medications currently. Her primary care doctor initially suggested iron supplementation, but she says iron was not started because her serum iron panel returned within the normal range. Which of the following is correct about iron supplementation for RLS?

A. Iron is best taken with food to avoid constipation and discoloration of stool.

B. Iron is best taken on an empty stomach with vitamin C to aid absorption.

C. Iron is not recommended unless the patient has a hematocrit in the anemic range.

D. Iron is not recommended unless iron deficiency is seen with ferritin levels less than 15.

11. You see a business man in sleep clinic for chronic onset and maintenance insomnia. He is obese, has already survived one heart attack, and is known to have severe sleep apnea, but he has declined therapy to improve his breathing, as he is instead focused on his insomnia symptoms and wants to discuss medication therapy. Which of the following is the most appropriate response?

A. Starting a selective serotonin reuptake inhibitor (SSRI) antidepressant agent will help, since most insomnia is secondary to depression.

B. Starting a REM-suppressing antidepressant agent will help, since most OSA is REM dominant and thus both OSA and insomnia will improve.

C. Starting trazodone is suggested since breathing is not worsened by nonbenzodiazepine agents.

D. Optimizing breathing will increase options, as many insomnia agents are sedating and may worsen sleep disordered breathing.

12. Stimulant prescriptions are used in several circumstances in sleep medicine, including treatment of the primary hypersomnias, as well as in treatment refractory sleepiness in patients with sleep apnea. Which of the following is true regarding management of chronic stimulant therapy?

A. Following blood pressure is not necessary unless hypertension was already present.

B. Liver function should be followed with any amphetamine-class stimulant due to hepatic metabolism.

C. Proton pump inhibitor use, via the CYP2A19 pathway, creates potential interaction with modafinil, which is a substrate of that pathway.

D. Because caffeine acts via a distinct pathway, monitoring concurrent caffeine use is not necessary in regard to side effects of prescription stimulants.

13. For some patients reporting excess sleepiness, workup may include MSLT. However, certain medications may impact interpretation of the MSLT results. Which of the following is most accurate regarding medication considerations when ordering MSLT testing?

A. Stimulants, including caffeine, should be avoided for approximately 2 weeks prior to MSLT; continuing up to the day of MSLT could result in rebound sleepiness and false positive latencies.

B. REM-suppressing medications should always be discontinued several weeks before MSLT[1] to avoid false negative findings of REM sleep during the naps.

C. If REM agents cannot be discontinued for clinical reasons, then blood or cerebrospinal fluid testing replaces the MSLT for diagnosing narcolepsy without cataplexy.

D. Prescription amphetamine-class agents should be replaced by transmitter reuptake inhibitor based stimulants, such as atomoxetine, to avoid impacting the MSLT results.

14. Patients with narcolepsy experience REM physiology intrusion into wakefulness. Accordingly, many antidepressants have been used clinically to address these symptoms in patients with narcolepsy. Which of the following antidepressants are not thought to reduce REM sleep in prior polysomnography studies?

A. Trazodone

B. Trimipramine

C. Bupropion

D. Selegiline

15. A primary care colleague contacts you because a patient of his, after using a consumer sleep monitor to track sleep using a "headband EEG," stated that he knew his antidepressant

was working because the device reported increased REM sleep. Which of the following is the most appropriate response to your colleague?

A. Consumer sleep monitors are totally useless and patients should never use them.

B. The result is plausible, since depression has been linked to reduced REM sleep.

C. The finding may be related to increased eye movements that occur with certain antidepressants, especially the SSRI class, that could confuse a scoring algorithm.

D. The patient could try several different sleep monitors, and different antidepressants, to see if the association can be confirmed.

16. A 31-year-old woman presents with sleepiness, and her workup reveals the most likely diagnosis to be idiopathic hypersomnia. You discuss treatment options and decide on modafinil. Which of the following is most accurate regarding this medication?

A. Modafinil has increased risk of Stevens-Johnson reaction when combined with oral contraceptive agents.

B. Modafinil should only be taken in the morning due to its long half-life.

C. Modafinil lowers the blood levels of oral contraceptives.

D. Modafinil should not be used because the patient does not have narcolepsy.

17. Which of the following statements is true about caffeine?

A. Caffeine undergoes renal excretion.

B. Caffeine does not enter breast milk.

C. Caffeine is pregnancy class B.

D. Caffeine exhibits interindividual variability in clinical effect and pharmacokinetics.

18. Which of the following drugs is classified as pregnancy class D?

A. Methylphenidate

B. Pramipexole

C. Lorazepam

D. Trazodone

19. Which is the most accurate statement about the effect of alcohol on sleep?

A. It improves sleep because it is a slow wave enhancer.

B. Effects include fragmented sleep and worsening of sleep apnea.

C. It prolongs sleep latency.

D. Its sedating effects reduce the chance of parasomnia.

20. Which of the following has the best evidence for treatment of nightmares in patients with PTSD?

A. Prazosin

B. Melatonin

C. Trazodone

D. Zolpidem

21. Occasionally physicians may opt to use drugs on an off-label basis for treating insomnia symptoms. Which of the following scenarios represents a reasonable off-label approach?

A. Using gabapentin in a patient with comorbid pain disorder

B. Using quetiapine in a patient who is overweight

C. Using trazodone in a patient with headaches and a history of prolactinoma

D. Using diphenhydramine in a patient with mild cognitive impairment to enhance sleep-related memory consolidation

22. You follow a 56-year-old man with RLS, who has been effectively treated with pramipexole. He explains that his symptoms are worse in the last 6 months. Which of the following is most likely regarding his worsening RLS?

A. The pramipexole resulted in iron deficiency anemia.

B. Augmentation is unlikely, since it is only seen with short acting levodopa formulations.

C. The patient began taking mirtazapine.

D. The patient began taking cetirizine.

23. Which of the following medications given for general medical reasons would be most likely to cause insomnia?

A. Atorvastatin

B. Prednisone

C. Warfarin

D. Atenolol

24. A 71-year-old man presents with chronic insomnia, but in the course of the evaluation, you gather the history of episodes of dream enactment. Although he has not fallen out of bed, some of the events have involved hitting his wife. His wife reports that if she awakens him he usually recalls the content of the dream, which his wife says seems to resemble his behavior. You make the presumptive diagnosis of REM behavior disorder (RBD). Because of his comorbidities of coronary artery disease, hypertension, and obesity, you also order a PSG to evaluate for occult OSA, and to confirm the RBD diagnosis. Which of the following would be an appropriate next step?

A. Since no serious injuries have occurred, you should recommend a course of CBT for his insomnia, and provide a bedroom safety handout and a weight loss handout.

B. Although clonazepam would be useful for the dual effect of treating insomnia and reducing RBD events, it is contraindicated since his PSG revealed OSA.

C. Offer the patient treatment for OSA, which may help consolidate his sleep, and then once treated, pharmacotherapy with melatonin and/or clonazepam can be considered.

D. Start an antihistamine sedative to treat his insomnia, because other sedatives are contraindicated in patients with OSA.

25. A 27-year-old man complains of several years of severe difficulty falling asleep. After seeing his primary care doctor, several hypnotics were tried, unsuccessfully, to treat his complaint under the presumptive diagnosis of sleep onset insomnia. Because he has to wake up early for a 9 AM–5 PM job during the week, he does not sleep much weeknights, and then catches up on the weekends, often sleeping until noon or 1 PM, and he feels much better when sleeping on this schedule. Which of the following pharmacological approaches is reasonable in this patient?

A. Use a long-acting benzodiazepine at the desired bedtime to last throughout his long sleep onset problem.

B. Melatonin at 11 PM and fixed schedule of 11 PM–7 AM

C. Melatonin at 9 PM and a fixed schedule of 11 PM–7 AM

D. Gradual shifting of sleep-wake times from 4 AM–12 noon, over the course of ~2 weeks, with melatonin given ~2.5 hours prior to bedtime

26. A patient with bipolar depression and chronic insomnia is given a medication to treat both the mood and insomnia symptoms after failing a first-line trial of CBT for insomnia. After initiating this medication, the patient developed worsening of RLS symptoms. Which of the following is the most likely medication?

A. Eszopiclone

B. Quetiapine

C. Clonidine

D. Bupropion

27. Which of the following is true of over-the-counter remedies for insomnia?
    A. Many contain sedating antihistamines.
    B. They are not FDA regulated because the safety profiles are low risk.
    C. Valerian improves sleep to a greater extent than melatonin.
    D. Because magnesium is a natural antagonist of NMDA-type glutamate receptors, it has the best efficacy of over-the-counter sleep aids.

28. Which of the following is true of receptor targets of drugs used to treat insomnia?
    A. Suvorexant is a synthetic agonist of orexin receptors.
    B. Benzodiazepines enhance GABA-B receptor function.
    C. The "z-drugs" are nonbenzodiazepine in chemical structure, but bind to benzodiazepine binding sites in the brain.
    D. Antihistamines block the H2 subtype receptors in the brain to cause sleepiness.

29. Gabapentin is a drug used for several indications clinically, including seizures and chronic pain, and gabapentin enacarbil is approved for use in RLS. Which of the following is true of gabapentin?
    A. It undergoes hepatic metabolism.
    B. It is a strong inhibitor of CYP3A4.
    C. Side effects include cognitive complaints, mood change, and peripheral edema.
    D. Its mechanism of action involves GABA receptors in the brain and periphery.

30. Suvorexant is a new hypnotic belonging to a distinct mechanistic class. Which of the following is true of this drug?
    A. Suvorexant undergoes hepatic CYP3A4 metabolism and undergoes renal excretion.
    B. Suvorexant is pregnancy class B.
    C. Cataplexy is a very common side effect.
    D. The final FDA approved dosing was similar to the doses using in phase 3 clinical trials.

31. Dopamine signaling is involved in many brain circuits and behaviors. Which of the following statements about the role of dopamine signaling in sleep medicine is most accurate?
    A. Neuroleptic drugs are preferred in patients with comorbid insomnia and sleep apnea.
    B. Treatment of restless legs symptoms versus periodic limb movements requires distinct targeting of dopamine receptor subtypes.
    C. Iron is a cofactor in the endogenous biosynthesis of dopamine.
    D. Stimulant drugs act in part by antagonizing dopamine signaling in the frontal cortex.

32. A 48-year-old patient with chronic insomnia transfers her care to your practice. She has been maintained on 10 mg of zolpidem nightly for several years. She has no new concerns, and asks for you to take over her prescription. Which of the following is the most appropriate response?
    A. Because she is tolerating the dosage well, there is no concern about continuing it.
    B. You insist that the patient sign a release stating her understanding that long-term hypnotic use is not recommended.
    C. You should tell the patient that she can only have refills if she agrees to CBT for insomnia referral.
    D. You counsel the patient regarding FDA warnings of the maximum dose of zolpidem in women and the risk of

morning car accident risk, even if the patient does not subjectively feel hung over.

33. A 25-year-old man with insomnia since college presents to you for a second opinion. His first sleep consultation recommended zolpidem after a failed trial of CBT for insomnia. Although he reported improvement in the insomnia, he noticed evidence in the morning of sleep eating for which he is amnestic. There is no psychiatric history or eating disorder history. On further review, he may have had some episodes prior to the zolpidem, and since stopping the drug he is still having episodes, and is noting symptoms of restless legs as well. What is the most appropriate course of action?
    A. Consider a course of topiramate.
    B. Have the patient lock the refrigerator and cabinets at night.
    C. Increase the dose of zolpidem to prevent arousals and thus reduce this parasomnia.
    D. Refer to psychiatry for evaluation of potential underlying reasons for sleep eating.

34. Which of the following medications are no longer recommended due to side effects that compromise the risk-benefit ratio for treatment of insomnia?
    A. Chloral hydrate
    B. Phenobarbital
    C. Bromide
    D. Triazolam

Answers

1. **The correct answer is B.**
   The z-drugs target mainly the alpha-1 subunit of GABA-A receptors, while other alpha subtypes are involved in the broader effects of benzodiazepines.[2] A is not correct: Z-drugs tend to be shorter acting, especially zaleplon, but several traditional benzodiazepines are also shorter acting (e.g., triazolam). C is not correct, as Z-drugs and benzodiazepines both act on GABA-A receptor chloride channels, not GABA-B metabotropic receptors. D is not correct, as individual drugs in each of these classes differ in P450 metabolism and renal versus hepatic pathways (Table 42.1), but the receptor subtype targeting is thought to underlie the clinical effect differences.

2. **The correct answer is C.**
   Stimulant therapy is an appropriate first choice in this patient.[3] A is not correct, as the hallucinations may be disturbing and warrant therapy, but quetiapine would not be chosen for hallucinations in this (nonpsychosis) setting. B is not correct: although venlafaxine would be appropriate for peri-REM phenomena, this should not be the sole initial plan, given the importance clinically of the hypersomnia and venlafaxine is not a stimulant in this regard. D is not correct, as sodium oxybate should be second line, for example, to be considered if the initial therapeutic plan was not successful.

3. **The correct answer is B.**
   Patients who wish to take a pill for middle of the night awakenings run the risk of morning hangover. Thus short acting agents would be preferred to mitigate this risk. Although zaleplon is approved for onset insomnia, it is not the pattern in this patient, and thus taking the ultra-short-acting zaleplon at bedtime is unlikely to provide symptom relief, and thus A is not correct. The FDA warning regarding morning blood levels refers to increase in women, not men, prompting the lower dosage recommendation,[4] and thus C is not correct. Eszopiclone is the longest acting of the three (see Table 42.1),

TABLE 42.1	**Pharmacology of Hypnotic Medications**		
Drug	Metabolism	Half-Life (h)	Pregnancy
Alprazolam	Hepatic (CYP3A4; glucoronidation); Renal	6–27	D; enters breast milk
Clonazepam	Hepatic (CYP3A4)	17–60	D; enters breast milk
Diazepam	Hepatic (CYP3A4 and 2C19; glucoronidation)	44–48	D; enters breast milk
Lorazepam	Hepatic (glucoronidation); Renal	12	D; enters breast milk
Oxazepam	Hepatic (glucoronidation)	6–11	?; enters breast milk
Temazapam	Hepatic (minor CYP; phase 2 metabolism); Renal	3–18	X; enters breast milk
Triazolam	Hepatic (CYP3A4; glucoronidation); Renal	2–6	X; expected to enter breast milk
Zaleplon	Hepatic (aldehyde oxidase, CYP3A4)	1	C; enters breast milk
Zolpidem	Hepatic (CYP3A4; 2C9)	1.5–4.5 (oral)	C; enters breast milk
(es)Zopiclone	Hepatic (CYP2E1, 3A4)	6	C; unknown but expected to enter breast milk

Data are from UpToDate (accessed May 2016).

and thus D is not correct due to concerns about the hangover effect even if the patient does not drive at all.

4. **The correct answer is C.**

Ramelteon is approved for sleep onset insomnia,[5] and may have a better risk profile in this setting.[6] A is not correct, as diphenhydramine can cause hangover and memory complaints. B is not correct, as clonazepam can lead to fall risk, cognitive changes, and dependence. D is not correct, as quetiapine may increase metabolic and lipid abnormalities (including weight gain) and is in general not recommended for insomnia.

5. **The correct answer is C.**

Nicotine may produce subjective calming effects in smokers, while objective sleep disturbance has been observed in polysomnography evaluations.[7] The effects may occur in part due to microwithdrawal owing to the ultrashort half-life of nicotine, and thus A is not correct. Nicotine interacts with a subset of acetylcholine receptors in the brain, and thus B is not correct. D is not correct, as REM suppression (not enhancement) has been demonstrated in such studies.

6. **The correct answer is B.**

Polymorphisms in the adenosine pathway have been linked to human sleep homeostasis.[8,9] Caffeine is an antagonist of adenosine action in the brain, which accounts for its wake-promoting effects,[10,11] and thus A is incorrect. C is incorrect because both A1 and A2A adenosine receptors are implicated in sleep physiology.[12] D is incorrect because sedating antidepressants do not likely operate via enhanced adenosine action, but may act via antihistamine off-target action.[13]

7. **The correct answer is A.**

Melatonin may increase the INR in patients taking warfarin.[14] Ramelteon is a synthetic melatonin agent approved by the FDA for sleep onset insomnia that acts on MT1 and MT2 subtype receptors,[5,15] and thus B is incorrect. Over-the-counter preparations of melatonin are not regulated by the FDA, and may exhibit heterogeneous bioavailability; doses greater than 1 mg are likely to be supraphysiological,[16–18] and thus C is incorrect. D is incorrect because light suppresses endogenous melatonin production, not levels from exogenous delivery.

8. **The correct answer is C.**

Sodium oxybate is strongly sedating, and therefore caution is necessary regarding comorbid sleep apnea. It is a naturally occurring neurotransmitter but not chemically related to neurosteroids, and thus A is incorrect. B is incorrect: its mechanism of action is not well understood but may operate via a specific GHB receptor,[19] not GABA-A receptors. This treatment may improve sleepiness as well as reduce cataplexy, and thus D is incorrect.

9. **The correct answer is D.**

PLMS are not uncommon in this demographic, and may contribute to sleep disturbance and/or nonrefreshing sleep. It is therefore reasonable to choose therapies aimed at the PLMS as the initial approach. Diphenhydramine can worsen motor restlessness,[20] and also has potential memory impact, especially in this age group,[21] and thus A is incorrect. Although mirtazapine is not known to worsen breathing, it has also been linked to increased restlessness,[22] and thus B is incorrect. C is incorrect, as zolpidem is not known to increase leg symptoms (also note the FDA has lowered the recommended dose in women to 5 mg).[4]

10. **The correct answer is B.**

Iron supplementation is best taken between meals, with vitamin C concurrently, to aid absorption.[23] Although constipation and darkened stools may occur with iron supplementation, A is incorrect, as taking with food reduces absorption (though it may reduce intolerance). C is incorrect, as iron can be used in patients with relative iron deficiency, even without frank anemia. D is incorrect: for RLS, ferritin levels less than 50 are recommended for supplementation, which may be considered normal from an anemia standpoint, and thus it would be prudent to check the actual value rather than the report that it was "normal."

11. **The correct answer is D.**

Given the history and comorbidities, emphasizing OSA treatment is important, and will increase options for him to treat the insomnia. In fact, OSA and insomnia are often comorbid, and some data suggest that treating OSA may improve sleep disturbance symptoms.[24,25] A is not correct, as it is not

TABLE 42.2 Pharmacology of Stimulants			
Drug	Metabolism	Half-Life (h)	Pregnancy
Dexmethylphenidate	Hepatic (de-esterification)	2–5	C; unknown if enters breast milk
Dextroamphetamine	Hepatic (CYP2D6); Renal	10–12	C; enters breast milk
Dextroamphetamine and amphetamine	Hepatic (CYP2D6); Renal	8–14	C; enters breast milk
Lisdexamfetamine	Red blood cell hydrolysis; renal (pro-drug; becomes dextroamphetamine)	10–13	C; enters breast milk
Methylphenidate	Hepatic (de-esterification)	3–4	C; low breast milk levels
Modafinil	Hepatic (CYP3A4 substrate)	15	C; unknown if enters breast milk
Armodafinil	Hepatic (CYP3A4 substrate)	15	C; unknown if enters breast milk

Data are from UpToDate (accessed May 2016).

appropriate to assume that the patient's insomnia is depression-related, especially given the known untreated OSA. B is incorrect, as there is no evidence that pharmacological reduction in REM percentage is an effective therapy for even REM dominant OSA. Although a nonbenzodiazepine sleeping pill may be preferred to a benzodiazepine due to the latter's risk of worsening OSA, even agents such as trazodone may worsen OSA in patients with airway compromise by raising the arousal threshold in certain patients,[26] and thus C is incorrect.

12. **The correct answer is C.**
The cytochrome P450 systems may underlie important potential drug-drug interaction,[27,28] and may include common agents such as proton pump inhibitors and modafinil as shared 2A19 substrates. A is incorrect: hypertension is a potential risk of long-term stimulant use, and should be tracked even if no independent history of hypertension is present. Not all stimulants are metabolized by the same pathway (Table 42.2), and routine liver function screening is not indicated; thus B is incorrect. D is not correct, as caffeine may cause similar side effects as prescription stimulants, despite having distinct brain targets.

13. **The correct answer is A.**
To properly interpret the MSLT, it is important that REM suppressing agents and stimulants be discontinued to avoid false negative (REM suppression agents), or false positive (rapid discontinuation of stimulants resulting in rebound sleepiness).[29] This includes new generation activating reuptake inhibitors, and thus D is incorrect. However, for some patients, the risk of discontinuation may be prohibitive, such as psychiatric instability, or functional compromise without stimulant therapy, and thus clinical correlation is necessary. Thus B is incorrect, as clinical judgment should be used in regard to the safety of stopping psychiatric medications. C is not correct, as HLA *0602 and low orexin levels in the spinal fluid have been much more strongly associated with narcolepsy with cataplexy than narcolepsy without cataplexy.

14. **The correct answer is B.**
REM suppression is commonly seen in many antidepressants, including trazodone and bupropion, and thus A and C are incorrect. Trimipramine has not shown this effect, and nor has nefazodone, which may actually increase REM sleep. REM suppression is especially prominent with the monoamine oxidase inhibitors such as selegiline,[13] and thus D is incorrect. The

clinical relevance of these differences in REM suppression is not well understood.

15. **The correct answer is C.**
Antidepressants, especially SSRI class, may increase the velocity of "slow eye movements," making them resemble rapid eye movements.[30] Headband-based sensors that track eye movements in their staging algorithm may over-classify REM sleep as a result. In fact, most antidepressants suppress REM sleep, and depression has mixed data suggesting earlier/increased REM physiology (and thus B is incorrect), though it remains unknown whether this physiological effect has relevance for mood therapy success. Consumer monitors are not validated for clinical decision making; however, your colleague could benefit from more than the discounting response in A, to help council patients to focus more on their symptoms and less on uncertain data from consumer devices. Because of the uncertain relevance of these findings, encouraging comparison with other consumer devices not validated for clinical use should not be recommended, and thus D is not correct.

16. **The correct answer is C.**
Modafinil has been shown to lower blood levels of some oral conceptive preparations, and thus patients taking OCPs should be counseled to use a second method concurrently. There is no evidence that the Stevens-Johnson reaction is increased by OCPs, and thus A is incorrect. B is not correct: modafinil can be taken twice per day, though the second dose should not be taken too late in the day as it might interfere with sleep. D is not correct, as prescription stimulants are recommended for idiopathic hypersomnia as well as narcolepsy.[3,31]

17. **The correct answer is D.**
Susceptibility to the alerting and adverse effects of caffeine can vary substantially across individuals, in part due to genetic variations.[32–36] It undergoes hepatic metabolism, and thus A is incorrect. B is incorrect, as caffeine does enter breast milk.[37] Caffeine is pregnancy class C, and thus C is incorrect. Pregnancy class A indicates no risk in controlled human studies. Class B indicates no evidence of risk in animal or uncontrolled human studies. Class C indicates risk cannot be ruled out (animal studies may show risk but data is inconclusive or unavailable in humans). Class D indicates positive evidence of risk in humans, but benefit may outweigh in certain circumstances (such as emergency circumstances). Class X indicates contraindicated in pregnancy.

18. **The correct answer is C.**

Lorazepam is pregnancy class D. The other agents are pregnancy class C,[37] and thus are incorrect. Pregnancy class A indicates no risk in controlled human studies. Class B indicates no evidence of risk in animal or uncontrolled human studies. Class C indicates risk cannot be ruled out (animal studies may show risk but data is inconclusive or unavailable in humans). Class D indicates positive evidence of risk in humans, but benefit may outweigh in certain circumstances (such as emergency circumstances). Class X indicates contraindicated in pregnancy.

19. **The correct answer is B.**

Alcohol has several deleterious effects on sleep, including brief awakenings, reductions in REM and slow wave activity, and worsening of sleep disordered breathing.[38,39] A is incorrect, as alcohol does not increase N3. Many individuals with insomnia self-medicate with alcohol because it can be sedating and reduce sleep latency to some extent (and thus C is incorrect), but the risks outweigh any small benefit in that regard. Alcohol can increase the risk of parasomnia,[40] especially if taken in combination with certain hypnotic agents acting on the benzodiazepine receptor complex, and thus D is incorrect.

20. **The correct answer is A.**

Prazosin has the best evidence for efficacy in nightmares from PTSD.[41] The other drugs have not been well studied for this, and may in fact present a risk of vivid dreams and/or nightmares,[42] and thus B, C, and D are not correct.

21. **The correct answer is A.**

Gabapentin, though initially designed and approved to treat seizures, is well understood to have utility in chronic pain, which itself is often comorbid with sleep disturbance,[43] and thus taking advantage of its off-label sedating properties in a pain patient is not unreasonable. B is not correct, as quetiapine, like other neuroleptics, may be associated with weight gain and would not be appropriate in an obese patient for weight loss.[44] Trazodone has been suggested to increase prolactin levels,[45] and thus C is not correct. Although improving sleep could theoretically improve cognitive function, the risk of memory disturbance from centrally acting antihistamines should preclude use in this setting, and thus D is not correct.

22. **The correct answer is C.**

Antidepressants, especially older generation examples such as mirtazapine, may worse motor restlessness and RLS symptoms.[22,46] Although iron deficiency is linked to RLS, it is not related to therapy with dopamine agents, and thus A is not correct. Augmentation[47] could be occurring here as well, but it is not true that it is limited to levodopa, it can happen with other dopamine agents, and thus B is not correct. D is not correct: centrally acting antihistamines may worsen RLS, but this would be less likely with newer agents like cetirizine that do not act centrally.[48]

23. **The correct answer is B.**

Systemic steroid exposure has been associated with insomnia most commonly of the choices here. Although anecdotal evidence sometimes suggests statins can cause insomnia, a meta-analysis did not support this,[49] and thus A is not correct. C is not correct, as warfarin has not been associated with sleep disturbance. Insomnia may be seen in the more lipophilic beta blockers (e.g., propranolol, metoprolol) than in hydrophilic agents that are less likely to cross the blood brain barrier (e.g., atenolol), and thus D is not correct.

24. **The correct answer is C.**

If the patient has OSA, which is likely given the demographic and comorbidities, it should be treated, which then increases the therapeutic options for the RBD. Clonazepam and melatonin are best studied, either alone or in combination, but the former should be used with caution in this demographic due to cognitive risk, fall risk, and suppression of breathing if occult or untreated OSA is present. Bedroom safety should be discussed with RBD patients, but in this case the behavior is concerning, and it would not be prudent to place RBD and OSA as a lower priority with handouts only (though they may be helpful adjuncts) while making CBT the priority, and thus A is not correct. It is true that clonazepam should not be used in patients with untreated OSA, but in this case OSA therapy should be offered, after which clonazepam could be safely introduced, and thus B is not correct. D is not correct, as antihistamine therapy would not be indicated, especially in this age group, as it may cause memory problems and hangover, can worsen motor restlessness, and does not address the RBD or the OSA.

25. **The correct answer is D.**

This patient is likely to have delayed sleep phase syndrome based on the demographic and the history.[50,51] Hypnotic medications do not address the primary root cause, and thus A is not correct. Neither of the fixed schedule responses of B or C are likely to succeed because of the severity of the delay, and the inability thus to rapidly shift, regardless of the melatonin timing options. In fact, such a rapid shift could paradoxically perpetuate the delayed phase syndrome by exposing the patient to light during his biological "night."

26. **The correct answer is B.**

Quetiapine is a dopamine antagonist that can exacerbate RLS symptomatology.[52] There is no evidence that eszopiclone or clonidine would induce RLS, and in fact the latter has some evidence of effectiveness for RLS treatment,[53] and thus A and C are not correct. Although many antidepressants have been associated with RLS and PLMS, bupropion may be an exception,[54,55] and thus D is not correct.

27. **The correct answer is A.**

Centrally acting antihistamines are used for their sedating properties in sleeping remedies, either alone or often in combination with analgesics in "PM" formulations. B is not correct: over-the-counter agents for sleep are not regulated by the FDA, but it is not because risk review concluded they are low risk, and in fact risk concerns are not uncommon due to side effects or even drug-drug interactions.[56] There is no evidence that valerian is superior to melatonin, and in fact existing studies are mixed in terms of valerian effectiveness for insomnia,[57] and thus C is incorrect. Although many natural remedy sources list magnesium as a potential sleep aid, there is little evidence, and the mechanism is unlikely to be linked to NMDA receptors, and thus D is incorrect.

28. **The correct answer is C.**

The new generation benzodiazepine ligands are so named because they bind to subsets of the traditional benzodiazepine sites on GABA-A receptor channels, but the term benzodiazepine refers to the chemical structure, which is not shared by the z-drugs. Suvorexant is an orexin antagonist, not agonist, and thus A is incorrect. Benzodiazepines bind to and enhance the activity of GABA-A receptors (which are chloride channels), not GABA-B receptors (which are metabotropic G-protein coupled receptors), and thus B is not correct. Centrally acting antihistamines bind to and block the activity mainly of the H1 subtype (the H2 subtype are mainly involved in stomach acid secretion; the H3 subtype is a presynaptic autoreceptor), and thus D is not correct. See Table 42.3 and Fig. 42.1 for a summary of various neurotransmitters and their relevance to sleep-wake physiology.

29. **The correct answer is C.**

Cognitive effects, mood instability, and peripheral edema are among the side effects of gabapentin, which also include nystagmus or diplopia. Gabapentin undergoes renal excretion, not hepatic metabolism, and thus A is not correct. It does not appreciably interact with cytochrome P450 systems, and thus B is incorrect. D is not correct: its mechanism of action is unrelated to GABA receptor, despite its structural similarity to GABA; rather, it is thought to interact with calcium channels.[59]

TABLE 42.3	Sleep-Wake Circuitry Overview	
Nucleus	Neurotransmitter	Function
Ventrolateral preoptic	GABA	Sleep-promoting
Basal forebrain	Acetylcholine	Wake-promoting
Lateral hypothalamus	Orexin	Wake-promoting
Laterodorsal and pedunculopontine	Acetylcholine	Wake-promoting; REM-promoting
Locus coeruleus	Norepinephrine	Wake-promoting
Parabrachial	Glutamate	Wake-promoting
Raphe	Serotonin	Wake-promoting
Tuberomammillary	Histamine	Wake-promoting

For further details, see Saper et al.[58]

Wakefulness

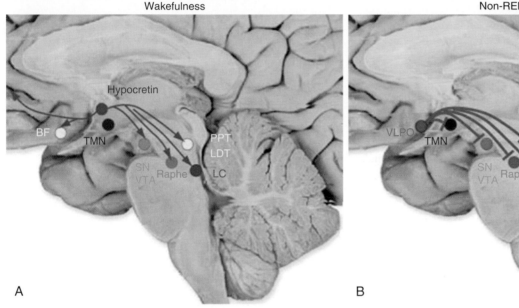

A

Non-REM sleep

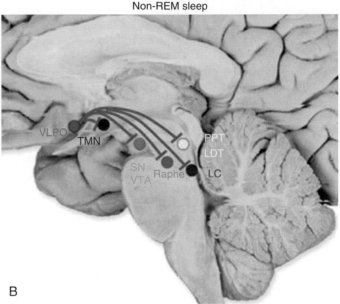

B

REM sleep

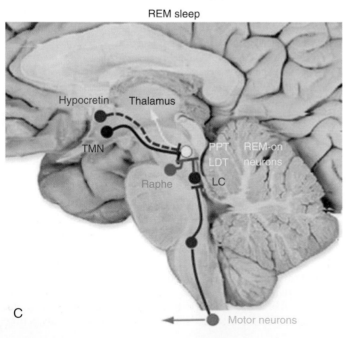

C

• **Figure 42.1** Schematic location of sleep-related circuitry Midsagittal view is shown with superimposed schematic representation of circuits most relevant for wakefulness **(A)**, non-REM sleep **(B)**, and REM sleep **(C)**. In wakefulness, hypocretin/orexin neurons project to, and excite, the other wake-promoting brainstem nuclei, as well as the basal forebrain, and widely throughout the cortex (*red arrows*). During non-REM sleep, the VLPO projects to, and inhibits, the wake-promoting nuclei (*green lines*). During REM sleep, the LDT and PPT cholinergic neurons lack the wake-inhibition (from hypocretin/orexin, TMN, raphe, and LC), and excite the thalamus (*yellow*). Medullary interneurons inhibit motor neurons, causing atonia in REM. *BF*, Basal forebrain; *LC*, locus coeruleus; *LDT*, laterodorsal tegmentum; *PPT*, pedunculopontine nucleus; *SN*, substantia nigra; *TMN*, tuberomammillary nucleus; *VLPO*, ventrolateral preoptic nucleus; *VTA*, ventral tegmental area. (Adapted from Nishino S. Neurotransmitters and neuropharmacology of sleep/wake regulations. *Encyclopedia Sleep*; 2013: 395–406.)

30. The correct answer is A.

Suvorexant undergoes hepatic metabolism, via CYP3A4, and is renally excreted. It is pregnancy class C, and thus B is incorrect. Although cataplexy was a theoretical concern at higher than the FDA approved doses, it is not commonly reported as a side effect, whereas parasomnia, and in particular next day sleepiness, was a major concern, and thus C is not correct. The FDA approved doses are in the lower half of those tested in clinical trials, due to concern about dose-dependent side effects that altered the risk-benefit balance, and thus D is not correct.

31. The correct answer is C.

Iron is a co-factor in the rate-limited step of dopamine biosynthesis, via the enzyme tyrosine hydroxylase. Neuroleptic agents are not recommended for insomnia, because of adverse risk profile, but are sometimes used at night if there is psychiatric indication and coexisting insomnia; there is no reason to believe them to be helpful in the presence of comorbid sleep apnea, and in fact with weight gain as a potential risk, this is an additional argument against their use, and thus A is not correct. RLS and PLMS are both linked to iron and dopamine; there is no evidence that distinct receptor subtypes are preferentially involved, and thus B is not correct. Stimulant drugs such as modafinil may act via dopamine systems, but through enhancement, not antagonism, and thus D is not correct.

32. The correct answer is D.

The FDA has released warnings about zolpidem, which lingers in the circulation on morning blood sampling more so in women than in men, prompting a recommendation to lower the maximum dose in women from 10 to 5 mg. The warning also addresses the potential risk of morning motor vehicle accident after taking zolpidem the prior night, due to lingering effects that the patient may not be aware of. Thus A is not correct, as the fact that the patient has no concerns does not preclude the need for a candid risk-benefit discussion. The long-term use of hypnotics is not recommended, but the discussion should focus on shared decision making rather than legal release forms, and thus B is not correct. Similarly, while emphasis of the benefits of CBT for insomnia should be routinely offered, it would be more appropriate to engage the patient in shared decision making rather than withholding her current therapy to coerce her into CBT, and thus C is not correct. For review of behavioral and pharmacological management of chronic insomnia, see Buysse (2013)[60] and Buscemi et al.[61]

33. The correct answer is A.

Although there are no FDA approved drug therapies for sleep eating,[62] some studies suggest that off-label use of topiramate is effective.[63] However, it is not tolerated in some patients, so close follow-up is needed. Restricting access with locks would not be the first line approach, and thus B is not correct. There is no evidence that increasing zolpidem dose would suppress the behavior, and might even worsen the clinical situation or cause hangover, and thus C is not correct. Psychiatric referral can be considered for certain patients, but in this case for amnestic events and no clear psychiatric history, such referral could be deferred to next line, and thus D is not correct.

34. The correct answer is D.

Although triazolam is not commonly used in modern practice compared with other more recently available agents, it has not been associated with as prominent risks as the other medications on this list. Chloral hydrate, and especially barbiturates and bromides, are not recommended due to overall poor risk profile, and thus A–C are not correct.

Suggested Reading

Buscemi N, Vandermeer B, Friesen C, et al. The efficacy and safety of drug treatments for chronic insomnia in adults: a meta-analysis of RCTs. *J Gen Intern Med*. 2007;22(9):1335-1350.

Buysse DJ. Insomnia. *JAMA*. 2013;309(7):706-716.

Luyster FS, Buysse DJ, Strollo PJ Jr. Comorbid insomnia and obstructive sleep apnea: challenges for clinical practice and research. *J Clin Sleep Med*. 2010;6(2):196-204.

Lynch T, Price A. The effect of cytochrome P450 metabolism on drug response, interactions, and adverse effects. *Am Fam Physician*. 2007;76(3):391-396.

Sarris J, Byrne GJ. A systematic review of insomnia and complementary medicine. *Sleep Med Rev*. 2011;15(2):99-106.

43

Polysomnography Pearls

LAURA A. LINLEY, RITA BROOKS, RICHARD S. ROSENBERG*

Questions, 642

Answers, 650

Suggested Reading, 657

Channel Key: REOG, right electrooculogram; LEOG, left electrooculogram; ECG, electrocardiogram; CHIN, chin electromyogram; RLEG, right leg electromyogram; LLEG, left leg electromyogram; SNORE, snoring microphone; THERM, nasal-oral thermal airflow sensor; PRESS, nasal pressure sensor; CHEST, chest effort belt recording; ABD, abdominal effort belt recording; O_2 Sat, pulse oximeter oxygen saturation; EEG, electroencephalogram; M1, Left mastoid electrode location (Reference Electrode); M2, Right mastoid electrode location (Reference Electrode); C3 and O1, left central and left occipital respectively; C4 and O2, right central and occipital respectively; F4, Right frontal electrode location.

Electroencephalogram signals use International 10–20 System identification.

Questions

1. In the following tracing (2-minute window) (Fig. 43.1), the electroencephalogram (EEG) channels contain significant artifact. How should the recording be improved?
   A. Apply a 60-Hz filter.
   B. Reapply the M1 (A1) electrode.
   C. Turn the temperature down in the room.
   D. Turn the channel sensitivity down.
2. In the following tracing (30-second window) (Fig. 43.2), artifact is so large that the signal cannot be read. Which of the following actions is most likely to reduce the artifact?
   A. Remove the nasal thermistor.
   B. Ask the patient to use the bathroom.
   C. Switch the recording to bipolar mode.
   D. Cool the room.
3. During calibrations we ask patients to close their eyes for 30 seconds for us to see sinusoidal activity coming from the occipital leads with a frequency of 8–13 Hz that is called _____ and is a sign of stage _____.

*For the American Association of Sleep Technologists

A. Theta, N1
B. Alpha, W
C. Spindles, N2
D. Delta, N3

4. This respiratory pattern in the following epoch (2-minute window) (Fig. 43.3) is representative of the recording from the start until midnight. What action might a recording technologist need to take?
   A. Start continuous positive airway pressure (CPAP) if split-night criteria is met.
   B. Turn down the low frequency filter.
   C. Reattach the leg electrodes to reset the signal.
   D. Begin cardiopulmonary resuscitation (CPR).
5. Which is the most appropriate initial response of the sleep technologist to an asystole lasting more than 8 seconds?
   A. Wake the patient and ask if he or she is OK.
   B. Call the sleep center medical director.
   C. Call the patient's referring physician.
   D. Wait and see if it happens again.
6. In this recording from a 47-year-old man (Fig. 43.4), the epoch previous to the following 30-second epoch shown is scored as stage N2. The waveforms in the oval:
   A. Result in the scoring of this epoch as stage R sleep
   B. Indicate this epoch is stage N3
   C. Are supportive of stage R sleep
   D. Occur when the patient is having a brief electrical seizure
7. End the scoring of stage N2 sleep when:
   A. There are no sleep spindles or K complexes for 30 seconds
   B. There are no sleep spindles or K complexes for 2 epochs
   C. The EEG meets criteria for scoring of stage N1 for more than 15 seconds
   D. There are 6 seconds or more of slow waves in an epoch
8. In Fig. 43.5, the respiratory event in the rectangular box can be scored as:
   A. An apnea
   B. An hypopnea using rule 1A or 1B
   C. An hypopnea only when using rule 1A
   D. An hypopnea only when using rule 1B
9. If electing to score a respiratory effort–related arousal (RERA), the event must contain:
   A. At least a 90% reduction of the thermal flow signal amplitude
   B. At least a 4% oxygen desaturation
   C. An arousal
   D. A significant reduction of respiratory effort

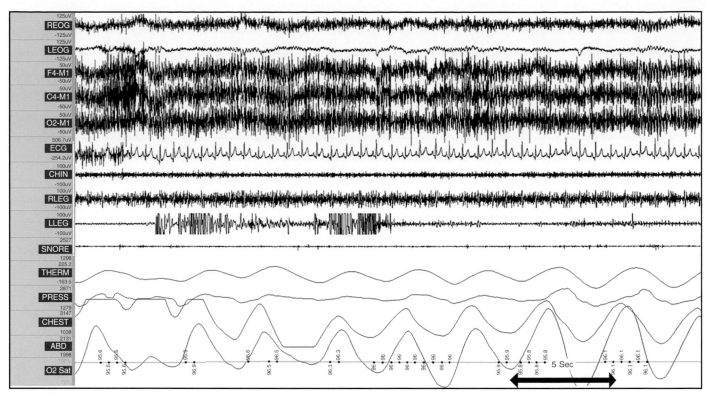

• Figure 43.1

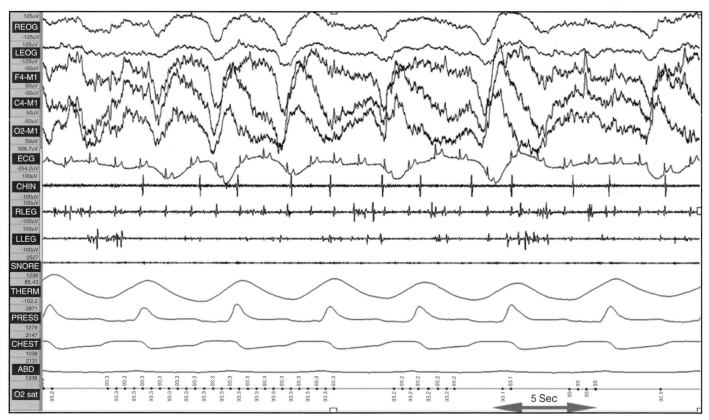

• Figure 43.2

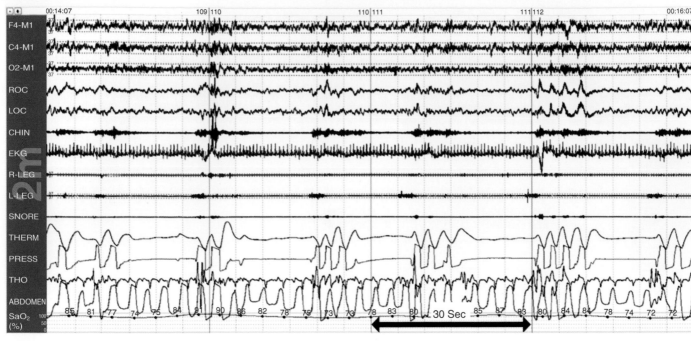

• **Figure 43.3**

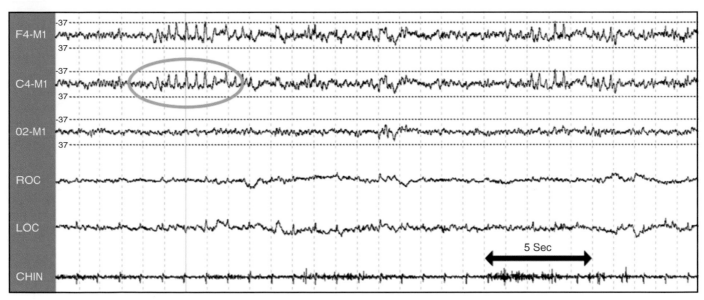

• **Figure 43.4**

10. According to the American Academy of Sleep Medicine (AASM) Scoring Manual, how many periodic limb movements (LMs) are scored in the following 2-minute figure (Fig. 43.6)?
    A. 6
    B. 9
    C. 12
    D. None of the events meet criteria for scoring

11. The recommended placement of electrocardiographic (ECG) recording electrodes during a sleep study differs from standard placement in that:
    A. One electrode is placed on the xiphoid process
    B. Both electrodes are on the torso

    C. Both electrodes are below the level of the nipple
    D. Both electrodes are on the arms

12. The following 10-second tracing (Fig. 43.7) is representative of a patient with:
    A. Excessive fragmentary myoclonus
    B. Hyperexplexia
    C. Alternating leg muscle activation
    D. Rhythmic movement disorder

13. The following 10-second tracing (Fig. 43.8) contains:
    A. No scorable cardiac events
    B. Atrial fibrillation
    C. Pacemaker artifact
    D. Narrow complex tachycardia

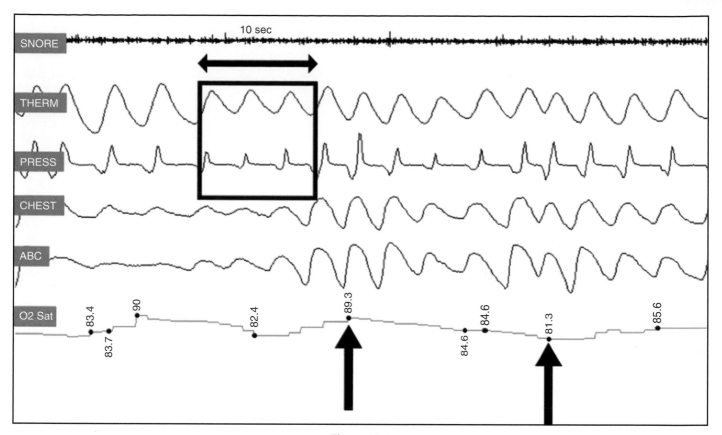

• Figure 43.5

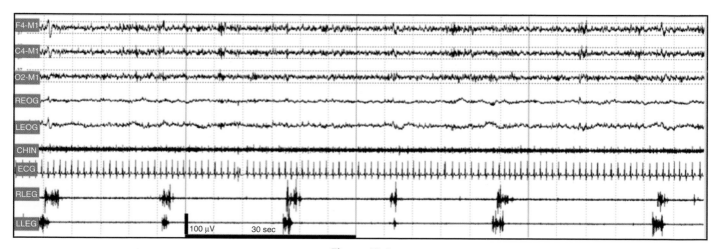

• Figure 43.6

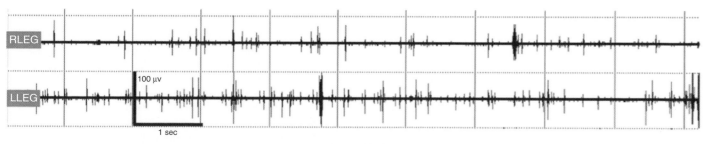

• Figure 43.7

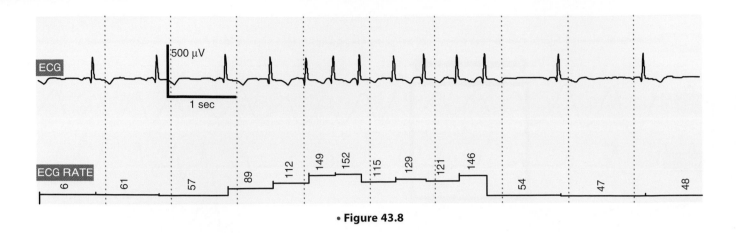

• **Figure 43.8**

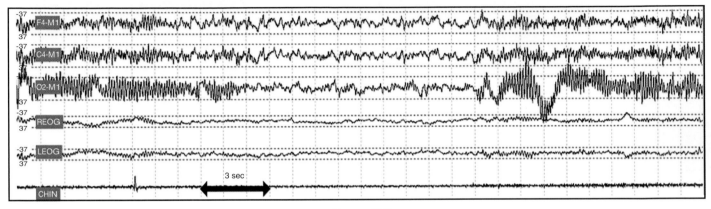

• **Figure 43.9**

14. Does the following 30-second epoch (Fig. 43.9) contain an arousal?
    A. No, it must have a 1-second increase in chin electromyogram (EMG).
    B. No, the epoch is scored as wake.
    C. No, the EEG frequency must increase for at least 3 seconds.
    D. Yes, it meets all criteria for scoring as an arousal.

15. The following 30-second epoch (Fig. 43.10) contains:
    A. Posterior slow waves of youth
    B. Paroxysmal spike and wave activity
    C. Frontal rhythmic delta activity
    D. Hypnagogic hypersynchrony (HH)

16. The minimum digital resolution of polysomnography (PSG) signals required by the AASM Scoring Manual is 12 bits per sample. This determines:
    A. The number of levels of voltage range that can be represented
    B. The fastest frequency that can be resolved by visual analysis
    C. How bright the display screen appears during scoring
    D. The effects of a digital filter on slow wave activity in the EEG

17. The 60-second epoch in Fig. 43.11 is consistent with a diagnosis of hypoventilation because:
    A. It contains variability of the nasal pressure signal
    B. The amplitude of the chest and abdominal signals is low
    C. The measure of carbon dioxide is elevated
    D. The oxygen saturation is low

18. The respiratory event index (REI) as defined by the AASM Manual underestimates the severity of sleep apnea compared with the apnea-hypopnea index (AHI) because:
    A. The REI requires a 4% oxygen desaturation for each hypopnea event
    B. The REI does not use a measure of flow
    C. The denominator for the REI is monitoring time, which is always longer than sleep time
    D. The REI includes RERAs even though there is no measure of arousal

19. In the home sleep apnea testing (HSAT) tracing (Fig. 43.12), the channel "XSUM" is:
    A. The sum of the amplitude of all of the other channels
    B. A valid substitute for the flow signal
    C. An indicator of snoring volume
    D. Derived by adding the nasal pressure and thermal flow signals

20. When HSAT is performed using peripheral arterial tone (PAT) devices, the device must allow:
    A. A trial of auto-adjusting positive airway pressure (PAP)
    B. At least one EEG channel for scoring of sleep stages
    C. A thermal flow channel
    D. Ability to display raw data for review

21. The EEG as recorded from the scalp most likely arises from:
    A. Excitatory and inhibitory postsynaptic potentials
    B. Action potentials traveling through axons
    C. Current leakage at the nodes of Ranvier
    D. Sequestration of neurotransmitters in synaptic vesicles

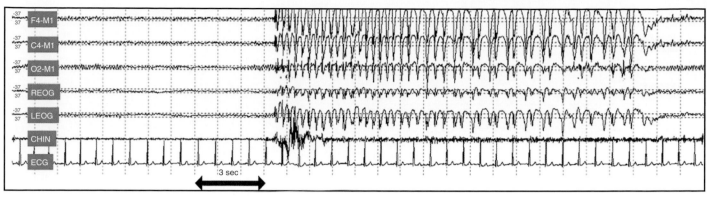

• Figure 43.10

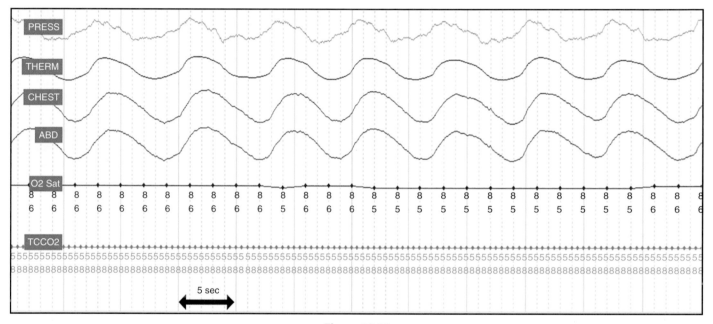

• Figure 43.11

22. The most appropriate response of a sleep technologist to the event shown in Fig. 43.13 is:
    A. Begin CPR immediately
    B. Administer an anticonvulsant, preferably diazepam
    C. Reassure the patient and parent that everything is OK
    D. Replace the ground electrode and check impedances

23. An LM occurs just before the end of an obstructive apnea. A scorable arousal occurs 4 seconds after the LM (Fig. 43.14). What movement event should be scored?
    A. Periodic LM without arousal
    B. Periodic LM with arousal
    C. Isolated LM
    D. No event

24. The tracing in Fig. 43.15 is the CPAP flow channel from a titration study. The black box contains:
    A. A hypopnea only if accompanied by an oxygen desaturation or arousal
    B. An apnea

C. A signal that cannot be used to define a respiratory event
D. Evidence of hypoventilation

25. A sequence of epochs is recorded as follows: Epoch A has a sleep spindle at the 10-second mark and elevated chin EMG throughout. Epoch B has low-amplitude, mixed frequency EEG without spindles or K complexes and elevated chin EMG throughout. Epoch C has low-amplitude, mixed frequency EEG without spindles or K complexes and low chin EMG throughout. Epoch D has low-amplitude, mixed frequency EEG without spindles or K complexes low chin EMG throughout and a rapid eye movement (REM) at the 5-second mark. The first epoch of REM sleep is:
    A. Epoch A
    B. Epoch B
    C. Epoch C
    D. Epoch D

26. The following tracing (Fig. 43.16) is from a 2-month-old male born at 36 weeks' gestation, and according

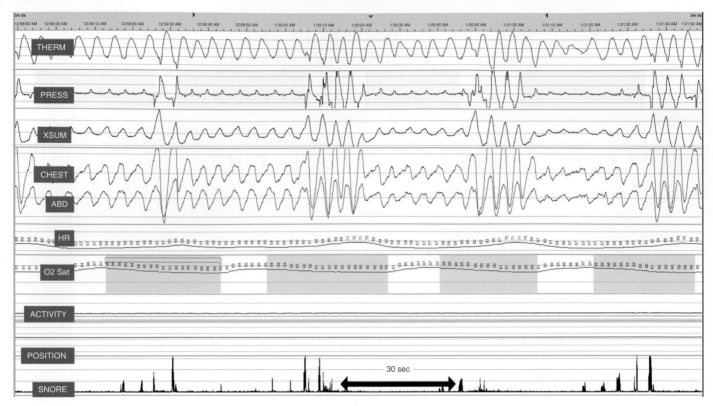

• **Figure 43.12**

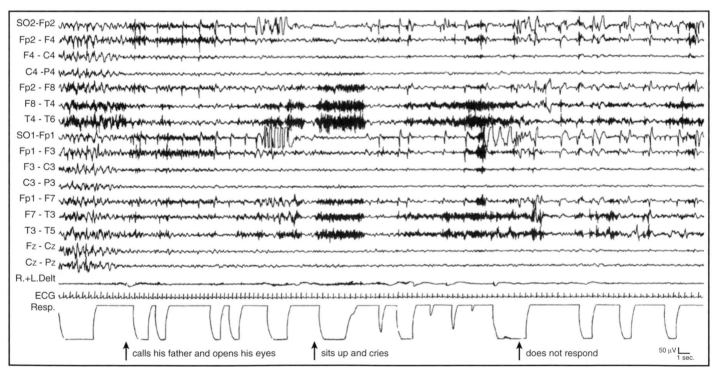

• **Figure 43.13** (From Chokroverty S, Zucconi M, Provini F, Manconi M. *Atlas of Sleep Medicine*. 2nd ed. Philadelphia: Saunders Elsevier; 2014.)

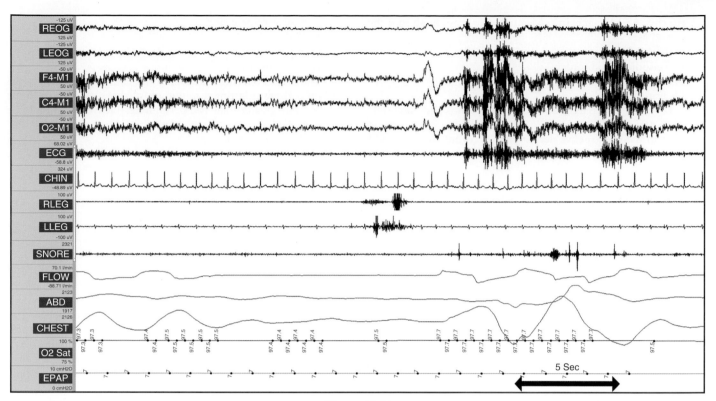

• Figure 43.14

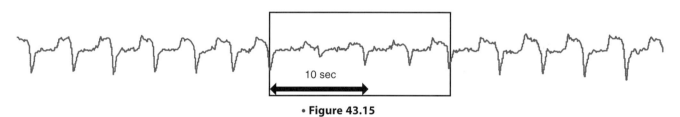

• Figure 43.15

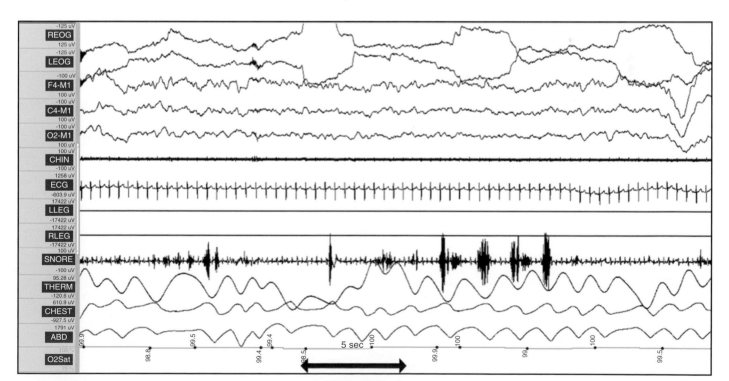

• Figure 43.16

to the AASM Scoring Manual the epoch should be scored as:

A. REM sleep

B. Periodic LM disorder

C. N sleep

D. Transitional sleep

27. A K complex with a duration of 0.75 seconds and amplitude of 65 µV from peak to peak is recorded from a 75-year-old woman with obstructive sleep apnea. According to the AASM Scoring Manual, should this waveform be scored as a slow wave?

A. Yes.

B. No, it does not meet the frequency requirements for a slow wave.

C. No, it does not meet the amplitude requirements for a slow wave.

D. No, K complexes are never scored as slow waves.

28. The recommended duration for each nap opportunity of the maintenance of wakefulness test (MWT) when the sleep clinician requires objective data to assess an individual's ability to remain awake is:

A. 8 minutes

B. 12 minutes

C. 20 minutes

D. 40 minutes

29. Movement and muscle artifact obscure the EEG for more than half of an epoch to the extent that the sleep stage cannot be determined. Three seconds of unambiguous alpha activity is seen. The epoch preceding the epoch is scored as stage N2. The epoch following the epoch is scored as N2. The epoch in Fig. 43.17 should be scored as:

A. Indeterminate sleep

B. Wake

C. Stage N2

D. Movement time

30. The AASM Scoring Manual recommends scoring tachycardia for a rhythm lasting a minimum of three consecutive beats at a rate greater than 100 per minute. Tachycardia should be identified as:

A. Atrial or ventricular

B. Slow or fast

C. Wide or narrow complex

D. Elevated or depressed T waves

Answers

1. **Answer B. Reapply the M1 (A1) electrode.**

The impedance of all three of the electrodes at F_4, C_4, and O_2 electrodes may be high. This would indicate failure of multiple electrodes and is not the most parsimonious answer. More likely, the M1 electrode may have high impedance. This is an electrode that is used as the reference signal in all three EEG channels. It is much more likely that the high impedance comes from the electrode common to the three channels than to each of the three separate electrodes. Replace or reapply M1 to reduce the noise.

Applying a 60-Hz filter (Answer A) will not eliminate the effect of high impedance on the reference electrode, cooling the room (Answer C) will have no effect on artifact that is caused by high impedance. Reducing channel sensitivity (Answer D) will only reduce the size of the signal.[1]

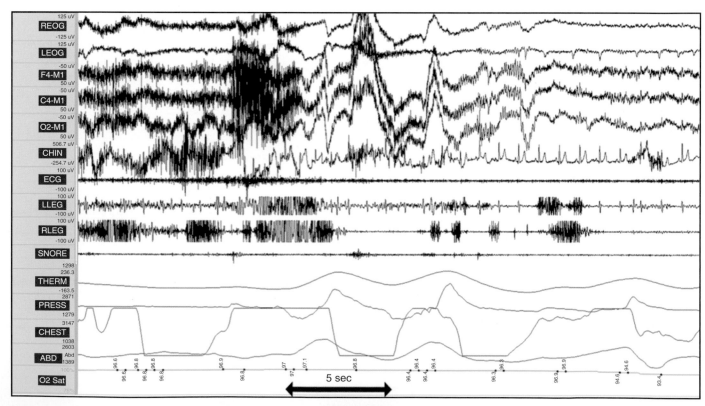

• Figure 43.17

2. **Answer D. Cool the room.**

Although the electrode application process includes cleaning of the scalp, patients continue to produce oils and sweat during the night. At times this results in an artifact that can grow into a problem over time. Sweat and oils can increase the electrode impedance, but usually sweat artifact looks different than the 60-Hz noise. Sweat artifact is usually very low frequency, producing a "wandering" signal. This is an example of sweat artifact.

At times, the sweat artifact can become so large that the signal cannot be read. There are several things that can be done to reduce sweat artifact:

1. Cool the room
2. Use a fan to increase airflow in the room
3. Use a towel to dry off the patient's scalp
4. Change the low frequency filter to eliminate the "wandering"

Option 4 should be used only as a last resort. Changing the low filter frequency eliminates signal as well as noise. Slow wave activity may be at the same or almost the same frequency as sweat artifact. Changing the filter would reduce the amplitude of the slow wave activity, possibly resulting in fewer waves meeting the 75-µV amplitude criterion and a reduction in the scoring of slow waves and therefore stage N3 sleep.

Answer A is incorrect. The nasal thermistor measures airflow at the nose and is not related to the artifact seen on the EEG channels. Getting the patient up to the bathroom (Answer B) may increase sweating and worsen the artifact, and switching to a bipolar mode (Answer C) will not affect the appearance of sweat artifact in the recording.[1]

3. **Answer B. Alpha, W.**

Alpha rhythm is defined as trains of sinusoidal 8–13 Hz activity recorded over the occipital region with eye closure, attenuating with eye opening. Score epochs as stage W when more than 50% of the epoch contains alpha rhythm over the occipital region.

Answer A is incorrect because theta activity does not arise from occipital leads. It is seen at a frequency of 4–7 Hz and is most prominent during stage N1 sleep. Sleep spindles (Answer C) occur at a frequency of 12–14 Hz, are seen during stage N2 sleep, and are most prominent in the central and frontal channels. Finally, delta activity (Answer D) occurs at a frequency of 0.5–2 Hz in the frontal derivations and is seen during stage N3 sleep. None of these waveforms would be seen in awake patients asked to close their eyes for 10 seconds. Fig. 43.18 shows a tracing from a patient asked to close and later open his eyes. Alpha rhythm is present especially in the occipital channel with eyes closed.[2]

4. **Answer A. Start CPAP if split-night criteria are met.**

For CPAP titration, a split-night study (initial diagnostic PSG followed by CPAP titration during PSG on the same night) is an alternative to one full night of diagnostic PSG followed by a second night of titration if the following criteria are met:

a. An AHI of at least 40 is documented during a minimum of 2 hours of diagnostic PSG.

b. An AHI of 20–40, based on clinical judgment (e.g., if there are also repetitive long obstructions and major desaturations).

1. However, at AHI values less than 40, determination of CPAP pressure requirements, based on split-night

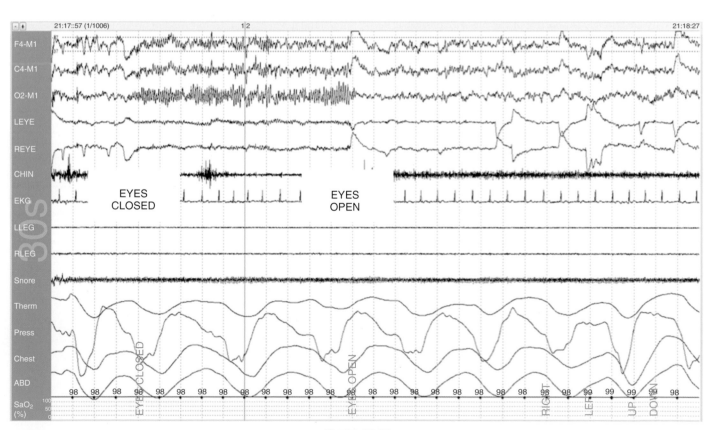

• **Figure 43.18**

studies, may be less accurate than during a full-night titration.

Reducing the low frequency filter (Answer B) will serve only to reduce the size of the waveforms. Answer C is also incorrect—the leg electrodes record EMG and in this example appear to be working appropriately. There is no need for CPR (Answer D) in a patient exhibiting classic signs of obstructive sleep apnea with a normal heart rate.[3]

5. **Answer A. Wake the patient and ask if he or she is OK.**
The technologist response to asystole depends on the duration. An 8-second asystole requires intervention (see Fig. 43.19 for an example of a >8-second asystole). The technologist should check to be sure that the flat portion of the recording is not a technical problem. For example, if ECG artifact continues in other channels when the ECG signal goes flat, there may be a problem with the ECG electrodes. Intervention for asystole usually begins with waking the patient and asking if they have any symptoms.

Sleep center protocol may require the technologist to call the sleep center medical director (Answer B) who may notify the referring physician (Answer C); however, the technologist's primary responsibility is to assure the patient is safe. If the patient has symptoms when awakened the first call should be to activate emergency medical services (EMS). It is never appropriate to wait and see if the asystole reoccurs without waking and checking the patient (Answer D).[1]

6. **Answer C. Are supportive of stage REM sleep.**
The waveforms are sawtooth waves, described in the AASM Scoring Manual as "trains of sharply contoured or triangular, often serrated, 2-to-6 Hz waves maximal in amplitude over the central head regions and often, but not always, preceding a burst of rapid eye movements." Subsequently in the Notes section the Manual states, "Sawtooth waves or transient muscle activity are strongly supportive of the presence of stage R sleep and may be helpful when the stage is in doubt, however, they are not required for scoring stage R."

Stage R sleep cannot be scored based solely on the presence of sawtooth waves (Answer A), the waveforms exhibited are classic sawtooth waves that do not meet criteria for slow waves that would be required for the scoring of stage N3 sleep (Answer B). Sawtooth waves may be confused with ictal (seizure) activity but are not considered to be epileptogenic in origin (Answer D).[2]

7. **Answer D. There are 6 seconds or more of slow waves in an epoch.**
The scoring of stage N2 sleep continues after the appearance of a K complex or sleep spindle even during epochs where these waveforms are absent. This includes epochs that meet criteria for scoring as stage N1. Therefore lack of sleep spindles or K complexes for 30 seconds (Answer A) or 2 epochs (Answer B) does not indicate the end of stage N2, nor does the appearance of 15 seconds of stage N1 sleep (Answer C).

The criteria for ending a bout of stage N2 include a transition to wake, arousal, or major body movement followed by low-amplitude, mixed frequency EEG, transition to stage REM or transition to N3 sleep. Six seconds of slow wave activity are sufficient to score an epoch as stage N3. Therefore the 6 seconds of slow wave activity in an epoch should lead to the end of scoring of stage N2. A transition from N2 to N3 is shown in Fig. 43.20.[2]

8. **Answer B. A hypopnea using rule 1A or 1B.**
The event shown is not accompanied by a 90% or greater drop in the thermal flow signal amplitude and therefore cannot be scored as an apnea (Answer A). It lasts more than 10 seconds and has a drop of amplitude in the pressure sensor channel of more than 30%. It is accompanied by an oxygen desaturation from 89.3% to –81.3% *(arrows)*. Rule 1A requires at least a 10-second event, 30% reduction in pressure sensor amplitude and a 3% oxygen desaturation or an arousal. The event meets these criteria. Rule 1B requires at least a 10-second event, 30% reduction in pressure sensor amplitude, and 4% oxygen

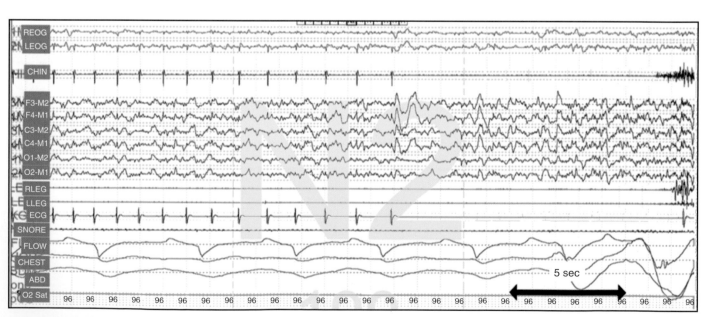

• **Figure 43.19**

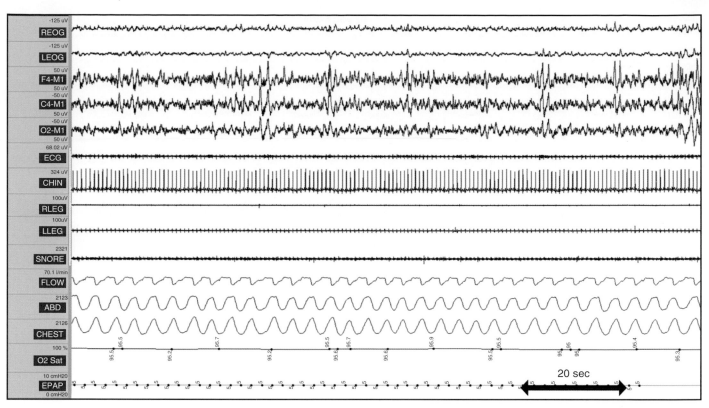

• **Figure 43.20**

desaturation. The event meets both of these criteria, and therefore both answers C and D are incorrect. The event can be scored a hypopnea using either scoring rule.[2]

9. **Answer C. An arousal.**

A RERA cannot meet criteria for an apnea or hypopnea. The only requirements for scoring are that the event contain a sequence of breaths lasting 10 seconds or more with increasing respiratory effort or flattening of the inspiratory portion of the nasal pressure waveform in a diagnostic study and that the event leads to an arousal from sleep.

A 90% reduction in the thermal flow signal amplitude indicates an apnea, therefore answer A is incorrect. There is no desaturation requirement for scoring a RERA, meaning that answer B is incorrect. There is no requirement for a reduction in respiratory effort, therefore answer D is also incorrect.[2]

10. **Answer A. 6.**

Each of the bursts of muscle activity from the right and left leg meet criteria for scoring as a LM based on amplitude and duration. This means that answer D is incorrect. The interval between LMs is more than 5 seconds and less than 90 seconds, and there are more than four LMs in the 2-minute record fragment. Leg movements on two different legs separated by less than 5 seconds between movement onsets are counted as a single leg movement, meaning that answers B and C are both incorrect.[2]

11. **Answer B. Both electrodes are on the torso.**

The usual placement of lead II electrodes is on the right arm and left leg. This was thought to increase the risk of displacement with the patient moving during sleep. Placement of both electrodes on the torso reduces the risk of displacement while preserving an adequate signal.

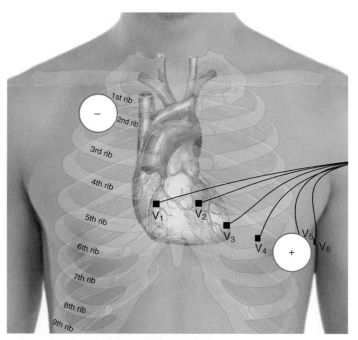

• **Figure 43.21**

ECG recording electrode placement is standardized for PSG and electrodes are not appropriately placed if they are on the arms (Answer D) or xiphoid process (Answer A) or if both of the electrodes are below the level of the nipple (Answer C). Correct placement is shown in Fig. 43.21.[2]

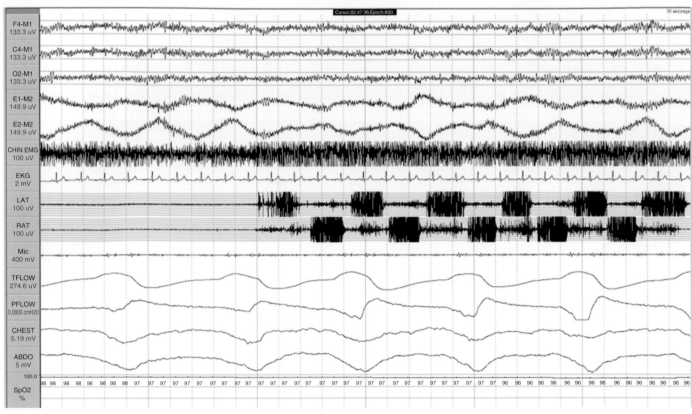

• **Figure 43.22**

12. **Answer A. Excessive fragmentary myoclonus.**

Excessive fragmentary myoclonus consists of brief (usually less than 150 seconds) electrical potentials recorded from EMG electrodes. In many cases it is not associated with visible movements. When present, movements are similar to those seen in REM sleep. It is a benign movement phenomenon with no clinical consequences reported.

Hyperexplexia (Answer B) is a rare condition of exaggerated startle reflex triggered by noise, movement, or touch that often resolves during sleep. Alternating leg muscle activation (Answer C) is typically seen as alternating periodic LMs of sleep events. An example is shown in Fig. 43.22. Rhythmic movement disorder (Answer D) is typically seen in the EEG recording as a repetitive rhythmic movement artifact and not in the LM recording.[2]

13. **Answer D. Narrow complex tachycardia.**

The AASM Scoring Manual includes criteria for sustained and nonsustained tachycardia. Sustained tachycardia is defined as a rate of greater than 90 beats per minute lasting more than 30 seconds. The tracing does not meet this criterion but has a rate greater than 100 beats per minute for at least three consecutive beats. This meets scoring criteria for nonsustained tachycardia, which is subdivided into narrow (less than 120 msec) or wide (greater than 120 msec) complex based on QRS duration.

This is a scorable cardiac event—answer A is incorrect. Atrial fibrillation appears as an irregularly irregular ventricular rhythm associated with replacement of consistent P waves

with rapid oscillations, and therefore answer B is incorrect. Pacemaker artifact is typically nonsustained and brief, and therefore answer C is incorrect.[2]

14. **Answer D. Yes, it meets all criteria for scoring as an arousal.**

The arousal rule requires an abrupt shift of EEG frequency that lasts at least 3 seconds with at least 10 seconds of stable sleep preceding the change. More than half of this epoch consists of alpha rhythm activity, and it is correctly scored as wake. However, arousals meeting all scoring criteria but occurring during an awake epoch in the recorded time between "lights out" and "lights on" should be scored and used for computation of the arousal index.

An increase in chin EMG is required only for an arousal occurring during REM sleep. REMs are not seen in this epoch, and REM cannot be scored. This means that answer A is incorrect. An arousal may be scored during an epoch of wake, as long as 10 seconds of sleep precede the arousal. The portion of the recording without alpha rhythm exceeds the 10-second requirement, and therefore answer B is incorrect. The increase in EEG frequency at the end of the epoch in this example meets the 3-second requirement, and therefore answer C is incorrect.[2]

15. **Answer B. Paroxysmal spike and wave activity.**

The activity in the EEG occurs abruptly; the patient is awake at the start of the epoch with alpha rhythm activity in the occipital channel. The pattern of the electrical activity is generalized (appearing in all of the EEG channels at the same time), and the waveform is a spike and wave discharge. The frequency starts at three cycles per second and slows

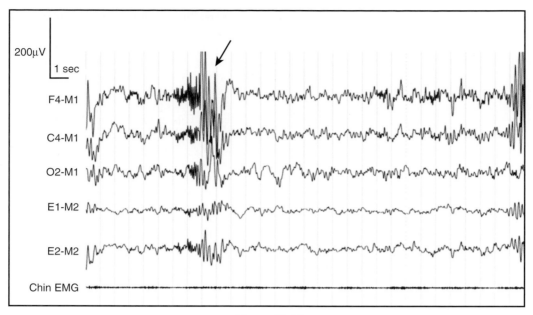

• **Figure 43.23**

progressively through the event. This is typically associated with primary generalized epilepsy.

Posterior slow waves of youth (Answer A) and frontal rhythmic delta activity (Answer B) occur during slow wave sleep and are not likely to arise during an epoch of wake. In contrast, HH (Answer D) is a distinctive EEG pattern of drowsiness and stage N1, characterized by paroxysmal runs or bursts of diffuse bisynchronous 75–350 µV, 3–4.5 Hz waves often maximal over the central, frontal, or frontocentral derivations. HH often disappears with deeper stages of nonrapid eye movement (NREM) sleep. An example is shown at the arrow in Fig. 43.23.[1,4]

16. **Answer A. The number of levels of voltage range that can be represented.**
The vertical resolution of a signal is dependent on the number of binary bits used to represent the digital values. The amplitude of the signal is assigned to a level that is defined by the number of bits available. A 12-bit system allow for identification of 4096 levels for the signal. Fewer bits result in voltage changes that are not detected.

The digital resolution does not affect frequency analysis (Answer B)—this is determined by the sampling frequency. It does not affect display brightness (Answer C) or the effects of digital filters (Answer D).[5]

17. **Answer C. The measure of carbon dioxide is elevated.**
According to the AASM Manual, scoring of hypoventilation is based entirely on increases of arterial PCO_2 or a surrogate. An increase to a value greater than 55 mmHg for 10 minutes or more or an increase of 10 mmHg greater than an awake supine value to a value exceeding 50 mmHg for 10 minutes or more qualifies for scoring of hypoventilation. Surrogate measures of PCO_2 include arterial PCO_2, transcutaneous PCO_2 ($TcCO_2$), or end-tidal PCO_2 ($ETCO_2$). The transcutaneous method is usually considered more accurate than the end-tidal method.

Changes in flow (Answer A) and effort (Answer B) channels are not part of the definition of hypoventilation. Oxygen saturation may be low in patients with hypoventilation but is not a diagnostic feature (Answer D).[2]

18. **Answer C. The denominator for the REI is monitoring time, which is always longer than sleep time.**
The REI is defined by the AASM Scoring Manual as the number of respiratory events times 60 divided by the monitoring time, whereas the definition of AHI is the number of apneas and hypopneas times 60 divided by sleep time. Monitoring time includes time spent awake after the start of the study (time to sleep onset, nocturnal awakenings and early morning awakening) and is therefore longer than the measure of sleep time used for AHI. Because the denominator is larger for the REI, the estimate of apnea severity will always be smaller.

Scoring of respiratory events during HSAT is essentially the same as for PSG. Therefore a 4% or 3% requirement would apply for both HSAT and in-laboratory studies (Answer A is incorrect). At least one measure of flow is required for HSAT; therefore answer B is incorrect. Scoring of respiratory events during HSAT does not include the option of scoring RERAs; therefore answer D is incorrect.[2]

19. **Answer B. A valid substitute for the flow signal.**
HSAT requires at least one measure of flow. Measures of heart rate and oxygen saturation must also be included. Ideally both an oronasal thermal sensor and a nasal pressure transducer should be used. However, alternative sensors that include tidal volume sensors such as respiratory inductance plethysmography sum (RIPsum) may be used. The signal is derived by adding the chest and abdominal effort signals and does not include flow, snoring, or ECG signals (Answers A and D are incorrect). The sum channel does not provide an adequate measure of snoring (snoring monitoring requires an acoustic sensor, piezoelectric sensor, or nasal pressure transducer, and therefore Answer C is incorrect).[2]

20. **Answer D. Ability to display raw data for review.**
Standards require that the PAT device must have the ability to display raw data for review, manual scoring, or editing of automated scoring.

Auto-adjusting PAP devices may be used for treatment of patients diagnosed with HSAT, but are not a substitute for the diagnostic test (Answer A). Sleep wake and REM sleep times may be estimated from an actigraphy signal. Therefore EEG signals are not a required part of HSAT using PAT (Answer B). The PAT signal may be used as a surrogate for airflow and effort, eliminating the need for the thermal flow channel (Answer C).[2]

21. **Answer A. Excitatory and inhibitory postsynaptic potentials.**

Excitatory and inhibitory postsynaptic potentials last much longer and induce more extensive voltage changes in extracellular space and are the most likely cause of the EEG.

EEG activity does not appear to be caused by individual or summed action potentials (Answer B), which are too short and have a limited distribution, or by changes in the axon as the action potential travels and is refreshed at the nodes of Ranvier (Answer C). Activity within the cell, such as neurotransmitter sequestration, is also unlikely to cause a recordable change in the scalp potential (Answer D).[6]

22. **Answer A. Reassure the patient and parent that everything is OK.**

The record fragment shows an apparent sleep terror. The sleep study of patients with NREM parasomnia disorders such as sleep terrors often shows abrupt arousals from stage N3 sleep. The sleep study may be requested to rule out a seizure disorder and typically includes extra EEG channels.

The ECG tracing is stable, and there is no indication of respiratory distress, making answer A incorrect. The record fragment does not contain abnormal EEG activity suggestive of a seizure, and therefore use of an anticonvulsant (Answer B) is not indicated. Documentation of the level of consciousness during the event and the recall for the event afterward may be helpful for evaluation of the event. After the event the recording shows typical wakefulness, and there does not appear to be a need to replace electrodes or check impedances (Answer D).[7]

23. **Answer D. No event.**

LM events should not be scored when associated with apnea. The rule is stated in note 4: "An LM should not be scored if it occurs during a period from 0.5 seconds preceding an apnea, hypopnea, RERA or sleep-disordered breathing event to 0.5 seconds following the event." Arousals may be associated with an LM if they occur together or if the interval between the end of one event is less than 0.5 seconds from the start of the other event.

This means that the LM, even though it meets amplitude and duration criteria, should not be scored. Even if the event is part of a series, it occurs during an apnea and should not be scored either without (Answer A) or with (Answer B) an arousal. It should also not be scored if it is an isolated event (Answer C).[2]

24. **Answer A. A hypopnea only if accompanied by an oxygen desaturation or arousal.**

The event in the box is a reduction of the flow signal by more than 30% but less than 90%. It may meet criteria for scoring as hypopnea if (rule 1A) "There is a ≥3% oxygen desaturation from pre-event baseline or the event is associated with an arousal" or (rule 1B) "There is a ≥4% oxygen desaturation from pre-event baseline."

The event in the box does not meet criteria for scoring as an apnea (Answer B), which requires a reduction in the amplitude of the signal by 90% or more for 10 seconds or

more. The CPAP flow signal may be used "During positive airway pressure (PAP) titration … to identify apneas or hypopneas." This means that answer C is incorrect. Identification of hypoventilation during sleep requires monitoring of carbon dioxide levels and cannot rely on a flow signal alone (Answer D).[2]

25. **Answer C. Epoch C.**

Epoch D is "definite" stage R because it contains a REM, has low chin EMG, and the EEG is low-amplitude, mixed frequency activity without K complexes or sleep spindles. Segments of the recording "preceding and contiguous with an epoch of definite stage R" are scored as stage R when:

a. The EEG shows low-amplitude, mixed frequency activity without K complexes or sleep spindles
b. The chin EMG tone is low (at the stage R level)
c. There is no intervening arousal
d. Slow eye movements following an arousal or stage W are absent

Epoch A must be scored as stage N2 because it contains a spindle in the first half of the epoch and elevated chin EMG (Answer A). Because the chin EMG continues to be elevated in epoch B, it cannot be scored as stage R (Answer B is incorrect; see rule b, described previously). Epoch C is scored as REM because it is preceding and contiguous with an epoch of definite REM sleep (making epoch D the second epoch of REM sleep, and therefore answer D is incorrect).[2]

26. **Answer A. REM sleep.**

According to the AASM Scoring Manual, recordings from infants between 37 and 48 weeks conceptional age (age from the time of conception) should be scored using infant scoring rules. These recommend a score of REM sleep in epochs with irregular respiration and REMs with two of the following three features: Low chin EMG, mouthing, sucking, twitches or brief head movement, and EEG exhibits a continuous pattern without sleep spindles.

There are no LMs present in this record fragment, and therefore answer B is incorrect. NREM (N) sleep is scored with regular respiration and no eye movements (Answer C is incorrect). Transitional sleep is scored when at least one feature of sleep stages is discordant (Answer D is incorrect).[2]

27. **Answer C. No, it does not meet the amplitude requirements for a slow wave.**

Although there was discussion on this issue, the amplitude requirements for a slow wave are the same for all age groups. The requirement is "Waves of frequency from 0.5 Hz-to-2 Hz and peak-to-peak amplitude >75 μV, measured over the frontal regions referenced to the contralateral ear or mastoid (F_4-M_1, F_3-M_2)." The peak-to-peak amplitude of 65 μV does not meet the slow wave amplitude criterion.

Because the amplitude is inadequate, the waveform should not be scored as a slow wave, and answer A is incorrect. The duration of 0.75 msec is a frequency of 1.33 Hz, which is in the range for a slow wave (Answer B is incorrect). The AASM Scoring Manual states: "K complexes would be considered slow waves if they meet the definition of slow wave activity." This means that answer D is incorrect.[2]

28. **Answer D. 40 minutes.**

According to the AASM Practice Parameter, "The MWT 40 minute protocol is recommended when the sleep clinician requires objective data to assess an individual's ability to remain awake." Shorter protocols suffer from a "ceiling effect" in which many of the subjects are able to stay awake for the entire nap.

This impairs the ability of the clinician to separate normal and abnormal findings on this test.

Durations of 8 and 12 minutes are never used for the MWT (Answers A and B are incorrect). The Practice Parameter does not recommend a 20-minute nap opportunity (Answer C) in the standard MWT protocol. The MWT is used as an objective assessment of patients unable to remain awake.[8]

29. **Answer B. Wake.**
The AASM Scoring Manual states: "If alpha rhythm is present for part of the epoch (even <15 seconds duration), score as stage W." In the absence of alpha rhythm, the epoch is scored as W if an epoch of W either precedes or follows the epoch. If neither of these conditions applies, "score the epoch as the same stage as the epoch that follows it."

Transitional or indeterminate sleep (Answer A) is scored in infants but not in adults. The epoch cannot be scored as stage N2 (Answer C), due to the presence of alpha rhythm. Movement time (Answer D) was scored in older scoring manual schemes but is not used in the current AASM Scoring Manual.[2]

30. **Answer C. Wide or narrow complex.**
The AASM Scoring Manual Task Force noted that sinus tachycardia is defined as a rate of greater than 100 beats per minute, and "By standard convention, narrow-complex and wide-complex tachycardias can be differentiated by a 120 msec QRS duration."

The Task Force noted limitations of scoring using a single lead. "A further potential shortcoming of the single ECG channel relates to the widened QRS complex. There are limited data to suggest that limb leads without an accompanying precordial lead, such as V1, pose limitations for differentiating ventricular from supraventricular origin in evaluating wide complex tachycardias." This means answer A is incorrect. The identification of tachycardia requires a rate of at least 100 beats per minute and is not further subdivided into slow or fast rates (Answer B). Limitations of the single channel recording also included an inability to accurately identify the source of ST segment fluctuations (Answer D is incorrect).[9]

Suggested Reading

American Association of Sleep Technologists. *A Technologist's Guide to Performing Sleep Studies*. 2nd ed. Darien, IL: American Association of Sleep Technologists; 2014.

Berry RB, Brooks R, Gamaldo CE, et al. *The AASM Manual for the Scoring of Sleep and Associated Events: Rules, Terminology and Technical Specifications, Version 2.2*. Darien, IL: American Academy of Sleep Medicine; 2015. www.aasmnet.org.

Littner MR, Kushida C, Wise M, et al. Standards of Practice Committee of the American Academy of Sleep Medicine. Practice parameters for clinical use of the multiple sleep latency test and the maintenance of wakefulness test. *Sleep*. 2005;28(1):113–121.

Rosenberg R. *A Technologist's Introduction to Sleep Disorders*. 2nd ed. Darien, IL: American Academy of Sleep Medicine; 2015.

44

Sleep Stage Scoring

LAURA A. LINLEY, RITA BROOKS, RICHARD S. ROSENBERG*

Channel Key

Channel key for figures used in this chapter are as follows: L outer canthus (LOC): E1- M2, R outer canthus (ROC): E2 - M2, Chin EMG; Frontal EEG: F4-M1 F3-M2, Central EEG: C4-M1 C3-M2, Occipital EEG: O2-M1 O1-M2

Questions

Waveform Recognition

1. What is the waveform in the gray box (Fig. 44.1)?
   A. Vertex sharp wave
   B. Sleep spindle
   C. Alpha rhythm
   D. K complex
2. What is the waveform in the gray box (Fig. 44.2)?
   A. K complex
   B. Vertex sharp wave
   C. Sleep spindle
   D. Spike and wave discharge
3. What is the waveform in the gray box (Fig. 44.3)?
   A. Alpha rhythm
   B. Mu rhythm
   C. Sawtooth waves
   D. Sleep spindle
4. What is the waveform in the gray box (Fig. 44.4)?
   A. Sleep spindle
   B. Alpha rhythm
   C. Slow wave activity
   D. Sawtooth waves

5. What is the frequency of the waveform in Fig. 44.5?
   A. 6 Hz
   B. 3 Hz
   C. 1.5 Hz
   D. 0.5 Hz
6. What is the frequency of the waveform in Fig. 44.6?
   A. 3 Hz
   B. 9 Hz
   C. 10 Hz
   D. 13 Hz
7. What is the waveform in the gray box (Fig. 44.7)?
   A. Sleep spindle
   B. Vertex sharp wave
   C. Low amplitude, mixed frequency
   D. Sustained alpha rhythm activity
8. What is the waveform in the gray box (Fig. 44.8)?
   A. K complex recorded in eye movement channels
   B. Lateral rectus spike
   C. Blink artifact
   D. Saccadic eye movement such as is seen during reading
9. What is the waveform in the gray box (Fig. 44.9)?
   A. Blink artifact
   B. Slow eye movement
   C. Rapid eye movement (REM)
   D. Reading eye movement
10. What is the waveform in the gray box (Fig. 44.10)?
    A. K complex
    B. Spike and wave discharge
    C. Positive occipital sharp transient (POST)
    D. Vertex sharp wave

Stage Scoring

11. What sleep stage should be scored for the 30-second epoch shown in Fig. 44.11?
    A. W
    B. N1
    C. N2
    D. N3
    E. R
12. What sleep stage should be scored for the 30-second epoch shown in Fig. 44.12?
    A. W
    B. N1
    C. N2
    D. N3
    E. R

---

*For the American Association of Sleep Technologists

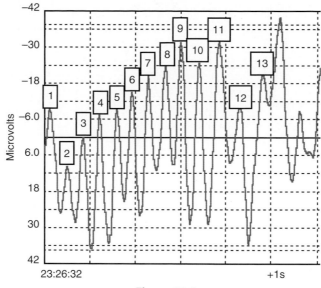

• **Figure 44.1**

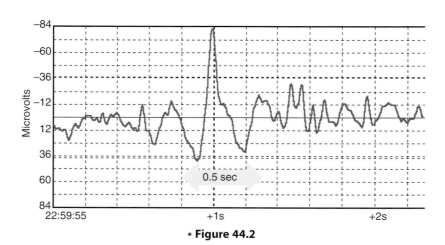

• **Figure 44.2**

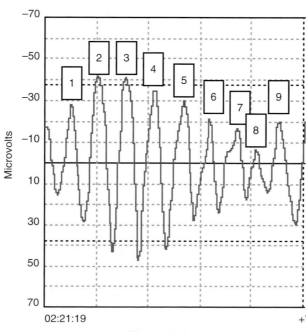

• **Figure 44.3**

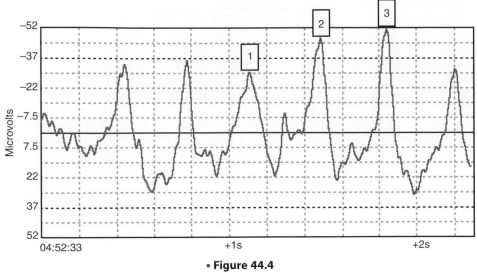

• Figure 44.4

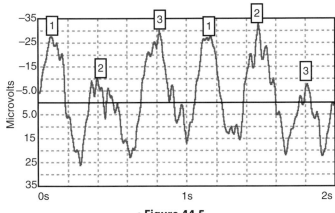

• Figure 44.5

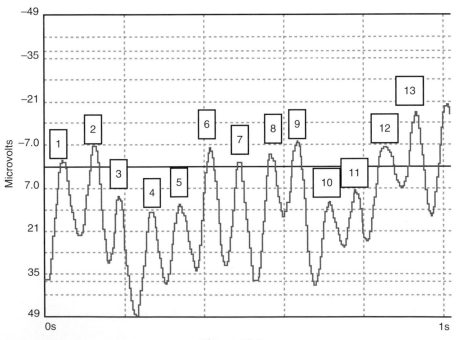

• Figure 44.6

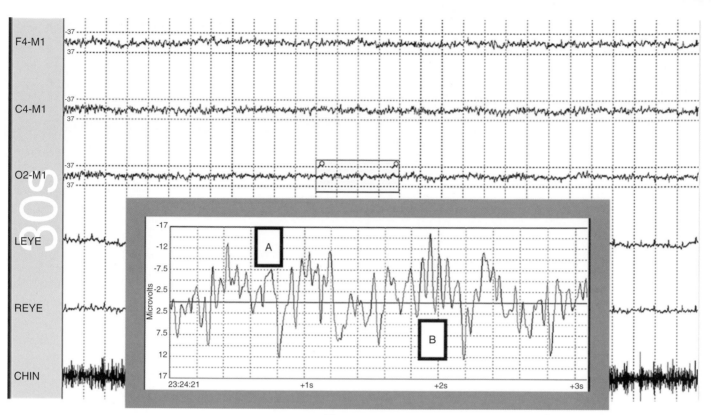

• **Figure 44.7**

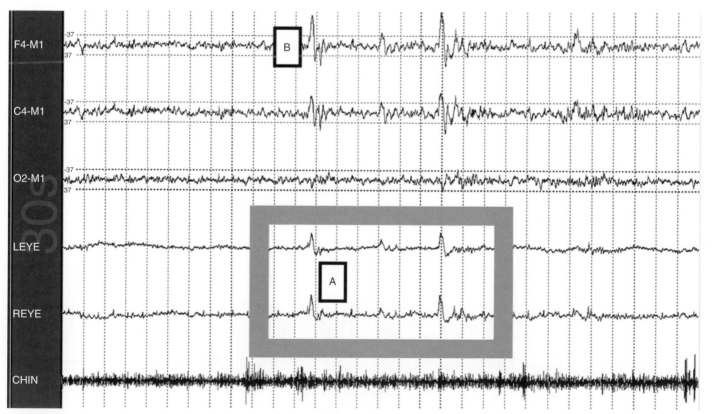

• **Figure 44.8**

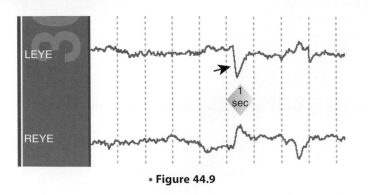

• **Figure 44.9**

13. What sleep stage should be scored for the 30-second epoch shown in Fig. 44.13?
   A. W
   B. N1
   C. N2
   D. N3
   E. R

14. What sleep stage should be scored for the 30-second epoch shown in Fig. 44.14?
   A. W
   B. N1
   C. N2
   D. N3
   E. R

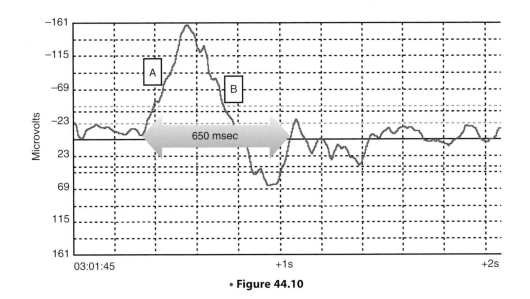

• **Figure 44.10**

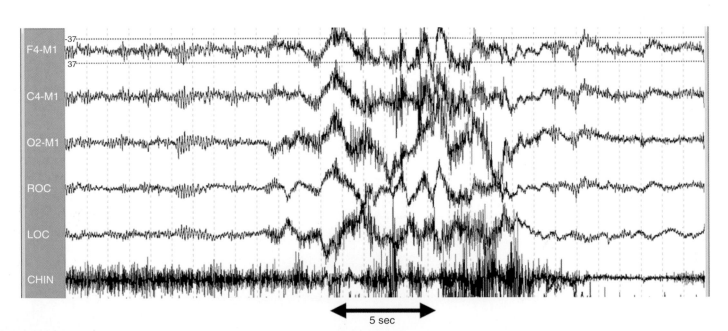

• **Figure 44.11**

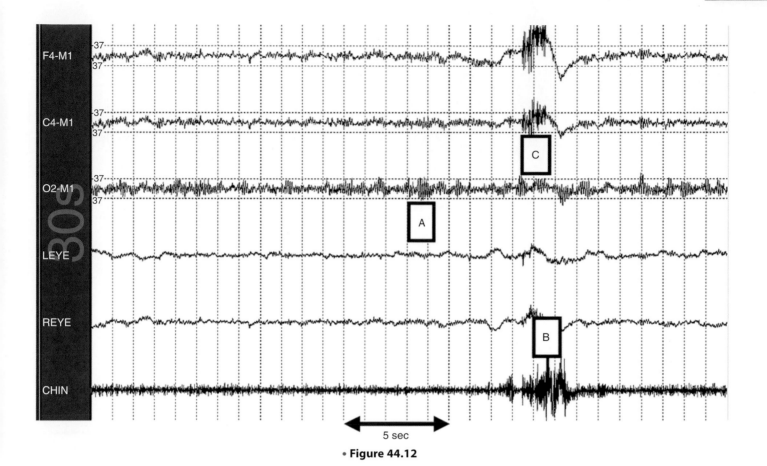

• Figure 44.12

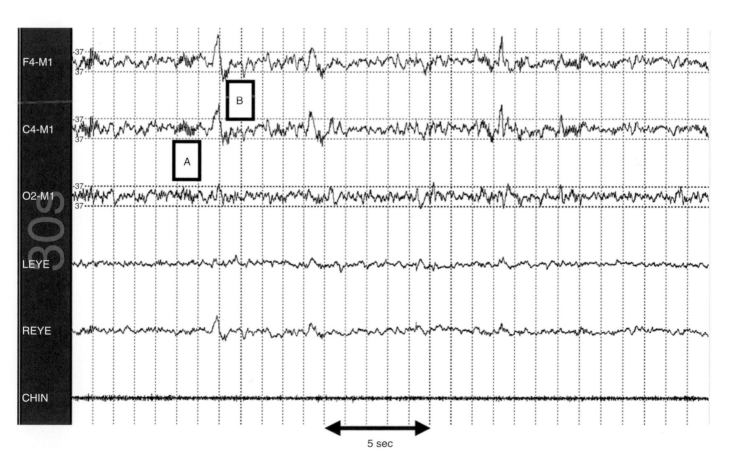

• Figure 44.13

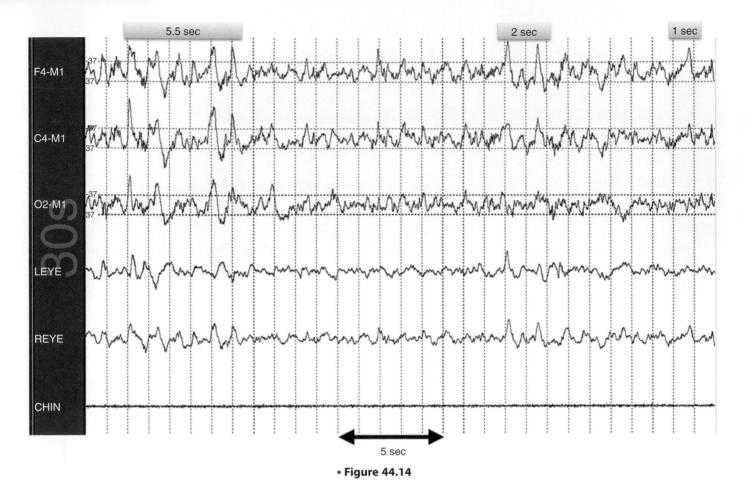

• **Figure 44.14**

15. What sleep stage should be scored for the 30-second epoch shown in Fig. 44.15?
    A. W
    B. N1
    C. N2
    D. N3
    E. R

16. What sleep stage should be scored for the 30-second epoch shown in Fig. 44.16?
    A. W
    B. N1
    C. N2
    D. N3
    E. R

17. What sleep stage should be scored for the 30-second epoch shown in Fig. 44.17?
    A. W
    B. N1
    C. N2
    D. N3
    E. R

18. What sleep stage should be scored for the 30-second epoch shown in Fig. 44.18?
    A. W
    B. N1
    C. N2
    D. N3
    E. R

19. What sleep stage should be scored for the 30-second epoch shown in Fig. 44.19?

    A. W
    B. N1
    C. N2
    D. N3
    E. R

20. What sleep stage should be scored for the 30-second epoch shown in Fig. 44.20?
    A. W
    B. N1
    C. N2
    D. N3
    E. R

Events

21. Is there an arousal in the epoch in Fig. 44.21 at the point marked by arrow A?
    A. Yes
    B. No, because the chin electromyogram (EMG) does not increase in amplitude
    C. No, because it is not preceded by 10 seconds of stable sleep
    D. No, because the electroencephalogram (EEG) frequency does not increase

22. What is the waveform in the gray box (Fig. 44.22)?
    A. K complex with arousal (K arousal)
    B. Spike and wave discharge
    C. K complex with sleep spindle
    D. Bruxism artifact

Text continued on p. 669

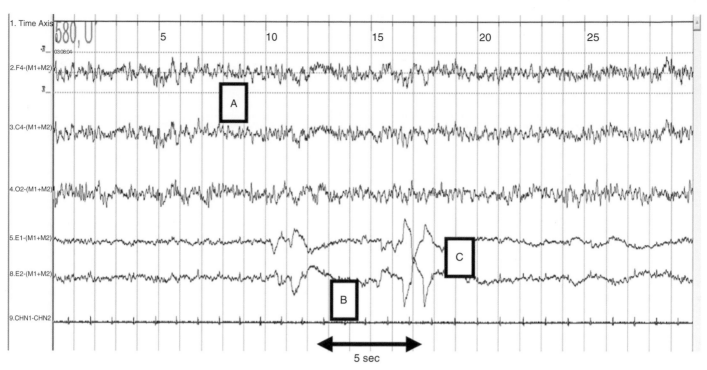

• **Figure 44.15**

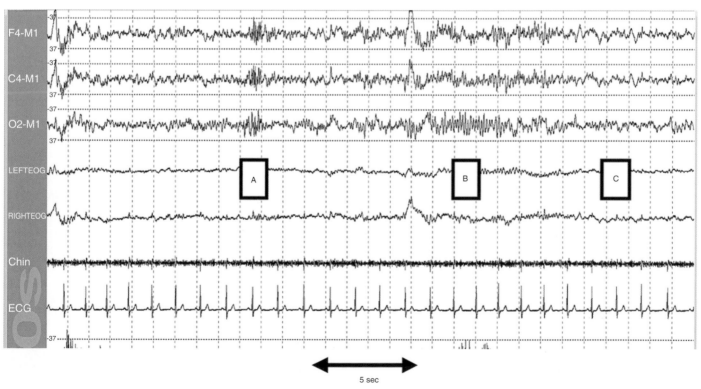

• **Figure 44.16**

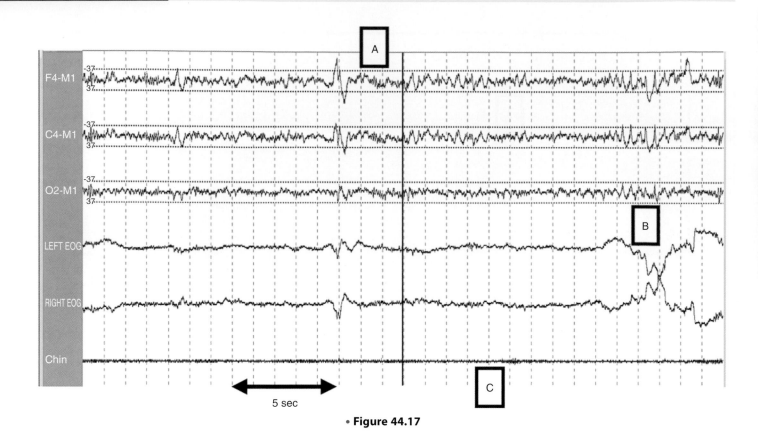

• **Figure 44.17**

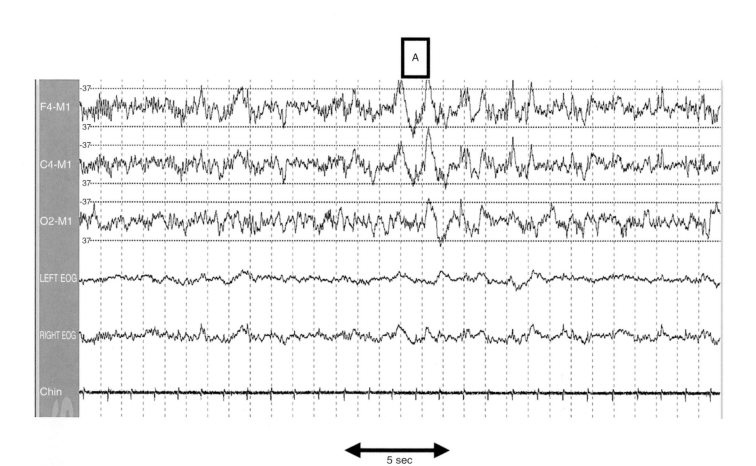

• **Figure 44.18**

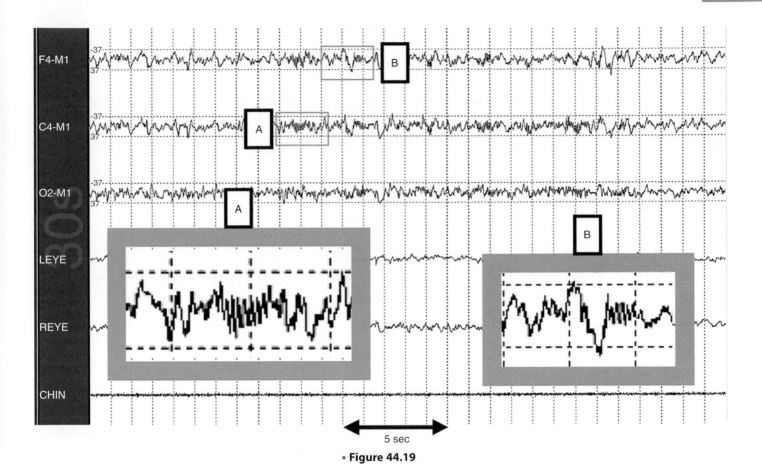

• **Figure 44.19**

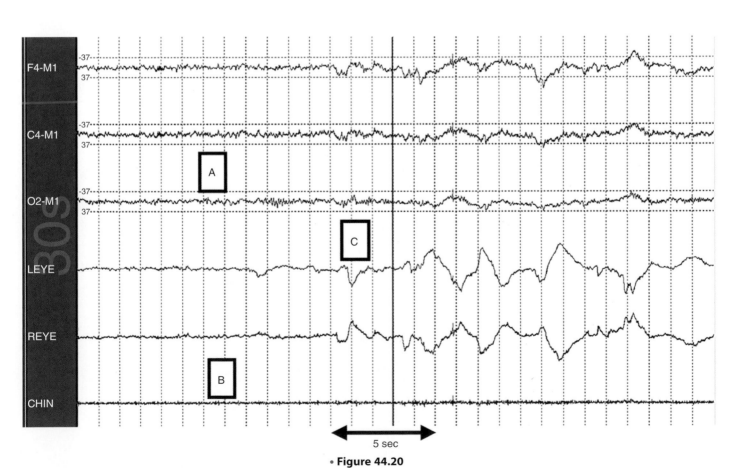

• **Figure 44.20**

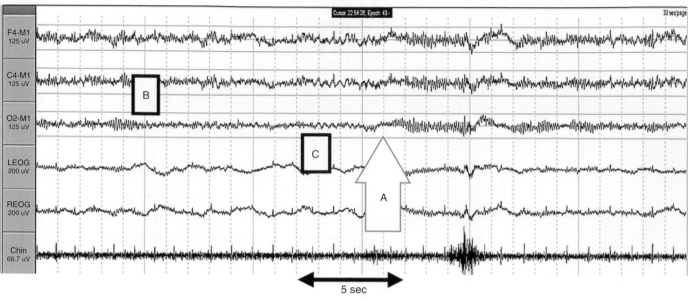

• **Figure 44.21**

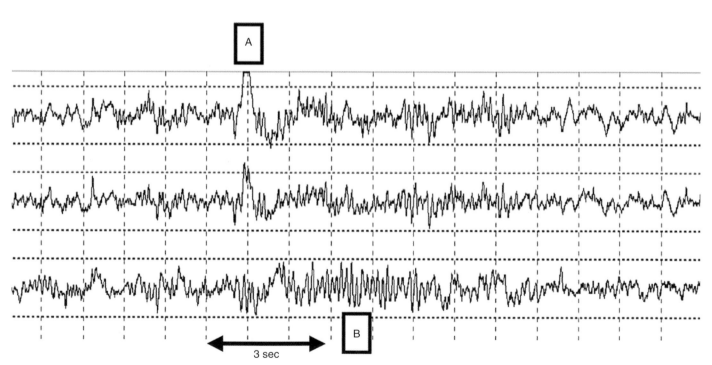

• **Figure 44.22**

23. What occurs during the portion of the recording in the gray box (Fig. 44.23)?
    A. Intrusion of sleep activity during wake (microsleep)
    B. Absence seizure
    C. Temporary artifact from ground electrode falling off
    D. Suppression of alpha rhythm with eye opening

24. At what point does "attenuation of alpha activity" first occur in Fig. 44.24?
    A. Point A
    B. Point B
    C. Point C
    D. Point D

25. The epoch in Fig. 44.25 contains three stages. They are:
    A. W, N1, N2
    B. N1, N2, N3
    C. W, N1, R
    D. N1, N2, R

Multi-Epoch Scoring (Scoring in Context)

26. What sleep stage should be scored for 30-second epoch #3 (shown in the gray box; Fig. 44.26)?
    A. W
    B. N1
    C. N2
    D. N3
    E. R

27. What sleep stage should be scored for 30-second epoch #3 (shown in the gray box; Fig. 44.27)?
    A. W
    B. N1
    C. N2
    D. N3
    E. R

28. What sleep stage should be scored for 30-second epoch #4 (shown in the gray box; Fig. 44.28)?
    A. W
    B. N1
    C. N2
    D. N3
    E. R

29. What sleep stage should be scored for 30-second epoch #3 (shown in the gray box; Fig. 44.29)?
    A. W
    B. N1
    C. N2
    D. N3
    E. R

30. What sleep stage should be scored for 30-second epoch #4 (shown in the gray box; Fig. 44.30)?
    A. W
    B. N1
    C. N2
    D. N3
    E. R

Text continued on p. 675

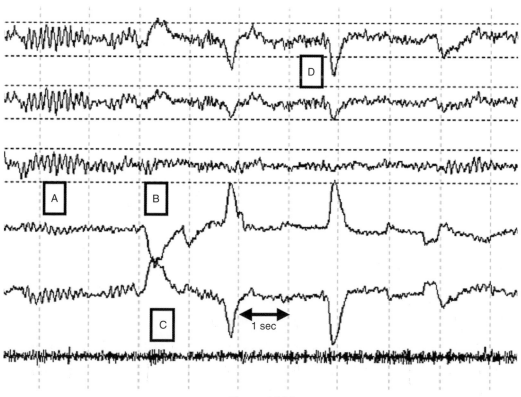

• **Figure 44.23**

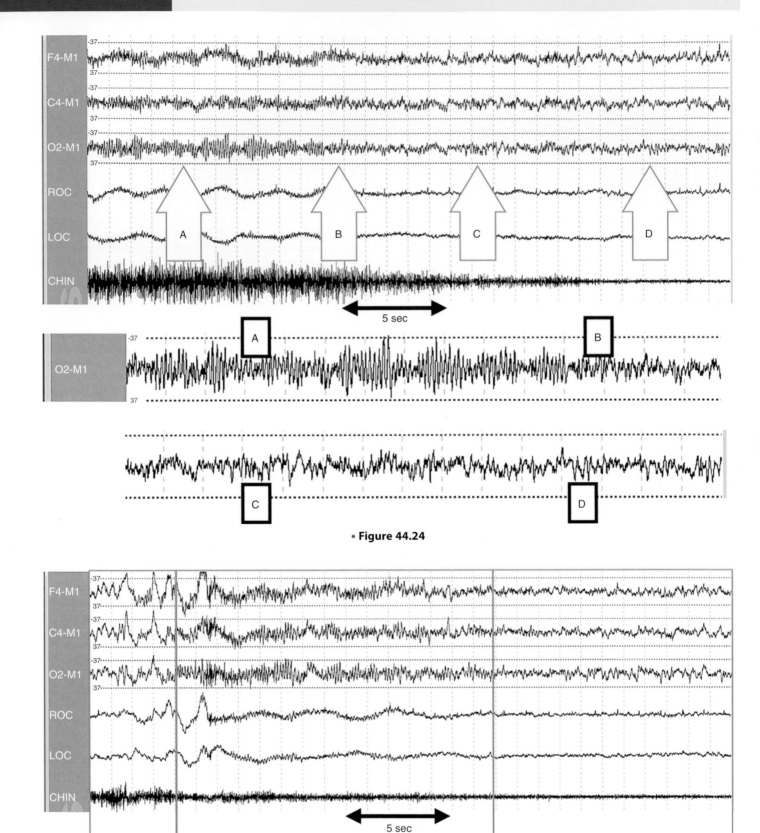

• Figure 44.24

• Figure 44.25

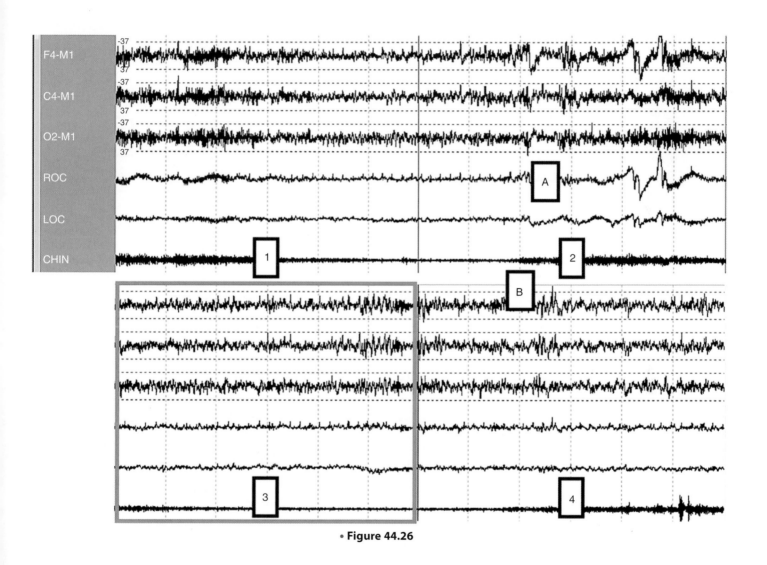

• **Figure 44.26**

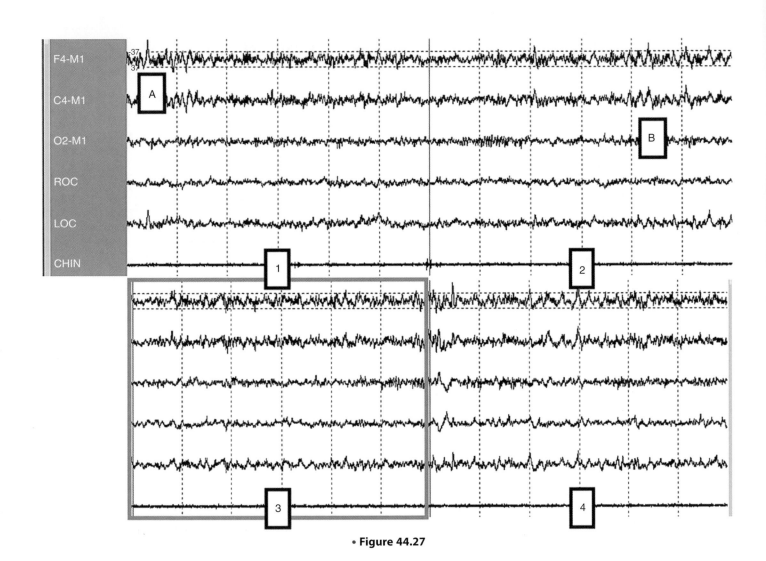

• Figure 44.27

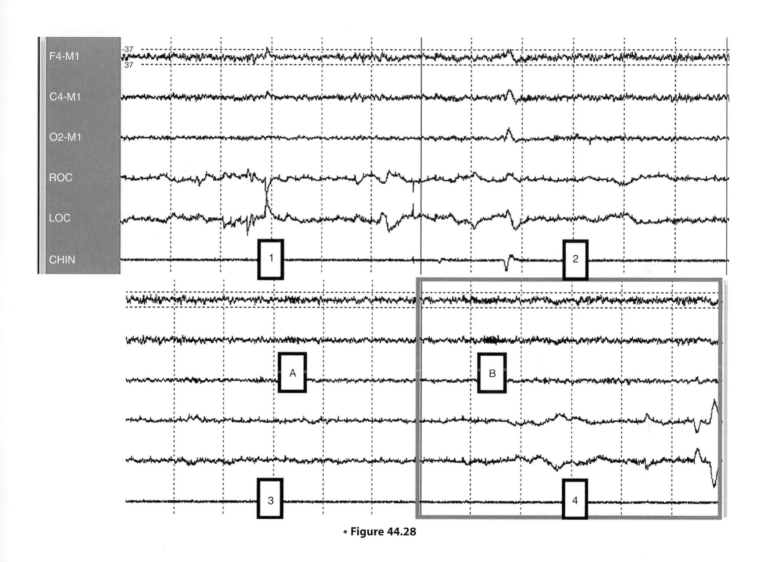

• **Figure 44.28**

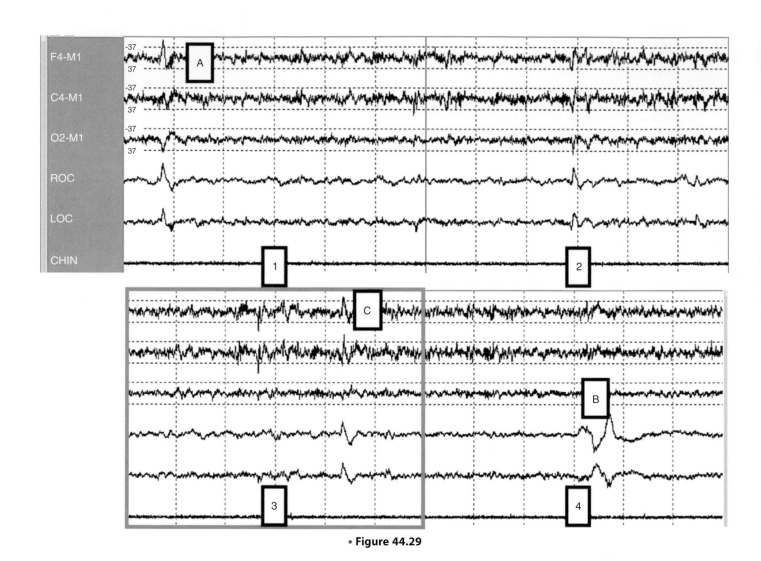

• **Figure 44.29**

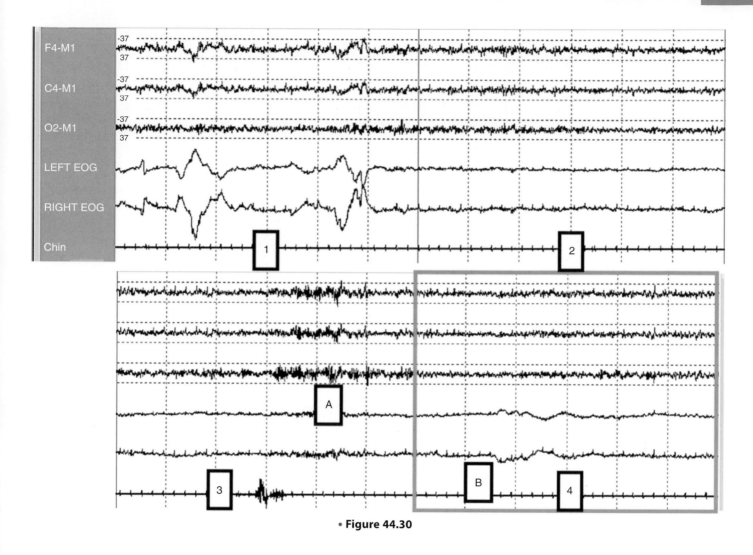

• **Figure 44.30**

Answers

Waveform Recognition

1. **Answer B. Sleep spindle.**

   A count of the peaks of the waveform puts the frequency at 13 Hz (Fig. 44.31). The waveform is maximal in the C4-M1 derivation (central derivation). This meets the criteria for scoring of a sleep spindle: "A train of distinct waves with frequency of 11-to-16 Hz (most commonly 12–14 Hz) with a duration ≥0.5 seconds, usually maximal in amplitude in the central derivations."[1]

   Answer A is incorrect. The waves seen are sinusoidal and occur in a train. In contrast, vertex sharp waves are: "Sharply contoured waves with duration <0.5 seconds (as measured at the base of the wave), maximal over the central region and distinguishable from the background activity. They are most often seen during transition to stage N1 sleep but can occur in either stage N1 or N2 sleep."[1] Answer C is incorrect. The waves seen are maximal over the central region. Alpha rhythm is: "An EEG pattern consisting of trains of sinusoidal 8-to-13 Hz activity recorded over the occipital region with eye closure and attenuating with eye opening."[1] Answer D is incorrect. The waves seen are sinusoidal and occur in a train. A K complex is: "A well-delineated, negative, sharp wave immediately followed by a positive component standing out from the background EEG, with total duration ≥0.5 seconds, usually maximal in amplitude when recorded using frontal derivations."[1]

2. **Answer B. Vertex sharp wave.**

   Vertex sharp waves are defined as "Sharply contoured waves with duration <0.5 seconds (as measured at the base of the wave), maximal over the central region and distinguishable from the background activity. They are most often seen during transition to stage N1 sleep but can occur in either stage N1 or N2 sleep."[1] The waveform in the gray box is sharply contoured with a duration of approximately 300 msec (0.3 sec) and is most evident in the central channel (Fig. 44.32).

   Answer A is incorrect. The vertex sharp wave is distinguished from a K complex by the duration of the waveform. A K complex is defined as "A well-delineated, negative, sharp wave immediately followed by a positive component standing out from the background EEG, with total duration ≥0.5 seconds, usually maximal in amplitude when recorded using frontal derivations."[1] Answer C is incorrect because the waveform does not meet the criteria for scoring of a sleep spindle, defined as "A train of distinct waves with frequency of 11-to-16 Hz (most commonly 12-to-14 Hz) with a duration ≥0.5 seconds, usually maximal in amplitude in the central derivations."[1] It does not occur in a train and the frequency is approximately 3 Hz. Answer D is incorrect. The duration of the waveform

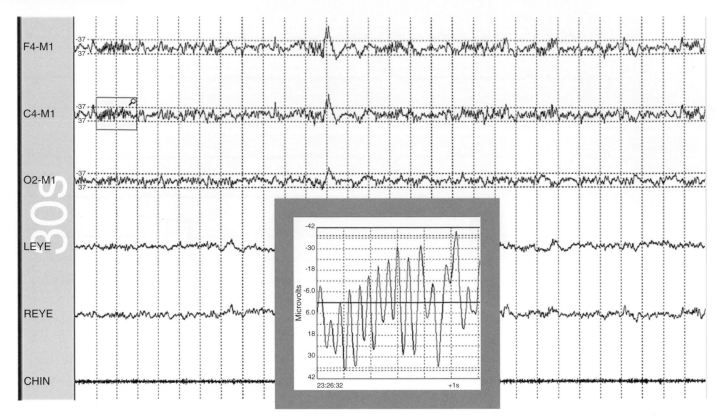

• **Figure 44.31**

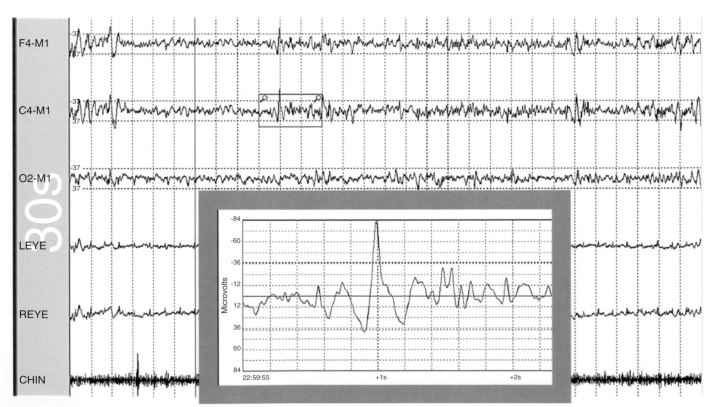

• **Figure 44.32**

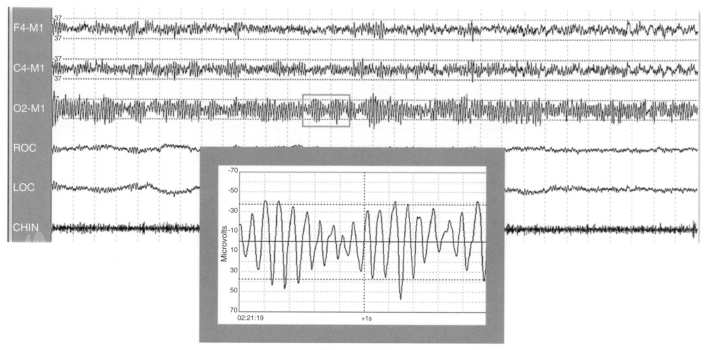

• **Figure 44.33**

is appropriate, but it is not preceded by a spike. Spikes must have a duration of less than 70 msec.[2]

3. **Answer A. Alpha rhythm.**

Alpha rhythm is: "An EEG pattern consisting of trains of sinusoidal 8-to-13 Hz activity recorded over the occipital region with eye closure and attenuating with eye opening."[1] The waveform in the figure has a frequency of 9 Hz and is maximal in the occipital channel, although it is easily seen in all EEG channels (Fig. 44.33).

Answer B is incorrect. Mu rhythm may be confused with alpha rhythm but differs in a number of features. It occurs during wake but is centrally predominant and has an "archiform" or "comb-like" wave shape rather than the sinusoidal shape of alpha rhythm. It is reactive to the movement of the contralateral hand.[2] Answer C is incorrect. Sawtooth waves are an EEG pattern consisting of trains of sharply contoured or triangular, often serrated, 2–6 Hz waves maximal in amplitude over the central head regions and often, but not always, preceding a burst of REMs.[1] Answer D is incorrect. Sleep spindles are defined by the American Academy of Sleep Medicine (AASM) Manual as: "A train of distinct waves with frequency of 11-to-16 Hz (most commonly 12-to-14 Hz) with a duration ≥0.5 seconds, usually maximal in amplitude in the central derivations."[1] This waveform is too slow to be a sleep spindle and is predominant in the occipital channel rather than in the central channel.

4. **Answer D. Sawtooth waves.**

"Sawtooth waves are an EEG pattern consisting of trains of sharply contoured or triangular, often serrated, 2-to-6 Hz waves maximal in amplitude over the central head regions and often, but not always, preceding a burst of rapid eye movements."[1] The waveforms in this figure are sharply contoured and have a frequency of approximately 3 Hz. They are best seen in the central EEG channel (Fig. 44.34).

Answer A is incorrect. Sleep spindles are defined by the AASM Manual as: "A train of distinct waves with frequency

of 11-to-16 Hz (most commonly 12-to-14 Hz) with a duration ≥0.5 seconds, usually maximal in amplitude in the central derivations."[1] This waveform is too slow to be a sleep spindle. Answer B is incorrect. Alpha rhythm is: "An EEG pattern consisting of trains of sinusoidal 8-to-13 Hz activity recorded over the occipital region with eye closure and attenuating with eye opening."[1] The waveform in the figure has a frequency of 3 Hz and is maximal in the central channel. Answer C is incorrect. Slow wave activity consists of waves of frequency 0.5–2 Hz and peak-to-peak amplitude greater than 75 μV, measured over the frontal regions referenced to the contralateral ear or mastoid (F_4-M_1, F_3-M_2).[1]

5. **Answer B. 3 Hz.**

Although there are faster frequencies mixed in, the prominent waveforms have a frequency of 3 Hz. This is counting the number of waveform peaks in the 2-second sample and dividing by 2. There are six peaks, yielding a frequency of 3 Hz (Fig. 44.35).

6. **Answer D. 13 Hz.**

The figure is a 1-second sample of recording. The frequency is determined by counting the number of peaks in the 1-second sample. Thirteen peaks are seen (Fig. 44.36).

7. **Answer C. Low amplitude, mixed frequency.**

Low-amplitude, mixed-frequency (LAMF) EEG is described as "low-amplitude, predominantly 4-to-7 Hz activity" (Fig. 44.37).[1] At A, slower frequencies are seen. Faster frequencies such as alpha rhythm are seen at B. The admixture of faster and slower waveforms is a hallmark of LAMF EEG.

Answer A is incorrect. Sleep spindles are defined by the AASM Manual as: "A train of distinct waves with frequency 11–16 Hz (most commonly 12-to-14 Hz) with a duration ≥0.5 seconds, usually maximal in amplitude in the central derivations."[1] The sample recording does not contain a train of distinct waves. Answer B is incorrect. Vertex sharp waves are: "Sharply contoured waves with duration <0.5 seconds (as measured at the base of the wave), maximal over the central region and distinguishable

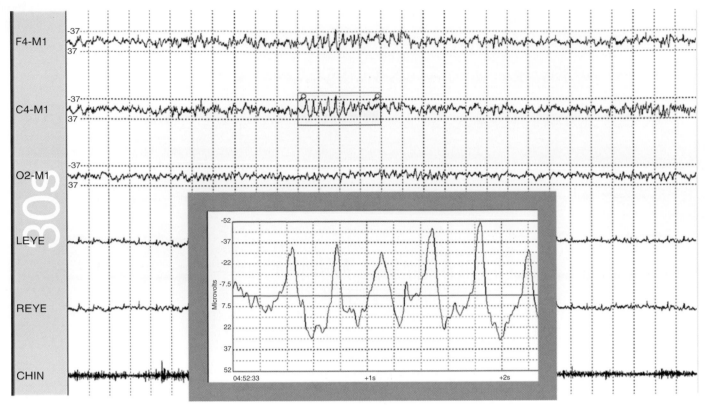

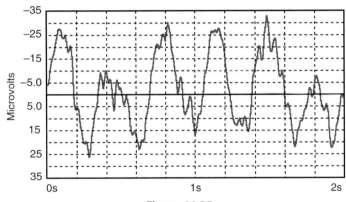

• Figure 44.34

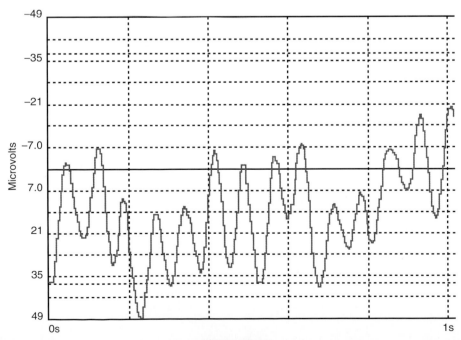

• Figure 44.35

• Figure 44.36

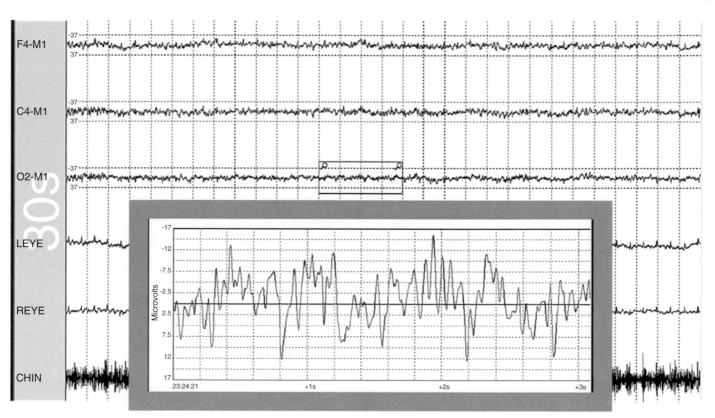

• **Figure 44.37**

from the background activity. They are most often seen during transition to stage N1 sleep but can occur in either stage N1 or N2 sleep."[1] Although some sharply contoured waves are present in the sample, they cannot be distinguished from the background activity. Answer D is incorrect. Alpha rhythm is: "An EEG pattern consisting of trains of sinusoidal 8-to-13 Hz activity recorded over the occipital region with eye closure and attenuating with eye opening."[1] The waveform in the figure has a frequency of 3 Hz and is maximal in the central channel. Some waveforms in this frequency range are seen in the sample, and the sample is taken from the occipital channel. However, the activity is not sustained.

8. **Answer A. K complex recorded in eye movement channels.**

Eye movement electrodes are in close proximity to frontal EEG leads and may record changes caused by K complexes due to volume conduction. The waves shown in the electrooculography (EOG) channels are in phase, that is the left eye channel shows a negative deflection at the same time as the right channel (at A) (Fig. 44.38). This could indicate a vertical eye movement, but as it occurs synchronously with a K complex in the F₄-M₁ channel (at B) it is more likely to be caused by the electrical activity of the brain rather than an eye movement.[2]

Answer B is incorrect. Lateral rectus spikes must have a duration of less than 70 msec.[2] Answer C is incorrect. Blinks occur during waking, and the presence of a K complex and spindle activity in this epoch indicate that the patient is asleep.[2] Answer D is incorrect. Reading eye movements also occur during waking and have a characteristic slow initial out-of-phase deflection as the patient scans across the page, followed by an abrupt opposite phase deflection as the eyes move to the beginning of the line.[2]

9. **Answer C. Rapid eye movement (REM).**

According to the AASM Manual, "Eye movements recorded in the EOG derivations consisting of conjugate, irregular, sharply peaked eye movements with an initial deflection usually lasting <500 msec."[1] The initial deflection in this example (at *arrow*) is brief, lasting approximately 100 msec and therefore meeting the duration requirement for a REM (Fig. 44.39).

Answer A is incorrect. Eye blinks are "Conjugate vertical eye movements at a frequency of 0.5-to-2 Hz present in wakefulness with the eyes open or closed."[1] The eye movements in the example are lateral (because the deflections are out of phase) and the low-voltage, mixed-frequency EEG and decreased chin EMG amplitude suggest that the patient is in REM sleep. Answer B is incorrect. Slow eye movements are "Conjugate, reasonably regular, sinusoidal eye movements with an initial deflection that usually lasts >500 msec. Slow eye movements may be seen during eyes closed wake and stage N1."[1] Answer D is incorrect. Reading eye movements are "Trains of conjugate eye movements consisting of a slow phase followed by a rapid phase in the opposite direction as the individual reads."[1] These eye movements are not part of a train and consist of a rapid initial deflection.

10. **Answer A. K complex.**

A K complex is: "A well-delineated, negative, sharp wave immediately followed by a positive component standing out from the background EEG, with total duration ≥0.5 seconds, usually maximal in amplitude when recorded using frontal derivations" (Fig. 44.40).[1] The waveform shown begins with a negative sharp wave (at A) which is followed by a positive component (at B). The waveform stands out from the LAMF EEG that precedes and follows. The duration of the waveform,

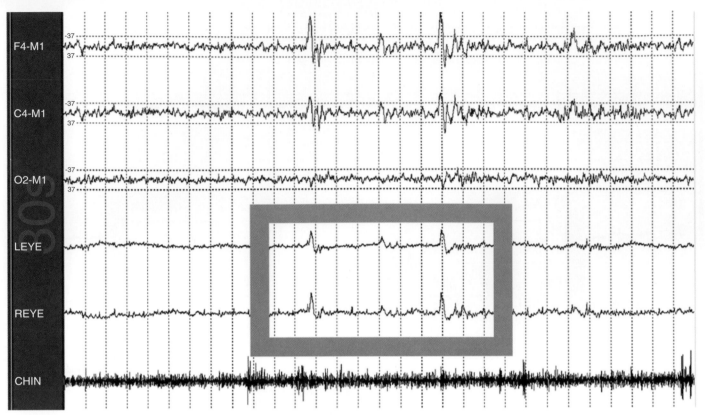

• Figure 44.38

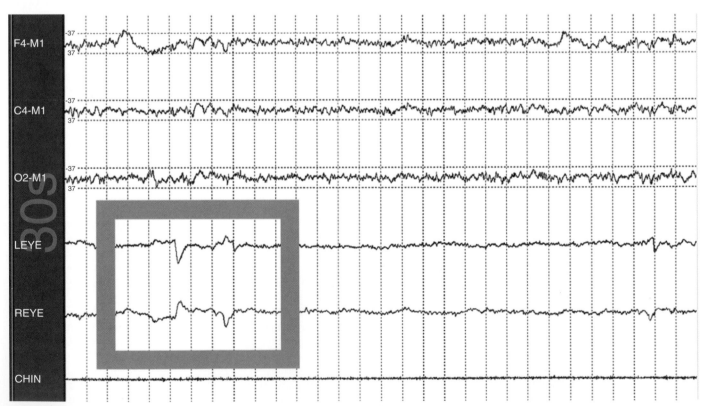

• Figure 44.39

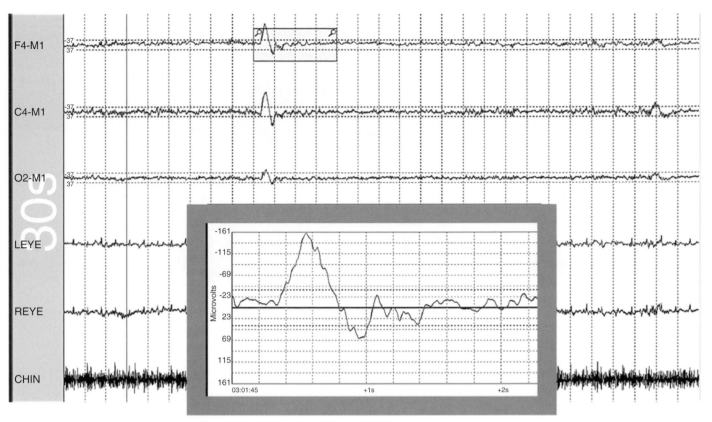

• **Figure 44.40**

measured here using a zero-crossing method, is 650 msec, and therefore exceeds the 500-msec minimum duration.

Answer B is incorrect. The duration of the waveform is appropriate, but it is not preceded by a spike. Spikes must have a duration of less than 70 msec.[2] Answer C is incorrect. POSTs "are sharp waves that can occur normally non-rapid eye movement (NREM) sleep. They are most prominent in the occipital derivations and are positive. Therefore in O_1-M_2 they would be downward deflections." The waveform in this example is highest in the frontal channel and negative in all channels. Answer D is incorrect. Vertex sharp waves are: "Sharply contoured waves with duration <0.5 seconds"[1] The waveform exceeds 0.5 seconds (500 msec).

Stage Scoring

11. **Answer A. W.**
The epoch contains a major body movement (at A) which obscures the EEG for a portion of the epoch (Fig. 44.41). According to the AASM Manual, "If alpha rhythm is present for part of the epoch (even <15 seconds duration), score as stage W."[1] Portions of the recording contain clear alpha rhythm (such as at B), and the epoch is therefore correctly scored as stage W. A single sleep stage should be assigned to each epoch.[1] This means that once a stage score of stage W has been assigned to the epoch, answers B, C, D, and E are incorrect.

12. **Answer A. W.**
The epoch contains alpha rhythm activity (at A and for more than half of the epoch) (Fig. 44.42). According to the AASM Manual, "Score epochs as stage W when more than 50% of the epoch contains … Alpha rhythm (posterior dominant rhythm) over the occipital region."[1] Elevated chin EMG tone (at B) and muscle artifact in the EEG (at C) are also suggestive of an awake patient but are not part of the scoring rules. A single sleep stage should be assigned to each epoch.[1] Once a stage score of W has been assigned to the epoch, answers B, C, D, and E are incorrect.

13. **Answer C. N2.**
The epoch contains multiple sleep spindles (e.g., at A) and K complexes (e.g., at B) (Fig. 44.43). The scoring rules state "Begin scoring stage N2 (in absence of criteria for N3) if EITHER OR BOTH of the following occur during the first half of that epoch or the last half of the previous epoch:
a. One or more K complexes unassociated with arousals
b. One or more sleep spindles

Because the epoch has both spindles and K complexes in the first half of the epoch, the score of N2 is assigned to the epoch. A single sleep stage should be assigned to each epoch."[1] Once a stage score of N2 has been assigned to the epoch, answers A, B, D, and E are incorrect.

14. **Answer D. N3.**
The AASM Manual rule is to "Score stage N3 when ≥20% of an epoch consists of slow wave activity, irrespective of age."[1] Sleep scoring epochs are 30 seconds long. Therefore 20% of the epoch is 6 seconds. Waves must exceed the 75-μV criterion in the F_4-M_1 channel, shown as dotted horizontal lines. Using a zero crossing method for determination of wave duration, the first zero crossing starts the wave, the second zero crossing occurs in the transition from a negative wave to a positive wave, and the third zero crossing ends the wave. Gray bars indicate the portions of the epoch that consist of slow waves (Fig. 44.44). There is a bout of slow wave activity lasting

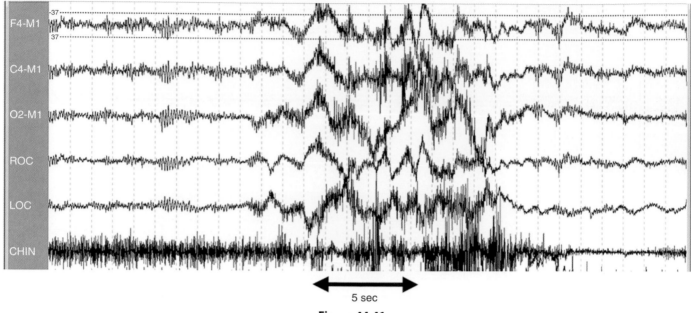

• **Figure 44.41**

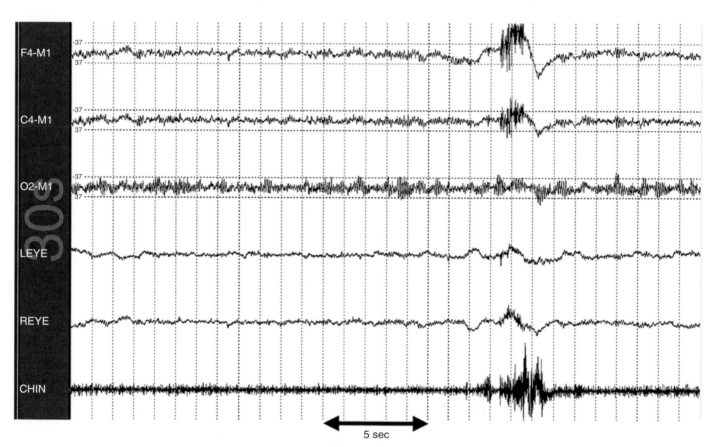

• **Figure 44.42**

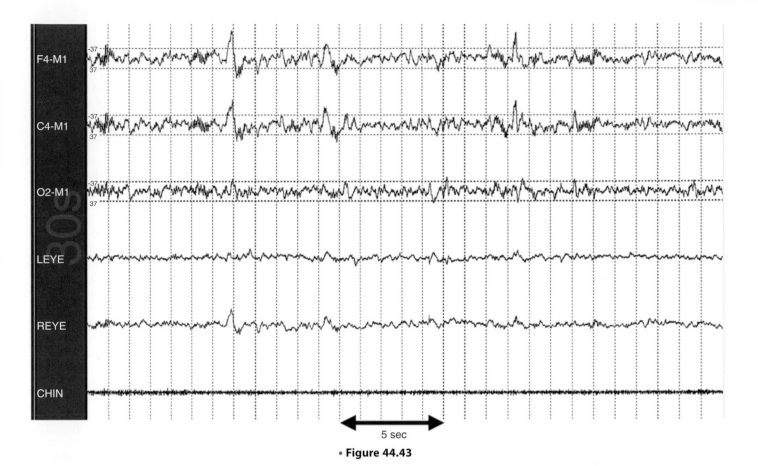

• Figure 44.43

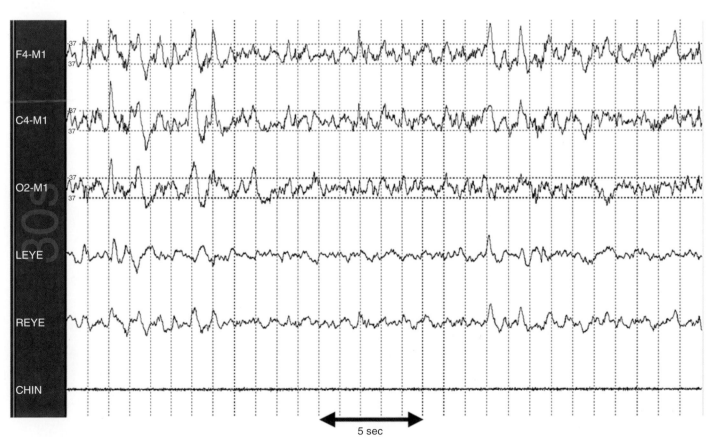

• Figure 44.44

5.5 seconds, two waves that add 2 seconds to the total, and a final slow wave near the end of the second for a total of 8.5 seconds of slow wave activity. Because the epoch consists of more than 6 seconds of slow wave activity, it is scored as N3 sleep. Once a stage score of N3 has been assigned to the epoch, answers A, B, C, and E are incorrect.

15. **Answer E. R.**

This epoch is an example of "definite REM sleep."[1] It meets criterion I2, which states: "Score stage R sleep in epochs with ALL of the following phenomena (definite stage R):"

a. LAMF EEG activity without K complexes or sleep spindles

b. Low chin EMG tone for the majority of the epoch and concurrent with REMs

c. REMs at any position within the epoch[1]

The epoch has LAMF EEG (at A), low chin EMG tone (at B), and a robust burst of REMs (at C) (Fig. 44.45). The epoch is assigned a score of stage R. Once a stage score of R has been assigned to the epoch, answers A, B, C, and D are incorrect.

16. **Answer C. N2.**

This epoch contains three stages (Fig. 44.46). Stage N2 with spindles (at A) and K complexes is seen at the start of the epoch. There is an arousal at B, which includes a transition to alpha rhythm for more than 3 seconds. A brief episode of N1 is seen at the end of the epoch (at C) after the arousal. The Manual states that "When three or more segments of an epoch meet criteria for different stages (stage W, N1, N2, N3, R):

i. Score the epoch as sleep if the majority of the epoch meets criteria for stage N1, N2, N3, or R.

ii. Assign the sleep stage that occurs for the majority of sleep within the epoch."[1]

Since N2 comprises the majority of the epoch, a score of N2 is assigned to the epoch. Once a stage score of N2 has

been assigned to the epoch, answers A, B, D, and E are incorrect.

17. **Answer E. R.**

This challenging epoch begins with N2 sleep, as evidenced by the K complex and spindle (at A) (Fig. 44.47). At the end of the epoch there is a burst of REMs and a run of sawtooth waves (at B). The scoring rules state "If the majority of an epoch contains a segment of the recording meeting criteria for stage R (I.2, I.3, I.5), the epoch is scored as stage R. Stage R rules take precedence over stage N2 rules."[1] The dark vertical line indicates the midpoint of the epoch, with the features of N2 sleep absent just before the line and therefore the majority of the epoch is consistent with REM sleep. The chin EMG remains low throughout the epoch (at C) and does not influence the score. Once a stage score of R has been assigned to the epoch, answers A, B, C, and D are incorrect.

18. **Answer C. N2.**

Several waveforms meeting the frequency criteria for slow wave activity are seen (Fig. 44.48). However, most do not reach the 75-μV peak-to-peak amplitude requirement, and the duration of the waveforms meeting amplitude criteria (at A) do not exceed the 6-second requirement. Slow wave activity consists of "Waves of frequency 0.5 Hz to 2 Hz and peak-to-peak amplitude >75 μV, measured over the frontal regions referenced to the contralateral ear or mastoid (F_4-M_1, F_3-M_2)."[1] Epochs such as this are scored N2 even if they follow an epoch scored as N3. "Epochs following an epoch of stage N3 that do not meet criteria for stage N3 are scored as stage N2 if there is no intervening arousal and the epoch does not meet criteria for stage W or stage R."[1] Once a stage score of N2 has been assigned to the epoch, answers A, B, D, and E are incorrect.

19. **Answer C. N2.**

This is an unambiguous epoch of N2 sleep: "An epoch of stage N2 meeting criteria in rule G.2 is termed definite stage

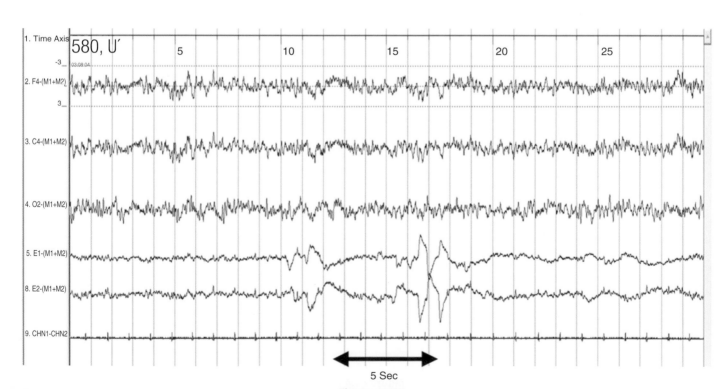

• **Figure 44.45**

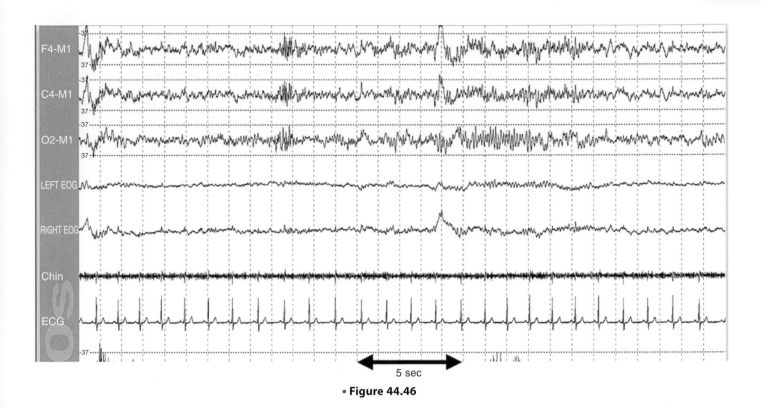

• **Figure 44.46**

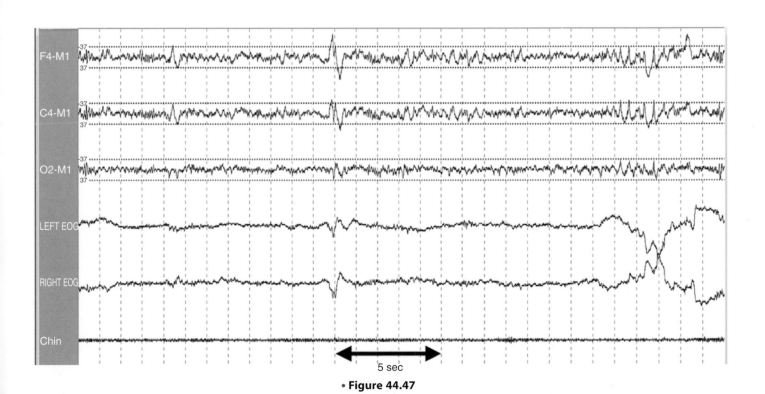

• **Figure 44.47**

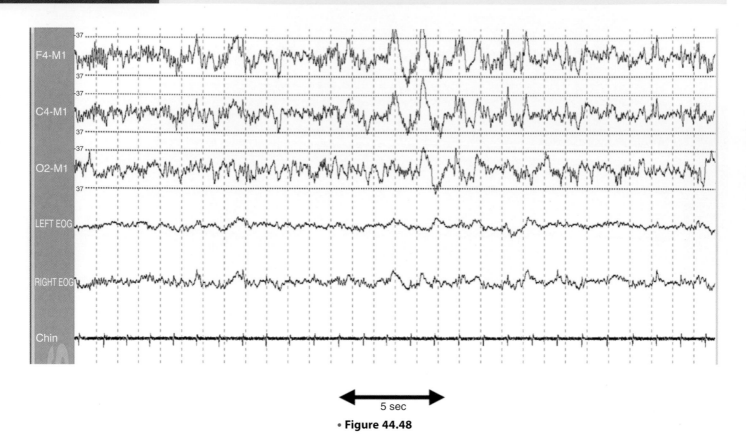

5 sec

• **Figure 44.48**

N2" (Fig. 44.49).[1] A clear sleep spindle is seen at A, and a poorly formed K complex with spindle attached is seen at B. Both occur in the first half of the epoch. Once a stage score of N2 has been assigned to the epoch, answers A, B, D, and E are incorrect.

20. **Answer E. R.**

This epoch is an example of "definite REM sleep."[1] It meets criterion I2, which states: "Score stage R sleep in epochs with ALL of the following phenomena (definite stage R):"
a. LAMF EEG activity without K complexes or sleep spindles
b. Low chin EMG tone for the majority of the epoch and concurrent with REMs
c. REMs at any position within the epoch[1]

The epoch has LAMF EEG (at A), low chin EMG tone (at B), and a robust burst of REMs (at C) (Fig. 44.50). The eye movements begin before the end of the first half of the epoch (solid vertical line). The epoch is assigned a score of stage R. Once a stage score of R has been assigned to the epoch, answers A, B, C, and D are incorrect.

Events

21. **Answer A. Yes.**

The arousal rule requires "Score arousal during sleep stages N1, N2, N3, or R if there is an abrupt shift of EEG frequency including alpha, theta and/or frequencies greater than 16 Hz (but not spindles) that lasts at least 3 seconds, with at least 10 seconds of stable sleep preceding the change. Scoring of arousal during REM requires a concurrent increase in submental EMG lasting at least 1 second."[1] This epoch meets these criteria (Fig. 44.51). An increase in chin EMG is not required because the epoch is not REM sleep (answer B is incorrect). The epoch

begins with stage W, but at B changes to N1 sleep. N1 persists for more than 10 seconds and ends at arrow A. Therefore answer C is incorrect. The EEG does increase in frequency, from the slower waveforms at C to the faster alpha rhythm that begins at arrow A. Therefore answer D is incorrect.

22. **Answer A. K complex with arousal (K arousal).**

A clear K complex is seen (at A) followed by occipitally prominent alpha rhythm activity (at B) (Fig. 44.52). This meets criteria for a K arousal: "For an arousal to be associated with a K complex, the arousal must either be concurrent with the K complex or commence no more than 1 second after termination of the K complex."[1] The K complex is not preceded by a spike and therefore does not have the morphology of a spike and wave discharge (answer B is incorrect). There is some faster frequency activity after the K complex, but it is not in a train and does not have sustained activity in the frequency range of 11–16 Hz to qualify for scoring of a sleep spindle (answer C is incorrect). Bruxism artifact is not seen and would be expected in the frontal and central channels with high frequency and high amplitude (answer D is incorrect).

23. **Answer D. Suppression of alpha rhythm with eye opening.**

At the beginning of the epoch the patient is awake with prominent alpha rhythm activity (at A) (Fig. 44.53). There are prominent REMs at B, and these are associated with suppression of alpha rhythm activity. These are unlikely to be associated with REM sleep because the chin EMG remains high (at C). Blink artifacts are seen at D. Taken together, these suggest that the patient briefly opened his or her eyes and looked around the room. Suppression of alpha activity with eye opening is a feature used to define the rhythm: "An EEG pattern consisting of trains of sinusoidal 8-to-13 Hz activity recorded over the occipital region with eye closure and

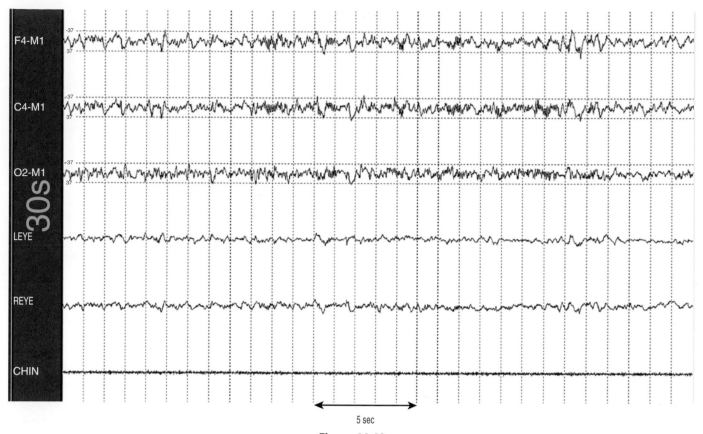

• **Figure 44.49**

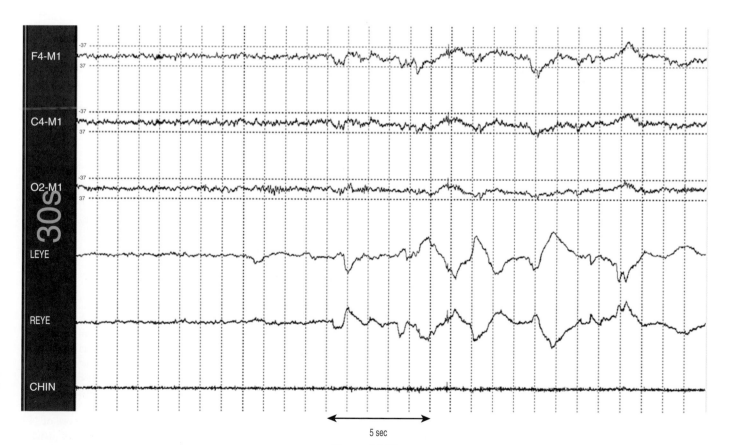

• **Figure 44.50**

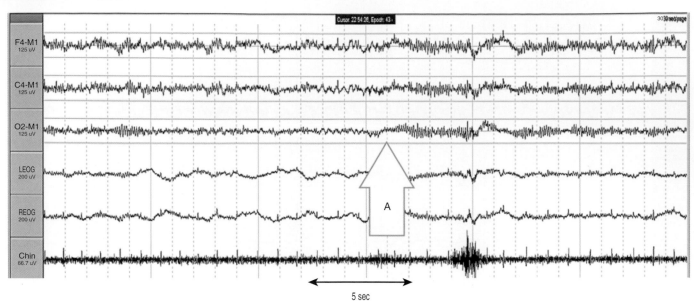

• Figure 44.51

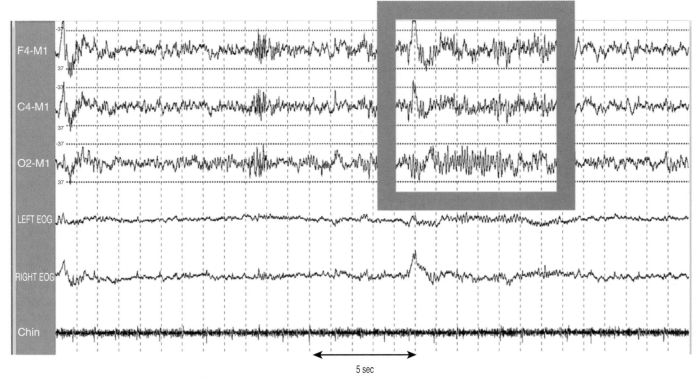

• Figure 44.52

attenuating with eye opening."[1] Sleep waveforms are not seen during the period of alpha suppression, and therefore answer A is incorrect. Similarly, there is no evidence of seizure activity in the EEG, and answer B is incorrect. Temporary artifact from the ground electrode falling off would cause high-amplitude line frequency activity in all channels. This is not seen, and answer C is incorrect.

24. **Answer B. Point B.**
Scoring of stage N1 requires that "alpha rhythm is attenuated and replaced by low-amplitude, mixed-frequency activity for more than 50% of the epoch."[1] This implies that both attenuation

and replacement with LAMF activity occur at the same time, but this is not always the case (Fig. 44.54). The prominent alpha rhythm activity in A is attenuated at B. This means that Answer A is incorrect, and Answer B is correct. Replacement with LAMF activity occurs at C and continues at D, but because the attenuation occurs first at B, Answers C and D are incorrect.

25. **Answer A. W, N1, N2.**
Prominent K complexes and a spindle lead to a score of N2 for the first 4 seconds of the epoch (Fig. 44.55). An arousal with alpha rhythm activity and muscle artifact in the EEG lead to a score of stage W for the middle 15 seconds of the epoch.

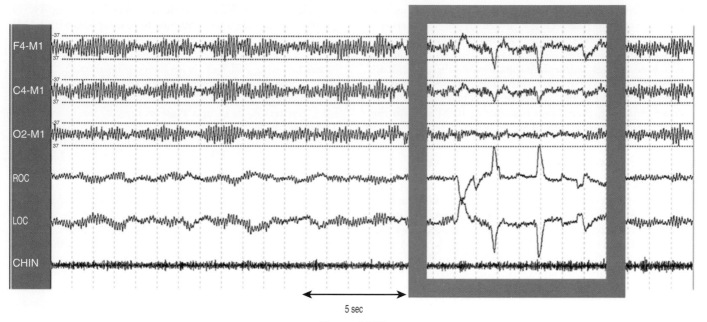

• Figure 44.53

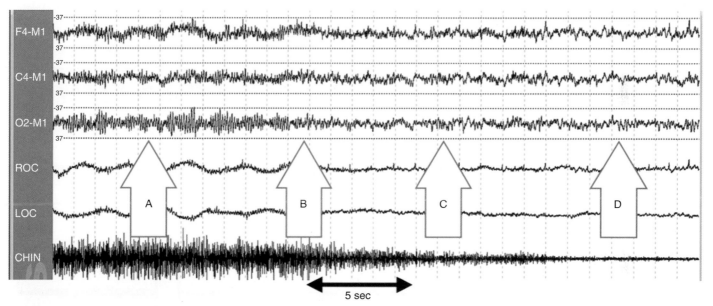

• Figure 44.54

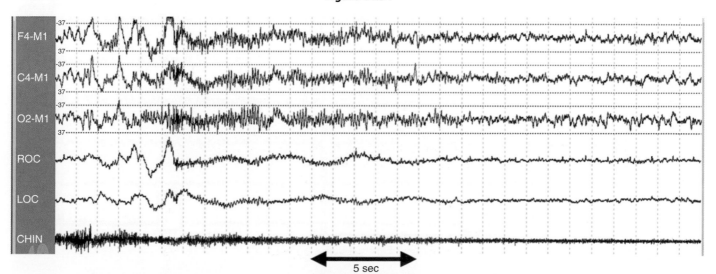

• Figure 44.55

After the arousal N1 is scored until a K complex or spindle is seen. The scoring rule requires "When an arousal interrupts stage N2 sleep, score subsequent segments of the recording as stage N1 if the EEG exhibits LAMF activity without one or more K complexes and/or sleep spindles until there is evidence for another stage of sleep."[1] Answer B is incorrect because stage W is scored in the middle of the epoch and N3 is not scored. Similarly, there is no evidence of REM sleep in this epoch, and answers C and D are incorrect.

Multi-Epoch Scoring (Scoring in Context)

26. **Answer B. N1.**

Epoch 1 appears to be stage W, with decreasing EMG activity in the second half of the epoch (Fig. 44.56). An arousal occurs at A, with an increase of chin EMG. Epoch 3 is sleep onset with LAMF EEG and reduced chin EMG. According to the Manual, "epochs with an EEG showing LAMF EEG activity are scored as stage N1 until there is evidence for another sleep stage (usually stage W, stage N2 or stage R)."[1] K complexes are not apparent until epoch 4 (at B). Once a stage score of N1 has been assigned to the epoch, answers A, C, D, and E are incorrect.

27. **Answer C. N2.**

Epochs 1 and 2 contain K complexes and spindles and are scored as N2 sleep (e.g., at A and B). Even in the absence of

these waveforms N2 sleep continues to be scored (Fig. 44.57). The Manual rule is to "Continue to score epochs with LAMF EEG activity without K complexes or sleep spindles as stage N2 if they are preceded by epochs containing EITHER of the following and there is no intervening arousal:

a. K complexes unassociated with arousals
b. Sleep spindles"[1]

Answers A, B, D, and E are incorrect.

28. **Answer E. R.**

Epochs 1 and 2 are unambiguous REM sleep due to the presence of REMs, LAMF EEG, and reduced chin EMG (Fig. 44.58). A sleep spindle appears in the second half of epoch 3 at A, and another sleep spindle occurs at B. According to the scoring manual, epochs such as these are scored based on "segments" of the recording. This segment of the recording between A and B is scored as N2 sleep, due to the presence of spindles and the absence of REMs, but the remainder of epoch 4 is scored as stage R, and epoch 4 is assigned a score of stage R because REM occupies the greatest portion of the recording. The rule is: "Score segments of the record with low chin EMG activity and a mixture of REMs and sleep spindles and/or K complexes as follows:

a. Segments between two K complexes, two sleep spindles, or a K complex and sleep spindle without intervening REMs are considered to be stage N2.

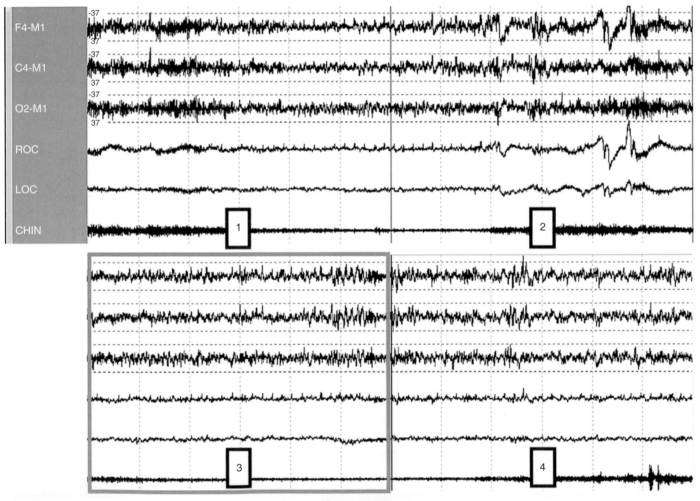

• **Figure 44.56**

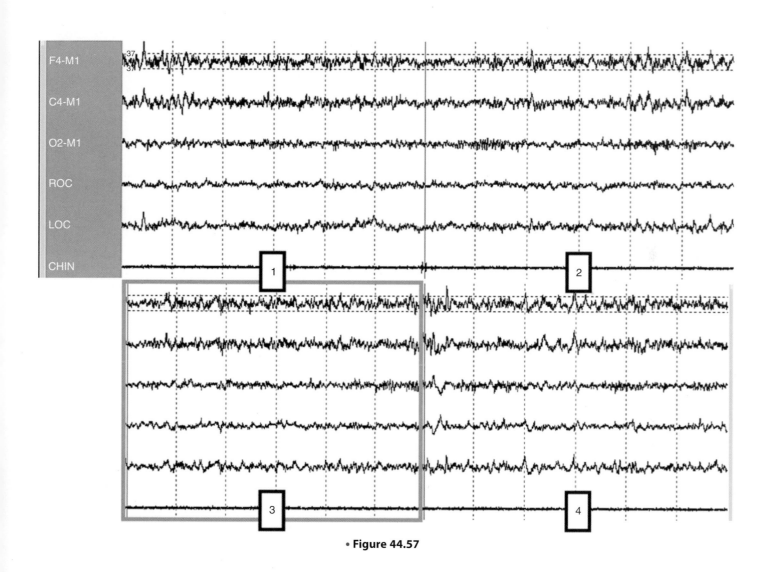

• Figure 44.57

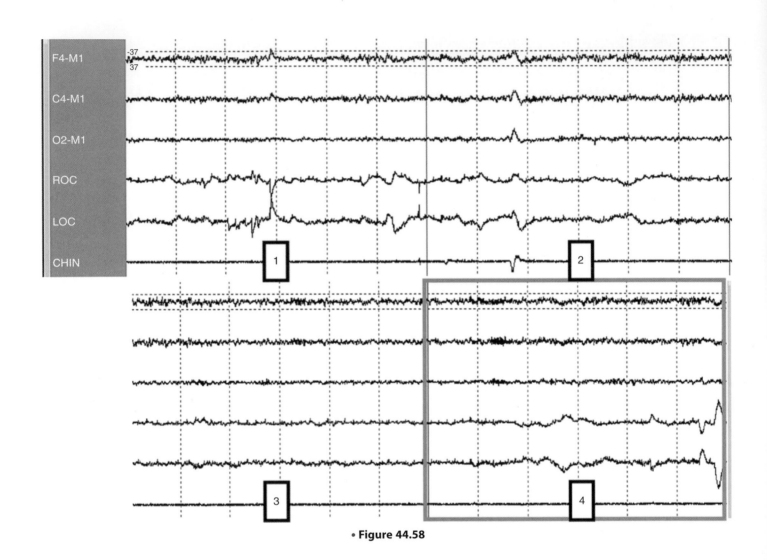

• **Figure 44.58**

b. Segments of the record containing REMs without K complexes or sleep spindles and chin tone at the REM level are considered to be stage R.

c. If the majority of an epoch contains a segment considered to be stage N2, it is scored as stage N2. If the majority of an epoch contains a segment considered to be stage R, it is scored as stage R."[1] Once a stage score of R has been assigned to the epoch, answers A, B, C, and D are incorrect.

29. **Answer C. N2.**

Epochs 1 and 2 show K complexes (such as at A) and spindles and are scored as N2 sleep (Fig. 44.59). REM is seen in epoch 4 (at B) and indicates the onset of REM sleep. The "look back" rule scores segments of the epochs as stage R that are contiguous with unambiguous REM (as in epoch 4) with the following rule: "Score segments of sleep preceding and contiguous with an epoch of definite stage R (as defined in I.2), in the absence of REMs, as stage R if ALL of the following are present: (see Figs. 44.10–44.12)

a. The EEG shows LAMF activity without K complexes or sleep spindles."[1] However, in this case the last K complex occurs in the second half of epoch 3 (at C) and the epoch is therefore scored as N2 because the majority of the epoch is scored as N2. Once a stage score of N2

has been assigned to the epoch, answers A, B, D, and E are incorrect.

30. **Answer B. N1.**

This series of epochs begins with stage R sleep in epoch 1, as indicated by REMs, LAMF EEG, and low chin EMG (Fig. 44.60). Epoch 2 is also scored as stage R because it is contiguous with an epoch of unambiguous REM. At A, there is an arousal, meeting the required increase of EEG frequency lasting at least 3 seconds and the increase of chin EMG lasting at least 1 second. The arousal is followed by slow eye movements (at B). According to this rule, this results in a score of N1 for epoch 4: "End scoring stage R sleep when ONE OR MORE of the following occur:

a. There is a transition to stage W or N3

b. An increase in chin EMG tone above the level of stage R is seen for the majority of the epoch and criteria for stage N1 are met

c. An arousal occurs followed by LAMF EEG and slow eye movements (score the epoch as stage N1; if there are no slow eye movements and chin EMG tone remains low, continue to score as stage R)"[1] Rule c results in a score of N1 for epoch 4. Once a stage score of N1 has been assigned to the epoch, answers A, C, D, and E are incorrect.

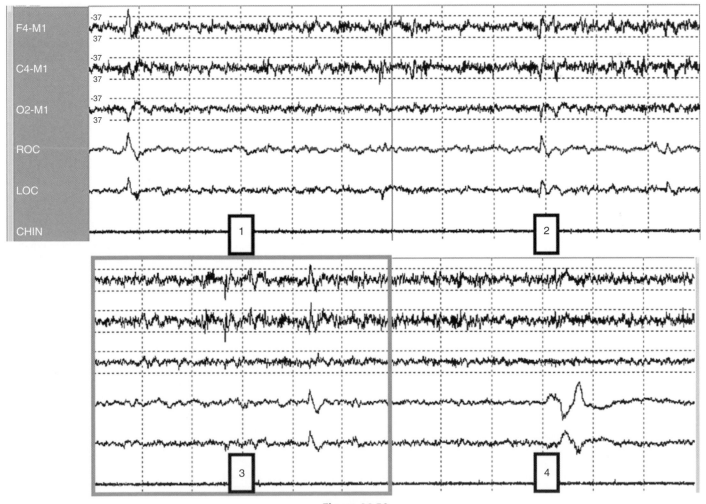

• **Figure 44.59**

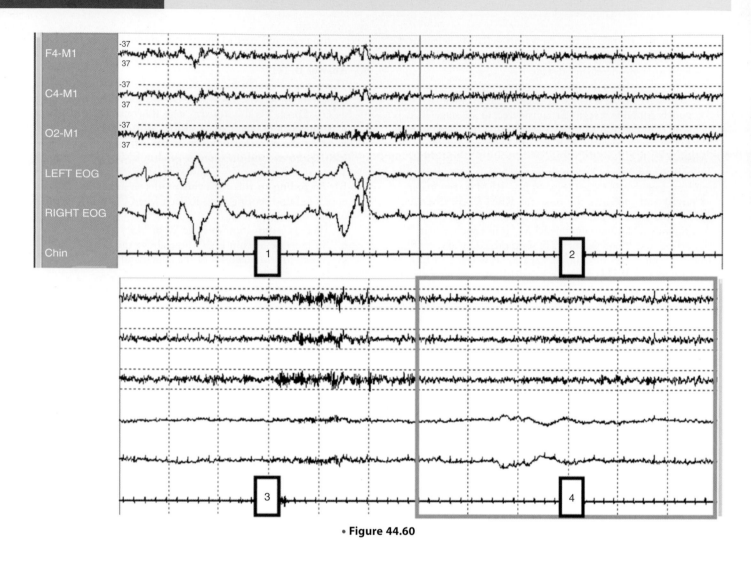

• Figure 44.60

Suggested Reading

Barry R, Wagner H. *Sleep Medicine Pearls*. 3rd ed. Fundamentals, Chapter 19 (Parasomnias). Philadelphia, PA: Elsevier/Saunders; 2014.

Berry R, Brooks R, Gamaldo C, et al. *The AASM Manual for the Scoring of Sleep and Associated Events: Rules, Terminology and Technical Specifications. Version 2.2*. Darien, IL: American Academy of Sleep Medicine; 2015. www.aasmnet.org.

Hershkowitz M, Moore C, Hamilton C, et al. Polysomnography of adults and elderly: sleep architecture, respiration and leg movement. *J Clin Neurophysiol*. 1992;9(1):56-62.

International Classification of Sleep Disorders (3rd ed) ICSD-3. American Academy of Sleep Medicine; 2014.

Littner MR, Kushida C, Wise M, et al. Practice parameters for clinical use of the multiple sleep latency test and the maintenance of wakefulness test. Standards of Practice Committee of the American Academy of Sleep Medicine. *Sleep*. 2005;28(1):113-121.

45

Artifacts

JAMES D. GEYER, PAUL R. CARNEY

Questions

1. A 38-year-old woman with a body mass index (BMI) of 35 kg/m^2 returns to the sleep laboratory for reevaluation of her sleep. Her initial sleep study was unremarkable. She reports that she has had at least a 35-pound weight gain over the past year. The phenomenon in Fig. 45.1 denoted by the black stars was identified on the polysomnogram (PSG). What is this characteristic of?
   A. Respiratory artifact
   B. Seizure activity
   C. Electrocardiogram (ECG) artifact
   D. Electrode pop artifact
   E. Rectus spikes related to extraocular muscle activity

2. A 52-year-old man with a BMI of 29 kg/m^2 presented to the sleep laboratory for evaluation of excessive daytime sleepiness. What artifact is denoted by the stars in Fig. 45.2?
   A. Seizure activity
   B. Respiratory artifact
   C. Swallow artifact
   D. Electrode pop artifact
   E. Ocular artifact

3. A 30-year-old woman presented to the sleep center for a nocturnal PSG. The patient is under a severe amount of stress because of caring for her mother who is suffering from dementia. She has been told that she snores loudly. She reports morning jaw and tooth pain. What is the most likely etiology of the artifact seen in Fig. 45.3?
   A. Bruxism and jaw movement artifact
   B. Generalized epileptiform activity
   C. Sweat artifact
   D. Respiratory artifact

4. A 67-year-old man with a BMI of 42 kg/m^2 presents for a sleep medicine clinical evaluation. He has a past history of lung cancer status postsurgery chemotherapy and radiation therapy, gastroesophageal reflux disease, and hypertension. His sleep complaints include excessive daytime sleepiness, leg twitching while asleep, and loud snoring. To combat his daytime sleepiness, he has been drinking numerous energy drinks throughout the day, afternoon, and even into the evening. During the recording of a nocturnal PSG, the nighttime technician observes unusual activity noted by the question marks in Fig. 45.4. What is this activity?
   A. Cough
   B. Swallow artifact
   C. ECG artifact
   D. Nocturnal myoclonus

5. A 53-year-old obese truck driver with a reported history of severe daytime sleepiness underwent polysomnography and was found to have obstructive sleep apnea. He presented for titration of positive airway pressure (PAP) therapy. Early during the study, the recording revealed a pattern identified in Fig. 45.5. What is the most likely explanation?
   A. The patient is sweating and technologist should apply a slow-frequency filter.
   B. The patient is sweating, so an electric fan must be turned on immediately and pointed toward the patient's face to eliminate this artifact.
   C. The patient has dementia resulting in slowing of the background rhythms.
   D. The patient is in slow wave sleep.
   E. This is a respiratory artifact.

For Questions 6–9, please match the following cases with the possible PSG fragment (Figs. 45.6–45.9) that corresponds with the scenario illustrated:

6. *Patient A*, a 44-year-old man with significant work-related problems, underwent a nocturnal PSG for evaluation of snoring and excessive daytime sleepiness, and witnessed episodes of apnea during sleep. He also had a history of chronic sleep-onset insomnia as well as sleep maintenance insomnia. On the night of his study, he tried to fall asleep by reading, as is his usual habit. Which PSG best corresponds to the clinical scenario illustrated?
   A. Fig. 45.6
   B. Fig. 45.7
   C. Fig. 45.8
   D. Fig. 45.9

Text continued on p. 704

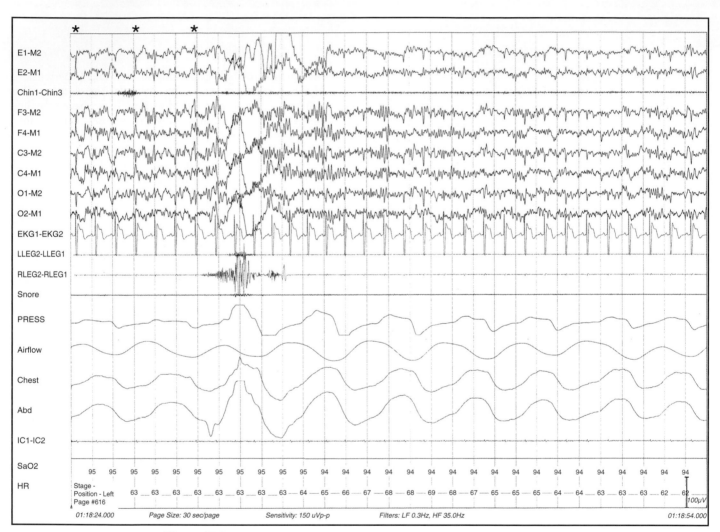

• **Figure 45.1** (Copyright James Geyer and JNP Media [2016]. Used with permission.)

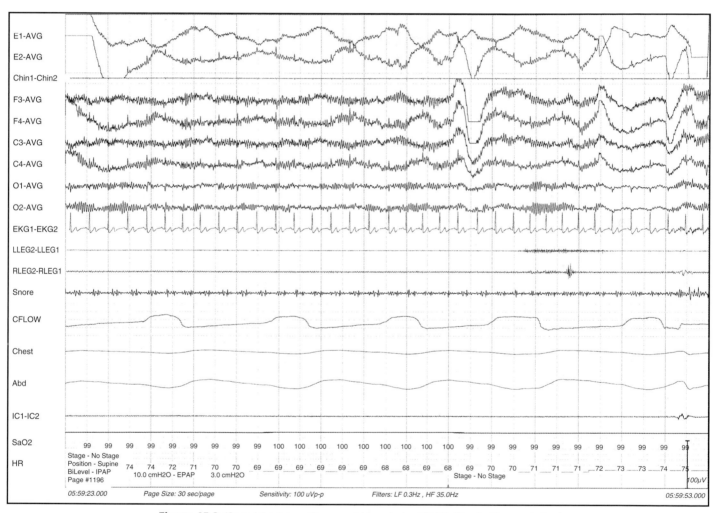

• **Figure 45.2** (Copyright James Geyer and Neurotexion [2016]. Used with permission.)

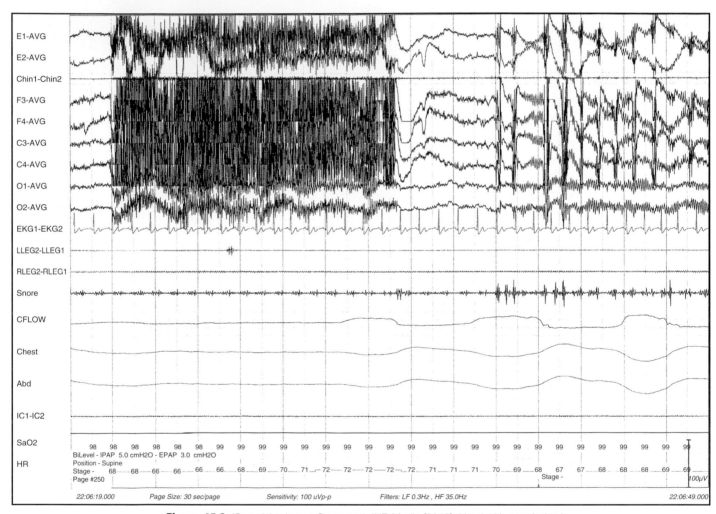

• **Figure 45.3** (Copyright James Geyer and JNP Media [2016]. Used with permission.)

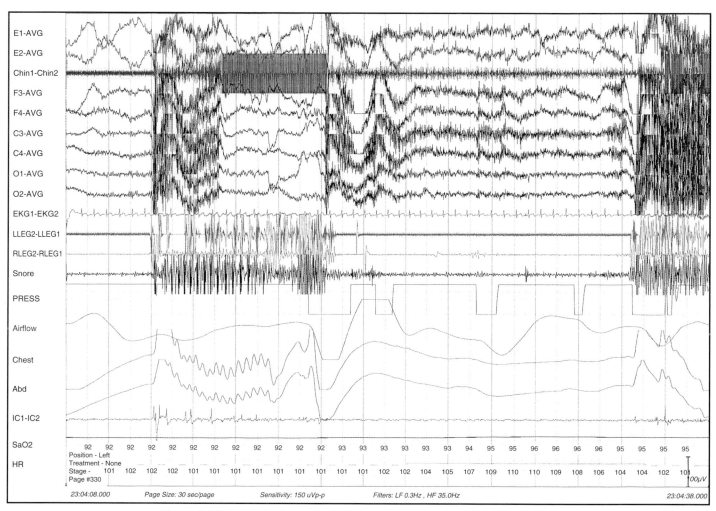

• **Figure 45.4** (Copyright James Geyer and JNP Media [2016]. Used with permission.)

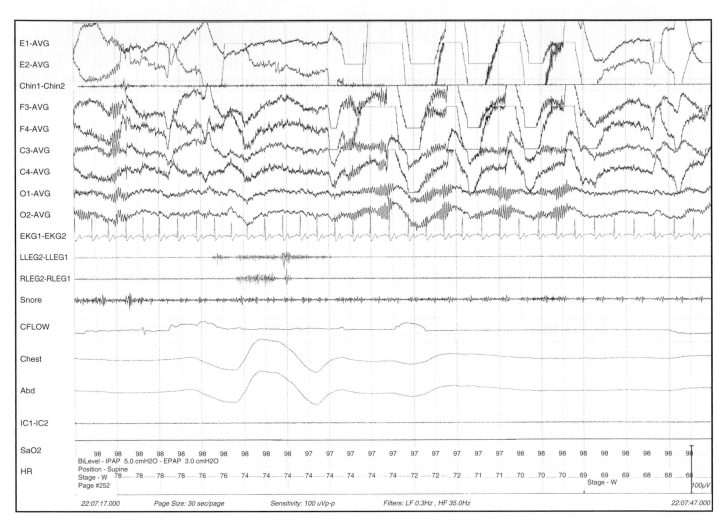

• **Figure 45.5** (Copyright James Geyer and JNP Media [2016]. Used with permission.)

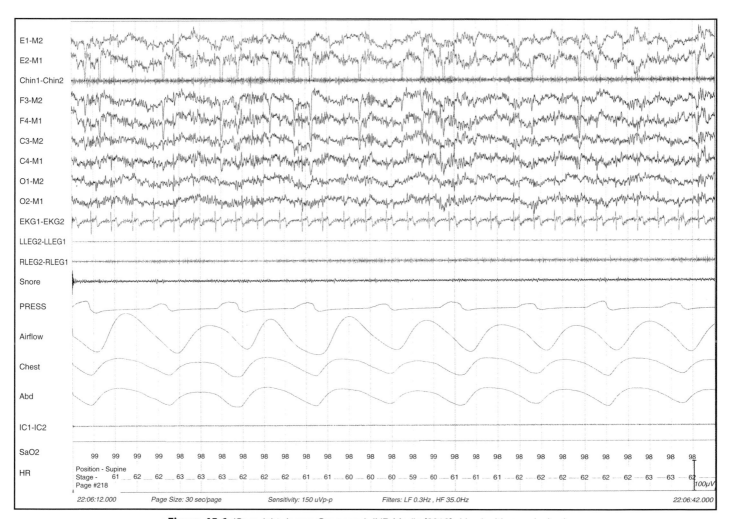

• **Figure 45.6** (Copyright James Geyer and JNP Media [2016]. Used with permission.)

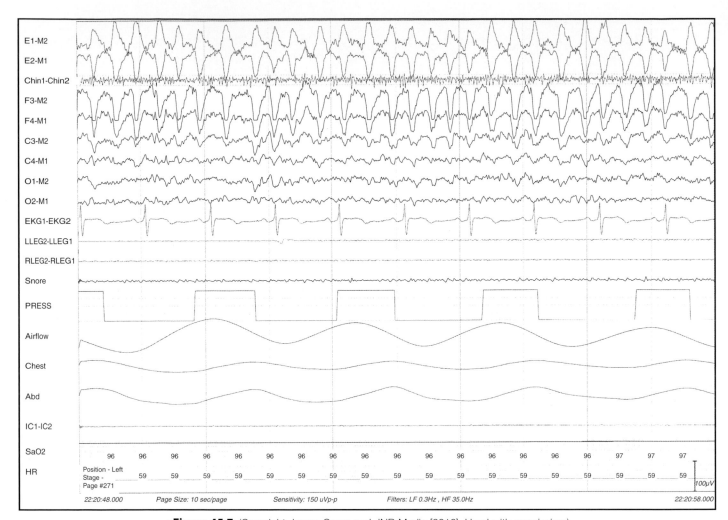

• **Figure 45.7** (Copyright James Geyer and JNP Media [2016]. Used with permission.)

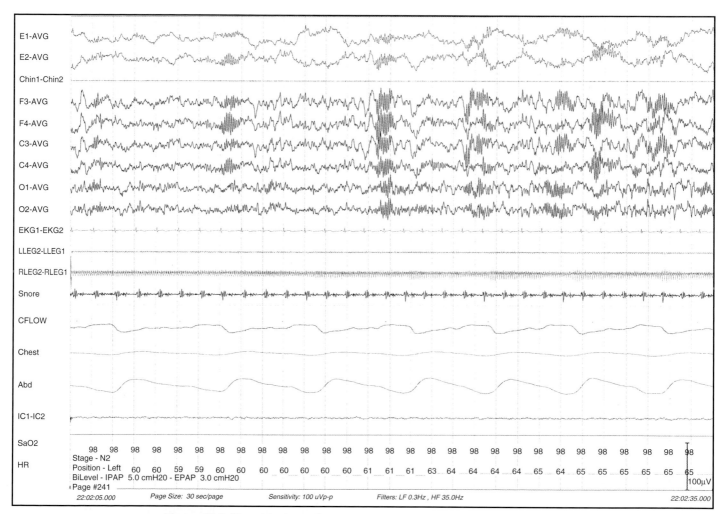

• **Figure 45.8** (Copyright James Geyer and JNP Media [2016]. Used with permission.)

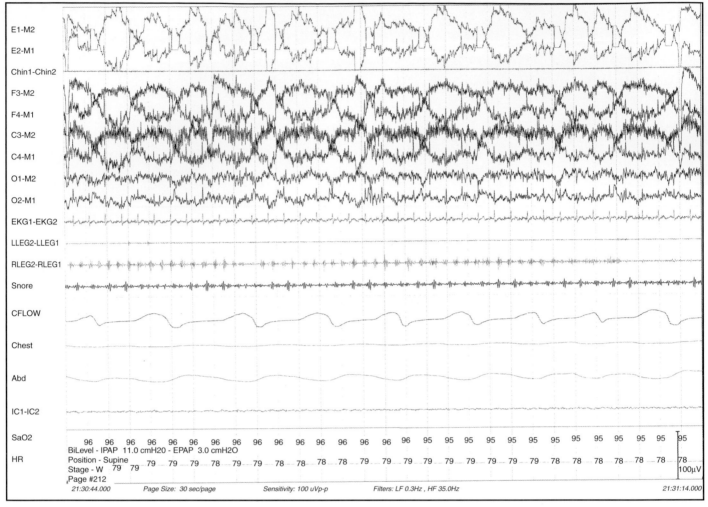

• **Figure 45.9** (Copyright James Geyer and JNP Media [2016]. Used with permission.)

7. *Patient B*, a 68-year-old man with a history of multisystem atrophy (MSA), was evaluated because of recent unusual behavior at night in which he screams, punches, and kicks his legs. The video portion of his nocturnal PSG demonstrated punching movements involving both arms associated with screaming. He is a combat veteran who was injured by an improvised explosive device explosion. Which PSG best corresponds with the clinical scenario illustrated?
   A. Fig. 45.6
   B. Fig. 45.7
   C. Fig. 45.8
   D. Fig. 45.9

8. *Patient C*, a 36-year-old woman with a past medical history of hypertension, rheumatoid arthritis, and depression, presented for evaluation of severe daytime sleepiness. Her medications include methotrexate, ibuprofen, and a selective serotonin reuptake inhibitor (SSRI). Which PSG tracing best corresponds with the clinical scenario illustrated?
   A. Fig. 45.6
   B. Fig. 45.7
   C. Fig. 45.8
   D. Fig. 45.9

9. *Patient D*, a 50-year-old man, is being evaluated for witnessed apneas and daytime sleepiness. The patient had a history of generalized anxiety and panic attacks. The neurological examination was unremarkable. He described feeling very anxious at the time of this tracing. Which PSG tracing is most consistent with the described clinical history and physical examination?
   A. Fig. 45.6
   B. Fig. 45.7
   C. Fig. 45.8
   D. Fig. 45.9

10. A diagnostic PSG was performed in a 63-year-old man for evaluation of possible obstructive and central sleep apnea based on reports from nursing staff during a recent hospitalization. The patient is obese and has a history of hypertension, diabetes mellitus type 2, coronary artery disease, and congestive heart disease. The sleep technologist reported seeing a bizarre ECG pattern (Fig. 45.10, noted by the star). What might be the explanation?
   A. The pattern probably represents polyspike and wave complexes originating in the electroencephalogram (EEG).
   B. The pattern is normal QRS pattern and probably represents amplification of the ECG signal.
   C. The patient most likely has a biventricular implantable cardioverter-defibrillator, which is used for cardiac resynchronization therapy.

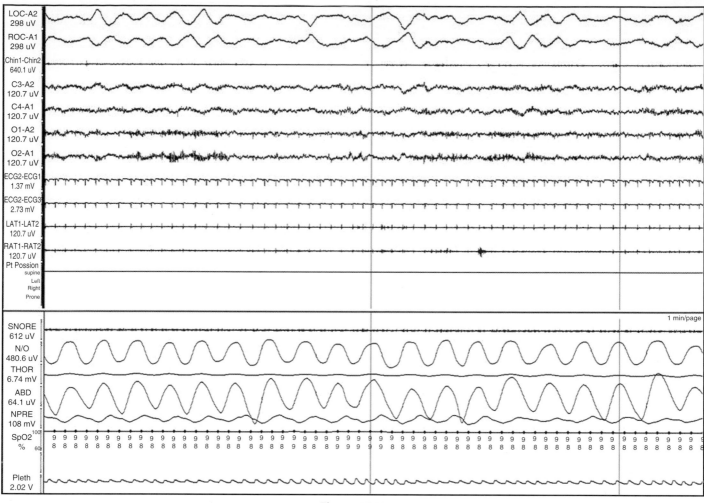

• **Figure 45.10**

D. It represents an electrode pop.

E. The sleep technologist applied the ECG electrodes incorrectly and the signal actually represents a normal ECG with reversed polarity.

F. It is a bimetallic artifact.

11. A 45-year-old man with recently diagnosed obstructive sleep apnea presents for a PAP titration study. The patient required increasing pressure levels for control of residual snoring. What is the artifact identified by the arrows in the mask flow channel (Mflo) on the PSG tracing in Fig. 45.11?

   A. Respiratory artifact
   B. Snore artifact
   C. CPAP mask leak artifact
   D. ECG artifact

12. What is the most likely explanation for the finding noted in the stars shown in Fig. 45.12?

   A. Alzheimer's type dementia can result in a slowing of the background rhythms and in some cases can result in a relatively high amplitude slow wave activity, especially in patients with a superimposed metabolic encephalopathy.

   B. The patient is in slow wave or delta sleep, which is characterized by 20% or more of the epoch consisting of synchronous slow waves, with a frequency between 0.5 and 2 Hz and an amplitude of 75 μV or greater over the frontal regions.

   C. This is a respiratory artifact, which correlates with the respiratory activity noted in the thoracic and abdominal channels and corresponds to movement of the electrode as a result of inhalation and exhalation.

   D. The process is caused by a chemical reaction in the conductive gel of the electrode cups.

13. A 42-year-old bank executive arrives at the sleep center for evaluation of excessive daytime sleepiness and snoring. He informs the sleep technologist that he is cold and quite nervous about undergoing medical testing. After lights out, one of the scalp electrodes begins to itch, and he scratches that region. What is the possible cause of the artifact indicated in Fig. 45.13?

   A. Shiver artifact
   B. Chewing artifact from the patient eating
   C. Movement artifact from the patient getting settled
   D. 60-Hz signal caused by a poorly attached electrode
   E. Swallow artifact

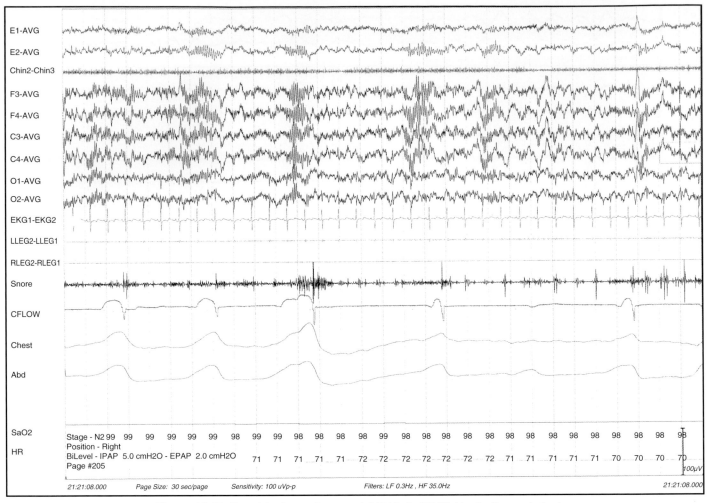

- **Figure 45.11** (Copyright James Geyer and JNP Media [2016]. Used with permission.)

14. Fig. 45.14 (30-sec epoch) is a recording from a 17-year-old male patient with a medical history that includes difficulty falling asleep on most nights. He then has difficulty sleeping late into the morning. What is the nature of the activity in the snore channel?
    A. ECG artifact
    B. Snoring
    C. Pulse artifact
    D. Talking
    E. Loose electrodes

15. A 24-year-old patient presents for evaluation of snoring. During the recording the technician observes the following unusual activity. What is the best explanation for the findings in Fig. 45.15?
    A. Restless legs syndrome
    B. Sucking artifact
    C. Chewing artifact
    D. Glossokinetic artifact
    E. Muscle artifact resulting from seizure activity

16. A 33-year-old female patient with a neck circumference of 17 inches and BMI of 37 kg/m² presents for evaluation of loud snoring and witnessed apneas. A fan was started to decrease the sweat artifact. The nasal/oral (N/O) airflow signal was described as erratic. What is the most likely cause of the disruption in the N/O signal (identified by the star on the tracing) in Fig. 45.16?
    A. The thermocouple signal is not being displayed at the correct sensitivity.
    B. The thermocouple is malfunctioning because of a loose connection.
    C. The thermocouple is displaying flow limitation because of snoring.
    D. The thermocouple is not picking up the necessary temperature differential.
    E. The thermocouple leads were incorrectly referenced.

17. A 16-month-old girl has episodes of possible pauses in breathing during sleep reported by her parents. She had difficulty falling asleep with the monitors in place. Fig. 45.17 demonstrates which of the following?
    A. Suck artifact
    B. Patting artifact
    C. Generalized spike and wave seizure activity
    D. Sweat artifact
    E. Rhythmic movement disorder

Text continued on p. 712

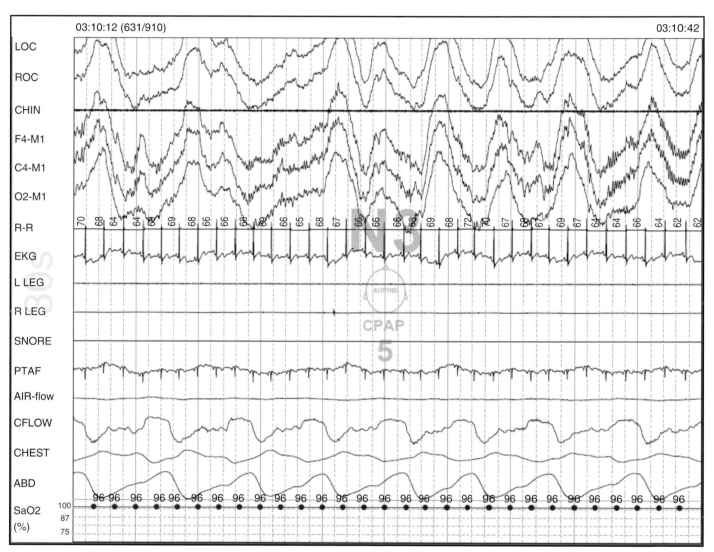

• **Figure 45.12** (Copyright Alon Avidan.)

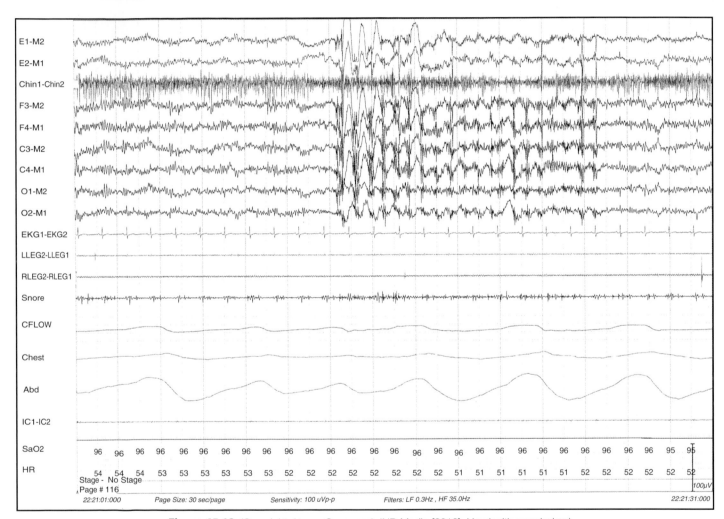

• **Figure 45.13** (Copyright James Geyer and JNP Media [2016]. Used with permission.)

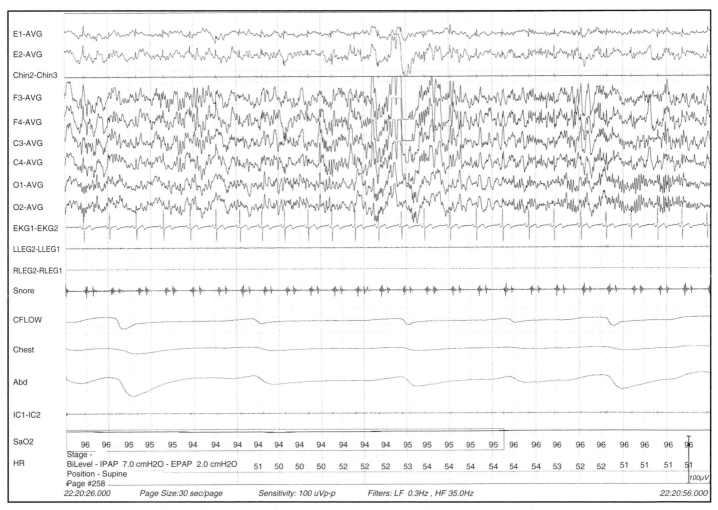

• **Figure 45.14** (Copyright James Geyer and JNP Media [2016]. Used with permission.)

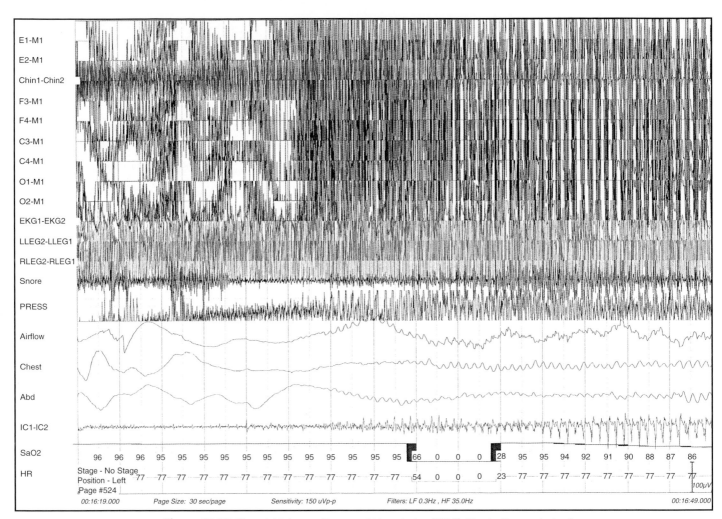

• **Figure 45.15** (Copyright James Geyer and Neurotexion [2016]. Used with permission.)

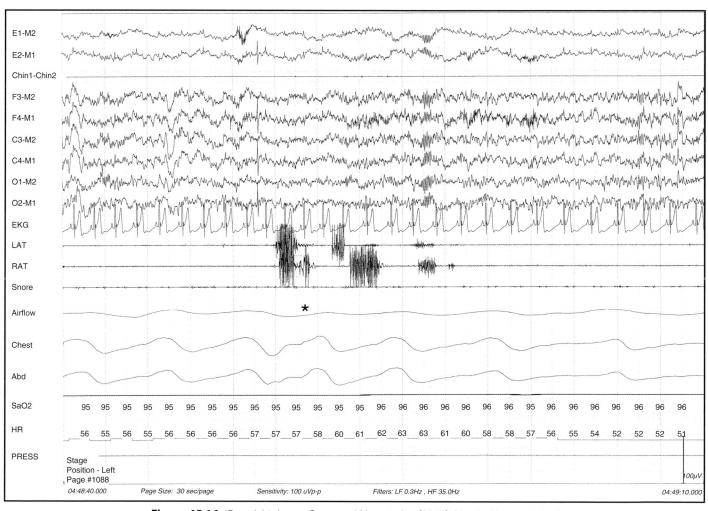

• **Figure 45.16** (Copyright James Geyer and Neurotexion [2016]. Used with permission.)

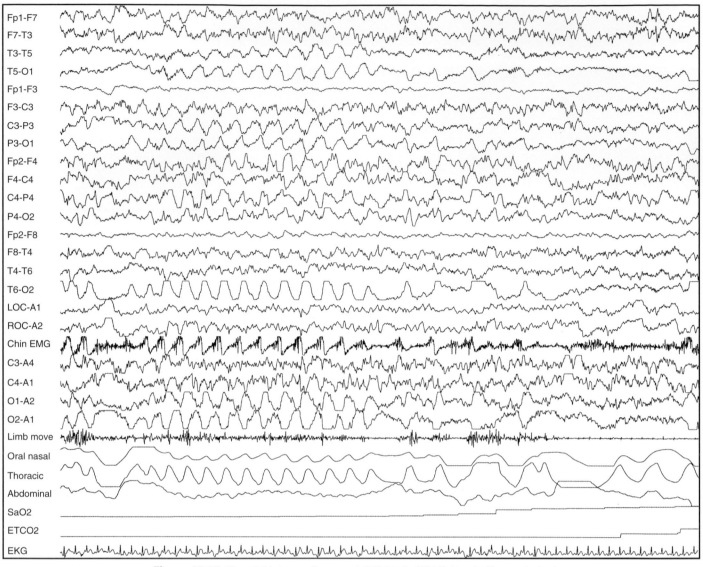

• **Figure 45.17** (Copyright James Geyer and JNP Media [2016]. Used with permission.)

18. A 40-year-old woman had a PAP titration. She preferred a cold room and also requested the ceiling fan be run throughout the study. What is the etiology of the activity demonstrated in the Mflo channel in Fig. 45.18?
    A. Bruxism
    B. Condensation artifact in the tubing
    C. ECG artifact
    D. Mask leak
    E. Shiver artifact

19. A 60-year-old male patient with a past a medical history of chronic obstructive pulmonary disease and Parkinson's disease was evaluated for frequent nocturnal awakenings and morning headaches. The history was suggestive of a sleep-related breathing disorder. A baseline nocturnal PSG was performed. A sample of the recording is displayed in Fig. 45.19. What is the best description of the artifact illustrated in the epoch (indicated by the stars)?
    A. Physiological artifact
    B. Instrumental artifact

C. Environmental artifact
D. Reading artifact

20. A 29-year-old morbidly obese man was referred for a nocturnal PSG for the evaluation of possible sleep apnea and possible obesity hypoventilation syndrome. The sleep technologist noted an unusual finding in the thoracic belt effort recording. What is the artifact noted by the arrows in Fig. 45.20?
    A. Scratching artifact
    B. Hiccup artifact
    C. Cardioballistic artifact
    D. Loose respiratory effort belt

Answers

1. **C. ECG artifact.**
   ECG artifact is a common physiological artifact arising from ECG electrical potentials. ECG artifact can be encountered at any location in the body, especially depending on the active to reference electrode distance and location. Pulse artifact is

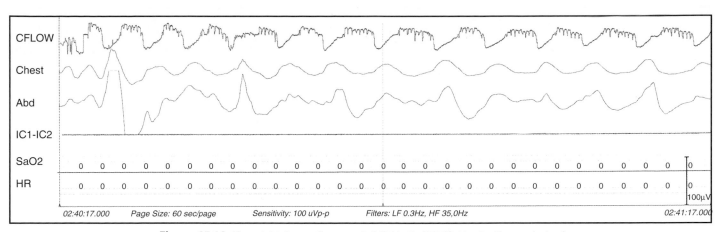

• **Figure 45.18** (Copyright James Geyer and JNP Media [2016]. Used with permission.)

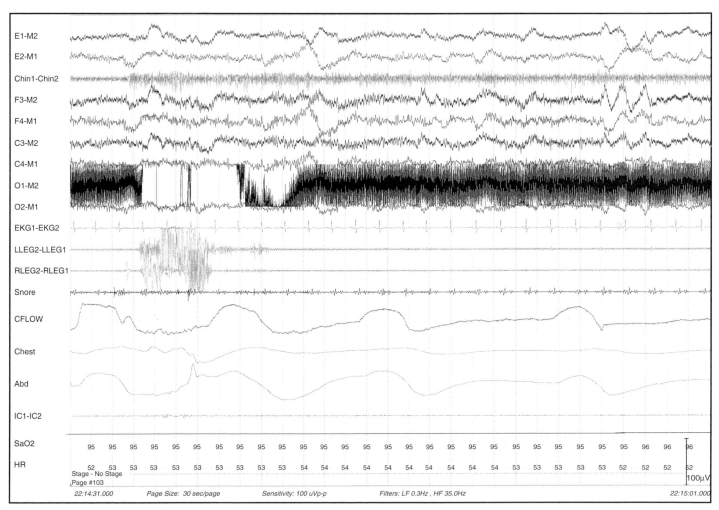

• **Figure 45.19** (Copyright James Geyer and JNP Media [2016]. Used with permission.)

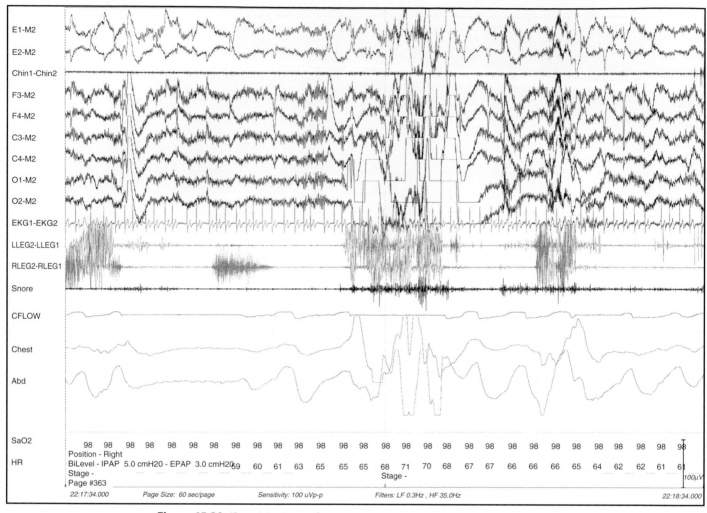

• **Figure 45.20** (Copyright James Geyer and JNP Media [2016]. Used with permission.)

more common when electrodes are located in close proximity to large blood vessels. Fig. 45.1 has an ECG artifact in the EEG, EOG, and chin EMG. These sharply contoured waveforms can be confirmed as an ECG artifact by their correlation with the ECG channel. ECG artifact may be minimized by repositioning the electrode or electrodes in which it seems to be appearing. It can also be minimized in the EEG leads by double referencing A1 and A2. The idea behind using the A1 + A2 reference is that the differential amplifier will receive a similar ECG signal from both A1 and A2 and cancelling at least a portion of the ECG signal in these derivations. The difficulty with linking A1 and A2 is that it may introduce or make the recording more vulnerable to more generalized artifacts if one or the other of the leads malfunctions.

The example demonstrated is not consistent with an electrode pop artifact, which is caused by an electrode that may be unstable because of insufficient conductive paste, poor or intermittent contact of the electrode with the skin, or a faulty electrode cup or wire. This creates a capacitance effect. This is shown in Fig. 45.21, where the P4 electrode is loose. The artifact could not be respiratory in origin because there is no evidence of synchronization with the breathing pattern. The record does not demonstrate any seizure activity. A rectus spike would originate from an eye movement and is not correlated with the ECG signal.

2. **E. Ocular artifact.**

An eye movement artifact, otherwise known as an ocular artifact, is seen in Fig. 45.2, as demarcated by the stars. Figs. 45.22 and 45.23 demonstrate the source of this artifact. The eye is a charged dipole (much like a battery). The positive pole is at the cornea, and the negative pole is at the retina (see Fig. 45.23). The EOG consists of a bipolar linkage from the ROC electrode, 1 cm lateral and 1 cm superior to one outer canthus, to the LOC electrode, 1 cm lateral and 1 cm inferior to the other outer canthus. The electrode toward which the eyes move becomes relatively positive and the other relatively negative. As the eyes move during both wake and sleep, they produce corresponding changes in the electrical field and a parallel change in potential in the EEG electrodes. This can be verified by noting corresponding movements in the EOG channels. The EOG can become actively involved when eye movements are common, such as during rapid eye movement (REM) sleep, while reading, and while awake. The pattern is not consistent with a respiratory artifact, snoring artifact, or repetitive paroxysmal polyspike seizure activity.

3. **A. Bruxism and jaw movement artifact.**

Fig. 45.3 is consistent with bruxism, which is a prevalent type of *parafunctional oromotor activity*[1] and in the sleep literature is categorized as a sleep-related movement disorder. Sleep bruxism is a stereotyped movement disorder characterized by

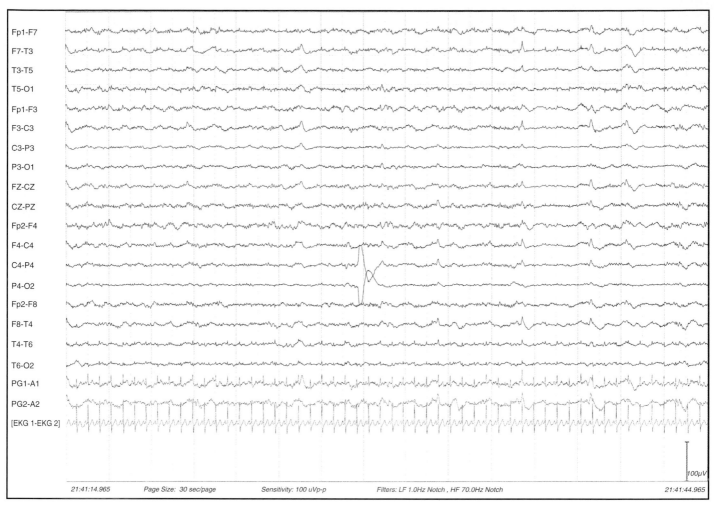

| 21:41:14.965 | Page Size: 30 sec/page | Sensitivity: 100 uVp-p | Filters: LF 1.0Hz Notch , HF 70.0Hz Notch | 21:41:44.965 |

• **Figure 45.21** (Copyright James Geyer and Neurotexion [2016]. Used with permission.)

grinding or clenching of the teeth during sleep.[2] The sounds made by friction of the teeth are perceived by an observer as unpleasant.[3] The disorder is typically brought to medical attention to eliminate the disturbing sounds, although the first signs of the disorder may be recognized by a dentist. Bruxism can lead to abnormal wear of the teeth, damage to periodontal tissue, or jaw pain, as it did in this patient.[3,4] In some cases, the patient can actually break off pieces of teeth because of the bruxism.

Although PSG monitoring is rarely indicated, when it is performed, it demonstrates increased rhythmic masseter and temporalis muscle activity during sleep. Bruxism may occur in all stages of sleep but is somewhat more common during stage N2 sleep.[4] Bruxism has a high night to night variability, creating a high false-negative rate on PSG.[5] A follow-up EEG or a PSG with a full EEG montage may be indicated if a seizure disorder is suspected as a cause for the bruxism. The other options, sweat artifact, respiratory artifact, and seizure activity, do not fit the characteristic checkerboard-type morphology that easily identifies the bruxism movement artifact as rhythmic clenching of the jaw that originates in the chin EMG electrode, with spread to the other EEG electrodes. Bruxism often follows hypopneas and apneas[6,7] and possibly represents autonomic arousal.

4. **D. Cough.**

The patient has a history of lung cancer status postsurgery, chemotherapy, and radiation therapy, which predispose patients to experiencing coughing. The findings associated with a cough relate in part to the forcefulness of the cough.

A hiccup has some similarities but occurs with a sudden contraction of the muscles of inspiration and closure of the glottis, which produces the characteristic sound.[8] The hiccup reflex consists of an afferent pathway via the vagus, phrenic, and sympathetic branches of T6–12 nerves and an efferent pathway via the phrenic nerve to the glottis, diaphragm, and external intercostal muscles.[9] Hiccups are common and can occur secondary to a large number of disorders and physiological factors.[10] Potential etiologies include luminal distention of the esophagus and stomach, gastroesophageal reflux disease, sarcoidosis, lung cancer, radiation therapy, and so on.[11]

The other options are incorrect. Nocturnal myoclonus refers to periodic limb movement disorder, which is characterized by periodic episodes of repetitive stereotypic limb movements that occur during sleep and are associated with sleep disturbance that cannot be accounted for by another primary sleep disorder. The modern term for nocturnal myoclonus is periodic limb movements during sleep (PLMS), which are usually determined on a PSG. PLMS require a series of at least four limb

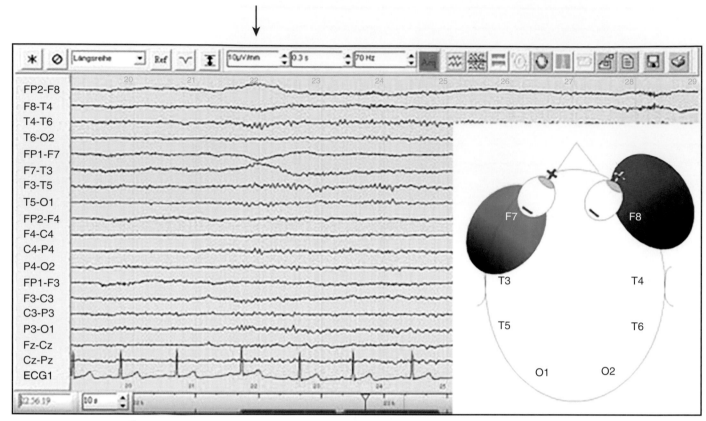

• **Figure 45.22** (From Hartmut Baier. Artefakterkennungund–beseitigungimEEG. *Neurophysiol Lab.* 2013;35:75–86.)

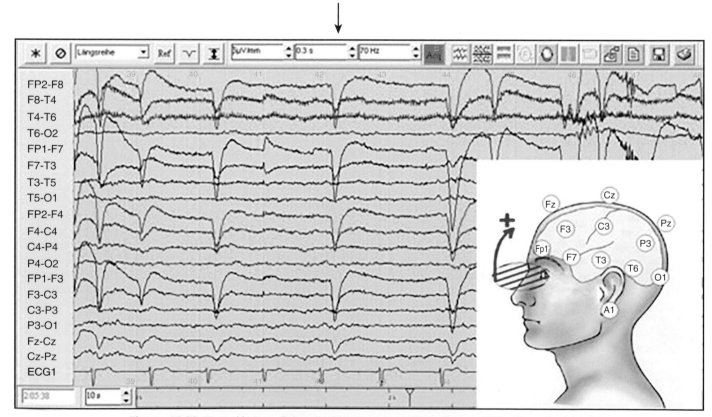

• **Figure 45.23** (From Hartmut Baier. Artefakterkennungund–beseitigungimFEG. *Neurophysiol Lab.* 2013;35:75–86.)

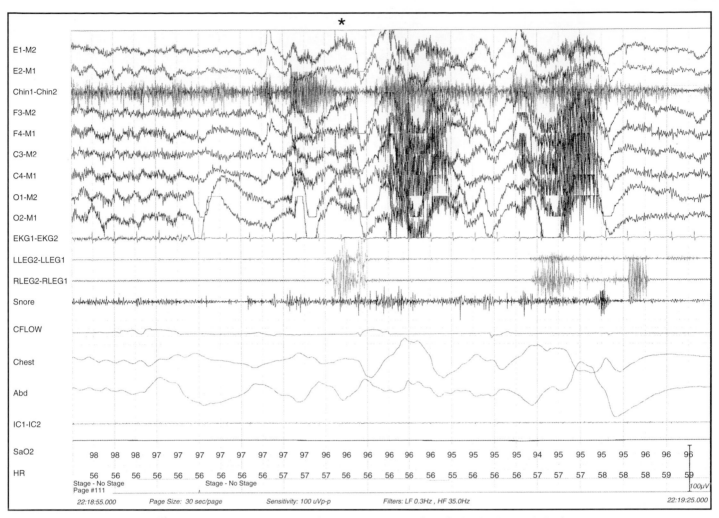

• **Figure 45.24** (Copyright James Geyer and JNP Media [2016]. Used with permission.)

movements (measured as electromyogram [EMG] bursts) recurring every 5–90 sec with a burst duration of 0.5–5 sec.[12] The ECG frequency does not correlate with the cough artifact. Swallow artifact has a different pattern correlating with tongue movement as exhibited in Fig. 45.24.

5. **B. The patient is sweating.** The most appropriate response is for the sleep technologist to reduce the room's thermostat setting or start a fan to cool the patient, thereby eliminating this artifact.

Sweat artifact is identified by a high amplitude and slow frequency waveforms, typically with superimposed EEG activity.[13] This may sometimes be erroneously labeled as slow wave sleep (stage N3) by an inexperienced technologist or polysomnographer. The electrooculogram (EOG) and EEG electrodes are the regions most frequently affected by sweat artifact.[13] The slow frequencies seen with sweat artifact are typically much slower than stage N3 and usually have superimposed faster frequencies.[7] Sweat artifact may also be referred to as sway artifact or slow wave artifact. The term slow wave artifact is obviously a misnomer and should never be used. The most appropriate way to correct the artifact is by cooling the patient, removing the electrode or electrodes affected by sweating and drying the area, or even applying an antiperspirant. Cooling the patient may be achieved by either using a fan or lowering the thermostat setting. Although it is customary

practice to use a fan during the night and this option is not necessarily incorrect, it is perhaps a less correct choice because it introduces an electrical appliance into the recording environment and could result in a 60-Hz artifact, as seen in Fig. 45.25. Having a ceiling fan hardwired into the room on a separate circuit will eliminate this potential for 60 Hz artifact. A 60-Hz artifact occurs when an electrode malfunctions and picks up frequencies from the environment in the form of electrical nose. In the United States, the frequency used by most electrical devices is at this frequency range.[13] If one applies a low-frequency filter, it is possible to filter out the sweat artifact, but also other critically important slow wave activity signals, such as slow wave sleep as well as the possibility of slow wave activity associated with disorders such as epilepsy, which is an incorrect option. These waveforms are also not consistent with the slowing seen in some patients with dementia.

6. **D. Fig. 45.9.**

Patient A's PSG (see Fig. 45.9) demonstrates an EOG pattern consistent with reading. The unique feature of this artifact is demonstrated by the repetitive rhythmic pattern compatible with reading.[14,15] Fig. 45.26 shows a patient reading with poor focus on the paper. Notice that the eye movements have two different slope morphologies: one that is faster returning to

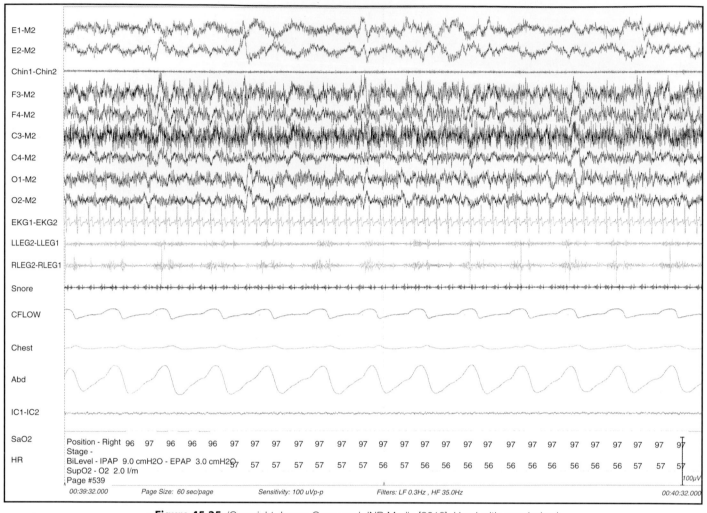

• **Figure 45.25** (Copyright James Geyer and JNP Media [2016]. Used with permission.)

the next line, and another that is slower as the line is read. A reading artifact can usually be confirmed by viewing the corresponding video image.

7. **A. Fig. 45.6.**

Patient B had left artificial eye with metallic components and also has eyelid dysfunction. An ocular prosthesis results in a loss of the dipole and therefore the loss of the left EOG signal (arrow in Fig. 45.6). This can be confirmed by reviewing the biocalibration data at the time of setup and reviewing the technician notes describing the abnormality. Some recordings of previous records from patients with prosthetic eyes have been encountered, in which the prosthetic hardware contains metallic components that may act as a dipole generating a typically smaller electrical potential that may appear as a low-amplitude eye movement when compared with the normal eye.

The patient experiences dream enactment behavior and probably has REM sleep behavior disorder (RBD). This is indeed confirmed by the abnormally elevated EMG activity in both the chin and limb leads as demarcated by the stars. The *International Classification of Sleep Disorders*, 3rd Edition (ICSD-3), has noted that RBD is the only parasomnia for which a diagnostic PSG is required for confirmation.[2]

The ICSD-3 diagnostic criteria for RBD are as follows[2]:
1. PGS abnormality—elevated EMG tone during REM sleep in either the submental or limb leads
2. Either a history of dream enactment behavior or observation of abnormal REM sleep behavior during the PSG
3. Absence of EEG epileptiform activity during REM sleep
4. The disturbance not able to be explained by another sleep, medical, neurological, or mental disorder, and not related to medication/substance use

The PSG reveals abnormal muscle augmentation REM sleep exceeding the normal REM sleep–related phasic EMG twitches. These motor phenomena may be complex (limb and trunk movements; repeated punching, kicking, or shouting) and are often associated with emotionally charged utterances.[16–19] When awoken from a dream enactment spell, patients may occasionally exhibit dream mentation that correlated with the observed behavior.

8. **C. Fig. 45.8.**

Patient C's tracing reveals abnormal eye movements related to SSRI use (originally termed "Prozac eyes"), revealed in the EOG channels (see Fig. 45.8). Prominent eye movements are seen during non-REM (NREM) stage N2 sleep. These abnormal eye movements during NREM sleep have been

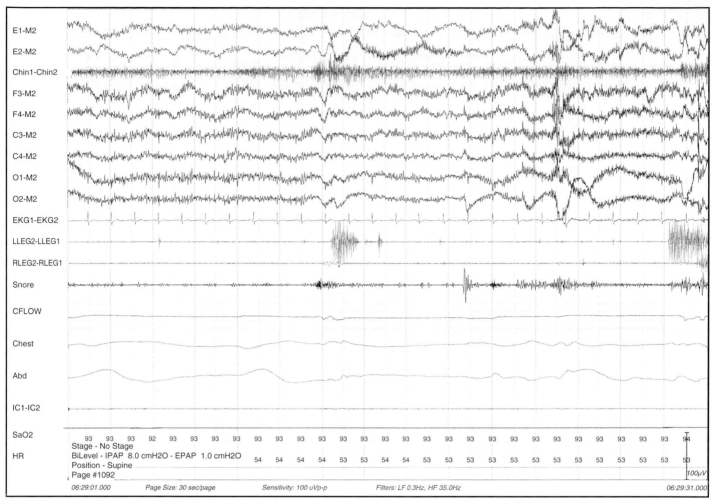

E1-M2	
E2-M2	
Chin1-Chin2	
F3-M2	
F4-M2	
C3-M2	
C4-M2	
O1-M2	
O2-M2	
EKG1-EKG2	
LLEG2-LLEG1	
RLEG2-RLEG1	
Snore	
CFLOW	
Chest	
Abd	
IC1-IC2	
SaO2	
HR	

93 93 93 92 93 93 93 93 93 93 93 93 93 93 93 93 93 93 93 93 93 93 93 93 93 93 93 94
Stage - No Stage
BiLevel - IPAP 8.0 cmH2O - EPAP 1.0 cmH2O   54 54 54 54 53 53 54 54 53 53 53 53 53 53 53 53 53 53 53 53 53
Position - Supine
Page #1092

06:29:01.000   Page Size: 30 sec/page   Sensitivity: 100 uVp-p   Filters: LF 0.3Hz, HF 35.0Hz   06:29:31.000

• **Figure 45.26** (Copyright James Geyer and JNP Media [2016]. Used with permission.)

described in patients taking SSRIs such as fluoxetine, paroxetine, citalopram, and escitalopram.[20] NREM eye movements are not necessarily associated with any symptomatology. The effect of fluoxetine on NREM eye movements is postulated to derive from potentiation of serotonergic neurons that inhibit brainstem "omnipause neurons," which in turn inhibit saccadic eye movements and thus result in disinhibited release of saccadic eye movements.[21] This interesting phenomenon may even persist after cessation of SSRI use.[21] NREM eye movements may also occur, though at a much lower prevalence, in patients using other mood stabilizers, neuroleptic agents, and even benzodiazepines.[22] SSRI eyes can also be seen during REM sleep, but are much more difficult to detect in this stage of sleep.

9. **B. Fig. 45.7.**

Patient D's tracing (see Fig. 45.7) reveals eye flutter. This may be seen with certain ocular disorders and in psychiatric conditions including anxiety and panic. There is no associated seizure activity.

10. **B. The patient most likely has a biventricular implantable cardioverter-defibrillator, which is used for cardiac resynchronization therapy.**

The patient has an implanted cardioverter-defibrillator with left ventricular–based pacing used as an adjunct to medical therapy for severe heart failure.[23] The resultant ECG

"defibrillator pattern" is appreciated better in the amplified box in Fig. 45.27. A pacemaker artifact typically produces sharp spikes preceding the remainder of the ECG complex that are characteristic of a paced rhythm (indicated by the stars). On-demand pacemakers may only result in an intermittent pattern of discharges. The patient's history should be reviewed to confirm the presence of a pacemaker. Other artifacts can be ruled out by changing the derivation of the input signal and by verifying the integrity of the electrode and its application by checking the impedances. A bimetallic artifact, which is usually manifested as an abrupt high-voltage signal seen in the chin EMG and EEG channels, is thought to be caused by dissimilar metals in dental work. The pattern is not the typical pattern of an electrode pop or poor electrode application. The epoch does not represent polyspike and wave complexes originating in the EEG associated with epilepsy, because there is no evidence of ictal activity in the EEG leads since the morphology does not fit and there is no evidence of filtering adjustments made. Incorrectly applied ECG would create a reversed polarity, and not the implanted cardioverter defibrillator pattern seen in the tracing.

11. **C. CPAP mask leak artifact.**

The tracing in Fig. 45.11 depicts the typical artifact seen with a mask flow artifact. The morphology of the Mflo displays the characteristic sharp dip at the end of each breath below

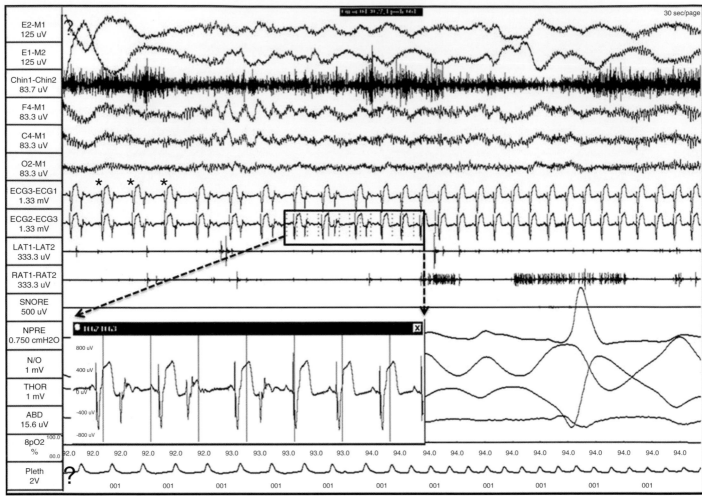

• **Figure 45.27**

the baseline level, as noted by the arrows. There is no correlation with the ECG tracing. There is no association with the snoring.

12. **D. The process is caused by a chemical reaction in the conductive gel of the electrode cups.**

Sweat artifact characteristically consists of a slow, undulating change in the EEG and EOG baseline wave signal activity with a wandering baseline, sometimes mistaken as stage N3, slow wave sleep.[24] Sweat consists of high sodium chloride and lactic acid levels, which may react with the exposed metal of the electrode and generate electrical potentials that combine with the skin and sweat gland potentials.[24]

Sweating can cause a barrier between the scalp and an electrode. In addition to the slow wave/sway artifact, higher-amplitude, faster-frequency "popping" artifact may also occur. A respiratory artifact is a more rhythmic, slow-frequency signal correlating (or in phase) with the patient's breathing and is usually at a faster frequency than a sweat artifact is. Sometimes the recording may have both sweat and slow wave artifact simultaneously, which can present a challenge to novice interpreting physicians.[24] Fig. 45.28 demonstrates a 60-sec recording of a sweat artifact.[24] It is important to remember that patients with obstructive sleep apnea are more likely to sweat.

13. **B. Chewing artifact from the patient eating.**

The artifact shown in Fig. 45.13 is chewing motion while awake that originates in the chin (star) with spread to the other EEG electrodes, which is similar to the pattern seen in association with bruxism. The other choices are incorrect; movement artifact from the patient getting settled is likely to result in a pattern shown in Fig. 45.29, which consists of motor activity that does not represent any specific rhythm, but that of the patient's normal movement at the time of recording. An example of a 60-Hz signal caused by a faulty/"bad" electrode is shown in Fig. 45.25. This would have been the correct epoch correlating with the option of the patient scratching his head and resulting in a loose/damaged electrode. Noted in this figure is the appearance of ECG artifact in the limb EMG leads.

14. **A. Pulse artifact in the snore channel.**

The patient's history is consistent with delayed sleep phase disorder, which is probably contributing to his sleepiness. The activity seen in Fig. 45.14 is consistent with pulse artifact in the snore lead. It comes after each QRS complex. It is not at the exact time of the QRS, and it has a longer duration, making ECG artifact incorrect. Snoring is incorrect, since the waveforms do not correlate with the

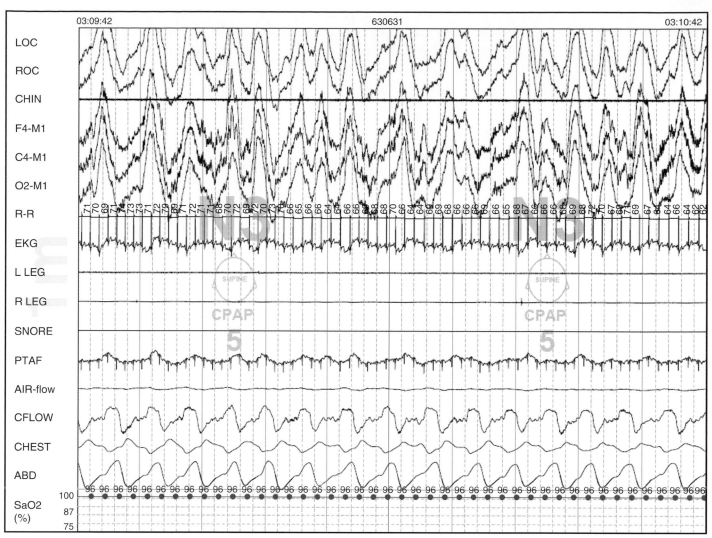

• **Figure 45.28** (Copyright Alon Avidan. Used with permission.)

respiratory cycle. This finding is not consistent with talking-related artifacts.

15. **E. Muscle artifact caused by seizure activity.**

On initial impression of the pattern seen in Fig. 45.15, this pattern might be mistaken for simple rhythmic movements such as chewing or sucking. However, the EEG tracing has a polyspike and wave morphology. A swallow or glossokinetic artifact is shown in Fig. 45.24. Like the eyeball, the tongue also functions as a dipole, with the tip being negative (−) with respect to the base (+). The tip of the tongue is relatively more mobile with respect to the tongue base.[25] The resulting artifact has a broad potential field that is attenuated from the frontal to the occipital areas, with amplitude potentials greater inferiorly than in the parasagittal regions and a corresponding delta frequency range (noted by the star), and it occurs synchronously when the patient is instructed to say "Lah-lah-lah-lah" or "Lilt-lilt-lilt-lilt."[25]

16. **D. The thermocouple is not picking up the necessary temperature differential.**

The N/O signal is derived from a thermocouple and is qualitative as opposed to quantitative; it allows recording of the fluctuations in temperature that occur during inspiration of relatively cooler air and expiration relatively warmer air. It is therefore important that the sensor be secured directly under the nose and be strategically positioned in the line of airflow from the mouth. Even with correct positioning, the thermocouple will have difficulty sensing temperature fluctuations if the expired air is being blown away by a fan and replaced by cooler air. A similar problem arises when the patient places bedcovers over the head and mouth. One would expect to observe a more uniform sinusoidal recording pattern in cases in which snoring was interfering with the signal or the displayed sensitivity was reduced. A loose connection or head box connection failure typically produces an erratic faster-frequency signal artifact.

17. **B. Patting artifact.**

Patting artifact is identified by the stars in Fig. 45.17. The artifact is seen primarily in the ECG, chest effort, abdominal effort, and to some degree in the EEG channels.

Suck artifact is typically seen primarily in the chin EMG with waxing and waning followed by swallowing. Such behavior is seen in infants and toddlers when sucking on a pacifier or

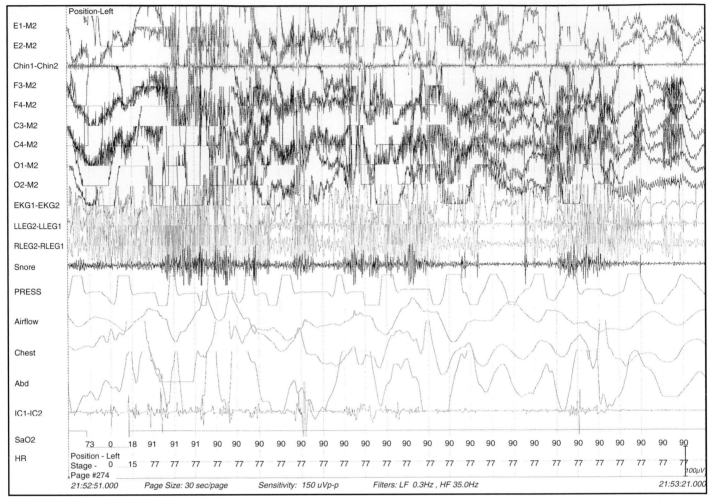

• **Figure 45.29** (Copyright James Geyer and JNP Media [2016]. Used with permission.)

bottle, or when breastfeeding. Less frequently this may be seen in patients with developmental delay or in older patients with dementia. Fig. 45.30 demonstrates a suck artifact. Sweat artifact has a much slower undulating frequency. The pattern is not consistent with generalized spike and wave activity or rhythmic movement disorder, the latter of which has a much more dramatic impact on the rest of the recording electrodes.

18. **B. Condensation artifact in the tubing.**
Condensation in the PAP system tubing can result in a reverberating pattern in the Mflo. The size of the reverberation on inspiration depends in part on the amount of condensation and on the mask flow.

A mask leak results in a dip in the mask flow tracing at the end of inspiration. ECG artifact would not be isolated to the inspiratory phase and would be unlikely to register in the Mflo. Bruxism would not appear in this channel and be isolated to inspiration.

19. **B. Instrumental artifact.**
These artifacts are caused by malfunctioning or faulty equipment used in recording the PSG, such as electrodes and head boxes. The tracing in Fig. 45.19 indicates a loose connection

at the O1 electrode. Noise artifacts are also related to faulty or malfunctioning equipment and fall in the category instrumental artifacts. A wide array of electrical and magnetic objects and machines can create an electrical field, resulting in an environmental artifact. Physiological artifacts are related to the patient—for instance, other sources of electrical potential emanating from the patient, such as ECG, EMG, swallow, suck, scratch, and sweat artifacts. This example is not typical of reading, as previous described.

20. **C. Cardioballistic artifact.**
Cardioballistic artifact is depicted in Fig. 45.20 during an episode of central sleep apnea. A cardioballistic artifact corresponds to cardiac pulsations, which are transmitted through the rib cage and are typically most apparent in the thoracic channel. It may also be picked up by the EEG electrodes, EOG, and esophageal pressure recording. Note that the airway is still occluded and the fluctuations in the thoracic lead do not represent airflow.

Illustrated in Figs. 45.31–45.55 are additional examples without corresponding questions for the reader's interest:

Text continued on p. 745

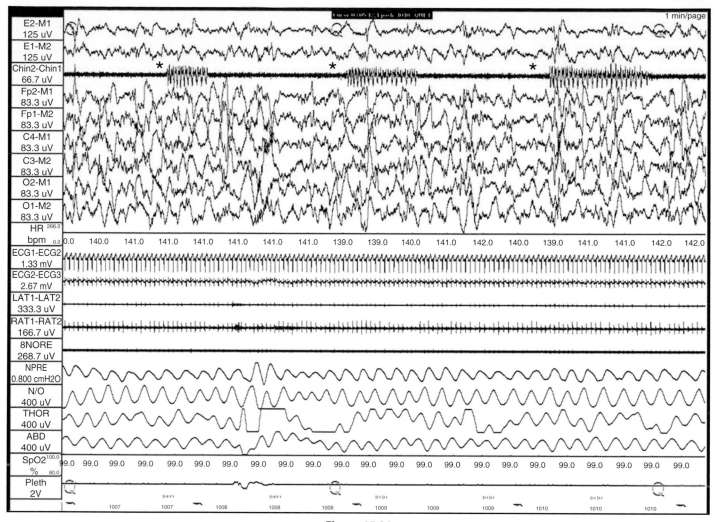

• **Figure 45.30**

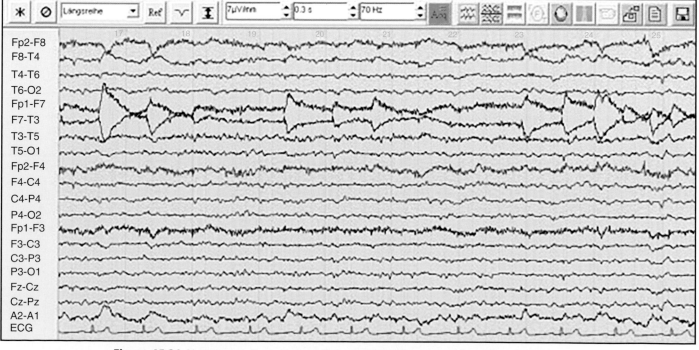

• **Figure 45.31** Nystagmus. (From Hartmut Baier. Artefakterkennungund–beseitigungimEEG. *Neuro-physiol Lab.* 2013;35:75–86.)

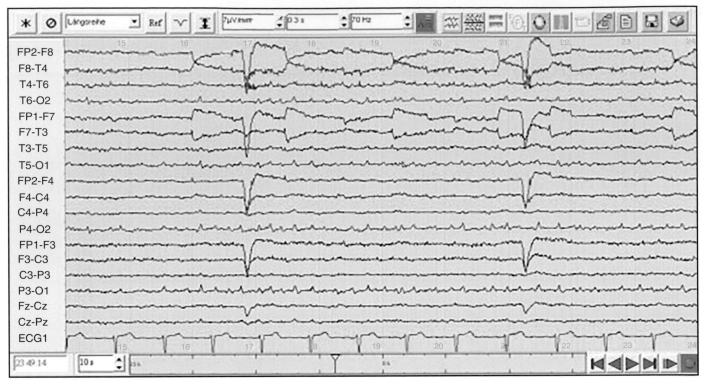

• **Figure 45.32** Rectus Spikes. (From Hartmut Baier. Artefakterkennungund–beseitigungimEEG. *Neurophysiol Lab.* 2013;35:75–86.)

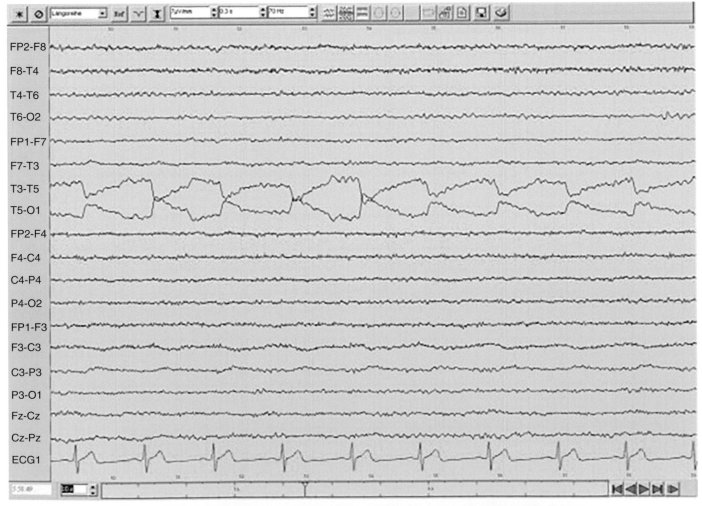

• **Figure 45.33** Pulse Artifact. (From Hartmut Baier. Artefakterkennungund–beseitigungimEEG. *Neurophysiol Lab.* 2013;35:75–86.)

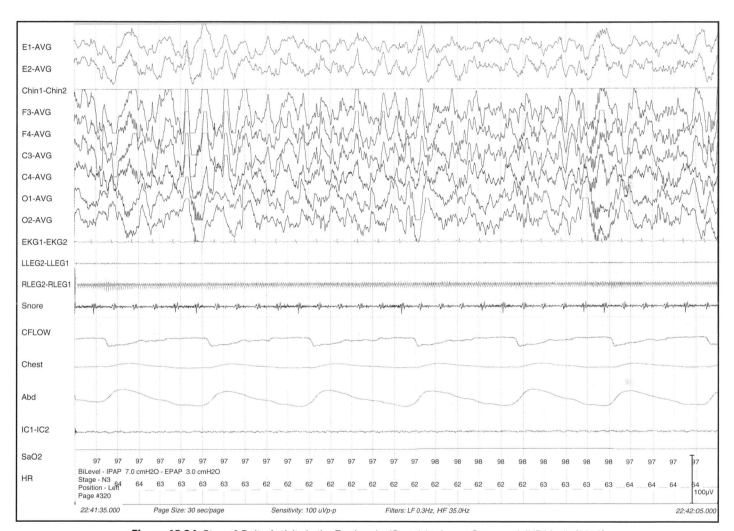

• **Figure 45.34** Stage 3 Delta Activity in the Eye Leads. (Copyright James Geyer and JNP Media [2016]. Used with permission.)

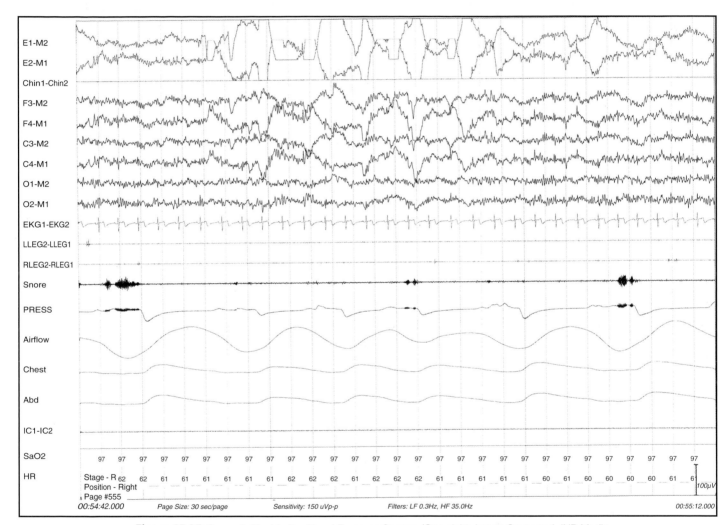

• **Figure 45.35** Snore Artifact in the Nasal Pressure Sensor. (Copyright James Geyer and JNP Media [2016]. Used with permission.)

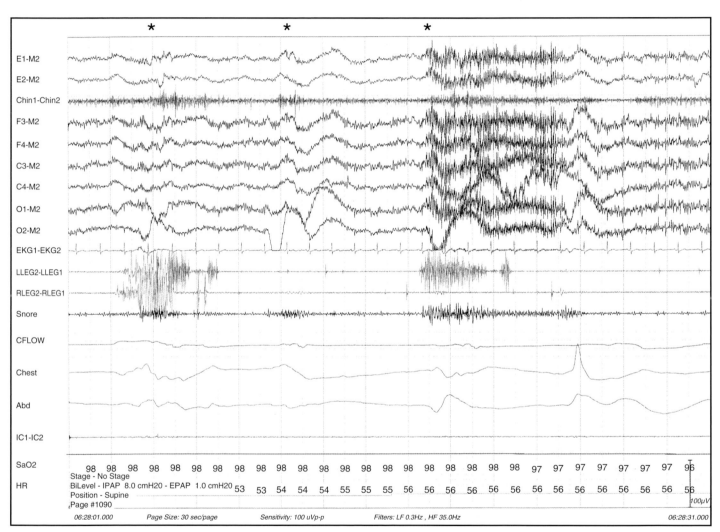

• **Figure 45.36** Scratching. (Copyright James Geyer and JNP Media [2016]. Used with permission.)

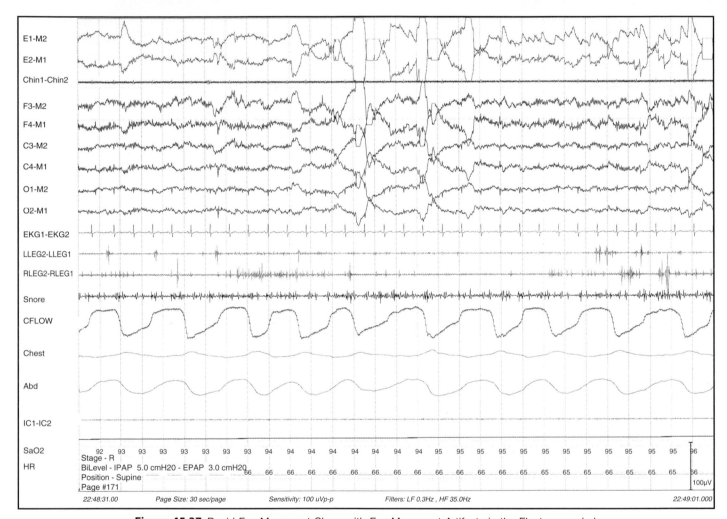

• **Figure 45.37** Rapid Eye Movement Sleep with Eye Movement Artifacts in the Electroencephalogram Channels. (Copyright James Geyer and JNP Media [2016]. Used with permission.)

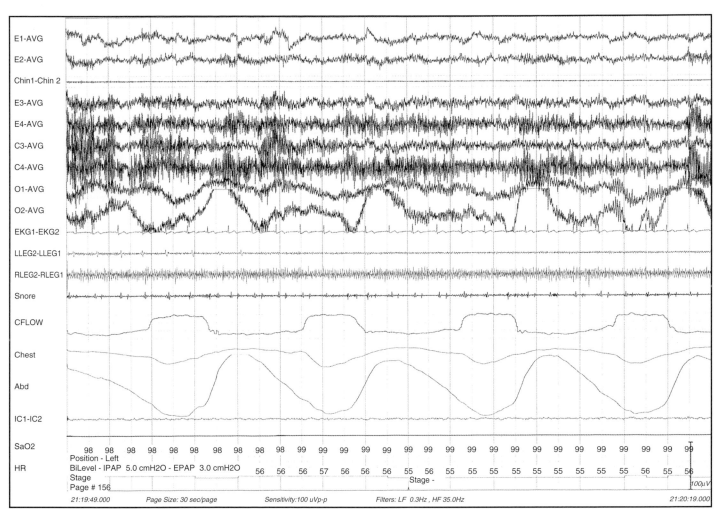

• **Figure 45.38** Respiratory Artifact in the Occipital Leads. (Copyright James Geyer and JNP Media [2016]. Used with permission.)

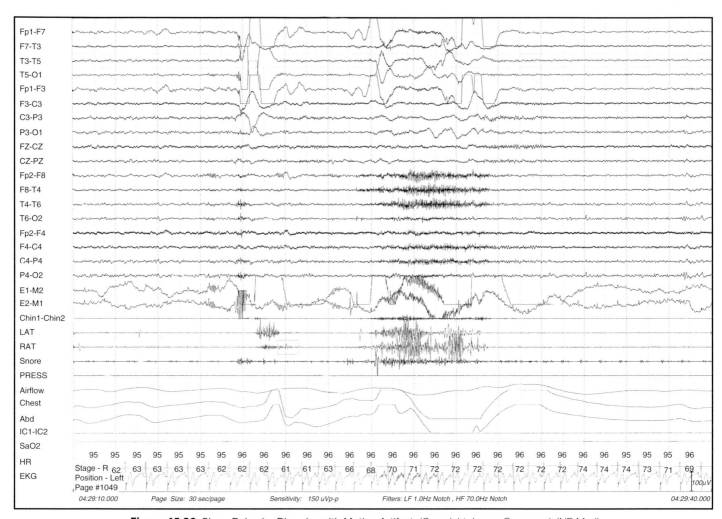

• **Figure 45.39** Sleep Behavior Disorder with Motion Artifact. (Copyright James Geyer and JNP Media [2016]. Used with permission.)

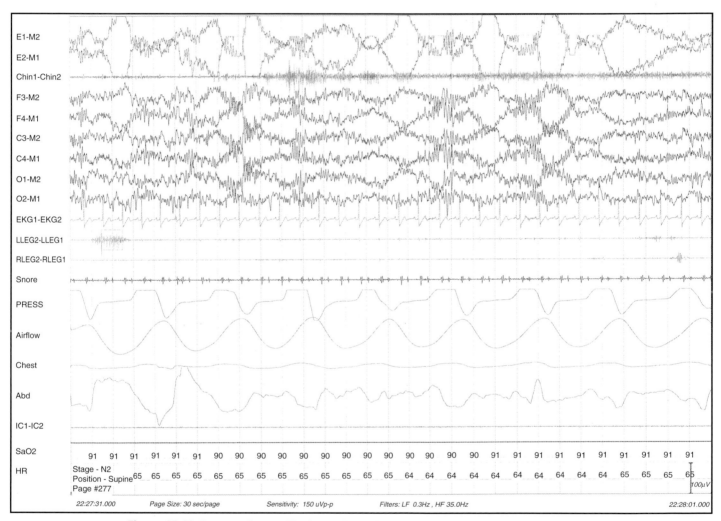

• **Figure 45.40** Pressure Sensor Clipping Artifact. (Copyright James Geyer and JNP Media [2016]. Used with permission.)

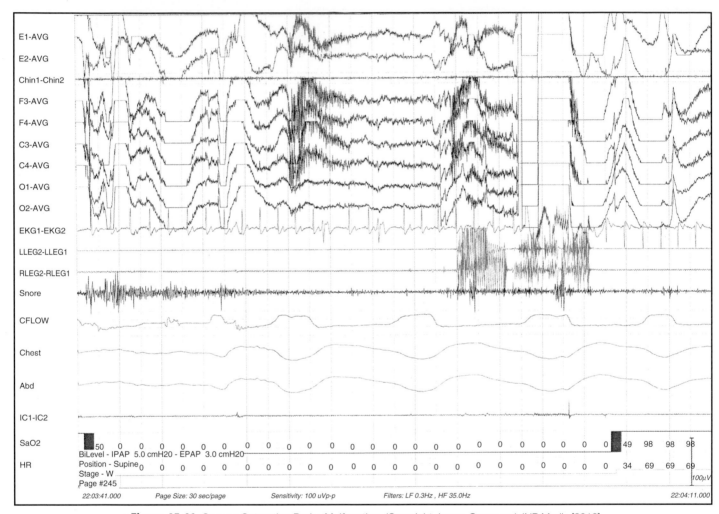

• **Figure 45.41** Oxygen Saturation Probe Malfunction. (Copyright James Geyer and JNP Media [2016]. Used with permission.)

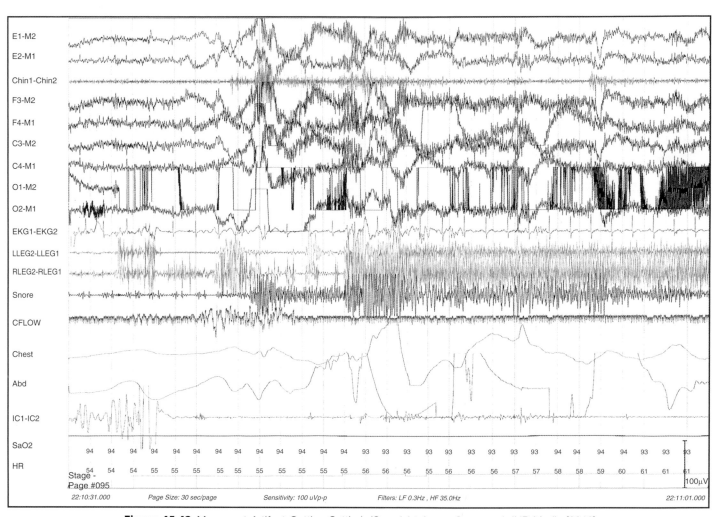

• **Figure 45.42** Movement Artifact Getting Settled. (Copyright James Geyer and JNP Media [2016]. Used with permission.)

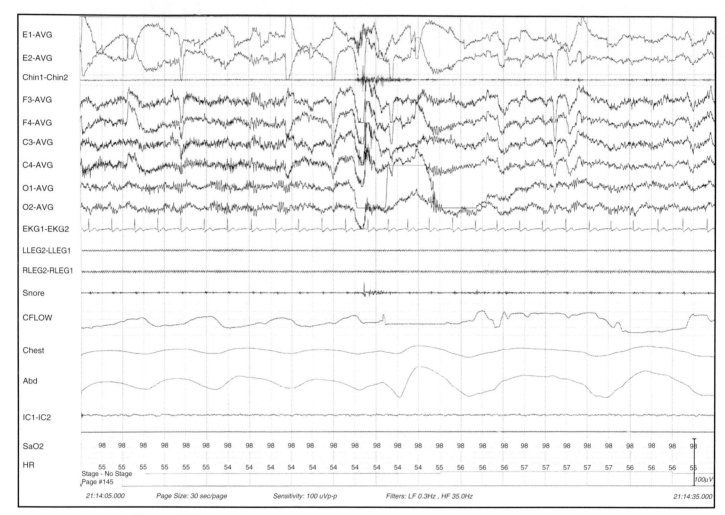

• **Figure 45.43** Loss of Mask Flow with Motion Artifact. (Copyright James Geyer and JNP Media [2016]. Used with permission.)

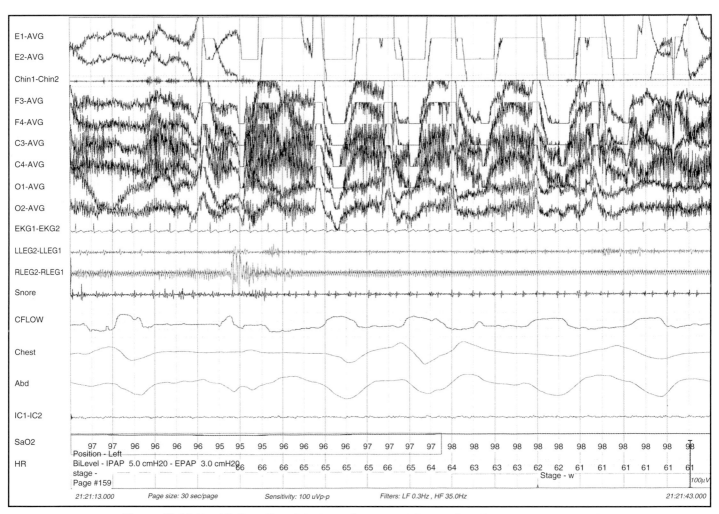

• **Figure 45.44** Head Rolling. (Copyright James Geyer and JNP Media [2016]. Used with permission.)

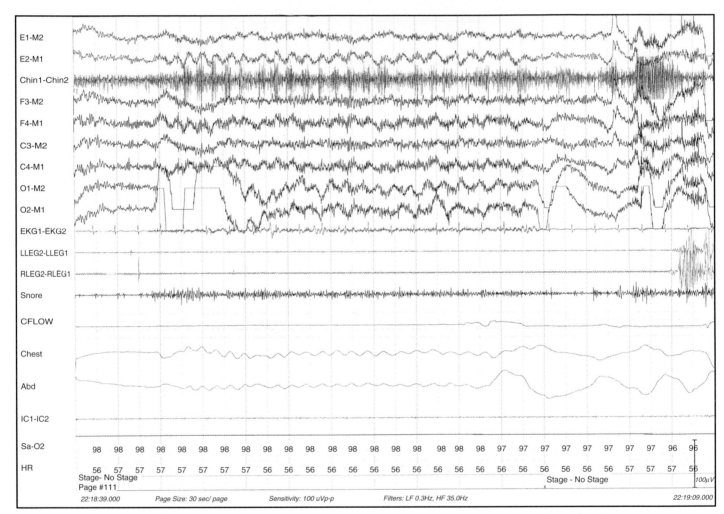

• **Figure 45.45** Face Rubbing. (Copyright James Geyer and JNP Media [2016]. Used with permission.)

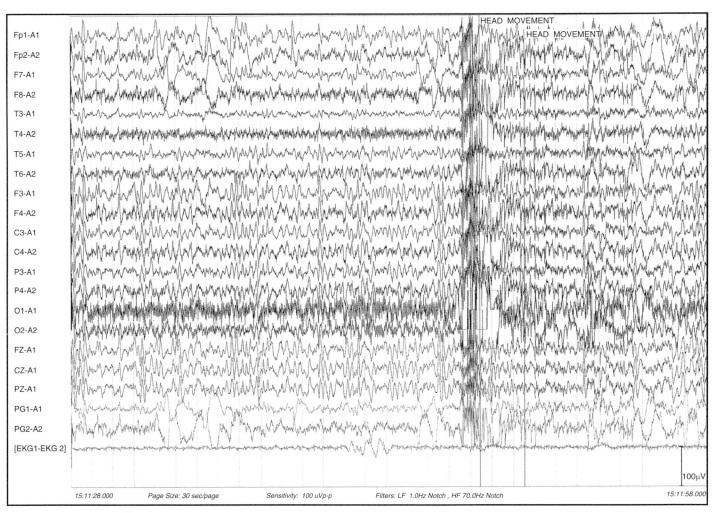

• **Figure 45.46** Awake Slowing in a Patient with Dementia. (Copyright James Geyer and Neurotexion [2016]. Used with permission.)

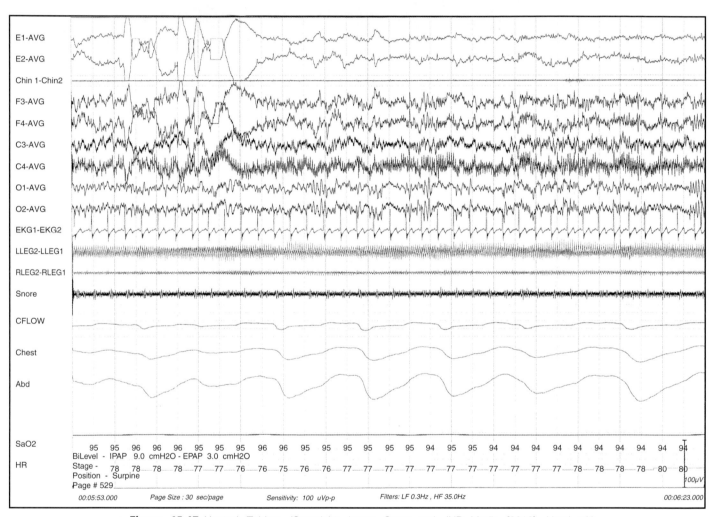

- **Figure 45.47** Heated Tubing. (Copyright James Geyer and JNP Media [2016]. Used with permission.)

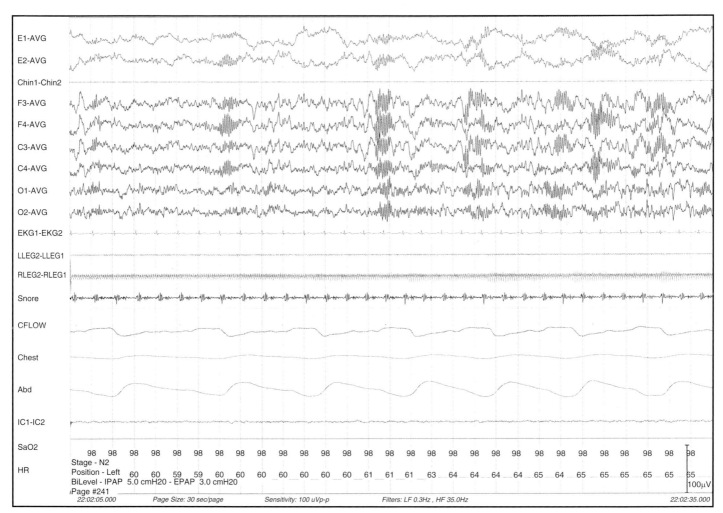

• **Figure 45.48** Sleep Spindles in the Electrooculogram. (Copyright James Geyer and JNP Media [2016]. Used with permission.)

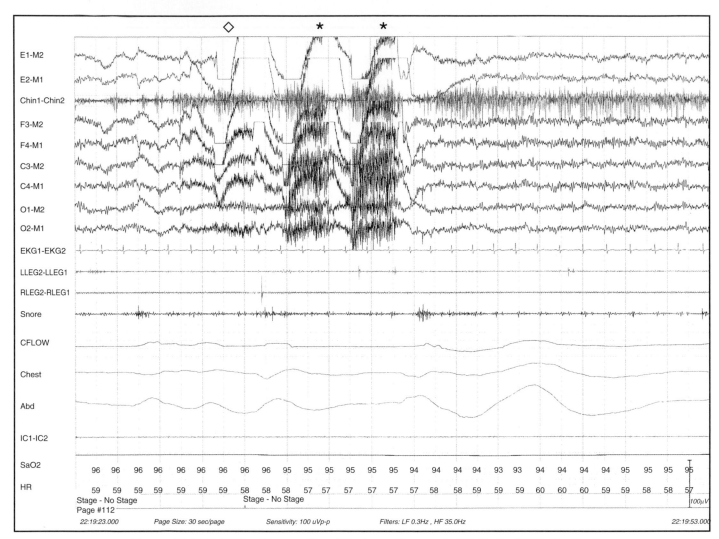

• **Figure 45.49** Tight Eye Closure. (Copyright James Geyer and JNP Media [2016]. Used with permission.)

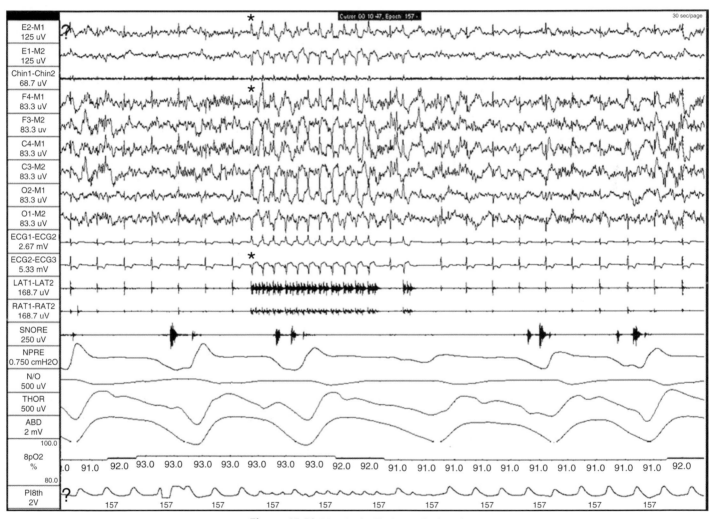

• **Figure 45.50** Ventricular Tachycardia *(stars)*.

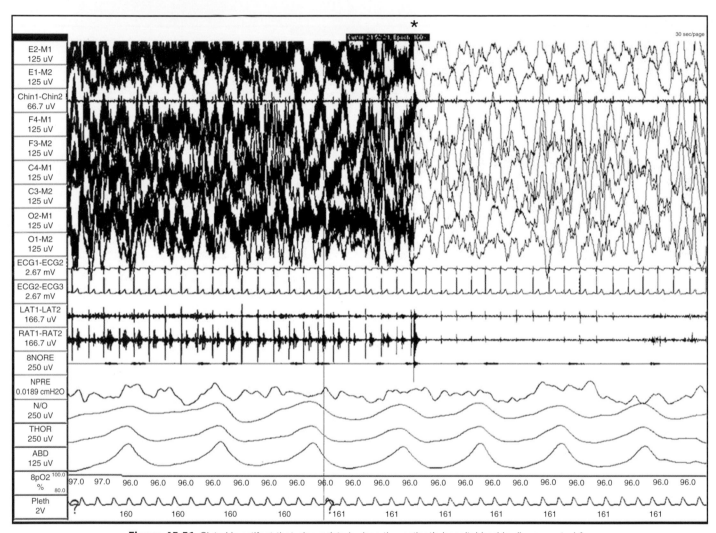

• **Figure 45.51** Sixty-Hz artifact that clears *(star)* when the patient's hospital bed is disconnected from the power supply (30-sec epoch).

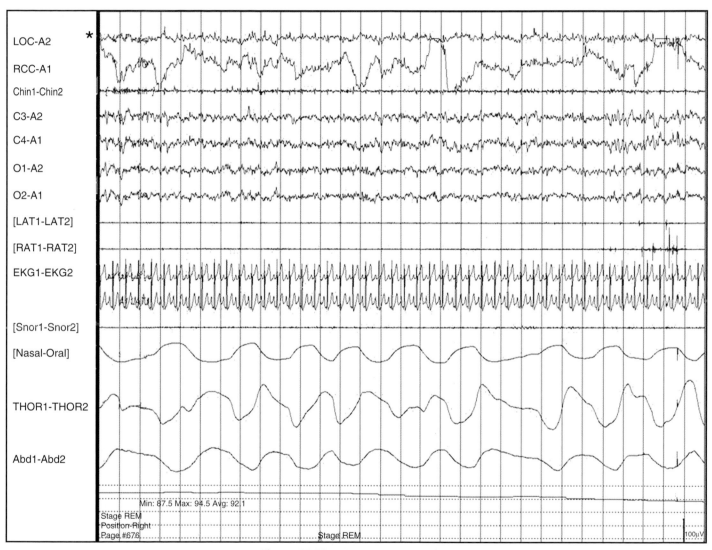

• **Figure 45.52** Left Eye Prosthesis *(star)*.

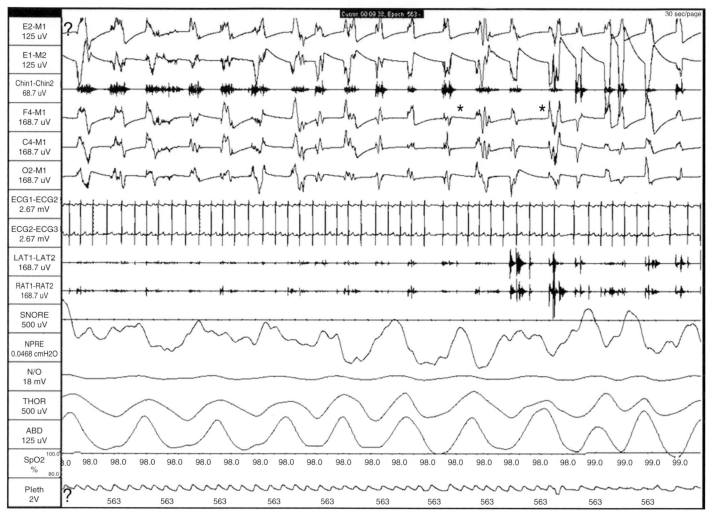

• **Figure 45.53** Ground Artifact *(stars).*

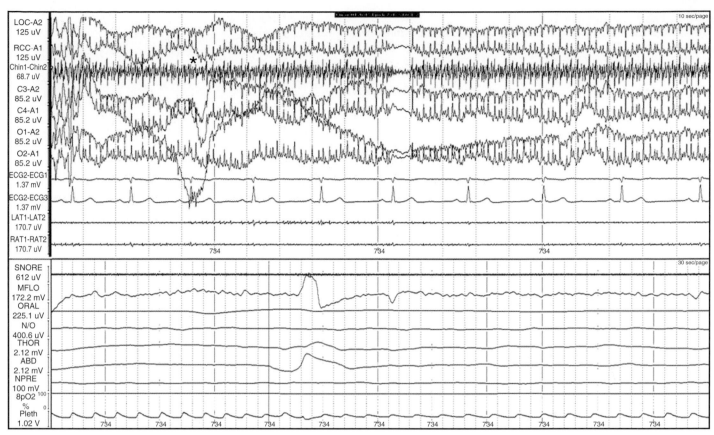

• **Figure 45.54** Vagus nerve stimulator (VNS) firing at about 13 Hz (*star*). VNS artifact frequency can vary depending on the settings of the VNS system. The artifact is intermittent because the VNS system fires on an intermittent basis. It is possible to disable the VNS, which will eliminate the artifact. This should not be done without the permission of the managing neurologist/epileptologist.

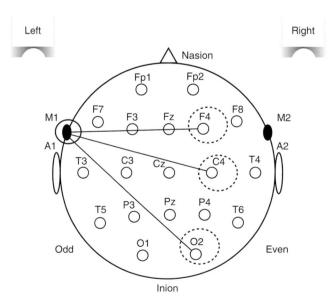

• **Figure 45.55** International 10-20 System of Electrode Placement.

Channel Key

The standard PSG montage was used and included the following:

Electrooculogram (left: LOC-A2, right: ROC-A1): LOC and ROC, left and right outer canthus EOG electrodes

EEG: C3-A2, C4-A1, O1-A2, and O2-A1, left central, right central, left occipital, and right occipital; electrode location: ground (FPZ), reference (CZ), and A1 and A2 (mastoids)

E1: Left outer canthus eye electrode

E2: Right outer canthus eye electrode

Chin1-Chin 2: submental EMG signal

M1: Left mastoid electrode location

M2: Right mastoid electrode location

C3 and O1: Left central and occipital EEG electrodes

C4 and O2: Right central and occipital EEG electrodes

EMG electrodes: LAT1-LAT2 and RAT1-RAT2, left and right lower limb electrodes

Two standard ECG leads are included: ECG1-ECG2, ECG2-ECG3

SNORE: Snore sensor sound

N/O: Nasal/oral thermistor

ORAL/N/O AIR-flow: Nasal-oral airflow

NPRE: Nasal pressure signal

THOR/CHEST and ABD: Chest and abdominal walls motion effort

MFLO: Mask flow of CPAP

PCO_2: mm Hg of carbon dioxide

SpO_2: Percent oxygen desaturation by pulse oximetry with a finger probe

Pt Position: Patient position (supine, left, right, prone)

NPRE: Nasal pressure

Pleth: Plethysmography

EEG electrodes:

Fp: Frontopolar or prefrontal

F: Frontal

C: Central

T: Temporal

P: Parietal

O: Occipital

A: Ear or mastoid

F3: Left midfrontal

P3: Left parietal

T4: Right temporal

A1: Right ear

Cz: Vertex

Suggested Reading

Benbadis S, Reilo D EEG artifacts. *eMedicine*; 2010.

Huynh N, Lavigne GJ, Okura K, et al. Sleep bruxism. *Handb Clin Neurol.* 2011;99:901-911.

International Classification of Sleep Disorders. 3rd ed. Illinois, IL, Westchester: American Academy of Sleep Medicine; 2014.

Spriggs WH. *Essentials of Polysomnography: A Training Guide and Reference for Sleep Technicians.* Carrollton, Texas: Sleep ed; 2008.

The Atlas Task Force. Recording and scoring leg movements. *Sleep.* 1993;16(8):748-759.

46

Use of Statistics in Sleep Medicine: Exam Questions

RON D. HAYS, HONGHU LIU

Questions

A sample of 1003 people completed a self-reported sleep problem measure with a possible score of 0–100; higher scores represented more problems. In addition, polysomnogram readings were used to identify any sleep disorder. Consider the self-reported measure to be a screener and classification of sleep disorders, with polysomnography as the gold standard.

Of the sample, a total of 152 people were identified as having a sleep disorder (15% prevalence rate). Use of a cut point of greater than 35 on the self-reported sleep problem measure yielded the contingency table shown in Table 46.1.

1. The frequencies observed for the four cells shown in Table 46.1 are 693, 37, 158, and 115. The expected frequencies, assuming independence between sleep disorder and the self-reported measure, for these four cells can be estimated from the marginal distributions (i.e., row totals and column totals) by multiplying the corresponding row and column totals for each cell and dividing the product by the total number of observations. The expected frequencies for Table 46.1 are approximately 619, 111, 232, and 41. The sum of the expected frequencies equals:
   A. 851
   B. 152
   C. 730
   D. 273
   E. 1003

2. The Pearson chi-square statistic for the data in Table 46.1 depicting the association between sleep disorder and the sleep-reported measure is 212.19, with a probability of less than 0.0001. This means that:
   A. Sleep disorder and the self-reported measure are independent of one another.
   B. Sleep disorder and the self-reported measure are not associated with one another.
   C. Sleep disorder and the self-reported measure are associated with one another.

   D. Sleep disorder and the self-reported measure are causally related to one another.
   E. The sum of observed frequencies differs from the sum of expected frequencies.

3. What is the sensitivity of the self-reported measure to sleep disorder at a cutoff of greater than 35?
   A. 42%
   B. 72%
   C. 76%
   D. 81%
   E. 95%

4. What is its specificity?
   A. 42%
   B. 72%
   C. 76%
   D. 81%
   E. 95%

5. What is the positive predictive value?
   A. 42%
   B. 72%
   C. 76%
   D. 81%
   E. 95%

6. What is the negative predictive value?
   A. 42%
   B. 72%
   C. 76%
   D. 81%
   E. 95%

7. What would be the positive predictive value if the prevalence of sleep problems was 39% instead of 15%?
   A. 42%
   B. 72%
   C. 76%
   D. 81%
   E. 95%

8. What would be the negative predictive value if the prevalence of sleep problems was 57% instead of 15%?
   A. 42%
   B. 72%
   C. 76%
   D. 81%
   E. 95%

TABLE 46.1	Self-Reported Sleep Problems by Polysomnogram-Defined Sleep Disorder		
	No Sleep Disorder	With Sleep Disorder	Row Totals
≤35 on self-report	693	37	730
>35 on self-report	158	115	273
Column totals	851	152	1003

TABLE 46.2	Stroke or Death by Apnea		
Apnea-Hypopnea Index	No Stroke or Death	Stroke or Death	Row Totals
AHI ≤3	258	13	271
AHI >36	216	34	250

AHI, Apnea-hypopnea index.

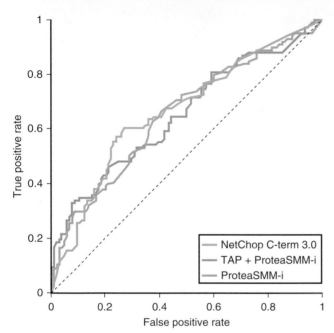

• **Figure 46.1** Receiver operating curve of three different human immunodeficiency virus epitope predictors. (Image from Wikipedia.)

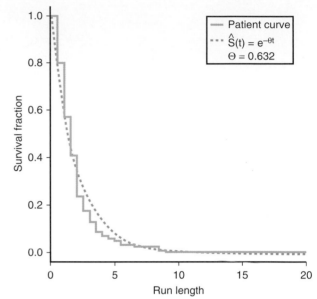

• **Figure 46.2** Fit of survival regression curve based on exponential distribution. The *solid line* shows the Kaplan-Meier survival curve in one subject with severe sleep-disordered breathing. The *dashed line* is the fitted survival regression curve. For this subject, the value of theta is 0.632, which provides a unidimensional measure of sleep continuity.

Receiver operating characteristic (ROC) curves are shown in Fig. 46.1. From Wikipedia: http://en.wikipedia.org/wiki/File:Roccurves.png. Fig. 46.1 shows three different human immunodeficiency virus (HIV) epitope predictors.

9. The ROC curve plots sensitivity on the *y*-axis. What does the *x*-axis represent?
   A. True-positive rate
   B. True-negative rate
   C. False-positive rate
   D. 1 − specificity
   E. Both C and D

Sleep stage records from full nocturnal polysomnography were used to define contiguous epochs of sleep (sleep runs). A run started with a change from wakefulness to any stage of sleep. A run ended when there was a change from stages 2, 3, 4, or rapid eye movement (REM) sleep to either stage 1 or wakefulness or from stage 1 to wakefulness. Fig. 46.2 shows a distribution of sleep runs (in minutes) for an individual with severe sleep-disordered breathing.[1] The solid curve is a Kaplan-Meier survival curve. The dashed line is a fitted survival regression curve.

10. A sleep duration of 5 minutes or longer was observed for what proportion of runs?

A. 0%
B. <20%
C. ≈40%
D. ≈60%
E. ≈80%

Table 46.2 shows incidents of stroke or death by apnea-hypopnea index (AHI).[2]

11. What is the *odds ratio* for stroke or death in those with a higher versus lower AHI score?
   A. 1.25
   B. 2.84
   C. 3.12
   D. 4.07
   E. 5.52

12. What is the *relative risk* for stroke or death in those with a higher versus lower AHI score?
   A. 1.25
   B. 2.84
   C. 3.12
   D. 4.07
   E. 5.52

A small study of six people finds that the three who are obese are more likely to have sleep apnea than the three who

TABLE 46.3	Obesity by Apnea	
Apnea	No Obesity	Obesity
No	2	0
Yes	1	3

are not obese (Table 46.3). That is, all three of the obese individuals have apnea but only one of the nonobese does. The product-moment correlation between obesity and sleep apnea in this sample is 0.707, and the two-tailed probability is 0.1161.

13. What is the independent variable?
    A. Obesity
    B. Apnea
    C. The six people in the study
    D. The three people in the obese group
    E. The three people in the nonobese group

14. How much variance in common do the obesity and apnea variables share in this sample?
    A. 10%
    B. 25%
    C. 50%
    D. 71%
    E. 84%

15. Are obesity and apnea statistically significantly associated at a probability of less than 0.05 in this sample?
    A. No
    B. Yes, using a one-tailed test of significance
    C. Yes, using a two-tailed test of significance
    D. Yes, using a three-tailed test of significance
    E. Yes, using any test of significance

Answers

1. **The correct answer is E. 1003.**
   The sum of expected frequencies is 619 + 111 + 232 + 41 = 1003. Note that the sum of expected frequencies equals the sum of observed frequencies. The similarity in observed and expected frequencies within the four cells indicates a lack of association between the two variables. Differences between the observed and expected frequencies beyond chance indicate a significant association.

2. **The correct answer is C. Sleep disorder and the self-reported measure are associated with one another.**
   The chi-square test evaluates whether the association between the two variables is statistically significant beyond what would be expected by chance. The formula for chi-square is the summation of (Observed frequency − Expected frequency)^2 ÷ (Expected frequency). Because the chi-square statistic is statistically significant, it means that the two variables are associated with one another. One cannot, however, conclude from this information that they are causally related to one another.

3. **The correct answer is C. 76%.**
   The numerator for sensitivity is the number of "true positives," or times that the screener (i.e., self-reported measure) exceeds the cut point *and* the gold standard (i.e., polysomnogram) indicates that the person has a sleep disorder (i.e., number of true positives = 115). The denominator is the sum of true

positives (i.e., 115) and false negatives (i.e., 37), or the number of times that the gold standard indicates that the person has a sleep disorder (i.e., 152). So the sensitivity is 115 ÷ 152 = 76%.

4. **The correct answer is D. 81%.**
   The numerator for specificity is the number of "true negatives," or times that the screener (i.e., self-report measure) is below the cut point *and* the gold standard (i.e., polysomnogram) indicates that the person does not have a sleep disorder (i.e., number of true negatives = 693). The denominator is the sum of true negatives (i.e., 693) and false positives (i.e., 158), or the number of times that the gold standard indicates that the person does not have a sleep disorder (i.e., 851). So the specificity is 693 ÷ 851 = 81%.

5. **The correct answer is A. 42%.**
   The positive predictive value is the proportion of persons with positive screener or test results who are correctly labeled as having the underlying condition. The numerator for the positive predictive value is the number of "true positives," or times that the screener (i.e., self-reported measure) exceeds the cut point *and* the gold standard (i.e., polysomnogram) indicates that the person has a sleep disorder (i.e., number of true positives = 115). The denominator is the sum of true positives and false positives, or the number of times that the screener exceeds the cut point (i.e., 273). So the positive predictive value is 115 ÷ 273 = 42%.

6. **The correct answer is E. 95%.**
   The negative predictive value is the proportion of persons with negative screener or test results who are correctly labeled as not having the underlying condition. The numerator for the negative predictive value is the number of "true negatives," or times that the screener (i.e., self-reported measure) is below the cut point *and* the gold standard (i.e., polysomnogram) indicates that the person does not have a sleep disorder (i.e., 693). The denominator is the sum of true negatives and false negatives (i.e., 37), or the number of times that the screener is below the cut point (i.e., 730). So the negative predictive value is 693 ÷ 730 = 95%.

7. **The correct answer is B. 72%.**
   The Bayes[3] formula for positive predictive value is

$$\frac{\text{Specificity} \times \text{Prevalence}}{(\text{Sensitivity} \times \text{Prevalence}) + [(1 - \text{Specificity}) \times (1 - \text{Prevalence})]}$$

   Because the sensitivity is 0.76, the prevalence 0.39, and the specificity is 0.81, the positive predictive value is 72%.

8. **The correct answer is B. 72%.**
   The Bayes[3] formula for negative predictive value is

$$\frac{\text{Specificity} \times (1 - \text{Prevalence})}{[\text{Specificity} \times (1 - \text{Prevalence})] + [(1 - \text{Sensitivity}) \times \text{Prevalence}]}$$

   Because the specificity is 0.81, the prevalence is 0.57, and the sensitivity is 0.76, the negative predictive value is 72%.

9. **The correct answer is E. Both C and D.**
   Plotted on the *x*-axis is 1 − specificity, or the false-positive rate—these are the same. The dotted line indicates what would be expected by chance alone, whereas the curves above the dotted line indicate improvements over chance (true-positive rate exceeding the false-positive rate).

10. **The correct answer is B. <20%.**

The fraction of runs that are 0 minutes or longer is 1.0 by definition (represented in the top left of Fig. 46.2). About 0.20 of the runs are around 3 minutes or longer. The patient curve flattens out well below the survival fraction of 0.20, and is a little above the survival fraction of 0.0 for run lengths of 5–20 minutes. Run lengths of 5 minutes or longer do occur, but they constitute less than 0.20 of the total number of run durations (survival times).

11. **The correct answer is C. 3.12.**

The odds ratio is the relative odds for stroke or death for the two groups of people (those with AHI >36 vs. AHI ≤3). The odds for those with an AHI greater than 36 is 34 ÷ 216 = 0.16; the odds for those with an AHI ≤3 is 13 ÷ 258 = 0.05. The odds ratio is (34 × 258) ÷ (216 × 13) = 3.12.

12. **The correct answer is B. 2.84.**

The relative risk (also known as the risk ratio) is the ratio of the probability of stroke or death in two groups of people (those with AHI >36 vs. AHI ≤3). The probability of stroke or death for those with an AHI >36 is 34 ÷ 250 = 0.14; the probability for those with an AHI ≤3 is 13 ÷ 271 = 0.05. The relative risk is (34 × 271) ÷ (250 × 13) = 2.84.

13. **The correct answer is A. Obesity.**

The independent variable is the variable that theoretically influences or has an effect on the dependent variable. In this study, obesity is considered the independent variable because it is expected to lead to or cause sleep apnea rather than vice versa.

14. **The correct answer is C. 50%.**

The correlation indicates the relationship between two variables. Correlations range from −1.00 to 1.00, with −1.00 representing a perfect negative correlation and 1.00 representing a perfect positive correlation φ. A correlation of 0.00 indicates no relationship between the variables.

As stated, the correlation between obesity and apnea is r = 0.707. The correlation between two dichotomous variables is a phi coefficient. If "a" represents the number in the upper left cell (2), "b" the number in the upper right cell (0), "c" the number in the lower left cell (1), "d" the number in the lower right cell (3), "e" the total of the first row (2), "f" the total of the second row (4), "g" the total of the first column (3), and "h" the total of the second column (3), then phi (φ), is

$$(a \times d) - (b \times c) \div \sqrt{e \times f \times g \times h} =$$
$$(2 \times 3) - (0 \times 1) \div \sqrt{2 \times 4 \times 3 \times 3} = 6 \div 8.485 = 0.707$$

The variance shared in common is the correlation squared. Hence, the variance in common between obesity and apnea is 0.707 × 0.707 = 0.50, or 50%.

15. **The correct answer is A. No.**

The two-tailed significance level is noted to be 0.1161. This is larger than the cutoff level of 0.05 for statistical significance. The one-tailed significance level is 0.1161 ÷ 2 = 0.058. This is also larger than the probability cutoff level of 0.05. A three-tailed test of significance does not exist. Because the two-tailed and one-tailed tests of significance indicate lack of significance, choice E is also incorrect.

Commonly Used Statistical Terms

- **Chi-square distribution:** A variable is said to have a chi-square (χ^2) distribution with K degrees of freedom if it is distributed like the sum of the squares of K independent random variables, each of which has a normal distribution with a mean of 0 and a variance of 1.
- **Cut point:** An arbitrarily chosen point or value in an ordered sequence of values that is used to separate the whole into parts.
- **False negative:** Negative test result in a person who possesses the attribute for which the test is conducted. Labeling of a diseased person as healthy when screening for the detection of disease.
- **False positive:** Positive test result in a person who does not possess the attribute for which the test is conducted. Labeling of a healthy person as diseased when screening for the detection of disease.
- **Gold standard:** A method, procedure, or measurement that is widely accepted as being the best available. It is often used for comparison with a new method.
- **Kaplan-Meier estimate:** A nonparametric method of compiling life or survival tables. It combines calculated probabilities of survival and estimates to allow censored observations, which are assumed to occur randomly.
- **Negative predicted value:** The proportion of patients with negative test results in whom the condition is correctly diagnosed.
- **Odds:** The ratio of the probability of occurrence of an event to that of nonoccurrence, or the ratio of the probability that something is so to the probability that it is not so.
- **Odds ratio:** The ratio of the odds in favor of exposure among cases to the odds in favor of exposure among noncases.
- **Pearson product-moment correlation coefficient:** Widely used in the sciences as a measure of the strength of linear association between two variables.
- **Positive predicted value:** Proportion of patients with positive test results in whom the condition is correctly diagnosed.
- **Prevalence:** The number of events in a given population at a designated time.
- **ROC curve:** Graphic means for assessing the ability of a screening test to discriminate between healthy and diseased persons.
- **Relative risk:** Ratio of the risk for disease or death among the exposed to the risk among the unexposed. Alternatively, the ratio of the cumulative incidence rate in the exposed to the cumulative incidence rate in the unexposed.
- **Sensitivity:** Proportion of truly diseased persons in the screened population who are identified as diseased by the screening test. It is a measure of the probability of correctly diagnosing a condition or the probability that any given condition will be identified by the test.
- **Specificity:** Proportion of truly nondiseased persons who are so identified by the screening test. It is a measure of the probability of correctly identifying a nondiseased person with a screening test.

47

Knowing Your Sleep Practice Parameters

KIMBERLY NICOLE MIMS, DOUGLAS BENJAMIN KIRSCH

AASM Practice Parameter Review Questions

1. A 6-year-old boy is brought to the clinic by his mother for episodes occurring during sleep. She describes episodes of repetitive jerking of the body that last 1–2 minutes and are sometimes associated with him yelling. He is unaware of the episodes, and he had a normal routine electroencephalogram (EEG) with no sleep recorded. The next most appropriate step is:
   A. Order magnetic resonance imaging (MRI)
   B. Order multiple sleep latency test (MSLT)
   C. Order polysomnography with expanded EEG montage
   D. Order polysomnography with extra arm electromyography (EMG) leads

2. A 12-year-old girl presents after developing bedwetting after resolution of bedwetting at the age of 4. She also snores and her teachers complain that she often falls asleep during classes. The most appropriate next step in her care is:
   A. Order polysomnography
   B. Order polysomnography with MSLT
   C. Refer to urology for complex bedwetting
   D. Start desmopressin for enuresis

Secondary Causes of Nocturnal Enuresis

Urinary tract infection	Bladder dysfunction	Chronic renal failure
Constipation	Diabetes insipidus	Diabetes mellitus
Hyperthyroidism	Obstructive sleep apnea	Pinworm infection
Psychological stress	Seizure disorder	Sickle cell disease

Aurora RN, Lamm CI, Zak RS, et al. Practice parameters for the non-respiratory indications for polysomnography and multiple sleep latency testing for children. *Sleep.* 2012;35(11):1467–1473.

3. A 13-year-old boy complains of growing pains and fragmented sleep during the night. Mom reports noticing excessive leg movements while he is asleep. His sleep study demonstrates no sleep-disordered breathing and a periodic limb movement index of 15 events per hour. Which of the following is most specific for a diagnosis of restless legs syndrome (RLS) in this patient?
   A. Patient report of growing pains
   B. Patient report of fragmented sleep
   C. Report of excessive leg movements during sleep
   D. Periodic limb movement index greater than 5 events per hour

4. A 5-year-old boy presents with his mother complaining of the child's irritability and decreased attention. His mother notes that he snores heavily at night and seems to be restless during sleep. His tonsils are enlarged and he has mild retrognathia. A polysomnogram reveals an apnea-hypopnea index (AHI) of 10 events per hour. The most appropriate therapy is:
   A. Adenotonsillectomy
   B. Oral appliance
   C. PAP therapy
   D. Tracheostomy

5. Two young parents present with their 4-year-old girl because of her sleep disturbance. She often wakes during the night and cries loudly. She usually will not stop crying unless a parent comes into the room, at which point the crying stops immediately. The most appropriate next step is:
   A. Advising the parents to taper their response to her crying
   B. Advise the parents to let the child sleep in their bed
   C. Order a polysomnogram with expanded EEG montage
   D. Start melatonin to help with sleep maintenance insomnia

6. A 58-year-old man presents to sleep clinic complaining of difficulty falling asleep due to his racing mind. He has no comorbid illnesses and does not take any medications other than over the counter sleep aids. He feels too exhausted to engage in activities after work, but rarely dozes during the daytime or in the evening. His workup should include which of the following first steps:
   A. Actigraphy
   B. Blood work
   C. Polysomnography
   D. Sleep diary

7. The best initial management of the above patient includes: (linked to question 6 above)
   A. Cognitive behavioral therapy
   B. Meditation
   C. Quetiapine
   D. Sleep hygiene

8. A 46-year-old woman presents to clinic complaining of difficulty falling asleep and staying asleep. Her medication list includes insulin, allopurinol, loratadine, and citalopram. The medication most likely to be contributing to insomnia is:
   A. Allopurinol
   B. Citalopram
   C. Insulin
   D. Loratadine

9. A 34-year-old woman complains of difficulty falling asleep. She is interested in nonpharmacologic therapy. Her mind races when she has trouble falling asleep, and she often relives the day or starts thinking about the coming day. You recommend:
   A. Biofeedback
   B. Relaxation therapy
   C. Sleep hygiene
   D. Sleep restriction

10. A 22-year-old woman presents with complaints of excessive daytime sleepiness. She sometimes falls to the ground if she laughs too hard or gets overly excited. She describes episodes of feeling like "a witch is riding me" sometimes as she is waking out of sleep. After testing confirms her diagnosis, the most appropriate pharmacologic therapy is:
    A. Amitriptyline
    B. Dextroamphetamine
    C. Methylphenidate
    D. Modafinil

11. A sleep consultation is requested on a 27-year-old man while in rehabilitation after being hospitalized following a flu-like illness with prolonged episodes of sleepiness, irritability, childish behavior, and excessive food intake. During episodes, he has difficulty being awoken and his family is frustrated due to his difficulty participating in rehabilitation. The most appropriate pharmacological treatment of this disorder is:
    A. Armodafinil
    B. Citalopram
    C. Lithium carbonate
    D. Sodium oxybate

12. A female patient with narcolepsy is trying to get pregnant. The best therapy for sleepiness in a patient with narcolepsy during pregnancy is:
    A. Amphetamine
    B. Modafinil
    C. Napping
    D. Protriptyline

13. A 64-year-old man presents with his wife complaining of dream enactment episodes. His wife describes him as jumping out of bed, screaming and yelling, and occasionally grabbing her arm or pushed her out of bed. He once had to go to the ED because he kicked the wall so hard while sleeping he fractured one of his toes. If his wife wakes him, he remembers dreaming, usually about being chased or trying to fight someone or something. He does not have any bowel or bladder incontinence associated with the episodes. He does not have a history of seizures, head trauma, or strokes. During exam, you check for:

A. Intention tremor
B. Nail pitting
C. Peripheral edema
D. Reduced facial expression

14. A 32-year-old man presents complaining of leg discomfort at night. He describes it as a tingling or numbness sensation temporarily relieved by moving his legs. He can try to avoid moving his legs but eventually the urge becomes so great that he cannot resist moving his legs. The symptoms are worse at night. What other symptom confirms the suspected diagnosis?
    A. Daytime sleepiness
    B. History of diabetes
    C. Relief with dopaminergic agents
    D. Symptoms that worsen with rest

15. After establishing the correct diagnosis in the above patient (linked to Q14 above), the most appropriate next step is:
    A. Confirm the diagnosis with actigraphy
    B. Confirm the diagnosis with polysomnography
    C. Start levodopa with dopa decarboxylase inhibitor
    D. Start a dopamine agonist

16. A 54-year-old man presents complaining of limb discomfort and feeling like there is "popcorn" in his legs when he lies down to sleep at night. He achieves temporary relief by rubbing or smacking his legs. He also has hypertension. He has tried ropinirole, gabapentin, and pramipexole without relief. His iron studies, including ferritin, are normal. The next most appropriate therapy is:
    A. Clonidine
    B. IV Iron
    C. Mirtazepine
    D. Pergolide

17. Home sleep apnea testing must monitor, at a minimum, the following factors:
    A. Blood oxygen, airflow, and respiratory effort
    B. Blood oxygen, airflow, and heart rate
    C. Electroencephalography, respiratory effort, and airflow.
    D. Electroencephalography, heart rate, and airflow

18. A 68-year-old man presents to clinic complaining of excessive sleepiness, particularly in the evening. He finds it difficult to maintain wakefulness after dinner. He also finds it challenging to return to sleep after 4 AM, so he typically gets up for the day at that time. He snores lightly but does not have witnessed apneas. He wakes 1–2 times/night. He does not fall asleep during work hours. The best next step in his care is to order:
    A. A hypnotic medication
    B. Actigraphy for 7 days
    C. Home sleep apnea testing
    D. In-lab polysomnography

19. A mother brings her 15-year-old boy to the office, complaining that she cannot seem to get her son to go to bed or wake at a reasonable hour. She thinks he goes to bed at 11 PM but when you question him without mom in the room, he reports he does not fall asleep until 1 AM–2 AM. He must wake for school at 6:30 AM but on the weekends, he often stays up quite late and sleeps until 11 AM. His mother reports rare snoring, no apneic spells. Your next step is to use:
    A. 7-day Actigraphy
    B. In-laboratory polysomnography
    C. Home sleep apnea testing
    D. A hypnotic medication

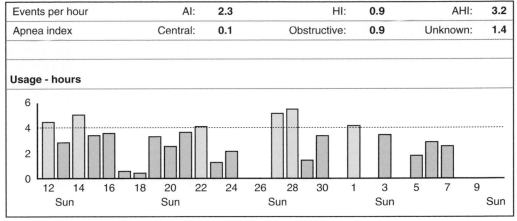

| Events per hour | | AI: | **2.3** | | HI: | **0.9** | AHI: | **3.2** |
| Apnea index | | Central: | **0.1** | | Obstructive: | **0.9** | Unknown: | **1.4** |

• **Figure 47.1** Download data from CPAP at 9 cmH₂O. *AI*, Apnea index; *HI*, hypopnea index; *AHI*, apnea-hypopnea index. Usage graph shows *X*-axis: time in days, *Y*-axis: time in hours.

20. A 24-year-old man presents complaining of excessive daytime sleepiness. He often falls asleep at work and cannot stay awake when watching movies. He voluntarily relinquished driving because of his significant other's concern about his dozing at the wheel. He complains of some sleep disruption as well but does not have difficulty returning to sleep after an awakening. Sometimes when he laughs, his head starts to feel heavy and falls to his chest. To further diagnose his condition, you order:
    A. Blood work including human leukocyte antigen (HLA) typing for narcolepsy
    B. Full-head EEG during his periods of muscle weakness
    C. Polysomnography with a maintenance of wakefulness test
    D. Polysomnography with a MSLT
21. A 32-year-old man comes to clinic complaining of difficulty falling asleep. He finds it difficult to fall asleep before 2 AM. He also has trouble getting up in the morning and often dozes at work in the morning. He does not complain of daytime sleepiness on his weekends when he is able to sleep in. A sleep diary reveals he sleeps from 2 AM–7 AM on weekdays and from 2 AM–10 AM on weekends. You suggest (see Fig. 47.1):
    A. Melatonin administered at A
    B. Light administered at B
    C. Melatonin administered at C
    D. Light administered at D
22. A 54-year-old man with congestive heart failure (CHF) presents with difficulty maintaining sleep. He often develops swelling in his legs at night and sleeps with at least three pillows. An overnight sleep study reveals an overall AHI of 36 events per hour and a central apnea index (CAi) of 24 events per hour. The next most appropriate step is:
    A. Start Servo-Ventilation
    B. Start Auto-titrating CPAP
    C. Start BPAP with spontaneous timed mode
    D. Start CPAP therapy
23. A 36-year-old patient diagnosed with obstructive sleep apnea (OSA) presents to clinic complaining of difficulty using CPAP therapy. She often develops nasal congestion that limits her ability to tolerate her nasal mask. The recommended solution to her congestion is:

CORE BODY TEMPERATURE (CBT)

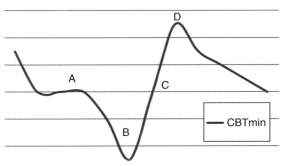

• **Figure 47.2** Core body temperature graph. *X*-axis: time; *Y*-axis: temperature from 36.5–38 degrees Celsius. *CBTmin*, Core body temperature minimum.

    A. Diphenhydramine daily
    B. Stop CPAP use during periods of rhinitis
    C. Fluticasone nasal spray daily
    D. Neosynephrine nasal spray daily
24. A 54-year-old woman presents for evaluation of snoring and nighttime awakenings. A sleep study demonstrates an AHI of 28 events per hour. After explaining the results of the study to her, you recommend CPAP therapy and:
    A. Follow-up in 3 days
    B. Follow-up in 3 weeks
    C. Follow-up in 3 months
    D. Follow-up at 1 year
25. A 45-year-old woman presents after starting CPAP therapy with cold Passover at 9 cm of water and her download looks like the figure below. She has no difficulty with pressure tolerance. Which of the following options is most likely to increase her CPAP use? (Fig. 47.2)
    A. Change interface to a full-face mask
    B. Increase pressure settings to 12 cm
    C. Initiate heated humidification
    D. Start temazepam to improve sleep quality

26. A 68-year-old postmenopausal lady presents after being diagnosed with obstructive sleep apnea. She continues complaining of fatigue despite adequate CPAP therapy. She developed high cholesterol and weight gain and always feels cold. Her hairstylist also has noted hair loss. The next most appropriate step is:
    A. Order an oral glucose tolerance test
    B. Order TSH and Free T4 levels
    C. Start estrogen replacement therapy
    D. Start daily modafinil therapy

27. A 56-year-old patient with a history of severe obstructive sleep apnea presents complaining of increased tiredness despite continued PAP therapy use. When he first started CPAP, he felt like "a million bucks" but now often requires a nap during his lunch break. After confirming no changes to his sleep history otherwise, the next best step is to perform:
    A. Actigraphy
    B. In-laboratory sleep test
    C. Home Sleep Apnea Testing
    D. Start modafinil therapy

28. A new sleep technologist calls to ask for clarification on appropriate technique for a PAP titration on a 45-year-old gentleman with severe sleep apnea. Yo u remind him that an optimal titration includes a RDI less than 5 events per hour for 15 minutes and observation of which of the following:
    A. NREM sleep
    B. Supine-REM sleep
    C. Any REM sleep
    D. Lateral-REM sleep

Answers

1. **Answer C.**
   A polysomnogram using an expanded EEG montage is indicated in a child with atypical or potentially injurious parasomnias or to differentiate a parasomnia from sleep-related epilepsy after an inconclusive clinical evaluation and standard EEG. If a parasomnia has any of the following characteristics, then a polysomnogram with expanded EEG is indicated: (1) unusual or atypical age of onset, time, duration, or frequency of occurrence of behavior or the motor patterns are stereotypical, repetitive, or focal, (2) if the activity is potentially injurious or caused injury to the patient or others, and/or (3) it could be seizure-related but the initial evaluation and standard EEG are inconclusive. In this case, the patient displays repetitive motor activity suspicious for seizure with an inconclusive EEG, so a polysomnogram with expanded EEG is indicated. An MSLT would not be indicated, and a MRI would not characterize the patient's events.[1]

2. **Answer A.**
   Recurrence of enuresis after 5 years, when nocturnal bladder continence is developmentally expected, can indicate obstructive sleep apnea, particularly with a supportive history, such as snoring or obesity, or is resistant to standard treatments. An MSLT is not indicated at this time. It would appear unlikely, based on the current history, that this is truly urologic problem. Desmopressin is a treatment for enuresis, but it would not necessarily be used until likely secondary causes had been ruled out.[1]

3. **Answer D.**
   Several studies demonstrated that PLM index greater than 5 events per hour is often helpful to diagnose children with RLS. In one study, complaints of growing pains, poor sleep, and parental history of RLS only provided a positive predictive value of 38% compared with overnight PSG with elevated periodic limb movements of sleep (PLMS). Similarly, parental report of a child kicking during sleep had a positive predictive value of only 10% for PLMS index greater than 5 events per hour.[1]

Diagnostic Criteria for Restless Legs Syndrome in Pediatrics

RLS Criteria	Urge to move the legs or leg discomfort Urge to move the legs or leg discomfort worsens during periods of inactivity Urge to move or leg discomfort relieved by movement Urge to move the legs or leg discomfort only occurs or worsens in evenings
Special considerations for diagnosis of RLS in pediatrics	Child describes RLS symptoms in own words Significant impact on sleep, mood, cognition, and function identified (impairment often manifests in behavioral and educational domains)
Associated findings commonly supporting diagnosis of pediatric RLS	PLMS > 5 per hour Family history of RLS in first degree relatives Family history of PLMS > 5 per hour Family history of PLMD in first degree relatives

PLMS, Periodic limb movements of sleep; *RLS*, restless legs syndrome.
Picchietti DL, Bruni O, de Weerd A, et al. Pediatric restless leg syndrome diagnostic criteria: an update by the International Restless legs syndrome study group. *Sleep Med.* 2013;14(12):1253–1259.

4. **Answer A.**
   The most appropriate treatment of children with large tonsils and mild obstructive sleep apnea is adenotonsillectomy. A following polysomnogram is also indicated if symptoms of sleep disruption persist and/or if the child has moderate to severe obstructive sleep apnea, obesity, craniofacial anomalies obstructing the upper airway, or neurologic disorders. Oral appliances are not first-line therapy for children due to maxillary expansion. PAP therapy is not indicated for children before adenotonsillectomy presuming they have no contraindications to surgery. If PAP therapy is utilized, an in-lab titration is indicated. Tracheostomy is not a first-line therapy for OSA, but if used, a polysomnography prior to decannulation is recommended in children to assess recurrence of sleep-related breathing disorders.[2]

5. **Answer A.**
   Usually this is done as graduated extinction as unmodified extinction has limited parental acceptance. Graduated extinction involves ignoring the child's crying and tantrums for specified periods and progressively lengthening the intervals (i.e., 5 minutes, then 10 minutes) to avoid reinforcing protest behavior.

TABLE 47.1	Definitions of Behavioral Treatment in Children with Night Wakings
Term	**Definition**
Unmodified extinction	Parents put child to bed at designated bedtime and ignore child until morning (while continuing to monitor for issues such as safety or illness)
Graduated extinction	Parents ignore bedtime crying and tantrums for scheduled periods before briefly checking on the child with progressive checking schedule (i.e., 5 minutes, then 10 minutes) intervals
Positive routines/ Faded bedtime with response cost	Bedtime routine characterized by enjoyable and quiet activities developed to establish a behavioral chain leading to sleep onset. Faded bedtime involves temporarily delaying bedtime to coincide with child's natural sleep time then fading it earlier as the child gains success falling asleep quickly. Response cost involves removing child from bed briefly if child does not fall asleep. These behavioral interventions focus on stimulus control.
Scheduled awakenings	Parents preemptively awaken the child prior to typical spontaneous awakening and provide "usual" responses such as feeding, rocking, soothing as if child awakened spontaneously
Parent education/ prevention	Educating parents to prevent development of sleep problems and incorporating behavioral intervention into these parent education programs

Morgenthaler TI, Owens J, Alessi C, et al. Practice parameters for behavioral treatment of bedtime problems and night wakings in infants and young children. *Sleep*. 2006;29(10): 1277–1281.

Children should not be encouraged to sleep with parents. A polysomnogram is not necessary as this child demonstrates behavior well suited to behavioral modification. Melatonin is also generally not indicated because behavioral therapy is the most effective treatment of bedtime problems and nighttime wakings in young children. For other behavioral treatments see Table 47.1. No single behavioral treatment or combination of treatments is more effective.[3]

6. **Answer D.**
Sleep diary data should ideally be collected prior to and during treatment of insomnia. A sleep log can help identify general patterns of sleep-wake times and day-to-day variability. Patients should also complete a general medical/psychiatric questionnaire and an Epworth Sleepiness Scale to assess comorbid disorders of sleepiness. Measures of subjective sleep quality, psychological assessment scales, daytime function, quality of life, and dysfunctional beliefs and attitudes can also be useful in treating the patient with chronic insomnia. Actigraphy may be useful in characterizing sleep patterns in patients who may have a circadian rhythm disorder, but is not necessary in the initial

workup of all insomnia patients. Blood work is not indicated unless there is a suspicion of comorbid medical disorders. Polysomnography is not indicated unless the initial diagnosis is uncertain, treatment fails, or arousals occur with violent or injurious behavior.[4]

7. **Answer A.**
Cognitive behavioral therapy for insomnia (CBTi) includes stimulus control therapy with relaxation therapy, or the combination of cognitive therapy, stimulus control therapy, sleep restriction therapy with or without relaxation therapy. Other aspects of CBTi are sleep restriction, paradoxical intention, and biofeedback therapy. When an initial psychological/behavioral treatment has been ineffective, combination therapy including CBTi with use of medication or an alternative therapy is recommended. Meditation alone has not been shown to be effective as a treatment for insomnia. Short-term hypnotic therapy can be supplemented with behavioral and cognitive therapies when possible but short-intermediate acting benzodiazepine receptor agonists or ramelteon are recommended initially over antidepressants, antipsychotics similar to quetiapine, or antiepileptics. Sleep hygiene is important and should be encouraged, but there is insufficient evidence indicating efficacy of sleep hygiene alone in improving insomnia.[4]

8. **Answer B.**
Medications are commonly associated with insomnia.

Medications Associated with Insomnia

Corticosteroids (e.g., prednisone and cortisone)	SSRIs (e.g., citalopram and fluoxetine)	MAOIs (e.g., selegiline)
Some TCAs (protriptyline, nortriptyline)	Stimulants (e.g., methylphenidate, dextroamphetamine, and caffeine)	Decongestants (e.g., pseudoephedrine)
Narcotic analgesics (e.g., oxycodone)	Beta blockers (e.g., propranolol and atenolol)	Alpha receptor blockers (e.g., doxazosin and tamsulosin)
Diuretics (e.g, furosemide)	Lipid lowering agents (e.g., pravastatin and rosuvastatin)	Cholinesterase inhibitors (e.g., donepezil and rivastigmine)

MAOIs, Monoamine oxidase inhibitors; *SSRIs*, selective serotonin reuptake inhibitors; *TCAs*, tricyclic antidepressants.
Schutte-Rodin S. Clinical guideline for the evaluation and management of chronic insomnia in adults. *J Clin Sleep Med*. 2008;4(5):487–504; Armon Neel. 10 Types of Meds that Can cause insomnia. <http://www.aarp.org/health/drugs-supplements/info-04-2013/medications-that-can-cause-insomnia.html> Accessed 27.04.16.

9. **Answer B.**
Relaxation therapy is designed to reduce somatic tension and/ or intrusive thoughts at bedtime that interfere with sleep (e.g., progressive muscle relaxation or autogenic training).

Psychological and Behavioral Treatments for Insomnia

Stimulus control therapy	Instructions provided to reassociate the bedroom with sleep including: (1) Only in bed when sleepy, (2) out of bed when unable to sleep, (3) use bed for sleep only, (4) arise at same time each morning, (5) no napping
Sleep restriction therapy	Curtail time in bed to amount of sleep time Periodic adjustments to sleep window made contingent upon sleep efficiency until optimal sleep duration achieved
Relaxation training	Techniques aimed at decreasing somatic tension or intrusive thoughts at bedtime (i.e., progressive muscle relaxation, autogenic training, imagery training, meditation)
Cognitive therapy	Techniques engineered to challenge and change misconceptions about sleep and erroneous beliefs about insomnia and its daytime consequences
Cognitive behavioral therapy	Combination of any of the above behavioral (i.e., stimulus control, sleep restriction, relaxation) and cognitive procedures (i.e., changing misconceptions about sleep)
Sleep hygiene	General guidelines geared to improving health practices (i.e., diet, exercise, substance use) and environmental factors (i.e., avoidance of light, noise, exposure to screens) that promote sleep
Paradoxical intention	Instruct patient to remain passively awake and avoid effort to fall asleep (goal to eliminate performance anxiety)
Biofeedback	Visual or auditory feedback used to help patients control physiologic parameters (i.e., muscle tension) to reduce somatic arousal

Morgenthaler T, Kramer M, Alessi C, et al. Practice parameters for the psychological and behavioral treatment of insomnia: an update. An American academy of sleep medicine report. *Sleep.* 2006;29(11):1415–1419; Morin CM, Bootzin RR, Buysse DJ, Edinger JD, Espie CA, Lichstein KL. Psychological and behavioral treatment of insomnia: update of the recent evidence (1998–2004). *Sleep.* 2006;29(11):1398–1414.

10. **Answer A.**
The patient describes having cataplexy and sleep paralysis in addition to her excessive daytime sleepiness. Pharmacologic therapy found to improve cataplexy and sleep paralysis symptoms includes tricyclic antidepressants (such as amitriptyline), venlafaxine, and sodium oxybate. While modafinil, dextroamphetamine, and methylphenidate may improve daytime sleepiness, they tend to have little effect on cataplexy symptoms. Selegiline may also be used to treat cataplexy, but because of potential drug interactions and diet-induced interactions, using it should be done with caution.[5]

11. **Answer C.**
This patient has Kleine-Levin syndrome based on the description of the patient's symptoms. Though only based on a case series, lithium carbonate reduced duration of hypersomnia episodes in patients with Kleine-Levin syndrome and eliminated some of the troublesome behavioral symptoms during episodes of sleepiness. Limited data on methylphenidate and modafinil does not suggest similar outcomes. Sodium oxybate is not currently indicated for patients with this disorder.[5]

12. **Answer C.**
All typical pharmacotherapy for patients with narcolepsy are in pregnancy category C. Napping can be used to improve daytime sleepiness associated with narcolepsy in pregnancy but pharmacotherapy should be avoided if possible (if risk of treatment outweighs possible benefit). Counseling is important when discussing pharmacotherapy in female patients with narcolepsy of childbearing age and should include caution of utilizing any pharmacotherapy while pregnant. It is also unknown whether most medications are excreted in breast milk. Three notable exceptions are amphetamine, fluoxetine, and venlafaxine; these medications are excreted in breast milk and should not be used in patients who are breast-feeding.[6] In addition, sodium oxybate was initially listed as pregnancy category B but was later changed to class C.

13. **Answer D.**
REM behavior disorder (RBD) is often associated with synucleinopathies and an estimated 38%–65% of patients with RBD develop a synucleinopathy such as Parkinson's disease (PD) or dementia with Lewy body (DLB) disease between 10 and 29 years after presentation. Conversely, RBD can be found in 70% of patients with multiple system atrophy, 40% of patients with DLB, and 15%–33% of patients with PD. Therefore in patients presenting with symptoms suggestive of RBD, it is important to assess cognitive and extrapyramidal signs. The tremor seen in PD is described as a pill-rolling, resting tremor. Intention tremors are seen with purposeful action and are usually benign. Nail pitting is not a symptom of a synucleinopathy (seen in Reiter's syndrome and psoriasis). Peripheral edema is associated with volume overload and seen most commonly in patients with heart dysfunction.[7]

14. **Answer D.**
The four cardinal symptoms of RLS include (1) an urge to move the limbs associated with paresthesia or dysesthesia, (2) symptoms that start or become worse with rest, (3) at least partial relief of symptoms with physical activity, and (4) worsening of symptoms in the evening or at night. Daytime sleepiness is a nonspecific symptom of many different sleep disorders. A history of diabetes does not confirm RLS although RLS-like symptoms are often seen in patients suffering from diabetic neuropathy. RLS is treated with dopaminergic agents, but this is not a cardinal diagnostic feature.[8]

15. **Answer D.**
Actigraphy would not be a common confirmatory test for RLS. RLS is a clinical diagnosis and does not require polysomnography confirmation for diagnosis, although 80%–90% of RLS patients demonstrate an increase in PLMS on polysomnography. Levodopa with dopa decarboxylate inhibitor is indicated for intermittent RLS but is more likely to be associated with augmentation if used nightly compared with dopamine agonists such as pramipexole and ropinirole. Pramipexole and ropinirole are dopamine agonists and are the recommended initial primary therapies to treat RLS.[8]

16. **Answer A.**
Clonidine, while not recommended as a first-line agent, may be effective in combination or as a second line agent and would not be contraindicated in patients with hypertension.

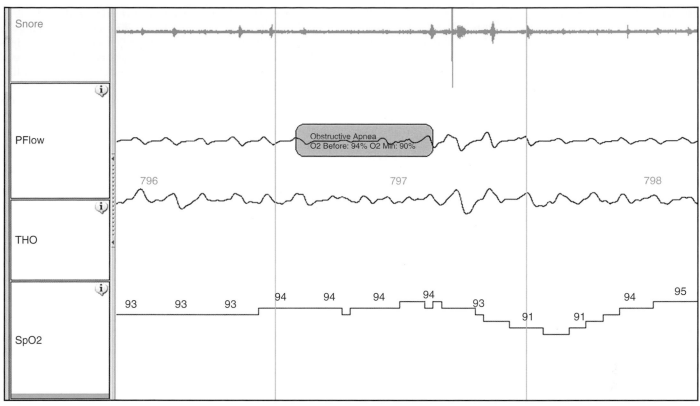

• **Figure 47.3** A 90-second image of a Philips Respironics Night One HSAT. The leads from top to bottom: snore, nasal pressure, effort, oxygen saturation. There is evidence of an obstructive apnea in the middle of the image.

Side effects are usually mild and include dry mouth, decreased cognition, lightheadedness, sleepiness post dose, constipation, and decreased libido. IV Iron is only recommended in patients with low ferritin levels. Mirtazepine may increase RLS symptoms, although the evidence is not sufficient to justify a recommendation against it in patients with RLS. Pergolide has been removed from the United States market due to the side effect of heart valve dysfunction.[8]

17. **Answer A.**

Home sleep apnea testing requires at least oximetry, airflow, and respiratory effort. Many home sleep apnea devices also monitor heart rate and body position, but these parameters are unnecessary to meet criteria for a type 3 portable monitoring device. While EEG improves the denominator (i.e., sleep time) used to generate the AHI, few studies demonstrated improved accuracy of OSA diagnosis with EEG monitoring. Ideally, home sleep apnea monitoring includes both an oronasal thermal sensor to detect apneas and a nasal pressure transducer to detect hypopneas. Calibrated or uncalibrated inductance plethysmography is recommended to identify respiratory effort. A pulse oximeter with appropriate signal averaging time and accommodation for motion artifact is recommended to detect blood oxygen level (Fig. 47.3).[9]

18. **Answer B.**

The patient does not have symptoms suggestive of obstructive sleep apnea or other sleep disorders justifying an in-lab polysomnography. His lack of sleep apnea symptoms also means home sleep apnea testing is not indicated. Starting a hypnotic medication would not likely be the most effective treatment for advanced sleep phase syndrome, from which the patient

likely suffers. Actigraphy is indicated to assist in evaluation of patients with circadian rhythm disorders, shift work sleep disorders, jet lag, and non-24-hour sleep/wake syndrome. It can also be used to monitor treatment in the above patients and in patients being treated for insomnia. Actigraphy may also be useful in characterizing and monitoring sleep and circadian rhythm patterns and outcome in older nursing home residents where traditional sleep monitoring may be challenging.[10]

19. **Answer A.**

Actigraphy would be the best way to assess his sleep schedule for delayed sleep phase syndrome, particularly given the discordance between his report and his mother's report. Home sleep apnea testing and in-laboratory polysomnography would not be the appropriate place to start, given his low risk for obstructive sleep apnea. As the patient likely suffers from a circadian rhythm disorder, using a sleep aid is not ideal therapy.[10]

20. **Answer D.**

A maintenance of wakefulness test is used to document maintenance of wakefulness, not propensity to fall asleep. An EEG might document normal, awake brainwaves during an episode of cataplexy but would not diagnose narcolepsy. To diagnose narcolepsy, a full overnight polysomnogram with cardiorespiratory channels and anterior tibialis EMG monitoring is recommended to eliminate other untreated sleep disorders that may cause daytime sleepiness. After an overnight polysomnogram, an MSLT performed with recommended test protocol and EEG, EOG, chin EMG, and EKG recording is recommended. HLA typing is not indicated as a replacement test for the MSLT because HLA typing lacks specificity in the diagnosis of narcolepsy.[11]

21. **Answer A.**
Best evidence suggests patients with delayed sleep phase syndrome respond to melatonin at 7 PM–9 PM with resulting improvement in total sleep time and sleep latency. Light administered at the core body temperature minimum (CBTmin) would have little effect and might even delay sleep phase. Melatonin administered at C would cause daytime sleepiness and might further delay his circadian rhythm. Light administered at D would have little effect on the circadian rhythm and light exposure tends to be less effective if the patient receives sufficient light exposure during the day.[12]

22. **Answer D.**
CPAP is the only therapy listed in this question with a standard recommendation for treatment of central sleep apnea secondary to CHF. BPAP with spontaneous timed (ST) mode should only be considered if there is no response to CPAP, ASV, and oxygen therapies because BPAP in ST mode may exacerbate central apneas. ASV is currently not advised for patients who have CHF, predominantly moderate to severe central sleep apnea, and whose left ventricular ejection fraction (LVEF) is less than 45%. Alteration of the recommendation occurred secondary to a Field Safety Notice issued by Resmed in May 2015 after a study designed to treat CHF in patients with predominantly central sleep apnea syndromes with an EF less than 45% revealed increased mortality in the treatment group. Not discussed in the question above, but relevant: oxygen therapy is also indicated for the treatment of central sleep apnea in patients with CHF, though stringent Medicare requirements may limit its use after a diagnosis of sleep apnea is obtained. A repeat sleep study is recommended in patients with central sleep apnea related to CHF after oxygen initiation to verify appropriate resolution of central apneas with oxygen.[13]

23. **Answer C.**
Topical corticosteroids like fluticasone may improve the AHI in patients with OSA and concurrent rhinitis and improve tolerance of CPAP use. This therapy is recommended as adjunctive to primary OSA therapies. In one study, fluticasone spray improved AHI from 20 to 12 events per hour. Diphenhydramine is systemic and therefore exposes the patient to more side effects than a topical nasal corticosteroid. Cessation of CPAP use when rhinitis occurs would not be recommended. Short-acting nasal decongestants such as neosynephrine are not recommended long-term because of risk of rebound vasodilation that would adversely affect nasal patency and total sleep time.[14]

24. **Answer B.**
Close follow-up for PAP usage is recommended; however, follow-up 3 days after PAP therapy may not allow enough opportunity for the patient to acclimate to CPAP. Ideally, the patient should be seen within the first few weeks of PAP usage and especially within the first few months.[15]

25. **Answer C.**
Several studies indicate that heated humidification increases CPAP adherence compared with patients using unheated or nonhumidified CPAP. In some studies, nasal masks proved to increase compliance compared with full face mask, although in smaller studies, there was no significant difference between the two types of masks. Adjusting pressure settings has little to no dependence on subsequent adherence based on most study results published assessing this relationship. Sleep aids would not be indicated over a trial of heated humidification when comparing the risk:benefit ratio of each intervention.[15]

26. **Answer B.**
This patient has symptoms of hypothyroidism and should be evaluated and treated as treatment of hypothyroidism significantly reduces AHI. Prior to alleviating OSA related to weight loss, patients should be treated with PAP until the OSA is documented as fully reversed. An oral glucose tolerance test evaluates for acromegaly, of which this patient does not demonstrate symptoms. Estrogen replacement therapy does not significantly improve AHI in postmenopausal woman in several studies, and with an increasing number of adverse effects associated with hormonal replacement therapy, estrogen replacement therapy should be avoided. Modafinil is not indicated if hypothyroidism explains the continued fatigue and treating the hypothyroidism improves the fatigue.[16]

27. **Answer B.**
In laboratory sleep testing is indicated for assessment of treatment results of patients on CPAP after substantial weight loss, substantial weight gain, when clinical response is insufficient, or symptoms recur despite appropriate initial response to CPAP. Actigraphy is unlikely to yield significant insight to the patient's condition. Repeating diagnostic sleep apnea testing is unnecessary. Modafinil is not indicated if PAP therapy is subtherapeutic.[17]

28. **Answer C.**
An optimal titration reduces RDI less than 5 per hour for at least 15 minutes, includes supine REM sleep, and is not continually interrupted by spontaneous arousals or awakenings. A good titration reduces RDI less than 10 or by 50% of baseline RDI less than 15 and should include supine REM sleep that is not interrupted by spontaneous arousals or awakenings. A repeat titration should be considered if optimal or good are not achieved.[18]

Suggested Reading

Collop NA, Anderson WM, Boehlecke B, et al. Clinical guidelines for the use of unattended portable monitors in the diagnosis of obstructive sleep apnea in adult patients. *J Clin Sleep Med.* 2007;3(7):737-747.

Kushida CA, Littner MR, Morgenthaler T, et al. Practice parameters for the indications of polysomnography and related procedures: an update for 2005. *Sleep.* 2005;28(4):499-521.

Littner MR, Kushida C, Wise M, et al. Practice parameters for clinical use of the multiple sleep latency test and the maintenance of wakefulness test. *Sleep.* 2005;28(1):113-121.

Schutte-Rodin S. Clinical guideline for the evaluation and management of chronic insomnia in adults. *J Clin Sleep Med.* 2008;4(5):487-504.

Wise MS, Arand DL, Auger RR, et al. Treatment of Narcolepsy and other hypersomnias of central origin. *Sleep.* 2007;30(12):1712-1727.

48

Quality Measures in Sleep Medicine

LYNN MARIE TROTTI, ROCHELLE ZAK, DENISE SHARON

Questions

1. In 2015 the American Academy of Sleep Medicine (AASM) published a series of quality measures for the care of patients with sleep disorders. These quality measures included which type(s) of measures?
   A. Structure measures only, as these relate to site accreditation
   B. Outcome measures only, as the main concern is the patient's overall health status and not whether good clinical practices were followed
   C. Process and outcome measures, because quality care involves not only maximizing clinical outcomes but also following best practices
   D. Structure, process, and outcome measures, because these quality measures assess not only patient outcomes and best practices but also can be used to evaluate site-specific characteristics such as staff-to-patient ratios

2. In the measurement of quality, process measures have the following characteristics:
   A. They refer to the health state of a patient resulting from clinical care.
   B. They are less sensitive to demographics, socioeconomics, and disease burden differences in the patient population than outcome measures.
   C. Adherence to process measures can only be assessed once the clinical outcome is clear, which may not be seen for several years after treatment.
   D. Best process measures do not include processes linked to desired outcomes.

3. Characteristics of outcome measures include the following:
   A. They are the result entirely of the processes of care and, thus, can be used to accurately compare the quality of practice at different institutions.
   B. They are easy to assess, as outcomes are apparent within a short period of time.
   C. The systematic use of outcome measures can lead to the identification of gaps in care that may be amenable to changes in processes to achieve the desired health care objectives.
   D. Completion of the Insomnia Severity Index (ISI) at a follow-up visit would be an outcome measure.

4. The AASM identified five conditions for which quality measure sets were developed, including obstructive sleep apnea (OSA) in adults and children, insomnia, restless legs syndrome (RLS), and narcolepsy. Of these conditions, existing quality measures were only available for adult obstructive sleep apnea. In order to be consistent with existing measures, the AASM OSA quality measures workgroup chose to exclude which of the following outcomes:
   A. Improve disease detection and categorization
   B. Improve quality of life
   C. Improve functional status
   D. Reduce cardiovascular risk

5. A heavy, bearded, 23-year-old male comes to you after a near-miss crash. His bed partner reports snoring since they met 2 months ago. The patient denies sleepiness and tells you the other car was at fault. You would like to comply with the recommended AASM quality measures. What will you include in your evaluation plan?
   A. Sleepiness and snoring assessment, weight and blood pressure check, quality of life assessment, and objective disease severity assessment within 2 months
   B. Epworth Sleepiness Scale, weight check, home sleep apnea testing (HSAT) within 3 months, overnight oximetry
   C. Airway and physical exam, blood pressure check, quality of life assessment, in-lab sleep study within 2 months
   D. Sleepiness and snoring assessment, weight check, overnight oximetry, sleep apnea study within 1 month

6. The same patient has an ESS score of 11, weighs 285 lbs, has a blood pressure of 125/80, and demonstrates large tonsils and elongated uvula on airway examination. On home sleep apnea testing, the REI is 20. After discussion of results, he refuses PAP therapy and opts instead for treatment with a mandibular advancement oral appliance (OA). Considering the quality measures, what will be the best long-term management plan for this patient on OA therapy?
   A. Yearly follow-up, including sleepiness report, quality of life assessment, weight and blood pressure measurements, and discussion regarding management of abnormal measurements
   B. Yearly follow-up, including sleepiness assessment, repeat sleep study, and weight and blood pressure check
   C. Follow-up every 6 months, including OA adherence based on patient report, Epworth Sleepiness Scale, and pharmacologic management of abnormal weight and blood pressure measurements
   D. Referral to dentist for long-term follow-up and management

7. In order to improve patient's quality of life, the following evidence-based therapies can be utilized. Please choose the most comprehensive answer:
   A. CPAP/BPAP treatment, OA, weight loss, and positional therapy
   B. CPAP treatment, OA, surgery, and cognitive-behavioral therapy (CBT)
   C. APAP treatment, OA, weight loss, and surgery
   D. PAP treatment, OA, surgery, and positional therapy

8. According to the AASM adult OSA quality measures, which of the following are acceptable ways to assess adherence to OSA treatment:
   A. Bed partner report on adherence to PAP or non-PAP therapies
   B. PAP download or subjective adherence report for non-PAP therapies
   C. PAP download or objective adherence report for non-PAP therapies
   D. Epworth Sleepiness Scale score

9. Per the AASM OSA adult quality measures, which of the following need to be checked at every visit, not just annually?
   A. Weight and blood pressure
   B. Adherence to treatment and weight
   C. Quality of life and adherence to treatment
   D. Adherence to treatment and blood pressure

10. The overall goal of developing quality measures for the care of pediatric patients with OSA was:
    A. To promote high quality patient-centered care
    B. To provide ideal standards of care
    C. To facilitate billing
    D. To promote evidence-based research

11. A pediatrician tells you about one of his patients, who is a 13-year-old, highly functioning boy with Down syndrome and a history of snoring and large tonsils. The pediatrician was not sure whether the patient snores three or more times per week, so he obtained an overnight oximetry recording that was interpreted as being in the normal range. The pediatrician tells you that his plan is to follow up with the patient at his next annual visit. In keeping with the AASM quality measures, what is your preferred management plan?
    A. The same as the pediatrician's
    B. Schedule a diagnostic polysomnography (PSG)
    C. Refer for immediate adenotonsillectomy
    D. Schedule an HSAT

12. The outcome measures indicate that reassessment of OSA signs and symptoms needs to be performed within 12 months of initiating a management plan. The 12-month frame was chosen because:
    A. It may take up to 12 months to complete all testing, analysis, intervention, and reassessment, but ideally it might be completed sooner.
    B. 12 months is the minimum amount of time needed to elapse for a reassessment to be performed, to allow adequate time for changes in symptoms.
    C. 12 months is the ideal amount of time for a reassessment to be performed.
    D. Insurance companies will pay only for annual reassessment.

13. The diagnosis and treatment of pediatric OSA poses several challenges, including:

A. AASM accreditation requirements
B. It is technically challenging to perform a PSG in children because of increased impedances.
C. The diagnosis depends on the integration of symptoms, physical findings, and descriptive nature of sleep.
D. There is a lack of consensus over which criteria should be used in the pediatric population (ages 2–12).

14. Objective documentation of PAP adherence in children should include:
    A. Average number of hours of use per night
    B. Percentage of nights per week that the device is used
    C. Percentage of nights per months that the device was used for at least 6 hours per night
    D. Percentage of nights per month that the device was used for at least 2 hours per night

15. How often should adherence of children to PAP therapy ideally be assessed?
    A. Every encounter
    B. Within 3 months of starting PAP
    C. Within 6 months of starting PAP
    D. Within 12 months of starting PAP

16. Quality measures were developed and graded based on the strength of evidence linking each process measure with its desired outcome. For the insomnia measures, the level of evidence grading for the majority of measures was:
    A. Nearly all Level 1 (i.e., highest level)
    B. Predominantly Levels 1 and 2
    C. Predominantly Levels 3 and 4
    D. Nearly all Level 4 (i.e., lowest level)

17. In the AASM quality measures for the care of patients with insomnia, a key process measure is the proportion of patients diagnosed with insomnia who receive an assessment of sleep satisfaction or quality. An acceptable tool for the measurement of sleep satisfaction or quality includes which of the following:
    A. The Epworth Sleepiness Scale score
    B. In-laboratory polysomnography
    C. The patient's report of sleep quality
    D. Actigraphy

18. A 37-year-old woman developed acute onset of insomnia following a period of increased stress at work. Although the stressor has since resolved, she continues to report a sleep latency of 2 hours and difficulty returning to sleep after awakening in the night. She tends to remain in bed worrying about her family and her lack of sleep, although she sometimes will watch TV in bed to try to prevent herself from focusing on these negative thoughts. On a typical night, she spends 11 hours in bed but estimates she sleeps only 6 hours. In the insomnia quality measures, which of the following is rated as a Level 1 (i.e., highest evidence) long-term treatment option?
    A. Sleep restriction therapy
    B. Stimulus control therapy
    C. Paradoxical intention therapy
    D. Doxepin

19. A 24-year-old man reports difficulty with falling and staying asleep for the last year. He has developed a feeling of dread when he thinks about trying to sleep, because he is very anxious about his inability to sleep. He sleeps better when he stays at his girlfriend's house, but does this infrequently. As a result of his poor sleep, he has difficulty concentrating in class, and his grades have declined. Which aspect of this patient's presentation is part of the ICSD-3 diagnostic criteria for chronic insomnia?

A. Difficulty with both sleep onset and sleep maintenance

B. Anxiety about sleep resulting in an inability to sleep

C. Falling asleep more easily when he is not at home

D. Impaired concentration and academic performance

20. In addition to sleep satisfaction and quality, assessment of which of the following at each visit is a recommended process measure in the AASM insomnia quality measures?

A. Side effects of insomnia medications

B. Side effects of cognitive-behavioral therapy

C. Side effects of both insomnia medications and cognitive-behavioral therapy

D. Sleep-related quality of life

E. Subjective sleep latency and sleep duration

21. A 72-year-old male complains of restlessness at night. When he lies down in bed, he experiences a pins-and-needles sensation in his right leg that is relieved when he changes position, and he is then easily able to fall asleep. The symptom does not recur during the night nor in the morning. He awakens refreshed in the morning and does not have any daytime dysfunction. Which of the following is true about this patient's clinical condition?

A. He has a variant of RLS characterized by numbness without the urge to move.

B. He has RLS because he has a dysesthesia in his leg that occurs at night and is relieved with movement.

C. He does not have RLS because he does not have daytime dysfunction from his leg symptoms.

D. He is experiencing a mimic of RLS with positional discomfort that occurs at night because of positioning and not because of circadian rhythmicity.

22. Assessment of iron stores is one of the AASM RLS process measures intended to result in improved accuracy of RLS diagnosis. Which of the following is sufficient for assessing iron stores in patients with RLS?

A. Serum ferritin level, with a full iron panel when possible

B. Hemoglobin and hematocrit

C. Iron, TIBC, and percent saturation

D. Haptoglobin

23. The overarching goal of the RLS Quality Measures is to promote high quality patient-centered care. Thus the RLS Quality Measures recommended certain initial and follow-up evaluations. Which of the following accurately reflects some of these recommendations?

A. Patients on dopaminergic medication should be counseled about the risk of augmentation only at the initiation of dopaminergic therapy.

B. Patients on dopaminergic medication should be counseled about the risk of developing or exacerbating impulse control disorders only at the initiation of dopaminergic therapy.

C. Patients on dopaminergic medications should be asked about impulse control disorders and augmentation at every visit.

D. To decrease the likelihood of side effects, physicians should not counsel patients about side effects when prescribing a new medication.

24. Which of the following are considered satisfactory assessments of RLS symptom severity?

A. Only the International RLS Study Group Rating Scale (IRLS)

B. A measure of severity of RLS symptoms combined with an assessment of at least one RLS-associated domain (sleep

quality, daytime sleepiness/tiredness, daytime function, or mood)

C. The Patient Global Impression (PGI) scale

D. Free-text documenting at least one RLS-associated domain (sleep quality, daytime sleepiness/tiredness, daytime function, or mood)

25. According to the RLS Quality Measures, processes aimed at decreasing RLS symptom severity include which of the following?

A. Assessment of iron stores

B. Assessment of medication side effects

C. Use of accepted diagnostic criteria

D. Assessment of symptom severity and delivery of evidence-based treatment

26. In the AASM quality measures for the care of patients with narcolepsy, a key outcome measure is the proportion of patients diagnosed with narcolepsy whose sleepiness improved from baseline. Acceptable tools for the measurement of sleepiness for this outcome include which of the following:

A. Validated measure of subjective sleepiness (e.g., Epworth Sleepiness Scale)

B. Patient self-report of sleepiness

C. Maintenance of wakefulness test

D. Driving safety record

27. Per the AASM narcolepsy quality indicators, patients diagnosed with narcolepsy should be directed to begin pharmacologic, behavioral, or combination treatment within what timeframe after the multiple sleep latency test (MSLT) is performed?

A. 1 week

B. 1 month

C. 3 months

D. 6 months

28. A 23-year-old man with a 12-month history of sleepiness presents to you for evaluation. You elicit a history of persistent daytime sleepiness despite average sleep times of nearly 8 hours per night, with regular 10 PM bedtime and 6 AM wake-up time. Typical cataplexy is present but rare. He denies snoring or witnessed apneas. He has a history of depression treated with venlafaxine and high blood pressure treated with lisinopril. Physical examination, including neurologic examination, is unremarkable. PSG demonstrates total sleep time of 400 minutes, apnea-hypopnea index of 3, and REM latency of 60 minutes. Next-day MSLT demonstrates a mean sleep latency of 4 minutes, with two sleep-onset REM periods. In addition to documenting the above, which of the following should be documented in the medical record to meet the narcolepsy process measures that promote the outcome of improved diagnostic accuracy?

A. No history of prior head injury

B. No history of episodic neurologic symptoms suggestive of multiple sclerosis

C. Laboratory testing to exclude anemia and hypothyroidism

D. MSLT was performed following standard protocols, including tapering off venlafaxine prior to the study

29. The AASM narcolepsy quality measures advise follow-up of treated patients at least how often:

A. Every 3 months

B. Every 6 months

C. Every 9 months

D. Every 12 months

30. An 18-year-old woman returns to your clinic to discuss the results of her recent PSG and MSLT testing. Her nocturnal study demonstrated a sleep latency of 5 min, a REM latency of 11 min, a sleep efficiency of 85%, and a total sleep time of 380 min. Next-day MSLT demonstrated a mean sleep latency of 3.5 min and one sleep onset REM period. Based on the narcolepsy quality measure processes, which of the following aspects of clinical counseling should be performed:
    A. Reasonable accommodations in school and in the workplace
    B. Age-appropriate safety measures
    C. Pregnancy and breast-feeding considerations
    D. Future risk of developing cataplexy

Answers

1. **Answer C. Process and outcome measures, because quality care involves not only maximizing clinical outcomes but also following best practices.**
    Each quality measure set commissioned and approved by the AASM includes process and outcome measures but not structure measures (Answers A, B, and D are incorrect). *Structure measures* evaluate the setting and system in which health care is delivered, and include factors such as practice volume, staff-to-patient ratios, and use of information technology. As such, structure measures tend to be variable from site to site. Key structure measures are addressed by AASM accreditation standards, and were judged by AASM leadership to be outside the purview of the quality measure development process.[1] Instead, quality metric task forces were instructed to assemble sets of both outcome and process measures (Answer C is correct). *Outcome measures* capture the "health state of a patient resulting from health care"[2]—that is, they are measures designed to reflect the degree to which overall goals of health care, such as decreased mortality or improved quality of life, are being achieved. *Process measures* capture the steps of practice in the course of clinical care that promote and are necessary precursors to the outcomes measures.[1]

2. **Answer B. They are less sensitive to demographics, socio-economics, and disease burden differences in the patient population than outcome measures.**
    Process measures capture individual clinical processes—that is, steps taken in the care of individual patients such as the measurement of blood pressure or assessment of sleepiness. Their completion or lack of completion may be relatively easy to document (depending on the process measure), which can allow comparison of care delivery within or across health care systems. Completion of a process measure is independent of the clinical outcome (Answers A and C are incorrect). Unlike outcome measures, which may be affected by differences in patient populations at different sites, process measures are relatively unaffected by differences in underlying population (Answer B is correct). Whether or not the processes were followed can be easily and immediately assessed at the time of completion, without the need to wait for a clinical outcome that may be considerably delayed (Answer C is incorrect). Characteristics of good process measures include those that have a strong link to desired outcomes (Answer D is incorrect).[1]

3. **Answer C. The systematic use of outcome measures can lead to the identification of gaps in care that may be amenable to changes in processes to achieve the desired health care objectives.**
    Outcome measures (OMs) provide an assessment of the adequacy of management of the medical condition. Although this concept is simple, many challenges arise when using OMs as the sole measure of adequacy of clinical care or as the comparison metric across different institutions. Although the steps taken in the care of the patient (i.e., the processes) clearly impact the course of disease, other factors beyond the control of the medical care provider also have an impact on the disease process, including socioeconomic factors, hereditary conditions, and cultural beliefs that may render a particular process less effective in certain situations. Outcome measures tend to reflect a combination of the processes followed by the health care provider and the patient-specific factors that are outside a health care provider's control. Thus, although OMs can be useful for internal benchmarking, complex and sometimes inadequate risk adjustments need to be made in order to compare medical care at different institutions (Answer A is incorrect). After an appropriate health care intervention, improvement in disease severity is not always immediately apparent (e.g., the process of recommending aspirin use following stroke will reduce the incidence of future strokes, but the outcome of stroke prevention is not immediately apparent). Outcomes may lag processes by years or decades. This can lead to difficulty in assessing delayed outcomes, as patients may move, be lost to follow-up, or develop comorbid diseases that also affect the outcomes (Answer B is incorrect). In contrast, using OMs to systematically follow outcomes over time and comparing them with the different processes used to treat and evaluate medical disorders can identify inadequacies in various processes of care and gaps that need to be resolved (Answer C is correct). OMs delineate the patient's state of health or disease, and are not an action that is completed. Thus, while the change in ISI score with treatment could be an outcome measure, its administration is a process measure (Answer D is incorrect).[1] A summary of some of the benefits and limitations of the three different types of quality measures can be found in Table 48.1.[3]

4. **Answer C. Improve functional status.**
    In their quest to identify one to three outcome measures that were patient-oriented, easily applicable, and well supported by the current literature and expert opinion, the OSA workgroup initially considered improvement in quality of life, improvement in functional status, and cardiovascular risk reduction. However, because OSA measures were already developed in conjunction with the American Medical Association's Physician Consortium for Performance Improvement (AMA-PCPI), the AASM OSA workgroup sought consistency with existing measures. Thus the final outcomes chosen by the OSA quality measure workgroup are improved disease detection and categorization (Answer A is incorrect), improved quality of life (Answer B is incorrect), and reduced cardiovascular risk (Answer D is incorrect). Improvement in functional status was not included in the final outcome measures (Answer C is correct).[4]

5. **Answer A. Sleepiness assessment, weight and blood pressure check, quality of life assessment, disease severity assessment within 2 months.**
    Because OSA remains considerably underdiagnosed and undertreated, one of the outcomes selected by the adult OSA workgroup was improvement in disease detection and categorization. Snoring and daytime sleepiness are two of the most common symptoms of OSA, and assessment of both of these

TABLE 48.1 Benefits and Limitations of Different Types of Quality Metrics

Measure of Quality	Example	Benefits	Limitations
Outcome measure	Decrease in severity of RLS symptoms over time	Face validity Patient-oriented Obvious alignment with patient goals of care	Impacted by multiple factors beyond provider or health care system control Duration between action and outcome may be very long Does not provide information about specifically how to change practice to improve outcome
Process measure	Measurement of RLS severity	Not stigmatizing Less impacted by features of patient population than are outcomes Can be measured at the time of the patient encounter Most providers or systems have room for improvement on some measures	Not necessarily directly important to patients
Structure measure	Patient volume of provider caring for RLS patients	In general, easy to measure	Not subject to change by individual care providers Not necessarily directly important to patients

Table reprinted from Trotti LM. Toward a definition of quality care for patients with restless legs syndrome. *Sleep Med Clin.* 2015;10:293-301, xiii.

• BOX 48.1 The Epworth Sleepiness Scale

The Epworth Sleepiness Scale is a 0–24 point scale in which individuals self-report their likelihood of falling asleep under the following eight specific situations (0 = no chance of dozing; 3 = high chance of dozing):

- Sitting and reading
- Watching TV
- Sitting quietly after lunch (without alcohol consumption)
- Talking to someone
- Riding as a passenger in a car for an hour without a break
- Driving a car, stopped for a few minutes in traffic
- Lying down to rest in the afternoon
- Sitting in a public place while inactive

Johns MW. A new method for measuring daytime sleepiness: the Epworth sleepiness scale. Sleep. 1991;14:540-545.

---

symptoms at initial evaluation is a recommended process measure (Answer C is incorrect). For this process measure, the Epworth Sleepiness Scale (ESS; Box 48.1) may be used, but other assessments of subjective sleepiness are also permitted.

Furthering the outcome of improved disease detection and categorization, objective testing for sleep apnea severity, through PSG or HSAT, is recommended within 2 months of initial evaluation for suspected sleep apnea (Answers B and D are incorrect). Quantification of sleep apnea severity may use any one of a variety of measures, including apnea-hypopnea index, respiratory disturbance index, or respiratory event index (the latter reflecting home sleep apnea testing). Early case identification (i.e., within 2 months of the identification of sleep apnea symptoms) and treatment are important, given that patients with moderate or severe OSA are at higher risk for cardiovascular diseases, neurocognitive dysfunction, lower quality of life, and other comorbid conditions.

Improving quality of life was chosen as an outcome, because quality of life is considered one of the most fundamental patient-reported outcomes in health care. There have been a number of studies demonstrating improved quality of life after adequate treatment of OSA with positive airway pressure, oral appliances, and upper airway surgery. Because change in quality of life is a measured outcome, it is necessary to assess quality of life at baseline and within 1 year of starting treatment for sleep apnea (Answers B and D are incorrect).

Obesity and hypertension are both common in patients with OSA and are known cardiovascular risk factors. Assessment of both of these parameters at every visit are process measures that support the outcome of reducing cardiovascular risk (Answers B, C, and D are incorrect). Nocturnal oxygen saturation level (overnight oximetry) is a helpful but incomplete instrument in assessing severity of OSA and treatment effects. While overnight oximetry may be used in selected cases, the Adult OSA Workgroup decided not to include it as a measure needed in all patients (Answers B and D are incorrect). Airway and physical exams, though important in clinical assessment, were not included as process measures (Answer C is incorrect). Answer A is correct in this case because all components are included as process measures (assessment of sleepiness and snoring, measurement of weight and blood pressure, objective assessment of severity with PSG or HSAT within 2 months) or support outcome measures (assessment of quality of life at baseline to allow measurement of change in quality of life with treatment).[4]

6. **Answer A. Yearly follow-up, including sleepiness report, quality of life assessment, weight and blood pressure measurements, and discussion regarding management of abnormal measurements.**
Once OSA is accurately diagnosed and categorized based on severity, the remaining outcome goals of the AASM quality measures are improving quality of life and reducing cardiovascular risk. Follow-up with the dentist who customized the oral appliance is an important piece of care for patients with sleep apnea treated with oral appliance, but does not replace health care provider assessment and follow-up (Answer D is incorrect). The health care provider is expected to continue to assess quality of life, sleepiness, and cardiovascular risk in order to achieve the remaining two outcome goals of the AASM quality measures (Answer A is correct). Sleepiness should be assessed at least annually, but a sleep study does not need to be repeated annually in the absence of specific clinical indications (Answer B is incorrect). Although blood pressure

TABLE 48.2	Strength of Evidence Supporting Obstructive Sleep Apnea Treatment Efficacy	
Treatment Modality	Evidence Level*	Treatment Effects
CPAP	1	Self-reported sleepiness
CPAP	3	Quality of life
CPAP	4	Functional outcome of severe OSA patients
OA	3, 4	Alertness
OA	3, 4	Improved quality of life
Airway surgery	3	Quality of life
Airway surgery	3	Alertness
Positional therapy	3, 4	Quality of life and function

*Evidence level is graded with 1 = highest level of evidence and 4 = lowest level of evidence.
OA, Oral appliance; OSA, obstructive sleep apnea.
Aurora RN, Collop NA, Jacobowitz O, Thomas SM, Quan SF, Aronsky AJ. Quality measures for the care of adult patients with obstructive sleep apnea. *J Clin Sleep Med.* 2015;11:357-383.

TABLE 48.3	Outcome and Process Measures for Quality Care of Adult Patients with Obstructive Sleep Apnea
Outcome or Outcome Measure	Processes That Support the Outcome
Improve disease detection and disease categorization	Assessment of OSA symptoms (at least snoring and sleepiness) at initial visit Quantification of OSA severity (by apnea-hypopnea-index, respiratory disturbance index, or respiratory event index) within 2 months of initial visit
Improve quality of life	Prescription of evidence-based treatment after diagnosis Assessment of treatment adherence at least annually Assessment of sleepiness at least annually Assessment of motor vehicle crashes or near-misses at initial evaluation
Reduce cardiovascular risk	Assessment of weight at every visit Discussion of weight status or referral to weight management specialist at least annually for those with BMI > 25 Assessment of blood pressure at every visit Discussion of blood pressure at every visit in which blood pressure is elevated

OSA, Obstructive sleep apnea.
Aurora RN, Collop NA, Jacobowitz O, Thomas SM, Quan SF, Aronsky AJ. Quality measures for the care of adult patients with obstructive sleep apnea. *J Clin Sleep Med.* 2015;11:357-383.

and weight should be measured at each follow-up visit (Answer A is correct), treatment of abnormal measurements can be appropriately referred to another provider (e.g., to a bariatric clinic), and the adult OSA process measures require only discussion of abnormal weight at least annually and discussion of elevated blood pressure at each visit in which it is elevated (Answer C is incorrect).[4]

7. **Answer D. PAP treatment, OA, surgery, and positional therapy.** Evidence-based treatments for OSA, highlighted in the AASM OSA quality measures,[4] include PAP therapies (CPAP, BPAP, APAP), oral appliances (OA), surgery, and positional therapy (Answer D is correct; Table 48.2). Weight loss, even though beneficial, was considered an adjunctive therapy rather than primary therapy by the OSA workgroup (Answers A and C are incorrect). CBT may be helpful in improving adherence to OSA treatment but is not considered a primary treatment for OSA (Answer B is incorrect).

8. **Answer B. PAP download or subjective adherence report for non-PAP therapies.** Currently in the United States, the only widely available objective measurements of adherence to OSA treatments are for PAP therapies, and monitoring of adherence to PAP is therefore expected to include objective information from a PAP download. Subjective adherence report to PAP therapies is not an acceptable way to assess adherence to OSA treatment (Answer A is incorrect). Objective measurements of adherence to OA are in development, but presently are not widely available, and there are currently no objective measures of adherence to positional therapy (Answer C is incorrect). Therefore subjective report of adherence to non-PAP therapy is considered acceptable (Answer B is correct, combining objective adherence measures for PAP and subjective adherence report for non-PAP therapies). Assessment of sleepiness (e.g., with the Epworth Sleepiness Scale) is an important component of management

of the OSA patient, but is not an acceptable surrogate for adherence (Answer D is incorrect).

9. **Answer A. Weight and blood pressure.** Weight and blood pressure are to be checked at every registered encounter because of their potential impact on cardiovascular risk (Answer A is correct). Moreover, documentation of a discussion regarding blood pressure elevations is required at every occurrence of an elevated reading. Even though weight needs to be measured at every encounter, a weight management discussion should occur at least annually. Quality of life and adherence to treatment need to be checked at least once a year (Answer B, C, and D are incorrect), although they may need to be checked more frequently if problems arise.[4] The full set of outcome and process measures for the care of adult patients with OSA is summarized in Table 48.3.

10. **Answer A. To promote high-quality patient-centered care.** The development of quality measures for the care of children with OSA is part of the AASM strategic plan to promote high-quality patient-centered care (Answer A is correct).[5] The pediatric OSA workgroup recognized that there are various types of providers (pediatricians, sleep specialists, otolaryngologists) who have slightly different guidelines for managing pediatric OSA in different settings (academic, clinic, sleep lab). Therefore the quality measures have to be widely applicable to each type of health provider or setting, while still ensuring that minimal practice standards are maintained (Answers B and D are incorrect). Even though insurers might use these quality measures, the goal was not to facilitate billing (Answer C is incorrect).

11. **Answer B. Schedule a diagnostic PSG.**

This question addresses two of the processes supporting the outcome of improved detection of pediatric OSA: (1) assessment of OSA symptoms or risk factors in children who snore; and (2) referral for PSG or to sleep/sleep apnea specialist (for objective t.esting) in children with complex medical conditions that increase risk of sleep apnea (e.g., Down syndrome) and who have signs or symptoms of sleep apnea.[5] Symptoms, signs, and risk factors of pediatric OSA are in Box 48.2 and include frequent snoring (three or more times per week). The presence of frequent snoring in a child should prompt a more detailed assessment for other OSA symptoms and risk factors. In otherwise healthy children in whom OSA is suspected, there are multiple evidence-based treatment options supported by clinical practice guidelines, including watchful waiting, adenotonsillectomy, polysomnography, or referral to a sleep/sleep apnea specialist (and use of such evidence-based recommendations are also included as a process measure in the AASM pediatric OSA quality measures). However, in patients with complex medical conditions associated with sleep apnea, neither watchful waiting nor adenotonsillectomy without preceding PSG are considered appropriate (Answers A and C are incorrect). In patients with such medical conditions (as detailed in Box 48.3), an AASM process measure details the need for objective assessment of OSA, either through

---

> ● **BOX 48.2 Symptoms, Signs, and Risk Factors of Pediatric Obstructive Sleep Apnea**

Daytime Symptoms:
- Sleepiness
- Attention deficit hyperactivity disorder symptoms
- Learning or behavioral problems
  Nocturnal Symptoms:
- Snoring at least 3 nights/week
- Labored breathing, snorting/gasping noises, witnessed apneas
- Bedwetting (especially secondary)
- Sleeping with neck hyperextended or in a seated position
- Cyanosis
- Morning headaches
  Clinical features:
- Increased weight and body mass index
- Elevated blood pressure

Kothare SV, Rosen CL, Lloyd RM, et al. Quality measures for the care of pediatric patients with obstructive sleep apnea. J Clin Sleep Med. 2015;11:385-404.

> ● **BOX 48.3 Complex Medical Conditions Associated with Pediatric Obstructive Sleep Apnea**

- Achondroplasia
- Craniofacial abnormalities
- Down syndrome
- Mucopolysaccharidoses
- Neuromuscular diseases
- Obesity
- Prader-Willi syndrome
- Sickle cell disease

Kothare SV, Rosen CL, Lloyd RM, et al. Quality measures for the care of pediatric patients with obstructive sleep apnea. J Clin Sleep Med. 2015;11:385-404.

---

polysomnography or referral to a specialist who can obtain polysomnography (Answer B is correct). Ambulatory testing including HSAT, oximetry, and nap PSG have been studied in children and have been shown to have a low negative predictive value. Therefore these tests are not the standard of care in the evaluation of pediatric sleep disordered breathing (Answer D is incorrect).

12. **Answer A. It may take up to 12 months to complete all testing, analysis, intervention, and reassessment, but ideally it might be completed sooner.**

Limited pediatric resources to complete highly specialized testing and interventions in a shorter period of time dictated the 12 months frame for reassessment (Answer A is correct).[5] In ideal conditions, reassessment should be completed sooner (Answers B and C are incorrect), and payment from the insurance company was not a criterion in the development of this process measure (Answer D is incorrect).

13. **Answer C. The diagnosis depends on the integration of symptoms, physical findings, and descriptive nature of sleep.**

The pediatric OSA workgroup recognized several challenges in the diagnosis and treatment of pediatric OSA. These challenges included the need to integrate in the diagnosis symptoms, physical findings, and descriptive nature of sleep (Answer C is correct), the challenges of performing PSG in children who do not tolerate monitoring (but not because of high impedances; Answer B is incorrect), and the lack of consensus over using pediatric versus adult criteria in children 13–18 years old (Answer D is incorrect). AASM accreditation criteria were not considered a challenge (Answer A is incorrect). Because of these challenges, the quality measures were designed to help providers implement at least a basic acceptable level of care required for diagnosing and managing pediatric OSA.[5]

14. **Answer A. Average number of hours of use per night.**

The pediatric OSA workgroup reached the conclusion that the objective assessment of PAP adherence is by itself an attainable and useful measure of reducing signs and symptoms of OSA. This measure should include documentation of the average numbers of hours of use per night (Answer A is correct), percentage of nights per month that the device is used (Answer B is incorrect), and percentage of nights per months that the device is used for at least 4 hours (Answers C and D are incorrect). However, the workgroup acknowledged that the threshold for optimum PAP use in children has yet to be determined.[5]

15. **Answer A. Every encounter.**

The pediatric OSA Workgroup specified that PAP adherence in children should ideally be assessed at every encounter (Answer A).[5] However, at a minimum (but not ideal), it must be measured within 3 months of starting PAP therapy (Answer B is incorrect). Six- and 12-month assessment periods were considered too long between measurements of PAP adherence in children (Answers C and D are incorrect). As a related issue, the process of growth may affect PAP needs in children. Even though this effect has not been fully established, reassessment of the need for and possible changes in pressure might be needed every year or two. The full set of pediatric OSA outcome and process measures are summarized in Table 48.4.

16. **Answer C. Predominantly Levels 3 and 4.**

Although AASM quality measure development followed a structured process designed to incorporate the highest level of available evidence, the insomnia workgroup found that existing practice guidelines were based largely on expert

TABLE 48.4	Outcome and Process Measures for Quality Care of Pediatric Patients with Obstructive Sleep Apnea
Outcome or Outcome Measure	**Processes That Support the Outcome**
detection of pediatric OSA	Assessment of at least one OSA symptom or risk factor in pediatric patients with snoring Use of an evidence-based management plan within 12 months of the detection of OSA symptoms or signs (including watchful waiting/medical management, surgical management, referral for polysomnography, referral to a sleep specialist, or a sleep apnea specialist) Referral for polysomnography or to a sleep or sleep apnea specialist for all pediatric patients with complex medical conditions that increase risk of OSA and who have signs and symptoms of sleep apnea
Reduce signs and symptoms of OSA	Reassessment of abnormal OSA signs and symptoms within 12 months of starting treatment for OSA Assessment of CPAP adherence within 3 months of starting CPAP therapy

OSA, Obstructive sleep apnea.

TABLE 48.5	Strength of Evidence Supporting Insomnia Quality Measure Indicators	
Grade	**Strength of Evidence**	**Description**
Level 1	Strongest evidence	Process measure reflects an evidence-based guideline's highest level of recommendation
Level 2	Moderately strong evidence	Process measure reflects an evidence-based guideline's mid-level or moderate level of recommendation
Level 3	Weak evidence	Process measure reflects a single randomized controlled trial with a large effect size or a consensus-level recommendation from an evidence-based guideline
Level 4	Workgroup consensus, may be informed by lower grade evidence	Process measure reflects the consensus of the quality measures workgroup, a single randomized controlled trial with a small effect size, or observational studies

consensus, other than for recommendations regarding behavioral or pharmacologic treatment. As a result, the majority of the process measures were graded level 3 or 4 (Answer C is correct; see Table 48.5 for measure evidence grading).[3] This highlights the need for more research specifically evaluating clinical processes and measurement of quality.

17. **Answer C. The patient's report of sleep quality.**
In developing the process measure requiring assessment of sleep satisfaction and sleep quality, the workgroup considered a variety of validated questionnaires for assessing insomnia severity or sleep quality, including the Pittsburgh Sleep Quality Index, the Insomnia Severity Index (Fig. 48.1), the Children's Sleep Habits Questionnaire, and the Sleep Self-Report. (The Epworth Sleepiness Scale is a measure of daytime sleepiness, not insomnia; Answer A is incorrect.) Many of these insomnia measures have been used to document treatment benefits in controlled clinical trials, and as such seem likely to be useful for measuring change with treatment in clinical practice. However, there were concerns among workgroup members that providers in primary care and other nonsleep specialty settings would not have access to or infrastructure support for the administration of such questionnaires. Thus, by consensus, the decision was made that all measures of sleep quality and satisfaction, including insomnia questionnaires, sleep diaries, and simple patient reports, are acceptable tools for this measure (Answer C is correct). However, the workgroup noted that the global clinician impression of patient reports may be particularly subject to bias, such that validated measures of patient-reported outcomes are preferred whenever possible.[6] Objective verification of sleep time or sleep efficiency was considered by the workgroup, but in light of the overall goal of improving patient satisfaction with sleep across a variety of practice settings, objective measures of sleep or rest/activity patterns were not selected as measures of sleep satisfaction and quality (Answers B and D are incorrect).

18. **Answer B. Stimulus control therapy.**
According to the Spielman 3-P model of insomnia, acute insomnia may be triggered by precipitating factors (acute stressors) in those with predisposing characteristics, while chronic insomnia develops and is maintained as a result of perpetuating factors (in general, behaviors adopted in an attempt to manage the insomnia, such as spending long amounts of time in bed; Fig. 48.2). Behavioral approaches to treatment can target some of these perpetuating factors.

In the insomnia quality measures,[6] recommendations for evidence-based treatment options were drawn from existing clinical practice guidelines,[7,8] which affirm Level 1 support for stimulus control therapy, cognitive behavioral treatment for insomnia, and relaxation therapy (Answer B is correct). Sleep restriction therapy and paradoxical intention are supported by Level 2 evidence (Answers A and C are incorrect). Doxepin, short-acting benzodiazepine receptor agonists, and ramelteon are supported by Level 3 evidence, via the consensus recommendation in the AASM Clinical Guideline (Answer D is incorrect).[7]

19. **Answer D. Impaired concentration and academic performance.**
The ICSD-3 criteria for chronic insomnia (Box 48.4) emphasize the presence of daytime dysfunction as a key aspect of the diagnosis of insomnia (ICSD-3). This daytime dysfunction can take many forms, including impairments in concentration and social, family, occupational, or academic performance (Answer D is correct). In the ICSD-2, the diagnostic criteria for psychophysiologic insomnia required evidence of

INSOMNIA SEVERITY INDEX (ISI)

Subject ID: _____   **Date:** _____

For each question below, please circle the number corresponding most accurately to your sleep patterns in the **LAST MONTH.**

For the first three questions, please rate the **SEVERITY** of your sleep difficulties.

1. Difficulty falling asleep:

None	Mild	Moderate	Severe	Very severe
0	1	2	3	4

2. Difficulty staying asleep:

None	Mild	Moderate	Severe	Very severe
0	1	2	3	4

3. Problem waking up too early in the morning:

None	Mild	Moderate	Severe	Very severe
0	1	2	3	4

4. How **SATISFIED**/dissatisfied are you with your current sleep pattern?

Very Satisfied	Satisfied	Neutral	Dissatisfied	Very Dissatisfied
0	1	2	3	4

5. To what extent do you consider your sleep problem to **INTERFERE** with your daily functioning (e.g., daytime fatigue, ability to function at work/daily chores, concentration, memory, mood).

Not at all Interfering	A little Interfering	Somewhat Interfering	Much Interfering	Very much Interfering
0	1	2	3	4

6. How **NOTICEABLE** to others do you think your sleeping problem is in terms of impairing the quality of your life?

Not at all Noticeable	A little Noticeable	Somewhat Noticeable	Much Noticeable	Very much Noticeable
0	1	2	3	4

7. How **WORRIED**/distressed are you about your current sleep problem?

Not at all	A little	Somewhat	Much	Very much
0	1	2	3	4

Guidelines for scoring/interpretation:

Add scores for all seven items   = _____
Total score ranges from 0–28

0–7	= No clinically significant insomnia
8–14	= Subthreshold insomnia
15–21	= Clinical insomnia (moderate severity)
22–28	= Clinical insomnia (severe)

• **Figure 48.1** The Insomnia Severity Index. (From Doghramji K. The evaluation and management of insomnia. *Clin Chest Med.* 2010;31[2]:327–339.)

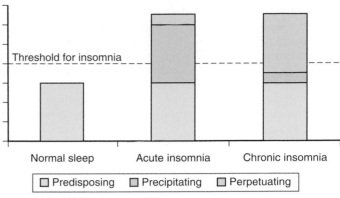

• **Figure 48.2** The 3-P Model of Insomnia. (From Galion A, Martin JL. Ontogeny of Insomnia. In: Kushida C, ed. *Encyclopedia of Sleep.* Amsterdam: Elsevier/Academic Press; 2013:171–176.)

• **BOX 48.4   International Classification of Sleep Disorders, Third Edition, Diagnostic Criteria for Chronic Insomnia**

A. Resistance to going to bed, difficulty with onset or maintenance of sleep, waking too early, or requiring parent or caregiver assistance to fall asleep
B. Daytime dysfunction (reported by the patient or caregiver) related to insomnia, including:
   a. Fatigue, sleepiness, or reduced energy/lack of motivation
   b. Impairments in cognition (memory, attention, concentration)
   c. Impairments in performance (social, family, work, or school); errors or accidents
   d. Mood changes
   e. Behavior changes (aggression, impulsivity, hyperactivity)
   f. Lack of satisfaction with sleep
C. Sufficient time and circumstances to allow sleep
D. Sleep and daytime symptoms present ≥ 3 times/week
E. Sleep and daytime symptoms present ≥ 3 months
F. Not better explained by another disorder
All six of the above criteria must be met.

American Academy of Sleep Medicine. International Classification of Sleep Disorders. *3rd ed. Darien, IL: American Academy of Sleep Medicine; 2014.*

---

conditioned sleep difficulty, which could be manifest by excessive anxiety about sleep or ease of falling asleep in locations or at times different than the typical pattern, among other features. However, this conditioned sleep difficulty is not a core component of the current chronic insomnia diagnosis criteria (Answers B and C are incorrect). Chronic insomnia may manifest as difficulty falling asleep, difficulty staying asleep, waking early, resistance to going to bed, or need for parent/caregiver support in order to sleep (Answer A is incorrect).

The insomnia quality measures were designed to emphasize the importance of assessing and improving insomnia-related daytime dysfunction through both an outcome measure (proportion of patients with improvement in daytime functioning after treatment) and a process measure (proportion of patients who receive an assessment of daytime function at each insomnia-related visit). The authors of the quality measures note that insomnia treatment often focuses only on nocturnal sleep, without targeting daytime dysfunction, while daytime dysfunction may be the symptom that motivates people to seek treatment, and may be an important determinant of satisfaction with treatment.[6]

20. **Answer C. Side effects of both insomnia medications and cognitive-behavioral therapy.**
   The proportion of treated patients receiving an assessment of side effects is an insomnia process measure.[6] While assessment of side effects of medications is common practice, the authors of the insomnia quality measures point out that behavioral treatments of insomnia may also have side effects, and these should also be systematically evaluated. In particular, sleep

restriction may result in daytime sleepiness and impairments in vigilance that may be clinically important (Answer C is correct; Answers A and B are incorrect). While improvement in quality of life is an overall goal of insomnia care, quality of life measures are not explicitly mandated to be collected at every patient encounter (Answer D is incorrect). Subjective sleep latency and sleep duration can be collected as part of sleep satisfaction and quality (Answer E is incorrect).

A summary of the full set of AASM insomnia quality measures is presented in Table 48.6.

21. **Answer D. He is experiencing a mimic of RLS with positional discomfort that occurs at night because of positioning and not because of circadian rhythmicity.**

There are a number of mimics of RLS, including positional discomfort, leg cramp, and arthritis.[9] Thus, prior to considering treatment for RLS, it is important the clinician be as certain of the diagnosis as possible, and ascertain whether or not the patient meets the standard criteria for RLS. Recently, there have been new diagnostic criteria drafted by the AASM (through the ICSD), the International RLS Study Group, and the American Psychiatric Association (through the DSM). They all agree on core features, but with some differences in emphasis on ruling out mimics, clinical consequences, and frequency/duration (Table 48.7).[13]

This patient does not have RLS for multiple reasons (Answer D is correct). First, he does not experience an urge to move his leg—he has a dysesthesia but without the urge to move, which is not sufficient for an RLS diagnosis (Answer A is incorrect). Although his discomfort occurs at night and is relieved with movement, it is relieved with a single position change and does not require the additional or continual movement that characterizes RLS (Answer B is incorrect). Although patients with RLS often (and, per ICSD-3, must) have a concern or disturbance of sleep or daytime dysfunction, the presence of that criterion alone is insufficient to diagnose RLS (Answer C is incorrect). This patient has positional discomfort, possibly caused by vascular compression.

22. **Answer A. Serum ferritin level, with a full iron panel when possible.**

An association between RLS and iron deficiency has been recognized since the 1950s.[14] The exact relationship is complicated,[15] but low systemic iron states can exacerbate or cause RLS,[16] and iron supplementation is recommended for patients with RLS with ferritin levels below 50 or 75 mcg/L.[17,18] Thus the workgroup concluded that every patient with RLS should undergo assessment of systemic iron stores at the time of diagnosis. Serum ferritin is the most sensitive and specific test of iron deficiency,[19] so the workgroup recommended that serum ferritin at a minimum should be checked (Answer A is correct and Answer C is incorrect). If a ferritin level has been done within a year prior to the diagnosis and there is no reason to suspect a change in iron status, the ferritin level does not need to be repeated to comply with this process measure. Because ferritin can be elevated with systemic inflammation,[20] the full iron panel is recommended although not required by this process measure. Hemoglobin and hematocrit are insufficient, as RLS patients may have low iron stores without anemia (Answer B is incorrect).[16] Haptoglobin is a protein that is used to screen for and monitor hemolysis (Answer D is incorrect).

TABLE 48.6	Outcome and Process Measures for Quality Care of Patients with Insomnia
Outcome or Outcome Measure	**Processes That Support the Outcome**
Proportion of patients with improved sleep satisfaction or quality	Assessment of sleep quality at each visit Provision of evidence based treatment
Proportion of patients with improvement in daytime functioning after treatment	Provision of evidence-based treatment Assessment of daytime function at each visit Assessment of side effects at each visit

Edinger JD, Buysse DJ, Deriy L, et al. Quality measures for the care of patients with insomnia. *J Clin Sleep Med.* 2015;11:311-334.

TABLE 48.7	Diagnostic Criteria for Restless Legs Syndrome		
	International Classification of Sleep Disorders, Third Edition[10]	**Diagnostic and Statistical Manual, Fifth Edition**[11]	**International Restless Legs Syndrome Study Group**[12]
Urge to move	Mandatory	Mandatory	Mandatory
Worsening at rest	Mandatory	Mandatory	Mandatory
Improvement with movement	Mandatory	Mandatory	Mandatory
Worsening in the evening/night	Mandatory	Mandatory	Mandatory
Ruling out mimics	Mandatory	Mandatory	Mandatory
Presence of concern, distress, impairment, or sleep disturbance related to symptoms	Mandatory	Mandatory	Can be specified as clinically significant but not mandatory for diagnosis
Duration and frequency of symptoms	No minimums required	Diagnosis requires symptoms at least three times per week for at least 3 months	No minimums required, although can be specified as chronic-persistent or intermittent

23. **Answer C. Patients on dopaminergic medications should be asked about impulse control disorders and augmentation at every visit.**

Adverse drug events are reduced when clinicians counsel patients about potential medication side effects, and in fact, the Agency for Healthcare Research and Quality recommends that clinicians counsel not just patients but also their caregivers about potential side effects (Answer D is incorrect). Although the workgroup agreed that counseling patients about side effects was only mandatory at the initiation of a new medication, the consensus was that impulse control disorders (ICDs) and augmentation needed to be evaluated at every visit for patients on dopaminergic therapy (Answers A and B are incorrect; Answer C is correct). ICDs are regarded as a serious treatment complication in RLS, and both the International RLS Study Group[21] and the RLS/Willis-Ekbom Disease Foundation[17] have endorsed screening patients on dopaminergic therapy for ICDs at every follow-up visit. In addition, ICDs may not be evident early in treatment, with the average onset of ICD occurring 9.5 months after the initiation of dopamine agonist therapy, thereby necessitating clinical suspicion for the onset of ICDs well after a patient has started a dopaminergic medication.[22] Augmentation, a progressive worsening of RLS symptoms with continued or increased dopaminergic therapy, is also considered a severe and delayed complication of therapy that requires careful vigilance by the clinician and frequent assessment. It is recommended that augmentation be defined based on criteria accepted at the time the patient is evaluated. At the time of the publication of the AASM RLS Quality Measures, the criteria in widespread use were the Max Planck diagnostic criteria (Box 48.5).[23] In contrast, counseling about potential medication side effects in general is recommended at the time a new medication is started, without specification of how frequently it needs to be repeated at subsequent visits, leaving this up to the clinician's discretion.[13]

24. **Answer B. A measure of severity of RLS symptoms combined with an assessment of at least one RLS-associated domain (sleep quality, daytime sleepiness/tiredness, daytime function, or mood).**

Process Measure 3 instructs the clinician to assess RLS severity at every visit. It further states that the assessment should include both a global measure of severity and an assessment of at least one RLS-associated domain, including sleep quality, daytime sleepiness/tiredness, daytime function, or mood. A free-text assessment of both is sufficient (e.g., "the patient reports that the RLS symptoms continue to be mild and sleep quality has remained stable and is improved compared with initial presentation"). The IRLS contains both, through questions relating to severity of disease as well as its impact on sleep quality and daytime functioning, but is not the only acceptable method of assessment (Answer A is incorrect). The PGI only assesses overall severity and not clinical impact (Answer C is incorrect), and documenting impact without an overall assessment of severity is also insufficient (Answer D is incorrect). A measure of severity of RLS symptoms combined with an assessment of at least one RLS-associated domain (sleep quality, daytime sleepiness/tiredness, daytime function, or mood) is recommended, and includes the IRLS or the combination of the PGI, with an assessment of clinical impact on an RLS-associated domain being sufficient (Answer B is correct).[13]

25. **Answer D. Assessment of symptom severity and delivery of evidence-based treatment.**

• BOX 48.5 Max-Planck-Institute Criteria

Preamble

Augmentation is a worsening of RLS symptom severity experienced by patients undergoing treatment of RLS. The RLS symptoms in general are more severe than those experienced at baseline.

A. Basic features (all of which need to be met):
   1. The increase in symptom severity was experienced on 5 out of 7 days during the previous week.
   2. The increase in symptom severity is not accounted for by other factors, such as a change in medical status, lifestyle, or the natural progression of the disorder.
   3. It is assumed that there has been a prior positive response to treatment.

   In addition, B, C, or both have to be met:

B. Persisting (although not immediate) paradoxic response to treatment: RLS symptom severity increases some time after a dose increase, and improves some time after a dose decrease.

C. Earlier onset of symptoms:
   1. An earlier onset by at least 4 hours.

   Or:

   2. An earlier onset (between 2 and 4 hours) occurs with one of the following compared with symptom status before treatment:
      a. Shorter latency to symptoms when at rest
      b. Spreading of symptoms to other body parts
      c. Intensity of symptoms is greater (or increase in periodic limb movements if measured by polysomnography or the suggested immobilization test)
      d. Duration of relief from treatment is shorter

   Augmentation requires criteria A and B, A and C, or A and B and C to be met.

From Garcia-Borreguero D. Dopaminergic augmentation in restless legs syndrome/Willis-Ekbom disease: identification and management. Sleep Med Clin. 2015;10:287-292.

In order to manage RLS symptoms effectively, the workgroup recognized that there needs to be a systemized measure of severity and incorporated Process Measure 3, assessment of symptom severity at every visit, into the quality measures. This assessment ensures that the severity of RLS will be evaluated at each and every visit relating to RLS and will have both a global measure of severity as well as an assessment of the impact of RLS on the quality of sleep or daytime functioning, thus providing a measure that can be followed from visit to visit. In addition, a therapeutic intervention is recommended in the form of delivery of evidence-based treatment, Process Measure 4 (Answer D is correct). Of note, emphasis was made that the choice of treatment should follow the current evidence-based guidelines at the time the patient is evaluated and treated. Thus, although the non-ergot dopamine agonists and the alpha-2-delta calcium-channel ligands in general were regarded as first-line treatments for RLS at the time of the publication of the RLS Quality Measures, recognition was given that different medications may become the preferred initial treatment or be the appropriate treatment in any particular patient. Assessment of iron stores and use of accepted diagnostic criteria are process measures intended to improve the accuracy of RLS diagnosis (Answers A and C are incorrect). Assessment of medication side effects is a process measure for minimizing treatment complications (Answer B is incorrect).[13] The full set of RLS quality outcome and process measures is summarized in Table 48.8.

TABLE 48.8	Outcome and Process Measures for Quality Care of Patients with Restless Legs Syndrome
Outcome or Outcome Measure	**Processes That Support the Outcome**
Improve accuracy of RLS diagnosis	Use of accepted diagnostic criteria at initial evaluation Assessment of serum ferritin and other measures of iron stores at initial evaluation
Decrease severity of RLS symptoms	Assessment of severity of RLS symptoms at every visit Use of evidence-based treatment once diagnosis is made
Minimize treatment complications	Counseling on potential medication side effects at medication initiation Assessment for impulse control disorders at every follow up visit (for patients on dopaminergic medications) Assessment for augmentation at every follow up visit (for patients on dopaminergic medications)

RLS, Restless legs syndrome.
Trotti LM, Goldstein CA, Harrod CG, et al. Quality measures for the care of adult patients with restless legs syndrome. *J Clin Sleep Med.* 2015;11:293-310.

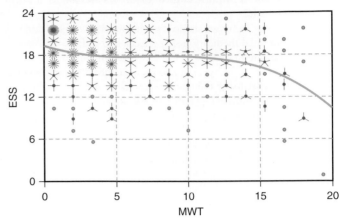

SCATTER-PLOT: ESS AND MWT
522 DRUG-FREE PATIENTS WITH NARCOLEPSY

• **Figure 48.3** Discrepant subjective and objective measures of sleepiness in patients with narcolepsy. (From Sangal RB, Mitler MM, Sangal JM. Subjective sleepiness ratings [Epworth sleepiness scale] do not reflect the same parameter of sleepiness as objective sleepiness [maintenance of wakefulness test] in patients with narcolepsy. *Clin Neurophysiol.* 1999; 110[12]:2131–2135).

• **BOX 48.6** Validated Scales for the Assessment of Subjective Sleepiness in Patients with Narcolepsy

Epworth Sleepiness Scale*
Stanford Sleepiness Scale
Karolinska Sleepiness Scale
Cleveland Adolescent Sleepiness Questionnaire
Visual Analog Scales of sleepiness

*Although the Epworth had not been formally validated in children at the time of the quality measures publication, this scale has been used extensively in clinical and research settings in children ages 6–16 and was judged acceptable for use in this population.
Krahn LE, Hershner S, Loeding LD, et al. Quality measures for the care of patients with narcolepsy. J Clin Sleep Med. 2015;11:335.

26. **Answer A. Validated measure of subjective sleepiness (e.g., Epworth Sleepiness Scale).**
This outcome measures the proportion of patients with improvements in subjective sleepiness. Objective tools, such as the maintenance of wakefulness test, may be very useful in the management of patients with narcolepsy, but were judged by the narcolepsy task force as overly burdensome for incorporation in a quality measure and for repeated measures in routine clinical practice (Answer C is incorrect).[24] The task force acknowledged that subjective and objective measures may measure different aspects of daytime sleepiness in patients with narcolepsy, in whom measures on subjective and objective tests may be only modestly correlated (Fig. 48.3). Reduction of risk of motor vehicle accidents and improving safety are implicitly contained in outcome 3 (reduce adverse events), but driving safety is not recommended as an acceptable tool for measurement of sleepiness (Answer D is incorrect).
In contrast to some of the other disease-related quality measures (e.g., insomnia, RLS), the narcolepsy quality measures mandate the use of a validated measure of subjective sleepiness rather than allowing patient-reported symptoms without validated quantification (Answer A is correct; Answer B is incorrect). The process measure for assessment of sleepiness requires assessment of subjective sleepiness using a validated scale at every visit. Other validated scales for the assessment of sleepiness in patients with narcolepsy are listed in Box 48.6.

27. **Answer B. 1 month.**
The AASM narcolepsy quality measures include a process measure evaluating the proportion of patients diagnosed with narcolepsy who are advised to begin treatment within 1 month

of the date of the diagnostic MSLT (or CSF hypocretin testing, if this is performed in lieu of MSLT; Answer B is correct). The rationale behind this time frame, which was based on expert consensus, was that the sleepiness caused by narcolepsy has severe implications for patients while untreated, including impairments in occupational and educational performance and increased risk of accidents and injury.[24] The taskforce acknowledged that some practice types may not be optimally set up to allow follow-up and treatment initiation within this time frame; in such cases, a phone call or approved electronic communication with the patient to discuss results and treatment options was deemed an acceptable alternative to a face to face visit.

28. **Answer D. MSLT was performed following standard protocols, including tapering off venlafaxine prior to the study.**
One of the three outcomes in the quality measures for narcolepsy is an improvement in the accuracy of narcolepsy diagnosis. This is supported by the process measures of performing a comprehensive sleep history and examination and

performing objective sleep assessment. A comprehensive sleep history must include sleep-wake patterns, evaluation for sleep apnea symptoms, and current medication use. Evaluation for a history of traumatic brain injury, multiple sclerosis, and other secondary causes of sleepiness and cataplexy is encouraged but not specifically mandated by the quality measures (Answers A and B are incorrect). Exclusion of secondary causes of sleepiness via blood tests may be indicated in some cases, but is not part of the process measures for narcolepsy diagnosis (Answer C is incorrect). Objective sleep assessment (i.e., PSG/MSLT) must be performed according to standardized protocols, which includes weaning off of antidepressants for at least 2 weeks or five half-lives,[25] and the use of a standardized protocol should be explicitly documented (Answer D is correct).[24] The workgroup acknowledged that, in some cases, antidepressants cannot safely be discontinued for testing. In such situations, the deviation from established protocols should be noted, the reason for this deviation explained, and an assessment of the diagnostic implications (e.g., change in number of sleep onset REM periods) should be reported.

29. **Answer D. Every 12 months.**
The narcolepsy task force recommended follow-up of patients to occur at least annually (Answer D is correct). However, they emphasized that an optimal follow-up schedule may involve considerably more frequent visits than this (e.g., every 3 months in some cases), but that 1 year was a minimally acceptable threshold for quality care. The need for regular follow-up in patients with narcolepsy is driven by several concerns: (1) ensuring sleepiness and other narcolepsy symptoms are appropriately treated; (2) evaluating for comorbid diseases that are common in people with narcolepsy (e.g., sleep disordered breathing, psychiatric disease, and obesity, the latter especially in children near disease onset);

TABLE 48.9 **Serious Side Effects of Medications Used for Treatment of Narcolepsy**

Medication*	FDA Schedule	Potentially Serious Side Effects Highlighted in the Narcolepsy Quality Measures[24]**
Stimulants	Schedule 2	Abuse, tolerance
Sodium oxybate	Schedule 3 (but with a Risk Evaluation and Mitigation Strategy program from the FDA)	Respiratory depression, coma, death
Antidepressants	Not scheduled	Risk of suicidality in people ≤ 24 years old
Modafinil, armodafinil	Schedule 4	Interaction with hormonal birth control to reduce effectiveness

*Some listed medications reflect off-label use in patients with narcolepsy.
**Medications may have other serious side effects not listed here.
FDA, US Food and Drug Administration.

TABLE 48.10 **Narcolepsy Medications and Their Pregnancy Categories**

Medication	FDA Pregnancy Category	EMA SPC Pregnancy and Lactation Statements
Modafinil/armodafinil	C	Modafinil should not be used during pregnancy and lactation
Sodium oxybate	C	GHB is not to be recommended during pregnancy or breast-feeding
Methylphenidate	C	Methylphenidate is not recommended for use during pregnancy unless a clinical decision is made that postponing treatment may pose a greater risk to the pregnancy. A risk to the suckling child cannot be excluded.
Dextroamphetamine	C	Dextroamphetamine is contraindicated during pregnancy. Dexedrine passes into breast milk.
Selegiline	C	It is preferable to avoid the use of selegiline in pregnancy. Selegiline should not be used during breast-feeding.
Venlafaxine	C	Venlafaxine must only be administered to pregnant women if the expected benefits outweigh any possible risk. A risk to the suckling child cannot be excluded.
Atomoxetine	C	Atomoxetine should not be used during pregnancy unless the potential benefit justifies the potential risk to the fetus. Atomoxetine should be avoided during breast-feeding.
Clomipramine	C	No information available
Fluoxetine	C	Not recommended during pregnancy and lactation
Protriptyline	C	No information available

EMA, European Medicines Agency; *FDA*, US Food and Drug Administration; *SPC*, summary of product characteristics.
Table reproduced from Thorpy M, Zhao CG, Dauvilliers Y. Management of narcolepsy during pregnancy. *Sleep Med.* 2013;14:367-376.

(3) addressing psychosocial needs that may develop in people with narcolepsy (e.g., work or school accommodations); and (4) assessment of adverse effects of medications. Although the task force chose not to delineate a full list of side effects to be addressed, both because of the ongoing development of new drugs and because of off-label use of medications to treat narcolepsy symptoms, they highlighted the fact that treatments for narcolepsy have potentially serious risks that should be regularly assessed (Table 48.9).

30. **Answer B. The narcolepsy quality measures contain two process measures designed to promote patient counseling.**

The first requires counseling about medication side effects and drug-drug interactions, and the second requires counseling about safety risks faced by people with narcolepsy (Answer B is correct). Safety concerns for patients with narcolepsy vary by age, but include issues with driving, household chores (e.g., cooking over a stove), and workplace safety.[24] Appropriate counseling about the presence of these risks and strategies to reduce them is a key process of quality care of the patient with narcolepsy.

The remaining answers may be part of appropriate counseling in some cases, but were not identified by the task force as a specific process measure for quality care of narcolepsy patients (Answers A, C, and D are incorrect). Some patients with narcolepsy require and benefit from accommodations at school or work, particularly use of scheduled, short naps. Women with narcolepsy face similar issues as women with other chronic medical conditions (e.g., epilepsy) regarding decision-making about medication management during preconception, pregnancy, and breast-feeding. Safety data regarding narcolepsy treatment during pregnancy are limited. Approved and commonly used medications are universally rated pregnancy class C by the US Food and Drug Administration (FDA; i.e., meaning that human data are insufficient to determine risk and that animal data are either insufficient or suggest increased risk; Table 48.10). The full set of AASM outcomes and process measures for quality care of patients with narcolepsy are summarized in Table 48.11.

TABLE 48.11	Outcome and Process Measures for Quality Care of Patients with Narcolepsy
Outcome or Outcome Measure	**Processes That Support the Outcome**
Proportion of patients with decreased subjective sleepiness after treatment	Assessment of sleepiness at each visit Provision of treatment within 1 month of MSLT or CSF hypocretin result
Improved diagnostic accuracy	Comprehensive sleep history and physical at or before diagnostic testing (including sleep-wake patterns, evidence for sleep-disordered breathing, current medications, and general and neurologic examinations) PSG/MSLT via standardized AASM protocols (exclusion from this measure if diagnosed by CSF hypocretin)
Decreased number of adverse events	Follow-up visit at least annually Counseling about medication side effects and interactions Counseling about safety risks relevant to patients with narcolepsy

AASM, American Academy of Sleep Medicine; *MSLT,* multiple sleep latency test; *PSG,* polysomnography;
Krahn LE, Hershner S, Loeding LD, et al. Quality measures for the care of patients with narcolepsy. *J Clin Sleep Med.* 2015;11:335.

Suggested Reading

Aurora RN, Collop NA, Jacobowitz O, et al. Quality measures for the care of adult patients with obstructive sleep apnea. *J Clin Sleep Med.* 2015;11:357-383.

Edinger JD, Buysse DJ, Deriy L, et al. Quality measures for the care of patients with insomnia. *J Clin Sleep Med.* 2015;11:311-334.

Kothare SV, Rosen CL, Lloyd RM, et al. Quality measures for the care of pediatric patients with obstructive sleep apnea. *J Clin Sleep Med.* 2015;11:385-404.

Krahn LE, Hershner S, Loeding LD, et al. Quality measures for the care of patients with narcolepsy. *J Clin Sleep Med.* 2015;11:335.

Morgenthaler TI, Aronsky AJ, Carden KA, et al. Measurement of quality to improve care in sleep medicine. *J Clin Sleep Med.* 2015;11:279-291.

Trotti LM, Goldstein CA, Harrod CG, et al. Quality measures for the care of adult patients with restless legs syndrome. *J Clin Sleep Med.* 2015;11:293-310.

49

Normal Sleep

BRANDON R. PETERS, CLETE A. KUSHIDA

Questions

1. On a cold, wintry night, an otherwise healthy 9-year-old boy is discovered by a police officer to be wandering the street near his school in his pajamas. He is initially confused and inappropriately responsive. After being vigorously awakened, he begins crying and complains about his painful bare feet that appear to have early signs of frostbite. When he later presents to the sleep clinic for further evaluation, his mother asks how he could have walked nearly a mile from home through the snow without being awakened. Which of the following *best* accounts for this phenomenon?
   A. An underdeveloped nervous system may allow for the acting out of dreams during rapid eye movement (REM) sleep.
   B. Sleep is characterized by a reversible state of perceptual disengagement and relative insensitivity to the environment.
   C. Given his confusion and lack of normal sensation, it is likely that he has an underlying seizure disorder.
   D. The perception of nociceptive pain is uniquely masked during slow wave sleep.

2. A 33-year-old congenitally blind man presents for evaluation of chronic insomnia and daytime sleepiness that seems to be cyclical in nature, gradually fluctuating in intensity over several months. He has slept poorly for most of his life. Given prior failures, he refuses to consider the use of any medications (including melatonin) as sleep aids. He reports no perception of light, but after reading about benefits to other similar patients, you recommend that he keep a regular sleep schedule with 30 min of sunlight exposure upon awakening. He returns several months later and reports improvement in his condition. What is the *correct order* of the anatomical pathway that must be preserved for a response to phototherapy in blind people with non-24-hour sleep-wake disorder?
   A. Rods, retinohypothalamic tract, suprachiasmatic nucleus (SCN) in the anterior hypothalamus, paraventricular nucleus of the hypothalamus, preganglionic sympathetic neurons, superior cervical ganglion, pineal gland

   B. Intrinsically photosensitive retinal ganglion cells (ipRGC), retinohypothalamic tract, SCN in the posterior hypothalamus, paraventricular nucleus of the hypothalamus, preganglionic sympathetic neurons, superior cervical ganglion pineal gland
   C. ipRGC, retinohypothalamic tract, SCN in the anterior hypothalamus, paraventricular nucleus of the hypothalamus, preganglionic sympathetic neurons, superior cervical ganglion, pineal gland
   D. Extrinsically photosensitive retinal ganglion cells (epRGC), retinohypothalamic tract, SCN in the anterior hypothalamus, paraventricular nucleus of the hypothalamus, preganglionic sympathetic neurons, superior cervical ganglion, pineal gland

3. Fig. 49.1 is a 30-sec epoch of sleep from a polysomnogram that you are reviewing. In which of the following situations would this particular stage of sleep be considered to be an abnormal finding?
   A. Within the first 15 min of sleep in a 2-month-old infant
   B. Occurring once during a nap opportunity as part of a multiple sleep latency test (MSLT) with a mean sleep latency of 7 min on a normal adult with excessive daytime sleepiness complaints
   C. Constituting an increased proportion of sleep on the second night of recovery after sleep deprivation
   D. Increasing in duration with adequate positive airway pressure (PAP) titration during the latter half of a split night study that was initially positive for severe obstructive sleep apnea

4. As part of his pioneering research into sleep-wake mechanisms in 1935–1936, Dr. Frédéric Bremer studied the electrical rhythms of sleep and wakefulness in cat brains through precise anatomical dissection. Using his original descriptors, which of the following is *improperly* paired with the corresponding brainstem anatomy and/or observed function?
   A. *Encéphale*: Section in the lower part of the medulla, used for the study of cortical electrical rhythms responsive to various sensory impulses
   B. *Encéphale isolé*: Demonstrated an alternating pattern between the waking and sleeping state
   C. *Cerveau isolé*: electroencephalogram (EEG) of this section demonstrated a sleeping state; it effectively suppresses nerve impulses necessary for the waking state of the telencephalon.
   D. *Chronic cerveau isolé*: Demonstrated the features of quiet sleep are located in the lower brainstem and modulated by forebrain structures

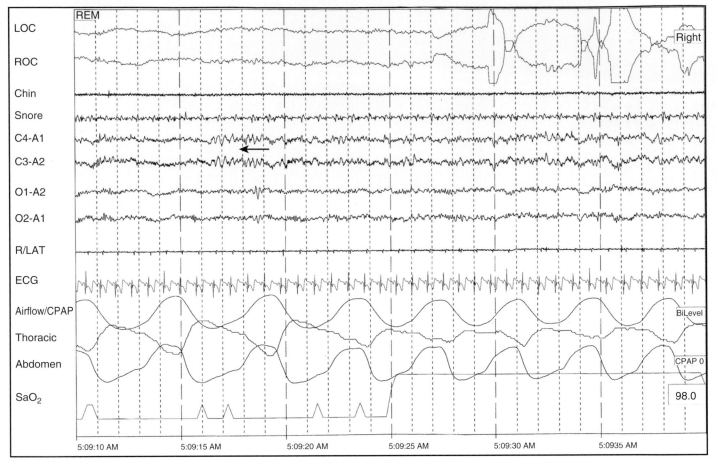

• **Figure 49.1** Thirty-second epoch. *C4-A1/C3-A2,* Right/left central electroencephalogram (*EEG*) leads; *ECG,* electrocardiogram; Chin electromyogram (*EMG*); *LOC/ROC,* left/right outer canthus; *O1-A2, O2-A1,* left/right occipital EEG leads; *R/LAT,* right/left leg EMG.

5. Concerned about their child's development, anxious first-time parents of a 3-month-old girl present to the clinic to assess her sleep. She is well appearing with an uncomplicated birth history and, to this point, has met normal developmental milestones. She sleeps approximately 15 hours in a 24-hour period, taking three to four naps per day and waking briefly 2–3 times at night. She cries briefly after nocturnal awakenings and is able to fall back asleep without further intervention. Her parents question whether she is sleeping normally. Which of the following is *false* regarding pediatric sleep at the age of 3 months?

   A. K complexes would be present on a sleep electroencephalogram (EEG).

   B. Sleep spindles would be present on a sleep electroencephalogram (EEG).

   C. It may be difficult to differentiate the stages of non-REM sleep based on the electroencephalogram (EEG).

   D. The average total sleep need may normally exceed 15 hours and includes multiple daytime naps.

6. There is a homeostatic balance that contributes to the transitions between states of sleep and wakefulness. Which of the following neuroanatomical structures important to the regulation of wakefulness is *improperly* paired to its function?

   A. *Lateral hypothalamus*: Releases orexin (hypocretin), stabilizes wakefulness

   B. *Tuberomammillary nucleus (TMN)*: Releases histamine, feedback to hypothalamus

   C. *Locus coeruleus*: Releases norepinephrine (NE), feedback to hypothalamus

   D. *Dorsal raphe*: Releases dopamine, feedback to hypothalamus

7. While acclimating at the north base camp of Mt. Everest in Tibet at 5150 meters (16,900 feet), a group of sleep researchers decide to evaluate the changes that occur in sleep. Beyond the periodic breathing that can be observed, what specific changes occur in relation to sleep?

   A. Total sleep time is significantly reduced.

   B. Slow wave sleep is relatively preserved.

   C. REM sleep is relatively preserved.

   D. The arousal index decreases.

8. In reviewing the results of a recent diagnostic polysomnogram with a patient in clinic, the 63-year-old woman patient becomes concerned with whether her distribution of sleep on the hypnogram is normal and interrupts to ask, "What is the deepest stage of sleep and what is its role?" Which of the following statements is true?

   A. There is no appreciable difference in the depth of sleep between the various sleep stages.

   B. REM sleep is the deepest stage of sleep and has a role in memory consolidation.

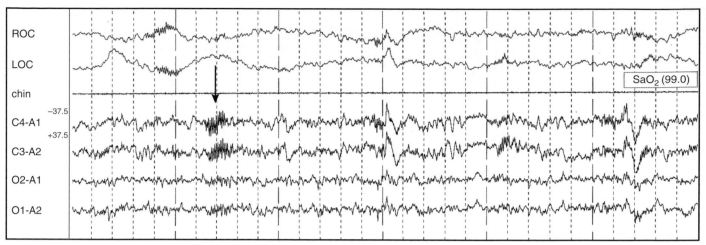

• **Figure 49.2** Thirty-second epoch. *C4-A1/C3-A2,* Right/left central electroencephalogram (*EEG*) leads; *ECG,* electrocardiogram; Chin electromyogram (*EMG*); *LOC/ROC,* left/right outer canthus; *O1-A2, O2-A1,* left/right occipital EEG leads; *R/LAT,* right/left leg EMG.

C. Slow wave sleep (N3) is the deepest stage of sleep and has roles in growth hormone release and long-term memory consolidation.

D. Stage 2 (N2) sleep is the deepest stage of sleep in older adults as slow wave sleep no longer occurs, but its role is unknown.

9. It is late June, and as part of the orientation training for new interns and residents, you have been invited to give the mandatory lecture on the importance of adequate sleep and its effects on medical-decision making. Which of the following statements is *not* true?

A. Performance impairments in working memory capacity are exacerbated by night call.

B. Attending physicians are not impacted by sleep deprivation due to acclimatization that occurs as part of training.

C. Residents who average five or fewer hours of sleep per night have more problems with accidents/injuries, professional staff conflict, alcohol, stimulant medications, and medical errors.

D. Extended work hours in trainees are linked to an increase in driving risk and vehicle crashes after longer shifts.

10. Researchers have studied the sleep of animals for more than a century. Though there are many similarities with the sleep of humans, some clear distinctions are noteworthy. Which of the following statements is *not* true about the unique characteristics of sleep in animals as compared with sleep in humans?

A. Unihemispheric sleep is limited to birds and the following mammals: dolphins (of the order Cetacea), eared seals, and manatees.

B. Slow wave (N3) sleep is a unihemispheric phenomenon in most animals but synchronously affects both hemispheres in humans.

C. All mammals experience REM sleep.

D. Parakeets do not have sleep spindles as part of N2 sleep.

11. In training a new sleep technologist, the lead technologist is flipping through an atlas of old polysomnographic tracings and discovers the image shown in Fig. 49.2. Though there is a lack of frontal leads, as currently recommended, the epoch does demonstrate an important finding in the electroencephalogram (EEG) at the arrow. It is used to quiz the trainee:

What is it, where anatomically is this finding generated, what stage of sleep is it associated with, and which EEG leads will *best* demonstrate it visually?

A. Sleep spindle—thalamus—N2 sleep—central leads

B. Sawtooth waves—thalamus—N2 sleep—frontal leads

C. Sleep spindle—hypothalamus—N2 sleep—central leads

D. Ponto-geniculo-occipital (PGO) spikes—pons—REM sleep—central leads

12. It is known as the main sleep switch. Its cells become active during sleep. It exerts its control by releasing galanin (Gal) and gamma-aminobutyric acid (GABA). It acts by inhibiting cell groups in the locus coeruleus, raphe nucleus, and the TMN. What is the anatomical structure referenced?

A. SCN

B. Pineal gland

C. Thalamus

D. Ventrolateral preoptic nucleus (VLPO)

13. A 79-year-old man presents to the sleep clinic with a large bandage across an abrasion on his left elbow. He reports that several nights ago he woke up from a dream in which he was fighting off an intruder. He fell off the side of the bed and injured his arm. He has had prior movements in sleep, and his wife has slept in another room for years after he hit her in the face one night. What feature would be expected to be observed on a polysomnogram, and what is the cause of the phenomenon?

A. Tonic REM due to loss of cholinergic neurons in the laterodorsal (LD) and pedunculopontine tegmental (PPT) nuclei

B. Phasic REM due to unopposed overactivity of the reticular activating system (RAS)

C. Absence of REM atonia due to loss of activation of dorsolateral pontine reticular formation neurons ventral to the locus coeruleus

D. Sleep paralysis due to loss of inhibition of motor neurons in the spine by both glycinergic and GABAergic mechanisms

14. In 1964 Dr. William C. Dement was present in San Diego as 17-year-old Randy Gardner attempted to set the world record for the longest period a human has gone without sleep

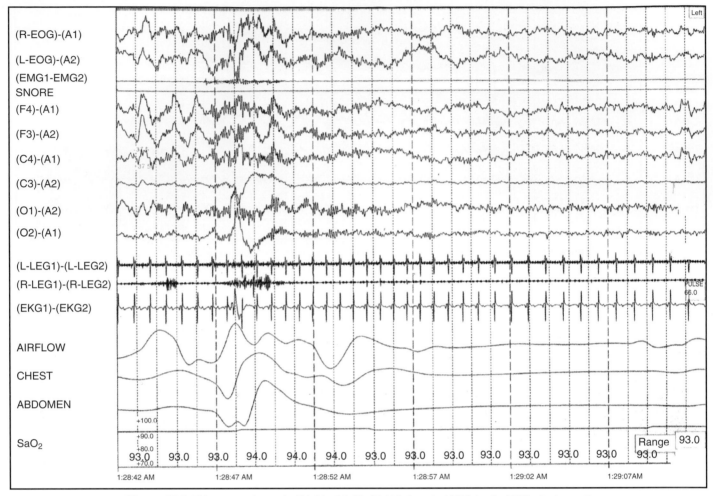

• **Figure 49.3** Thirty-second epoch. *C4-A1, C3-A2,* Right/left central EEG leads; *ECG,* electrocardiogram; *EMG1-EMG2,* chin electromyogram; *F4-A1/F3-A2,* right/left frontal electroencephalogram (EEG) leads; Left/Right leg EMG; *O1-A2, O2-A1,* left/right occipital EEG leads; *R-EOG/L-EOG,* right/left electrooculogram; Snore microphone. Each vertical dotted line demarcates 5 sec.

without the use of stimulants. With careful monitoring, and a lot of basketball and pinball games, the high school student managed to stay up for 264.4 hours (11 days 24 min). Which of the following physiological changes has *not* been observed with chronic sleep deprivation in humans?

A. Hyperactive deep tendon reflexes but sluggish corneal reflexes

B. Suppression of the sex hormones (testosterone, estrogen, and progesterone)

C. Increased secretion of ghrelin and reduction in leptin hormones, leading to increased appetite

D. Increase in delta and theta activity in the awake state

15. A woman's sleep is uniquely subject to the impacts of hormonal fluctuations, including infradian rhythms like the menstrual cycle, as well as changes that occur during the trimesters of pregnancy and the transition of menopause. Which of the following statements does *not* accurately describe some of the features associated with women's sleep?

A. Premenopausal women have a better sleep efficiency compared with men, but have greater subjective sleep complaints.

B. Pregnant women tend to note improved sleep during the second trimester.

C. The risk of sleep apnea increases nearly 10-fold in women at menopause, but this risk is mitigated by hormone replacement therapy.

D. At all ages, women have a higher incidence of insomnia compared with men.

16. A 34-year-old otherwise healthy man has been referred for a diagnostic polysomnogram for evaluation of loud snoring and daytime sleepiness. He has no history of (or symptoms consistent with) heart failure, narcotic use, or brainstem pathology. In reviewing the scoring of the study, the epoch seen in Fig. 49.3 is properly interpreted as which of the following?

A. A respiratory effort-related arousal (RERA) that should be scored, as it may contribute to his presenting symptoms

B. A central apnea indicating an unstable respiratory pattern and that is likely secondary to an unrecognized medical condition

C. A postarousal central apnea that is caused by brief hyperpnea and is a normal finding

D. A central apnea due to ventilatory changes that results when carbon dioxide levels exceed the CO_2 set point

17. A 46-year-old obese man is referred to the sleep clinic for evaluation of persistent nocturnal reflux symptoms associated

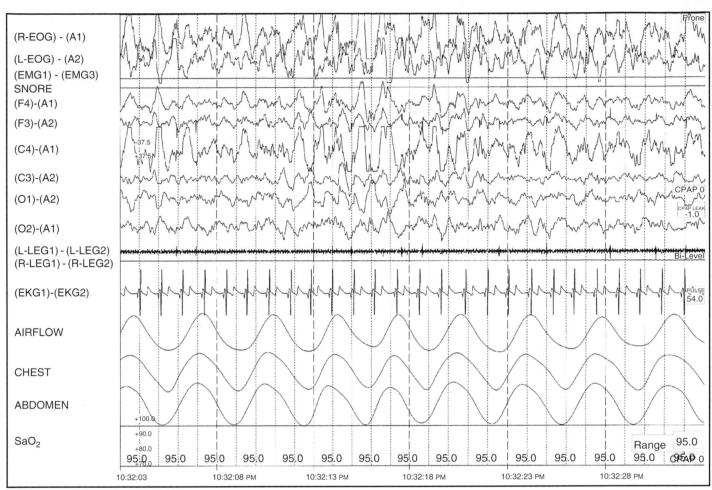

(R-EOG) - (A1)
(L-EOG) - (A2)
(EMG1) - (EMG3)
SNORE
(F4)-(A1)
(F3)-(A2)
(C4)-(A1)
(C3)-(A2)
(O1)-(A2)
(O2)-(A1)
(L-LEG1) - (L-LEG2)
(R-LEG1) - (R-LEG2)
(EKG1)-(EKG2)
AIRFLOW
CHEST
ABDOMEN
SaO₂

- **Figure 49.4** Thirty-second epoch. *C4-A1, C3-A2,* Right/left central EEG leads; *ECG,* electrocardiogram; *EMG1-EMG3,* chin electromyogram; *F4-A1/F3-A2,* right/left frontal electroencephalogram (EEG) leads; Left/Right leg EMG; *O1-A2, O2-A1,* left/right occipital EEG leads; *R-EOG/L-EOG,* right/left electrooculogram; Snore microphone. Each vertical dotted line demarcates 5 sec.

with heartburn complaints. Despite optimization of his diet and the use of multiple proton pump inhibitors, he remains symptomatic. The secretion of gastric acid is normally increased secondary to the stimulation of food intake with meals. There also seems to be reliable findings regarding gastric acid secretion during sleep. Which of the following accurately describes the relationship of gastric acid secretion to sleep?

A. Gastric acid secretion increases much more in REM sleep compared with NREM sleep.

B. The peak of gastric acid secretion occurs early in the night with a circadian periodicity.

C. Gastric acid secretion follows the pattern of cortisol release, peaking in the morning just before awakening.

D. Gastric acid secretion is minimal at night and remains stable throughout sleep due to the lack of food intake.

18. A 9-year-old boy with allergic rhinitis, ADHD, and failure to thrive presents to the sleep clinic for evaluation of snoring, night sweats, and persistent enuresis. He was born at term and was at the 60th percentile for length and weight. By the age of 7, he had dropped to the 10th percentile for height and the 20th percentile for weight without significant improvement in the subsequent 2 years. After a diagnostic polysomnogram, it was discovered that he had pediatric sleep apnea,

and he was referred for tonsillectomy and allergy treatment. He had a repeat postoperative polysomnogram that showed normal proportions of the sleep stage shown in Fig. 49.4 and that his breathing had normalized. By the age of 13, he had improved to the 65th percentiles for both height and weight. What *best* accounts for these changes?

A. By treating his obstructive sleep apnea, he has had normalization of the amount of N3 sleep he obtains with corresponding increases in growth hormone release.

B. Chronic sleep deprivation from his obstructive sleep apnea had decreased the release of ghrelin and increased the release of leptin in N3 sleep, with normalization after treatment.

C. Treatment of his obstructive sleep apnea had favorable effects on the release of testosterone, improving his growth.

D. Though treatment of obstructive sleep apnea may have modestly improved his symptoms, it has no impact on growth in children.

19. After infection with bacteria, a normal host responds with several biochemical changes, including altered sleep regulation. These changes may partially explain the increased sleep requirements that occur when recovering from an illness. Which of

the following *best* describes the response of the host's sleep due to bacterial challenge?

A. Endotoxin from bacterial cell walls is only somnogenic at higher concentrations.

B. The amount of NREM sleep increases in duration and intensity, and REM sleep is inhibited.

C. Much like viral infections, replication within the host is required to alter sleep regulation.

D. Cytokines such as IL-4 and IL-10 are examples of sleep regulatory cytokines that strongly promote NREM sleep.

20. To evaluate the differing effects of acute sleep deprivation on hormones in subjects based on age, a researcher has developed an experimental design with two groups: young adults (aged 20–40 years) and older adults (aged 50–70 years). While monitoring hormone levels through a period of total sleep deprivation, the subjects were allowed several nights of recovery sleep. Which of the following observations is *most unlikely*?

A. Total sleep disruption blunts the secretion of growth hormone and prolactin, with rebound secretion observed during recovery sleep.

B. Though initially blunted during sleep deprivation, adrenocorticotropic hormone (ACTH) rebounds with recovery sleep.

C. Cortisol is unchanged during sleep deprivation, but it decreases more in young adults on the recovery night due to a stronger rebound of N3 sleep.

D. Cortisol and ACTH increase during sleep deprivation, and growth hormone and prolactin rebound during recovery sleep.

21. The days of pulling an all-nighter to cram for a test are long since passed. In preparation for the sleep board examination, you have explained the importance of getting adequate sleep to your companions. Though you have been committing yourself to adequate study and review, you have also ensured that you are consistently meeting your sleep needs to optimize the retention of the material learned. Which of the following statements does *not* describe an important function of sleep in memory consolidation and learning?

A. Visual learning is enhanced by sleep and impaired by sleep loss.

B. Memorization of facts, known as declarative memory, is enhanced by N3 sleep.

C. Memory encoding is dependent on N3 and REM sleep, but not on N1 or N2 sleep.

D. Learning is impaired when sleep and wakefulness are misaligned to the circadian rhythm.

22. It is August, and a 16-year-old boy presents to clinic with concerns about the upcoming school year. Last year he developed complaints of difficulty initiating sleep and problems waking for school. He began to suffer from extreme sleep deprivation, often only getting 5 hours of sleep per night, and his grades and attendance at school fell precipitously. He wants to ensure he can sleep normally this academic year, and he needs to be up for school at 7 AM. His current bedtime is 3 AM, and wake time is 11 AM. In order to treat his delayed sleep phase syndrome in preparation for school, based on his likely minimum core body temperature, what is the recommended time that he should start waking up to get morning sunlight?

A. He should get up at 7 AM, as this is when school starts.

B. He should get up at 8 AM, approximately 1 hour before his minimum core body temperature.

C. He should get up at 9 AM, at his minimum core body temperature.

D. He should get up at 10 AM, approximately 1 hour after his minimum core body temperature.

23. A colleague in cardiology asks for a curbside consult in reviewing the long-term cardiac monitoring tracing for a patient with complaints of palpitations. She has noted that the patient periodically has accelerations and irregularities in the cardiac rhythm overnight, often at intervals of several hours and predominately in the last one-third of the night. She asks for a reasonable explanation for this phenomenon. What is the *best* explanation for this noted variation?

A. Peripheral vascular resistance decreases towards morning, and this evokes arrhythmias.

B. Systemic blood pressure decreases during REM sleep, and this stresses cardiac function.

C. Cardiac output progressively declines through the night with the lowest level in the last period of REM, and this reveals underlying arrhythmias.

D. The heart rate normally fluctuates due to phasic heart rate changes associated with REM sleep.

24. Even among normal subjects, respiratory changes occur in sleep that may lead to subtle changes in carbon dioxide and oxygen levels overnight. The interpretation of sleep-related arterial blood gases in normal patients, as well as those with pulmonary and sleep disorders, is important. Minute ventilation changes are observed in the transition from wakefulness to sleep, with further alterations occurring in REM sleep. Which of the following changes in sleep compared with wakefulness have been noted in the arterial blood gas measurement of normal subjects?

A. Elevation in $PaCO_2$ by 2-to-8 mmHg

B. Elevation in PaO_2 by 3-to-5 mmHg

C. Decrease in $PaCO_2$ by 2-to-4 mmHg

D. Decrease in PaO_2 by 15 mmHg

25. A basic understanding of the role of neurotransmitters in sleep is required to appreciate the mechanisms of action of existing and novel pharmacological agents used in the treatment of sleep disorders, as well as the impacts of substances that are consumed. Control of the sleep-wake cycle can also be understood in the context of these neurotransmitters. Which of the following statements is true?

A. Serotonin (5-HT) has its highest activity during the waking state.

B. Acetylcholine has its lowest activity during NREM and REM sleep.

C. NE has higher activity during REM sleep and wakefulness.

D. Orexin has its lowest activity during the waking state.

Answers

1. **Answer B. Sleep is characterized by a reversible state of perceptual disengagement and relative insensitivity to the environment.**

Sleep can be defined in terms of behavior, physiology, and electrical changes of the brain, as measured by electroencephalography (EEG). It is an active process characterized by a reversible behavior state of perceptual disengagement and relative insensitivity to the environment (Answer B is correct). Sleep is usually accompanied by a recumbent posture, closed eyes, decreased muscle activity, specific physiological changes, and absent or only slight mobility.[1] Of significance, there is a loss of sensory input to the brain from other parts of the body. This occurs due to an electrically reversible deafferentation of the cerebral cortex. Sleep is subdivided into two broad categories: nonrapid eye movement (NREM) and REM sleep with distinct characteristics.

Although his nervous system is likely underdeveloped, somnambulism (sleepwalking) is a NREM parasomnia and not related to REM sleep (Answer A is incorrect). Given his underlying health and quick normalization of cognition with vigorous awakening, this does not likely represent a postictal state as may occur in epilepsy (Answer C is incorrect). Nociceptive pain may be sharp, throbbing, or aching, and occurs due to damage of body tissues, but it is not unique among the perceptions masked during sleep (Answer D is incorrect).

2. **Answer C. ipRGC retinohypothalamic tract SCN in the anterior hypothalamus paraventricular nucleus of the hypothalamus preganglionic sympathetic neurons superior cervical ganglion pineal gland.**

In the absence of effective synchronization to the natural light-dark cycle, an individual's innate circadian rhythm (called *tau*) will become expressed.[2] Without constraint, this typically results in a cyclical pattern of successively delayed sleep onset and wake time. The propensity for sleep and wakefulness will continually shift around the actual 24-hour clock. As a result, an affected individual with a free-running rhythm or non-24-hour sleep-wake disorder who attempts to observe a standard schedule will gradually experience profound daytime sleepiness with significant nocturnal insomnia every few weeks as the misalignment unfolds.[3] This condition affects 50%–73% of the totally blind.[4] It is possible for some who are totally blind to have an intact anatomical pathway that preserves the response to phototherapy.[5]

Light activates the ipRGC, which contact the photopigment melanopsin (Answers A and D are incorrect). The retinohypothalamic tract extends from the retina to the SCN in the anterior hypothalamus (Answer B is incorrect). The relay from the SCN to the pineal gland includes the paraventricular nucleus of the hypothalamus, preganglionic sympathetic neurons in the spinal cord, and the superior cervical ganglion (Answer C is correct). Low doses of properly timed oral melatonin can be a highly effective treatment in this population.[6,7]

3. **Answer B. Occurring once during a nap opportunity as part of a MSLT, with a mean sleep latency of 7 min on a normal adult with excessive daytime sleepiness complaints.**

This epoch demonstrates the classic findings of REM or stage R sleep. Sawtooth waves of theta frequency can be seen at the arrow, approximately 6–8 sec into the epoch. There is an absence of sleep spindles and K complexes. The EEG shows a low-amplitude, mixed-frequency pattern with desynchronized brain activity. REM sleep is associated with vivid dreaming, skeletal muscle atonia (with the exception of eye and diaphragm muscles), memory processing, and learning. As such, the chin and leg EMG signals show minimal muscle activity. In the last 10 sec of the epoch, the REMs become clearly apparent.

In older children and adults, REM sleep normally occurs at intervals of 90–110 min, starting 80–100 min after the onset of sleep.[8] Young adults have four to five REM periods in 8 hours of nocturnal sleep, with periods becoming more prolonged towards morning, linked to the circadian rhythm.

TABLE 49.1	Causes of Sleep-Onset Rapid Eye Movements Periods

- Infants <3 months of age
- Sleep deprivation
- Flying across more than three time zones (without a period to synchronize circadian rhythms to the new environment before travel)
- Narcolepsy
- Idiopathic hypersomnia
- Acute withdrawal from a REM-suppressant medication (e.g., tricyclic antidepressant)
- Chronic non-REM suppressant antidepressants
- Shift workers (male > female)
- Apnea patients with desaturations (male > female)

REM, Rapid eye movement.

REM (or active) sleep represents 50% of the sleep in infants, and this proportion gradually decreases through childhood until it reaches the normal adult level of 20%–25% of sleep.[9] It is considered abnormal for children older than 3 months of age and adults to enter sleep through REM (Answer A is incorrect). There are a number of causes of sleep-onset REM (SOREM) periods (Table 49.1).[10]

The first night of recovery sleep after total sleep deprivation is predominated by slow wave (N3) sleep, but the second night demonstrates a normal rebound of REM sleep (Answer C is incorrect).[11,12] A rebound of REM sleep may also occur with resolution of sleep apnea as part of adequate PAP titration, corresponding with the naturally increased concentration of REM sleep towards morning (Answer D is incorrect).

One of the causes of REM sleep that is observed as part of a MSLT is idiopathic hypersomnia. The affected person has an irrepressible need to sleep with daytime lapses into sleep for more than 3 months that is not better explained by insufficient sleep time or another sleep disorder.[13] Unlike in narcolepsy type 1, cataplexy is absent. Fewer than two SOREM periods are observed during the MSLT. For the diagnosis of idiopathic hypersomnia, the mean sleep latency of the MSLT must also be ≤ 8 min, or the total 24-hour sleep time observed must be ≥ 660 min, as observed by 24-hour polysomnographic monitoring or by wrist actigraphy in association with a sleep log (averaged over at least 7 days with unrestricted sleep; Answer B is correct).

4. **Answer D. *Chronic cerveau isolé*: Demonstrated the features of quiet sleep located in the lower brainstem and modulated by forebrain structures.**

Though it may seem relatively unimportant to understand the anatomy of the cat's brainstem, these early studies by Dr. Frédéric Bremer laid the groundwork for our contemporary understanding of the structures that are integral to the physiology of sleep and wakefulness.[14,15] It is important to have a working knowledge of the centers for wakefulness, primary sleep, and REM sleep, as well as the predominant corresponding neurotransmitters (Table 49.2).[16]

Beyond the details provided in the correctly paired sections (Answers A, B, and C), the *cerveau isolé* also isolated the study of the olfactory and visual impulses. In addition to the sleeping state noted on electroencephalogram (EEG) within the *cerveau isolé* section, correspondingly the eyes turned downward with

TABLE 49.2	Sleep Neuroanatomy and Primary Neurotransmitters
Wakefulness Centers	
Locus coeruleus	Norepinephrine
Tuberomammillary nucleus	Histamine
Pedunculopontine (PPT) and laterodorsal tegmental (LDT) nuclei of pons	Acetylcholine
Median and dorsal raphe nuclei	Serotonin
Substantia nigra	Dopamine
Lateral/posterior hypothalamus	Orexin
Reticular activating system	Glutamate
Primary Sleep Center	
Ventrolateral preoptic (VLPO) area	GABA
REM Sleep Center	
Pedunculopontine (PPT) and laterodorsal tegmental (LDT) nuclei of pons	Acetylcholine
Reticular magnocellularis nucleus	Glycine

TABLE 49.3	Comparing Sleep Stages in Infants, Young Adults, and Elderly		
	Infants	Young Adults	Elderly
Wake after sleep onset	<5%	<5%	10%–25%
Sleep efficiency	>90%	>90%	75%–85%
Stage N1	Quiet sleep	2%–5%	5%–8%
Stage N2	Quiet sleep	45%–50%	57%–67%
Stage N3	Quiet sleep	13%–23%	6%–17%
Stage R	50%	20%–35%	17%–20%
Stage R/NREM ratio	50:50	20:80	20:80
Timing of stage R cycle intervals	45–60 min	90–110 min	90–110 min
Total sleep time	14–16 hours	7–8 hours	7 hours

progressive miosis. The suppression of nerve impulses necessary for the waking state of the telencephalon led to the conclusion that sleep is a reversible de-afferentation of the cerebral cortex. Answer D is incorrect because the *chronic cerveau isolé* demonstrated the features of paradoxical (active or REM) sleep are located in the lower brainstem and modulated by forebrain structures.[17] By understanding the basic neuroanatomical localization of the centers of sleep and wakefulness, it is possible to answer the question without familiarity with the historical context.

5. **Answer A. K complexes would be present on a sleep electroencephalogram (EEG).**
Fortunately, this child is sleeping quite normally, without even sleep-onset association behavioral insomnia of childhood occurring.[13] Sleep spindles begin to appear around 6–8 weeks of age, and would be expected in this child's sleep electroencephalogram (EEG) (Answer B is incorrect).[18,19] On the other hand, K complexes do not appear until 4–6 months of age, and would not likely be present in this 3-month-old girl (Answer A is correct).[20] It is difficult to identify the stages of non-REM sleep until around 3–6 months of age. This sleep staging relates to dendritic growth (and the frequently observed delta waves represent hypersynchrony of pyramidal cells of the cerebral cortex).[21] Given her age, it may still be too early to differentiate the non-REM stages (Answer C is incorrect). Prior to this transition, the sleep of infants may be classified as quiet (non-REM equivalent) or active (REM equivalent) sleep. Indeterminate or transitional sleep may not clearly be identified as either type, and often disappears with maturation. The amount of sleep obtained, and the presence of naps is normal for her age (Table 49.3; Answer D is incorrect).

6. **Answer D. *Dorsal raphe*: Releases dopamine, feedback to hypothalamus.**
Beyond the RAS and the brainstem, there are major subcortical structures that are also important to the regulation of wakefulness. The excitatory neuropeptides orexin A and B (also known

as hypocretin 1 and 2) are produced by neurons in the lateral and posterior hypothalamus, and have a central role in sustaining wakefulness (Answer A is incorrect).[22,23] Orexin levels are highest during wakefulness.[24] Located at the base of the posterior hypothalamus, the TMN is a small cluster of cells that innervate much of the forebrain and brainstem and are the sole source of histamine in the brain (Answer B is incorrect).[16] Antihistamines, such as the H_1 receptor antagonists like diphenhydramine, promote NREM and REM sleep by blocking histamine signals.[25] An elongated structure located beneath the floor of the fourth ventricle, the locus coeruleus is the major source of NE in the forebrain with maximal activity during wakefulness (Answer C is incorrect).[26] Although dopamine promotes wakefulness, especially when a subject is highly motivated or physically active, it is unclear which neurons actually promote arousal and a population of neurons in the ventral periaqueductal gray of the pons may have a role.[27] Serotonin (5-HT), not dopamine, is produced by neurons in the dorsal raphe nucleus, with innervations extending to the preoptic area, basal forebrain, hypothalamus, and thalamus (Answer D is correct).[16]

7. **Answer C. REM sleep is relatively preserved.**
Sleep has been well studied by researchers at altitude. As a rule, sleep is noted to become more fragmented with increased arousals and lighter sleep (Answer D is incorrect). Periodic breathing likely contributes to this phenomenon, as increases in both are correlated, with arousals occurring during the hyperpnea phase. These changes diminish over time. There is an increase in stage N1 sleep at progressively higher elevations and a significant reduction in stage N3 (slow wave sleep; Answer B is incorrect). Stage N2 is also reduced, but REM sleep is believed to be relatively preserved (Answer C is correct). Despite these changes, the total sleep time is unchanged at altitude (Answer A is incorrect).[28,29]

8. **Answer C. Slow wave sleep (N3) is the deepest stage of sleep and has roles in growth hormone release and long-term memory consolidation.**
Constituting the largest portion of sleep during the night, NREM is characterized by decreased blood flow to the brain and skeletal muscle, as well as decreases in heart rate, blood pressure, and respiratory volumes. By current nomenclature,

NREM is subdivided into stages N1, N2, and N3 (formerly stages 3 and 4 of sleep).[30] N3 sleep is also sometimes called slow wave sleep or delta sleep, with the latter descriptor recognizing the slow speed of the brain waves occurring at a delta frequency (1–4 Hz). Sequentially, these stages are associated with progressively deepening sleep with higher arousal thresholds (Answer A is incorrect). This is due to increased synchronization of the cortex.

Stage N1 involves slow-rolling eye movements and partial relaxation of voluntary muscles. It is a very light stage of sleep and is often subjectively misinterpreted as wakefulness, contributing to complaints of paradoxical insomnia. Stage N2 shows characteristic patterns on the electroencephalogram (EEG), including K complexes and sleep spindles. The K complex is a high-amplitude negative waveform, followed by a positive waveform lasting 0.5 sec or more. Sleep spindles are closely spaced high frequency (11–16 Hz) waves. Stage N2 constitutes about 50 percent of adult sleep, but it is not the deepest stage, as N3 still occurs in adults (Answer D is incorrect). Stage N3 shows high amplitude, slow wave activity on EEG. It is the deepest stage of sleep, making it difficult to respond to external stimuli, and is associated with growth hormone release and long-term memory consolidation (Answer C is correct).[31] It is relatively easier to wake someone from REM sleep, especially when compared with N3 sleep (Answer B is incorrect).

9. **Answer B. Attending physicians are not impacted by sleep deprivation due to acclimatization that occurs as part of training.**
In 1984 a landmark case ruled that medical error resulted in the death of Libby Zion in a New York hospital, due to physician negligence in her care, and that both sleep deprivation and a lack of attending supervision played a role.[32] This created the impetus for changes in physician work hours. The Association of American Medical Colleges (AAMC) initially recommended that the work week for resident physicians be limited to 80 hours in 2003, with at least one 24-hour period of nonworking time per week. Starting in 2011, more stringent restrictions were implemented by the Accreditation Council for Graduate Medical Education (ACGME). These changes were made based on research linking medical errors to inadequate rest among residents.

Residents who average 5 or fewer hours of sleep per night have been shown to have more problems with accidents/injuries, professional staff conflict, alcohol, stimulant medications, and medical errors (Answer C is incorrect).[33] Mistakes in intensive care unit (ICU) care have been linked to intern fatigue. These errors can be reduced with a more limited schedule and shorter shifts.[34] Night call seems to exacerbate performance impairments in working memory capacity (Answer A is incorrect).[35] When the shift has ended, there is a higher risk of vehicle crashes after extended work hours and longer shifts (Answer D is incorrect).[36]

Inadequate sleep among resident physicians in training has serious consequences. There are impacts on quality of life, health, work performance, job satisfaction, mental health, and alcohol/drug abuse. There must be a balance among work hours, sleep needs, and personal time outside of work. With work hour restrictions, there may be improvements in these domains, but the impacts on patient care and education and training time (especially in highly demanding training programs) may be mixed. Increased hand-offs may also impact

patient safety if information is not communicated effectively. Trainees may also face pressures to document compliance without full adherence to the guidelines.[37] Unfortunately, attending physicians are not able to acclimate to sleep deprivation and are affected similarly, as are nurses and other allied health professionals (Answer B is correct).

10. **Answer C. All mammals experience REM sleep.**
Although nearly all mammals exhibit NREM (slow wave sleep, inactive, or "quiet" sleep) and REM (paradoxical, active, or desynchronized sleep), the percentages vary from species to species.[38] Notably, REM sleep is absent in dolphins (Answer C is correct),[39] but contrary to prior research, the spiny anteater (echidna) does enter REM sleep. Birds experience both NREM and REM sleep, and REM occurs in both hemispheres. Sleep spindle density also varies considerably, from high-density 12–16 Hz range in primates to the absence of spindles in parakeets (Answer D is incorrect).[40] Among animals, N3 sleep may occur exclusively in one hemisphere, or in both (as occurs in humans; Answer B is incorrect).

Unihemispheric sleep is characterized by electroencephalogram (EEG) evidence of one hemisphere demonstrating N3 sleep, while the other hemisphere simultaneously exhibits wakefulness. Unihemispheric sleep in mammals is limited to dolphins (of the order Cetacea), eared seals, and manatees (Answer A is incorrect).[41] This adaptation may be a protective feature: allowing for continuous monitoring of the environment, facilitating ease of movement (especially for migratory species) and sensory processing, and permitting surfacing to breathe in aquatic mammals.[42] Birds also experience unihemispheric sleep, even during flight, and keep the eye open on the same side as the awake hemisphere (which also is protective against predation).[43,44] Body temperature changes, as well as the timing of the release of growth hormone and melatonin, may differ in animals (Table 49.4).

11. **Answer A. Sleep spindle—thalamus—N2 sleep—central leads.**
The finding is a sleep spindle, and it is generated within the thalamus and consistent with N2 sleep (Answer C is incorrect). A sleep spindle is a train of distinct sinusoidal waves with frequency of 11–16 Hz (most commonly 12–14 Hz) and a duration of ≥0.5 sec, usually maximal in amplitude in the central derivations.[30] As such, it will be seen most prominently in the central or parietal (midline) leads, though it can also be picked up subtly in the occipital leads in the figure (Answer A is correct). These sinusoidal waves shift to more central regions by the end of the night. The faster range of spindles (14–16 Hz) predominate in the centroparietal region, whereas slower range spindles (11.5–14 Hz) are seen more in anterior leads.[45]

Sawtooth waves are strongly supportive of the presence of REM sleep, and K complexes are the finding more prominent in frontal leads (Answer B is incorrect).[46,47] PGO spikes appear 30–60 sec before other signs of REM sleep. PGO spikes are generated within the pons and extend to the lateral geniculate nucleus (LGN) of the thalamus and to the visual occipital cortex. They are measures with implanted electrodes.[48]

12. **Answer D. VLPO.**
The VLPO is the main sleep switch, releasing Gal and GABA to inhibit cell groups in the locus coeruleus, raphe nucleus, and the TMN (Answer D is correct). The SCN controls the circadian timing of sleep and wakefulness, with inputs from ipRGC (containing the photopigment melanopsin) via the retinohypothalamic tract (Answer A is incorrect). The pineal

TABLE 49.4	Contrasting Human Sleep and Animal Sleep	
	Humans	**Animals**
Sleep spindles	12–14 Hz (cycles per second)	Not detected in parakeets
N3 sleep	Bilateral hemispheric production	Unihemispheric production in cetaceans (dolphins and whales)
R sleep	20%–25% of adult sleep	Present in mammals (except for lack of recording evidence in dolphins)
Body temperature	Can drop by 1°C (in a nonhypothermic state), which can still be normal during sleep	Hibernating bears may have reductions of 4–5°C
Growth hormone	Secreted maximally during N3 sleep	Secreted in the awake state of dogs
Melatonin	Maximal secretion during sleep	Maximal secretion during the awake state of nocturnal animals

TABLE 49.5	Defining Tonic Versus Phasic Rapid Eye Movements Characteristics
Tonic REM	**Phasic REM**
Lack of rapid eye movements on EOG Skeletal muscle atonia	Rapid eye movements on EOG — Muscle twitches on EMG Middle ear muscle activity Diaphragm muscle activity Skeletal muscle atonia

EMG, Electromyogram; *EOG*, electrooculography; *REM*, rapid eye movement.

gland responds to input from the SCN and serves as the site of melatonin production, with an increase in melatonin production occurring 2 hours before the onset of sleep (Answer B is incorrect). The cells of the thalamus are active in sleep, and it is the site of sleep spindle generation, but it is not the primary sleep switch (Answer C is incorrect).[16]

13. **Answer C. Absence of REM atonia due to loss of activation of dorsolateral pontine reticular formation neurons ventral to the locus coeruleus.**

The man described in the clinical scenario is experiencing REM sleep behavior disorder with dream-enactment behaviors, and a polysomnogram is likely to demonstrate a loss of muscle atonia in REM sleep (Answer C is correct).[13] The primary REM-generating center is located in the brainstem, isolated chiefly to the cholinergic neurons of the LD and PPT nuclei at the junction of the pons and midbrain (Answer A is incorrect).[49] REM sleep is characterized by a desynchronized, low-amplitude activity pattern on the electroencephalogram (EEG) that is similar to wakefulness (without alpha activity noted). The electrooculography (EOG) shows REMs in phasic REM, whereas these are absent in tonic REM (Answer B is incorrect; Table 49.5). Muscle atonia (lack of muscle tone) noted on electromyography (EMG) occurs after the activation of the dorsolateral pontine reticular formation neurons ventral to the locus coeruleus. Sleep paralysis occurs due to inhibition of motor neurons in the spine by both glycinergic and GABAergic mechanisms, and this would lead to a lack of movement during the transition from REM sleep to wakefulness (Answer D is incorrect).

14. **Answer B. Suppression of the sex hormones (testosterone, estrogen, and progesterone).**

Humans who have been observed after undergoing more than 200 hours of complete sleep deprivation have important physiological changes. These changes affect the neurological system, hormones, metabolism, temperature regulation, and the immune system (Table 49.6). Subjects are noted to have brisk gag and hyperactive deep tendon reflexes, but sluggish corneal reflexes (Answer A is incorrect). In addition, chronic sleep deprivation contributes to intermittent slurred speech, ptosis (eyelid droop), hand tremors, and mild nystagmus.[50,51] There are also important impacts on neurocognitive function. Impaired psychomotor performance is noted with chronic sleep deprivation.[52] One study noted 48 healthy adults experiencing 4–6 hours of sleep over 14 consecutive days had deficits in cognitive performance, similar to those with 2 nights of total sleep deprivation.[53] They were subjectively unaware of these deficits by sleepiness ratings (perhaps suggesting a lack of insight that could have societal implications). The danger of neurocognitive effects with chronic partial sleep deprivation, largely unrealized by the individual, may exacerbate the risk for occupational hazards, compromised public safety (drivers, etc.), and lost productivity. Psychiatric symptoms, including visual hallucinations, are associated with sleep deprivation.[54]

Sleep deprivation leads to electroencephalogram (EEG) changes during wakefulness. There is a linear reduction in alpha activity as sleep deprivation becomes more prolonged. There is an increased intrusion of delta and theta waves during the wake state (Answer D is incorrect). The ability to sustain alpha activity (even with eye closure) is also diminished.[55] Transient microsleep periods, correlating with brief EEG slowing (sometimes lasting only seconds), may be associated with deficits in performance. Some research suggests that older people may tolerate sleep deprivation better, with faster reaction times, fewer lapses in performance, and less frequent unintentional sleep periods than younger subjects.[56]

There are several important hormonal changes that occur with sleep deprivation. Thyroid hormones (thyrotropin, thyroxine, and triiodothyronine) are increased. There is a reduction in the secretion of prolactin, growth hormone, and noradrenaline. However, there are no effects on the sex hormones (testosterone, estrogen, and progesterone; Answer B is correct). In addition, metabolism and appetite are impacted by elevated secretion of ghrelin and reduction in leptin, hormone changes leading to increased appetite (Answer C is incorrect).[57]

TABLE 49.6 Effects of Acute Human Sleep Deprivation

Neurological changes	Hand tremor Mild nystagmus Intermittent slurred speech Ptosis Hyperactive deep tendon reflexes Hyperactive gag reflex Slowed corneal reflexes
EEG changes	Linear reduction in alpha activity as hours of sleep loss increase Increase in delta and theta activity in the awake state Intermittent microsleep EEG slowing during the awake state
Hormone changes	Thyrotropin, thyroxine, and triiodothyronine are increased Reduction in secretion of prolactin, growth hormone, and noradrenaline
Metabolic changes	Increased secretion of ghrelin and reduction in leptin hormones
Thermoregulation	0.3–0.4°C decrease in body temperature (very mild heat retention deficits)
Immune system changes	Inflammatory changes occur but the results are conflicting, depending on the level of sleep deprivation and the model used Increased risk of rhinovirus infection

EEG, Electroencephalogram.

15. **Answer D. At all ages, women have a higher incidence of insomnia compared with men.**

There are some important gender differences in sleep that impact the proper diagnosis and treatment of sleep disorders like insomnia and obstructive sleep apnea. Infant girls have more total sleep and less frequent awakenings than infant boys, and they also have less REM sleep and more NREM sleep.[58] Adolescent girls have longer sleep-onset latencies, sleep longer, and have a better sleep efficiency compared with adolescent boys. Premenopausal women have better sleep efficiency, greater subjective sleep complaints, greater delta power, shorter sleep-onset latencies, and longer total sleep times (Answer A is incorrect).[59,60] Overall, women have a greater prevalence of insomnia (50% higher than men), but a decade-by-decade breakdown of prevalence across the lifespan showed that men had a greater prevalence of insomnia for the decade 30–39 years (Answer D is correct).[61]

Pregnancy has significant impacts on sleep quantity and quality. In the first trimester, around week 10 of pregnancy, the total sleep time increases with a longer sleep period at night and frequent daytime naps. Sleep becomes less efficient, with frequent awakenings, decreased amount of slow wave (N3) sleep, and more frequent complaints about sleep quality. Within the second trimester (weeks 13–28), sleep tends to improve with better sleep efficiency and less time spent awake after going to sleep at night (Answer B is incorrect). By the end of the second trimester, however, the number of awakenings during the night again increases. Women in their final trimester of pregnancy experience more nighttime awakenings and spend more time awake at night, with decreased sleep efficiency and more daytime naps. In addition, sleep is lighter with more frequent N1 and N2 sleep.[62]

Menopause leads to a reduction in sleep efficiency, especially in those with vasomotor symptoms of hot flashes and night sweats. This may be related to the increased risk of obstructive sleep apnea. The prevalence of sleep apnea is lowest in premenopausal women at 0.6%, intermediate in those postmenopausal women on hormone replacement therapy (1.1%), and highest in postmenopausal women not on hormone replacement at 5.5% (Answer C is incorrect).[63]

16. **Answer C. A postarousal central apnea that is caused by brief hyperpnea and is a normal finding.**

The epoch of sleep presented in Fig. 49.3 shows findings consistent with an arousal, followed by a respiratory pattern that suggests a central sleep apnea event, and this is a normal finding in sleep (Answer C is correct). According to the scoring guidelines, an arousal is scored during sleep if there is an abrupt shift of EEG frequency, including alpha, theta, and/or frequencies greater than 16 Hz, that lasts at least 3 sec, with at least 3 sec of stable sleep preceding the change. In the context of REM sleep, there must also be an increase in submental EMG lasting at least 1 sec.[30] Though the respiratory signals are suggestive of a central apnea event, the context (following the arousal) and the unremarkable patient history make a diagnosis of central sleep apnea inappropriate (Answers B and D are incorrect).

RERAs may be identified if a sequence of breaths lasting ≥10 sec are characterized by increasing respiratory effort or by flattening of the inspiratory portion of the nasal pressure (diagnostic study) or PAP device flow (titration study) waveform, leading to an arousal from sleep. These events do not meet the criteria to be scored as either a hypopnea or apnea event. Considering that the epoch does not show the respiratory pattern prior to the arousal, this would not be possible to identify, given the information provided (Answer A is incorrect).

17. **Answer B. The peak of gastric acid secretion occurs early in the night with a circadian periodicity.**

It is known that unstimulated gastric acid secretion peaks between 10 PM and 2 AM and follows a circadian periodicity (Answer B is correct).[64] When 24-hour collections of gastric acid secretions were performed, researchers discovered the greatest rate of secretion occurred in the evening, and the lowest secretion was noted toward morning (Answer C is incorrect). Compared with the waking states, the overall levels of gastric acid secretion are lower, but they do not remain

TABLE 49.7	Sleep Regulatory Cytokines	
Somnogenic (Promote NREM Sleep)	**Antagonistic to Sleep**	
IL-1α and IL-1β	Anakinra (IL-1β receptor antagonist)	
TNF-α and TNF-β	Etanercept (TNF-α receptor antagonist)	
Acidic fibroblast growth factor		
Epidermal growth factor	IL-4	
Nerve growth factor	IL-10	
IL-2, IL-6, IL-8, IL-15, and IL-18 (promote sleep after activation by NFκB)		

IL, Interleukin; *NFκB,* nuclear factor κB; *NREM,* nonrapid eye movement sleep; *TNF,* tumor necrosis factor.

TABLE 49.8	Effects of Acute Human Sleep Deprivation
First night of recovery sleep	**Normal young adults:** Decreased sleep latency, increased N3 rebound, decreased N1, decreased N2, decreased R, increased R sleep latency **Normal elderly:** Increased N3 rebound but with less pressure than young, normal N2, decreased R sleep latency
Second night of recovery sleep	**Normal young adults:** N3 nears normal, increased R rebound **Normal elderly:** Trend toward normal
Third night of recovery sleep	Sleep architecture normalizes to baseline values

constant in sleep (Answer D is incorrect). These levels are not affected by any specific sleep stage (Answer A is incorrect). Gastric acid output seems to increase in association with arousals and awakenings, and this may be vagally mediated.[65] Nocturnal reflux symptoms may also be associated with obstructive sleep apnea. Gastric motility is preserved during sleep, with myoelectric activity occurring at about 3 cycles per minute with no clear differences based on sleep stage.[66]

18. **Answer A. By treating his obstructive sleep apnea, he has had normalization of the amount of N3 sleep he obtains with corresponding increases in growth hormone release.**
The figure shows N3 sleep with greater than 20% of the epoch demonstrating slow wave activity, consisting of waves with a 0.5–2-Hz frequency and a peak-to-peak amplitude greater than 75 μV, as measured over the frontal regions referenced to the contralateral mastoid lead.[30] Growth hormone release is strongly associated with N3 sleep, and children with untreated obstructive sleep apnea are likely to have both compromised, with normalization with effective treatment (Answer A is correct).[67] A major pulse of growth hormone occurs just after the onset of sleep, and this reaches maximal levels within minutes of the onset of N3 sleep. Awakenings from sleep, sleep fragmentation, and inadequate N3 sleep suppress growth hormone secretion (Answer D is incorrect). Though chronic sleep deprivation can indeed affect hormones related to appetite regulation, ghrelin levels would increase and leptin levels would decrease (both stimulating appetite; Answer B is incorrect).[57] The effects of growth hormone in relation to N3 sleep, not testosterone, would account for the changes observed in his growth (Answer C is incorrect).

19. **Answer B. The amount of NREM sleep increases in duration and intensity, and REM sleep is inhibited.**
After a bacterial challenge, there are increases noted in the duration and intensity of NREM sleep, and REM sleep is inhibited (Answer B is correct). The timing of these changes is very dependent on the type of bacteria and the route of inoculation. There are a number of cytokines that have somnogenic properties, and others (like IL-4 and IL-10) are antagonistic to sleep (Table 49.7; Answer D is incorrect).[68] Unlike in a viral infection, the bacteria do not need to replicate within the host to induce changes in sleep (Answer C is incorrect). Somnogenic molecules within the bacterial cell wall induce the same effects, even when killed bacteria or purified cell walls are introduced to the host. Muramyl peptides

from the cell walls are relatively nontoxic and induce sleep, even at very high concentrations. In contrast, endotoxin is somnogenic at lower doses, but at higher concentrations results in shock (Answer A is incorrect).[69]

20. **Answer D. Cortisol and ACTH increase during sleep deprivation, and growth hormone and prolactin rebound during recovery sleep.**
In the setting of sleep deprivation, there are clear differences in the response of young and older adults, especially as observed in the period of recovery sleep (Table 49.8). On the first night of recovery sleep, slow wave sleep (N3) predominates in young adults, with a subsequent reduction in sleep latency and in N1, N2, and REM, but a prolonged REM sleep latency. Among the normal elderly, there is less slow wave sleep pressure. There is nevertheless an increase in the amount of slow wave sleep with a normal amount of N2 sleep and reduced REM sleep latency. On the second night of recovery sleep, slow wave sleep normalizes and REM rebound occurs. By the third night of recovery sleep, the sleep architecture normalizes with near baseline values.[55]

Beyond these observed changes in sleep architecture during recovery sleep, there are clear alterations in hormone levels during acute sleep deprivation. Researchers have evaluated these changes in healthy young men receiving a constant glucose infusion while being observed during nocturnal sleep, nocturnal sleep deprivation, and daytime recovery sleep. Fig. 49.5 illustrates the resulting patterns observed in plasma growth hormone, cortisol, thyroid-stimulating hormone, prolactin, glucose, and insulin secretion rates.[70]

Total sleep disruption can blunt secretion of sleep-linked hormones (growth hormone and prolactin), with rebound secretion during recovery sleep (Answer A is incorrect).[55,71] ACTH also rebounds higher with recovery sleep (Answer B is incorrect).[72] Cortisol is unchanged during sleep deprivation, but it decreases on the recovery night due to a rebound of N3 sleep (Answer D is incorrect).[73] As such, given the increased rebound of N3 in young adults, this would likely be further suppressed in this population (Answer C is incorrect).

21. **Answer C. Memory encoding is dependent on N3 and REM sleep, but not on N1 or N2 sleep.**
Memory and learning are closely associated with sleep, and inadequate sleep quantity or quality affects both.[74] Memory consolidation allows for the retention of daily experiences initially encoded as new memories, learning (including studying

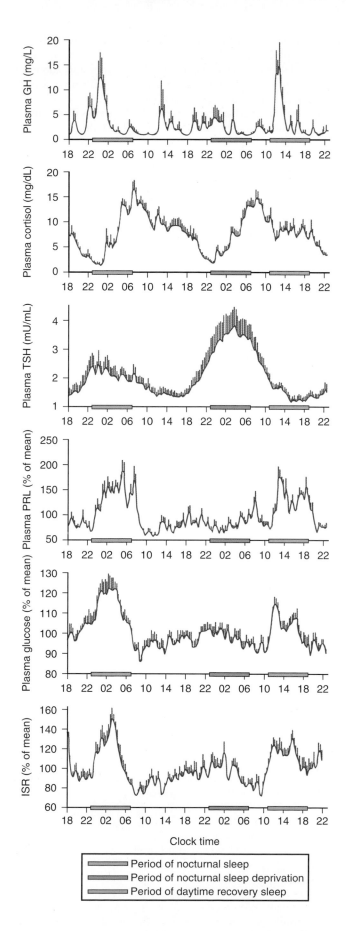

Clock time

Period of nocturnal sleep
Period of nocturnal sleep deprivation
Period of daytime recovery sleep

• **Figure 49.5** From top to bottom: Mean 24-hour profiles of plasma growth hormone (GH), cortisol, thyrotropin (TSH), prolactin (PRL), glucose, and insulin secretion rates (ISR) in a group of eight healthy young men (20–27 years old) studied during a 53-hour period, including 8 hours of nocturnal sleep, 28 hours of sleep deprivation, and 8 hours of daytime sleep. The vertical bars on the tracings represent the standard error of the mean (SEM) at each time point. The green bars represent the sleep periods. The blue bars represent the period of nocturnal sleep deprivation. The orange bars represent the period of daytime sleep. Caloric intake was exclusively in the form of a constant glucose infusion. Shifted sleep was associated with an immediate shift in release of GH and PRL. In contrast, the secreto profiles of cortisol and TSH remained synchronized to the circadian time. Both sleep-dependent and circadian input can be recognized in the profiles of glucose and ISR. Note: the green bar mentioned in this original figure caption correlates to the first bar seen on the x-axis when reading from left to right, the blue bar is in the center, and the orange bar is on the right. (Adapted from Van Cauter E, Spiegel K. Circadian and sleep control of endocrine secretions. In: Turek FW, Zee PC, eds. *Neurobiology of Sleep and Circadian Rhythms*. New York, NY: Marcel Dekker; 1999; and Van Cauter E, Blackman JD, Roland D, Spire JP, Refetoff S, Polonsky KS. Modulation of glucose regulation and insulin secretion by sleep and circadian rhythmicity. *J Clin Invest*. 1991; 88:934-942; The figure and caption are reprinted from Van Cauter E, Tasali E. Endocrine physiology in relation to sleep and sleep disturbances. In: Kryger MH, Roth T, Dement WC, eds. *Principles and Practice of Sleep Medicine*. 5th ed. St Louis: WB Saunders; 2011:292.)

for a sleep board examination), and programming of innate behavior. To learn a new task or skill, training must be followed by encoding, review, refinement, and consolidation to retain the memory. Sleep may also allow for the elimination of unimportant memories and irrelevant observations. Memory encoding depends on N2, N3, and REM sleep (Answer C is correct).[75,76] In particular, slow wave sleep (N3) is important to reinforce novel declarative memory, such as the memorization of facts for a test (Answer B is incorrect). The emotion linked to episodic memory is better recalled after REM sleep. Visual learning is enhanced by sleep and impaired by sleep loss (Answer A is incorrect).[77] Learning is optimal when the efforts are synchronized with the individual's circadian clock (Answer D is incorrect).[78] Chronic sleep deprivation causes all types of memory to deteriorate, with an associated decline in long-term performance.

Sleep targets prior neuronal activity in areas that worked most during wakefulness. Localized functional effects of sleep deprivation evident on functional magnetic resonance imaging (fMRI) depend upon which cognitive tasks were performed in the period before sleep.[79] Refinement of synaptic connections occurs by reinforcing needed and used pathways and integrating new neuronal firing patterns. This has an important role in brain plasticity.[74]

22. **Answer C. He should get up at 9 AM, at his minimum core body temperature.**
Human core body temperature follows a sinusoidal circadian periodicity. Among those with an in-phase circadian rhythm and normal sleep timing, there is a peak in body temperature that occurs at about 9 PM, with a minimum body temperature trough around 5 AM (Fig. 49.6). As a rule of thumb, the minimum core body temperature occurs 2–3 hours before the natural waking time. When light exposure occurs after this minimum, an advance in the sleep phase occurs (with an

earlier sleep onset and offset). It has the most powerful effect when this light exposure occurs as soon as possible after the minimum. To achieve a delay in sleep timing, whereby the phase is shifted later, light exposure ideally occurs just prior to this minimum.

As body temperature decreases, sleep latency also diminishes. Sleep is terminated as the body temperature starts to rise toward morning, just after the core body temperature minimum occurs. The preoptic anterior hypothalamus is important in thermoregulation and integrates at the spinal cord level. There is afferent input from thermoreceptors, the skin, and the spinal cord. Neural projections from the SCN also innervate this site of thermoregulation and directly influence the regulation of core body temperature.[80]

Therefore, in the case presented, light exposure should occur at or just after his minimum core body temperature, upon awakening at 9 AM (2 hours before his current natural wake time; Answer C is correct). Light exposure at 7 AM or 8 AM would cause a further delay of his sleep timing and disrupt his ability to adjust his schedule to begin school (Answers A

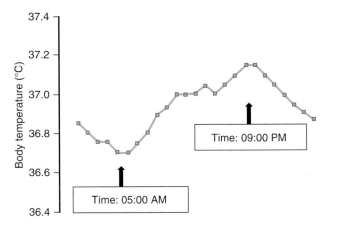

• **Figure 49.6** The core body temperature of humans follows a sinusoidal rhythm with a circadian periodicity. Among those with a normal circadian rhythm, the peak occurs at approximately 9 PM and the core body temperature minimum occurs at approximately 5 AM. Phase advance and delay with light exposure depends on the timing in reference to the minimum core body temperature.

and B are incorrect). Although light exposure at 10 AM would be helpful, it would have the greatest effect if he can wake at 9 AM (Answer D is incorrect). This would also allow him sufficient time to continue incremental adjustments in his wake time prior to starting school.[81]

23. **Answer D. The heart rate normally fluctuates due to phasic heart rate changes associated with REM sleep.**
There are a number of important hemodynamic changes that occur during sleep, affecting cardiac function and peripheral vascular blood flow (Table 49.9). These effects can be distinguished by considering the role of the autonomic nervous system, with parasympathetic tone predominating in non-REM (NREM) sleep and sympathetic tone increasing in REM sleep. NREM is characterized by increases in parasympathetic discharge associated with heightened baroreceptor sensitivity.[82] There is a simultaneous decrease in sympathetic discharge that results in reduced heart rate, blood pressure, cardiac output, and systemic vascular resistance. In contrast, REM sleep demonstrates an increase in sympathetic tone that results in bursts of heart rate and coronary blood flow, and an overall reduction in peripheral blood circulation. It is common to observe sinus pauses and arrhythmias during the transition from NREM to REM sleep, due to surges in vagus nerve activity.[83]

These changes impact the blood supply of various systems. In muscles, blood flow does not change between wakefulness and NREM sleep. When REM sleep occurs, blood flow is decreased due to vasoconstriction of the skeletal muscle and cutaneous vascular beds (especially during phasic REM).[84] Splanchnic blood flow increases as a result of vasodilation, leading to an overall decrease of peripheral vascular resistance in REM sleep. Coronary blood flow is increased during REM sleep and decreases between wakefulness and NREM sleep.[85]

Although peripheral vascular resistance decreases in association with REM sleep, which predominates toward morning, this alone is unlikely to evoke arrhythmias (Answer A is incorrect). Systemic blood pressure fluctuates in REM sleep, but it decreases further in NREM sleep (Answer B is incorrect). It is true that cardiac output progressively declines through the night, reaching a nadir during the last REM period and perhaps contributing to adverse cardiovascular events, but this is unlikely to contribute to the findings noted on the cardiac monitoring (Answer C is incorrect). As noted, due to the

TABLE 49.9	Vascular Blood Flow and Hemodynamic Changes During Sleep	
	NREM Sleep	**REM Sleep**
Muscular and cutaneous blood flow	Relatively unchanged	Decreases
Cerebral blood flow	Decreases	Increases
Peripheral vascular resistance	Unchanged or slightly decreases	Decreases
Heart rate	Decreases	Increases and decreases because of phasic heart rate changes
Systemic blood pressure	Decreases	Fluctuates
Cardiac output	Decreases progressively throughout sleep with the lowest level during the last REM period of the night	—

NREM, Nonrapid eye movement; *REM*, rapid eye movement.

influence of the sympathetic nervous system, the heart rate normally fluctuates due to phasic changes associated with REM sleep, and this may be noted on extended rhythm monitoring (Answer D is correct).

24. **Answer A. Elevation in PaCO$_2$ by 2–8 mmHg.**

At the transition between wakefulness and sleep, there is a normal reduction in minute ventilation by about 0.5–1.5 L/min. This sleep-related hypoventilation causes a slight increase in PaCO$_2$ by about 2–8 mmHg (Answer A is correct and Answer C is incorrect). There is also a concomitant reduction in PaO$_2$ by 3–10 mmHg (Answers B and D are incorrect). Periodic breathing may be observed as an individual transition between wakefulness and N1 sleep. If the PaCO$_2$ falls below the PaCO$_2$ threshold, this is sensed at the level of the medullary chemoreceptor, which induces hypoventilation or apnea until the PaCO$_2$ rises enough to trigger resumption of ventilation. Breathing is relatively stable in N3 sleep, though minute ventilation is still less than occurs during the waking state.[86]

Automatic control of ventilation is centered in the pons and medulla of the brainstem, which control breathing regardless of state of consciousness. The pons pneumotaxic center (or pontine respiratory group) is located at the rostral pons in the area of the parabrachial nucleus and Kölliker-Fuse nuclei. The dorsolateral lower pons is known as the apneustic center, and may be the location of the inspiratory off switch for medullary inspiratory neurons. Within the nucleus tractus solitarius, the dorsal regulatory group controls the medullary responses for inspiration. Both inhalation and exhalation are controlled by the medullary ventral respiratory center in the nucleus ambiguus and caudal nucleus retroambiguus. This ventral respiratory group is the center for the generation of the intrinsic respiratory rhythm at the pre-Bötzinger complex.[87]

25. **Answer A. Serotonin (5-HT) has its highest activity during the waking state.**

Neurotransmitters may be excitatory or inhibitory, promoting wakefulness or promoting sleep, with the same substance sometimes having differing effects, depending on the neuroanatomical location (due to negative feedback loops; Table 49.10).[88] These neurotransmitters may also vary in concentration and activity in specific regions, depending on whether there is a state of wakefulness, NREM, or REM sleep (Table 49.11).[16]

Glutamate is one of the main excitatory neurotransmitters in the brain, and it is found in the highest concentrations in the reticular formation of the brainstem. Agonists of glutamate can induce seizures (due to excessive excitation), while antagonists like ketamine work as an anesthetic. Acetylcholine is primarily found in the basal forebrain and dorsal brainstem,

TABLE 49.10 Generalized Neurotransmitter Activities

Wake Promoting
Acetylcholine
Norepinephrine
Histamine
Serotonin
Dopamine
Orexin/Hypocretin
NREM Sleep Promoting
GABA
Galanin
REM Sleep Promoting
Acetylcholine
Monoamines
GABA
Melanin-concentrating hormone (MCH)

This table is simplified and further exploration of this subject with other references is recommended.

TABLE 49.11 Neurotransmitter Activity in Sleep and Wakefulness

Neurotransmitter	Neurons of Highest Concentration	NREM Sleep	REM Sleep	Waking State
Acetylcholine	Basal forebrain and dorsal brainstem	Lowest activity	High activity	High activity
Dopamine	Ventral tegmental area of the midbrain and substantia nigra	Not as clear in activity in these different states; extracellular dopamine is increased in the waking state, and dopamine agonists reduce sleep.	—	—
Histamine	Tuberomammillary nucleus of the posterior hypothalamus	Lower activity	Lowest activity	High activity
Norepinephrine (Noradrenergic)	Locus coeruleus of the rostral pontine reticular formation	Lower activity	Lowest activity	High activity
Orexin/Hypocretin	Perifornical region of the lateral and posterior hypothalamus	Lower activity	Controversy over activity in human REM sleep	Highest activity
Serotonin (5-HT)	Dorsal/median raphe nuclei in the midline region of the brainstem reticular formation	Lower activity	Virtually inactive	High activity

NREM, Nonrapid eye movement; *REM,* rapid eye movement.
This table is simplified with a much more complicated neuronal projections that can be presented in this fashion, and further exploration of this subject with other references is recommended.

and is involved in vigilance and attention (with highest levels during wake and REM sleep; Answer B is incorrect). Histamine predominates in the TMN of the posterior hypothalamus and promotes wakefulness. Serotonin is released from the median and dorsal raphe nuclei, with highest levels in wakefulness, lower activity during NREM sleep, and virtually no activity during REM sleep (Answer A is correct). NE is found in the locus coeruleus of the rostral pontine reticular formation and has its highest activity during wakefulness (Answer C is incorrect). Orexin (or hypocretin) is concentrated in the perifornical region of the lateral and posterior hypothalamus, and is noted to have its highest activity during the waking state (Answer D is incorrect).

Suggested Reading

Amlaner CJ, Fuller PM, eds. *Basics of Sleep Guide*. 2nd ed. Westchester, IL: Sleep Research Society; 2009.

Berry RB, Brooks R, Gamaldo CE, et al. *The AASM Manual for the Scoring of Sleep and Associated Events: Rules, Terminology and Technical Specifications, Version 2.2*. Darien, IL: American Academy of Sleep Medicine; 2015. www.aasm.org.

España RA, Scammell TE. Sleep neurobiology from a clinical perspective. *Sleep*. 2011;34(7):845-848.

Kryger MH, Roth T, Dement WC, eds. *Principles and Practice of Sleep Medicine*. 6th ed. Philadelphia, PA, Pennsylvania: Elsevier; 2017.

The International Classification of Sleep Disorders. *American Academy of Sleep Medicine*. 3rd ed.; 2014.

50

Mechanisms of Sleep Neuroscience: Putting It All Together

CHRISTOPHER J. WATSON

Questions

1. In the flip-flop switch model of arousal state control, neurons localized in this brain region inhibit wake-promoting brain regions, such as the dorsal raphé nucleus, locus coeruleus, and tuberomammillary nucleus (TMN) to switch from wakefulness to non-rapid eye movement (NREM) sleep.
   A. The ventrolateral preoptic area (VLPO)
   B. The lateral hypothalamus
   C. The laterodorsal pontine tegmentum
   D. The pedunculopontine tegmentum

2. In 1930 Constantin von Economo published a report that linked specific brain regions to sleep regulation. Based on the postmortem examination of brains from patients with *encephalitis lethargica*, von Economo concluded that the mechanisms regulating sleep and wakefulness were localized in the hypothalamus. In modern anatomical nomenclature terms, which of the following was one of von Economo's conclusions?
   A. Groups of sleep-promoting neurons were localized to the posterior and lateral hypothalamus.
   B. Groups of sleep-promoting neurons were localized to the anterior and lateral hypothalamus.
   C. Groups of wake-promoting neurons were localized to the posterior and lateral hypothalamus.
   D. Groups of wake-promoting neurons were localized to the anterior and lateral hypothalamus.

3. Fibromyalgia is considered to be the prototypical centralized pain phenotype. More than 90% of patients with fibromyalgia report some form of sleep disturbance, and sleep disturbances are correlated to patient pain severity. In polysomnographic recordings, this sleep abnormality is common among patients with fibromyalgia.
   A. A prominent α-frequency during NREM sleep
   B. A prominent α-frequency during rapid eye movement (REM) sleep
   C. The presence of K complexes and sleep spindles throughout REM sleep
   D. A prominent δ-frequency during REM sleeps

4. In humans, systemic administration of muscarinic acetylcholine receptor agonists or acetylcholinesterase inhibitors has been shown to have this effect on arousal state.
   A. It causes an increase in NREM sleep.
   B. It causes an increase in REM sleep.
   C. It causes an increase in wakefulness.
   D. It has no effect on arousal state.

5. Studies conducted to elucidate the mechanisms underlying the ongoing obesity epidemic have found an association between sleep disorders and metabolic syndrome. A possible link between these two conditions is the hormone leptin, which suppresses appetite and may modulate arousal state. Leptin modulates arousal state by:
   A. Decreasing the number of arousals and stage shifts during sleep.
   B. Increasing the total amount of NREM sleep during a 24-hour period.
   C. Increasing the total number of sleep episodes.
   D. Increasing the total amount of REM sleep during a 24-hour period.

6. Neurons that discharge with the highest frequency during REM sleep are considered REM-on cells. These neurons typically play a role in the mechanisms underlying REM generation and maintenance. Which of the below brain regions contains REM-on cells?
   A. The TMN
   B. The VLPO
   C. The dorsal raphé nucleus
   D. The laterodorsal pontine tegmentum

7. All mammals display theta (θ)-rhythms (4.5–8.0 Hz) during REM sleep. θ Rhythms also occur during attention or memory tasks in humans and during times of movement in rodents. Which brain region acts as the pacemaker for and drives the hippocampal θ-rhythms?
   A. The oral part of the pontine reticular formation (PRF)
   B. The hippocampus
   C. The medial septum
   D. The supermammillary nucleus

8. Wakefulness promoting neurons in the ventral tegmental area and the substantia nigra pars compacta (SNC) display

state-independent firing and signal other arousal regulating brain regions with this neurotransmitter.
A. Hypocretin/orexin
B. Norepinephrine
C. Serotonin
D. Dopamine

9. Symptoms of night eating syndrome include excessive eating and frequent awakenings due to hunger. This peptide likely plays a role in this syndrome.
A. Met-enkephalin
B. Ghrelin
C. Leptin
D. Nociceptin

10. Caffeine is perhaps the most self-prescribed psychoactive compound for the treatment of daytime sleepiness and to increase alertness. In what brain region does caffeine inhibit the activity of NREM sleep-promoting neurons?
A. The prefrontal cortex
B. The VLPO
C. The basal forebrain (BF)
D. The sublaterodorsal nucleus

11. Based on the 1949 paper by Moruzzi and Magoun, this neurotransmitter is contained in projection neurons arising from the ascending reticular activating system (ARAS).
A. Norepinephrine
B. Hypocretin/orexin
C. Galanin
D. Dopamine

12. Systemic administration of gamma-aminobutyric acid (GABA)-mimetic drugs causes sedation, sleep, and general anesthesia. However, enhancing GABAergic transmission locally within this brain region increases wakefulness and decreases sleep.
A. The laterodorsal pontine tegmentum
B. The dorsal raphé nucleus
C. The locus coeruleus
D. The PRF

13. Opioids are commonly used to treat surgical pain, but they can also adversely affect arousal state. Name one effect that systemic opioid administration may have on states of sleep and wakefulness.
A. Increases stage N3 NREM sleep
B. Increases REM sleep
C. Increases stage N2 NREM sleep
D. Increases NREM and REM sleep

Use the following case description to answer questions 14 and 15. A 25-year-old man has difficulty coming to complete wakefulness almost every morning, and this is accompanied by confusion, disorientation, poor motor coordination, slow movements, and repeated return to sleep. He also reports abnormally deep and prolonged sleep and frequently being overcome by sleepiness during the day.

14. What is the most likely diagnosis?
A. Somnambulism
B. Narcolepsy
C. Sleep drunkenness
D. Pavor nocturnus

15. The underlying cause of this disorder has not been determined, but which of the following could be considered the most likely mechanism?
A. An abnormality in the VLPO
B. An abnormality in dopamine signaling

C. An abnormality in the sublaterodorsal nucleus
D. An abnormality in the hypocretin/Orexin system

16. Neurons localized to the TMN contain histamine. Scientists have developed a genetically modified mouse that does not express histamine. What would be the most likely physiological effect caused by the loss of histaminergic signaling?
A. Hyper-arousal
B. Fragmented sleep
C. Somnolence
D. Decreased REM sleep

17. Although coordinated electrical activity in the cortex is the primary source of the waves that are observed on the electro-encephalography (EEG), the thalamus and the cortex act together to drive cortical waves. Why does the reticular nucleus of the thalamus have an important role in the generation of cortical activity?
A. K complexes represent rapid depolarization of thalamic reticular nucleus cells.
B. δ waves are generated by neurons in the thalamic reticular nucleus.
C. GABAergic projection neurons from the thalamic reticular nucleus inhibit components of the ascending activating system (AAS).
D. Thalamocortical network oscillations require neurons of the thalamic reticular nucleus.

18. A deficiency in this neurotransmitter system is a common trait in patients with narcolepsy.
A. Dopamine
B. Hypocretin/orexin
C. Galanin
D. Acetylcholine

19. The suprachiasmatic nucleus (SCN) is a major center for setting the circadian clock, and entrainment of this clock is primarily dependent on photic signals. Which pathway transfers photic input to the SCN?
A. From the retinal ganglion cells through a GABAergic projection
B. From the median forebrain bundle through a glutamatergic projection
C. From the lateral geniculate nucleus through a serotoninergic projection
D. From the intergeniculate leaflet through a neuropeptide Y projection

20. When GABA$_A$ receptor agonists are administered to discrete brain regions, the sleep/wake effects are dependent upon the specific brain region. What are the effects of GABA$_A$ receptor agonists when given systemically?
A. A prolonged increase in wakefulness
B. An overall increase in sleep
C. An increase in the duration of REM sleep
D. A pronounced fragmentation of NREM sleep

21. Electrical field potentials that become synchronized between the pons, the lateral geniculate nucleus, and the occipital cortex are called ponto-geniculo-occipital (PGO) waves. PGO waves are an electrographic sign of which arousal state?
A. Wakefulness
B. Stage N1 NREM sleep
C. Stage N2 NREM sleep
D. REM sleep

22. Although this brain region is known to play in arousal state control, mechanistic studies regarding the neurochemical makeup of this region have not been performed in rodents.

A. The BF
B. The thalamus
C. The VLPO
D. The PRF

23. Pregabalin is an α-2-δ ligand that is approved for the treatment of neuropathic pain, fibromyalgia, partial onset seizures, and general anxiety disorder. The analgesic, anxiolytic, and anti-convulsant properties of pregabalin have been extensively studied. Patients with chronic pain or anxiety often experience disrupted sleep. What effect, if any, does pregabalin have on arousal state?
    A. Increases the amount of slow wave sleep (SWS)
    B. Increases the amount of wakefulness
    C. Increases the number of REM sleep episodes
    D. Does not have a statistically significant effect on arousal state

24. In humans, melatonin is an important regulator of the cir-cadian pacemaker system, and the functions of the secreted hormone have been well characterized. Measurement of melatonin secretion across the circadian cycle was of particu-lar importance, because it revealed functional roles for the hormone. How does melatonin secretion change across the circadian cycle?
    A. It occurs in pulses.
    B. Its onset occurs in the early morning.
    C. It varies from day to day.
    D. It is greater during NREM sleep than during REM sleep.

Use the following case description to answer questions 25 and 26: A 22-year-old male patient presents with the following symptoms: inability to stay awake at any time of the day, difficulty falling sleep, fragmented sleep, and early morning awakening. He reports being in a car accident 6 months prior that resulted in a minor head injury. His medical history reveals that recovery from the head injury was complete with all neurological and medical signs being normal. This includes a recent computed tomography scan. When questioned, the patient reports that his sleep problems began to worsen in the last couple of months, and in the immediate post-accident period, he was sleeping normally.

25. Based on this evidence, what area of the brain would you consider most likely to be affected in this patient?
    A. Thalamus
    B. Basal ganglia
    C. Hypothalamus
    D. Locus coeruleus

26. Which test would be the best first step in developing a treatment plane for this patient?
    A. Cerebrospinal fluid (CSF) hypocretin/orexin levels
    B. CSF angiotensin-converting enzyme levels
    C. Multiple sleep latency test (MSLT)
    D. Beck Depression Inventory II

27. During stage N3 NREM sleep, the cortical EEG is characterized by the presence of slow waves (oscillations with frequencies of less than 4 Hz). These oscillations have two distinct com-ponents, δ-waves (1–4 Hz) and a slower oscillation with a frequency below 1 Hz. This slow oscillation does not show a decrease with continued sleep. Furthermore, δ-waves and the slow oscillation are dependent on different processes. In which brain structure is the less than 1-Hz slow oscillation generated?
    A. The cortex
    B. The thalamus

C. The hippocampus
D. The PRF

28. GABAergic mechanisms play a role in the generation of REM sleep, and significant changes in the discharge pattern of GABA-containing neurons during REM sleep have been described. What is an important GABAergic influence that could be responsible for the generation of REM sleep?
    A. Continuous GABAergic inhibitory drive on pontine monoaminergic neurons except during REM sleep
    B. Induction of REM sleep by GABA agonists administered in the sublaterodorsal nucleus (SLD) nucleus
    C. Inhibition of orexin/hypocretin neurons during REM sleep by GABAergic interneurons
    D. Activity of all GABAergic neurons in the ventrolateral periaqueductal gray matter during REM sleep

29. Sleepiness and fever are hallmarks of an infectious disease. The CSF levels of several cytokines and hormonal factors are increased in this state and have also been shown to be sleep factors. They are thus likely candidates to mediate the increased sleepiness associated with infection. Which of the following would mediate the increased sleepiness of an infectious disease?
    A. Tumor necrosis factor-α (TNF-α)
    B. Interleukin-10 (IL-10)
    C. Corticotropin-releasing hormone
    D. Transforming growth factor-β (TGF-β)

30. Intravenous administration of the acetylcholinesterase inhibitor physostigmine into a patient during NREM sleep induces REM sleep with a short latency. This is one example of the importance of cholinergic systems in the control of REM sleep. In animal studies, to determine the location of the REM sleep induction area for this effect, acetylcholinesterase inhibi-tors are infused directly into certain brain regions. In which brain region would the most rapid induction of REM sleep by compounds such as physostigmine be expected?
    A. The lateral hypothalamus
    B. The VLPO
    C. Peri-locus coeruleus-α (peri-LC-α)
    D. Laterodorsal pontine tegmentum

31. It has been estimated that chronic insomnia affects approxi-mately 25% of adults in the United States. Several conventional treatments for insomnia also have significant side effects that may include the following: drug dependence and tolerance, rebound insomnia, cognitive impairment, and increased feelings of anxiety. In an effort to reduce the side-effect profile associated with the treatment of insomnia, new classes of drugs targeting this neurotransmitter system have been developed.
    A. Norepinephrine
    B. Serotonin
    C. Dopamine
    D. Hypocretin/orexin

32. Mechanistic studies in animals have demonstrated that individual components of REM sleep (e.g., electroencepha-lographic activation, PGO waves, and muscle atonia) can be dissociated. Which brain region functions in REM sleep to specifically inhibit spinal neurons (resulting in muscle atonia)?
    A. The ventral gigantocellular reticular nucleus
    B. The lateral geniculate nucleus
    C. The PRF
    D. Ventrolateral preoptic nucleus (VLPO)

33. Between 60% and 90% of patients with major depressive disorder report sleep disturbances. Which of the following may be a unique biomarker for depression?

A. Decreased latency to NREM sleep onset

B. Increased total sleep time

C. Decreased latency to REM sleep onset

D. Increased SWS duration

34. Glutamate is the main excitatory neurotransmitter in the mammalian brain, and it is localized to many projection neurons throughout the central nervous system. Which of the following cell types does not contain glutamate?

A. Lateral hypothalamus neurons that project to histaminergic cells in the TMN

B. Corticothalamic neurons that project to glutamatergic cells in the thalamus

C. Mesencephalic reticular formation neurons that project to the GABAergic cells in the thalamus

D. VLPO neurons that project to noradrenergic cells in the locus coeruleus

35. Increased power in the δ range (1–4 Hz) in the EEG occurs in stage N3 NREM sleep and is associated with sleepiness. What neurotransmitter accumulates during wakefulness and is likely the cause of increased sleepiness?

A. Melatonin

B. Adenosine

C. Serotonin

D. Histamine

36. Natural sleep and states of surgical anesthesia share some common mechanisms for their onset, maintenance, and offset. This results in natural sleep and anesthetic states sharing certain traits. Which of the following is common to both during the maintenance phase of each?

A. The possibility of dreaming and/or amnesia

B. The duration is dependent on prior wakefulness or circadian rhythms

C. The depth or stage of each can be held constant for long periods

D. Maintenance is altered by environmental factors

37. Fatal familial insomnia is a rare prion disorder that results in gliosis and neurodegeneration of the thalamus. In postmortem studies, this thalamic nucleus shows the most significant cell loss.

A. The nucleus reticularis

B. The dorsomedial thalamus

C. The zona incerta

D. The ventromedial thalamus

38. Animal studies have shown that specific brain lesions can create a pathology that mimics REM sleep behavior disorder and includes over oneiric behavior appearing during episodes of REM sleep. A lesion to which brain region creates this pathology in animals?

A. The perifornical hypothalamus

B. The intralaminar nucleus of the thalamus

C. The brainstem region ventral to the locus coeruleus

D. The brainstem region lateral to the dorsal raphé nucleus

39. The average duration of a REM sleep episode is constant. Which of the following is most likely to affect the duration of a REM sleep episode?

A. Metabolic rate

B. The hypocretin/orexin system

C. Circadian time

D. Sleepiness

40. Norepinephrine maintains the sleep-promoting neurons of the preoptic area of the BF under an inhibitory during

wakefulness. What is the mechanism for inhibition of these neurons by norepinephrine?

A. Presynaptic effect at the β-adrenoceptor

B. Postsynaptic action at the α-adrenoceptor

C. Activation of GABAergic inhibitory neurons

D. Local generation of adenosine

Answers

1. **Answer A. The VLPO.**
   As shown in Fig. 50.1, the VLPO uses the inhibitory neurotransmitters GABA and galanin to inhibit wake-promoting brain regions that include the dorsal raphé nucleus, locus coeruleus, and TMN.[1] The lateral hypothalamus plays (Answer A) is incorrect, because neurons in this region play a role in the onset of wakefulness and provide a balance between the wakefulness/NREM sleep switch and the NREM/REM sleep switch. Both the laterodorsal pontine (Answer C) and pedunculopontine tegmentum (Answer D) are incorrect because neurons in these brain regions play a role in the generation and maintenance of REM sleep.

2. **Answer C. Groups of wake-promoting neurons were localized to the posterior and lateral hypothalamus.**
   In 1930 von Economo linked specific brain regions to sleep regulation.[2] Postmortem analysis of brains from patients with encephalitis lethargica and presenting with insomnia revealed lesions localized to the anterior hypothalamus and the preoptic area, suggesting that one or both of these regions play a role in generating and/or maintaining sleep. In similar patients presenting with hypersomnia, lesions were localized to the posterior hypothalamus, which suggests that this region plays a role in generating and/or maintaining wakefulness. Answer C is correct, and answer D is incorrect, because von Economo hypothesized that wake-promoting neurons were localized in the posterior and lateral hypothalamus. Answers A and B are incorrect because von Economo hypothesized that sleep-promoting neurons are localized to the anterior and medial portions of the hypothalamus (Fig. 50.2).[89] These findings have since been replicated using preclinical lesioning studies.[3]

3. **Answer A. A prominent α-frequency during NREM sleep.**
   A prominent α-frequency during NREM sleep is often denoted as α-intrusion[4,5] or alpha-delta (α-δ) sleep.[6] α-Intrusions originate in the frontal cortex,[7] and may represent a state of awakening.[8] Since α-intrusions occur during NREM sleep, answer B is incorrect (Fig. 50.3). Other sleep disturbances observed in patients with fibromyalgia include a decrease in the duration of stage 2 NREM sleep,[9] a decrease in the number of sleep spindles,[10] and an increase in the number of sleep and wakefulness stage transitions.[11] The presence of K complexes and sleep spindles throughout REM sleep (Answer C), and a prominent δ-frequency during REM sleep (Answer D) have not been reported as sleep disturbances in patients with fibromyalgia, so both C and D are incorrect. For a detailed review of the interactions between sleep, pain, and fibromyalgia.[12]

4. **Answer B. It causes an increase in REM sleep.**
   Intravenous administration of the muscarinic acetylcholine receptor agonist arecholine to healthy human volunteers shortens the latency to REM sleep onset and also increases the number of episodes of REM sleep.[13,14] Conversely, administering the muscarinic receptor antagonist scopolamine to the same volunteers decreases the number of REM episodes

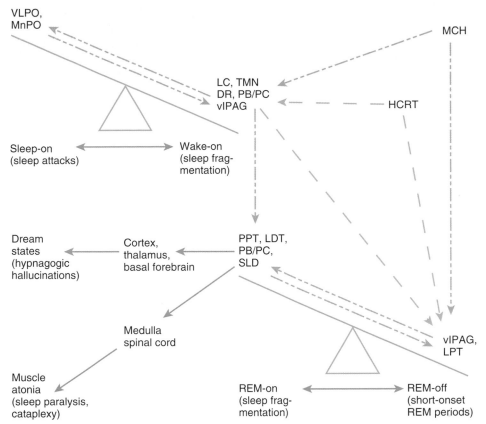

• **Figure 50.1** Schematic Linking the Wake/NREM Flip-Flop Switch and the NREM/REM Flip-Flop Switch. The wake/NREM sleep switch is in the upper left of the schematic, and the NREM sleep/REM sleep switch is in the lower right portion of the schematic. The dashed lines represent inhibitory projections, while the two-dot dashed lines represent excitatory projections. Monoaminergic wake-promoting neurons inhibit NREM-on neurons during wakefulness. These neurons also inhibit REM-on and excite REM-off neurons in the NREM/REM switch, which makes a transition from wakefulness directly to REM sleep nearly impossible. In patients with narcolepsy, hypocretin/orexin signaling is lost. This causes a destabilization of both switches and may lead to the symptoms listed in parentheses. *DR*, dorsal raphe nucleus; *LC*, locus coeruleus; *LDT*, laterodorsal pontine tegmentum; *LPT*; *MCH*, melanin-concentrating hormone; *MnPO*, median preoptic area; *NREM*, non-rapid eye movement; *ORX*, orexin/hypocretin; *PB*, parabrachial nucleus; *PC*, paracoeruleus; *PPT*, pedunculopontine tegmentum; *REM*, rapid eye movement; *SLD*, sublaterodorsal nucleus; *TMN*, tuberomammillary nucleus; *vlPAG*, ventrolateral periaqueductal gray; *VLPO*, ventrolateral preoptic area. (Modified from Saper CB, Fuller PM, Pedersen NP, Lu J, Scammell TE. Sleep state switching. *Neuron.* 2010;68:1023–1042.)

and prolongs the onset of REM sleep. The selective M₁ receptor agonist RS-86 or the acetylcholinesterase inhibitor donepezil shortens the time to REM sleep onset or increases the duration of REM sleep, respectively, when given orally to humans.[15] Systemic administration of acetylcholinesterase inhibitor physostigmine to healthy volunteers during NREM sleep also induces or increases REM sleep.[16,17] The laterodorsal (LDT) and pedunculopontine tegmentum (PPT). The LDT and PPT have "REM-on" and wake-on and REM-on neurons. Systemic administration of these cholinergic drugs act on these neurons (Fig. 50.4). Based on the above evidence, the answers of causing: an increase in NREM sleep (B), an increase in wakefulness (C), or having no effect on arousal state (D) are incorrect. For reviews on the cholinergic modulation of REM sleep.[13,16,18]

5. **Answer A. Decreasing the number of arousals and stage shifts during sleep.**
Genetic mouse models of obesity have been used to investigate a link between metabolic syndrome, sleep disruptions, and leptin signaling. One study demonstrated that *ob/ob* mice

(obese mice with a leptin deficiency) had increased arousals and stage shifts compared with wild-type (healthy) controls.[19] The *ob/ob* mice also showed an increase in total sleep time during a 24-hour period with no increase in the amount of REM sleep. Similar results were observed when the sleep patterns of *db/db* mice (obese mice with a leptin resistance) were compared with those of wild-type mice.[20] In healthy humans, short sleep duration has been associated with decreased circulating levels of leptin compared with healthy patients with normal circulating levels of leptin.[21,22] The evidence above supports the interpretation that the presence of normal circulating levels of leptin (compared with reduced levels of leptin or disruption of leptin signaling presented above) plays a role in sleep consolidation by decreasing the number of arousal and stage shifts during sleep (Answer A). The absence of leptin causes an increase in total sleep time but no change in REM sleep, so normal levels of leptin would not increase NREM sleep (Answer B) or decrease REM sleep (Answer D). Since normal circulating levels of leptin help consolidate sleep,

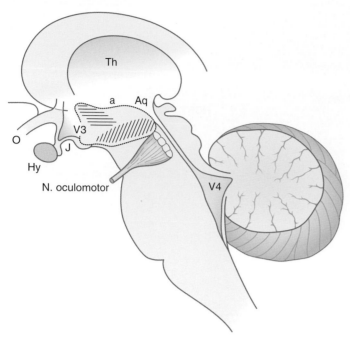

• **Figure 50.2** The Results of Von Economo's Landmark Study. A representation of von Economo's boundaries indicating lesions in the anterior and posterior regions of the marking of the boundary of the field in the transition between the diencephalin and the mesecephalin (*dotted line* a).[2] If lesions are localized to the anterior portion (denoted by *horizontal lines*), the result is insomnia. If the lesions are localized to the posterior portion (denoted by *slanted lines*) the resulting affect sleep. *Aq*, aqueduct; *Hy*, hypophysis; *J*, infundibulum; *O*, optic chiasm; *Th*, optical thalamus; *V3*, third ventricle; *V4*, fourth ventricle. (Reprinted with permission from Lazaros C. Triarhou. The percipient observations of Constantin von Economo on encephalitis lethargica and sleep disruption and their lasting impact on contemporary sleep research. *Brain Res Bull.* 2006;69[3]:244–258.)

increasing the total numbers of episodes (Answer C) would also be an incorrect answer.

6. **Answer D. The laterodorsal pontine tegmentum.**
The laterodorsal pontine tegmentum and the pedunculopontine tegmentum each have a subset of neurons that have the highest discharge rate during REM sleep and are termed "REM-on" neurons.[23] The LDT and PPT (Fig. 50.5; see also Fig. 50.4) also have a second subset of neurons that have the highest discharge rates during wakefulness and REM sleep and are termed "Wake-on/REM-on" neurons.[24] Answer A is incorrect because neurons in the TMN fire with a "Wake-on" discharge pattern and promote wakefulness.[25] Answer B is incorrect because neurons localized to the ventrolateral preoptic nucleus increase discharge rate during the transition from wakefulness and NREM sleep (i.e., NREM-on), and maintain an elevated discharge rate (compared with wakefulness) during NREM and REM sleep.[26] Answer C is incorrect because neurons originating in the dorsal raphé nucleus have the highest discharge rate during wakefulness, and decrease discharge frequency during NREM and REM sleep.[27]

7. **Answer C. The medial septum.**
When neurons in the oral part of the pontine reticular formation (PnO) fire in a tonic manner, glutamatergic neurons projecting from the PnO to the supermammillary (SMN) nucleus excite SMN neurons. This results in a rhythmic/oscillating firing of SMN neurons. Glutamatergic signaling

from the SMN causes activation of GABAergic and cholinergic neurons in the medial septum and the vertical limb of the diagonal band (MS/vDB). Excitation of the MS/vDB acts as the pacemaker, or drive, for hippocampal θ rhythms (4.5–8.0 Hz). Based on the data description, answer C (the medial septum) is the correct answer because it uses cholinergic and GABAergic projection neurons to excite and inhibit the hippocampus. The PnO (Answer B) is incorrect. Although tonic firing of the PnO may initiate the process of θ rhythm generation, PnO do not drive θ rhythm via a direct projection. Instead, the PnO creates a rhythmic firing in the SMN. The SMN (Answer D) is also incorrect because also does not directly signal the hippocampus, but instead activates neurons of the MS/vDB. The hippocampus (Answer B) is also incorrect because it is actually driven by the MS/vDB during θ rhythm firing.[28]

8. **Answer D. Dopamine.**
Each of the answers are wake-promoting neurotransmitters, but only dopamine neurons that promote wakefulness are localized in the ventral tegmental (VTA) are and the SNC (Fig. 50.6). Amphetamines, cocaine, and methylphenidate are stimulants that increase wakefulness and decrease hypersomnia by increasing endogenous levels of dopamine (reviewed in Boutrel and Koob[29]). The wake-promoting drug modafinil, which is used to treat narcolepsy and other sleep disorders, blocks dopamine transporters and increases endogenous levels of dopamine.[30] Hypocretin/orexin (Answer A) cell bodies are localized to the lateral hypothalamus and not the VTA and SNC. Likewise, neurons that release norepinephrine (Answer B) and serotonin (Answer C) are localized to thc locus coeruleus and dorsal raphé nucleus, respectively, and not the VTA and SNC.

9. **Answer B. Ghrelin.**
Ghrelin (sometimes called the "hunger hormone") stimulates hunger and is normally secreted when the stomach is empty. A case study showed that a nonobese patient with night eating syndrome had increased nighttime levels of ghrelin compared with healthy controls.[31] A second study compared ghrelin levels between healthy people with normal weight, healthy overweight individuals, patients with nighttime eating syndrome (NES) and normal weight, and patients with NES and overweight.[32] Patients with NES and normal weight had lower nighttime levels of ghrelin than healthy people with normal weight. Fig. 50.7 shows that in both groups, overweight individuals had lower levels of ghrelin compared with their normal weight match.[33] These studies suggest that ghrelin acts as a wake-promoting hormone. Met-enkephalin (Answer A) is incorrect, because it acts on endogenous opioid receptors and mainly plays a role in pain processing and not hunger. Leptin (Answer C; sometimes called the "satiety hormone") is released by adipose tissue and inhibits hunger. Thus, leptin would not be the cause of night eating syndrome. Nociceptin (Answer D), also known as orphanin FQ, acts at nociception receptors and is grouped in the opioid family of endogenous peptides, but it does not act at classical μ-, κ-, and δ-opioid receptors. Nociceptin does not modulate hunger, but it is thought to have hyperalgesic effects.[34]

10. **Answer B. The VLPO.**
Adenosine is a breakdown product of adenosine-5′-triphosphate and the gradual increase in adenosine levels within the BF correspond with the amount of time awake (Fig. 50.8). Caffeine is an A_1 and A_{2A} adenosine receptor antagonist and inhibits

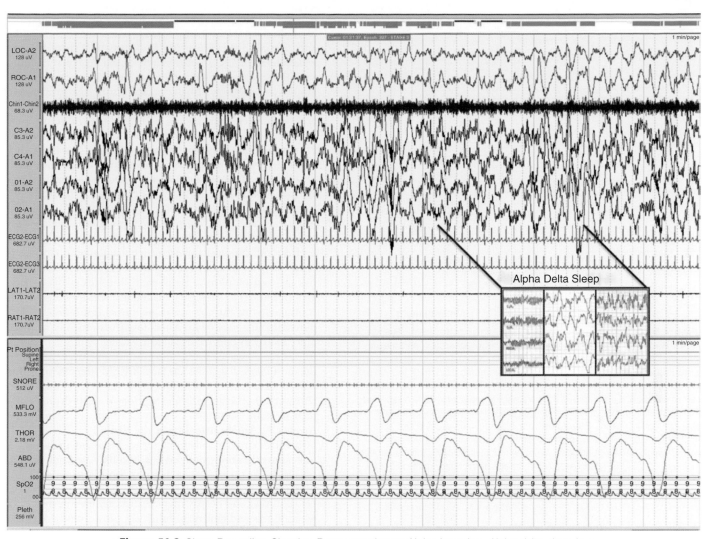

• **Figure 50.3** Sleep Recording Showing Representative an Alpha Intrusion. Alpha-delta sleep in a patient with fibromyalgia. Polysomnogram fragments from a 53-year-old woman who complained of fatigue despite obtaining 8.5 hours of sleep per night. The electrographic abnormalities in these patients are characterized by an abnormal alpha-wave intrusion during slow-wave sleep, termed alpha-delta sleep. (Reprinted from Kryger M, Avidan AY, Berry R, eds. *Atlas of Clinical Sleep Medicine.* Philadelphia: Elsevier; 2013.)

the sleep-inducing effects of adenosinergic signaling at these receptor subtypes. Numerous studies support the idea that adenosine promotes sleep (reviewed in Watson et al.[27]). Caffeine most likely decreases signaling from sleep-promoting neurons within the VLPO, so answer B is correct. Caffeine most likely increases wakefulness by increasing signaling from wake-promoting neurons within the BF, so answer C is not correct. When administered to the prefrontal cortex (PFC), adenosinergic antagonists caused an increase in both acetylcholine release and wakefulness, suggesting that caffeine would increase the activity of wake-promoting neurons.[35] Neurons in the SLD are REM-promoting neurons, so caffeine in the SLD would work on NREM sleep-promoting neurons, making answer D incorrect.

11. **Answer A. Norepinephrine.**

The classic work by Moruzzi and Magoun[36] used the *cerveau isolé* preparation in cat to demonstrate that an arousal center located in the pons below the level of transection. Using electrical stimulation of discrete brain regions, they showed

that the pontine reticular system plays a critical role in generation and maintenance of arousal and wakefulness. This system, which they termed the *ARAS*, has projections that innervate the midbrain and the cortex (Fig. 50.9). With the advent of bioanalytical techniques, it is now known that cell bodies within the pontine reticular system portion of the AAS, as it is now called, contain acetylcholine, glutamate, norepinephrine, and serotonin. Neurons containing norepinephrine are localized to the locus coeruleus, which is part of the AAS, so answer A is correct. Neurons containing hypocretin/orexin (Answer B) act on neurons of the AAS, but are not considered to be part of the AAS, so answer B is incorrect. Similarly, answer C is incorrect, because neurons from the VLPO use GABAergic/galaninergic projection neurons to modulate cell activity in the AAS, but they are not thought to be part of the AAS. Answer D is incorrect because dopaminergic neurons that modulate arousal are localized to the ventral tegmental area and substantia nigra pars compacta, neither of which are considered to be part of the AAS.

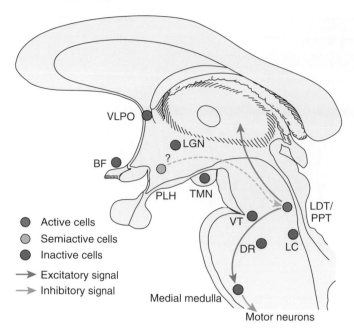

- **Figure 50.4** Schematic Showing Hypocretin and Cholinergic Regulation of Rapid Eye Movement (REM) Sleep. The generation and maintenance of REM sleep is controlled by an interaction of cholinergic laterodorsal tegmental and pedunculopontine areas (LDT/PPT, *red circle* and *arrows*) with aminergic brainstem neurons. Neurons from the postlateral hypothalamus (PLH, *gray circle*) are semiactive during REM sleep. The gray dotted line indicates that it is unclear whether this projection is excitatory or inhibitory. Structures with black circles are inactive during REM sleep. Reduced levels of hypocretin/orexin are commonly associated with a narcoleptic phenotype. *BF*, basal forebrain; *DR*, dorsal raphe nucleus; *LC*, locus coeruleus; *LGN*, lateral geniculate nucleus; *TMN*, tuberomammillary nucleus; *VLPO*, ventral lateral preoptic area; *VT*, ventral tegmental area. (Reprinted from Baumann CR, Bassetti CL. Hypocretins (orexins) and sleep-wake disorders. *Lancet Neurol.* 2005;4:673–682.)

12. **Answer D. The PRF.**
    The PRF, as a component of the AAS, contributes to the generation of REM sleep. Directly administering drugs that increase GABAergic transmission to the PRF causes an increase in wakefulness and a decrease in sleep (reviewed in Watson et al.[27]). Increasing GABAergic transmission within the laterodorsal pontine tegmentum (Answer A), dorsal raphé nucleus (Answer B), and locus coeruleus (Answer C) would inhibit the activity of these wake-promoting neurons and thus likely increase sleep.

13. **Answer C. Increases stage N2 NREM sleep.**
    Pain and opioid treatment for pain both cause sleep disruptions, and sleep disruptions exacerbate pain, which leads to an increased need for opioid treatment for pain.[37–39] Systemic administration of morphine causes an increase in stage N2 NREM sleep and a decrease in both stage N3 NREM sleep and REM sleep,[40,41] which means that answer C is correct and answers A (increasing stage N3 NREM sleep), B (increases REM sleep), and D (increases NREM and REM sleep) are incorrect. Chronic opioid can also lead to ataxic breathing (Fig. 50.10).[42] Opioids decrease levels of adenosine in the BF and PRF, two regions where adenosine is known to have sleep-promoting effects.[43] Direct administration of morphine to the PRF of rat or cat causes an increase in wakefulness and a decrease in REM sleep.[44,45]

14. **Answer C. Sleep drunkenness.**
    Sleep drunkenness is characterized as a period of disorientation and partial alertness during the transition from sleep to wakefulness.[46,47] It is occasionally considered in the clinical semiology of confusional arousal, although the latter is an arousal disorder that usually occurs during the early part of the night with rapid awakening from SWS. Patients who experience sleep drunkenness report that the symptoms in the case definition occur at almost every awakening and last for 15–60 minutes, occasionally longer. Approximately, a third of patients who suffer from hypersomnia also exhibit sleep drunkenness, most of whom are idiopathic, but a small percentage have been described with neurological involvement, including, notably, one report of encephalitis.[48] A familial history in some of the idiopathic cases suggests a genetic basis, and no difference in the severity of symptoms with age has been found. Nocturnal electroencephalographic records are essentially normal, and except for extended sleep, no abnormalities in sleep patterns are observed. The lack of REM sleep abnormalities (i.e., sleep paralysis and hallucinatory experiences) combined with the absence of nocturnal insomnia enables a differential diagnosis with narcolepsy (Answer B) to be made. Since the symptoms reported are associated with the transition from sleep to wakefulness, somnambulism (Answer A) is not the most likely diagnosis. The lack of REM sleep abnormalities would also rule out a diagnosis of pavor nocturnus (Answer D). For an early description of sleep drunkenness, refer to Roth.[49]

15. **Answer A. An abnormality in the VLPO.**
    Switching between wakefulness and sleep and then back to wakefulness has been modeled as a "flip-flop" neuronal circuit.[1] Fig. 50.1 illustrates the concept of a flip-flop circuit. Mutual inhibition of the VLPO and the AAS provides such a circuit between wake and sleep, with gradual accumulation/dissipation of sleepiness and circadian influences providing the factor or factors that abruptly tip the balance in this circuit from one state to the other. The evolutionary advantage of such a circuit is evident by avoiding a prolonged partially awake, yet drowsy state. The symptoms of sleep drunkenness can be likened to a description of what would happen if the VLPO-AAS circuitry were imbalanced toward the sleep side, thus suggesting a VLPO circuitry abnormality as a possible cause of the disorder. The other mechanisms listed can be eliminated from consideration, because they have already been characterized in the cause of other disorders (i.e., Parkinson disease with dopamine deficiency [Answer B], REM sleep behavior disorder with SLD pathology [Answer C], and narcolepsy with hypocretin/orexin deficiency [Answer D]).

16. **Answer C. Somnolence.**
    Histamine neurons originate in the TMN and project throughout the forebrain. The discharge profile for histaminergic neurons is "wake-on" (highest during wakefulness, less in NREM sleep, and silent during REM sleep). Histamine is a component of the AAS; therefore, reduced arousal and wakefulness would be expected in a mouse that does not express histamine. Scientists have generated this mouse model,[50] and the phenotype can be summarized as showing behavioral and electroencephalographic signs of somnolence, most particularly at times when a normal mouse is active (i.e., at the time of transition to the awake period at lights off and during exploration of a novel environment). Other parameters of NREM and REM sleep are not significantly changed in this mouse,

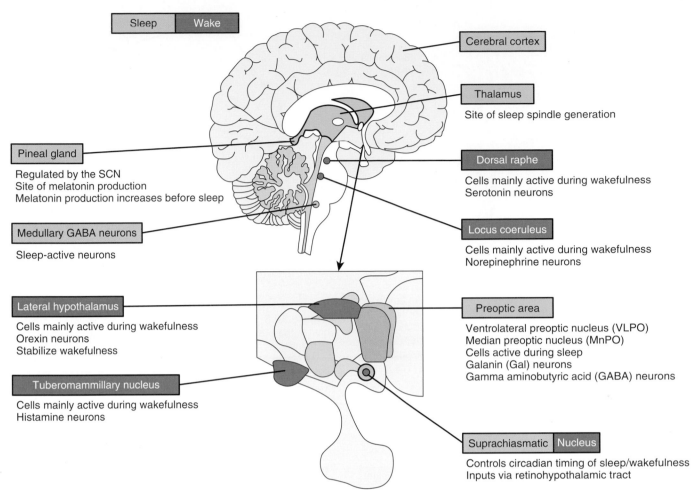

• **Figure 50.5** Schematic Representation of the Principal Components for Arousal State Control. The basic circuitry, including key "nodes," that underlies the regulation of sleep and wakefulness and the transitions between these states in mammals. Current models of wakefulness and sleep hold that wakefulness is maintained by the combined excitatory influence of forebrain-projecting noradrenergic (locus coeruleus), histaminergic (tuberomammillary nucleus), serotoninergic (dorsal raphe), and cholinergic (not shown) cell groups located at or near the mesopontine junction. Sleep, on the other hand, is initiated and maintained by neurons in the median preoptic (MnPO) and ventrolateral preoptic (VLPO) nuclei via inhibitory projections to the more rostrally situated wakefulness-promoting cell groups. Hypocretin (orexin) neurons located in the lateral hypothalamus reinforce activity in the brainstem arousal pathways and stabilize both sleep and wakefulness. Disruption of the hypocretin system leads to narcolepsy. The suprachiasmatic nuclei (SCN) determine the timing of the sleep-wake cycle and help to "consolidate" these behavioral states. The pineal gland, located in the epithalamus, produces melatonin, a hormone thought to function as a hypnotic signal. The cerebral cortex and medullary brainstem also contain subpopulations of γ-amino butyric acid (GABA)-ergic sleep-active neurons. (From Kryger M, Avidan AY, Berry R, eds. *Atlas of Clinical Sleep Medicine*. 2nd ed. Philadelphia: Saunders; 2013.)

although the direction of change is as expected, toward increased and consolidated sleep. Histaminergic receptor antagonists are commonly used as over-the-counter sleep aides. Based on these data, hyper arousals (Answer A), fragmented sleep (Answer B), and decreased REM sleep (Answer) would not be correct answers. Fig. 50.5 displays a schematic representation of the principal components of the AAS, including the histamine projection from the TMN.

17. **Answer D. Thalamocortical network oscillations require neurons of the thalamic reticular nucleus.**
Spindle oscillations are an example of oscillations generated by the thalamic reticular nucleus and transferred through the

thalamocortical network (Fig. 50.11).[24,51] The thalamocortical network, which includes neurons of the reticular nucleus, synchronizes δ waves that are generated by thalamic and cortical neurons. In each example, the network synchronizes the discharge of large populations of cortical neurons to produce the volume conduction that is observed as the electroencephalographic signal (for review, see Steriade et al.[52]). Therefore, although both answers B and D can be considered correct, answer D is the correct answer because it is more complete (accounts for both δ waves and spindles). Answer A is incorrect, because although the formation of K complexes is not well understood, it is thought to involve a rapid and coordinated

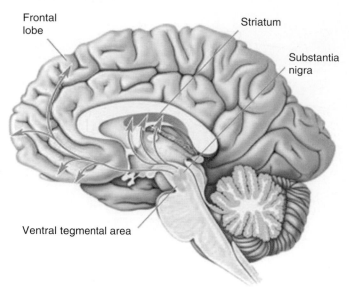

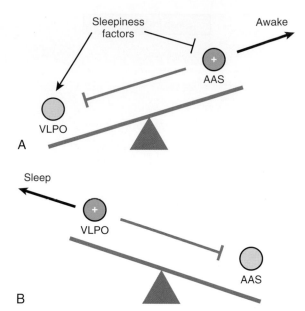

• **Figure 50.6** Projections of Dopaminergic Neurons. Wake promoting dopaminergic neurons originate in the substantia nigra and the ventral tegmental area. Although these neurons do not change discharge rate across states, they are wakefulness promoting. (Reprinted from Weng J, Paslaski S, Daly J, VanDam C, Brown J. Modulation for emergent networks: serotonin and dopamine. *Neural Netw.* 2013;41:225–239.)

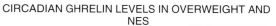

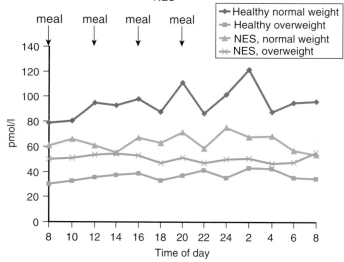

• **Figure 50.7** Graph of Circadian Ghrelin Levels. Ghrelin levels were quantified (pmol/L) in healthy individuals and individuals with night eating syndrome *(NES)*. For each group, they compared ghrelin levels between normal weight and overweight. For each group, there was a significant lowering of ghrelin associated in the samples for the overweight groups. (Reprinted from Birketvedt GS, Geliebter A, Kristiansen I, Firgenschau Y, Goll R, Florholmen JR. Diurnal secretion of ghrelin, growth hormone, insulin binding proteins, and prolactin in normal weight and overweight subjects with and without the night eating syndrome. *Appetite.* 2012;59:688–692.)

• **Figure 50.8** Diagrammatic illustration of a "flip-flop" circuit that controls the onset of non–rapid eye movement (NREM) sleep. During wakefulness (A), components of the ascending activating system (AAS) are active and inhibiting the sleep-promoting cells of the ventrolateral preoptic area (VLPO). Homeostatic and circadian sleepiness factors that influence both the VLPO and AAS are gradually changing during this period such that the AAS is being subjected to a gradually increasing inhibitory influence. Concurrently, the VLPO is being subjected to a gradually increasing level of excitation. When AAS activity drops below a critical level, the inhibition from the AAS onto the VLPO is removed. The VLPO then rapidly completes the inhibition of AAS (B) components, and the switch flips to the opposite pole to produce sleep. This circuit arrangement therefore allows a rapid state transition without an intermediate drowsy phase. A similar process then occurs in reverse to flip the switch back to wakefulness. This takes place when the homeostatic and circadian drives are sufficient to re-inhibit VLPO activity so that it now falls below the critical level necessary to maintain sleep. (Reprinted from Sinton CM. Mechanisms of sleep neuroscience. In: Avidan AY, Barkoukis TJ, eds. *Review of Sleep Medicine.* 3rd ed. Philadelphia: Elsevier Saunders; 2012:368–386.)

decline in cortical network activity at a frequency related to the slow oscillation in the cortex. Answer C is incorrect, because neurons within the reticular nucleus of the thalamus project within the thalamus and not to portions of the AAS.

18. **Answer B. Hypocretin/orexin.**
Hypocretinergic/orexinergic neurons are localized to the lateral hypothalamus and project to all major arousal-regulating brain regions.[53,54] These neurons have the highest discharge rate during active wakefulness, and little, if any, discharge activity during states of sleep.[55,56] As reviewed in Watson et al.,[27] dogs with a narcoleptic phenotype also have a mutation in the hypocretin 2 receptor gene. Levels of hypocretin mRNA and the hypocretin peptide are significantly reduced in patients with narcolepsy, and patients with narcolepsy-cataplexy have significantly lower levels of CSF hypocretin compared with healthy controls. As shown in Fig. 50.1, patients with narcolepsy due to a disruption of hypocretinergic signaling may experience other sleep-related symptoms including sleep fragmentation or short-onset sleep bouts. Fig. 50.4 also shows how a deficiency in the hypocretin/orexin system would play a role in REM sleep via a project from the lateral hypothalamus to the laterodorsal and

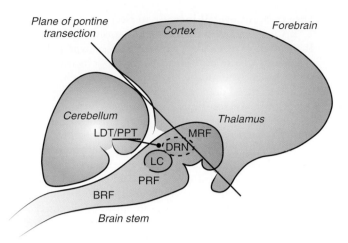

• **Figure 50.9** Diagram Depicting the Plane of Transection Used to Create the *Cerveau Isolé* Preparation of a Mammalian Brain (Cat) Showing the Location of Nuclei Especially Important for Rapid Eye Movement Sleep. The locus coeruleus *(LC)* contains norepinephrine. *DRN*, dorsal raphé nucleus; *BRF*, *PRF*, and *MRF*, bulbar, pontine, and mesencephalic reticular formation; *LDT/PPT*, laterodorsal tegmental and pedunculopontine areas. (Reprinted from McCarley RW. Neurobiology of rapid eye movement and non-rapid eye movement sleep. In: Chokroverty S, ed. *Sleep Disorders Medicine: Basic Science, Technical Considerations, and Clinical Aspect.* 3rd ed. Cambridge: Elsevier; 2009:29–58.)

pedunculopontine tegmental areas A deficiency in the dopamine system (Answer A) would result in chronic depression and fatigue, so this answer is not correct. Answer C is incorrect, because deficiency in the galaninergic system would likely cause a deficit in neuropathic or pain behaviors.[57] Acetylcholine (Answer D) would be incorrect, because a deficiency in this neurotransmitter system would likely have symptoms that include muscle weakness, fatigue, and cognitive impairments.

19. **Answer D. From the intergeniculate leaflet through a neuropeptide Y projection.**

The primary photic input to the SCN is from retinal ganglion cells through the retinohypothalamic tract, which is a glutamatergic pathway. A secondary multisynaptic and indirect pathway by which photic information reaches the SCN is through the lateral geniculate nucleus and thence via the geniculohypothalamic tract. This tract contains neuropeptide Y as its neurotransmitter. These pathways that transfer photic information to the SCN are schematically represented in Fig. 50.12. Answer A is incorrect, because the retinal ganglion cells signals the SCN via the retinohypothalamic tract and is a glutamatergic pathway. Answer B is incorrect, because neither primary nor secondary tract from the retinal ganglion to the SCN contains medium forebrain bundle neurons. Answer C, is incorrect because the lateral geniculate nucleus signals the SCN via the geniculohypothalamic tract.

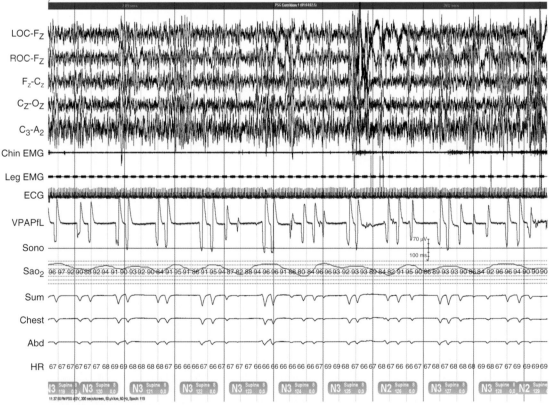

• **Figure 50.10** Chronic Opioid Use and Ataxic Breathing. A typical polysomnogram showing ataxic breathing in a patient with chronic opioid use. Each epic *(vertical lines)* is 30 sec long and the polysomnogram shows 10 epics of non-rapid eye movement sleep (shown at the bottom of the polysomnogram). (Reprinted from Junna MR, Selim BJ, Morgenthaler TI. Medical sedation and sleep apnea. *Sleep Med Clin.* 2013;8:43–58.)

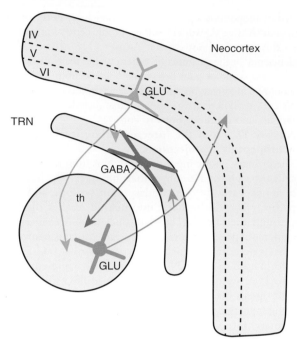

• **Figure 50.11** The Sleep Spindle Circuitry of the Thalamic Reticular Nucleus (*TRN*). This nucleus between the neocortex (top) and the parts of the thalamus (lower left). Both the thalamus and the neocortex use glutamate to signal the two other brain regions (*blue* and *green arrows*). The TRN signals the remainder of the thalamus via a GABAergic projection neuron. (Reprinted by permission of Elsevier from Reduced Sleep Spindles in Schizophrenia: A Treatable Endophenotype that Links Risk Genes to Impaired Cognition? By Manoach DS, Pan JQ, Purcell SM, Stickgold R, *Biol Psychiatry* 80[8], 599–608, 2016 by the Society of Biological Psychiatry.)

20. **Answer B. An overall increase in sleep.**

GABA is the main inhibitory neurotransmitter in the brain. The activation of $GABA_A$ receptors causes hyperpolarization of neurons due to an influx of chloride ions into the cells. When given systemically, various $GABA_A$ receptor agonists result in increased sleep, sedation, or general anesthesia. Multiple classes of pharmaceuticals that target the $GABA_A$ receptors are used as sleep aids and general anesthetics. One example of this is a report demonstrating that the positive allosteric modulator EVT 201 decreases sleep latency and the wake after sleep onset in a dose-dependent manner (Fig. 50.13).[58] It also increases total sleep time in a dose-dependent manner and determined that this compound is safe for adults with primary insomnia. For this reason, answer B is correct, and answers C and D are incorrect. While systemic administration of $GABA_A$ receptor agonists causes an overall increase in sleep, actions of the $GABA_A$ agonists at the level the PRF would try to cause an increase in wakefulness, meaning answer C is incorrect (i.e., systemic administration of $GABA_A$ receptor agonist would disrupt REM sleep).[27]

21. **Answer D. REM sleep.**

Typically, a single high-amplitude PGO wave occurs just prior to the onset of REM sleep and then bursts of lower amplitude PGO waves occur during episodes of REM sleep.[24] Since PGO waves are specifically associated with REM sleep, answers A (wakefulness), B (stage N1 NREM sleep), and C (stage N2 NREM sleep) are incorrect. Multiple lines of evidence support the idea that the formation of PGO waves requires cholinergic input into the thalamus from brain stem nuclei (reviewed in Brown et al.[28]). Stimulation of the central nucleus of the amygdala, which signals the brain stem nuclei, during REM

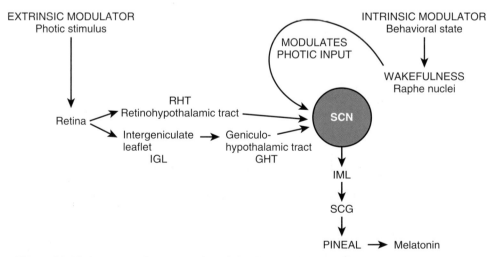

• **Figure 50.12** Schematic Representation of the Principal Input to the Suprachiasmatic Nucleus (SCN). Inputs into the SCN include extrinsic modulation (i.e., photic information from the retina, which reaches the SCN through the retinohypothalamic tract [RHT] and the geniculohypothalamic tract [GHT]) and intrinsic modulation (i.e., serotoninergic innervation, which ascends from the raphé nuclei to modulate the photic input at the level of the SCN). A significant output from the SCN descends via the intermediolateral (IML) nucleus of the spinal cord and the superior cervical ganglia (SCG) to innervate the pineal gland, where it modulates the secretion of melatonin. *IGL*, intergeniculate leaflet. (Reprinted from Sinton CM. Mechanisms of sleep neuroscience. In: Avidan AY, Barkoukis TJ, eds. *Review of Sleep Medicine*. 3rd ed. Philadelphia: Elsevier Saunders; 2012:368–386.)

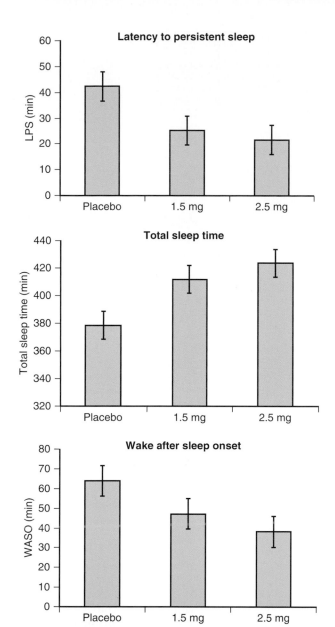

Latency to persistent sleep

Total sleep time

Wake after sleep onset

• **Figure 50.13** Dose-Dependent Effects of a Positive Allosteric Modulator for GABA_A Receptors. EVT 201 has been shown to be a safe and effective treatment for the adult patients with primary insomnia. Error bars on the figure give the 95% confidence interval of the results. In addition to significantly increasing total sleep time, this compound also significantly decreased latency to sleep onset and wake after sleep onset. (Reprinted from Walsh JK, Thacker S, Knowles LJ, Tasker T, Hunneyball IM. The partial positive allosteric GABA(A) receptor modulator EVT 201 is efficacious and safe in the treatment of adult primary insomnia patients. *Sleep Med.* 2009;10:859–864.)

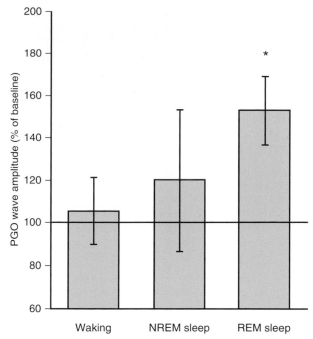

• **Figure 50.14** Rapid Eye Movement (REM) Sleep and Ponto-Geniculo-Occipital (PGO) Waves. Electrical Stimulation of the central nucleus of the amygdala during REM sleep caused a significant increase (~50% over baseline) in PGO waves. The data are graphed and percent over control, and the error bars represent standard error. *p < 0.05, n = 5″. (Reprinted from Deboer T, Sanford LD, Ross RJ, Morrison AR. Effects of electrical stimulation in the amygdala on ponto-geniculo-occipital waves in rats. *Brain Res.* 1998;793:305–310.)

sleep significantly increased PGO waves compared with electrical stimulation during NREM sleep or wakefulness (Fig. 50.14).[59] Experiments in rats have revealed that the pontine component of PGO waves is generated via noncholinergic neurons in the subcoeruleus and parabrachial nucleus.[60–62]

22. **Answer C. The VLPO.**
Sampling techniques for the quantification of neurotransmitters include microdialysis, push-pull perfusion, multielectrode arrays, and carbon fiber microelectrodes (reviewed in Watson

et al.[3]). Due to the size of some brain regions, such as the VLPO (Fig. 50.15), quantifying levels of neurotransmitters is a technological challenge. Because the sampling regions of both microdialysis probes and microelectrode arrays are significantly larger than the VLPO, they do not have the required special resolution to adequately reflect levels of neurotransmitters within the VLPO. Microelectrode arrays also have the drawback of quantifying one neurotransmitter at a time. While the spatial resolution of push-pull perfusion probes may allow for sampling from very small brain regions, the time resolution of this technique can be prohibitive. The main drawback to carbon fiber microelectrodes, which have adequate spatial and temporal resolution for small brain regions, is that they can only monitor natively electroactive species. Future studies should focus on decreasing the sampling area of microdialysis probes to better understand the mechanisms within the VLPO that underlie its regulation of arousal state. The BF (A), the thalamus (B), and the PRF (D) are incorrect, because area of each region is large enough for each sampling technique to have the spatial resolution necessary to quantify neurotransmitters discretely from each.

23. **Answer A. Increases the amount of SWS.**
Patients taking pregabalin for the treatment of chronic pain, general anxiety, or restless legs syndrome report improved sleep quality, and polysomnographic data reveal a significant increase in time to wake after sleep onset, a significant increase in the amount of NREM sleep, and a significant decrease amount of time spent in stage N1 NREM sleep (Fig. 50.16).[63]

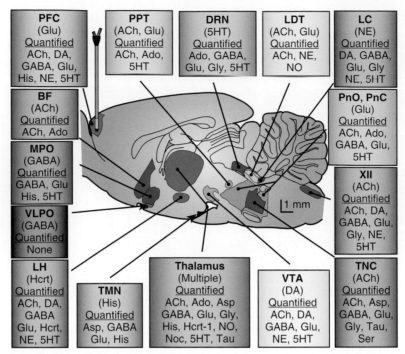

• **Figure 50.15** Brain Regions That Modulate States of Arousal. A sagittal drawing of the rat brain schematizes the location, shape, and size of brain regions known to regulate sleep and wakefulness. The name of each brain region is in bold print, the primary signaling neurotransmitters are in parentheses, and neurotransmitters measured in a brain region are listed under the header "Quantified." The microdialysis probe depicted in the prefrontal cortex is drawn to scale. *ACh*, Acetylcholine; *Ado*, adenosine; *Asp*, aspartate; *BF*, basal forebrain; *DA*, dopamine; *DRN*, dorsal raphé nucleus; *GABA*, γ-aminobutyric acid; *Glu*, glutamate; *Gly*, glycine; *Hcrt*, hypocretin; *His*, histamine; *LC*, locus coeruleus; *LDT*, laterodorsal tegmental nucleus; *LH*, lateral hypothalamus; *MPO*, medial preoptic area; *NE*, norepinephrine; *NO*, nitric oxide; *Noc*, nociceptin; *PFC*, prefrontal cortex; *PnC*, pontine reticular formation, caudal part; *PnO*, pontine reticular formation, oral part; *PPT*, pedunculopontine tegmental nucleus; *Ser*, serine; *Tau*, taurine; *TMN*, tuberomammillary nucleus; *TNC*, trigeminal nucleus complex; *VLPO*, ventrolateral preoptic area; *VTA*, ventral tegmental area; *XII*, hypoglossal nucleus; *5HT*, serotonin. (Reprinted from Watson CJ, Baghdoyan HA, Lydic R. Neuropharmacology of sleep and wakefulness: 2012 update. *Sleep Med Clin.* 2012;7:469–486.)

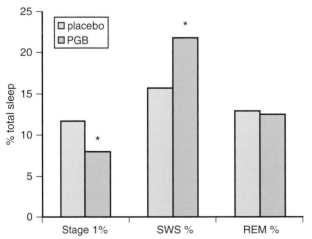

• **Figure 50.16** The Effect of Pregabalin Treatment on Slow Wave Sleep (SWS). When administered to patients with insomnia, pregabalin significantly decreased stage 1 non-rapid eye movement sleep and significantly increased SWS. Data reported as percent of total sleep time. *p < 0.05 compared to placebo. (Reprinted from Bazil CW, Dave J, Cole J, Stalvey J, Drake E. Pregabalin increases slow-wave sleep and may improve attention in patients with partial epilepsy and insomnia. *Epilepsy Behav.* 2012;23:422–425.)

Pregabalin treatment relating to partial onset seizures showed no significant alterations in sleep measures in this population. Analyses of the sleep data reveal that treatment with pregabalin has a direct effect on measures of sleep that is distinct from the drug's analgesic and anxiolytic properties. There were no significant effects on REM sleep reported. These data are reviewed in Roth et al.[64] Based on these clinical studies, answers B-D are incorrect because: pregabalin would not increase wakefulness (B), or the number of REM episodes (C), and it has been shown to significantly alter sleep (D).

24. **Answer A. It occurs in pulses.**

In humans, the pineal gland secretes melatonin primarily during the night. Melatonin is secreted in a pulsatile manner and at a constant rate across sleep stages.[65] As Fig. 50.17 shows, the correlation between the nocturnal increase in melatonin and the timing of the sleep phase indicates that melatonin may be important for sleep regulation. The onset of melatonin secretion occurs approximately 2 hours prior to bedtime and corresponds with the onset of evening sleepiness, indicating that answer B (onset in early morning) is incorrect. In other words, the transition from wakefulness and arousal to increased sleep propensity coincides with the nocturnal rise in endogenous melatonin. Endogenous levels of melatonin can vary widely

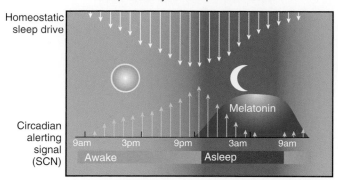

Sleep-wake cycle: two-process model

Homeostatic sleep drive

Melatonin

Circadian alerting signal (SCN)

9am 3pm 9pm 3am 9am

Awake Asleep

• **Figure 50.17** The Two-Process Model of the Sleep-Wake Cycle. As nighttime falls, homeostatic sleep drive increases and circadian alerting signal from the suprachiasmatic nucleus (SCN) decrease. An increase in melatonin is associated with process, indicating that importance of melatonin as a sleep-promoting hormone. (From Edgar DM, Dement WC, Fuller CA. Effect of SCN lesions on sleep in squirrel monkeys: evidence for opponent processes in sleep-wake regulation. *J Neurosci.* 1993;13:1065–1079.)

from individual to individual, but in any individual the secretion of melatonin remains constant over time,[66] demonstrating that answer C (varies from day to day) is incorrect. Answer D (greater in NREM sleep than REM sleep) is incorrect because melatonin release is constant across sleep stages.

25. **Answer B. Hypothalamus.**

The most likely diagnosis for this individual is posttraumatic narcolepsy without cataplexy. Posttraumatic hypersomnia remains a possible diagnosis, though unlikely, because it is typically most severe immediately after trauma and then gradually remits. Narcolepsy can be induced in a susceptible individual by head injury, and nocturnal insomnia and fragmented sleep are symptoms of the disorder. On the basis of this diagnosis, the brain area that is most likely to be affected is the hypothalamus, specifically the region around the lateral hypothalamus where the hypocretin/orexin cell bodies are uniquely located.[53] Also, because narcolepsy shows a high association with deficiencies in hypocretinergic/orexinergic neurons of the lateral hypothalamus, answers A (thalamus), B (basal ganglia), and D (locus coeruleus) would be incorrect.

26. **Answer C. MSLT.**

Because posttraumatic narcolepsy without cataplexy is probable, an MSLT would provide the best initial supportive evidence of a reduction in sleep latency and, importantly, the presence of sleep-onset REM (SOREM) periods. The SOREM period reflects fragmentation of the vigilance state, and an inability to maintain a prolonged period of either wakefulness or sleep is a characteristic of narcolepsy. However, SOREM periods may also result from reduced hypocretin/orexin function since there is evidence that this neuropeptide increases REM sleep latency, an effect that is independent of cataplexy.[67,68] Since there is no evidence of cataplexy, CSF analysis would be unlikely to reveal any evidence of significantly reduced hypocretin/orexin levels (i.e., <110 pg/mL).[69] A hypocretin/orexin level greater than 110 pg/mL would not be definitive, making answer A an incorrect choice. There is no evidence of sarcoidosis, and thus no reason to consider CSF angiotensin-converting enzyme measures (Answer B). Note that the MSLT would not be definitive, and in fact an early diagnosis of narcolepsy is difficult

to make. The diagnosis would therefore remain tentative for some time, but it is often missed in the early stages because it seems an unlikely possibility in the absence of cataplexy. Although the Beck Depression Inventory II test (Answer D) might provide additional information for the treatment of this patient, it would not be the appropriate initial test to run.

27. **Answer A. Cortex.**

In 1993, Steriade and colleagues[70–72] published a series of three papers that described a novel sleep-related slow oscillation in the EEG. The process that generates the slow (<1 Hz) oscillation on the EEG is separable from the process that generates waves in the δ (1–4 Hz) frequency band, although all frequencies lower than 4 Hz are observed during stage 3 NREM sleep. Isolation of the cortex in animal preparations revealed that the slow (<1 Hz) oscillations are generated in the cortex without any input from the thalamus, so answer B is not a correct answer. The authors proposed that the slow (<1 Hz) oscillations, δ-waves, and sleep spindles work in concert for certain neuronal populations where plasticity is vital. The hippocampus (Answer C) is associated with θ rhythms (4.5–8.0 Hz), and the PRF (Answer D) is associated with REM sleep and not with NREM sleep, during which these slow oscillations occur.

28. **Answer D. Activity of GABAergic neurons in the ventrolateral periaqueductal gray matter during REM sleep.**

The cell bodies of the AAS projections (e.g., pontine monoaminergic neurons) are inhibited during NREM sleep and REM sleep by GABA/galanin projections from the VLPO area, a center that coordinates inhibition of the AAS at sleep onset, so answer A is incorrect. Answer C is also incorrect because hypocretin/orexin neurons in the lateral hypothalamus are inhibited only partially during sleep and are inhibited by VLPO projection neurons. An additional inhibitory influence is provided by the neighboring MCH-containing neurons, in which GABA is co-localized.[73] Neither the MCH neurons nor the VLPO projections are interneurons. One significant pontine GABAergic influence during REM sleep affects the SLD nucleus (i.e., the peri-LC-α), which is under constant GABAergic inhibition that is lifted only during REM sleep, so answer B is correct (Fig. 50.18). Hence, local administration of GABA antagonists in this region induces REM sleep. Another REM sleep GABAergic mechanism implicates the ventrolateral periaqueductal gray area in which two mutually inhibiting populations of GABAergic cells are described. One of these is specifically active during REM sleep, but the other is not, making answer D incorrect. For a recent review of GABAergic mechanisms during REM sleep, refer to Fort and colleagues.[74]

29. **Answer A. TNF-α.**

TNF-α has been identified as a sleep factor and is a potent somnogen. Brain levels of this cytokine also vary with sleep propensity, being highest when sleep propensity is at a maximum, and levels of TNF-α also increase with sleep deprivation. Other proinflammatory cytokines such as IL-1 are also sleep factors and accumulate with increased wakefulness, thus suggesting that wakefulness may be a proinflammatory state. Infectious disease could therefore potentially be considered equivalent to prolonged wakefulness in terms of the effect on cytokine levels. In contrast, anti-inflammatory cytokines, including IL-10 (Answer B) and TGF-β (Answer D), are wakefulness promoting, a category that also includes the stress-related hormone corticotropin-releasing hormone (Answer C).[75]

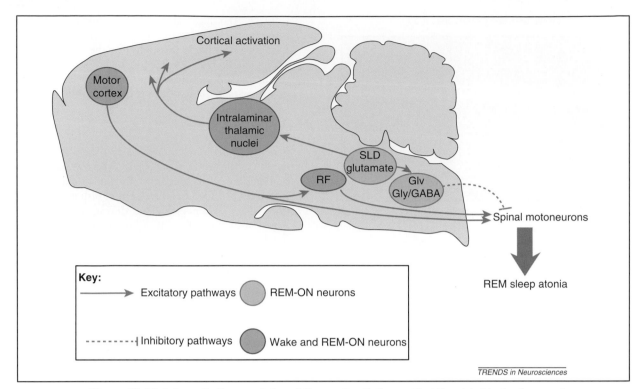

• **Figure 50.18** Schematic Representation of Descending Pathways That Regulate Mechanisms and Signs of Rapid Eye Movement (REM) Sleep. A critical area for the generation of signs of REM sleep is the sublaterodorsal (SLD) nucleus (also know as the peri-locus cocruleus-α (peri-LC-α). GABAergic inhibitory neurons from the ventrolateral periaqueductal gray (vlPAG, not shown) continuously inhibit the REM-on neurons of the SLD nucleus, except during REM sleep, when they begin to discharge. SLD neurons are glutamatergic and send excitatory projections to neurons of the ventral gigantocellular reticular nucleus portion of the pontine reticular formation (PRF). These neurons are, in turn, glycinergic/GABAergic neurons that project to spinal motor neurons (SM) to induce muscle atonia. (Reprinted from Srinivasan V, Pandi-Perumal SR, Trakht I, et al. Pathophysiology of depression: role of sleep and the melatonergic system. *Psychiatry Res.* 2009;165:201–214.)

30. **Answer C. peri-LC-α.**
    Initial studies demonstrated that local injections of physostigmine or neostigmine to cat[76] or mouse[77] PRF could trigger, with a short latency to onset, a state indistinguishable from natural REM sleep. Subsequently, systematic investigations using small quantities of acetylcholinesterase inhibitors or muscarinic receptor agonists these cholinergic agents described two areas within the PRF in which injections produce REM sleep with minimal latency to onset. One of these short-latency induction areas was in the dorsal pons in the region ventral to the locus coeruleus. This region was named the peri-LC-α in the cat and is equivalent to the SLD nucleus in the rat. Injection of cholinergic agents into the region of the cholinergic cell bodies in the LDT/PPT area also induce REM sleep, but at a longer latency, since this region is the source of cholinergic innervation to the cholinergic sensitive REM sleep induction areas in the PRF.[76] Because of the longer latency to REM sleep, the LDT (Answer D) is not correct. Answer A is incorrect, because the activation of the lateral hypothalamus would increase wakefulness. Due to the primary role of activating the NREM sleep portion of the wakefulness/NREM sleep switch (see Fig. 50.2), the VLPO would be an incorrect answer. For a review of cholinergic mechanisms regulating REM sleep, see reference.[16]

31. **Answer D. Hypocretin/orexin.**
    Selective orexin receptor antagonists (SORAs) and dual orexin receptor antagonists (DORAs) have been developed to inhibit hypocretin/orexin signaling thereby increasing sleep. The DORA compound MK-4305 (Suvorexant) received FDA approval in 2014 and reduces active wakefulness while increasing NREM and REM sleep. Minimal side effects have been observed in human studies. The phase III trials of the DORA ACT-78573 (Almorexant) were discontinued in 2013 due to tolerability issues and the side-effect profile. For a review of hypocretin/orexin receptors antagonists as a treatment for insomnia,[78] many antidepressants, such as selective serotonin reuptake inhibitors (SSRIs), serotonin-norepinephrine reuptake inhibitors (SNRIs), and tricyclic antidepressants (TCAs) all work on the serotonin and norepinephrine systems (Answers A and B), both of which inhibit REM sleep promoting cells and can cause an increase in latency to REM sleep onset and an overall decrease in REM sleep (refer to Fig. 50.5).[79] Stimulants, such as amphetamine, methamphetamine, and methylphenidate, work on the dopaminergic system (Answer D) and are wake promoting.

32. **Answer A. The ventral gigantocellular reticular nucleus.**
    Descending GABAergic and glycinergic neurons from the ventral gigantocellular reticular nucleus (a discrete part of the

a. Healthy Control

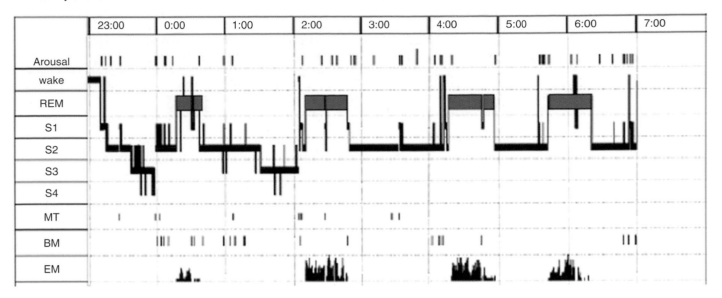

b. Depressed Patient

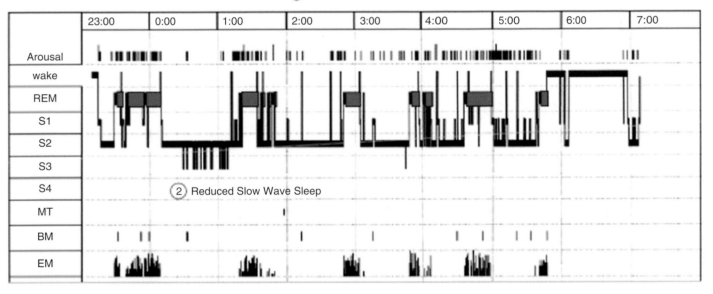

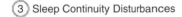

• **Figure 50.19** Polysomnographic Comparison of a Patient with Depression and a Healthy Control. Compared with the healthy control **(A)**, the patient with depression **(B)** has *(1)* shortened REM sleep latency, *(2)* Reduced slow wave sleep, and *(3)* sleep continuity disturbances. (Reprinted from Peever J, Luppi PH, Montplaisir J. Breakdown in REM sleep circuitry underlies REM sleep behavior disorder. *Trends Neurosci.* 2014;37:279–288.)

PRF) inhibit spinal motor neurons during REM sleep atonia (see Fig. 50.18), making answer A the most accurate answer.[74] Overall, the PRF, and specifically the SLD or the peri-LC-α, also plays a vital role in both the electroencephalographic activation and muscle atonia associated with REM sleep.[80] Because of the multiple roles the PRF plays in the formation of REM sleep traits, answer C is less accurate than answer B. The lateral geniculate nucleus (Answer B) functions in the

generation of PGO waves, not muscle atonia. Cells in the VLPO (Answer D) begin to discharge just prior to the onset of sleep and have no direct role in the generation of any sign of REM sleep.

33. **Answer C. Decreased latency to REM sleep onset.**
Sleep disturbances associated with depression can be divided into three categories (reviewed in Ref.[79]): (1) disturbances related to the continuity of sleep (Fig. 50.19). These disturbances

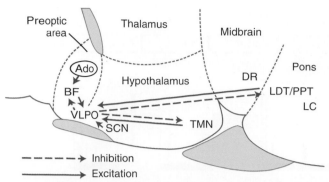

• **Figure 50.20** Schematic of a Sagittal Section of the Basal Forebrain (BF) and Hypothalamic Areas Showing Important Centers in This Region Involved in the Regulation of Sleep and Wakefulness. A pathway from the suprachiasmatic nucleus (SCN) innervates the sleep-active neurons of the ventrolateral preoptic area (VLPO) to modulate the discharge rate of VLPO neurons according to the circadian phase. The inhibitory influence of adenosine (Ado) within the BF couples homeostatic sleepiness with the activity of VLPO neurons. Thus, reciprocal projections between the BF and VLPO integrate circadian and homeostatic sleep to drive VLPO sleep-active neurons. GABAergic VLPO neurons and closely associated GABAergic neurons in the BF project to the tuberomammillary nucleus (TMN) and the brainstem nuclei involved in electroencephalographic activation and the rapid eye movement (REM) sleep cycle. These brainstem nuclei include the dorsal raphé nucleus (DR), laterodorsal/pedunculopontine tegmentum (LDT/PPT), and locus coeruleus (LC). Neurons in the DR and LDT/PPT send inhibitory projections back to the VLPO. The inhibitory GABAergic VLPO/BF projections are important for the coordinated decrease in discharge activity of ascending activating system neurons as NREM sleep begins and deepens. (Reprinted from Sinton CM. Mechanisms of sleep neuroscience. In: Avidan AY, Barkoukis TJ, eds. *Review of Sleep Medicine*. 3rd ed. Philadelphia: Elsevier Saunders; 2012:368–386.)

include increased NREM sleep latency, wake after sleep onset, and number of awakenings during the night. Sleep disturbances that fall into this category also include early morning awakenings, reduced total sleep time, and sleep efficiency; (2) disturbances of SWS that include decreased amount of SWS and an abnormal distribution of δ-activity; and (3) disturbances of REM sleep that manifest as shortened latency to REM sleep onset, and increased duration and density of REM sleep. Since disturbances falling into categories 1 and 2 can be associated with other disorders, disturbances of REM sleep may be the best sleep biomarker for major depressive disorder. Answer A is incorrect, because major depressive disorder is associated with an *increased* latency to NREM sleep onset (category 1). This disorder is also associated with a *decreased* total sleep time (category 1) and not increase (Answer B). Patients with major sleep disorder also show a decrease in SWS duration (category 2), as opposed to an increase (Answer D).

34. **Answer D. VLPO neurons that project to noradrenergic cells in the locus coeruleus.**
Neurons localized to the VLPO contain the inhibitory neurotransmitters GABA and galanin, but not the excitatory neurotransmitter glutamate. The inhibitory neurons of the VLPO project to all areas of the AAS (Fig. 50.20) and inhibit arousal at the onset of NREM sleep.[81] For the following reasons, answers A–C are incorrect. Certain projections from the lateral hypothalamus (Answer A), including the projection to the

histaminergic cells of the TMN, contain both hypocretin/orexin and glutamate.[82] These two neurotransmitters are packaged into separate vesicles, indicating that each can be released independently. Many cortical pyramidal cells that project to the thalamus (Answer B) utilize glutamate as their transmitter, and the Mesencephalic reticular formation neurons of the AAS contain a glutamatergic projection to the thalamus (Answer C).

35. **Answer B. Adenosine.**
Increased electroencephalographic power in the δ range (1–4 Hz) during sleep is an indicator of the depth of sleep and thus of the sleepiness that follows prolonged wakefulness. There is now considerable evidence supporting the idea that adenosine mediates this sleepiness via its inhibitory action on the BF wakefulness-promoting neurons. McCarley and colleagues hypothesize that, during prolonged wakefulness, adenosine accumulates selectively in the BF and promotes the transition from wakefulness to sleep by inhibiting, via the adenosine A_1 receptor, cholinergic and non-cholinergic wakefulness-promoting BF neurons.[83] Studies have shown a direct correlation between accumulation of adenosine in the BF and electroencephalographic δ power. Although melatonin (Answer A) release coincides with the onset of sleepiness, the hormone is degraded rapidly and does not accumulate, and levels have therefore not been correlated with electroencephalographic δ power. Serotonin and histamine (Answers C and D, respectively) do not accumulate during prolonged wakefulness, and serotonergic and histaminergic neurons of the dorsal raphe nucleus and tuberomammillary are mainly active during wakefulness.

36. **Answer A. The possibility of dreaming and/or amnesia.**
Dreaming and/or amnesia are both possible during states of sleep and anesthesia (Fig. 50.21). Answer B is incorrect, because while natural sleep is dependent on the duration of prior wakefulness or circadian rhythms, states of anesthesia are dependent on drug dose and are independent of duration of prior wakefulness or circadian rhythms. Answer C is incorrect, because the ability to maintain the depth or stage constant for long periods is unique to the anesthetic state. The natural sleep state oscillates between NREM sleep, REM sleep, and can include brief periods of wakefulness. Answer D is incorrect, because maintenance of the state being able to be altered by environmental factors is unique to the natural sleep state.[3]

37. **Answer B. The dorsomedial thalamus.**
Fatal familial insomnia is a rare disorder that is significant, because it affects our understanding of the involvement of the thalamus in sleep mechanisms. A genetically linked, prion protein disorder,[84] postmortem analysis of the thalamus has demonstrated that fatal familial insomnia is characterized by progressive and selective neurodegenerative atrophy of the anterior and dorsomedial thalamic nuclei. Thus, based on this analysis, answer B is correct, and answers A, C, and D are not correct. The onset of the disorder, frequently at about the age of 50 years, is signaled by sleep initiation insomnia, and this typically evolves within a few months to total insomnia that is refractory to treatment. Polysomnographic monitoring of these patients reveals a progressive decline in the duration of NREM and REM sleep that culminates in total insomnia, which progresses to stupor and then coma and death.

38. **Answer C. The brainstem region ventral to the locus coeruleus.**
Bilateral lesions in animals in an area ventral to the locus coeruleus and medial to the locus subcoeruleus in the dorsal

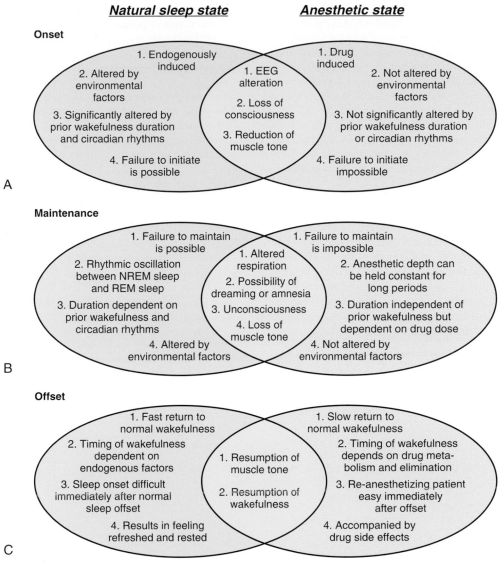

Natural sleep state   **Anesthetic state**

Onset

Natural sleep (Onset):
1. Endogenously induced
2. Altered by environmental factors
3. Significantly altered by prior wakefulness duration and circadian rhythms
4. Failure to initiate is possible

Intersection (Onset):
1. EEG alteration
2. Loss of consciousness
3. Reduction of muscle tone

Anesthetic (Onset):
1. Drug induced
2. Not altered by environmental factors
3. Not significantly altered by prior wakefulness duration or circadian rhythms
4. Failure to initiate impossible

A

Maintenance

Natural sleep (Maintenance):
1. Failure to maintain is possible
2. Rhythmic oscillation between NREM sleep and REM sleep
3. Duration dependent on prior wakefulness and circadian rhythms
4. Altered by environmental factors

Intersection (Maintenance):
1. Altered respiration
2. Possibility of dreaming or amnesia
3. Unconsciousness
4. Loss of muscle tone

Anesthetic (Maintenance):
1. Failure to maintain is impossible
2. Anesthetic depth can be held constant for long periods
3. Duration independent of prior wakefulness but dependent on drug dose
4. Not altered by environmental factors

B

Offset

Natural sleep (Offset):
1. Fast return to normal wakefulness
2. Timing of wakefulness dependent on endogenous factors
3. Sleep onset difficult immediately after normal sleep offset
4. Results in feeling refreshed and rested

Intersection (Offset):
1. Resumption of muscle tone
2. Resumption of wakefulness

Anesthetic (Offset):
1. Slow return to normal wakefulness
2. Timing of wakefulness depends on drug metabolism and elimination
3. Re-anesthetizing patient easy immediately after offset
4. Accompanied by drug side effects

C

• **Figure 50.21** Venn Diagrams Illustrating the Similarities and Differences Between Natural Sleep and an Anesthetic State. The intersections between the natural sleep and anesthetic state ellipses contain the similarities found between sleep and anesthesia during the onset **(A)**, maintenance **(B)**, and offset **(C)** of each state. Traits lying outside of the intersection and highlighted in the blue ellipses are unique to natural sleep state, and traits outside of the intersections and highlighted in yellow ellipses are unique to the anesthetic state. (Modified from Watson CJ, Baghdoyan HA, Lydic R. A neurochemical perspective of states of consciousness. In: Hudetz A, Pearce R, eds. *Suppressing the Mind: Anesthetic Modulation of Memory and Consciousness*. New York: Humana Press; 2010:33–80.)

PRF produce a preparation that shows all of the characteristic signs of REM sleep except muscle atonia.[85] In the cat, this area is denoted the peri-LC-α region, which is equivalent to the SLD in the rat nucleus. Because this transection study identified the peri-LC-α, answers A, B, and D are incorrect. These animal preparations thus exhibit REM sleep without muscle atonia, which is the symptom of REM sleep behavior disorder (RBD) in humans.[86] The complex dream-enacting behavior that these preparations exhibit is termed oneiric behavior, from the Greek oneiros (dream). Although neurodegeneration in the peri-LC-α region in the human disorder has not yet been demonstrated, the animal experiments have been important for understanding both the potential neuropathology in RBD and the mechanisms that control muscle atonia during REM sleep. For further information regarding the relative location of the SLD nucleus and PRF, refer to Fig. 50.6.

39. **Answer A. Metabolic rate.**

In cross-species examination of sleep parameters in a wide range of mammals, Siegel and colleagues noted that one of the most significant correlations was between the duration of the sleep cycle and body mass or brain size.[87] Smaller animals have a shorter sleep cycle (i.e., the time from onset of NREM sleep to the end of the following REM sleep period). Although the reason for this correlation is currently unknown, body mass is also highly correlated with the metabolic rate; therefore, it is possible that the metabolic rate (Answer A) determines sleep cycle duration and hence REM sleep bout length.

Discovery of the hypocretin/orexin and MCH systems in the lateral hypothalamus and their effect on REM sleep, combined with regulation of these systems by metabolic parameters, now provides a mechanism for this correlation. Hypocretin/orexin (Answer B) gates the onset of REM sleep as seen in patients with narcolepsy and animal models of narcolepsy; therefore, this neuropeptide affects the number of REM sleep episodes without changing their duration. In contrast, MCH, MCH in combination with hypocretin/orexin, or a currently unknown hypothalamic factor may, or may not, determine the REM sleep bout duration.[74] Neither circadian time (Answer C) nor sleepiness (Answer D) has been shown to affect the average duration of an episode of REM sleep.

40. **Answer B. A postsynaptic action at the α-adrenoceptor.** Norepinephrine acts at the α2-adrenoceptor to hyperpolarize and inhibit discharge of the cell. The sleep-promoting neurons of the VLPO express the α2-adrenoceptor and are therefore inhibited by norepinephrine, as displayed in Fig. 50.20.[88] When acting at the β-adrenoceptor (Answer A), norepinephrine primarily excites the cell, although weak inhibitory effects are also possible, for example, in the cortex. Answer C is incorrect, because the α2 adrenoceptors were localized to sleep-promoting projection neurons, not interneurons. Answer D is incorrect, because adenosine build-up in the BF precedes the transition from wakefulness to NREM sleep, and thus not promote wakefulness.

Acknowledgment

This work was supported by the Department of Anesthesiology. This work was not an industry-supported study, and the author has no financial conflicts of interest. The author would like to thank Christopher M. Sinton for writing a solid foundation for this chapter in previous editions of this review.

Suggested Reading

McCarley RW. Neurobiology of REM sleep. *Handb Clin Neurol.* 2011;98:151-171.

Saper CB. The neurobiology of sleep. *Continuum (Minneap Minn).* 2013;19(1 Sleep Disorders):19-31.

Schwartz MD, Kilduff TS. The neurobiology of sleep and wakefulness. *Psychiatr Clin North Am.* 2015;38(4):615-644.

Siegel JM. The neurobiology of sleep. *Semin Neurol.* 2009;29(4):277-296.

Watson CJ, Baghdoyan HA, Lydic R. Neuropharmacology of sleep and wakefulness. *Sleep Med Clin.* 2010;5(4):513-528.

Index

Page numbers followed by "*f*" indicate figures, "*t*" indicate tables, and "*b*" indicate boxes.